Brief Contents

Maternity, Newborn, and Women's Health Nursing

A CASE-BASED APPROACH

Maternity, Newborn, and Women's Health Nursing

A CASE-BASED APPROACH

Amy Mandeville O'Meara, DrNP, WHNP, AGNP

Associate Clinical Professor
Department of Nursing
College of Nursing and Health Sciences
University of Vermont
Burlington, Vermont

Women's Health Nurse Practitioner
Planned Parenthood of Northern New England
Vermont

Adult-Gerontology Nurse Practitioner
Appletree Bay Primary Care
Burlington, Vermont

Immediate Past President
Vermont Nurse Practitioners Association
Vermont

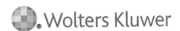. Wolters Kluwer

Philadelphia • Baltimore • New York • London
Buenos Aires • Hong Kong • Sydney • Tokyo

Vice President and Publisher: Julie K. Stegman
Senior Acquisitions Editor: Natasha McIntyre
Director of Product Development: Jennifer K. Forestieri
Senior Development Editor: Meredith L. Brittain
Freelance Development Editor: David R. Payne
Editorial Coordinator: Tim Rinehart
Marketing Manager: Brittany Clements
Editorial Assistant: Leo Gray
Design Coordinator: Terry Mallon
Art Director, Illustration: Jennifer Clements
Production Project Manager: Marian Bellus
Manufacturing Coordinator: Karin Duffield
Prepress Vendor: S4Carlisle Publishing Services

9 8 7 6 5 4 3

Printed in The United States of America

Library of Congress Cataloging-in-Publication Data

Names: O'Meara, Amy Mandeville, 1975– author.
Title: Maternity, newborn, and women's health nursing : a case-based approach
 / Amy Mandeville O'Meara.
Description: Philadelphia : Wolters Kluwer Health, 2018. | Includes
 bibliographical references.
Identifiers: LCCN 2018036241 | ISBN 9781496368218 (hardback)
Subjects: | MESH: Maternal-Child Nursing | Women's Health | Pregnancy
 Complications—nursing | Case Reports
Classification: LCC RG951 | NLM WY 157.3 | DDC 618.2/0231—dc23 LC record available at
 https://lccn.loc.gov/2018036241

CD122021

Dedication

To my children, Madeleine and Elizabeth, to whom I just recently had the opportunity to reintroduce myself after two packed years of book writing and editing. And to my students, whose wisdom and curiosity provide a template for learning.

About the Author

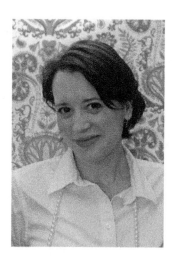

Amy Mandeville O'Meara, DrNP, WHNP, AGNP

Amy Mandeville O'Meara is a clinical associate professor in the Department of Nursing, College of Nursing and Health Sciences at the University of Vermont. She earned a bachelor of arts degree in anthropology with an emphasis in physical anthropology from Fresno State University. In 2006, she received her master of science in nursing degree, specializing in women's health, from Boston College as part of their direct-entry program. Soon after, she earned her women's health nurse practitioner certification through the National Certification Corporation. She earned her doctor of nursing practice degree, with a focus on nursing education, from Drexel University in 2014. That same year she returned to school for a postgraduate certificate from the University of Vermont that enabled her to earn her adult-gerontology nurse practitioner certification from the American Association of Nurse Practitioners.

Since 2011, Dr. O'Meara has been a member of the University of Vermont faculty. She teaches both undergraduate and graduate courses in maternity nursing and women's and gendered health, as well as health assessment, pathophysiology, nursing theory, and policy, politics, and ethics. She is the immediate past president of the Vermont Nurse Practitioners Association. In 2018, she won the Vermont Advocate State Award for Excellence from the American Association of Nurse Practitioners.

Dr. O'Meara practices as a nurse practitioner at Planned Parenthood of Northern New England as well as at Appletree Bay Primary Care, a clinic owned by the College of Nursing and Health Sciences at the University of Vermont and staffed by nurse practitioner faculty of the Department of Nursing. She previously practiced as a maternity visiting nurse, a medical assistant in a fertility center, and a nurse practitioner in a private practice caring for gynecology, urogynecology, and gynecologic oncology patients.

Dr. O'Meara is married to another Dr. O'Meara, John O'Meara, an astrophysicist who researches cosmic origins. Together they have two young daughters, Madeleine and Elizabeth. They share their home with a dog, two cats, and two parakeets, all of whom are named after Jane Austen characters. Dr. O'Meara enjoys painting, pottery, and cooking, despite her notable lack of talent or appreciable improvement over time.

Reviewers

Vicki Aaberg, PhD, MSN, BSN, RNC
Associate Professor of Nursing
Seattle Pacific University
Seattle, Washington

Kathy Adams, MSN, RNC-OB
Instructor/Clinical Supervisor
Missouri State University—School of Nursing
Springfield, Missouri

Sonya L. Allen, MSN ED, RN
Nursing Instructor
Augusta University
Athens, Georgia

Lydia Andrews, MSN, RN
Adjunct Professor
Oakwood University
Huntsville, Alabama

Debra Bacharz, PhD, MSN, RN
Professor of Nursing
University of Saint Francis
Fort Wayne, Indiana

Linda Baker, PhD, RN
Associate Professor
Columbia College of Nursing
Glendale, Wisconsin

Karen Balyeat, MSN, RN
Nursing Faculty
Gogebic Community College
Ironwood, Michigan

Nina M. Brown, MSN, RNC-OB
Assistant Professor
Department of Nursing
Prince George's Community College
Largo, Maryland

Kari Bunker, MSN-ED, RNC-OB
Obstetric Nursing Faculty
Glendale Community College
Glendale, Arizona

Barbara Butynskyi, MSN, RN, CPN
Nurse Educator
Jefferson College of Nursing
Philadelphia, Pennsylvania

Carol Caico, PhD, CS, NP
Associate Professor
New York Institute of Technology
Old Westbury, New York

M. Alice Colwell, RNC-NIC
Assistant Professor
Kent State University
Kent, Ohio

Georgina Colalillo, MS, RN, CNE
Professor
Queensborough Community College/CUNY
Queens, New York

Patricia D. Coyne, RNC-MNN, MS, MPA
Faculty
Montefiore School of Nursing
Mount Vernon, New York

Heather Denlinger, CNM, MSN
Assistant Professor
Harrisburg Area Community College
Lancaster, Pennsylvania

Bernadette Dragich, PhD, RN, CFNP
Professor of Nursing
Bluefield State College
Bluefield, West Virginia

For a list of the contributors and reviewers for the ancillaries,
please visit http://thepoint.lww.com/OMeara1e.

Jennifer Dunlap, MS, RN
Nursing Instructor
St. Elizabeth College of Nursing
Utica, New York

Melissa Dyer, MBA, MSN, RN
Associate Lecturer
Kent State University, School of Nursing
Kent, Ohio

Lisa C. Engel, MSN, RN, CNE
Assistant Professor
Harding University Carr College of Nursing
Searcy, Arkansas

Dr. Susan Hall, MSN, RNC-OB, CCE
Assistant Professor/Family and Community Health Area
Coordinator
Winston-Salem State University
Winston Salem, North Carolina

Betty Hennington, RN
Nursing Instructor
Meridian Community College
Meridian, Mississippi

Terri Hood-Brown, PhD(c), MSN, RN
Assistant Professor
Ohio University
Athens, Ohio

Charlotte S. Hurst, PhD, RN, CNM
Professor of Nursing
Dillard University
New Orleans, Louisiana

Margaret Johnson, MSN, RN
Assistant Professor
Indian River State College
Fort Pierce, Florida

Christine Kuoni, RN, MSN, CNE
Assistant Professor
San Antonio College
San Antonio, Texas

Francine Laterza, MSN, RN, PNP
Assistant Professor of Nursing
Farmingdale State College
Farmingdale, New York

Robyn Leo, MS, RN
Associate Professor
Worcester State University
Worcester, Massachusetts

Nikki Lee, PhD, RNC-OB
Assistant Professor of Nursing
University of Mississippi Medical Center
Jackson, Mississippi

Jeanne Linhart, RN-C, FNP-BC
Professor
Rockland Community College
Suffern, New York

Rebecca Luetke, PhD, RN
Professor of Nursing
Colorado Mountain College
Glenwood Springs, Colorado

Sue Mahley, MN, RN, CNE
Assistant Professor of Nursing and Coordinator of Clinical and
Faculty Resources
Research College of Nursing
Kansas City, Missouri

K. Shea Mobley, MSN, RN
Nursing Faculty
Wallace State Community College
Hanceville, Alabama

LaDonna Northington, DNS, RN, BC
Professor of Nursing
University of Mississippi School of Nursing
Jackson, Mississippi

Robin Oliver, MS, RNC-OB
Professor of Nursing
Rose State College Health Sciences Division
Norman, Oklahoma

Katherine A. Raker, MSN, CNM, RNC-OB
Assistant Professor
Bloomsburg University
Bloomsburg, Pennsylvania

Jacquelyn Reid, MSN, EdD
Professor Emeritus
Indiana University Southeast
New Albany, Indiana

Sheila A. Smith, PhD, RN
Associate Professor
Medical University of South Carolina
Charleston, South Carolina

Leigh A. Snead, RN, MSN
Assistant Professor of Nursing
University of Arkansas at Little Rock Department of Nursing
Little Rock, Arkansas

Heidi Stone, MS, RN-C OB, CNE
Clinical Assistant Professor
Towson University
Towson, Maryland

Denise Berry Talenti, DNP, CNE, CNM
Associate Professor
Elmira College
Elmira, New York

Maureen Tremel, MSN
Professor of Nursing
Seminole State College
Sanford, Florida

Rebekah L. Valdez, RNC, MSN
ADN Faculty
Lone Star College—CyFair Campus
Cypress, Texas

Dianna Vermilyea, MSN, RN
Assistant Professor of Nursing
Tennessee Wesleyan University Department of Nursing
Maryville, Tennessee

Laura J. Wallace, CNM, PhD
Associate Professor
Brenau University
Gainesville, Georgia

Josephine West, MSN
Professor, ADN Transition
San Jacinto College (South)
Pasadena, Texas

Pam Williams, PhD, RNC-AWHC
Assistant Professor
Widener University School of Nursing
Chester, Pennsylvania

Michele Wolff, RN, MSN
Nursing Instructor
Saddleback College
Mission Viejo, California

Preface

A Case-Based Approach: The Power of Storytelling

In a learning climate in which clinical placements are progressively shorter and harder to find, we often think of expensive simulation solutions as the best alternative. With these high-fidelity options and well-stocked labs, it's easy to forget as we run through our scenarios the power of the stories themselves. People learn by telling stories, by hearing stories, and by reading them. We remember the lessons of fables and legends because they are contextualized and compelling. We know that slow and steady can win the race because Aesop's tortoise and hare told us so. We learned from Icarus the folly of execution in the absence of adequate preparation. When dry facts fail, stories breathe into them meaning and importance. Stories are also the ancient and ultimate memory aid. Beowulf, an epic poem of 3,182 lines, was passed orally from person to person long before reading and writing were generally accessible and before anyone wrote it down.

Students often tell educators that everything they learn, they learn in clinical, which is a valid perception. What makes clinicals such an effective context for learning is not only the hands-on experience they offer but also the repetition of tasks and information a student experiences when caring for patients. Continually providing the same or similar information within fresh contexts and scenarios is what helps students retain information in a deep and lasting way. This book, borrowing from that phenomenon, strives to provide a similar dynamic learning experience.

What is often of immediate importance in the context of maternity care is not so much the physical tasks of nursing (which may, in some cases of routine care, be fairly limited), but the psychosocial care. As new learners, however, nursing students have a tendency to concentrate—appropriately—on the concrete. Will I hurt the patient? Can I remember how to set an infusion pump? What if I miss something important? Learning can be very task based while neglecting more subtle aspects of care, such as family relations, economic context, and cultural variations. A story-based approach helps learners to contextualize a patient and a patient's care in a safe space without immediate concern for correctly executed tasks. Patients become not just a series of problems and tasks but people and personalities. Students are compelled to learn because they want to know what happens next. And after engaging in this safe practice, they can bring that same curiosity to real patient scenarios.

A Unique, Customizable Organization

An Embedded Learning Solution

As with any text, the content of this book can be reordered as seen fit by the instructor. There is a learning solution, however, embedded in the progression of this book. Each of the 13 scenarios in Unit 1 focuses on a different aspect of maternity and newborn care and women's and gendered health. Greater breadth and depth of content emerges as the reader continues; Units 2 through 4, although still striving for compelling context, offer a more traditional text that provides a greater wealth of information. Through the case snippets in these units that ask students to recall patients from Unit 1, students can link these later units to those scenarios for improved recall through repetition.

As our curricula change, we know that some programs of study may be truncated. Classes such as maternity and newborn nursing, which some programs once may have taught over a semester, now may be taught over half a semester or over a single month. These shorter programs may find the organization of this text particularly helpful because Unit 1, which covers the full breadth of required information, may be used apart from the remainder of the text.

In addition, most students are in clinical at the same time they are taking the related course and may struggle to function in the clinical setting without the foundational knowledge essential to that clinical experience. By providing students at the very beginning of their clinical experiences with holistic patient overviews that span pregnancy from preconception to the postpartum period, this book better prepares students to optimize their time with patients.

Structure of the Book

Each chapter in Unit 1, Scenarios for Clinical Preparation, presents a patient scenario that highlights essential and often overlapping aspects of routine nursing care as well as more unusual conditions and complications of pregnancy. (These rare situations, which students are less likely to witness or recognize during the course of their brief clinical rotations, include postpartum hemorrhage, preeclampsia, gestational trophoblastic disease, cord prolapse, and shoulder dystocia, to name a few.) In this way, although not every scenario captures every aspect of care, related pieces from different scenarios come together as a coherent and familiar whole.

x

Unit 2, Maternity and Newborn Nursing for Uncomplicated Pregnancies, shifts from the story-based format of Unit 1 to a more traditional textbook approach and provides an overview of routine pregnancy, delivery, and newborn care. All the chapters in this unit frequently refer back to aspects of pregnancy-related care first illustrated in context in Unit 1. Students are reminded, for example, of the preconception care provided to Bess, Lexi, and Letitia, and that Tatiana's physician said the fact that she was 2 cm dilated at 39 weeks was a normal finding in late pregnancy. These references act as memory cues to reinforce content with context.

Unit 3, High-Risk Conditions and Complications, revisits issues and problems of pregnancy, delivery, and newborns found in Unit 1 while introducing some new ones. The chapters in Unit 3 are, as much as possible, ordered chronologically according to when problems are most likely to manifest in a pregnancy. Although some problems of pregnancy don't fit easily into a timeline, others do; for example, for molar pregnancy, gestational diabetes, and preeclampsia, the timeline is critical not only to understanding the problem but to recognizing it and successfully addressing it with a patient. Where relevant in this unit (as in Unit 2), characters from Unit 1 are reintroduced as "ticklers" to remind readers that they have had prior contextualized exposure to this information. This context reminder serves as an aid to memory and to facilitate comprehension of material that is often dense, complex, and difficult to access and retain.

Unit 4, Women's and Gendered Health, covers essential aspects of women's and gendered healthcare. As in Units 2 and 3, where appropriate, the experiences of the characters from Unit 1 are referenced in the chapters in Unit 4. This unit includes information about important aspects of subjects such as contraception and routine screening, and also includes essential information about caring for transgendered patients and patients seeking abortion care.

Accessible Writing Style

Another unique feature of this text is the author's casual, conversational writing style. Because jargon can be alienating to the student reader, this text avoids it as much as possible. However, great care has been taken to ensure the accuracy and currency of the content. Unit 1 is written as a series of accessible stories in the third person from the patient's point of view and in the present tense, which lends them immediacy. This approach allows the student to experience pregnancy from the patient's perspective, and thus to develop empathy for patients from many different backgrounds. Units 2 through 4, although written in a more traditional textbook format, still prioritize accessibility. Whenever possible, language and style are simplified while continuing to provide clear, concise, updated, and evidence-based information.

Features of This Book

Please refer to the User's Guide (which immediately follows this preface) for explanations of this book's features.

A Comprehensive Package for Teaching and Learning

To further facilitate teaching and learning, a carefully designed ancillary package has been developed to assist faculty and students.

Instructor Resources

Tools to assist you with teaching your course are available upon adoption of this text on thePoint° at http://thepoint.lww.com/OMeara1e.

- A **Test Generator** features National Council Licensure Exam (NCLEX)-style questions mapped to chapter learning objectives.
- An extensive collection of materials is provided for each book chapter:
  - **Prelecture Quizzes** (and answers) allow you to check students' reading.
  - **PowerPoint Presentations** provide an easy way to integrate the textbook with your students' classroom experience; multiple-choice and true/false questions are included to promote class participation.
  - **Discussion Topics** (and suggested answers) can be used in the classroom or in online discussion boards to facilitate interaction with your students.
  - **Assignments** (and suggested answers) include group, written, clinical, and Web assignments to engage students in varied activities and assess their learning.
  - **Case Studies** with related questions (and suggested answers) give students an opportunity to apply their knowledge to patient cases similar to those they might encounter in practice.
- **Answers to the Think Critically questions in the book** reinforce key concepts.
- Sample **Syllabi** are provided for 7-week and 15-week courses.
- **Maps Linking Cases with Chapters** provides a visual representation of the links between the content covered in Unit 1 and Units 2 through 4.
- A **Quality and Safety Education for Nurses (QSEN) Competency Map** identifies content and special features in the book related to competencies identified by the QSEN Institute.
- A **Bachelor of Science in Nursing (BSN) Essentials Competency Map** identifies book content related to the BSN Essentials.
- An **Image Bank** lets you use the photographs and illustrations from this textbook in your course materials.
- An **e-book** serves as a handy resource.
- Access to all **Student Resources** is provided, so that you can understand the student experience and use these resources in your course as well.

Student Resources

An exciting set of free learning resources is available on thePoint° to help students review and apply vital concepts in maternity nursing. Multimedia engines have been optimized so that students can access many of these resources on mobile devices. Students can access all these resources at http://thepoint.lww.com/OMeara1e using the codes printed in the front of their textbooks.

- **NCLEX-Style Review Questions** for each chapter help students review important concepts and practice for the NCLEX exam.
- **Journal Articles** offer access to current articles relevant to each chapter and available in Wolters Kluwer journals to familiarize students with nursing literature.
- **Learning Objectives** from the book are provided for convenience.

- **Interactive Learning Resources** appeal to various learning styles. Icons in the text direct readers to relevant resources:
  - **Practice & Learn Case Studies** present case scenarios and offer interactive exercises and questions to help students apply what they have learned.
  - **Watch & Learn Videos** reinforce skills from the textbook and appeal to visual and auditory learners.

Adaptive Learning Powered by PrepU

Lippincott's Adaptive Learning Powered by prepU helps every student learn more, while giving instructors the data they need to monitor each student's progress, strengths, and weaknesses. The adaptive learning system allows instructors to assign quizzes or students to take quizzes on their own that adapt to each student's individual mastery level. Visit http://thePoint.lww.com/prepU to learn more.

vSim for Nursing

vSim for Nursing, jointly developed by Laerdal Medical and Wolters Kluwer Health, offers innovative scenario-based learning modules consisting of Web-based virtual simulations, course learning materials, and curriculum tools designed to develop critical thinking skills and promote clinical confidence and competence. vSim for Nursing | Maternity includes 10 of the 12 cases from the Simulation in Nursing Education—Obstetric Scenarios, authored by the National League for Nursing. Students can progress through suggested readings, pre- and postsimulation assessments, documentation assignments, and guided reflection questions, and will receive an individualized feedback log immediately upon completion of the simulation. Throughout the student learning experience, the product offers remediation back to trusted Lippincott resources, including Lippincott Nursing Advisor and Lippincott Nursing Procedures—two online, evidence-based, clinical information solutions used in healthcare facilities throughout the United States. This innovative product provides a comprehensive patient-focused solution for learning and integrating simulation into the classroom.

Contact your Wolters Kluwer sales representative or visit http://thepoint.lww.com/vsim for options to enhance your maternity nursing course with vSim for Nursing.

Lippincott DocuCare

Lippincott DocuCare combines web-based academic electronic health record (EHR) simulation software with clinical case scenarios, allowing students to learn how to use an EHR in a safe, true-to-life setting, while enabling instructors to measure their progress. Lippincott DocuCare's nonlinear solution works well in the classroom, simulation lab, and clinical practice.

Contact your Wolters Kluwer sales representative or visit http://thepoint.lww.com/DocuCare for options to enhance your maternity nursing course with DocuCare.

A Comprehensive, Digital, Integrated Course Solution

Lippincott CoursePoint+ is an integrated digital learning solution designed for the way students learn. It is the only nursing education solution that integrates:

- **Leading content in context:** Content provided in the context of the student learning path engages students and encourages interaction and learning on a deeper level.
- **Powerful tools to maximize class performance:** Course-specific tools, such as adaptive learning powered by prepU, provide a personalized learning experience for every student.
- **Real-time data to measure students' progress:** Student performance data provided in an intuitive display lets you quickly spot which students are having difficulty or which concepts the class as a whole is struggling to grasp.
- **Preparation for practice:** Integrated virtual simulation and evidence-based resources improve student competence, confidence, and success in transitioning to practice.
  - vSim for Nursing: Co-developed by Laerdal Medical and Wolters Kluwer, vSim for Nursing simulates real nursing scenarios and allows students to interact with virtual patients in a safe, online environment.
  - Lippincott Advisor for Education: With over 8,500 entries covering the latest evidence-based content and drug information, Lippincott Advisor for Education provides students with the most up-to-date information possible, while giving them valuable experience with the same point-of-care content they will encounter in practice.
- **Training services and personalized support:** To ensure your success, our dedicated educational consultants and training coaches will provide expert guidance every step of the way.

Acknowledgments

This book is the product of tremendous effort but also of tremendous opportunity. Those opportunities I must credit to others, including my husband, John O'Meara, and my parents, Joyce and John Mandeville. I must also credit Greg Kinsky for inexplicably surmising I might be good at this, and Natasha McIntyre for trusting Greg's instincts. I gratefully acknowledge the patient persistence and work of Meredith Brittain, David Payne, the cohort of eagle-eyed reviewers, and the rest of the talented team at Wolters Kluwer.

I gratefully acknowledge the encouragement, mentorship, and hard work of so many who directly or indirectly made this work possible, including Genell Mikkalson, Sarah Pinard Rogers, Joellen Hawkins, Joan Rosen Bloch, Ellen Watson, and Barbara Rouleau. I acknowledge the considerable contribution of the dedicated and talented nurses and nurse practitioners at the University of Vermont Medical Center, Planned Parenthood of Northern New England, and Appletree Bay Primary Care. Finally, without the inspiration provided by my students, both past and present, none of this would be possible.

User's Guide

Maternity, Newborn, and Women's Health Nursing: A Case-Based Approach contains many accessible features to help students grasp the important content.

Case-Based Features

Chapter-long **Clinical Scenarios** make up each chapter of Unit 1, as mentioned in the preface. Each of the 13 scenarios in Unit 1 focuses on a different aspect of maternity and newborn care and women's and gendered health.

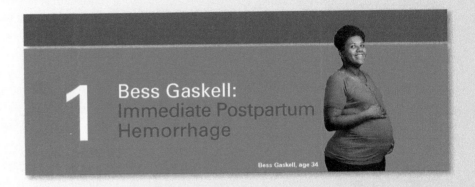

1

Bess Gaskell:
Immediate Postpartum
Hemorrhage

Bess Gaskell, age 34

Bess Gaskell, who was pregnant for the third time (Chapter 1), anticipated fatigue as a normal part of early pregnancy.

Greater breadth and depth of content emerge as the reader continues; Units 2 through 4, although still striving for compelling context, offer a more traditional text that provides a greater wealth of information. Through the case snippets in these units that ask students to recall patients from Unit 1, students can link these later units to those scenarios.

Unfolding Patient Stories, written by the National League for Nursing, are an engaging way to begin meaningful conversations in the classroom. These vignettes, which appear at the end of the first chapter in each unit, feature patients from Wolters Kluwer's vSim for Nursing | Maternity (co-developed by Laerdal Medical) and DocuCare products; however, each Unfolding Patient Story in the book stands alone, not requiring purchase of these products.

For your convenience, a list of all these case studies, along with their location in the book, appears in the "Case Studies in This Book" section later in this front matter.

Unfolding Patient Stories: Amelia Sung • Part 1

Amelia Sung is 36 years old and 8 weeks pregnant with her second child. She tells the nurse that she is considering an amniocentesis because of her age. What information would the nurse include when providing education on an amniocentesis? (Amelia Sung's story continues in Unit 3.)

Care for Amelia and other patients in a realistic virtual environment: ***vSim** for Nursing* (thepoint.lww .com/vSimMaternity). Practice documenting these patients' care in DocuCare (thepoint.lww.com /DocuCareEHR).

The Nurse's Point of View feature in Unit 1 changes the narrator from the patient to a knowledgeable nurse preceptor who picks up the story from the nursing perspective, including information about how and why particular aspects of care are provided to a character.

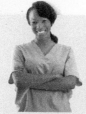

The Nurse's Point of View

Cara: It never does any good to judge anyone, or any person's situation. It would be easy for me to look at Loretta and say that she's foolish or weak or not worth my time. But the truth is much harder. Loretta has been taught by so many people in her life that she's not worth the trouble that she believes them. She doesn't trust because the people in her life don't have a track record of earning that trust.

The Partner's Point of View

Russ: There is a sign on the door to Rebecca's room with a leaf and a drop of water. One of the nurses told me it's the universal sign for stillbirth. To me, it is a mark of tragedy; a warning to anyone who passes that beyond this door lies an all-consuming sadness; a plea for sensitivity; a cue to not ask unprompted questions. I've heard someone use the term "angel baby," and I wish I could believe in heaven. But I don't want to hear that the baby is in a better place or with God. This is the place Rebecca and I made for her. This is where she belongs.

The Partner's Point of View feature, which appears in Chapter 6, conveys thoughts of the main character's partner.

Chapter-Beginning Features

Learning Objectives state clear and concise learning goals for each chapter.

Objectives

1. Identify current recommendations for Pap screening by patient age.
2. Recognize the diagnostic criteria for polycystic ovarian syndrome.
3. Recognize important risk factors and interventions for late (secondary) postpartum hemorrhage.
4. Distinguish between autosomal recessive and autosomal dominant genetic inheritance.
5. Identify signs of uterine atony and pertinent assessments.
6. Discuss the significance of Rh incompatibility.
7. Explain some of the noncontraceptive benefits of combined oral contraceptives.
8. Contrast true and false labor.
9. Identify infant feeding readiness cues.

Key Terms are listed at the beginning of each chapter, boldfaced on first use in the chapter text, and included in a glossary at the back of the book.

Key Terms

Autosomal dominant
Autosomal recessive
Bloody show
Braxton Hicks contractions
Colostrum
Combined oral contraceptive (COC)
Cystic fibrosis
Engorgement

False labor
Orthostatic hypotension
Polycystic ovarian syndrome (PCOS)
Rh_o (D) immune globulin
Stripping of the membranes
Tay-Sachs disease
Uterine atony

Features That Teach Skills and Concepts

For your convenience, a list of all the features that teach skills and concepts, along with their location in the book, appears in the "Special Features in This Book" section later in this front matter.

Analyze the Evidence compares sometimes conflicting and contradictory research that supports or challenges current maternity nursing practice.

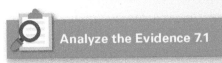

Analyze the Evidence 7.1 — Expedient Induction of Labor With Term or Near-Term Rupture of Membranes

Induction Within 24 h

- Pregnancies in group B streptococcus–positive women may benefit from induction rather than watchful waiting (Tajik et al., 2014).
- Induction of labor may reduce the incidence of neurodevelopmental delays at 2 y of age (Heyden et al., 2015).

Watchful Waiting as an Acceptable Alternative

- Induction of labor does not reduce the rate of neonatal sepsis or other neonatal outcomes and may slightly increase the risk for chorioamnionitis (Ham et al., 2012).
- Prolonged preterm rupture of membranes does not increase the risk of neonatal sepsis (Drassinower, Friedman, Običan, Levin, & Gyamfi-Bannerman, 2016).

Lab Values 9.1

Blood Glucose Parameters for Asymptomatic Neonates

- Within first 4 h of life, maintain plasma glucose levels >25 mg/dL (1.4 mmol/L).
- Between 4 and 24 h of life, maintain plasma glucose levels >35 mg/dL (1.9 mmol/L).
- Between 24 and 48 h of life, maintain plasma glucose levels >50 mg/dL (2.8 mmol/L).
- Greater than 48 h of life, maintain plasma glucose levels >60 mg/dL (3.3 mmol/L).

Data from Committee on Fetus and Newborn from the American Academy of Pediatrics. (2011). Postnatal glucose homeostasis in late-preterm and term infants. *Pediatrics, 127*(3), 575–579.

Lab Values includes normal values as well as the significance of out-of-range values and appropriate nursing interventions.

Patient Teaching includes important points nurses must cover with patients to effectively educate them.

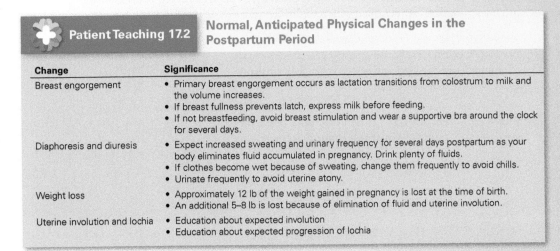

Patient Teaching 17.2 — Normal, Anticipated Physical Changes in the Postpartum Period

Change	Significance
Breast engorgement	• Primary breast engorgement occurs as lactation transitions from colostrum to milk and the volume increases. • If breast fullness prevents latch, express milk before feeding. • If not breastfeeding, avoid breast stimulation and wear a supportive bra around the clock for several days.
Diaphoresis and diuresis	• Expect increased sweating and urinary frequency for several days postpartum as your body eliminates fluid accumulated in pregnancy. Drink plenty of fluids. • If clothes become wet because of sweating, change them frequently to avoid chills. • Urinate frequently to avoid uterine atony.
Weight loss	• Approximately 12 lb of the weight gained in pregnancy is lost at the time of birth. • An additional 5–8 lb is lost because of elimination of fluid and uterine involution.
Uterine involution and lochia	• Education about expected involution • Education about expected progression of lochia

The Pharmacy provides must-know pharmaceutical information, including, where appropriate, dosing and common titration protocols as well as essential safety information.

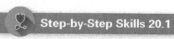

The Pharmacy 11.1	Sumatriptan
Overview	• Acute treatment for migraine and cluster headaches
Route and dosing	• Oral: 25-mg, 50-mg, or 100-mg single dose or second dose after 2 h, depending on the response • Intranasal powder: 11 mg in each nostril (total of 22 mg), single dose or second dose after 2 h, depending on the response • Intranasal solution: 5-mg, 10-mg, or 20-mg total single dose. May repeat in 2 h, depending on the response • Subcutaneous: dose depends on the product. More doses may be allowable when doses are separated by at least an hour. • Transdermal: one 6.5-mg patch. A second patch may be added after 2 h. Medication is delivered over 4 h per patch.
Care considerations	• Total daily dose no more than 200 mg by mouth • Total daily dose no more than 44 mg by intranasal powder • Total daily dose no more than 40 mg by intranasal solution • The safety of treating more than four headaches a month with sumatriptan is not established.
Warning signs	• Use is associated with cardiac events, stroke, elevated blood pressure, anaphylaxis, central nerve system depression, vasospasm, rare transient and permanent blindness, and serotonin syndrome

Step-by-Step Skills presents clear, easy-to-follow boxed tutorials of common nursing procedures with rationales.

Step-by-Step Skills 20.1
Blood Pressure Assessment
1. Have the patient sit or lie down, with the upper arm on one side level with heart and free of clothing. 2. If the patient is sitting, the legs should be uncrossed and the feet flat on the floor. 3. Position the blood pressure cuff snugly about an inch above the brachial pulsation. 4. Close the valve on the sphygmomanometer by turning it clockwise. 5. Palpate the radial or brachial pulse, inflate the cuff, note when the pulse can no longer be palpated, and inflate it 20 to 30 mm Hg higher. 6. Place the diaphragm of stethoscope over the brachial artery, and slowly deflate the cuff (2 to 3 mm Hg per second). 7. Listen for the appearance of sound (systolic) and the disappearance of sound (diastolic). 8. Deflate the cuff completely, and remove it from the arm.

In addition to the special boxes mentioned in this section, **Interactive Learning Tools** available online enrich learning and are identified with icons in the text:

 Practice & Learn Case Studies present case scenarios and offer interactive exercises and questions to help students apply what they have learned.

 Watch & Learn Video Clips reinforce skills from the textbook and appeal to visual and auditory learners.

Chapter-Ending Features

Think Critically offers short, often multipart questions requiring students to synthesize information found in the chapter. Suggested answers are available to instructors at http://thepoint.lww.com/OMeara1e.

Think Critically

1. You have a 43-year-old patient who is considering a pregnancy next year. What should you discuss with her in terms of pregnancy timing and risks?
2. You are caring for a newly pregnant patient who is considering cell-free DNA testing instead of amniocentesis. What points should you be careful to discuss when talking about the advantages and disadvantages to this approach?
3. You have a patient who has received no prenatal care and is presenting in the second trimester with hyperemesis gravidarum. She is diagnosed with a complete molar pregnancy. What additional complications do you know she is at risk for as a result of this diagnosis?
4. Your patient has just been diagnosed with a complete molar pregnancy. How do you describe to her the differences between a complete and partial molar pregnancy?
5. You have a patient who is trying to decide between a dilation and curettage and a hysterectomy with a molar pregnancy. How can you as the nurse help facilitate her decision-making?
6. Your patient was diagnosed with a molar pregnancy and treated with a dilation and curettage. She has had three assessments of her blood hCG level in a row, and the levels have been subclinical every time. When do you expect her next blood hCG test to be scheduled?

References cited are listed at the end of each chapter and include updated, current sources.

Suggested Readings include current evidence-based resources related to the key topics discussed in the chapter, so that students can expand and deepen their understanding of the content.

References

Berkowitz, R. S., & Goldstein, D. P. (2013). Current advances in the management of gestational trophoblastic disease. *Gynecologic Oncology, 128*(1), 3–5.

Elias, K., Shoni, M., Bernstein, M., Goldstein, D., & Berkowitz, R. (2012). Complete hydatidiform mole in women aged 40 to 49 years. *Journal of Reproductive Medicine, 57*(5–6), 254–258.

Soper, J. T., Mutch, D. G., & Schink, J. C. (2004). Diagnosis and treatment of gestational trophoblastic disease: ACOG Practice Bulletin No. 53. *Gynecologic Oncology, 93*(2), 575–585.

Vargas, R., Barroilhet, L. M., Esselen, K., Diver, E., Bernstein, M., Goldstein, D. P., & Berkowitz, R. S. (2014). Subsequent pregnancy outcomes after complete and partial molar pregnancy, recurrent molar pregnancy, and gestational trophoblastic neoplasia: An update from the New England Trophoblastic Disease Center. *Journal of Reproductive Medicine, 59*(5–6), 188–194.

Suggested Readings

American Cancer Society Medical and Editorial Content Team. (2016). *About gestational trophoblastic disease.* Retrieved from http://www.cancer.org/cancer/gestationaltrophoblasticdisease/detailedguide/gestational-trophoblastic-disease-what-is-g-t-d

March of Dimes. (2016). *Pregnancy after age 35.* Retrieved from http://www.marchofdimes.org/complications/pregnancy-after-age-35.aspx#

Monchek, R., & Wiedaseck, S. (2012). Gestational trophoblastic disease: An overview. *Journal of Midwifery and Women's Health, 57*(3), 255–259.

O'Connor, A., Doris, F., & Skirton, H. (2014). Midwifery care in the UK for older mothers. *British Journal of Midwifery, 22*(8), 568–577.

Contents

Unit 2
Maternity and Newborn Nursing for Uncomplicated Pregnancies   224

Unit 3
High-Risk Conditions and Complications 378

xxii   Contents

Unit 4
Women's and Gendered Health   600

Case Studies in This Book

Cases That Unfold Across Units

Special Features in This Book

Step-by-Step Skills

Unit 1
Scenarios for Clinical Preparation

1 Bess Gaskell: Immediate Postpartum Hemorrhage

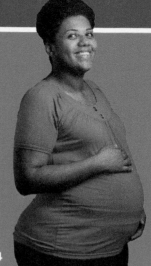

Bess Gaskell, age 34

Objectives

1. Identify risk factors for postpartum hemorrhage.
2. Identify appropriate management of immediate postpartum hemorrhage.
3. Recognize the signs of placental abruption.
4. Interpret some common fetal monitoring patterns.
5. Describe routine prenatal screening methods and examinations.
6. Analyze the roles of the nurses in the scenario.

Key Terms

Acceleration
Amniotic sac
Anencephaly
Biophysical profile
Body mass index (BMI)
Deceleration
Dilation and curettage (D&C)
Embryo
Endometrium
Fentanyl
Gestational sac
Human papillomavirus
Hysterectomy
Intrauterine system
Lanugo
Large for gestational age
Lochia
Naegele's rule

Neural tube defect
Nonstress test
Oxytocin
Pap test
Placenta
Placenta previa
Placental abruption
Premature rupture of membranes
Progestin
Reactive
Spina bifida
Tamponade
Tocodynamometer (toco)
Transvaginal transducer
Umbilical cord
Uterus
Variability
Yolk sac

Before Conception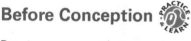

Bess is a woman with many roles and responsibilities. She is a 34-year-old optometrist and owns her own practice in partnership with three other optometrists. She is a coach for her 9-year-old daughter's after-school running group, and she shares the duties of parenting her and her son, a toddler, with her husband of 13 years, Jake. Every Friday she and Jake have a stay-at-home date night and share the cooking and the cleanup. She's struggled with her weight as she's grown older, and she sometimes has

2

trouble finding time to take care of herself. Her life is loud, busy, sometimes overwhelming, and mostly very happy.

The birth of her daughter, Annabelle, was uncomplicated and the pregnancy easy. Her son, Aiden, the younger child, was a different story. After Bess pushed for an hour, her labor and delivery nurse became concerned about the fetal heart rate changes she noted on the monitoring strip. The nurse worried about something called "late decelerations," which could indicate that the placenta wasn't doing a good job of getting oxygen to the baby anymore (Fig. 1.1). The nurse told Bess's physician about the changes. They tried turning her on her side and giving her oxygen, and it must have worked, because whatever was so concerning seemed to stop and Aiden was born vaginally less than half an hour later.

About a half-hour after the baby was born, the placenta was delivered. The team members checked the placenta and found that part of it was missing and was likely left behind in the uterus (Fig. 1.2). And Bess was still bleeding, causing them more concern. Within minutes, the team was performing a dilation and curettage, or D&C, to remove the pieces of the placenta that remained in her uterus. Once the pieces were gone, her uterus was able to contract to stop the bleeding. It was scary but quick, and the birth was otherwise uneventful.

She returned home a few days after the birth and was busy with the two kiddos. Aiden initially had some issues with breastfeeding that took some time, and then there was the matter of integrating a new baby into the family while keeping an older child happy. Six weeks after the birth, she went back to work part time, and 6 weeks after that she was back to work full time.

About 3 months after Aiden's birth, she had an intrauterine system (IUS) placed, which slowly releases the hormone progestin for up to 7 years (Fig. 1.3). The nurse practitioner, Rachel, who placed the IUS, told her that it worked primarily by keeping her cervical mucus thick so that sperm couldn't swim through it and fertilize an egg. As a bonus, Rachel told her, she could expect an overall 90% reduction in menstrual bleeding; in fact, about 20% of women with IUSs stop having their period altogether (Perriera et al., 2016). The insertion of the device took less than 15 minutes. Afterwards, Bess felt a little crampy. She liked the idea of not having to think about her birth control. After all, she couldn't forget to "take" her IUS in the morning (The Pharmacy 1.1).

Now, however, just 2 years after getting the IUS, she is feeling broody. She smiles at strangers' babies, and smells the heads of babies she knows. When little Annabelle got her first training bra and when Aiden insisted, precociously, on "making bubbles in the toilet just like daddy," she was equally sad and proud. She never quite gets around to taking all those perfect little infant pants and dresses to the charity shop in town. The crib is still in the garage. One day when they are driving somewhere together, Jake smiles at her and takes her hand.

"We're not going to stop funding the daycare center anytime soon, are we?" he asks.

She smiles back. "Just one more?"

Soon afterwards, Bess goes to the same nurse practitioner, Rachel, to have her IUS removed. Rachel tells her that about 88% of women will conceive within 12 months of removal of their IUS (Perriera et al., 2016). Rachel does advise her, however, to start taking a prenatal vitamin now, just in case.

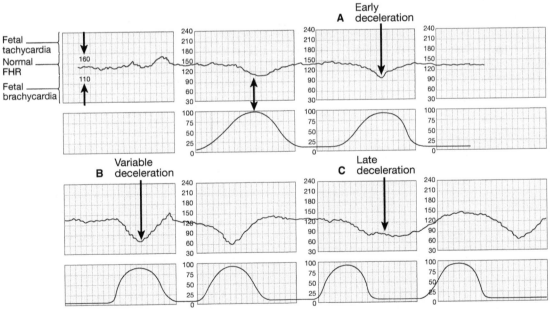

Figure 1.1. Fetal heart rate (FHR) with and without decelerations. (A) Early deceleration. Notice how the nadir of the deceleration occurs at the same time as the peak of the uterine contraction; they are mirror images of each other. **(B)** Variable deceleration. These decelerations may start before, during, or after a uterine contraction starts. **(C)** Late deceleration. The onset, nadir, and recovery of the deceleration occur, respectively, after the beginning, peak, and end of the contraction. (Reprinted with permission from Beckmann, C. R., Herbert, W., Laube, D., Ling, F., & Smith, R. [2013]. *Obstetrics and gynecology* [7th ed., Fig. 9.11]. Philadelphia, PA: Lippincott Williams & Wilkins.)

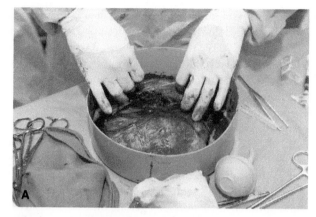

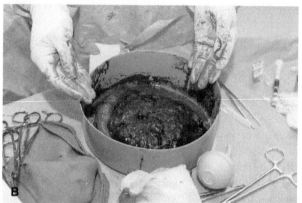

Figure 1.2. The placenta. The placenta is always examined after its delivery to ensure that it is intact. If pieces of it remain in the uterus, they may cause the uterus to not contract properly, which can cause severe maternal blood loss. **(A)** The membranous side, or "shiny Shultz," is the side that faces inward, toward the fetus. **(B)** The beefy-looking side, or "dirty Duncan," is the side that attaches to the maternal uterus. (Reprinted with permission from Chow, J., Ateah, C., Scott, S., Ricci, S., & Kyle, T. [2012]. *Canadian maternity and pediatric nursing* [Fig. 14.18]. Philadelphia, PA: Lippincott Williams & Wilkins.)

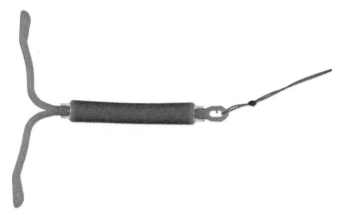

Figure 1.3. An intrauterine system (IUS). An IUS is placed in the uterus during a simple in-office procedure. An IUS is a highly effective method of contraception and lasts for 3 to 7 years, depending on the device. (Reprinted with permission from Berek, J. S. [2011]. *Berek and Novak's gynecology* [15th ed., Fig. 10.5]. Philadelphia, PA: Lippincott Williams & Wilkins.)

"The most important part of the prenatal vitamin for most women is the folic acid," Rachel says. "It helps to prevent **neural tube defects** such as **spina bifida** and **anencephaly**. That damage can happen before you even know you're pregnant, though, so it's best to start while you're trying to get pregnant, even if you think it's going to be a while."

Pregnancy

First Trimester

No one is more surprised than Bess when she has a positive home pregnancy test just 3 months later without even having a single period since her IUS was removed. She calls the office of the physician who delivered her two other children. The triage nurse she speaks with orders an ultrasound to confirm her pregnancy dating. She explains that when a woman is sure of the first day

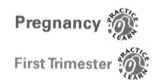

The Pharmacy 1.1	Intrauterine Devices	
	Copper IUD (ParaGard)	**Levonorgestrel IUS (Mirena, Skyla, Liletta)**
Mechanism of action	A sterile inflammatory reaction that impedes a sperm's ability to penetrate the egg	Thickening of cervical mucus, prohibiting passage of sperm; a secondary action may be the thinning of the uterine lining and inhibition of ovulation.
Composition	Copper wrapped around non-BPA plastic	Non-BPA plastic with a spine of levonorgestrel (a progestin) that releases over 3–7 y, depending on the device
Menstrual changes	Patients may complain of longer, heavier, crampier menstrual periods, especially during the first 6 mo.	Overall, 90% reduction of menstrual bleeding; up to 20% of women will cease menstruation after a year. Irregular unscheduled bleeding is possible.
Efficacy	99.2%	99.8%
Duration of efficacy	12 y or until removed	3–7 y, depending on the device

IUD, intrauterine device; IUS, intrauterine system; BPA, bisphenol A.

of her last period, calculating her due date is just a matter of subtracting 3 months from that date and adding 1 year and 7 days, a method called "Naegele's Rule" (Box 1.1). They also rely on ultrasound to estimate the due date, particularly when the date of the most recent period is less clear.

Bess goes the following week for the ultrasound, which is performed using a transvaginal transducer, which looks like a plastic stick, about a foot and a half long, that someone put a condom on to keep it clean. The ultrasound technician puts a lot of blue gel on the tip and then has Bess scoot her bottom a little further down the table before inserting the transducer into her vagina a few inches. It doesn't hurt, but it certainly feels weird. The tech asks if she'd like to know what she's seeing on the screen, and Bess says yes.

Everything on the screen is black, white, or gray, and it's all shifting around like static on a television screen. First the tech, Ellen, indicates a gray form in the shape of a papaya that takes up most of the image. She explains that this is the uterus. Running down the middle of the image is a lighter gray line, which Ellen explains is the inner lining of her uterus, the endometrium(called the decidua during pregnancy). In the larger, rounder part of the uterus, not quite centered with the lighter gray line, is a black circle that fills maybe 20% of the image. Ellen explains that this is the gestational sac, and that all of the other elements of the pregnancy that they'll be looking for will be contained in it.

As Ellen rotates the wand within the vagina, other structures come into view, such as a narrow white outline of a circle inside the gestational sac. Ellen explains that this is the yolk sac, which will form red blood cells for the pregnancy until the embryo can take over, after which it will become a part of the umbilical cord. Another move of the wand, and a short white rod resembling a grain of rice comes into view. Using a trackball on a console of the ultrasound machine, Ellen takes some measurements (Fig. 1.4).

"Six weeks," Ellen says. She points out the grain of rice. "That's the embryo."

Ellen points to a little flutter of movement at the center of the grain of rice.

"You see?" Ellen says. "A heartbeat."

Later that day, while Bess is with a client in her optometry office, the triage nurse from her physician's office calls and leaves a voice mail on her phone. She calls her back, and they agree, based on the ultrasound findings, to schedule an appointment for a month later. Because this is Bess's third baby, the triage nurse explains, she is less concerned about providing early pregnancy education. Bess has, after all, been around that block twice before.

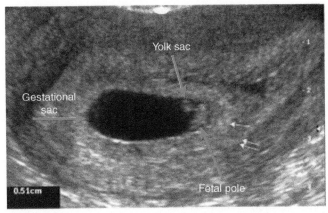

Figure 1.4. Structures of pregnancy at 6 weeks. A 6-week pregnancy should include the structures of a gestational sac, yolk sac, and fetal pole with heartbeat evident. (Reprinted with permission from Stephenson, S. R. [2015]. *Obstetrics and gynecology* [3rd ed., Fig. 13.9]. Philadelphia, PA: Lippincott Williams & Wilkins.)

When Bess comes to her visit the following month, she is glad to see that Dr. Phillips, who delivered her two other children, has not yet retired. The history taking is mostly a matter of informing Dr. Phillips that nothing has changed (Box 1.2). She has no new health concerns, no new medications. She's still married to the same guy, and the kids are doing great. Dr. Phillips does a quick physical exam, including a pelvic exam (Box 1.3). She had a Pap test 2 years ago with Rachel, her nurse practitioner, as well as testing for the human papillomavirus. Both tests were negative, so she won't need to take them again for more 3 years (Massad et al., 2013).

She tells Dr. Phillips that she feels pretty good, just a little tired and bloated. She doesn't have any morning sickness, but then she didn't with her other two pregnancies, either. She complains of some minor cramping right in the middle of her pelvis, but says she hasn't had any bleeding. She says the cramping is a little bit like period cramps, and she remembers it from prior pregnancies. Dr. Phillips confirms that this is a normal part of early pregnancy, as her body, particularly her uterus, starts to grow and change.

At the end of the history taking and exam, Dr. Phillips says his only real concern is her weight. He says that based on a calculation that included her height and weight, she has a body mass index (BMI) of 29, which puts her in the category of overweight (Box 1.4). Bess has never been a small person, but she admits that the weight she gained with her first two kids hasn't really gone away. In fact, if anything, she's added to it in the intervening years.

"Because your BMI is so high," says Dr. Phillips, "I'd really like you to limit your weight gain to between 15 and 25 pounds." So much for eating for two (Box 1.5).

Before Bess leaves, she discusses prenatal testing with Dr. Philips.

"How old are you now, Bess?" he asks, scrolling through her record on the computer. "Will you turn thirty five before the birth?"

Bess shakes her head and says, "I'll be a few months short of my thirty-fifth birthday on the baby's due date. Why do you ask?"

"Well, if you were, we'd consider you advanced maternal age. With advanced maternal age we know women are at increased risk for certain complications and that they're more likely to carry a fetus with a genetic defect."

Box 1.1 Calculating the Estimated Date of Delivery by Last Menstrual Period Using Naegele's Rule

Example

First day of LMP: June 6
Subtract 3 mo: March 6
Add 7 d: March 12
EDD = March 12

LMP, last menstrual period; EDD, estimated date of delivery.

Box 1.2 Elements of an Initial Prenatal Health History

- Information about current pregnancy
  - Last menstrual period
  - Pregnancy symptoms
  - Bleeding
  - Complaints and concerns
- Obstetric history
  - Number of pregnancies and births
  - Complications of pregnancy and delivery
  - Method of delivery
  - Newborn outcomes
  - Number of spontaneous and elective abortions
- Social history
  - Father of pregnancy
    - Age
    - Medical history
    - Substance use
    - Involvement in pregnancy
    - Family history of congenital disorders
  - Safety at home and in relationship
  - History of physical and/or sexual or emotional abuse
  - Support system
  - Living situation
- Gynecologic history
  - Papanicolaou smear history
  - Contraception
  - History of sexually transmitted infections, treatment, and complications
- Medical history
  - Past and current conditions
  - Chronic conditions such as asthma and diabetes
  - Hospitalizations
- Surgical history
  - Surgical indications, locations, and outcomes
  - Anesthesia
- Religious and cultural beliefs and preferences, preferred language
- Medications
  - Prescription
  - Over the counter
  - Vitamins
  - Herbal supplements
- Allergies, medication and other
- Substance use
  - Illegal drugs
  - Cannabis
  - Medications prescribed for others
  - Nicotine
  - Alcohol
- Nutrition
  - Diet
  - Eating disorder
- Family history
  - History of congenital defects
  - Ethnicity (sometimes useful for guiding genetic screening)
  - Family history of pregnancy or birth complications

Box 1.3 First Prenatal Visit Physical Exam

- Vital signs
- Height and weight
- Thyroid
  - Assessing for thyroid enlargement
- Breast exam
  - Assessing for masses
- Heart
  - Assessing rate and rhythm. *Note:* murmurs are not uncommon in pregnancy
- Abdomen
  - Tenderness, uterine size
- Pelvic exam
  - Uterine size
  - Normal pelvic exam findings in pregnancy:
    - *Chadwick's sign:* blue-violet discoloration of cervix and vagina in pregnancy
    - *Goodell's sign:* softening of cervix
    - *Hagar's sign:* softening of lower uterine segment

Box 1.4 What Is Body Mass Index?

BMI is a calculation between height and weight. As a tool, it was designed to assess body mass across populations, but has become a regularly used tool in clinical practice.

BMI classifications include the following:

- Normal: 18.5–24.9
- Underweight: <18.5
- Overweight: 25–29.9
- Obese: ≥30

It is important to keep in mind that BMI does not take into account bone structure or muscle mass. Bodybuilders, for example, may appear to be overweight according to the BMI calculation, when in fact their body fat is very low, and their muscle mass is quite high.

BMI, Body mass index

Box 1.5 Recommended Weight Gain in Pregnancy

By Prepregnancy BMI

Normal BMI (18.5–24.9): 25–35 lb
Underweight BMI (<18.5): 28–40 lb
Overweight BMI (25–29.9): 15–25 lb
Obese BMI (≥30): 12 lb or less

By Trimester

First trimester: 1–5 lb
Second and third trimesters: 1 lb/wk

BMI, Body mass index

"Hold up," Bess says. "Advanced maternal age? Seriously? I'm just two months off being labeled 'advanced maternal age'?"

Dr. Phillips smiles. "Advanced maternal age is just a risk factor for pregnancy complications. It's not a diagnosis. It just tells us we need to think about a pregnancy a little differently."

"But there still is a risk of a defect, even if I'm under thirty-five, right?" asks Bess.

Dr. Phillips nods. "We screened you for the genetic trait associated with sickle cell anemia and cystic fibrosis with your first pregnancy because you are of northern European and African descent. Those tests were negative. As far as you know, you do not have any Greek or Ashkenazi Jewish ancestry, do you?" Bess shook her head. "Based on what we know, I advise that we just do the standard first trimester and integrated screening, as we did with your last two pregnancies. If any of the results are concerning, we'll do further diagnostic testing to confirm. Sound good?" (Table 1.1; Fig. 1.5).

Before Bess leaves the office, she makes an appointment for a month from now, and then walks to the lab next door to drop

Table 1.1 Pregnancy Screening Recommendations for Congenital Defects

Disorder	At-Risk Population	Screening (Determines Who Is at Highest Risk)	Diagnostic Test (Confirms or Denies Conclusively Results of Screening)
Cystic fibrosis	Northern European, Ashkenazi Jewish, and Celtic	Analysis of maternal DNA for mutation of the CFTR gene; if the mother is a carrier, the partner will be tested. If both carry the trait, diagnostic testing of the fetus is indicated.	If both parents are positive, fetal DNA may be conclusively evaluated by amniocentesis or chorionic villi sampling.
Tay-Sachs disease	Ashkenazi Jewish, Cajun, and French Canadian	DNA mutation analysis or decreased serum hexosaminidase-A; the mother is usually screened first. If she is found to be at high risk, the partner will be tested. If both carry the trait, diagnostic testing of the fetus is indicated.	If both parents are positive, fetal DNA may be conclusively evaluated by amniocentesis or chorionic villi sampling.
Various (Tay-Sachs, cystic fibrosis, Canavan disease, familial dysautonomia, and others may be ordered as a four-panel test or an extended 11-panel test.)	Ashkenazi Jewish	DNA mutation carrier analysis of the mother and then of the partner of the pregnancy, as indicated; if both carry the trait, diagnostic testing of the fetus is indicated.	If both parents are positive, fetal DNA may be conclusively evaluated by amniocentesis or chorionic villi sampling.
Sickle cell anemia	African, Central or South American, Middle Eastern, Indian, and Caribbean	Presence of sickle cell hemoglobin and/or electrophoresis of maternal blood; the mother may be diagnosed with sickle cell anemia or may be a carrier. Positive results in the mother indicate screening of the partner. If both carry the trait, diagnostic testing of the fetus is indicated.	If both parents are positive, fetal DNA may be conclusively evaluated by amniocentesis or chorionic villi sampling.
Alpha and beta thalassemia	Alpha: Southeast Asian and Filipino; Beta: Italian and Greek	MCV less than 75%–80% and electrophoresis of maternal blood; the mother may be diagnosed with a form of alpha or beta thalassemia or may be a silent carrier of alpha thalassemia. Positive results in the mother indicate screening of the partner. If both carry the trait, diagnostic testing of the fetus is indicated.	If both parents are positive, fetal DNA may be conclusively evaluated by amniocentesis or chorionic villi sampling.

(continued)

Table 1.1   Pregnancy Screening Recommendations for Congenital Defects (continued)

First Trimester Screening for Trisomies
Recommended for all women

Blood Test Between 11 and 13 wk
PAPP-A: low in an abnormal test
hCG: high in an abnormal test

Ultrasound Between 11 and 13 wk
Nuchal translucency (measurement by ultrasound of space at the back of the fetal neck): thick in an abnormal test

Integrated Screening
Recommended for all women

- This is done in addition to first trimester screening.
- This is an additional blood test ideally performed at 15–16 wk but always before 22 wk.
- The additional test provides more accurate screening for trisomy 21 and trisomy 18, as well as screening for neural tube defects such as spina bifida.

Additional labs drawn at 15–16 wk (in addition to first trimester screening labs and ultrasound)

- MSAFP: high levels are associated with neural tube defects; low levels are associated with Down syndrome.
- hCG: high levels are associated with Down syndrome; low levels are associated with trisomy 18.
- uE3: low in Down syndrome and some neural tube defects V
- inhA: high in Down syndrome

Diagnostic Testing for Abnormal Screening Results

- High MSAFP concerning for neural tube defect: amniocentesis for amniotic fluid AFP and elevated acetylcholinesterase
- Results concerning for trisomy: DNA may be conclusively evaluated by amniocentesis or chorionic villi sampling.

MCV, maternal mean corpuscular volume; PAPP-A, pregnancy-associated plasma protein; hCG, human chorionic gonadotropin; MSAFP, maternal serum alpha-fetoprotein; uE3, unconjugated estriol; inhA, inhibin-A; AFP, alpha-fetoprotein.

off a urine sample and have routine pregnancy blood work done (Lab Values 1.1). If all goes well, she'll be spending a lot of time here over the next several months. Even a routine pregnancy involves quite a few office visits (Box 1.6).

Bess is glad to have a relatively nonexciting pregnancy so far. When her first trimester and integrated screen results come back, they're fine, suggesting that her chances of carrying a fetus with a trisomy or neural tube defect are very low. Just as with her

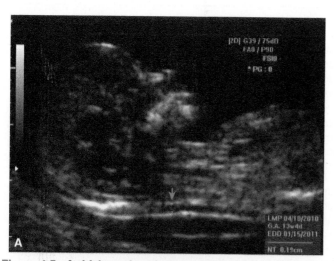
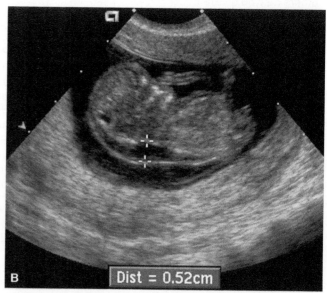

Figure 1.5. A thickened nuchal translucency. A thickened area at the back of the fetal neck viewed during an ultrasound nuchal translucency measurement may indicate a chromosomal defect of the fetus **(A)** A normal nuchal translucency. **(B)** A thickened nuchal translucency. (Reprinted with permission from Penny, S. M. [2017]. *Examination review for ultrasound* [2nd ed., Fig. 25.10B]. Philadelphia, PA: Lippincott Williams & Wilkins.)

Box 1.6 Routine Prenatal Visit Schedule

General Guidelines

- First visit typically in first trimester, especially for first pregnancies
- Once monthly through 27th week of pregnancy
- Every other week from 28–36 wk
- Weekly from 36 wk until birth

Exceptions

- Visits may be more frequent if the pregnancy is diagnosed as high risk.
- Not all providers follow this classic schedule. Some schedules include group visits, less frequent visits in the second trimester, and no first trimester visit, among others.

 Lab Values 1.1 Routine First Trimester Labs

Lab Test	Purpose	Normal Results	Bess's Results
Blood type and screen	To determine blood type, Rh factor, and any antibodies present in the blood from exposure to fetal blood. With certain blood types, such as a mother who is Rh−, a fetus with the opposite blood type (in this case Rh+) has the potential to promote maternal antibodies against that pregnancy.	A, B, O, AB Rh+ or Rh− Antibody negative	Not ordered this visit as Bess is known to be O+
CBC	To evaluate the blood for various kinds of anemia and infection	*RBC:* 4.2–5.4 million cells/µL *WBC:* 4,500–10,000 cells/µL *HCT:* 36.1%–44.3% *HGB:* 12.1–15.1 g/dL *MCV:* 80–95 fl *MCH:* 27–31 pg/cell *MCHC:* 32–36 g/dL	*RBC:* 4.3 million cells/µL *WBC:* 6,800 cells/µL *HCT:* 36.1% *HGB:* 12.1 g/dL *MCV:* 88 fl *MCH:* 28 pg/cell *MCHC:* 33 g/dL
Rubella	Rubella is a virus that is routinely vaccinated for in childhood. A rubella infection in pregnancy can be highly damaging to a fetus (teratogenic). Because vaccinations don't always work and sometimes wear off, pregnant women are often screened in pregnancy to see if they're susceptible. The rubella vaccine is a live virus and cannot be given during pregnancy. It is often given in the hospital during the postpartum period.	More than 10 IU/mL indicates immunity	Not drawn this visit as Bess has been vaccinated and her immune status was confirmed with prior blood work.
HBV	Many people are now vaccinated. A person may also have an acute or chronic infection or no exposure. HBV is *vertically transmitted,* which means it can be passed from mother to fetus. HBV can lead to liver cancer.	Anti-HBVs positive = immune from HBV	Not drawn this visit as Bess has been vaccinated and her immune status was confirmed with prior blood work.
Syphilis	Syphilis infection is also vertically transmitted from mother to fetus and is teratogenic.	Initial testing includes RPR and VDRL. A positive result would require additional testing to confirm the diagnosis	Negative

(continued)

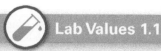

Lab Test	Purpose	Normal Results	Bess's Results
Gonorrhea and chlamydia	These are two of the most common sexually transmitted infections. Both can cause pregnancy complications and problems with future fertility. Urine test or swab.	Negative	Negative for both
HIV	HIV can also be transmitted to a fetus vertically. With treatment of the mother in pregnancy, however, transmission is reduced to a less than 2% chance. Finger stick, serum testing, or oral swab.	Negative	Negative
Urine dip	Tests for urinary tract infection; glucose in the urine, indicating high blood sugar; and protein in the urine, which may indicate kidney problems	*Protein:* negative *Glucose:* negative *Ketones:* negative *Nitrites:* negative *Leukocytes:* negative *Blood:* negative	*Protein:* negative *Glucose:* negative *Ketones:* negative *Nitrites:* negative *Leukocytes:* negative *Blood:* negative

RBC, red blood cell; WBC, white blood cell; HCT, hematocrit; HGB, hemoglobin; MCV, mean corpuscular volume; MCH, mean corpuscular hemoglobin; MCHC, mean corpuscular hemoglobin concentration; HBV, hepatitis B virus; RPR, rapid plasma reagin; VDRL, venereal disease research laboratory; HIV, human immunodeficiency virus.

previous pregnancies, she has had very little morning sickness. She's felt some initial fatigue with this pregnancy, just as she had with her other two, but it has pretty much lifted by the time her second trimester starts at 13 weeks (Box 1.7).

Second Trimester

At 20 weeks' gestation, Bess has her fetal survey, and the results are mostly fine (Box 1.8). The baby looks great. The only caution Dr. Philips gives her is that her placenta is lower than they'd like to see it.

"The location of the placenta in relation to the cervix can change as the uterus grows," explains Dr. Phillips. "When the placenta is very low—when it's over the cervix—a vaginal birth is impossible."

"But my placenta isn't *that* low, is it?" Bess asks. "I don't remember it being over the cervix."

"No," agrees Dr. Phillips. "That would be a condition called **placenta previa**, and you're correct that your placenta isn't quite that low (Fig. 1.6). We do like to see the placenta higher up in the uterus, however. It's the muscles of the uterus that stop the site of the placenta from bleeding after the birth, and there is a lot more muscle at the top of the uterus than at the bottom. When the placenta is attached low, there is a greater risk of bleeding after the birth."

"I bled after my last birth," says Bess.

Dr. Phillips nods. "I remember. That was different. Parts of your placenta were still attached to the wall of the uterus, which kept those muscles from contracting. Same end, different means. We'll keep an eye on it. We'll get a few more ultrasounds before

Box 1.7 Trimesters of Pregnancy

First trimester: Conception through week 12

Second trimester: Week 13 through week 28

Third trimester: Week 29 through week 40

Box 1.8 Aspects of Fetal Survey Ultrasound

Head, Face, and Neck
- Brain
- Upper lip

Chest
- All four chambers of the heart, as well as the outflow tracts, if possible

Abdomen
- Stomach
- Kidneys
- Bladder
- Umbilical cord insertion site
- Umbilical cord vessel number

Spine

Extremities
- Presence or absence of limbs

Sex
- If medically indicated (i.e., known sex-linked congenital disorder in the family) or according to patient preference (AIUS, 2013)

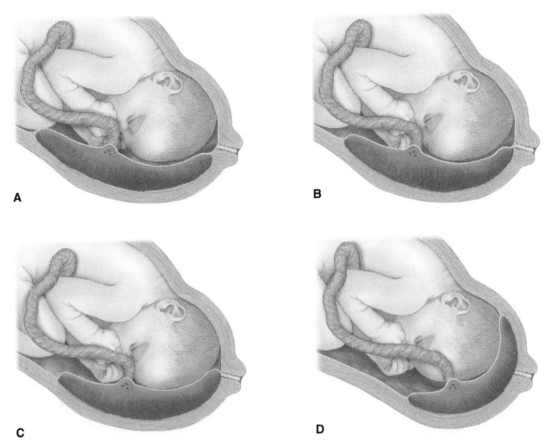

Figure 1.6. Placenta previa. A placenta oriented in the lower segment of the uterus poses a risk of hemorrhage for the mother. If the placenta overlies the cervix, it may rupture as the cervix dilates for birth. If the placenta is low but does not overlie the cervix, bleeding may occur after the birth because the lower part of the uterus is not as muscular as the fundus, or upper portion, and may not be able to adequately contract to stop bleeding from the site of placental attachment. **(A)** Low-lying placenta. **(B)** Marginal placenta previa. **(C)** Partial placenta previa. **(D)** Complete central placenta previa. (Reprinted with permission from Stephenson, S. R. [2015]. *Obstetrics and gynecology* [3rd ed., Fig. 18.9]. Philadelphia, PA: Lippincott Williams & Wilkins.)

the birth. Think of them as extra visiting hours with the fetus before the birth."

Her subsequent visits with Dr. Phillips are fine. Her vital signs, including her blood pressure, stay where they should be. The fetal heartbeat stays between 120 and 160 beats per minute (bpm), and her belly measurement is always in keeping with what would be predicted for the duration of her pregnancy.

At 24 weeks, Bess visits the lab again, this time for an oral glucose tolerance test to screen for gestational diabetes, a kind of diabetes that occurs only in pregnancy and resolves after the birth. She drinks 50 g of glucose in a solution that tastes like flat orange soda. The drink is syrupy, orangey sweet, and she thinks it's absolutely disgusting. She has her blood glucose checked an hour later, and she is a little anxious while she waits for the results. She knows that as long as her blood glucose level at the 1-hour mark is below 130 mg/dL, she does not have diabetes and will not have to undergo further testing for the condition (American College of Obstetricians and Gynocologists, 2013). Her glucose comes back at 126 mg/dL. She's relieved she won't ever have to drink the orange stuff again.

Third Trimester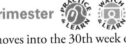

As Bess moves into the 30th week of her pregnancy, which is the beginning of the third trimester, she has another ultrasound to evaluate the position of the placenta. When following up with her about the ultrasound, Dr. Phillips says the placenta is still low but is not as close to the cervix as it was. This is good news but not great news, because it means that the placenta is still located in the lower, less muscular part of her uterus and that she will still need to be monitored very closely for bleeding.

And then, at 34 weeks of pregnancy, she does start to bleed. She notices it when she gets up to go to the bathroom late one night. It isn't a lot, but it is certainly blood. She suddenly feels tingly, frightened, and nauseous. Her abdomen is tender, particularly on the curve under her belly button. She feels a series of small, tightening contractions across her back and belly, like early labor. Jake calls a neighbor to stay with the kids and drives her straight to the hospital.

By the time they get to the hospital, the bleeding has stopped, and she tells the triage nurse who evaluates her that the contractions seem to be dissipating, as well. Her vital signs are fine, as usual, and the baby's heart beats along at a steady 140 bpm.

The triage nurse, Courtney, places what looks like a little pink hockey puck over her belly and cinches it into place with an elastic band. She positions it high up on her uterus near her ribs and explains that it is the **tocodynamometer**, or "toco," which detects any uterine contractions and monitors them. The information from the toco is graphed on a paper strip that continuously spews out of a machine, which Bess can see from her bed. The monitor shows a straight line. Courtney tells her that if she has a contraction, the line will form a little mountain.

As Courtney adjusts the toco, she explains that its location is important. It must be placed on the top part of the uterus, called the fundus, because this is where most of the action happens in terms of contractions. Bess says she's not feeling any contractions now, although she did earlier. Courtney says that sometimes the contractions are so small that the mother doesn't notice them but that they're still important to monitor. She says that if Bess does have some, Courtney will be able to evaluate how the baby's

heartbeat responds to them by looking at a second line on the monitor, above the toco line. Bess remembers this from Aidan's delivery—that the drops in his heart rate were important in relation to when the contractions occurred.

Before placing a second hockey puck, which she calls a transducer, Courtney feels all over Bess's belly and explains she is trying to figure out where the baby's back is, as that's the best place to monitor for the heartbeat (Fig. 1.7). As she palpates, she asks about tenderness, and Bess reports that she thinks it's a little better.

After Courtney has palpated for a few minutes more, she places the second transducer on her left side, just above the line of her pubic hair (Fig. 1.8). Courtney has been watching the monitor with its twin horizontal graphs as she places the second puck, and when she's done she explains what she's looking at.

Courtney says that the top line is the baby's heart rate and the bottom line, which has so far changed only in that the line dropped when the machine is adjusted, is monitoring contractions. She tells her that the baby's heart rate is averaging about 150 bpm,

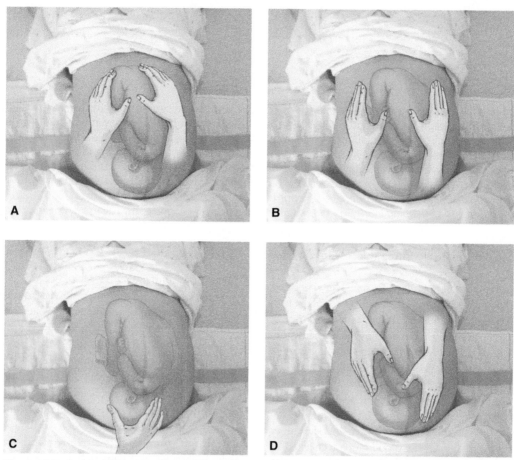

Figure 1.7. Leopold's maneuvers. (A) Feel the uterine fundus to determine the presence of the buttocks or head. **(B)** Place hands on the left and right sides of abdomen. Determine location of fetal back and fetal limbs. **(C)** Feel the area just above the pelvis and attempt to grasp fetal part (head or buttock depending on fetal position). Movement indicates fetus is not engaged in pelvis. **(D)** Slide hands down abdomen toward pelvis to determine if fetal head is flexed or extended. (Reprinted with permission from Stephen, T. C., Skillen, L., Day, R. A., & Jensen, S. [2011]. *Canadian Jensen's nursing health assessment* [1st ed., Fig. 27.11]. Philadelphia, PA: Lippincott Williams & Wilkins.)

with moderate **variability**. She explains that variability refers to the sawtooth pattern in the graph of the fetal heart rate, which indicates that it is going up and down. She says this is a good sign. She explains she's also looking for **decelerations**, or drops in the fetal heart rate, usually in relation to the contractions. She says sometimes these are a concern and sometimes they don't mean anything, but that she isn't having any right now, anyway (Fig. 1.9).

The on-call physician, Dr. Cates, arrives to evaluate Bess. She examines the fetal monitoring and toco strip and palpates all over Bess's belly, explaining that she's feeling the tone of the uterus. On the electronic health record, Dr. Cates is able to view the previous ultrasounds for placental position, and she can see the notes from her most recent visit. She measures Bess's abdomen and compares the measurement with that of 3 days previous, when she had her regularly scheduled visit with Dr. Philips. An ultrasound machine is wheeled in, and Dr. Cates does the ultrasound herself. She moves aside the straps with monitors for the contractions and fetus' heart rate and squirts warm blue gel over Bess's belly before running the transducer over it. She places an order for Bess's blood to be drawn to check for blood loss and coagulation (clotting) problems and a second order for an intravenous (IV) line to be placed in Bess's arm for hydration.

"I think you have a mild **placental abruption**," Dr. Cates says. "You don't seem to have any of the major risk factors, but sometimes these things just happen" (Fig. 1.10 and Box 1.9).

Bess looks at Jake, who appears similarly confused. Finally she asks, "What does that mean? Is the baby okay?"

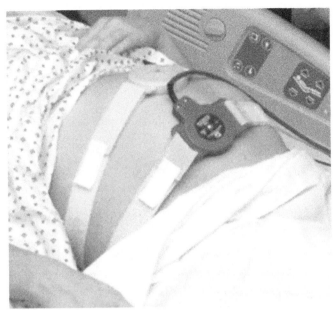

Figure 1.8. Electronic monitoring during labor. The tocodynamometer is placed higher on the maternal abdomen, toward the rib cage, and is over the top, or fundus, of the uterus. The location is important because the fundus is the most muscular part of the uterus and thus the best site for detecting a contraction. The Doppler ultrasound device is placed over the fetal back near the heart to detect fetal heart tones. This fetus is in the vertex (head down) position. (Reprinted with permission from Ricci, S. S. [2013]. *Essentials of maternity, newborn, & women's health nursing* [3rd ed., Fig. 14.5]. Philadelphia, PA: Lippincott Williams & Wilkins.)

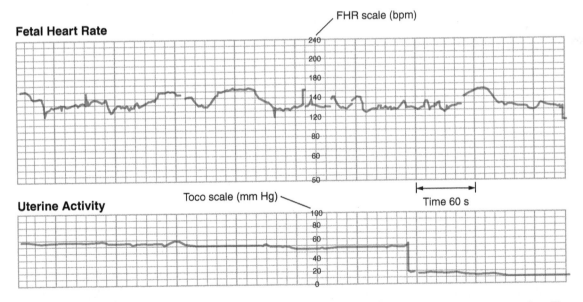

Figure 1.9. A fetal monitoring strip showing fetal heart rate (FHR) during a single contraction. The FHR is shown in the top of the image. Uterine contractions are shown in the bottom of the image. We can note several things from this fetal monitoring strip. (1) The baseline FHR is 150 beats per minute. (2) The FHR shows good variability. (3) There are no accelerations of the FHR. (4) There are no decelerations of the FHR. (5) There are no contractions. (Reprinted with permission from Suresh, M. [2012]. *Shnider and Levinson's anesthesia for obstetrics* [5th ed., Fig. 5.2]. Philadelphia, PA: Lippincott Williams & Wilkins.)

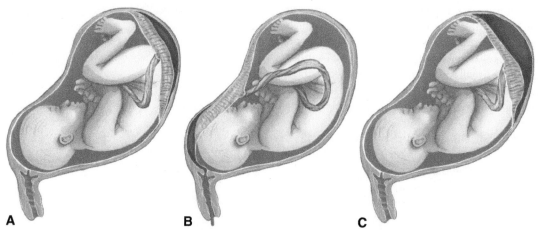

Figure 1.10. **Placental abruption. (A)** Partial abruption, concealed hemorrhage. **(B)** Partial abruption, apparent hemorrhage. **(C)** Complete abruption, concealed hemorrhage. (Reprinted with permission from Ricci, S. S. [2013]. *Essentials of maternity, newborn, & women's health nursing* [3rd ed., Fig. 19.5]. Philadelphia, PA: Lippincott Williams & Wilkins.)

"That means that part of the placenta peeled away from your uterus before it was supposed to. I'm reassured that your bleeding stopped, and the baby looks healthy. Your uterus doesn't seem very active at all" (Box 1.10).

"How much trouble are we in?" Jake asks. He takes Bess's hand in his own.

"It's too early to say for sure, but everything so far is reassuring. We'll need to admit you, Bess, and keep an eye on things. You're early enough in your pregnancy now that I'd like to avoid birth for a few more weeks, if possible. Sometimes these abruptions can heal spontaneously. I don't want you to get your hopes up just yet, but it's possible. Otherwise, we'll keep you here until the birth."

"We have six weeks left on the clock, Doc," says Jake.

Dr. Cates shakes her head. "You *had* six weeks left on the clock."

The week following the diagnosis of placental abruption goes slowly. At first, it seems like her vital signs are being checked every few minutes, and the toco and Doppler transducers never

---

Box 1.9   Risk Factors for Placental Abruption

- Maternal hypertension
- Maternal cigarette smoking
- Short umbilical cord
- Premature rupture of membranes
- History of placental abruption
- History of multiple pregnancies
- Advanced maternal age
- Abdominal trauma
- Cocaine use
- Multiple pregnancies (two or more fetuses)
- Blood clotting disorders

Box 1.10   Clinical Manifestations of Placental Abruption

- Vaginal bleeding (may be light or heavy; may be absent if concealed behind the placenta)
- Uterine tenderness (may be mild, acute, or localized)
- Frequent contractions with incomplete relaxation between contractions
- Back pain
- Hypovolemic shock of the mother
- Nonreassuring fetal heart rate patterns
- Increased fundal (uterine) height
- Hard maternal abdomen

---

leave her belly; they keep transmitting their information to the computer in her room and one at the nurses' station. She keeps the IV in for a few days.

After a while, however, it looks as though the danger is over. Her vital signs are stable, there are no contractions, the tenderness in her abdomen goes away entirely, and all the while the fetus seems fine. Eventually, the IV comes out, and the monitoring happens periodically on a schedule instead of continuously. When Bess asks why they were checking up on her so often and what they were looking for, the nurse tells her, gently, that they were making sure that she wasn't going into hypovolemic shock (Box 1.11).

"I don't know what that is," says Bess.

"Major blood loss," explains the nurse.

Finally, Dr. Phillips comes in with the news that she can go home but that she must rest, visit his office weekly, and call immediately if any changes occur.

After leaving the hospital, she now has **nonstress tests** (NSTs) with the fetal and contraction monitors weekly in Dr. Phillips'

Box 1.11   Clinical Manifestations of Hypovolemic Shock (Shock From Blood Loss)

Signs in the Mother

- Change in mental status (restlessness or trouble with concentration)
- Decreased (<30 mL/h) urinary output
- Thready (weak) pulse
- Decreased pulse rate
- Increased respiratory rate
- Decreased blood pressure (a late sign)
- Cool, moist, pale skin
- Decreasing hemoglobin and hematocrit

Signs in a Fetus With Maternal Hypovolemic Shock

- Nonreassuring fetal heart rate pattern, including:
  - Decreased variability
  - Tachycardia (heart rate > 160 beats per minute)
  - Late decelerations (fetal heart rate dips down *after* contraction)

office. During the NSTs, every time the baby moves, Bess notices that the little line representing the baby's heart rate goes up and then comes down. The nurse monitoring the NST, Liza, tells her that these little jumps are called **accelerations**, and that if the strip shows two accelerations in 20 minutes, the NST is referred to as **reactive**, which is considered a good thing (Fig. 1.11).

The NST is then added to an ultrasound to complete **biophysical profiles** (BPPs) (Table 1.2). The BPPs are done in the office, and it's almost like Dr. Phillips said it would be when checking for the position of the placenta: after a while, with all tests coming back fine, it is like having extra visiting hours with the baby. That is, extra visiting hours with a baby you're really worried about.

At 36 weeks, Dr. Phillips collects a rectal and vaginal swab to check for group B streptococcus. As with her last two pregnancies, the screening comes back negative. Because it is negative, Bess is told, she won't need antibiotics during labor to prevent the bacteria from being passed to the newborn (American College of Obstetricians and Gynecologists Committee on Obstetric Practice, 2013).

At 39 weeks, Bess wakes up wet again and panics, thinking that she's bleeding again, this time much more heavily. She turns on her bedside lamp and realizes the wetness is clear. For one confused second, she wonders why her blood is clear and where all of her red blood cells have gone before she realizes it's not blood at all. The **amniotic sac** surrounding the baby has sprung a leak. Her water has broken. She's relieved, excited, and buzzing with nerves. It's time for the baby to come. Jake wakes up alert, as though he's been expecting something to happen. He calls Dr.

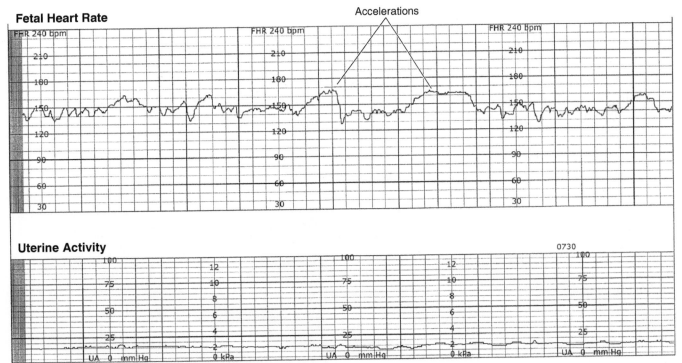

Figure 1.11. A reactive nonstress test. A nonstress test monitors fetal heart rate (FHR) but also uterine contractions. If contractions are present, the test is not a nonstress test but is instead a contraction stress test. A nonstress test is reactive or nonreactive. A reactive test is considered reassuring and includes at least two accelerations of FHR in 20 minutes. (Reprinted with permission from Gabrielli, A., Layon, A. J., & Yu, M. [2008]. *Civetta, Taylor, and Kirby's critical care* [4th ed., Fig. 101.4]. Philadelphia, PA: Lippincott Williams & Wilkins.)

Table 1.2 Biophysical Profile

Component	Normal (2 Points)	Abnormal (0 Points)
Nonstress test (done by evaluation of fetal and contraction monitoring strips)	At least two accelerations of fetal heart rate in 20 min	Less than two accelerations in 20 min
Fetal breathing movement by ultrasound	At least one episode of 30 s or more in 30 min of breathing movement	Fewer than 30 s of breathing movement in 30 min
Fetal activity by ultrasound	At least three general movements of body or limbs	Fewer than three movements of body or limbs
Fetal muscle tone by ultrasound	At least one episode of extending and then returning to flexion a limb, trunk, or hand	No movement, slow movement, or incomplete cycle
Amniotic fluid volume by ultrasound	At least one pocket of fluid with a vertical access equal to or greater than 2 cm	Largest pocket of fluid less than 2 cm

Recommended Management
Two or less: induce labor
Four: labor induction if >32 wk
  If <32 wk, repeat the BPP the same day, and deliver if the BPP stays <6.
Six: labor induction if >36 wk with normal amniotic fluid volume and favorable cervix
  If <36 wk with unfavorable cervix, repeat in 24 h and deliver if <6.
Eight: Labor induction indicated by amniotic fluid volume under 2 cm (oligohydramnios)

BPP, biophysical profile.

Phillips' office and then his mother, asking her to come over to watch over their sleeping children.

They are back in triage with a nurse named Pat, who wants to verify that Bess's waters have in fact broken and that she isn't having contractions. She first puts the toco up high on her belly under her ribs and then adds the Doppler to pick up fetal heart tones on the lower curve of her belly, off to one side. It's just like it was before. The baby is highly active, but there are no contractions.

Next, Pat places a speculum inside her vagina. She explains that it is sterile so that if her water has broken, the speculum won't introduce anything that could cause an infection. Pat looks to see whether any fluid is pooling in Bess's vagina. Finding some, she collects a sample. She explains that she will use Nitrazine paper to check the pH of the fluid (Fig. 1.12). If the paper turns blue, it is highly likely that Bess's membranes have ruptured and that the fluid is amniotic. She will also examine the fluid under a microscope (Fig. 1.13). If the fluid sample looks like little clear ferns, it is also a good indication that her water has broken. Lastly, Pat takes out the speculum and inserts a sterile-gloved hand into the vagina.

"You're about four centimeter dilated and fifty percent effaced," Pat says. "The baby's head is sitting nice and low. That's good." After helping Bess back to a seated position, Pat leaves to look at the fluid she has collected under the microscope. She returns a few minutes later and confirms that she had seen the little clear ferns consistent with amniotic fluid.

Dr. Phillips comes in a few minutes later looking fresh, like it isn't 2 AM.

"No contractions, eh?" he asks her. "And busted membranes." Bess agrees.

"Your contractions started all on their own with your first two, but this time we may have to help them out. When your waters break before you start having contractions it's called **premature rupture of membranes**. Back in the old days we'd

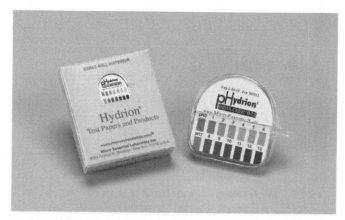

Figure 1.12. Nitrazine paper. (Reprinted with permission from Weber, J. R., & Kelley, J. H. [2014]. *Health assessment in nursing* [5th ed., figure in Table 3.1]. Philadelphia, PA: Lippincott Williams & Wilkins.)

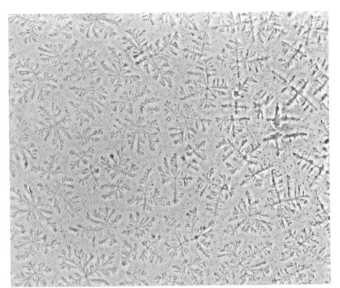

Figure 1.13. Ferning pattern of amniotic fluid. Urine and amniotic fluid can be distinguished by microscopic examination of a droplet of the fluid spread and dried on a microscope slide. The proteins in amniotic fluid give the appearance of ferning that is not observed with urine. (Reprinted with permission from McClatchey, K. D., Alkan, S., Hackel, E., Keren, D. F., Lewandrowski, K., Lee-Lewandrowski, E., & Woods, G. L. [2002]. *Clinical laboratory medicine* [2nd ed., Fig. 31-4]. Philadelphia, PA: Lippincott Williams & Wilkins.)

wait a day or two to see whether your contractions would start on their own. Unfortunately, we learned the hard way that this can give you and the baby a nasty infection, and we'd rather not risk it" (American College of Obstetricians and Gynecologists, 2016).

Bess and Jake both nod.

Dr. Phillips continues. "Now, Pat tells me that you're four centimeter dilated and about fifty percent effaced, which means that your cervix has been doing a nice job opening up and thinning out (Figs. 1.14 and 1.15). She also says that your baby is low in your pelvis, which is a very good thing, particularly as your water has broken. I'm going to check as well, but if your cervix seems as ripe to me as it does to Pat, I think we can start the **oxytocin** without doing anything extra to help soften up your cervix" (Analyze the Evidence 1.1).

Dr. Phillips' findings mirror Pat's. "Sometimes with a cervix that isn't as soft and open as yours we have to administer some additional medication to get the cervix ready before we start oxytocin to get the contractions going, but I think we're in pretty good shape here. Are you ready?" (The Pharmacy 1.2).

Bess looks at Jake and then back at Dr. Phillips. She takes a deep breath and swallows hard. She grabs Jake's hand and it's shaking, just like hers. "Do we have any other choice?"

Labor and Delivery

Dr. Phillips excuses himself, promising to check up on her later. Pat hangs the oxytocin on the same IV pole as the big bag of clear fluid that she started soon after Bess arrived. Pat says that she'll be starting the oxytocin at 1 mU/min and will check in every 15 minutes or so to increase the rate until the contractions are strong and regular. It takes a few hours, but the contractions finally start and slowly become stronger and more regular. Jake,

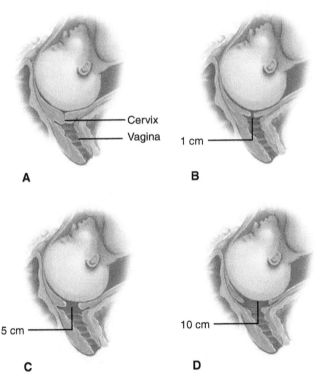

Figure 1.14. Cervical dilation. (A) Before labor: Cervix is not effaced or dilated. **(B)** Early effacement, early dilation to 1 cm. **(C)** Complete effacement, middilation to 5 cm. **(D)** Full dilation to 10 cm. (Reprinted with permission from Hatfield, N. T. [2014]. *Introductory maternity and pediatric nursing* [3rd ed., Fig. 8-3]. Philadelphia, PA: Lippincott Williams & Wilkins.)

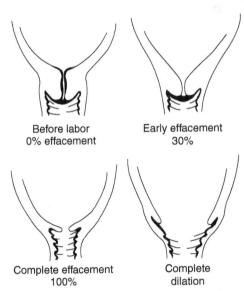

Figure 1.15. Cervical effacement. (Reprinted with permission from Evans, A. T., & DeFranco, E. (Eds.). [2014]. *Introductory maternity and pediatric nursing* [8th ed., Fig. 2-3]. Philadelphia, PA: Lippincott Williams & Wilkins.)

Analyze the Evidence 1.1 Use of the Bishop Score to Evaluate Cervical Ripeness

When a care team is deciding whether to induce labor in a pregnant woman, one important consideration is how favorable or "ripe" her cervix is. A favorable cervix is one that is more likely to efface and dilate to allow for passage of the fetus. An unfavorable cervix may not open sufficiently for fetal passage. How can we tell whether a cervix is favorable? For years the Bishop score has been the standard method for assessing for cervical ripeness. Recent evidence, however, has found this method may have limited ability to provide an accurate prediction of a successful labor induction. Two studies are listed here representing opposing viewpoints on whether the Bishop score should be used. Following that is the Bishop score tool, along with an explanation of how to interpret results.

Don't Use the Bishop Score

The Bishop score as a predictor of labor induction success: a systematic review. (Kolkman, et al., 2013)

Conclusion: "The Bishop score is a poor predictor for the outcome of induced labor at term and should not be used to decide whether to induce labor or not."

Use with Caution

Measures of success: Prediction of successful labor induction. (Gibson & Waters, 2015)

Conclusion: "Overall, if a patient has a favorable Bishop score, one could expect a successful induction. However, an unfavorable score does not adequately differentiate patients who will not deliver vaginally."

Bishop Score

	Score				Further Explanation
	0	1	2	3	
Position	Posterior	Middle	Anterior	–	The cervix moves to "point" toward the woman's front at the very end of pregnancy
Consistency	Firm	Medium	Soft	–	Prior to birth, a cervix may feel firm, like a chin. Women who have given birth previously have softer cervixes.
Effacement	0%–30%	40%–50%	60%–70%	80+%	At the beginning of labor, the cervix is about 3–4 cm thick. With full effacement, the cervix thins to become part of the lower uterus.
Dilation	Closed	1–2 cm	3–4 cm	5+ cm	Refers to how open the cervix is
Fetal station	−3	−2	−1, 0	+1, +2	Refers to the position of the fetus' head in relation to the distance from the ischial spines. These spines are part of the pelvis and are about 4 cm inside the vagina. When assessing fetal station, negative numbers mean the fetus is above the spines, and positive numbers mean the fetus is below the spines.

Recommended Management

Score of 5 or less: Labor likely not imminent without induction
Score of 9 or higher: Spontaneous labor likely
Score of 8 or higher: Possible greater likelihood of successful induction
Score less than 8: Induction may be less likely to be successful

Note: A successful induction is an uncomplicated vaginal delivery.

Bishop score adapted with permission from Bishop, E. (1964). Pelvic scoring for elective induction. *Obstetrics & Gynecology, 24* (2), 266–268.

The Pharmacy 1.2 Oxytocin

Guidelines	• Always administered through a pump, typically as a piggyback to the most proximal port • Standard concentrations typically range from 10 to 30 U in 500–1,000 mL. • Infusions start at 1 mU/min and are titrated up by 1–2 mU/min every 30–60 min, depending on response. • Goal: one contraction every 2–3 min lasting 80–90 s consistently, strong to palpation
Complications	• Uterine tachysystole (contractions too strong), placental abruption (placenta detaching before the birth of the infant), postpartum uterine hemorrhage, and rupture of the uterus • Uterine tachysystole, placental abruption, and uterine rupture can all result in insufficient oxygen reaching the fetus, which can be recognized by nurses viewing particular changes on the fetal monitoring strip.
Nursing Assessments	• Continuous fetal and contraction monitoring is required and should be reviewed every 15 min and with every change in dose. Fetal monitoring should be every 5 min during active pushing. • Maternal heart rate, blood pressure, and respirations should be monitored every half-hour to an hour and with dose changes. • Urine output should be at least 120 mL every 4 h. • Intravenous intake should not exceed 1,000 mL in 8 h.

who is paying close attention to the proceedings, tells her that it wasn't until the oxytocin was up to 9 mU/min that her labor really got started (Table 1.3).

Now that she is fully in labor, the birth experience becomes just like Bess and Jake remembered from prior births. Jake touches her shoulders and jaw so she'll remember to relax them. They listen to an MP3 of the ocean through a Bluetooth speaker linked to Jake's phone. Bess counts through her contractions, noting how long it takes to get to the worst part, the apex, knowing that afterwards it gets easier, like running down a hill, until the next contraction starts to build.

Her sense of time begins to change. It was feeling slow, as though everything were taking a long time, but now it feels like things aren't taking any time at all. Then things become really intense. She gets restless and wants to sit, then to lie down, then to stand up, and then to sit again.

Dr. Phillips returns to check on her. He tells her that she is in transition and that her cervix is so stretched it has almost disappeared; soon she'll be able to start pushing. And then the contractions stop, and she is able to rest and catch her breath.

What a marvelous invention of nature, she thinks: a final pit stop before the final push. Then, after 10 wonderful minutes of rest that feel like half an hour, the contractions start again, stronger than ever, and it is time to push.

The entire second stage, the pushing stage, is over in 20 minutes. Her first two births were quick pushes, as well, and at the end with

Table 1.3	**Stages of Labor**			
	First Stage	**Second Stage**	**Third Stage**	**Fourth Stage**
Results	Complete effacement and dilation of the cervix	Fetal expulsion	Delivery of the placenta	Initial bonding and recovery
Duration	*First birth:* Latent phase: 7–9 h Active phase: 6–18 h (cervical dilation 1.2 cm/h) Transition phase: 3.5 h *Subsequent birth:* Latent phase: 4–5.5 h Active phase: 2–10 h (cervical dilation 1.5 cm/h) Transition phase: 0–30 min	Average of 30 min–3 h for first births Average of 0–30 min for subsequent births	Up to 30 min	Up to first 4 h after birth

(continued)

Table 1.3	Stages of Labor (continued)			
	First Stage	**Second Stage**	**Third Stage**	**Fourth Stage**
Uterus and cervix	*Cervical dilation:* Latent phase: 0–3 cm Active phase: 4–7 cm Transition phase: 8–10 cm *Uterine contractions:* Latent phase: mild-to-moderate contractions lasting 30–40 s Active phase: contractions every 2–3 min lasting 40–60 s, moderate-to-strong Transition phase: every 2 min, lasting 60–90 s, strong	Uterine contractions: often a pause between transition and contractions of the second stage; shorter than transition phase contractions, 40–60 s Strong, usually every 40–60 s	Consistently and firmly contracted	Consistently and firmly contracted
Sensation	Pain often begins in the back and then wraps around to the front; it may refer down to the legs and buttocks.	Similar to the first stage plus an urge to bear down and a stretching sensation of the vagina and vulva, known as the "ring of fire"	Mild to no cramping	"Afterpains" similar to the first stage may be present, especially with breastfeeding and for women who have given birth previously
Behavior	A range of behaviors may occur in the first stage, from excited to anxious; the client is typically more focused in the active phase. Behavior may be erratic and uncontrolled in transition.	Intense concentration and lack of awareness of surroundings	Relieved, excited, and exhausted	Tired and excited

this baby, just as with her others, she feels strong and confident, as though she was made for giving birth. Their baby, a lovely boy, they find out, starts crying as soon as his body slithers out. Dr. Phillips puts him on Bess's belly, and Pat rubs him down with a warm flannel blanket and laughs as he pushes off with his feet, seeming to crawl.

Jake and Bess are fascinated by his scrunched angry face and the sparse dark hair plastered to his head. His nails have a bluish cast, which Bess remembers from her other babies as being normal and expected. Jake puts his finger in his son's hand, and his son grabs it.

Jake becomes aware of the activity before Bess does. People suddenly seem to be moving very quickly and appear very worried. She plays with the baby's little shell-shaped nails. She feels drowsy and peaceful and is glad not to be in pain.

"Am I bleeding?" she asks, only mildly curious.

"Yes," says Dr. Phillips. "You're bleeding."

Then everything fades away.

After Delivery

Bess wakes up in a room she doesn't recognize. She has an IV in each arm. One tube is clear and the other deep, dark red. It must be blood in that tube, she realizes. Jake is holding her hand.

"Hey lazy," he says. "You slept through all of the excitement."

"I feel awful," says Bess. "What happened? Where's the baby? What time is it?"

"The baby is fine," says Jake. "He's in the nursery. You're in the surgical intensive care unit recovering. It's 5:30 in the morning, and you had the baby yesterday afternoon. Bess, they couldn't stop the bleeding. I'm sorry. They had to take out your uterus."

"Oh," says Bess, still groggy. "Really? Does that mean we can't ever have sex again?"

Jake laughs, but a little sadly, a little cautiously. "They've got you drugged up good. They took out your uterus, not your vagina. We can still have sex, but no more babies."

"Okay," Bess says, closing her eyes again.

By the end of the day, much of the wooziness has worn off, and Bess has been transferred down to the regular postpartum floor. She finds she can do everything just fine if she does it cautiously. She discovers that a urinary catheter has been placed at some point that she doesn't remember. Once she's proven that she can walk to and from the bathroom twice without assistance, the catheter is removed.

When her head is clearer, Bess is curious about exactly what happened while she was out. Jake is sitting in a chair next to her bed and has just caught her up on how the kids are doing. Bess says, "Can you tell me more about what happened after the birth? I need to know. Everything turned out fine, right? We made it."

Jake agrees and is quiet a moment.

Then he says, "Dr. Phillips said that if the placenta didn't deliver within a half-hour of the birth of the baby, bleeding would be more likely to occur. So he waited that half-hour and then pulled on the umbilical cord—he called it 'applying traction.' That's when you started to bleed, and that's when people started rushing around" (Box 1.12).

"I remember that part," Bess says.

"Pat called for help, and some other nurses came in. One took the baby from you; another—I can't remember her name—took me to a corner of the room, out of the way. She was trying to explain what was going on. I was freaking out, but she just kept talking to me in a gentle way, and it helped calm me down. She was great."

"Pat put an oxygen mask on your face and kept checking your vitals on the computer. She added a pain med to your IV—I think fentanyl—while another nurse started a second IV in your other arm."

"They gave you a bunch of different drugs to try to make your uterus stop bleeding, but none of it worked" (The Pharmacy 1.3).

"That must have been scary," Bess says.

"That's not the worst of it," Jake says. "I saw Dr. Phillips put one hand into your vagina and with the other push down hard

---

Box 1.12   Risk Factors for Early Postpartum Hemorrhage

- Retained placenta (pieces of the placenta that are left behind in the uterus after the birth of the rest of the placenta during the third stage)
- Failure to progress in the second stage (the infant fails to move down the birth canal during the pushing stage)
- Placenta accreta (the placenta grows into the muscle of the uterus)
- Lacerations of the cervix, vagina, or vulva
- Instrumental deliveries (vaginal deliveries that include use of vacuum suction or forceps applied to the fetal head)
- Large for gestational age infant (infants over the 90th percentile for weight)
- Hypertensive disorders
- Induction of labor with oxytocin
- Augmentation of labor with oxytocin

Adapted from Sheiner, E., Said, L., Levy, A., Seidman, D., & Hallack, M. (2005, September). Obstetric risk factors and outcome of pregnancies complicated with early postpartum hemorrhage: A population-based study. *Journal of Maternal-Fetal & Neonatal Medicine, 18* (3), 149–154.

The Pharmacy 1.3   Fentanyl, Misoprostol, Methylergonovine

	Fentanyl	Misoprostol	Methylergonovine
Overview	Strong opioid analgesic, rapid onset, short half-life	Stimulates uterine contractions (off label use. Also prescribed as ulcer prophylaxis)	Stimulates uterine contraction; vasoconstrictive
Route and dosing	50–100 µg IV hourly. May also be used as part of an epidural	800–1,000 µg rectally. Onset rapid	IM: 0.2 mg every 2–4 h, max four doses. Onset 2–5 min Oral: 0.2–0.4 mg every 6–12 h. Onset 5–10 min IV: contraindicated, emergency only due to severe hypertension and stroke risk. 0.2 mg/min
Care considerations	• If used in epidural, it may cause pruritus (itching) • As with any opioid, may cause nausea and respiratory depression • In the case of overdose or severe respiratory depression, naloxone (Narcan) can reverse effects of opioid	Patient may experience headache, diarrhea, or abdominal pain	• Should never be used prior to birth of fetus because of potential for very strong, prolonged contractions • If used in third stage obstetric provider should be directly supervising • Smoking strongly discouraged because of vasoconstrictive properties of medication • Monitor for appropriate uterine firmness, fundal height, and lochia • Patient may have very strong cramping
Warning signs	Respiratory rate less than 12 breaths/min when at rest	Continuing uterine atony and profuse lochia indicate treatment failure	• Patient blood pressure should be carefully monitored for severe hypertension • Monitor for toxicity: chest pain, headache, nausea, muscle pain, general weakness, cold or numb digits, extremities tingling

IM, intramuscular; IV, intravascular.

over and over again on your belly. It looked like he was assaulting you, and I asked the nurse what he was doing to you. I was ready to go over and punch him. But the nurse explained that he was massaging your uterus so that it would contract and close off the blood vessels to stop the bleeding.

"They tried to get me to leave the room, because they could tell I was upset, but I wasn't about to leave you. Dr. Philips kept reaching deeper and deeper inside of you. He would pull out his arm, which was covered in blood, check his hand for something, and go back in. Pat drew some tubes of your blood and handed them off to someone.

"Then the anesthesiologist came in. He looked inside your mouth and asked about when you had last had something to eat or drink. Then I heard Dr. Phillips telling Pat to get ready for a blood transfusion. I saw them trade out an empty bucket for one that was filled with blood."

Jake gets choked up and has to stop. Bess just squeezes his hand and waits. "I've never been more afraid in my life," he says, after a moment.

"You don't have to keep going," says Bess.

"It's all right," says Jake. "It's good to talk about it—unless you don't want to hear anymore."

"I'd like to hear the rest," says Bess.

"Alright," he says. "It was right after that when another nurse came in and explained that you were bleeding badly and they weren't sure why. They wanted to put you under general anesthesia and see if they could stop the bleeding. The nurse said if they still couldn't stop the bleeding, they might have to remove your uterus... to do a **hysterectomy**. She asked me to sign some consents. I told her that you should sign them, but she said you were not in any condition to do that. It seemed like there was no other choice, so I signed them. I didn't even read them. And then they wheeled you out of the room and down the hall for surgery."

"Hey—everything's okay now," Bess says. "You did the right thing."

"I know," Jake says. He shakes his head and grins. "I'm not worried about that. Man, it's just so good to have you here, trying to make me feel better, like I'm the one who had the near-death experience."

The baby, Milo, is now rooming with her, sleeping in a clear plastic bassinette next to her bed. He is swaddled from neck to feet and wears a little knit cap with dark blue and kelly green stripes. Every now and then in his sleep he squeaks. Periodically,

a nurse, a different one every 8 hours or so, comes in to check her vital signs and Milo's. The nurse checks her abdominal wound, which doesn't looks as bad as Bess would have thought. She doesn't have any vaginal bleeding, or **lochia**, because she no longer has a uterus with a lining to shed. She cries a little bit, but not much. She thinks she's just being sentimental. After all, her uterus was the original residence of all three of her children.

A nursing student, Shoshi, comes to see her after Bess has been on the postpartum unit for nearly a week and is preparing to leave. Jake is there too. Shoshi tells them that Bess bled so much that she received more than 30 units of blood, that it was going out as quickly as they could get it in.

"For context," explains Shoshi, who has been doing a lot of reading on the topic, "The average human body contains four to five liters of blood, and in pregnancy you have about fifty percent more, so about six or seven liters."

"That's a lot of blood," says Jake.

"That's a lot of blood," agrees Shoshi.

"I feel like I slept through a near tragedy, like napping through a pile-up on the freeway," says Bess. "I think I'll be processing all of it for a while."

The Newborn

Milo is a big baby at birth: 8 lb, 5 oz, or 3,900 g (or 3.9 kg), to be exact. But he is not above the 90th percentile (Fig. 1.16), which would have made him **large for gestational age**. His head circumference is 34.2 cm, and he is 54 cm long, with his legs straightened out of their preferred flexed position. Bonnie, a nurse who works with Bess and baby Milo postpartum, tells Bess that he scored nine on his 1-minute Apgar test and nine again on his 5-minute Apgar (Table 1.4). Like most babies, Bonnie explains, he lost a point both times because his hands and feet had a bluish cast to them, but he is in excellent health. He is a round, brown baby with a light down of hair, called **lanugo**, swirled over his shoulders and temples, and a sweet pink raspberry of a mouth.

After Bess was moved from the surgical intensive care unit to the postpartum unit, Bonnie filled her in about Milo and all that had happened with him since his birth. She pointed out that the hospital ID bracelet around his ankle was identical to the bracelets Bess and Jake were wearing. When he arrived in the newborn nursery, on the same ankle he was given a security tag

The Nurse's Point of View

Shoshi: Although Bess doesn't remember it, I was in the operating room during the surgery. Bess was in very good hands during the surgery; everyone worked hard to stop the bleeding.

I watched first as the team tried a D&C, a dilation and curettage. During the procedure, the walls of the uterus were scraped to dislodge any placental fragments that might have been left behind. When pieces of the placenta remain in the uterus, the

uterus can't contract down on the blood vessels and stop the bleeding from the site where the rest of the placenta detached.

As I watched, no placental fragments were removed. Next, the team placed a device resembling a deflated balloon, called a tamponade, and inflated it. The purpose of the tamponade is to apply pressure to the walls of the uterus to compress the blood vessels and stop the bleeding. This, however, did not work completely, either, although it did slow the bleeding. Ultimately, the decision was made to perform a hysterectomy to stop the bleeding and save Bess's life.

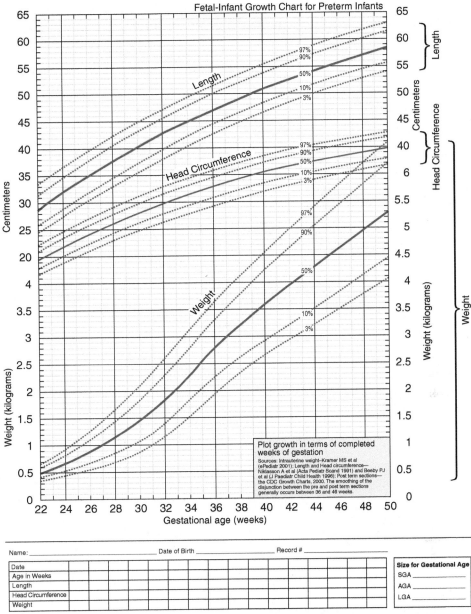

Figure 1.16. Neonatal growth chart. The gestational age depends on the duration of the pregnancy at the time of birth. Below the 10th percentile is considered small for gestational age (SGA). Above the 90th percentile is considered large for gestational age (LGA). AGA, appropriate for gestational age. (Reproduced with permission from Fenton TR; licensee BioMed Central Ltd. This is an open-access article: Verbatim copying and redistribution of this article are permitted in all media for any purpose, provided this notice is preserved along with the article's original URL. http://www.biomedcentral.com/1471-2431/3/13.)

that would trigger an alarm if anyone tried to remove him from the floor. She had scanned his feet for footprints, which loaded directly into the electronic health record.

Bonnie performed an initial physical assessment, noting the baby's general appearance and respiratory effort, his normal heart sounds and body movements, his soft, round belly and clear eyes, and normal-appearing penis and testes. His respiratory rate was 40 breaths a minute, which is normal for a newborn, and his heart, when she listened at its apex, was beating 140 bpm. His chest rose and fell symmetrically. She saved the axillary temperature for last, because babies hate having things put in their armpits,

and found it was a normal 37°C. In accordance with hospital protocol, no blood pressure was taken as there was no immediate reason to be concerned about the baby boy's heart.

She checked his reflexes. She inserted a finger into his mouth, and he sucked at it reflexively. When she lightly stroked his cheek, he turned to her finger as though rooting for his mother's breast. She startled him by creating the sensation that he was dropping, and he made the "baby jazz hands" sign and then brought his arms back tight to his chest, which is the Moro reflex. She inserted a finger into his hand, as his father had done, and he grabbed it, demonstrating the grasp reflex.

Table 1.4 APGAR Scoring of an Infant

	0 Points	1 Point	2 Points
Activity and muscle tone	Absent	Flexion of arms and legs	Active movement
Pulse	Absent	Below 100 bpm	Over 100 bpm
Grimace (reflex) with stimulation, such as suctioning of the nares	No response, floppy	Some extremity flexion or cry	Pulls away, sneezes, or coughs
Skin color (appearance)	Pale, blue body and extremities	Body pink, extremities blue	Body and extremities pink
Respirations	Absent	Slow and irregular	Robust cry

Done at 1 min and 5 min after birth, Apgar scoring is used to assess if an infant needs immediate medical care; it does not predict long-term outcomes.

APGAR Interpretation
- 0 to 3: Severely depressed: prompt resuscitation indicated
- 4 to 6: Moderately depressed: some assistance for breathing indicated
- 7 to 10: Excellent condition

bpm, beats per minute.

Within the first 24 hours after birth, Bonnie performed a second, more thorough head-to-toe exam. She weighed and measured him regularly. He was given a bath and had his hearing checked. His heel was stuck after 24 hours, and the blood was sent away for a battery of routine neonatal testing.

Now, as it is getting close to time for Bess and Milo to be discharged, a lactation consultant stops by and gives Bess some final guidance on breastfeeding. As Bess watches Milo successfully latch on, she is very grateful to have him and excited to be taking him home soon.

Think Critically

1. What if Bess had chosen a form of intrauterine contraception that did not contain hormones? What would your patient teaching include about side effects?
2. What, if any, risk factors did Bess have for immediate postpartum hemorrhage?
3. If Bess lost enough blood to go into hypovolemic shock, what signs and symptoms would you expect to see?

4. Compare the nursing considerations of two uterotonics, oxytocin and methylergonovine. How are they similar? How do they differ?
5. What newborn reflex looks like "baby jazz hands"? What are some other anticipated newborn reflexes?

Unfolding Patient Stories: Brenda Patton • Part 1

Brenda Patton is 18 years old at 24 weeks' gestation with her first child. During each prenatal visit, what questions would the nurse ask to evaluate fetal well-being? What factors can interfere with normal growth and development of the fetus? Describe the assessments the nurse performs to monitor fetal growth and development. (Brenda Patton's story continues in Unit 4.)

Care for Brenda and other patients in a realistic virtual environment: *vSim for Nursing* (thepoint.lww.com/vSimMaternity). Practice documenting these patients' care in DocuCare (thepoint.lww.com/DocuCareEHR).

Unfolding Patient Stories: Amelia Sung • Part 1

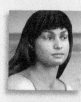

Amelia Sung is 36 years old and 8 weeks pregnant with her second child. She tells the nurse that she is considering an amniocentesis because of her age. What information would the nurse include when providing education on an amniocentesis? (Amelia Sung's story continues in Unit 3.)

Care for Amelia and other patients in a realistic virtual environment: *vSim for Nursing* (thepoint.lww.com/vSimMaternity). Practice documenting these patients' care in DocuCare (thepoint.lww.com/DocuCareEHR).

References

American College of Obstetricians and Gynecologists. (2013). *Gestational diabetes mellitus* (ACOG Practice Bulletin No. 137). Washington, DC: Author.

American College of Obstetricians and Gynecologists. (2016). Practice Bulletin No. 160 summary: Premature rupture of membranes. *Obstetrics and Gynecology, 127*(1), 192–194.

American College of Obstetricians and Gynecologists Committee on Obstetric Practice. (2013). *Prevention of early onset group B streptococcal disease in newborns* (Committee Opinion No. 485). Washington, DC: Author.

American Institute of Ultrasound in Medicine. (2013). *AIUM practice parameter for the performance of obstetric ultrasound examinations.* Laurel, MD: Author.

Gibson, K. S., & Waters, T. P. (2015, October). Measures of success: Prediction of successful labor induction. *Seminars in Perinatology, 39*(6), 475–482.

Kolkman, D., Verhoeven, C., Brinkhorst, S., van der Post, J., Pajkrt, E., Opmeer, B., & Mol, B. W. (2013). The bishop score as a predictor of labor induction success: A systematic review. *American Journal of Perinatology, 30*(8), 625–630.

Massad, L. S., Einstein, M. H., Huh, W. K., Katki, H. A., Kinney, W. K., Schiffman, M., . . . Lawson, H. W. (2013). 2012 Updated Consensus Guidelines for the Management of Abnormal Cervical Cancer Screening Tests and Cancer Precursors. *Journal of Lower Genital Tract Disease, 17*(5), S1–S27.

Perriera, L. K., Blumenthal, P. D., Stuart, G. S., Thomas, M. A., Gilliam, M., & Creinin, M. (2016). Return of spontaneous menses and fertility after removal of the liletta levonorgestrel intrauterine system. *Obstetrics & Gynecology, 127*.

Suggested Readings

George, T. P., DeCristofaro, C., Dumas, B. P., & Murphy, P. F. (2015). Shared decision aids: Increasing patient acceptance of long-acting reversible contraception. *Healthcare, 3*(2), 205–218.

Heavey, E., & Maher, M. D. (2015). Placental abruption: Are we going to lose them both? *Nursing, 45*(5), 54–59.

Macones, G. A., Hankins, G. D., Spong, C. Y., Hauth, J., & Moore, T. (2008). The 2008 National Institute of child health and human development workshop report on electronic fetal monitoring: Update on definitions, interpretation, and research guidelines. *Obstetrics and Gynecology, 37*(5), 510–515.

Main, E. K., Goffman, D., Scavone, B. M., Low, L. K., Bingham, D., Fontaine, P. L., . . . Levy, B. S. (2015). National partnership for maternal safety consensus bundle on obstetric hemorrhage. *Journal of Midwifery & Women's Health, 60*(4), 458–464.

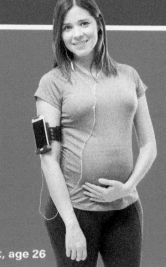
Objectives

1. Identify current recommendations for Pap screening by patient age.
2. Recognize the diagnostic criteria for polycystic ovarian syndrome.
3. Recognize important risk factors and interventions for late (secondary) postpartum hemorrhage.
4. Distinguish between autosomal recessive and autosomal dominant genetic inheritance.

5. Identify signs of uterine atony and pertinent assessments.
6. Discuss the significance of Rh incompatibility.
7. Explain some of the noncontraceptive benefits of combined oral contraceptives.
8. Contrast true and false labor.
9. Identify infant feeding readiness cues.

Key Terms

Autosomal dominant
Autosomal recessive
Bloody show
Braxton Hicks contractions
Colostrum
Combined oral contraceptive (COC)
Cystic fibrosis
Engorgement

False labor
Orthostatic hypotension
Polycystic ovarian syndrome (PCOS)
Rho (D) immune globulin
Stripping of the membranes
Tay-Sachs disease
Uterine atony

Before Conception

Tati Bennett, who's 26 years old, has a pretty good life with her husband, Caleb. They met in college their senior year and have been together ever since. Tati and Caleb married 2 years ago on the shore of a small lake in her hometown. It rained a little that day, and Caleb said that was good luck. Caleb works as a computer engineer and Tati works for a company that rents out studio space to different artists and craftspeople. They have a Maltese dog named Thor and a black-and-white cat named Jim. Last year they bought a small house with a real picket fence and rose bushes that take turns blooming throughout the summer.

Tati has been on a **combined oral contraceptive (COC)**, "the pill," since she was 19, and her menstrual cycle is as regular as clockwork. Before she started the pill, however, she would sometimes go months without getting her period. She did not have her first period until she was 16, long after most of her friends. She'd carried a little more weight than most of her friends for as long as she could remember, and her mother had thought maybe that was why she wasn't getting her period. Her mother was on the heavier side, as well.

A few years after her period finally started, when she was a freshman in college, she noticed that her skin seemed to be greasier than her friends' skin. Most of them had skin that was getting smoother and clearer as time went on. Once, when she was using a friend's new magnifying mirror, she was horrified to notice spiky, dark hairs on her chin, and even some on her upper lip. She went home to borrow her mother's tweezers and then asked her mother to make an appointment with Elsa, the nurse practitioner she'd been seeing since childhood

Elsa asked her all about her periods, and Tati told her that she sometimes went as long as 4 or 5 months without having one. She thought it was normal because she was still a teenager, but if anything she was getting fewer every year instead of more. She told Elsa about the oily skin and acne, and how she'd found the hairs on her chin and her upper lip, and how she even had some thick, coarse hairs sneaking up from her bikini line toward her belly button. Elsa said she'd like to do some blood tests, but that she was pretty sure Tati had **polycystic ovarian syndrome (PCOS)** (Box 2.1, Fig. 2.1, and Lab Values 2.1).

When all of the lab results were returned, Elsa said that she was confident that Tati had PCOS and that, though they could manage the condition, there wasn't a cure. She said there wasn't good agreement on what caused the condition but that Tati's symptoms were a classic presentation.

The first thing that Elsa recommended was a healthy diet and exercise to get her down to a healthy body mass index (BMI), between 18.5 and 24.9 (Moran, Hutchison, Norman, & Teede, 2011) (see Box 1.5). She explained that this could help reduce the extra male hormones, known as androgens, she had, which could reduce the acne and the extra hair and might help prevent her from developing diabetes in the future. It might also make her periods more regular.

Tati felt embarrassed. She'd never felt so fat or unattractive in her whole life. Here was Elsa telling her that the best thing she could do was lose weight because she had way too much "boy hormone" in her. She wanted to cry.

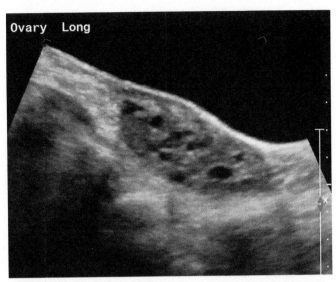

Figure 2.1. Ovarian cysts. Dark circles represent ovarian cysts. Although not independently diagnostic of polycystic ovary syndrome, they are a common finding. (Reprinted with permission from Iyer, R. S., & Chapman, T. [2015]. *Pediatric imaging: The essentials* [1st ed., Fig. 22.14B]. Philadelphia, PA: Lippincott Williams & Wilkins.)

Tati looked up and met Elsa's eye. "I feel like a big, gross blob," she said.

Elsa leaned toward her. "You're not a big, gross blob. You've just got your hormones in a twist. This is good news. We have a diagnosis to work with now. That means we can start to make you healthier."

Next, Elsa said she wanted to put her on a COC, birth control.

"I'm not even sexually active," said Tati. "I broke up with my boyfriend like a year ago and we maybe did it twice. We used condoms," she said quickly.

"I'm glad you're being safe, and as I'm sure you know from your sex education class, condoms are the best way to prevent the transmission of sexually transmitted infections, besides abstinence and regular screening." Elsa said. "But there's actually a couple of reasons I'd like to start you on the pill."

Elsa went on to explain that the pill would help keep her menstrual cycle regular and would also help with the acne and hair issues (Legro et al., 2013) (Fig. 2.2). She also told her that many people think a woman can't get pregnant if she has PCOS and that this wasn't true. Many women with PCOS still ovulate, but it can be a lot harder for them to tell when they're ovulating and thus fertile because of irregular menses (Durain & McCool, 2015).

"You may ovulate only once or twice a year and are fertile for only twenty-four hours each time, but we still have to consider you fertile until proven otherwise," said Elsa.

Tati had watched her mother put on weight as she'd grown older. She knew her mother now took medications for hypertension and high cholesterol. She had a grandmother who had such bad type 2 diabetes that she had to give herself insulin injections. Her father was overweight, and her mother said she thought she had some cousins with PCOS, as well. Tati had gained 12 lb in the first semester of college alone.

Box 2.1   Rotterdam Criteria for Diagnosis of PCOS

Two of the following three criteria are required for the diagnosis of PCOS:

- Oligo- or anovulation (either fewer than nine menstrual periods a year or no menstruation is considered evidence of this)
- Clinical and/or biochemical signs of hyperandrogenism (clinical signs may include male-pattern hair growth and acne; biochemical signs would include laboratory test results such as high testosterone level)
- Polycystic ovaries (as seen on ultrasound, polycystic ovaries are enlarged by many cysts; not present in every woman with PCOS)

PCOS, polycystic ovary syndrome.

Adapted from Rotterdam ESHRE/ASRM-Sponsored PCOS consensus workshop group. (2004). Revised 2003 consensus on diagnostic criteria and long-term health risks related to polycystic ovarian syndrome (PCOS). *Human Reproduction, 19*, 41.

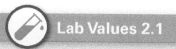

Lab Values 2.1 — Polycystic Ovary Syndrome

Lab Name	Rationale	Value
Labs to Evaluate for Hyperandrogenism		
Total testosterone	Evidence of hyperandrogenism	For adult women, normal values are 40–60 mg/dL (1.4–2.1 nmol/L).
		Women with PCOS commonly have values in the range of 20–150 ng/dL (1.0–5.2 nmol/L).
		Values over 200 ng/dL (6.9 nmol/L) suggest a testosterone-producing tumor.
Free testosterone	Alternate to total testosterone	The normal range for women is 0.06–1.08 ng/dL.
Labs to Rule Out Other Conditions		
DHEA-S	Tests for adrenal sources of hyperandrogenism, especially if changes are rapidly progressing	A value over 700 μg/dL (13.6 mmol/L) is suggestive of an androgen-producing tumor.
TSH	Thyroid hormones may alter menstruation. Hypothyroidism (high TSH) may result in more menstrual bleeding than usual. Hyperthyroidism (low TSH) may cause amenorrhea or oligomenorrhea and lighter menstrual bleeding.	The normal range for TSH level is 0.03–5.0 U/mL.
Serum cortisol	Rule out Cushing disease or cortisol resistance	A value less than 10 μg/dL (276 nmol/L) suggests that Cushing disease is not present.
Prolactin	Prolactin is produced by the anterior pituitary. Some medications, as well as tumors of the pituitary, can cause elevated prolactin levels, which can lead to amenorrhea and oligomenorrhea.	A value over 25 ng/mL suggests that a high prolactin level may be causing menstrual irregularities.
IGF-1	Elevation may indicate acromegaly (a rare syndrome of excess growth hormone produced by the anterior pituitary, causing gigantism).	The normal range varies by age (in years): • 182–780 ng/mL for ages 16–24 • 114–492 ng/mL for ages 25–39 • 90–360 ng/mL for ages 40–54 • 71–290 ng/mL for ages 55 and older
Labs to Monitor for Associated Conditions		
Fasting lipids	Women with PCOS often also have elevated cholesterol.	• Desirable total cholesterol level is under 200 mg/dL. • Optimal LDL level is less than 100 mg/dL. • Optimal HDL level is greater than 59 mg/dL. • Normal triglycerides level is less than 150 mg/dL.
Two-hour OGTT	Insulin resistance and type 2 diabetes are common in women with PCOS.	The normal range is less than 140 mg/dL (7.8 mmol/L). The prediabetic range is from 140 to 199 mg/dL (7.8–11.1 mmol/L). The diabetic range is 200 mg/d (12 mmol/L) and over.
Fasting glucose or hemoglobin A_{1c}	Alternate to OGTT	A fasting glucose level of 126 mg/dL (7 mmol/L) or higher on two different occasions indicates diabetes. Hemoglobin A_{1c}: • 4%–5.6%, normal • 5.7%–6.4%, increased risk of diabetes • 6.5% or higher, diabetes

Not all labs may be performed.
PCOS, polycystic ovary syndrome; DHEA-S, dehydroepiandrosterone sulfate; TSH, thyroid-stimulating hormone; IGF-1, insulin-like growth factor 1; LDL, low-density lipoprotein; HDL, high-density lipoprotein; OGTT, oral glucose tolerance test.
Adapted from Buggs, C., & Rosenfield, R. (2005). Polycystic ovary syndrome in adolescence. *Endocrinology Metabolism Clinics of North America, 34*, 677.

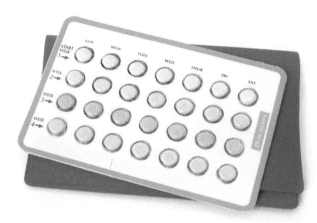

Figure 2.2. Combined oral contraceptive. Shown is a standard monthly dispenser package of a combined oral contraceptive that contains both estrogen and progestin.

Following that visit with Elsa, Tati began keeping a diary of all the food that she ate every day, along with calorie estimates. She started walking everywhere. She went to her school's gym and, finding it intimidating, she decided to run outside, instead. She didn't run far at first and mixed it with a lot of walking, but by the end of her freshman year, she'd lost the 12 lb she'd gained and another 15 on top of that. She could run 6 miles without stopping. She still took her pill every day, when she remembered, but she felt like it was really her hard work that had restored her period and given her nicer skin. She felt better. She felt good. And she kept it up.

By the time she met Caleb, she was eating mostly vegetarian, with the occasional cheeseburger to mark special occasions. She'd run three 10K races and one half marathon and was training for a full marathon that would happen a month after graduation. That's how they'd met, on the track when they were both interval training to improve their times. They trained together, graduated together, finished the marathon within a half hour of each other, and married at the end of the summer. The reception menu included cheeseburgers.

Now, 2 years after her wedding, Tati's health is excellent. Because of the PCOS, she has her cholesterol and fasting glucose levels checked every few years. The results are always great, and Elsa tells her to just keep doing what she's doing. And that's pretty much what she does. She runs most days and eats a balanced diet. She maintains her BMI in a healthy range. She takes her birth control pill—most of the time.

The truth is, Tati isn't great about taking her pill regularly. As disciplined as she is about most everything else in her life, something about taking that tiny pill every day trips her up. She has tried putting reminders in her phone. She has tried keeping her pill pack next to her toothbrush. She has tried having her pills delivered to her home automatically every 3 months so she wouldn't have to remember to pick them up from the pharmacy. Her mother, who wants grandchildren, jokes that it is her lizard brain, the primitive brain that answers to the basic biologic imperative of reproduction and sustaining of the species, that

causes her to forget to take her pill, because it wants most of all for her to reproduce.

Whatever, thinks Tati. When she forgets her pill, she doubles up like she is supposed to (Patient Teaching 2.1). Sometimes she misses more than one. She knows that she should use back-up, such as condoms or abstinence, when that happens. But she figures the PCOS is her safety net. Because, really, what are the chances she will get pregnant without some sort of help? It has to be close to zero.

Pregnancy

First Trimester

When she misses her period, it is for the first time since she was 19. Even as often as she missed taking her pill, she never completely skipped a period until now. Two thin blue lines appear on the display of the grocery store pregnancy test. She takes two more tests, just in case. The second test uses pink lines and the third has a digital display, but they all indicate the same result: she's pregnant (Fig. 2.3).

It isn't so much an unplanned pregnancy as a mistimed one. She and Caleb do want children—someday. They haven't talked much about when they want to have children, just that it would happen in the future. Tati has thought maybe she could have children after she isn't needed so much at work, when it would be easier to cut back on her hours for a while. Or maybe after she turns 30. But this is happening now.

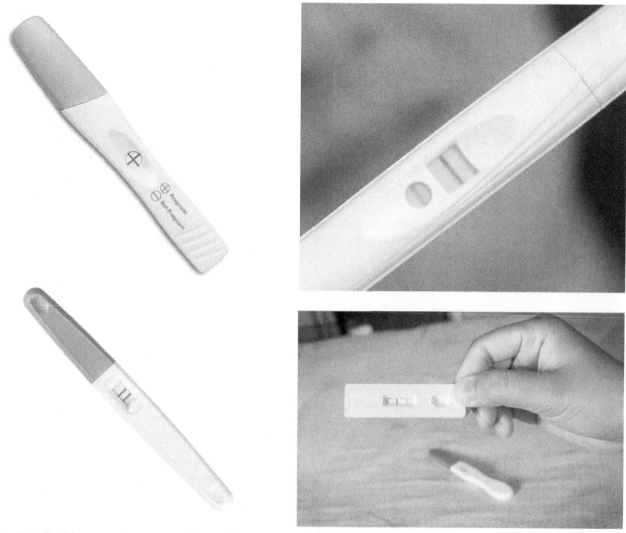

Figure 2.3. Positive pregnancy tests. Home urine pregnancy tests are now highly sensitive and accurate and may detect a pregnancy prior to missed menses. (The top right image is reprinted with permission from Pillitteri, A. [2002]. *Maternal and child health nursing: Care of the childbearing and childrearing family* [4th ed., figure from Chapter 5 opener]. Philadelphia, PA: Lippincott Williams & Wilkins.)

She and Caleb take stock. They have a house and jobs. They have a dog and a cat—at least they've managed to keep their pets alive. They have some savings, not a lot. Tati's mother lives half an hour from their little house. Maybe she could babysit sometimes.

"What do you think?" Tati asks Caleb.

"It's not what we planned," says Caleb. "I don't know if I'm ready."

"My mother says it's such a huge decision to have kids that you almost can't make it. It has to choose you."

"Or like you could choose not to take your birth control?" says Caleb. "I'm sorry. That was a jerk thing to say. I'm just kind of in shock."

Tati takes his hand. "He might look like you," she says.

He squeezes it. "If I'm incredibly lucky she will be just like you."

Tati meets Alice, a nurse practitioner working in an obstetrics and gynecology office she picks at random because it's closest to work. Alice explains that she will share Tati's care with another nurse practitioner and the two physicians, all of whom comprise the care providers in the practice.

Tati is transferred to an exam room and has her vital signs taken. Alice says they're excellent. She performs an initial history, asking about her family, her current living situation, her work, her health, and whether she feels safe in her home (see Box 1.2). They discuss her PCOS and past pregnancy history (Box 2.2).

"This is it," says Tati. "My first pregnancy."

"It's an exciting time," says Alice. "It can be a little nerve-wracking. Don't be shy about asking questions."

"I have an obvious one. I feel silly asking it," says Tati.

"Go ahead."

"I went on the pill originally for my PCOS. Now that I'm pregnant, should I still be taking it?"

Alice shakes her head. "You can stop taking it until after the pregnancy. You have some pretty great pregnancy hormones that will take over. However, don't worry if you've continued to take the pills. They won't hurt a pregnancy."

Box 2.2 Pregnancy and Birth Status

GTPAL

G: The number of pregnancies a woman has had in her lifetime

T: The number of pregnancies that have ended at term (37 wk plus)

P: The number of pregnancies that have ended preterm (20–37 wk)

A: The number of pregnancies that end by spontaneous or elective abortion before 20 wk

L: The number of living children

Tatiana is now *G*1 *T*0 *P*0 *A*0 *L*0

Gravidity and Parity

G: The number of pregnancies a woman has had in her lifetime

P: The number of pregnancies carried to viable gestational age (variously defined as 20–24 wk gestation)

Tatiana is now *G*1 *P*0

Patient Teaching 2.2

Cervical Cancer Screening With Pap Testing and HPV

Cervical Cancer Screening Guidelines

- The first Pap test should be performed at age 21 y, regardless of sexual history.
- A Pap test without screening for the HPV virus should be performed every 3 y through age 29 y. Between 25 and 29, HPV testing should be added in the case of a low grade Pap abnormality called ASCUS.
- A Pap test with HPV testing (cotesting) should be performed every 5 y between the ages of 30 and 64 y.
- No further screening is required for women 65 y and older with no history of an abnormal Pap test in the past 20 y.

Quick Pap Facts

- A Pap test refers to the evaluation of samples of cells scraped from the cervix for changes that may indicate cancerous or precancerous conditions of the cervix. The sample is taken during a speculum examination.
- HPV screening may be done at the same time as the Pap test. HPV is a sexually transmitted virus that causes cancerous and precancerous changes in the cervix.
- Although Pap screening was once recommended annually, newer research indicates that less frequent screening leads to fewer unnecessary interventions and better outcomes.

HPV, human papillomavirus.

Adapted from Saslow, D., Solomon, D., Lawson, H. W., Killackey, M., Kulasingam, S. L., Cain, J., . . . Waldman, J. (2012). American Cancer Society, American Society for Colposcopy and Cervical Pathology, and American Society for Clinical Pathology screening guidelines for the prevention and early detection of cervical cancer. *Journal of Lower Genital Tract Disease, 16*(3).

Alice performs a full head-to-toe exam (see Box 1.3). Tati cannot remember the last time she had a Pap test—more than 3 years ago, she thinks. She's never had an abnormal one as far as she knows. Alice explains that women in their 20s should have a screening Pap every 3 years, possibly more often if anything abnormal is found (Patient Teaching 2.2 and Analyze the Evidence 2.1).

Because she has taken her pill packs, each of which has four rows of seven pills, month after month for the past 7 years, Tati is really confident about when her last period was. It was a normal period, not any lighter or heavier than usual, and the cramping was the same as ever. She reports all this to Alice. Alice says that because she's confident about her last period, they'll be able to calculate how far along she is based on the first day of her last period. Alice says she can use a computer program to calculate her due date or a little simple math, but she prefers to do it "old school," with a pregnancy wheel (Fig. 2.4).

"They're all based on the same idea," Alice explains. "You take the first day of your last period, subtract three months, and add

seven days" (see Box 1.1). "Because your last period started on April 7th, you are five weeks and four days pregnant today. You are due January 14th."

Tati thinks about that for a second. "My period was five weeks and four days ago. I thought you couldn't get pregnant when you have your period."

Analyze the Evidence 2.1   Frequency of Pap Tests

Fewer Paps, Current Guidelines

- Human papillomavirus (HPV), the virus that causes the cervical changes that can lead to cervical cancer, is usually transient, and changes caused by HPV typically regress spontaneously.
- Studies have indicated no reduced efficacy in fewer screening Paps, but less risk of false positives and unnecessary interventions (Moyer, 2012).

Retaining Annual Paps

- There is concern that if guidelines recommending annual Pap tests are eliminated, patients may not return for annual gynecologic visits, which are important for health assessments other than Pap tests.
- There is concern that patients will be uncomfortable with new guidelines (Perkins, Anderson, Gorin, & Schulkin, 2013).

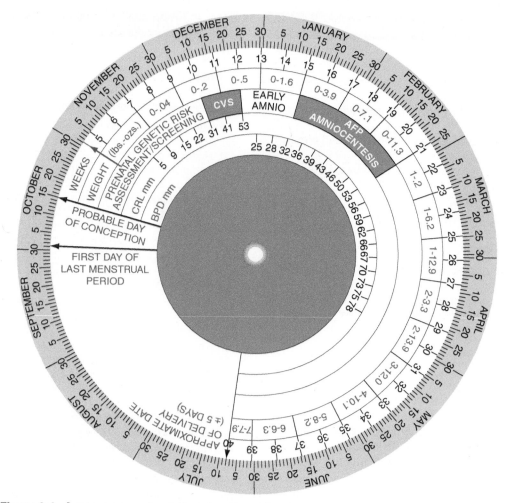

Figure 2.4. A pregnancy wheel. Based on Nagele's rule, pregnancy wheels are often still used for a quick way to identify the estimated date of delivery. (Reprinted with permission from Jensen, S. [2014]. *Nursing health assessment: A best practice approach* [2nd ed., Fig. 25.3]. Philadelphia, PA: Lippincott Williams & Wilkins.)

"I know it's confusing," says Alice. "So five weeks and four days ago isn't when you got pregnant. This calculation assumes you actually got pregnant three weeks and four days ago, but we talk about how long you've been pregnant as though you've been pregnant since the first day of your last period."

"That makes no sense," says Tati.

"I think it made more sense when they first came up with it," says Alice. "Before ultrasound, our best guesses had to be based on the first day of the last period. Because you've had PCOS since you were 19 and haven't always taken your pills on time, I'd like to do an ultrasound while you're here so we can get your date pinned down a little more precisely, just in case."

Because the fetus is still in the pelvis and not in the abdomen at this stage, Alice uses the vaginal ultrasound transducer. In the grainy image that looks like a snowstorm, she points out the gestational sac and the feathery outline of the yolk sac. She points to another tiny blob on the screen (Fig. 2.5).

"I can't be sure," says Alice, "but I think this is likely the fetal pole, which will become the fetus. If you were a little further on we'd be able to see the heartbeat to confirm that."

Alice then takes a series of measurements and explains that she's taking three measurements of the gestational sac from two different angles, or planes. She then adds the three numbers, divides the sum by three, and adds 30 to determine the gestational age in days (Butt & Lim, 2014).

"Looks like my earlier estimate was right on the money," says Alice. "You are at thirty-nine days, or five weeks, four days pregnant."

Alice and Tati discuss genetic screening recommendations. As far as Tati knows, her ancestors were all of northern European descent, though she does mention that her father's family identifies as French Canadian. Together they decide to order the genetic screening for **cystic fibrosis** because of the northern European part of the family, and genetic screening for **Tay-Sachs disease** because of the French Canadian side (see Table 1.1). They agree that she will also do the standard labs, such as blood typing and screening for sexually transmitted infections (see Lab Values 1.1). Later in the pregnancy she will have another ultrasound and more blood work for the integrated screening (see Table 1.1).

"Tell me how you've been feeling," Alice asks.

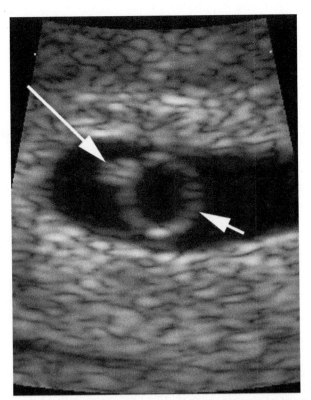

Figure 2.5. Ultrasound image of a gestational sac at 6 weeks. Shown are the embryo (long arrow) and yolk sac (short arrow). (Reprinted with permission from Doubilet, P. M., & Benson, C. B. [2011]. *Atlas of ultrasound in obstetrics and gynecology: A multimedia reference* [2nd ed., Fig. 1.6]. Philadelphia, PA: Lippincott Williams & Wilkins.)

"Not that different," says Tati. "My breasts have been really sore, like they are before my period starts but worse. I'm more tired than usual. I'm not nauseous at all, so that's good."

Alice tells her that the soreness in her breasts is normal and will improve over the next few weeks. The fatigue, she tells her, can last much longer and can return at the end of pregnancy. "Nausea may still occur, unfortunately" Alice says. "As for the fatigue, listen to your body. Rest when you can. You will get your energy back."

"What about exercise?" Tati asks. "I'm a runner. I'd like to keep doing it. I remember how hard it was to get into when I started. I'm worried that if I stop I'll never start again."

"There's no reason to stop," says Alice. "You were a runner before you got pregnant and you had a nice, normal exam today. This is another time to listen to your body. If you get too tired, slow down. Don't exercise so hard that you can't talk. Don't take up any exercise wherein you're likely to fall down or get hit in the abdomen. And don't quit. Healthy mothers make healthy babies" (The American College of Obstetricians and Gynecologists [ACOG] Committee on Obstetric Practice, 2015).

Within a week Alice calls her back with her blood test results.

"Two things," Alice says. "The first thing is, you came back as a carrier for cystic fibrosis. This doesn't mean that you have the disease. It does mean, however, that if your husband is also

a carrier you could pass the disease on to your offspring. How much do you know about cystic fibrosis?"

"Not much," says Tati. "It has something to do with thick mucus in the lungs. I think I read that it's not curable but it's more manageable now that it used to be. Don't they do lung transplants for people who have it? And, like, salt air treatments and stuff?"

"Sometimes," Alice says. "And it is more manageable than it once was, certainly."

"Alright," says Tati. "What now?"

"First, I want you to know it's not at all uncommon to be a carrier of the mutation," says Alice. "About one in twenty-seven people who are of European descent carry a cystic fibrosis mutation. Cystic fibrosis is autosomal recessive, which means that to actually get the disease, you need two copies of the mutation, one from each parent. The next thing we need to do is get some blood from Caleb and see whether he's a carrier, as well" (Fig. 2.6) (Zvereff, Faruki, Edwards, & Friedman, 2013).

"Alright," says Tati. "I'm panicking a little. Can I have Caleb come in today for the blood work? How long will it be until we know the results?"

"Usually within a week," says Alice. "No panicking. You have a twenty-six in twenty-seven chance of Caleb not being a carrier. If he is a carrier, you have a twenty-five percent chance of having a child with cystic fibrosis and a fifty percent chance of having a child who is a carrier. You'd also have a twenty-five percent chance of having a child without the disease who is not a carrier."

"But if he's negative there's no chance of passing it on?" asks Tati.

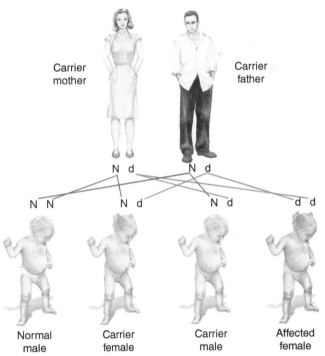

Figure 2.6. Autosomal recessive inheritance. (Reprinted with permission from Kyle, T., & Carman, S. [2016]. *Essentials of pediatric nursing* [3rd ed., Fig. 27.2]. Philadelphia, PA: Lippincott Williams & Wilkins.)

"Not quite," says Alice. "There would be no chance that the child would have cystic fibrosis, but there's a fifty percent chance with each pregnancy of passing on the mutation."

"What would the mutation do?" asks Tati.

"A single mutation does nothing by itself," says Alice. "It wouldn't hurt the baby. You have a single mutation and it doesn't hurt you. But that child, like you, would be at risk for passing on the mutation. If the child's future partner also had the mutation, there would be a twenty-five percent risk of your grandchild having cystic fibrosis."

"Alright," Tati says. "I'm not panicking anymore—worried, but not panicking."

"That's good. Do you have other questions?" asks Alice.

"You said there were two things," says Tati. "What's the second thing?"

Alice explains that Tati's blood work shows she is Rh negative, which isn't abnormal. In fact, she tells her, as many as 15% of people in some ethnic groups are Rh negative and that, as with cystic fibrosis, it is most common in people of European descent (American College of Obstetricians and Gynecologists [ACOG], 1999). She explains that women who are Rh negative can have completely normal pregnancies and healthy babies but that it is recommended that she have an injection at 28 weeks of pregnancy to ensure that she doesn't have an immune reaction to the fetus.

"I'm sorry, I don't understand," says Tati.

"Okay, because you have Rh-negative red blood cells, we ran another test to see whether you have any antibodies against Rh-positive red blood cells," says Alice. "If you have the antibodies, it would mean that you previously had a pregnancy with a fetus that was Rh positive and that you were exposed to the fetal blood."

"But I've never been pregnant before," says Tati.

"I know," says Alice. "But sometimes women have an early pregnancy loss before they're aware they're pregnant. You're considered at risk for sensitization to Rh blood if you're sexually active."

"What if Caleb is Rh negative, too?"

"If Caleb is Rh negative, then there'd be no chance of the fetus being Rh positive. If he's Rh positive, however, you'd have a fifty to one hundred percent chance of carrying an Rh-positive fetus, depending on whether he carries two Rh-positive genes or just one."

"I don't understand," says Tati. "With cystic fibrosis if he's a carrier there's a twenty-five percent chance of having a child with cystic fibrosis. Why would it be a fifty to one hundred percent chance with the Rh thing?"

"Good question," says Alice. "The difference is that cystic fibrosis is autosomal recessive. You need two copies, one from each parent, to have the disease. The Rh-positive trait is autosomal dominant. If you have one Rh-positive gene, you will be Rh positive. The Rh-negative trait is autosomal recessive. You'd need two Rh-negative genes to be Rh negative. So we know the only gene you can pass on is Rh negative. So, if Caleb is Rh positive and has one Rh-positive gene and one Rh-negative gene, you'd have a fifty percent chance of having an Rh-positive fetus because he might give the baby an Rh-positive gene or an Rh-negative gene. If he has two Rh-positive genes, you'd have a one hundred percent chance of carrying an Rh-positive fetus. We know that because you can give only Rh negative but he could give only Rh positive. Your

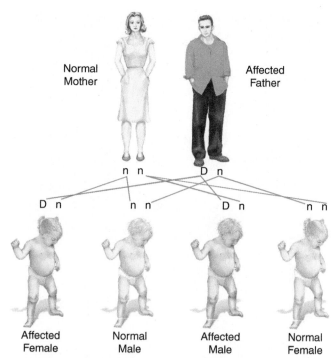

Normal Mother — Affected Father

n n — D n

D n — n n — D n — n n

Affected Female — Normal Male — Affected Male — Normal Female

Figure 2.7. Autosomal dominant inheritance. (Reprinted with permission from Kyle, T., & Carman, S. [2016]. *Essentials of pediatric nursing* [3rd ed., Fig. 29.1]. Philadelphia, PA: Lippincott Williams & Wilkins.)

baby would be guaranteed to have one Rh-positive gene and to, therefore, be Rh positive" (Fig. 2.7).

Alice suggests that they test Caleb's blood type at the same time that they screen him as a carrier for cystic fibrosis. If he is Rh positive, Tati would need an injection of **Rho (D) immune globulin**, often called by the brand name RhoGAM, at 28 weeks. They would then check the baby's blood type at birth. If the baby is also Rh positive, then Tati would need a second dose of the RhoGAM to prevent her from developing the antibodies against any Rh-positive blood she may have been exposed to during the birth process.

"Okay," Tati says slowly. "So the shot at twenty-eight weeks is about preventing my blood from attacking this pregnancy or any future pregnancy, and the shot after the birth is about preventing my body from attacking the next pregnancy."

"You got it," says Alice. "Almost all women who develop antibodies to Rh-positive blood do so after twenty-eight weeks" (ACOG, 1999).

"And this isn't about keeping me healthy, it's about making sure my body doesn't attack a fetus with a different blood type from mine," says Tati.

"Right again," says Alice.

"It's a wonder any of us manage to be born," says Tati.

"Tell me about it," says Alice.

Tati calls Caleb to tell him about her results, and he comes in and has his blood work done the same day. Within a week, they get the news that he is Rh negative and is not a carrier for cystic fibrosis. Tati will not need any RhoGAM injections, and no further testing is indicated to determine whether the fetus has cystic fibrosis.

Recommended Visits

- First visit typically in the first trimester, especially for first pregnancies
- Once monthly through the 27th week of pregnancy
- Every other week from 28 to 36 wk
- Weekly from 36 wk until birth

Exceptions

- Visits may be more frequent if the pregnancy is diagnosed as high risk.
- Not all providers follow this classic schedule. Some providers follow schedules that include group visits, less frequent visits in the second trimester, and no first trimester visit, among other variations.

Second Trimester

After a dramatic start to prenatal care, Tati falls into the regular schedule as outlined by Alice (Box 2.3). The visits have a comforting routine to them, and Tati finds that she looks forward to them. Sometimes Caleb comes, and they listen to the fetal heart tones together and look on as Tati's belly measures bigger and bigger (Box 2.4). Caleb, a science geek at heart, particularly likes the predictability of the belly measurements.

"Who figured that out," he asks, rhetorically. "Who figured out that if you measure from the pubic bone to the top of the uterus after sixteen weeks of pregnancy, the number of centimeters should match the number of weeks? Genius!" (Fig. 2.8).

In addition to the routine meetings with Alice and others with a second nurse practitioner, named Nina, and the two physicians, Joy and Philip, she has routine testing done throughout her pregnancy. She is told that all is well (Box 2.5). Considering that since she was 19 she has assumed that her PCOS might make even getting pregnant challenging, her pregnancy has been remarkably easy.

- Weight
- Vital signs
- Urine dip (protein, glucose, nitrites, and leukocytes)
- Fetal heart tones
- Fundal assessment (assessing how much the uterus has grown)
- Assessment of smoking use and exposure, alcohol use, and substance abuse
- Assessment of infant feeding plans and breastfeeding education

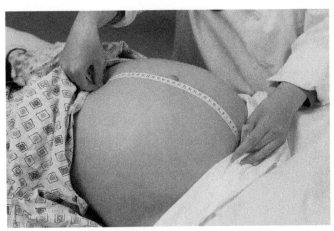

Figure 2.8. Symphysis-fundal height measuring. Starting in the 20th week of pregnancy, it is routine to measure the uterus from the pubic symphysis to the top of the uterine fundus to assess fetal growth. Measurement in centimeters should correspond with weeks of gestation. (Reprinted with permission from Weber, J. R., & Kelley, J. H. [2017]. *Health assessment in nursing* [6th ed., Fig. 29.11]. Philadelphia, PA: Lippincott Williams & Wilkins.)

One test, however, a vaginal and rectal swab, comes back positive for group B streptococcus (GBS).

"This isn't really a diagnosis," says Alice, who has just called her with the results. "It just tells us that you are colonized with the bacteria and that you and the baby are more at risk for certain infections. We'll start you on some intravenous, or IV, antibiotics, something called penicillin G, when you're admitted to the hospital and then we'll give you another dose every four hours until the delivery."

"Can't I just take some penicillin now?" Tati asks. "I was hoping I wouldn't have to have an IV."

"I'm sorry but no," says Alice. "Taking the antibiotic before delivery doesn't seem to be as helpful for avoiding an infection in the infant. By doing the IV antibiotic with delivery, we are able to get enough of the medicine into you that it gets into the amniotic fluid and the baby, as well" (Baecher & Gobman, 2008).

Third Trimester

Since she reached the 20-week mark, Tati has sometimes noticed some tightening of her abdomen. It doesn't really hurt, exactly, but it feels weird—almost as if her torso is making a fist. The tightening always goes away after a little while, and it usually stops if she walks around. Nina, one of the nurse practitioners in the practice, says that she is most likely experiencing **Braxton Hicks contractions**, or **false labor** (Patient Teaching 2.3). Tati starts to notice the contractions quite frequently in the final month of the pregnancy. Nina recommends that she drink some water or rest when they happen, or maybe take a warm bath. If they continue, Nina tells her, she can assess whether they're real labor contractions by remembering the "4-1-1" of contractions.

"When you start having contractions that are four minutes apart and last at least a minute each for at least an hour, that's

Box 2.5 Recommended Pregnancy Screenings

Screening for Trisomies: First Trimester

- Pregnancy-associated plasma protein A and hCG serum test at 11–13 wk
- Ultrasound of the back of the fetal neck at 11–13 wk

Screening for Trisomies and Neural Tube Defects: Integrated Screen at 15–16 wk

- Combined with first trimester screening
- Maternal serum alpha-fetoprotein, hCG, unconjugated estriol, and inhibin alpha serum testing (see Table 1.1)

Urinalysis

- Periodic clean-catch urine test
- Assessment for bacteria, white blood cells, and nitrites, which may suggest a urinary tract infection
- Assessment for glucose, which may suggest diabetes
- Assessment for protein, which may suggest preeclampsia

Second Trimester Ultrasound

- Assessment of fetal structure, placenta placement, and amniotic fluid volume
- An abdominal ultrasound (a full bladder is recommended to displace the uterus upward), usually done at 16–20 wk of gestation

One-Hour OGTT

- 24–28 wk to assess for gestational diabetes
- The patient drinks a glucose solution. A serum test is done an hour later to assess the blood glucose level.
- An elevated blood glucose level indicates the need for a 3-h OGTT.

Vaginal and Rectal Cultures

- Testing for group B streptococcus
- Performed at 35–37 wk

hCG, human chorionic gonadotropin; OGTT, oral glucose tolerance test.

when we start thinking you might be in labor," says Nina. "But listen to your body. Not everyone's the same. If you think it's time to go to the hospital, go to the hospital. The worst thing that will happen is that you'll be sent back home."

When she is just shy of 39 weeks, Tati has a visit with Joy, one of the physicians. Joy tells her that her cervix is pretty soft and that she is about 2 cm dilated.

"Two centimeters!" says Tati. "That means only eight more to go!"

"That's an excellent attitude," says Joy. "I like it. Although I do think it's only fair to tell you that many women can stay at two, three, or even four centimeters dilated for weeks before labor starts."

Tati makes a face. "I'm not sure about going on like this for weeks," she says. "I miss being able to lie on my stomach at night. I miss jeans. I miss being able to see my feet."

Joy suggests stripping Tati's membranes.

"That sounds horrible," Tati says. "What does it mean?"

Joy explains that **stripping of the membranes**, sometimes called sweeping of the membranes, would involve another pelvic exam. This time Joy would insert a finger right into the cervix and run her finger around the bottom part of her uterus to detach the fetal membranes from the uterine lining.

"Does it hurt?" asks Tati.

"Some women can get pretty crampy. It's probably not the most pleasant sensation," says Joy. "It's typical to get **bloody show** within about twenty-four hours of the stripping, as well, even if labor doesn't start."

"Bloody show?" Tati says. "That sounds even worse than stripped membranes. What does it mean?"

"Right now you have an accumulation of mucus in your cervix," explains Joy. "That's totally normal. But if I strip your membranes, I'll disrupt that mucus. Sometimes when it comes out it mixes with some blood from the cervix and is pink. This is called bloody show, and it usually indicates that labor will start within the next few days."

Tati decides against having her membranes stripped.

The next day, while she is at work, she feels the tightening in her abdomen again. It feels different this time, however—stronger. She finishes a letter to a donor she has been composing and shuts the door of her office to give herself some privacy. Every 5 minutes the contractions come, lasting for 30 seconds. And then every 4½ minutes, lasting almost a minute. After a half hour, she calls Caleb.

"I think this is it," she tells him. "I think it's time. Will you come get me?"

Patient Teaching 2.3 True Versus False Labor Contractions

Characteristic	True Labor Contractions	False Labor Contractions
Location felt	Lower back and abdomen, pressure in the pelvis	Abdomen
Quality of contractions	Regular, progressive; become stronger, closer together, and longer	Mostly irregular; may become regular for short periods of time
Effect of ambulation	Become more intense	May stop
Effect of rest and hydration	Do not resolve	Often resolve

"The baby?" he asks. And then quickly he says, "Yes the baby. Duh. I'll be right there."

It isn't far from her work to the hospital, maybe 5 miles, but by the time they get there the contractions are, if anything, less predictable. Sometimes they come 2 minutes apart, sometimes 6. By the time they see the triage nurse on the labor and delivery floor, she hasn't had a contraction in almost 10 minutes.

"It's a false alarm, I think," she tells the nurse, Judy. She's almost in tears saying it.

"Well, that happens," Judy says. "We make it sound like it's easy to tell the difference between true labor and false labor, but really, even experienced mothers can be fooled." She's a big woman and enthusiastic. "The only way to tell whether your labor is true or false is to see what your cervix is doing. With true labor, we'll see changes in your cervix. With false labor, your cervix doesn't change. We're lucky because you had an exam just yesterday, and we share the same records system as your obstetrics office. We can compare yesterday's exam to today's and see whether your cervix is opening."

"So I'll need an exam?" asks Tati.

"If those contractions come back you will," says Judy. "Right now I'd like to just check your vital signs and see how the baby's heart rate is doing."

First, Judy takes a set of Tati's vitals and listens for the baby's heartbeat. Judy says the fetal heart rate is 120, and that the baby is probably sleeping. She tells her that on average fetuses sleep 15.7 minutes at a time (Suwanrath & Suntharasaj, 2010). "Are you sure you're ready for a baby that sleeps for less than sixteen minutes at a stretch?" she asks, and everyone laughs.

Judy's hand is resting on Tati's belly as they talk. She asks about allergies (Tati has none) and whether she has any cold symptoms (she doesn't). She asks when she last ate (maybe a half hour ago? When was she *not* eating?). They discuss Tati's hopes for having an unmedicated birth, and how, if nothing else, she really doesn't want an epidural.

"There's something about the idea of having a needle stuck in my back," Tati says.

"I understand," says Judy. "It's not for everyone. The risks of major complications are low, but side effects are not uncommon. The important thing here is that you don't want one and you certainly don't have to have one" (Patient Teaching 2.4). Judy changes the subject. "So, Tati. I've had my hand on your belly for 15 minutes now and no action. Have you felt anything?"

"No. And I feel dumb. It's just more Braxton Hicks contractions. You'd think I'd know a Braxton Hicks when I felt one by now."

"Don't feel dumb," says Caleb. "It's not like you've ever done this before."

"Think of this as good news," says Judy. "You can go home, maybe soak in the tub. Maybe this husband of yours can make you a nice dinner. Maybe you can have some seltzer with some fresh lemon juice. You can rest in a place that's quieter and more comfortable than this hospital. We'll be here waiting when it's your time."

Tati doesn't want to rest and wait. She knows that she has only limited time off from work, and the clock is ticking. She loves her work and feels like she can make a real difference to

Patient Teaching 2.4

Potential Side Effects of Epidural and Spinal Anesthesia

- Maternal hypotension (occurs in as many as 50% of epidurals)
- Fetal heart rate changes, such as prolonged decelerations
- Transient increase in uterine tone
- Pruritus (itching; occurs in 50%–90% of women)
- Nausea and vomiting
- Urinary retention and bladder distension
- Respiratory depression
- Lower extremity numbness and weakness (occur only in epidurals)
- Headache (occurs in 1%–2% of combined spinal/epidural patients)
- Back pain
- Spinal cord injury (occurs in 0.06% of spinals and in 0.02% of epidurals)
- Maternal temperature above 38°C
- Increased risk of operative vaginal delivery

Adapted from Trout, K. K., & Eshkevari, L. (2015). Support for women in labor. In T. King, M. Brucker, J. Kriebs, J. Fahey, C. Gegor, & H. Varney (Eds.), *Varney's midwifery* (pp. 883–911). Burlington, MA: Jones & Bartlett Learning.

the arts community in town, but the benefits aren't great. She is one of only three employees, and she is the only one who works full time. That means that, according to the Family and Medical Leave Act, she has no right to any time off at all when the baby comes. If the company were bigger, if it had at least 50 employees and she'd worked there for a year, then she could have 12 weeks of leave—unpaid leave, that is (U.S. Department of Labor, Wage and Hour Division, 2012).

In spite of the law, her employers have been generous to her. They are planning to let her take a few weeks off after the birth, work part-time for a little while, and even bring in the baby sometimes. But she doesn't want to press her luck by taking off any more time than is necessary. She really wants to keep her job. Too bad she doesn't live in New Zealand, she thinks. She read recently that mothers in that country get 18 weeks of fully paid leave. The article also mentioned that, in France, a mother can stay home for 16 weeks at 70% pay after the birth, and, in Canada, 15 weeks at 55% pay (Addati, Cassirer, & Gilchrist, 2014).

Labor and Delivery

They don't have to wait long. Two days later, Tati is at work again when the contractions start. At first they feel like the tightening in her belly again—like the Braxton Hicks—and she tries to ignore them. She drinks some water and tries to concentrate. At 4:30, she notices that the pain is more in her back and that it wraps across the front. More than before, she thinks, it feels like pain. But maybe it's just wishful thinking. They have only one car, and Caleb picks her up in it shortly after 5:00. As they drive along, she makes a sharp, gasping noise.

"Contraction?" he asks.

"Maybe. I don't know which kind, though," she says. "It's definitely stronger than before."

"Should we head to the hospital instead of home?" Caleb asks.

"No way," says Tati. "Thor and Jim have been alone all day and need to be fed. I want to go home, have a little something to eat myself, and maybe take a warm bath. I'm waiting for the four-one-one of contractions before we go back to the hospital."

"The four-one-one?" Caleb says. "What does that mean?"

"It means when the contractions are 4 minutes apart, last for 1 minute, and have been going like that for one solid hour. I may even wait more than an hour."

"You don't have to be a hero," says Caleb. "We can go back to the hospital."

Tati refuses and they head to the house. By the time Jim and Thor have been fed and Thor has tick-ticked his way down the sidewalk with Caleb to do his business, she is beginning to change her mind.

"I think I'm going to throw up," she says.

"Okay," says Caleb. "That's cool." His eyes are wide and he stands there looking at her, like he's not sure what to do. "That's a normal thing to do in labor, right?"

"Yeah," says Tati. She retches into the sink. When she's done, she says, "Let's go to the hospital."

At the hospital, a labor and delivery nurse, Nadia, takes her vital signs and asks her many of the same questions Judy asked at her previous trip to the hospital. Tati forgot to rinse her mouth before she left the house, and Nadia gives her some mouthwash to gargle.

Rather than just listening to the fetus with the Doppler ultrasound, Nadia places two belts over her rotund abdomen. The first belt, she explains, the one above her belly button, is attached to a round, plastic device that will measure her contractions. The device attached to the lower belt will measure the fetal heart rate.

"Why not just use the Doppler thing to listen to the baby, like last time?" asks Caleb.

"We want to get a better view of what's going on," says Nadia. "I've been observing your contractions while you've been here. I'd say they're four minutes apart, maybe closer, and they must be lasting close to a minute. This machine is more precise than I am, though. Plus, this setup allows us to check the fetal heart rate and see how the baby is responding to the contractions. The Doptone, the way we've been listening before, isn't as accurate for giving us the second-to-second variations in fetal heart rate."

"Do I have to wear this the whole time?" Tati asks, referring to the belts.

"That's between you and your provider," Nadia says. "In this hospital, most women do. In other places, they sometimes just listen to the baby on a schedule, like every fifteen minutes or half hour, depending on what's happening."

By the time Joy arrives to check on her, Tati doesn't care much what is wrapped around her abdomen. She's completely focused on each contraction, as though she's trying to control them with her mind.

Nadia starts an IV in Tati's left wrist, securing it with several pieces of tape.

"I have bacteria in my vagina," says Tati, recovering from a contraction. She is feeling a little loopy, as though talking requires her to wake up from a vivid dream. "I'm supposed to have antibiotics."

Nadia nods. "We're starting that now. We'll give you a big dose of penicillin G now and then we'll give you more every four hours. It says in your chart no penicillin allergy. Is that accurate?" (The Pharmacy 2.1).

Tati nods. She closes her eyes as she waits for the next contraction.

In between contractions, Joy performs a pelvic exam on Tati.

"You've made a lot of progress," Joy says. "Your cervix has opened right up to about five centimeters. You're doing awesome."

Tati just nods. She is concentrating on taking deep, slow breaths, which she is counting. She knows that each contraction is lasting about 12 breaths, and that the contraction is strongest at six breaths and then starts to relax. It is just like running up a hill, turning around, and running back down.

"How much longer do you think?" asks Caleb.

✻ The Pharmacy 2.1   **Penicillin G**

Overview	• Antibiotic • First-choice medication for treatment of GBS colonization during labor and delivery
Route and dosing	• Initial dose of 5 million U IV, and then 2.5–3 million U IV every 4 h until delivery • Infuse over 15–30 min
Care considerations	• Patient education and reassurance • Penicillin allergies are common. It is essential to verify allergies with patients before administering any medication.
Warning signs	• Monitor for hypersensitivity (anaphylaxis), including shortness of breath, swelling of the tongue or throat, vomiting, itchy rash, low blood pressure, or lightheadedness.

GBS, group B streptococcus; IV, intravenous.
Adapted from Verani, J. R., McGee, L., & Schrag, S. J. (2010, November 19). Prevention of perinatal group B streptococcal disease: Revised guidelines from CDC, 2010. *Morbidity and Mortality Weekly Report*, 1–32.

"It's not something that's easy to guess," says Joy. "Right now I'd say she's in the active phase of the first stage. Because this is her first pregnancy, she should be dilating at the rate of a little over a centimeter an hour until she hits about seven centimeters dilated. Centimeters seven to ten are called the transition phase. That can go pretty fast, maybe a half hour or less, and be pretty intense. Then comes the pushing" (see Table 1.3).

"How long is that?"

Joy shrugs. "That can vary quite a bit. I think we'll all find that out at the same time. She's doing great. I'll be back to check on her soon."

Caleb tries his best to be helpful, but Tati's tolerance is low. He rubs her back until she can't stand it anymore and tells him not to touch her. He offers her water through a straw between contractions. She takes a few sips, but is irritated by the distraction and shakes her head when he offers it again. Time seems to compress and expand simultaneously. She zones out for a while.

Later, she seems to come out of a trance and sees Caleb sitting next to her eating a sandwich. Tati sits up and says, "I want a bath."

"Let's wait until after Joy has checked your cervix again," Nadia says.

Joy returns with Nadia within a few minutes and does another pelvic exam between contractions. "You've done fantastic," she tells Tati. "You're at ten centimeters, and that baby is down in your pelvis. How do you feel right now?"

Tati wrinkles her forehead. "I stopped contracting."

"You'll start again," Joy says. "When you do, it's going to be push time."

The contractions do start again. Tati has opted for a birthing bar that attaches to the bed and arches over it (Fig. 2.9), which allows her to hang in a squatting position, partially supported by her arms. The position opens her pelvis, giving the baby more room to descend, and lets gravity help. Between contractions, she lies back against Caleb, who is positioned behind her.

Tati does as she's told and tries not to hold her breath as she pushes. Several pushes in, she feels a mild, yet embarrassing release.

"I pooped," she says when the contraction has passed, to no one in particular.

"That's completely normal," says Nadia. "A lot of women poop during birth. It's already been cleared away."

With the next push, Tati feels a burning sort of pain. When did the pain move? When did it stop feeling like a giant trying to tear her spine out of her back and start feeling like, well, a ring of fire? She grits her teeth and grunts through the contractions, noticing that the pushing offers some relief, that the burning actually seems to get a little better when she is bearing down.

"You're doing amazing," Joy says. "I can see the baby's head. When you get your next contraction, I want little pushes. We want to avoid any tearing as much as we can."

In a different life those words would have sounded horrifying to her. In this life she just wants it over. Two more, and then three more contractions, and the baby's head is out. Tati knows mostly because people tell her it is.

"She has dark hair," says Caleb. "They're using a suction thing to get stuff out of her nose and mouth" (Fig. 2.10).

And then one more tremendous push and she feels the slither as the rest of the baby girl makes her way into the world.

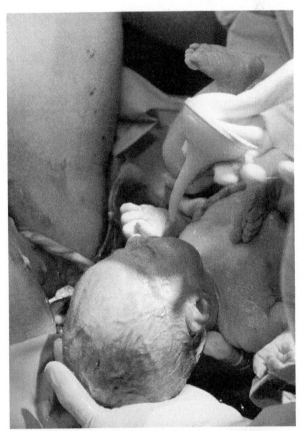

Figure 2.10. Suctioning the airways of a neonate. A bulb syringe is usually sufficient to clear mucus from the airways of the neonate. (Reprinted with permission from Evans, R. J., Brown, Y. M., & Evans, M. K. [2014]. *Canadian maternity, newborn, and women's health nursing* [2nd ed., Fig. 20-4]. Philadelphia, PA: Lippincott Williams & Wilkins.)

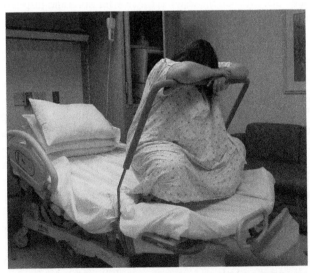

Figure 2.9. A birthing bar. Birthing bars are often available now with birthing beds. They are commonly used to help a patient assume a squatting position during the second stage of pregnancy. (Reprinted with permission from Irion, J. M., & Irion, G. L. [2009]. *Women's health in physical therapy* [1st ed., Fig. 15.9]. Philadelphia, PA: Lippincott Williams & Wilkins.)

After Delivery

The placenta is born soon after the baby is delivered, though Tati barely notices it. She is aware of calm activity in the room—of clean up and wind down. The tocodynamometer and Doppler device are removed from her abdomen. She feels cool washcloths applied between her legs and the changing of draw sheets. She relishes the delicious lack of pain. She watches her pink daughter with her little blue hands as she wriggles on Tati's chest, a warmed blanket over her, looking at the brand new world through dark gray eyes that squint because of the facial swelling brought on by the birth.

For the first hour after the birth, she notices that a nurse comes in and checks her about every 15 minutes. In the second hour, she is checked every half hour (Box 2.6).

Box 2.6   Schedule and Common Elements of Routine Maternal Postpartum Assessment

Schedule

1. First hour: every 15 min
2. Second hour: every 30 min
3. Hours 3–24: every 4 h
4. After 24 h: every 8–12 h

Assessment Elements

1. Maternal affect
2. Lung sounds
3. Uterine fundus
4. Lochia
5. Perineum
6. Pain
7. Intravenous site
8. Urinary output
9. Ambulation
10. Sensation and mobility (if epidural or other regional anesthesia is administered)
11. Urinary output
12. Abdominal incision (if any)

Vital Signs and Variations From Normal

1. *Blood pressure (BP):* BP should be equivalent to baseline (before labor). Increased BP may indicate pain, anxiety, or preeclampsia. Low BP is concerning for hemorrhage or severe dehydration. Orthostatic hypotension is common.
2. *Pulse:* Bradycardia (pulse of 50 beats per minute or less) may be normal. Tachycardia is concerning for pain, anxiety, and hemorrhage.
3. *Temperature:* A low-grade temperature is considered normal for the first 24 h. After 24 h, a temperature of 38°C is suspicious for infection.
4. *Respirations:* Respirations of 12–20 breaths/min are normal. Slower respirations with magnesium sulfate are concerning for magnesium toxicity. Slower respirations are also concerning for opioid overdose. Rapid respirations are concerning for pain, hemorrhage, pulmonary embolism, and anxiety.

During one of these assessments, about 3 hours after the baby's birth, her nurse, Geena, looks concerned as she feels Tati's uterus.

"When was the last time you emptied your bladder?" she asks.

Tati thinks. She's been napping and isn't sure when she fell asleep. She doesn't feel like she needs to urinate, and tells Geena so.

"Sometimes after a delivery women temporarily lose some of the sensation that tells them that they need to pee for a little while," says Geena. "If your bladder gets too full, it can push on your uterus in such a way that it can make it relax. A relaxed uterus is a bleeding uterus."

Tati looks down and gingerly feels her abdomen. To her eye, she still looks pregnant. "Is my uterus relaxed?" she asks.

"It's more relaxed than I want it to be," says Geena. "Let's get you up to the bathroom, and then we'll bring you back and check where you are."

Geena has her swing her legs over and sit on the edge of the bed for a minute before getting her on her feet. Geena explains that after giving birth women can get lightheaded and even faint if they stand up too fast. She calls it **orthostatic hypotension.**

"You also haven't been up for a little while, so you'll likely have some bleeding when you stand. It may look like a lot, but keep in mind that it's been pooling as you've been lying there," says Geena. Tati watches as Geena lays a trail of absorbent pads between the bed and the bathroom.

Tati stands up with Geena's help. She looks back on the bed and sees a pool of dark blood where she was sitting. "There's blood," she says.

"It's not unexpected," says Geena. "But it's more than I want to see. Let's get your bladder emptied and then assess you."

Geena keeps one arm around Tati's back on the way to the bathroom to stabilize her. Caleb is in a chair next to the bed and offers to help. He is holding the baby, and Geena tells him he can stay where he is.

Geena gets Tati to the bathroom and positions her on the toilet. She turns on the water in the sink for noise and inspiration and then leaves the room, discreetly closing the door behind her except for a few inches.

"I'm going to change your bedding while you're in there," Geena says when she steps out. "Don't try to get up without me."

Geena comes back a few minutes later and shows Tati a small squeeze bottle that she fills with warm water. "You'll use this to clean up," Geena explains. "It will feel soothing and won't get stuck like toilet paper. Make sure the water's warm, though. When it's too cold or too hot, it's not a nice surprise."

Next she shows her a pair of mesh panties and some large pads like the ones she's been wearing. She shows Tati how to put them on herself, and encourages her to change them often and keep track each time of how saturated the pad is.

Geena helps Tati back to the bed. Tati is feeling more steady, having made the first trip, and declines Caleb's support again. As promised, Geena has changed the bedding. She helps Tati into bed, and then feels again near her umbilicus for the fundus of her uterus. She is frowning again.

"No good?" asks Tati.

"It's still not as firm as I'd like it to be," says Geena. "When the uterus is soft like this, we call it **uterine atony**. It means the muscles aren't squeezing down like they should and so aren't squeezing the blood vessels closed. When this happens, you can bleed."

As Geena says this, Tati watches her position her hands on Tati's abdomen. After explaining to Tati what she plans to do, she scoots Tati's fresh pad and panties back down her so she can visualize the lochia as it exits her vagina. Already they can both see that the pad contains a pocket of rich, dark blood in its center.

"This is going to be uncomfortable," Geena says, and starts kneading Tati's abdomen with her hands.

"Ow!" Tati says. "What are you doing?"

"This is a uterine massage," Geena explains. "It should help your uterus to firm. We want it hard, like a softball."

They both watch as her pad fills with a few gushes of dark blood, and then a brief trickle, and then nothing. After a few minutes, Geena stops kneading and looks satisfied.

"All firmed up," she says. "I'll check again in a half hour, but don't worry. I won't massage again unless I have to."

As it turns out, she does have to massage Tati again, and again her uterus firms up. Then, when it's nearly 48 hours since she gave birth—a time by which she should have been home from the hospital already—Tati wakes up in a pool of blood so large that she pulls the cord to call the nurse. She feels anxious and slightly panicky. A nurse she hasn't met yet answers the call light, followed by three others.

The Nurse's Point of View

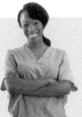

Angela: It's not uncommon for people to accidentally set off their call lights. It's an easy thing to do because they're attached to strings that are hooked to the bed and next to the toilet rail. Even though most of the time when someone pulls the emergency cord it's an accident, all available nurses on the floor still go running. A lot of people don't know this, but most of the time when women die from a complication of childbirth, it's after the birth. So though most times the alarm is an accident, when it's the real thing, we need a well-trained team there immediately.

I'm the first nurse in the room. When I see the blood, I immediately start uterine massage. Another nurse, Melanie, comes in right after me, then calmly leaves the room and comes back in with the supplies to start an IV, which she does with equal calmness, and then checks Tati's vital signs. A third nurse, Rachel, opens the computer and starts charting everything in real time. A fourth nurse, Janet, leaves and returns within 5 minutes with Joy, who is the on-call provider today and also happens to be the person who delivered Tati's baby.

I stop uterine massage and Joy checks Tati's uterus again. After she's done checking, I start massaging again. Joy looks up at Rachel, the nurse who came into the room with her. "Let's do a shot of methylergonovine maleate, 0.2 mg intramuscular," she says (The Pharmacy 2.2). "And I'd like to get a bedside ultrasound in here." Joy then turns to Tati. "I think you're hemorrhaging, which I know sounds terrifying, but it's a fancy way of saying you're bleeding more than we'd like you to. This happens sometimes. I think you may still have some placenta in your uterus that's keeping it from contracting and firming up. I want to use the ultrasound to check."

By the time the ultrasound arrives, the combination of the methylergonovine maleate and the massage is working. I can feel that Tati's uterus is firmer, and she is bleeding less. Melanie checks Tati's vital signs again, and notes her temperature is 37.9°C. I stop the uterine massage again as Joy performs the ultrasound with Caleb and Tati looking on.

"I'm not seeing much," Joy says finally. "It may be that you have endometritis, a common infection of the lining of your uterus, or it could be something else. We don't always know what causes uterine atony, which is what we call a soft uterus. I'd like to keep you here for another few days on some antibiotics" (The Pharmacy 2.3). "We'll give you the oral version of that medication we just gave you a shot of; you'll take it every six hours for the next day or two and we'll see how you do. Hopefully your uterus will stay firm" (Box 2.7).

"What if it doesn't?" asks Caleb.

"If it doesn't, then we'll figure out something else," says Joy. "The good news is, this happened while you're all still here and we have the resources available right away. It can be a different story if it happens later, when you're out of the hospital. We'll also keep a close eye on the baby. If this bleeding is due to an infection, it may be related to the GBS. If that was an ongoing problem even with the antibiotics we gave you during labor, it could be an issue for the baby, as well."

"What kind of issue?" asks Caleb.

"We worry about a lung infection most," says Joy.

"How would we know if that's happening?" Caleb says.

"If the baby starts making little grunting noises or has a bluish tone to the skin—not just the hands and feet, that's expected, but around the mouth—that would be a cause for concern. Sometimes babies with infections have temperatures that drop instead of go up, so your nurses will look for that, as well.

"Tati, I know we've been pressing on your uterus a lot. This might seem like a silly question, but is it sore at all now when I push on it?" asks Joy, pushing firmly.

"Ow, yes," says Tati. "It doesn't feel good."

"Have you noticed any odor?" asks Joy.

"Besides the smell of all the blood?" Tati asks. "I don't know, really. I've felt really sweaty, particularly at night."

"That can be normal," says Joy. "Women offload a lot of fluid after a birth, some of it by sweating. You have a mild fever. The antibiotics are a good idea."

The Pharmacy 2.2 | Methylergonovine Maleate

Overview	• Stimulates uterine contraction • Vasoconstrictive
Route and dosing	• IM: 0.2 mg every 2–4 h, maximum of four doses; onset in 2–5 min. • Oral: 0.2–0.4 mg every 6–12 h; onset in 5–10 min. • IV: contraindicated; for use in emergency only due to severe hypertension and stroke risk: 0.2 mg/min.
Care considerations	• This drug should never be used prior to the birth of the fetus because of its potential for very strong, prolonged contractions. • If used in the third stage, the obstetric care provider should be directly supervising administration. • Smoking is strongly discouraged while using this medication because of its vasoconstrictive properties. • Monitor for appropriate uterine firmness, fundal height, and lochia. • The patient may have very strong cramping.
Warning signs	• The patient's blood pressure should be carefully monitored for severe hypertension. • Monitor for toxicity: chest pain, headache, nausea, muscle pain, general weakness, cold or numb digits, or extremities tingling.

IM, intramuscular; IV, intravenous.

The Pharmacy 2.3 | Common IV Therapy for Endometritis

Gentamicin and Clindamycin

Overview	• The cure rate with combined treatment is 90%–97%. • Treatment continues until the patient is asymptomatic for 24 h. • IV ampicillin may also be included for a woman known to be GBS positive.
Route and dosing	• Gentamicin: 5 mg/kg IV every 24 h • Clindamycin: 900 mg IV every 8 h • *With GBS* • Additional ampicillin: 1–2 g every 4–6 h
Care considerations	• Provide comfort measures, including blankets, perineal care, hydration, and cool compresses. • Breastfeeding is encouraged during treatment. • Administer ampicillin over 10–15 min. • Administer clindamycin diluted over 10–60 min. • Administer gentamicin over 30–120 min.
Warning signs	• Ampicillin: Rapid infusion may cause seizures. • Clindamycin: Observe for bowel changes, as it can cause colitis (colon inflammation). • Gentamicin: May cause neurotoxicity. Monitor eighth cranial nerve (vestibulocochlear: hearing and balance) function. • All: Monitor for hypersensitivity (anaphylaxis), including shortness of breath, swelling of the tongue or throat, vomiting, itchy rash, low blood pressure, or lightheadedness.

IV, intravenous; GBS, group B streptococcus.

Box 2.7   Risks Factors for Postpartum Hemorrhage

Pregnancy-Related Risks*

• *Uterine atony (a failure of the uterus to stay contracted)*
• *Retained placenta or membranes*
• *Subinvolution (the uterus does not contract after birth)*
• Failure to progress during the second stage of labor (the pushing stage)

• Adherent placenta (the placenta does not detach from the uterine wall within half an hour)
• *Lacerations of the vulva, vagina, or cervix*
• Surgical vaginal delivery (forceps or vacuum)
• *Genital hematoma*
• Large for gestational age newborn (>4,000 g)

Box 2.7 Risks Factors for Postpartum Hemorrhage (continued)

- Hypertensive disorders (preeclampsia, eclampsia, and HELLP syndrome [hemolysis, elevated liver enzymes, and low platelets])
- Induction of labor with oxytocin
- Prolonged first or second stage of labor (the pushing stage)

Maternal Risk Factors[†]

- Personal history of postpartum hemorrhage
- Family history of postpartum hemorrhage
- Maternal obesity

- Multiple previous births
- Precipitous labor
- Uterine overdistension (macrosomia [large baby], multiple gestation [twins or more], or polyhydramnios [excess amniotic fluid])
- Uterine infection
- Asian or Hispanic ethnicity
- Uterine inversion
- *Coagulopathy (a defect of coagulation)*
- Uterine inversion (the uterus turns inside out so that the fundus exits the cervix as the placenta is removed)

Note: All risk factors apply to immediate (primary) postpartum hemorrhage. Italicized risk factors also apply to late (secondary) postpartum hemorrhage. Primary postpartum hemorrhage occurs in the first 24 hours after birth. Secondary postpartum hemorrhage may occur after 24 hours or for up to 12 weeks postpartum.
*Adapted from Sheiner, E., Sarid, L., Levy, A., Seidman, D., & Hallak, M. (2005). Obstetric risk factors and outcome of pregnancies complicated with early postpartum hemorrhage: A population-based study. *The Journal of Maternal-Fetal & Neonatal Medicine, 18*(3), 149.
[†]Adapted from Bateman, B., Berman, M., Riley, L., & Leffert, L. (2010). The epidemiology of postpartum hemorrhage in a large, nationwide sample of deliveries. *Anesthesia & Analgesia, 110*(5), 1368–1373.

As frightening as the bleeding is for Tati and Caleb, the nurses on the team make them feel safe and supported. A nurse has checked in with them hourly throughout Tati and the baby's stay, but they notice the nurses come even more often now, always ready to talk, answer questions, and reassure. Over the next 48 hours, Tati doesn't have any more frightening bleeding, and the tenderness in her uterus goes away completely. Her temperature goes down to 36°C and stays there.

The Newborn

The upside of this extended stay is the extra help Tati received with breastfeeding the baby (who still didn't have a name). She'd had an initial visit with a lactation consultant starting soon after the baby was born, but breastfeeding was tougher than she'd expected. Neither Tati nor Caleb had thought much about it prior to the birth. So much focus had been on the birth itself and the supplies—so many supplies!

"All you really need is a boob and a blanket," her mother had told her early in the pregnancy. Of course, when she'd visited, she'd brought gift bags full of those same supplies she'd deemed unnecessary, most in shades of pink.

Caleb and Tati had agreed that her mother's initial advice was solid, and yet they had a crib that the cat had been sleeping in for the past 3 months. They had an infant swing that was piled with tiny t-shirts. They had a stroller that folded down into a carriage and then folded again, origami-like, almost flat to slide into the back of the car. They had a breast pump, diapers, organic lotion, no-gas baby bottles, a diaper bag, cloth wipes, disposable wipes, a baby bath, a baby bucket, a bouncy seat, a sling carrier, a front carrier, and a back carrier. They had a book about how to breastfeed your baby that neither had thought about after Tati had unwrapped it at her baby shower until now. Now, watching their baby girl cry as she rooted, shoved her own fist into her mouth, and failed to find a nipple, they both wished very much they'd packed it for the hospital.

The first time Donna, the lactation consultant for the day, had checked in with the family within the first 24 hours of the birth, Tati was in tears. Caleb had gone out for supplies and she'd been trying to get the baby to latch onto her breast for half an hour.

"This is supposed to be natural," she said. "Mammals have survived for millennia by breastfeeding. What am I doing wrong?"

Donna perched on the edge of the chair next to the bed. "It is natural, but that doesn't mean it's automatic. We're going to work on this, all four of us: you, me, Dad, and baby."

"I don't even think my milk has come in," said Tati. "I think it's just that yellow stuff. What if I'm starving her?"

"Look at that beautiful baby," said Donna. "She's not starving. She's getting all that she needs from the colostrum, the yellow stuff. That's liquid gold (Box 2.8). We'll work on the latch to make sure she gets as much as she can. You're headed into day two after the birth now. Your milk should come in very soon."

"How will I know?" asked Tati.

"You'll know," said Donna. "When you feel your breasts now, they're very soft. As they begin to fill, you'll notice they'll feel fuller. Sometimes they can feel a little too full. We call that engorgement. Right now let's start with the basics. The best time to feed your baby is when she wants to eat."

Tati looked at her daughter, who was crying while trying to stick her entire tiny hand in her mouth. "She looks pretty ready to me," she said.

Donna agreed. "Maybe a little too ready. When the baby gets to the point of crying, it makes it much more challenging to get her to latch. You want to pay attention to earlier signs, like what she's doing with her hands and her mouth, licking her lips, or making sucking motions. Some babies will smack their lips. Almost all of them will root if you touch their cheek, regardless of how hungry they are, so sometimes that's a harder sign to work with." Donna paused and patted Tati's hand. "I know none of this feels natural right now. It will."

Box 2.8 Composition of Breast Milk

Lactogenesis I: Colostrum (Starts in Pregnancy and Lasts Through the First Few Days After Birth)

- Rich in immunologic components
  - Immunoglobulin A (helps protect the gastrointestinal tract)
  - Lactoferrin
  - Leukocytes
- Epidermal growth factor (responsible for repair of damage from low oxygen exposure)
- Laxative properties (help with excretion of meconium and bilirubin)
- Low in lactose compared with later milk
- High in magnesium, chloride, and sodium compared with later milk
- Low in calcium and potassium compared with later milk

Lactogenesis II: Transitional Milk (Starts on Day Two or Three and Lasts About 10 d)

- Lactose increases
- Immunologic components decrease
- Fat and calories increase

Lactogenesis III: Mature Milk

- Foremilk and hindmilk (foremilk may appear watery, whereas hindmilk appears creamier and has a higher fat content)
- 20 kcal/oz
- About 50% of calories are from fat
- Provides almost complete nutrition for the infant: carbohydrates, fat, protein, vitamins, minerals, and digestive enzymes.
- Only vitamin D is not provided in sufficient quantity. Supplementation with 400 IU daily is recommended.

Adapted from Ballard, O., & Morrow, A. L. (2013). Human milk composition: Nutrients and bioactive factors. *Pediatric Clinics of North America, 60*(1), 49–74.

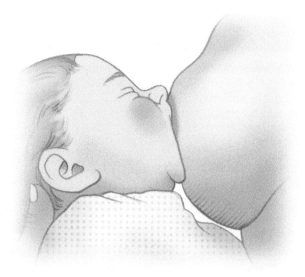

Figure 2.11. A perfect latch in breastfeeding. (Reprinted with permission from *Lippincott Procedures.* [2018, February]. Philadelphia, PA: Wolters Kluwer.)

Donna positioned Tati on the bed with pillows behind her back and supporting her arms. She unswaddled the baby and, after telling Tati what she planned to do and asking her permission, she opened her gown and positioned the baby against her, belly to belly, with the baby's face directly facing Tati's breast.

Next, Donna showed Tati how to hold her breast with her hand in the shape of the letter C, with her thumb on top, well back on the breast from the nipple and areola. The baby almost seemed to be paying attention and had calmed just a little. While Tati watched, Donna assisted her in brushing her nipple against the baby's lips. As she did so, the little girl opened her mouth wide and Donna quickly pushed her little mouth against the nipple. Tati felt a tug and watched, fascinated, as the baby's cheek began to move.

"Beautiful!" said Donna. "That's a lovely latch. Look at how much of the areola the baby has in her mouth. That's just what you want to see. And see how those lips are flanged out over the breast and not tucked in? That's just right" (Fig. 2.11).

Both adults watched as the baby settled into her own rhythm. After about 5 minutes, Donna spoke again.

"Listen," she said. "Do you hear that? That little clicking noise? That means that she's swallowing. Good job, Mom."

"How long should I feed her?" asked Tati.

"She'll let you know. Until she stops," said Donna. "If she's still awake after that, you'll know to switch her to the other breast."

They watched for a few minutes longer. Caleb came in quietly with a bag containing some extra clothing and a paper bag full of deli sandwiches.

"First cold deli meat after the birth," he said, holding up the bag.

"That roast beef best be rare," says Tati.

"Yes ma'am," said Caleb. Then he noticed the baby on the breast.

"You did it," he said quietly. "Nice job. What does it feel like?"

"I don't know," said Tati. "Strange. It makes me so sleepy. Like I could just nod off right here, right now."

"That's the prolactin and the oxytocin," said Donna. "I promise it won't always be like this, but it's really common, early on in particular, to feel really drowsy with breastfeeding. It's important to make sure the baby's back in her crib though, if you think you really will fall asleep."

Donna then turned to Caleb, and recruited him to monitor for Tati's sleepiness, and to take the baby if it seemed she would fall asleep. She explained to him the same points she'd explained to Tati about recognizing a hungry baby, and advised that he too could be instrumental in recognizing when it was a good time to feed.

"How often should she feed?" he asked.

"It varies," Donna said. "She may feed eight to twelve times a day for a while. Sucking helps with the production of the hormones that are making Tati so tired. Those hormones also help with milk production. The more the baby sucks, the better the milk supply."

Tati turned to Caleb. She looked drowsy but satisfied, like a cat having drunk a bowl of cream. "We can't just call her baby forever. She'll need a name."

"Tati Junior," Caleb proposed.

"Donna is a beautiful name," said Donna.

"Calebetta," said Tati. "Calebina."

"Don't worry," said Donna. "In this state they give you sixty days to decide. Go ahead and get to know her a little. It will come to you. I think you three are going to be just fine."

Think Critically

1. Write a brief script explaining to a patient in your care how she should correctly use COCs.
2. You have a patient with brown eyes who is carrying a child fathered by a man with blue eyes. You know that brown eyes are a dominant trait, whereas blue eyes are a recessive trait. How would you describe the chances of their child having blue or brown eyes?
3. How would you describe to a first-time mother the difference between true and false labor?
4. Why do we treat GBS during labor? What important question should you ask a patient before administering the medication?
5. Describe what behaviors would make you suspect a baby is hungry. How would you describe to a new mother what a good latch looks like?
6. What is uterine atony? What are the priority actions when you suspect it?
7. You are caring for a patient postpartum who is reluctant to get up to empty her bladder, stating she doesn't feel like she has to. How would you convince her it's a good idea?

References

Addati, L., Cassirer, N., & Gilchrist, K. (2014). *Maternity and paternity at work: Law and practice across the world.* Geneva, Switzerland: International Labour Office.

American College of Obstetricians and Gynecologists. (1999). *Prevention of RhD alloimmunization* (Practice Bulletin No. 4). Washington, DC: Author.

Baecher, L., & Gobman, W. (2008). Prenatal antibiotic treatment does not decrease group B streptococcus colonization at delivery. *International Journal of Gynecology & Obstetrics, 101*(2), 125–128.

Butt, K., & Lim, K. (2014, February). Determination of gestational age by ultrasound. *Journal of Obstetrics and Gynaecology Canada, 303,* 171–181.

Durain, D. C., & McCool, W. F. (2015). Menstrual cycle abnormalities. In T. L. King, M. C. Brucker, J. M. Kriebs, J. O. Fahey, C. L. Gegor, & H. Varney (Eds.), *Varney's midwifery* (pp. 353–370). Burlington, MA: Jones & Bartlett Learning.

Legro, R., Arslanian, S., Ehrmann, D., Hoeger, K., Murad, M., Pasquali, R., & Welt, C. K.; Endocrine Society. (2013). Diagnosis and treatment of polycystic ovary syndrome: An Endocrine Society clinical practice guideline. *The Journal of Clinical Endocrinology and Metabolism, 98*(12), 4565.

Main, E. K., Goffman, D., Scavone, B. M., Low, L. K., Bingham, D., Fontaine, P. L., . . . Levy, B. S. (2015). National partnership for maternal safety: Consensus bundle on obstetric hemorrhage. *Journal of Obstetric, Gynecologic, & Neonatal Nursing, 44*(4), 462–470.

Martins, H. E., Souza, M. D., Khanum, S., Naz, N., & Souza, A. C. (2016). The practice of nursing in the prevention and control of postpartum hemorrhage: An integrative review. *American Journal of Nursing Science, 5*(1), 8–15.

Moran, L., Hutchison, S., Norman, R., & Teede, H. (2011). Lifestyle changes in women with polycystic ovary syndrome. *Cochrane Database Systematic Review, 16*(2), CD007506.

Moyer, V. (2012). Screening for cervical cancer: U.S. Preventive Services Task Force recommendation statement. *Annals of Internal Medicine, 156*(12), 880–891.

Perkins, R. B., Anderson, B. L., Gorin, S. S., & Schulkin, J. A. (2013). Challenges in cervical cancer prevention: A survey of U.S. obstetrician-gynecologists. *American Journal of Preventative Medicine, 45*(2), 175–181.

Suwanrath, C., & Suntharasaj, T. (2010). Sleep–wake cycles in normal fetuses. *Archives of Gynecology and Obstetrics, 281*(3), 449–454.

The American College of Obstetricians and Gynecologists Committee on Obstetric Practice. (2015). *Physical activity and exercise during pregnancy and the postpartum period.* Washington, DC: Author.

U.S. Department of Labor, Wage and Hour Division. (2012). *Fact Sheet #28: The Family and Medical Leave Act.* Washington, DC: Author.

WomensHealth.gov. (2014, December 23). *Polycystic ovary syndrome (PCOS) fact sheet.* Retrieved from http://womenshealth.gov/publications/our-publications/fact-sheet/polycystic-ovary-syndrome.html

Zvereff, V. V., Faruki, H., Edwards, M., & Friedman, K. J. (2013). Cystic fibrosis carrier screening in a North American population. *Genetics in Medicine, 16,* 539–546.

Suggested Readings

Main, E. K., Goffman, D., Scavone, B. M., Low, L. K., Bingham, D., Fontaine, P. L., . . . Levy, B. S. (2015). National partnership for maternal safety: Consensus bundle on obstetric hemorrhage. *Journal of Obstetric, Gynecologic, & Neonatal Nursing, 44*(4), 462–470.

Martins, H. E., Souza, M. D., Khanum, S., Naz, N., & Souza, A. C. (2016). The practice of nursing in the prevention and control of postpartum hemorrhage: An integrative review. *American Journal of Nursing Science, 5*(1), 8–15.

WomensHealth.gov. (2014, December 23). *Polycystic ovary syndrome (PCOS) fact sheet.* Retrieved from http://womenshealth.gov/publications/our-publications/fact-sheet/polycystic-ovary-syndrome.html

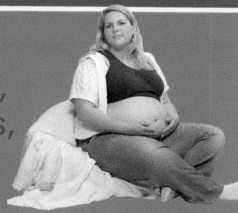

Susan Rockwell:
3 Gestational Diabetes, Deep Vein Thrombosis, and Postpartum Pulmonary Embolism

Susan Rockwell, age 27

Objectives

1. Discuss the mechanisms of gestational diabetes.
2. Outline the progression from risk factors to diagnosis to treatment for a patient with gestational diabetes.
3. Recognize risk factors and common signs and symptoms for pulmonary embolism and deep vein thrombosis.
4. Prioritize care considerations for a patient suspected of pulmonary embolism and deep vein thrombosis.
5. Consider the impact of obesity and low income on pregnancy.
6. Explain the mechanism for hypoglycemia in infants with macrosomia.
7. Identify key characteristics of the contraceptive shot.

Key Terms

Cesarean section
Compression ultrasound (CUS)
Crackles
Deep vein thrombosis
Depot medroxyprogesterone acetate (DMPA)
Dyspnea
Ectopic pregnancy
Gestational diabetes
Macrosomic

Normoglycemic
Oral glucose tolerance test
Pulmonary embolism
Rales
Tachycardic
Tachypneic
Type 1 diabetes
Type 2 diabetes

Before Conception

Susan Rockwell has a love–hate relationship with her contraceptive, the **depot medroxyprogesterone acetate (DMPA)** shot (The Pharmacy 3.1). On the one hand, it is convenient to go in and get her shot every 3 months (she likes to call it her "baby vaccine"); on the other hand, it is a painful shot she *has* to remember to get every 3 months. When she first started it 3 years ago when she was still in the hospital with her son, Robbie, she didn't really take the time to learn much about it. She doubts she would have even remembered to come back and get another shot if the receptionist at her physician's office didn't call to remind her.

In the last few years, though, she's started to wonder whether the DMPA might be part of the reason she still hasn't lost all that pregnancy weight. She gained 80 lb with Robbie. Eighty pounds! Every time she thinks of it, it sounds too big, too huge. Who gains that much weight? During the pregnancy she just ate and ate. She figured that she'd breastfeed, that a lot of it was water weight, and that she'd practically be back in her size 6 skinny jeans by the time she left the hospital. She was not. Breastfeeding lasted for less than a week, but she knows that this was only a fraction of the problem. She'd never tell her boyfriend Rob, but she still wears her maternity pants sometimes, 3 years after the birth. She likes the stretchy waistband.

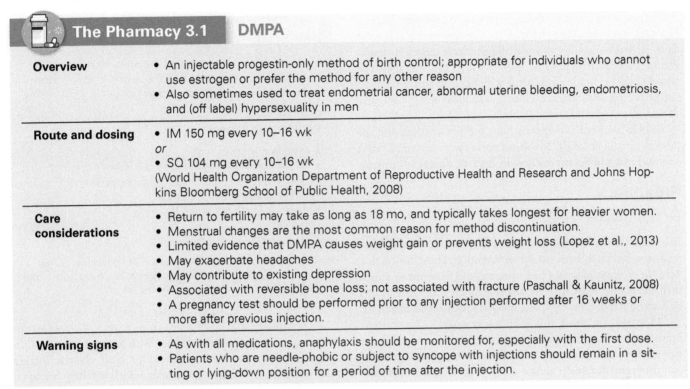

The Pharmacy 3.1 DMPA

Overview	• An injectable progestin-only method of birth control; appropriate for individuals who cannot use estrogen or prefer the method for any other reason
	• Also sometimes used to treat endometrial cancer, abnormal uterine bleeding, endometriosis, and (off label) hypersexuality in men
Route and dosing	• IM 150 mg every 10–16 wk
	or
	• SQ 104 mg every 10–16 wk
	(World Health Organization Department of Reproductive Health and Research and Johns Hopkins Bloomberg School of Public Health, 2008)
Care considerations	• Return to fertility may take as long as 18 mo, and typically takes longest for heavier women.
	• Menstrual changes are the most common reason for method discontinuation.
	• Limited evidence that DMPA causes weight gain or prevents weight loss (Lopez et al., 2013)
	• May exacerbate headaches
	• May contribute to existing depression
	• Associated with reversible bone loss; not associated with fracture (Paschall & Kaunitz, 2008)
	• A pregnancy test should be performed prior to any injection performed after 16 weeks or more after previous injection.
Warning signs	• As with all medications, anaphylaxis should be monitored for, especially with the first dose.
	• Patients who are needle-phobic or subject to syncope with injections should remain in a sitting or lying-down position for a period of time after the injection.

DMPA, depot medroxyprogesterone acetate; IM, intramuscular; SQ, subcutaneous.

She's tried to diet. She tries telling herself that she is making permanent life changes and that she isn't dieting. But it's dieting: Paleo, Weight Watchers, South Beach, and Scarsdale. She's done them all. Sometimes she loses a little bit and sometimes she doesn't, but the final result is always the same. She feels too tired to bother weighing her food or too poor to buy bushels of fresh cilantro and organic chicken breasts, too poor to pay the subscription fees for the diets. It doesn't help that she works in the deli of a convenience store. It's not like they are serving up celery sticks and raw almonds there.

And she is so hungry. What every diet seems to do successfully is crank up her desire to eat. She's tried exercising, but the gym is expensive and the streets around their apartment are too busy. She feels shy about running or walking on them. She feels as though people are staring and pointing at her. People walk past her on the sidewalk like she is standing still. Every time it is like a reminder that she is so big, things will always be harder for her. She'll always be bigger, she'll always be slower, she'll always be hungrier. The other thing she hasn't told Rob is that she's gained another 10 lb since Robbie was born.

To even get the DMPA, she has to visit a nurse practitioner at the clinic once a year in addition to the visits every 3 months to get the shot itself. Lisa, the nurse practitioner, told her that some studies showed weight gain with DMPA. Of course, she also said that some studies didn't show weight gain, but she mentioned she had patients who'd gained a lot of weight with DMPA, and it was her opinion that DMPA

played a role in that. They went over some other methods together, but none of them seemed quite right. She didn't like the idea of something being stuck in her arm or her uterus. She didn't think she could remember to take a pill. Lisa said she was too big for the patch, which apparently had a weight limit of 198 lb, which sounds pretty arbitrary. And there's no way Rob would do condoms.

So, she's stayed on the DMPA, but has been going in later and later to get the shot. It's just a hassle and it hurts, and with it being something she does only four times a year, it's just too easy to forget it. It's usually her body that remembers the shot before her brain does. She hasn't had a period since the pregnancy, thanks to the shot. When she is late for her shot now, however, she gets a little light bleeding, and that makes her remember to go back in to get it just to stop her period. She has a friend, a big woman like her, who says that she's been trying to get pregnant after stopping the DMPA for over a year with no luck. Susan thinks maybe that would be true for her, too. Maybe between the DMPA and her weight, she's screwed up her hormones badly enough that she can't get pregnant.

And would a pregnancy be so bad? She loves little Robbie with all her heart, and Rob is a good father. He picks up construction jobs when they are available, and he does some under-the-counter handyman work. He doesn't drink too much, and he's never laid a hand on either one of them. He is good with Robbie and looks after him just fine on days when they can't get childcare.

She gets some assistance through the state to cover her childcare expenses, but it isn't enough for all the days she works, and some days she works odd hours when the childcare center is closed. Her mother could fill in some, but she works, too. Her sister can afford to stay at home all the time with her kids and sometimes she helps, but she's made it clear that she isn't a free sitter and doesn't want to be taken for granted.

Robbie has been asking for a baby brother or sister, and she thinks he might be lonely. So she just doesn't go to her next DMPA appointment and doesn't reschedule. And she doesn't tell anyone.

Pregnancy

First Trimester

In less than 6 months after that missed DMPA appointment, she's pregnant. She's not sure how she feels about it. She tells Rob that her DMPA must have stopped working, and he seems to accept that. He doesn't react strongly one way or the other. She knows he'll come around, though. Her mother's reaction surprises her.

"How do you think this is going to work?" Tina, Susan's mother, asks. "You think I'm going to quit my job to help? Are you going to quit your own job? How are you going to eat and pay your rent? Robbie is almost ready to go to school now, and that's free. Now you want another five years of scrambling to pay for childcare? What are you thinking?"

"There's no point in arguing, Mom. There's going to be a baby and that's just what's going to happen. We'll figure it out. We've figured it out with Robbie, haven't we?"

"Susan, the reason you've been able to figure it out is that you've had me to help, and you've had your sister to help. Did you think about asking us about it before you decided to get pregnant? You won't be raising this baby by yourself, you know. You'll need all of us to help you out, and not one of us here isn't stretched thin already."

"This wasn't really a decision," Susan says. "It just sort of happened."

"You and me, we both know that's not true," says Tina. "You can pretend all you want with other people, but don't you do it with me."

Susan wishes she were rich. She wishes she could have kids and not worry about the cost. It seems like a pretty basic thing, having kids—all part of having a nice life, of having joy and a sense of purpose. It's hard having to worry whether it will fit in the budget. Susan isn't lazy. She's been working since she was 14, and she works 30 hours a week at the deli right now, but she's never had a job that paid better than $12 an hour. Rob's income is good when he can get work, but he has had long dry patches when they have had to count on what she makes alone. And still they make so little money that they all qualify for Medicaid to cover their healthcare costs. There have been really lean times, like when her hours were cut temporarily at the deli and she had to go to the local food shelf. She never told anyone about those visits.

Susan goes to see Lisa, the nurse practitioner, to get her prenatal vitamin prescription. Although she can buy them over the counter, she knows that if she gets the prescription kind, Medicaid will cover the cost. Susan tells Lisa her period has been pretty regular over the last 3 months, and Lisa estimates her due date using a program in her electronic health record. She is about 6

weeks pregnant. Lisa provides her with a confirmation of the pregnancy form that she can take to the local Women, Infants, and Children (WIC; Box 3.1) center, which will help her access good food during the pregnancy.

"Have you had any bleeding since your last period?" Lisa asks.

"I had a tiny bit of spotting when I thought I'd get my period, but nothing since then," says Susan.

"That's likely implantation bleeding," says Lisa. "The egg is usually fertilized up in the fallopian tube, between the ovary and the uterus. Sometime between six and twelve days after fertilization, the egg implants in the uterus. Some women get a little bit of spotting. Have you had any cramping?"

"A little bit," says Susan. "It's right in the middle of my belly. It feels like period cramps."

"That sounds normal, too," says Lisa. "As your uterus starts to grow, you can get some cramping like that. We worry, though, when the cramping is off to one side or the other, if it radiates to the shoulder, or you have more bleeding. Then we start to consider the possibility of an ectopic pregnancy."

"I don't know what that is," says Susan.

"An ectopic pregnancy happens when the fertilized egg implants somewhere other than the uterus. The most common place is in the fallopian tube," says Lisa. "I don't have any reason to think that's happening with you, however. Are you having any pregnancy symptoms?" (Box 3.2 and Fig. 3.1).

"Some," says Susan. "I'm really tired. When I get home, I just want to lie on the couch. My breasts are pretty sore. The smell of coffee is starting to bother me, and I'm getting some nausea. It usually goes away if I eat something."

By the time Susan visits the office of her obstetrics and gynecology provider, she is 10 weeks pregnant and feeling a little better. She still has some mild cramping in the lower middle of her belly, but she hasn't had any bleeding since that early spotting. The nausea is maybe a little better, or maybe she's just learned to manage it. She is still tired, but her sister has taken pity on her and is having Robbie over to play with his cousins more often.

Box 3.2 Clinical Manifestations of Ectopic Pregnancy

- Most commonly seen 6–8 wk after the first day of the last menstrual period but may be seen later
- Vaginal bleeding, light to very heavy (if ruptured); typically intermittent but may be continuous
- The quality of pain varies but is usually not crampy. The pain is classically off to one side but depends on the location of the ectopic pregnancy. Severe abdominal bleeding may cause referred shoulder pain.

A medical assistant named Gwen gives her a gown and leaves while she changes. It is too small, which makes her feel fat and exposed. Gwen returns and takes her vital signs. When it comes time to take her blood pressure (BP), Gwen tells her the BP cuff is too small and that she'll have to find a bigger one. It takes her a long time to come back. In the end, at least her BP is okay.

The physician she saw for Robbie is no longer with the practice. The new physician she sees, Raina Cheema, tells her that she will rotate through and see the four physicians who remain with the practice.

"We all take turns being on call, of course," says Dr. Cheema. "You could have any one of us at the delivery."

Dr. Cheema reviews Susan's chart with her and asks her questions about her health and previous pregnancy (see Box 1.2).

"Ah," says Dr. Cheema. "You had your first baby by cesarean section, is this correct?"

Susan nods. She labored for a long time. They watched the baby's heart the whole time on the monitor. After a while, when her cervix didn't open as fast as it should have, the baby's heart

rate started to worry her team and they were afraid the baby wasn't able to get what it needed from the placenta anymore. She consented to the cesarean section.

"We will schedule your cesarean section when we get closer to your due date," says Dr. Cheema. "Since you are having a cesarean section, you may be able to choose which physician performs the delivery."

"I can't try for a normal delivery this time?" asks Susan.

"Some women elect to attempt a vaginal birth after a cesarean section," says Dr. Cheema. "The hospital where we do deliveries, however, does not allow this. They feel it carries a greater risk to the mother and baby than simply repeating the cesarean. If you want to try a vaginal delivery, you would have to go to a different practice—one that uses a different hospital."

"Oh," says Susan. "Not really. I was just wondering."

"I notice," says Dr. Cheema, "That you are quite a bit heavier now than you were at the beginning of your last pregnancy. When we consider weight, we think about body mass index, or BMI, which is a calculation we make using height and weight. We like to see that number between 18.5 and 24.9 (see Box 1.4). Right now, your BMI is 38. This tells us that you are quite obese."

Susan feels sick with embarrassment. The way Dr. Cheema said it was so stark and unapologetic. She wasn't cruel, but her frankness stuns Susan. There she is, too big again—too poor and too big. She wants to cry. She wants to leave. Instead, she waits and tries to listen to Dr. Cheema.

"Having obesity when you are pregnant can lead to some very bad outcomes," says Dr. Cheema. "We will keep a very close eye on you, but you must know that you are at greater risk for complications with this pregnancy. We will test your blood today to make sure you are not diabetic already" (Boxes 3.3 and 3.4).

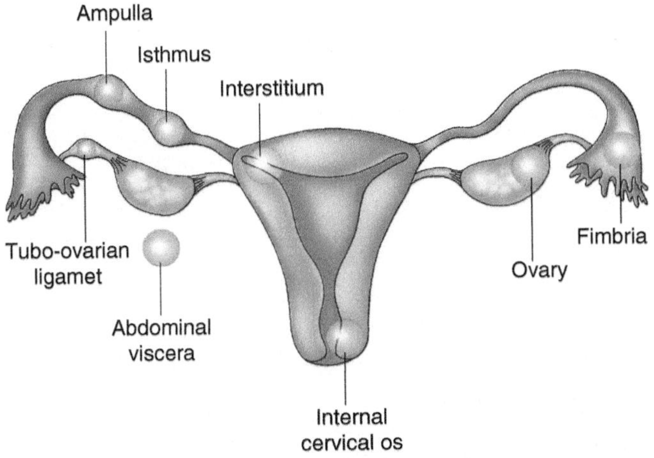

Figure 3.1. Common sites of ectopic pregnancy. In approximately 95% of patients with ectopic pregnancy, the ovum implants in part of the fallopian tube: the fimbria, ampulla, or isthmus. Other possible abnormal sites of implantation include the interstitium, ovarian ligament, ovary, abdominal viscera, and internal cervical os. Ectopic pregnancies are acutely dangerous for the mother and rarely viable. (Reprinted with permission from *Lippincott Advisor*. [2017, October]. Philadelphia, PA: Wolters Kluwer.)

Box 3.3 Obesity Risks in Pregnancy

Maternal Risks
- Gestational diabetes
- Gestational hypertension
- Preeclampsia
- Cesarean section
- Wound complications

Fetal Risks
- Neural tube defects
- Prematurity
- Stillbirth
- Congenital anomalies
- Macrosomia (high birth weight)
- Low birth weight

Child Risks
- Childhood obesity
- Hypertension
- Increased all-cause mortality

Adapted from ACOG Committee on Ethics. (2014). Committee opinion No. 600: Ethical issues in the care of the obese woman. *Obstetrics and Gynecology, 123*(6), 1388–1393.

"What can I do?" asks Susan. "I just want this baby to be healthy."

"You mustn't gain any more than twenty pounds, and you must exercise. Ideally you would have lost weight before the pregnancy, but we must now work with what we have."

Susan doesn't want to talk about it anymore. She just wants to be done. She doesn't ask any more questions. She doesn't tell Dr. Cheema about the trouble she has trying to lose weight or how hard it is to exercise or how tired she is all the time.

Dr. Cheema performs an exam (see Box 1.3). Then she advises her to change back into her clothes and tells her that a nurse will be coming in to draw her blood and talk with her about prenatal screening. Susan nods. Dr. Cheema tells her to stop by the front desk and schedule her next appointment for 1 month from now. Dr. Cheema finally leaves. Susan changes and waits in a plastic chair placed next to the sink.

Within minutes, a nurse comes into the room carrying a caddy full of needles, tubes, bandages, and alcohol swabs.

"Hi," she says. "I'm Valerie."

Susan nods at her and puts her arm out. "What are you testing for?" she asks.

"Well, the good news is we don't need as much as we did for your first pregnancy," says Valerie. "Some things, such as your blood type, never change, so we don't need to do that again. We tested you for genetic problems you could pass on with your first pregnancy. You didn't have any and that doesn't change, so no need to do that again. We do need to do an extra test for diabetes, though. Dr. Cheema ordered a hemoglobin A$_{1c}$. It's a test that will tell us how your blood sugar has been for the last two or three months and whether you're diabetic or at risk for diabetes" (Lab Values 3.1).

And now Susan finally does begin to cry.

 Lab Values 3.1 Susan's First Trimester Labs

Lab Test	Purpose	Normal Results	Susan's Results
Complete blood count	This test evaluates the blood for various kinds of anemia and infection.	RBC: 4.2–5.4 million cells/μL	RBC: 4 million cells/μL
		WBC: 4,500–10,000 cells/μL	WBC: 8,000 cells/μL
		HCT: 36.1%–44.3%	HCT: 36.1%
		HGB: 12.1–15.1 g/dL	HGB: 12.1 g/dL
		MCV: 80–95 fL	MCV: 80 fL
		MCH: 27–31 pg/cell	MCH: 27 pg/cell
		MCHC: 32–36 g/dL	MCHC: 32 g/dL
Syphilis	Syphilis infection is also vertically transmitted from the mother to the fetus and is teratogenic.	Initial testing includes RPR and VDRL. A positive result would require additional testing to confirm the diagnosis.	Negative
Gonorrhea and chlamydia	These are two of the most common sexually transmitted infections. Both can cause pregnancy complications and problems with future fertility. Assessment is by urine test or swab.	Negative	Negative for both
HIV	HIV can also be transmitted to a fetus vertically. With treatment of the mother in pregnancy, however, transmission is reduced to a less than 2% chance. Assessment is by finger stick, serum testing, or oral swab.	Negative	Negative
Urine dip	This test assesses for urinary tract infection, glucose in the urine indicating high blood glucose level, and protein in the urine, which may indicate kidney problems.	Protein: negative	Protein: negative
		Glucose: negative	Glucose: negative
		Ketones: negative	Ketones: negative
		Nitrites: negative	Nitrites: negative
		Leukocytes: negative	Leukocytes: negative
		Blood: negative	Blood: negative

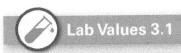

Lab Values 3.1   Susan's First Trimester Labs (continued)

Lab Test	Purpose	Normal Results	Susan's Results
Hemoglobin A$_{1c}$	This test provides an average of blood glucose level over the prior 2–3 mo.	4%–5.6% *Increased risk for diabetes:* 5.7%–6.4% *Diabetes:* 6.5%+	6%

RBC, red blood cell; WBC, white blood cell; HCT, hematocrit; HGB, hemoglobin; MCV, mean corpuscular volume; MCH, mean corpuscular hemoglobin; MCHC, mean corpuscular hemoglobin concentration; RPR, rapid plasma reagin; VDRL, venereal disease research laboratory; HIV, human immunodeficiency virus.

- *Blood type and screen* not drawn. Susan's blood type was determined to be O+ during her last pregnancy.
- *Rubella and hepatitis B* titers not drawn. Susan was determined to have been successfully immunized when screened during prior pregnancy.
- *Hemoglobin electrophoresis* not drawn. It was determined during her last pregnancy that Susan has no congenital abnormalities of her hemoglobin.

"Oh no," says Valerie, putting aside the equipment she is gathering and grabbing a box of tissues, "how can I help?"

Susan can't stop crying. Valerie lays a hand over hers and waits.

"I'm so fat," says Susan, finally. "I eat too much and I don't exercise and now I'm so fat I might hurt my baby. And I don't know how it happened or what to do and I'm so scared and feel so stupid."

"You're not stupid," says Valerie. "Obesity is a disease. What we need to do now is help you manage it so you and your baby can be as healthy as possible."

"I didn't know I was so big," says Susan. "I knew I was over-weight, but I didn't know I was obese."

"It's just a word," says Valerie. "It just tells us something about risk. We know that you and your baby are at higher risk for some things, so we'll look for those things and address problems as we come to them. 'Obese' isn't a judgment, it's a diagnosis. I don't

Box 3.4   Indications for Screening for Preexisting Type 2 Diabetes in Early Pregnancy

- Body mass index ≥ 30 (obese)
- Diagnosis of gestational diabetes with previous pregnancy
- Diagnosis of impaired glucose metabolism (increased risk for diabetes)
- Diagnosis of polycystic ovarian syndrome

Adapted from Legro, R., Arslanian, S., Ehrmann, D., Hoeger, K., Murad, M., Pasquali, R., & Welt, C. K.; Endocrine Society. (2013). Diagnosis and treatment of polycystic ovary syndrome: An Endocrine Society clinical practice guideline. *Journal of Clinical Endocrinology and Metabolism, 98*(12), 4565; ACOG Committee on Practice Bulletins, Obstetrics. (2013). Practice Bulletin No. 137: Gestational diabetes mellitus. *Obstetrics and Gynecology, 122*(2), 406–416.

want you to feel like you are any less worthy of anything because of it. Okay?"

Susan nods. She wipes at her eyes with the tissue and blows her nose. "You're so thin."

Valerie shrugs. "Just because I'm thin doesn't mean I can't understand about obesity. I'm not asthmatic either, but it doesn't mean I can't understand about asthma. Remember, it's a condition. It's not a judgment."

"Okay," says Susan.

"Okay," agrees Valerie. "Regardless of how your testing comes out, I'd like to talk with Dr. Cheema about referring you to a nutritionist, who can help you with your diet. Would that be okay with you?"

As it turns out, she isn't quite diabetic, although she is at risk for diabetes. Valerie has called to tell her, and says that this is good news, but she also cautions her that increased insulin resistance is a normal part of pregnancy.

"I'm sorry," said Susan. "I don't know what that means."

"So, think of the cells of your body having little doors they can open to let sugar in. When the little doors open easily, you're not insulin resistant and you don't have **type 2 diabetes**. When the little doors are harder to open, you're insulin resistant. When you're insulin resistant you end up with more sugar staying in your bloodstream than you should have. When you have type 2 diabetes, those doors really don't want to open, and you end up with way more sugar in your blood than is good for you in the long run."

"Okay," says Susan. "So if I'm at risk for diabetes that means the doors are already sticking. With the pregnancy, they'll be even harder to open so I could still end up with diabetes later during the pregnancy."

"That's exactly right. When the diabetes starts in pregnancy, it's called **gestational diabetes**."

"So this is good news but it's not great news," says Susan. "So—I'm sorry, I'm just trying to understand. So, gestational diabetes is similar to type 2 diabetes. What's **type 1 diabetes**?"

"Think of it this way. The fist that knocks on the doors to your body's cells to get them to open up and allow sugar to enter is insulin. Insulin is produced by the pancreas. When you're a type 1 diabetic, your pancreas doesn't make insulin, so the doors don't know when to open up to let the sugar in and the sugar stays in the blood."

"I think I get that," Susan says.

"On the other hand, when you have insulin resistance, such as in type 2 diabetes or gestational diabetes, you may have plenty of insulin being produced by your pancreas, and the fist is knocking on the doors, but your cells aren't as responsive to insulin—they're resistant."

"Is there anything I can do to make it better?"

"We know that exercise makes the cells more sensitive to insulin. I'd definitely recommend that. We've also made the referral to a nutritionist for you. That person should be able to help with the diet piece," says Valerie.

"I've been trying to lose weight since I had my little boy. That was almost five years ago," says Susan. "I'm so scared that I'm going to fail this time, too. You know, it's one thing to be obese when I'm not pregnant, because it's just me I'm hurting, but when I'm pregnant? It's just so much more pressure."

"What do you see as the major barriers to exercise and following a healthy diet?" asks Valerie.

"I don't know," says Susan. "Time, for one thing. I work a lot, and I have Robbie to take care of. I'm the only one who cooks and does stuff around the house. Good food, you know, vegetables and stuff, they're expensive. Plus, I'm so tired right now with the pregnancy and everything. That makes it harder to get up the energy to cook. On the plus side, I'm signed up with WIC now, so I can get some better food."

"That's great," says Valerie. "Is there anyone else in the house who can help with cooking or cleaning?"

"Not really. My Rob, he's a good guy and he'll babysit our son and stuff, but he doesn't go in for cooking or cleaning. But I was thinking maybe I could make a couple of really big meals early in the week and then have leftovers later in the week, so I'm not cooking every night. It could be easy stuff, healthy stuff."

"It's a good idea. But start out slow. You don't have to do everything at once. Walk for ten minutes instead of half an hour. Do you think you could do that?"

"Probably," says Susan. "Maybe on my breaks."

"Try it. But don't beat yourself up if you don't get out there every break or if you eat something you think you shouldn't have. Just start over. Do better next time. Take baby steps."

"Baby steps," says Susan. "I can try that."

A month later, Susan meets with the nutritionist, Janet. Janet tells her she likely wouldn't be able to prevent her getting gestational diabetes if it is going to happen, but she can help her to establish some good eating habits that will help her to limit her weight gain in pregnancy and keep her blood sugar in a healthier range (Box 3.5). She tells her she is hoping to give her the tools she'll need not only for this pregnancy but for her life after the pregnancy and her goal to get to a healthy weight.

Box 3.5 Nutritional Recommendations for Diabetics in Pregnancy

Caloric Intake

- BMI 18.5–30: 30 kcal/kg/d
- BMI > 30: 22–25 kcal/kg/d
- Morbid obesity*: 12–14 kcal/kg/d

  Susan weighs 200 lb with a BMI of 38. She should consume between 1,995 and 2,268 kcal/d.

Nutrient Distribution

- 40% of calories from carbohydrates, primarily fruits and vegetables; avoidance of simple carbohydrates such as candy and baked goods
- 40% of calories from fat, avoiding trans fats
- 20% of calories from protein

Timing of Calories

- Breakfast: 10% of calories
- Lunch: 30% of calories
- Dinner: 30% of calories
- Snacks: 30% of calories

*Morbid obesity is defined as BMI ≥ 40, or BMI ≥ 35 with obesity-related conditions, or ≥100 lb over ideal body weight.
BMI, body mass index.
Adapted from Viana, L., Gross, J., & Azevedo, M. (2014). Dietary intervention in patients with gestational diabetes mellitus: A systematic review and meta-analysis of randomized clinical trials on maternal and newborn outcomes. *Diabetes Care, 37*(12), 3345–3355.

It is hard. It is so much harder than any of the other diet plans she's been on. She has a list of common foods and their calorie counts that Janet gave her. She disciplines herself on the basics: she fills half of her plate with nonstarchy vegetables (she likes broccoli best but has vowed to try some others), a quarter with a starch, such as rice, peas, or potatoes, and another quarter with some sort of protein (American Diabetes Association, 2015). She usually has chicken for her protein because she can get big bags of frozen chicken breasts cheaply through work. She has an app on her phone that helps her keep track of her diet, as well. The hardest thing is the starch. It is cheap and satisfying and fills her up. It is tough trying to limit it.

The diet is pretty tedious, and Rob refuses to eat his chicken unless it's fried, which she isn't supposed to do anymore. Robbie, copying his father, sometimes puts up a fuss, as well. It means making more meals. It means counting every calorie and doing math for every meal. She is determined to get it right as much as she can, but some days, particularly when she's in the deli facing a row of candy bars for hours, it seems almost impossible. But every day it gets a little easier. She meets with Janet twice more and with Valerie after every prenatal visit. Both help her fine-tune her approach and both provide support, encouragement, and a helpful dose of faith in her.

She does as Valerie suggests and starts with 10-minute walks. Then every day she tries to walk one telephone pole further. She starts to look forward to it. She's never thought much about setting aside time for herself. It feels strange and indulgent.

At 12 weeks she returns to the office and has the blood work and ultrasound taken for the first trimester screening (see Box 2.5). She watches as the fetus—all arms and legs—moves inside her and even does a little flip.

Second Trimester

At 16 weeks, she returns for the blood work for the integrated screening. The results show that the fetus is healthy—there is no sign of trisomies or neural tube defects.

At 20 weeks, she goes to the radiology department at the hospital for the fetal survey (see Box 1.8 and Fig. 3.2). Rob has just started a job on a building site he hopes will last for several months, so Susan's mother, Tina, comes with her. Together they gaze at the ultrasound image and meet Susan's new baby, a boy. The two women hug, and the ultrasonographer hands over a box of tissues. They dab their eyes. On the way out Tina gives Susan a long hug.

"I'm sorry I was so hard on you," she says. "I just worry about you is all. I'm so proud of how you're taking care of yourself and your family. It'll work out."

At 24 weeks, Valerie calls to help set up an appointment for her **oral glucose tolerance test** and explain the process to her.

"You're going to drink a sweet orange solution they give you. It tastes like a flat orange soda. An hour later they'll check your blood glucose level. If it is less than 130, then you don't have gestational diabetes and no further testing is needed. If it is 130 or greater, then we'll need to do more testing" (Donovan et al., 2013).

Susan comes in for her appointment and drinks the sweet orange solution. Blue lettering on the side of the drink container reads "50 grams Glucose." She's had so little sugar over the prior months that the sweetness is overwhelming, and for much of the hour between finishing the drink and having her blood drawn she concentrates on not vomiting. Her mouth waters with the effort. Her blood glucose level is found to be 180.

"I've been trying so hard," Susan says to Valerie later when she calls to discuss the results. "I feel like I might as well have not bothered."

"Please don't think that," says Valerie. "We talked at the beginning about how diet and exercise would help but would likely not prevent gestational diabetes. Remember that your cells become more resistant to letting sugar in when you're pregnant. Even if you do get a diagnosis of gestational diabetes, which you don't have yet, it doesn't mean that you won't have better control of your blood sugar after the pregnancy is done. Try to think about the long term. I know it's hard, but you've made some really important changes."

"What now?"

"We have to do another, longer, test to see how your body responds to a higher dose of sugar over a longer period of time."

"Oh no," Susan says. "More orange drink?"

"I'm sorry," says Valerie. "I know it's hard. This test will be a little different. You didn't have to fast for the last one, but for this test you'll fast overnight and come to the lab first thing in the morning. They'll take a blood sample to check your fasting blood glucose level and then have you drink more of the orange solution—two bottles this time. They'll check your blood glucose level again at one hour, two hours, and three hours. So that's four checks of your blood glucose level during one test. If two or more of these levels are high, you'll be diagnosed with gestational diabetes" (Lab Values 3.2).

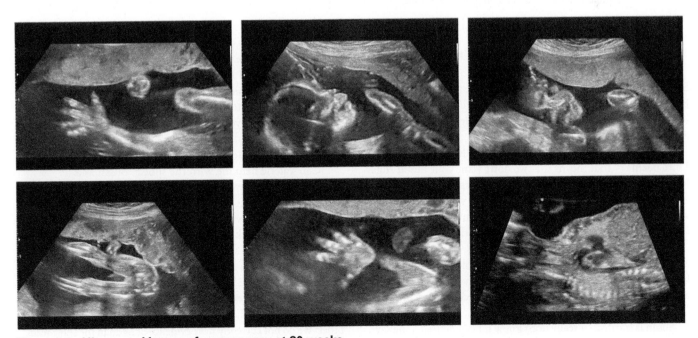

Figure 3.2. Ultrasound image of a pregnancy at 20 weeks.

Lab Values 3.2 Screening and Diagnosis of Gestational Diabetes

Standard Two-Step Screening*
Step 1: Standard screening at 24–28 wk

1. The patient is not fasting.
2. The patient drinks a solution containing 50 g of glucose.
3. An hour after the patient ingests the solution, the blood glucose level is measured.
   If the patient's blood glucose level is greater than 130 mg/dL based on the standard screening, diagnostic testing is indicated, as follows:

Step 2: Diagnostic testing

1. After an overnight fast, the patient's fasting glucose level is checked.
2. The patient drinks a solution containing 100 g of glucose.
3. At 1, 2, and 3 h after ingestion, the patient's blood glucose level is checked.
4. If two or more of the four measurements are elevated, as indicated by the levels below, gestational diabetes is diagnosed.
   a. Fasting: ≥95 mg/dL
   b. One hour: ≥180 mg/dL
   c. Two hours: ≥155 mg/dL
   d. Three hours: ≥140 mg/dL

Alternate Single-Step Combined Screening and Diagnosis Testing†

1. After an overnight fast, the patient's fasting glucose level is checked.
2. The patient drinks a solution containing 75 g of glucose.
3. The blood glucose level is checked again after 1 and 2 h.
4. If one value is elevated, as indicated by the levels below, gestational diabetes is diagnosed.
   a. Fasting: ≥92 mg/dL
   b. One hour: ≥180 mg/dL
   c. Two hours: ≥153 mg/dL

*Adapted from Donovan, L., Hartling, L., Muise, M., Guthrie, A., Vandermeer, B., & Dryden, D. (2013). Screening tests for gestational diabetes: A systematic review for the US Preventive Services Task Force. *Annals of Internal Medicine*, *159*(2), 115; NIH Consensus Development Program. (2013). *NIH development conference: Diagnosing gestational diabetes mellitus*. Bethesda, MD: US Department of Health and Human Services.
†Adapted from Sacks, D. A., Hadden, D. R., Maresh, M., Deerochanawong, C., Dyer, A. R., Metzger, B. E., . . . Trimble, E. R.; HAPO Study Cooperative Research Group. (2012). Frequency of gestational diabetes mellitus at collaborating centers based on IADPSG consensus panel–recommended criteria. *Diabetes Care*, *35*(5), 526–528.

"Twice as much?" Susan says. "Holy cow."

After the test, she's not surprised when she hears the results. She does have gestational diabetes. But it's still hard to hear. It just doesn't seem fair. It was just one more thing. She has a good, long cry. The next day she goes in for a visit with Dr. Cheema and Valerie to discuss the next steps.

"We want to keep you as **normoglycemic** as possible," says Dr. Cheema. "That means that we don't want your blood sugar level to go too high or too low. Most importantly, you must continue your diet and your exercise. Normally with this diagnosis, we recommend lifestyle changes, but as you are already eating correctly and exercising, we must now take the next steps."

Susan nods.

"We need you to start checking your blood sugar level at home with finger sticks. Valerie will show you how to do this after we are done speaking. You will also need to start injecting insulin at home."

Susan is startled. "I really don't know if I can do that," she says. "I'm not good with needles. My grandmother injects insulin, and I can't even watch. Can't I take a pill or something?"

"There are some noninsulin oral medications you could take, but we would like to avoid medication in pregnancy as much as possible, and we currently do not know the long-term effects on your fetus of the oral medications. Insulin occurs naturally in your body, and we do not have these safety concerns with it."

Valerie comes into the room then and gives her a friendly nod.

"Can Valerie help me with the shots?" Susan asks.

"Valerie will show you how to perform the injections, but she cannot perform them all. There will be too many," says Dr. Cheema. "You will need to learn how to do these at home."

Susan feels panicky. "I'm sorry, but I just don't think I can. If I have to stick myself all the time to check my blood sugar I just don't think I can do it with insulin as well. Do they know that the pills hurt babies?"

Dr. Cheema shakes her head. "We do not know this. We simply do not have the studies that tell us with certainty one way or the other. We do not currently have evidence of harm in the short term."

"Can I try that first? Can I just start out checking my blood sugar and taking a pill and then if that doesn't work, I do the insulin?"

Patient Teaching 3.1   Home Glucose Monitoring

Blood Glucose Target Levels*

- Fasting: <90 mg/dL
- Before lunch and before the evening meal: <90 mg/dL
- One hour after the first bite of a meal: <120 mg/dL

  Patients may be instructed to monitor their blood glucose level only twice, fasting and 1 h after the largest meal, if all readings are within range for a period of time.

How to Check Blood Glucose Level

1. Gather the glucose meter, a test strip, a lancet, and a cotton ball.
2. Wash your hands (you may use an alcohol-based hand sanitizer if soap and water are unavailable).
3. Use the lancet to puncture the skin on the side of a finger (some machines allow blood collected from other places, such as the thigh or forearm).
4. Wipe the first drop of blood away with the cotton ball.
5. Apply the test strip to the second drop of blood.
6. The result will appear on the readout of the glucose meter.

*Adapted from HAPO Study Cooperative Research Group. (2008). Hyperglycemia and adverse pregnancy outcomes. *New England Journal of Medicine, 358*(19), 1991–2002.

"Yes, we can try that if you truly feel that insulin is not an option for you at this time," Dr. Cheema says. "The drug I will start you on is called metformin. Sometimes it can upset people's stomachs. We will start with a smaller dose and then build up. You should know, however, that there is still a fifty-fifty chance you will need insulin still (Rowan, Hague, Gao, Battin, & Moore, 2008). Also, you must continue to track your eating in your food diary; keep it with you at all times. For now we will have you check your blood sugar six times a day. Check it when you first get up in the morning, one hour after the first bite of each meal, just before lunch, and just before dinner. Can you do this?"

Susan glances at Valerie, who gives her an encouraging smile. She nods.

"Good," says Dr. Cheema. "Valerie will teach you how to check your blood sugar" (Patient Teaching 3.1 and Fig. 3.3). "We will see you back in one week to check your diary and determine whether you are ready to increase your dose of metformin" (The Pharmacy 3.2). "After next week, you will come to see us every two or three weeks so we can monitor your diet and your blood sugar."

Third Trimester

Susan does just as she is told. She monitors her blood six times a day faithfully for almost a month, when Valerie tells her she can go down to twice a day. She is diligent about her diet and walks regularly. After nearly 2 months, her metformin dose is

The Pharmacy 3.2   Metformin

Overview	• The only medication in the category of biguanide; an antidiabetic agent. It works in two ways: it suppresses the production of glucose by the liver and increases the sensitivity of cells to insulin. • It is used frequently for treatment of type 2 diabetes and gestational diabetes.
Route and dosing	• Oral. It is typically started at a low dose, such as 250 mg or 500 mg once daily for a week, then twice daily for a week, and gradually titrated up stepwise to 2,000–2,550 mg or the highest dose tolerated by the patient. The time between dose titrations is typically 1–2 wk.
Care considerations	• Complaints of gastrointestinal side effects are common and typically improve with a lower dose. Diarrhea, flatulence, vomiting, and nausea are most common. • The drug should be discontinued temporarily prior to major surgery and use of iodine contrast.
Warning signs	• Risk for lactic acidosis is associated with use, especially with hepatic and renal impairment, alcohol abuse, dehydration, sepsis, and congestive heart failure. Signs of lactic acidosis include respiratory distress, malaise, myalgia, somnolence, abdominal pain.

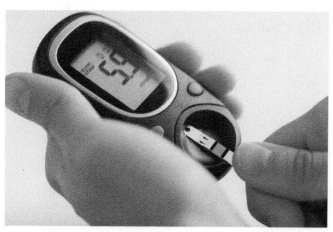

Figure 3.3. A glucometer. Glucometers are used for routine in-home glucose monitoring.

up to 1,000 mg twice daily, and she doesn't have any nausea or diarrhea. And she never has to start insulin. For the first time in a long time, she feels like someone who can win.

At 32 weeks, Dr. Cheema recommends she have a weekly nonstress test (Box 3.6) as well as an ultrasound to determine

---

Box 3.6 Nonstress Test Interpretation

A fetal nonstress test is an assessment of a fetus' heart rate reactivity to its own movements, when no stress is placed on the fetus. It is used to evaluate whether the fetus is receiving adequate blood flow and oxygen. It is typically initiated only after 26–28 wk of gestation, as the fetus is not neurologically mature enough prior to this time to initiate heart rate accelerations. The results of the test are characterized as either reactive or nonreactive, which are described below.

Reactive

- *Weeks 26 through 32:* at least two accelerations of at least 10 beats per minute (bpm) lasting at least 10 s over 20 min
- *Weeks 33 and later:* at least two accelerations of at least 15 bpm for at least 15 s over 20 min

Nonreactive

- The above standards have not been met.
- The fetal heart rate should be monitored for an additional 20–100 min.
- The fetus' lack of reactivity may be due to low oxygen, fetal sleep, fetal anomalies, maternal smoking, and other reasons.
- As many as 60% of nonreactive stress tests are false positives.
- The test may be repeated in 30 min, or additional testing may be ordered to confirm the results.

Adapted from Macones, G. A., Hankins, G. D., Spong, C. Y., Hauth, J., & Moore, T. (2008). The 2008 National Institute of Child Health and Human Development workshop report on electronic fetal monitoring: Update on definitions, interpretation, and research guidelines. *Journal of Obstetric, Gynecologic, and Neonatal Nursing, 37*(5), 510–515.

---

the volume of amniotic fluid in her uterus. Valerie explains that the amniotic fluid volume is important to measure because it can indicate if there's a problem with the placenta or the baby. When the fetus receives less oxygen from the placenta than it needs, the good, oxygenated blood is sent to critical organs such as the brain and heart, and diverted away from more minor organs, such as the kidneys.

"It's the kidneys, you see, that produce the amniotic fluid," says Valerie.

Susan pauses and thinks for a moment. "Do you mean to tell me that babies are floating in their own pee?"

Valerie nods. "So, a low volume of amniotic fluid may mean that less oxygenated blood is reaching the kidneys, which means that the baby is not receiving enough oxygen overall. With maternal diabetes we're more likely to see a high volume of fluid, polyhydramnios, though we're not really sure why."

"Holy cow," says Susan.

Susan is scheduled for delivery by cesarean section in her 39th week of pregnancy. All of her nonstress tests are normal, and her amniotic fluid volume is good. She is eating according to instructions and tries to exercise daily. She takes her metformin twice a day. She checks her blood sugar twice a day. Some days it comes really close to being high, but most of the time it is in the normal range. She is proud of all she's done for this pregnancy. And she is sick of being pregnant (Box 3.7).

At a visit with Dr. Cheema, Susan vents her frustration. "I'm on my feet all day at work. My ankles swell up and my legs cramp. I don't sleep well because the baby's moving all the time and I have to get up to pee ten times a night. I'm just done with being pregnant. Robbie was born at just 38 weeks. Can't you take this one early, as well?"

"When a woman has diabetes, the lungs of her fetus mature more slowly than in the fetus of a mother without diabetes," says Dr. Cheema. "You have been most excellent with your diabetes control, but the risk remains that if we take your baby earlier, it might have trouble with its breathing after the birth. I do not think it is worth the risk."

Labor and Delivery

Finally, her scheduled day arrives. The advantage of the planned cesarean, she supposes, is that Rob has been able to arrange for time off from the job site to be with her during delivery. Also, she's been able to arrange it so that her mother and sister will spend the day with Robbie so that he'll feel special and not feel completely overshadowed by his new baby brother.

Box 3.7 Common Discomforts of the Third Trimester of Pregnancy

- Increased urinary frequency and urgency
- Intensifying of Braxton Hicks contractions
- Increased shortness of breath
- Insomnia
- Leg cramps
- Ankle swelling (edema)
- Anxiety, ambivalence, and moodiness

She and Rob arrive at the hospital at seven in the morning, as scheduled. She has followed the instructions to not eat for 6 hours before hand and to not have anything fried or fatty for at least 8 hours before hand. She did eat a salad with some turkey on it close to midnight, knowing she'd be hungry in the morning. She was also allowed to have clear liquids and black coffee up to 2 hours before the surgery (American Society of Anesthesiologists Task Force on Obstetric Anesthesia, 2016). She has also not taken her metformin this morning, as directed.

It is so different arriving at the labor and delivery floor with a scheduled appointment instead of in an excited flutter of contractions and anxiety. It makes it feel businesslike, as though she were at work taking an order from a customer. It helps to soothe her nerves. A nurse named Reggie helps her change into a voluminous hospital gown and short socks with rubber traction strips on the bottom, which stretch over her swollen ankles. Reggie takes a set of vital signs and places a fetal heart rate monitor and a tocodynamometer over her belly. She checks her fasting glucose and tells them it is within the range of normal. Susan pumps her fist in the air at this news, and Rob whistles so loud that it makes Reggie jump. Rob holds her hand while an intravenous (IV) line is placed. Reggie confirms that Susan does not have any medication allergies and then right away adds some medications into the IV.

"What are those for?" asks Rob.

"One of them, ranitidine, is to help reduce the amount of acid in your stomach, to prevent acid reflux during the surgery," Reggie replies. "The other one is an antibiotic" (The Pharmacy 3.3).

After about 15 minutes, the anesthesiologist, who introduces himself as Dr. Ryan, arrives to place the epidural.

"We have to numb you up pretty far," he says, "all the way to your chest."

"I remember," says Susan. "I had to do this with my first baby, as well."

"Did you have any problems that time?" he asks.

"No," says Susan. "It makes me a little nervous thinking about having a needle in my back, but I didn't have any problems last time."

Just as she did with Robbie's birth, Susan sits at the edge of the bed, her back rounded forward, as Dr. Ryan instructs, so that he can get his needle between her vertebrae. Robbie squats in front of her and takes her hands.

"Don't be scared," he says. "You're in good hands here. You just look right in my eyes and don't move and it will be over quick."

The Pharmacy 3.3	Common Medications Given Prior to Initiating Anesthesia Before Cesarean Section	
Ranitidine		
Overview	• A histamine H2-receptor antagonist (H2-blocker) • Decreases stomach acid production	
Route and dosing	• May be given PO, IM, or IV • In the context of a surgical premedication, typical dosing is 50 mg IV 40–60 min prior to surgery	
Care considerations	• When given IV, it must be diluted. • Maximum administration rate is 10 mg/min (50 mg would take 5 min). • Effects last for 6–8 h after dosing	
Warning signs	• Rapid injection may cause bradycardia	
Cefazolin		
Overview	• Antibiotic, first-generation cephalosporin	
Route and dosing	• May be IV or IM, single dose • For a patient <120 kg: 2 g • For a patient ≥120 kg: 3 g • Should be administered at least 60 min before surgery. • IV: direct over 3–5 min or intermittent over 30–60 min • IM: deep into a large muscle	
Care considerations	Patients with a penicillin allergy may also be allergic to cephalosporins	
Warning signs	Monitor for hypersensitivity reaction, particularly in patients with a penicillin allergy	

Many different antibiotics may be selected. Cefazolin is often preferred, but any of the following combinations may be used: ampicillin-sulbactam; clindamycin or vancomycin plus gentamicin or aztreonam; or metronidazole plus gentamicin. All are typically given as a single dose of medication.

PO, per os (by mouth); IM, intramuscular; IV, intravenous.

It is over quick. Dr. Ryan injects some local numbing medication into her back that feels like a bee sting. After that, all she really feels is pressure, and then the application of tape over her shoulder as he affixes the tubing into place. Within minutes she is numb. Her BP is being checked regularly and is stable. She is wheeled into an operating room, with a goofily gowned Rob walking by her side and holding her hand.

She knows she must be completely numbed from the epidural because she is told that a urinary catheter is being placed but feels nothing. A drape is set up between her face and her belly. Because Dr. Cheema has ended up providing most of her prenatal care, she is scheduled to perform the delivery, as well. She enters the room, greets her, and tells her that the procedure should not be painful and will, in any case, be quick.

Once the surgery is under way, Susan's belly feels to her like a big purse that someone is rooting around in, looking for a pack of gum or some car keys. Rob holds her hand and pats her shoulder. He tries to peek around the blue drape a few times, but she swats at him and tells him to stop. There are some parts of her body he just doesn't need to see at the moment.

And then she hears a tiny cry from a deeply annoyed baby and is overwhelmed with relief.

"It's a boy!" says Dr. Cheema. Susan already knows this, but she still feels her eyes tear up on hearing it.

The little boy, still slimy from birth, is placed on her chest and vigorously rubbed with one warmed blanket and then covered with another. Rob pretends to have something stuck in his throat and Susan just cries.

"He's okay, it's okay," she says, again and again.

The placenta is born next, and then the layers of her body, first the uterus and last the skin, are stitched closed. She is taken back to the room where she started for a brief period of observation prior to being moved to the postpartum recovery floor.

Reggie adds another bag to her IV as Susan watches.

"Is that another antibiotic?" she asks.

"This one is oxytocin," Reggie says. "You'll have this going for another four to eight hours, depending on how you're doing, to keep your uterus contracted so you don't bleed more than you should."

After Delivery

She is transferred down to postpartum within a few hours of the baby's birth. Suddenly, she thinks of her blood sugar and wonders whether it's high. When she asks her new nurse, Betty, when her next fingerstick will be, Betty tells her that her fasting glucose will be checked a few times over the next 3 days.

"And after that?" Susan says.

"That's it. No more fingersticks."

"I don't understand. So I'm not diabetic anymore? No more medicine?" she asks.

"Most women go back to having a normal blood sugar level after delivery. You should know, though, it's not uncommon for

women with gestational diabetes to develop type 2 diabetes," Betty tells her. "Your physician will probably have you take another oral glucose tolerance test in six to twelve weeks, but for now you're in the all clear" (Lab Values 3.2).

"So that's it?" asks Susan. "I have to tell you, this has been such a source of stress since the pregnancy started. It feels almost like a letdown. I mean, I'm relieved and everything, but it gave me a motivation to do better with what I eat and stuff. It was like a goal I could work towards."

"It's still a good goal," says Betty. "Taking care of yourself."

"Yeah, I know, it's just different." says Susan. She thinks for a moment and then smiles. "No more finger sticks!"

She hates the compression system on her legs. Two cuffs are wrapped around her calves that rhythmically inflate and deflate to keep her from developing clots in her legs. She cooperates readily with Betty to get up and walk to the bathroom and back a few times just so she can take the cuffs off and get her catheter out.

The next day, the lower part of her left leg starts to hurt. It is warm—warmer than her right leg. It seems bigger, more swollen than her right leg, as well (Fig. 3.4). She has back pain, too, and her belly hurts. It's hard to tell, though, whether the pain is from the epidural, the surgery, or something else.

She doesn't know whether she should be worried. And then suddenly she is very, very worried. She can't catch her breath, and her chest hurts every time she tries to take a breath.

"Rob," she calls out, and then remembers he went home for the night. She presses her call button.

"Can't breathe," she tells Betty when she comes in. "I'm so scared."

Betty looks at her and pulls the emergency cord next to her pillow. "Things are going to start happening fast," she tells Susan. "You're in good hands."

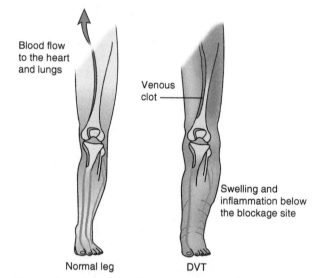

Figure 3.4. A normal leg compared with one with DVT. Approximately 90% of pregnancy-related deep vein thromboses occur in the left leg. DVT, deep vein thrombosis. (Reprinted with permission from Herzog, E. [2012]. *The cardiac care unit survival guide* [1st ed., Fig. 28.2]. Philadelphia, PA: Lippincott Williams & Wilkins.)

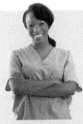

The Nurse's Point of View

Betty: People sometimes get a particular look when they have a pulmonary embolism. They suddenly can't breathe, and they become frightened and anxious. That's what Susan looked like when I walked in the door, and that's why I pulled her emergency cord before doing anything else. I wanted to make sure to have help if I need it.

I start oxygen from the wall right away at ten liters through a nonrebreather mask. Our goal is to keep her oxygen saturation at 90% or higher. I raise the head of the bed as well because this position can help improve lung capacity and breathing. Another nurse, named Katie, comes in, and I ask her to go get the on-call physician, Dr. Kahn, to evaluate a suspected pulmonary embolism.

"Susan," I say. "I know you're scared, but I need you to answer some questions."

Susan nods. She looks frightened. Another nurse from the floor, Madison, wraps a BP cuff around her arm and clips the oxygen saturation monitor to her finger.

"Do you have any leg pain?" I ask Susan.

Susan nods. "I woke up and it was all swollen," she says. Her words sound garbled because of the mask. "Then I couldn't breathe."

"I know it hurts and you're scared, but know this: you can breathe even though it feels like you can't get enough air. It's important that you stay calm. I'm going to check your leg."

I pull back the sheets and look at Susan's legs. "The left is certainly more swollen." I feel both Susan's legs with my hands. "It feels warmer, too."

I cover Susan's legs and listen to her heart and lungs with my stethoscope. A minority of people with a pulmonary embolism have tachycardia, rales, or reduced breath sounds. She has a mildly elevated heart rate and no abnormalities of lung sounds, but that doesn't rule out a pulmonary embolism. I open the computer on the wall of the room and chart my findings. Madison has already charted a set of vitals. The BP is consistent with past readings. Her oxygen saturation is 93%, which is lower than what it was previously but still within the range we want to see.

I'm glad to see Dr. Kahn when she comes in.

"This is Dr. Kahn," I tell Susan before turning to the physician.

"Suspected pulmonary embolism and deep vein thrombosis," I say. "Twenty-seven-year-old female, ten hours post delivery by cesarean section. Dyspnea and anxiety, left leg notably swollen and tender. Tachypneic and tachycardic. No rales, no wheezing. Breath sounds equal bilaterally. Normal heart sounds. Obese. History of gestational diabetes with this pregnancy. No known prior history of blood clots" (Boxes 3.8 and 3.9).

Dr. Kahn turns and smiles at Susan. "Susan," she says. "We are going to take good care of you. Does your chest hurt?"

"I can't breathe. My chest hurts. And my leg hurts," says Susan.

"How are her vitals?" Dr. Kahn asks me.

"Stable," I tell her.

Box 3.8 Signs and Symptoms of a Pulmonary Embolism

Symptoms (Ordered From Most to Least Common)
- Dyspnea
- Pleuritic pain (pain relating to the lining of the lung)
- Cough
- Orthopnea (shortness of breath when lying flat)
- Unilateral leg pain or swelling, redness, or tenderness (symptom of deep vein thrombosis)
- Wheezing
- Hemoptysis (coughing up blood)

Signs (Ordered From Most to Least Common)
- Tachypnea
- Unilateral leg swelling, redness, or tenderness; palpable cords in the leg
- Tachycardia
- Course crackles in the lung
- Accentuated second heart sound (S2)
- Jugular vein distention
- Fever

Warning: A minority of patients with pulmonary embolism will go into circulatory collapse that may manifest as minor hypotension or shock. For these patients, intubation, IV fluid resuscitation, vasopressors, and oxygen support may be warranted.

Adapted from Stein, P. D., Beemath, A., Matta, F., Weg, J. G., Yusen, R. D., Hales, C. A., . . . Woodard, P. K. (2007). Clinical characteristics of patients with acute pulmonary embolism: Data from PIOPED II. *The American Journal of Medicine, 120*(10), 871–879.

"Good. I need a bedside CUS, and let's start dalteparin subcutaneous two hundred units per kilogram daily. And let's do five milligrams of IV morphine. We need to calm her down."

Madison is standing at the ready, and I ask her to get the medications so I can stay with Susan (The Pharmacy 3.4).

Dr. Kahn turns again to Susan. "I think you have some blood clots. I think you have one in your leg and one in your lung. We're going to do something called a compression ultrasound, a CUS, on your leg to see if there's a clot in your leg. In the meantime, we're going to give you a shot of blood thinner to stop your blood from clotting so much. We're also going to give you some medication to help with the anxiety from the breathing."

"I don't care about my leg!" says Susan. "I want you to look at my lungs."

"I understand," says Dr. Kahn, "but it's much faster and easier to find a clot in the leg. The treatment is the same for the clot in the lung and the clot in the leg. If we confirm the clot in the leg, we have our answer about the lungs. Okay?"

Box 3.9 Risk Factors for Blood Clots in Pregnancy and Postpartum

Risk Factors During Pregnancy

- Diabetes
- Body mass index ≥ 30
- Multiple gestation (twins, triplets, etc.)
- Varicose veins
- Maternal age ≥ 35 y
- Urinary tract infection
- Inflammatory bowel disease (ulcerative colitis or Crohn disease)
- Antepartum hospitalization

Risk Factors Postpartum

- Cesarean delivery
- Body mass index ≥ 35
- Delivery prior to 36 wk of gestation
- Obstetric hemorrhage
- Postpartum infection
- Smoking
- Hypertensive disorders of pregnancy
- Diabetes
- Inflammatory bowel disease
- Varicose veins
- Urinary tract infection
- Cardiac disease

Adapted from Jacobsen, A. F., & Sandset, F. E. (2008). Incidence and risk patterns of venous thromboembolism in pregnancy and puerperium—A register-based case-control study. *American Journal of Obstetrics and Gynecology, 198*(2), 233.e1–233.e7; Sultan, A. A., Tata, L. J., West, J., Linda Fiaschi, K. M., Nelson-Piercy, C., & Grainge, M. J. (2013). Risk factors for first venous thromboembolism around pregnancy: A population-based cohort study from the United Kingdom. *Blood, 121*, 3953–3961.

"Okay," says Susan. I can see she's anxious and I'm guessing that, like most people, she just wants it fixed. She asks, "Can't you just do a blood test or something?"

There's a quick knock on the door, and a tech rolls in an ultrasound without waiting for a reply.

"It's a good question," says Dr. Kahn. This is one of the reasons I like Dr. Kahn. At times like this with frightened patients she keeps her cool. She sounds so calm, chatty, almost. "The blood clots more easily during and immediately after pregnancy. That's why women are about five times more likely to get a clot during these times. Because of this, the blood tests we'd normally do to check for clotting issues are not very useful." Dr. Kahn gestures at the person working on the machine. "Susan, this is Jeremy. He's going to do that ultrasound we talked about. It will not be painful" (Fig. 3.5).

While Jeremy is getting the machine ready, Madison returns.

"I'm going to give you a shot of dalteparin, a type of heparin," Madison says to Susan. In her hand is a syringe with a short, thin needle. "It's a blood thinner. It will keep you from getting more blood clots. I'll inject it into your abdomen, near your belly button. I'm also going to give you some morphine to help calm you down and ease your breathing. That one I'll put into your IV."

If anything, Susan looks more anxious, "I hate needles," she says.

"I'll be quick," Madison promises. She quickly cleans off a spot on Susan's belly and injects the dalteparin. "All done."

Susan opens her eyes, which she'd screwed shut while Madison was giving the injection. "Will I need surgery or something for the clots?" she asks.

"Unlikely," Dr. Kahn says. "Your vital signs are stable. Your oxygen levels are fine and your BP isn't low. I think these are small clots." She glances at the machine. "But we're getting a little ahead of ourselves. Let's see what Jeremy finds."

The Pharmacy 3.4 — An Example of Anticoagulant and Opioid Treatment for Pulmonary Embolism

Dalteparin	
Overview	• A low-molecular-weight heparin • An anticoagulant
Route and dosing	• Deep SQ injection • 200 units/kg/d single or split dose 12 h apart
Care considerations	• Risk for bleeding • Risk for thrombocytopenia • Protamine partially reverses the effects
Warning signs	• Signs and symptoms of bleeding include dark tarry stool, altered mental state, and others

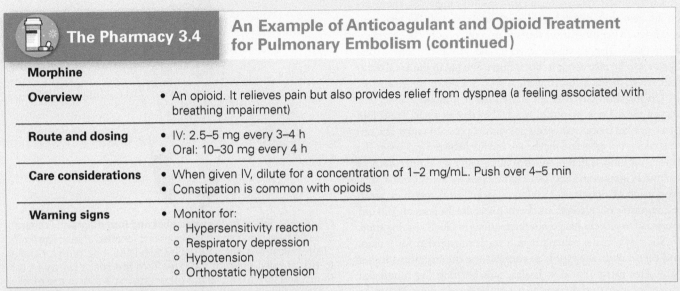

The Pharmacy 3.4 — An Example of Anticoagulant and Opioid Treatment for Pulmonary Embolism (continued)

Morphine

Overview	• An opioid. It relieves pain but also provides relief from dyspnea (a feeling associated with breathing impairment)
Route and dosing	• IV: 2.5–5 mg every 3–4 h • Oral: 10–30 mg every 4 h
Care considerations	• When given IV, dilute for a concentration of 1–2 mg/mL. Push over 4–5 min • Constipation is common with opioids

Warning signs	• Monitor for:
	  ○ Hypersensitivity reaction
	  ○ Respiratory depression
	  ○ Hypotension
	  ○ Orthostatic hypotension

SQ, subcutaneous; IV, intravenous.

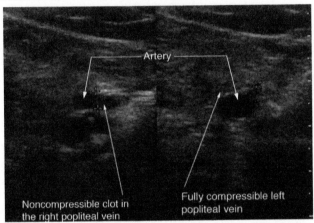

Figure 3.5. Compression ultrasound images of the leg. The image on the left demonstrates a noncompressible right popliteal vein, which indicates the presence of deep vein thrombosis. The image on right demonstrates a fully compressible left popliteal vein, which is normal. (Reprinted with permission from Cosby, K. S., & Kendall, J. L. [2013]. *Practical guide to emergency ultrasound* [2nd ed., Fig. 17.13D]. Philadelphia, PA: Lippincott Williams & Wilkins.)

It doesn't take Jeremy long at all to find a clot in the common femoral vein.

"So there it is," says Dr. Kahn. "Okay folks, we have a plan. Susan, we're going to continue the dalteparin shots to keep your blood thin. When you're in bed, keep the compressors on your legs. But I want you up and about and pacing these halls."

"Shouldn't I be staying in bed?," asks Susan. "I just had a baby, and my leg hurts."

"Sorry, but no," Dr. Kahn says. "We used to keep people on bed rest who had clots because we thought it would keep the clots from breaking free. Now we know it doesn't do any good keeping you in bed, and that your pain will get better faster by having you up and about" (Analyze the Evidence 3.1).

Analyze the Evidence 3.1 — Bed Rest for DVT

Pro	Con
• Bed rest has long been advised as part of the treatment for DVT • Providers feared that ambulation might dislodge a clot that could then travel to the lungs to form a PE or to the brain to provoke a stroke. • No evidence could be found in the current literature to support this practice.	• A meta-analysis of five different studies, including 3,048 patients with DVT, did not find increased risk of new PE from ambulation. • An overall lower rate of new PE and DVT and progression of PE and DVT was found. • An overall lower mortality rate was found for patients who were prescribed ambulation rather than bed rest. • Patients who ambulate report less pain than patients on bed rest.

DVT, deep vein thrombosis; PE, pulmonary embolism.

Data from Aissaouia, N., Martinsb, E., Moulyc, S., Webera, S., & Meune, C. (2009). A meta-analysis of bed rest versus early ambulation in the management of pulmonary embolism, deep vein thrombosis, or both. *International Journal of Cardiology, 137*(1), 37–41; Liu, Z., Tao, X., Chen, Y., Fan, Z., & Li, Y. (2015, April 10). Bed rest versus early ambulation with standard anticoagulation in the management of deep vein thrombosis: A meta-analysis. *PLoS One*. Retrieved from http://dx.doi.org/10.1371/journal.pone.0121388

Over the next few days, Susan's pain gradually improves. The nurses on different shifts watch her diligently, and they take her vital signs and listen to her lungs more times than could possibly be necessary, Susan thinks. They also make her get up and walk several times a shift. She tries to be nice about it, but it hurts. She has to use a walker, as well, which makes it embarrassing as well. But slowly she gets better.

On the third day after she started her first blood thinner, she starts a second one, warfarin, which she takes as a pill. She is told that once her blood test results are within a certain range, she can stop taking the shots and maybe she and her baby can go home. The new medication, warfarin, seems to come with a lot of rules. Because vitamin K intake can affect clotting time, she'll have to eat the same proportion of vitamin K–rich foods (green leafy vegetables, green tea, vegetable oil, alcohol, cranberry juice, the list goes on and on) every day to prevent dangerous fluctuations in blood clotting time.

She stays on the dalteparin and warfarin together for 5 days, and then finally she is able to stop getting the injections in her belly. Her nurse that day, Jessica, tells her that her blood test results indicate that the warfarin is at the correct dose. However, she should still have her blood checked daily until Dr. Cheema thinks it can be done less frequently.

"But I'm going home tomorrow," Susan says.

"You're going to be taking this medication for a while," says Jessica. "It depends on what your provider and you decide. Women who have clots like yours usually stay on warfarin for at least six weeks."

"Six more weeks of watching my diet and getting my blood checked?" asks Susan. "This stinks. I'm just so ready to be done with all of this. I worked so hard on my diet and had my finger stuck all through my pregnancy, and I still got diabetes. Then I got clots even though I did everything I was supposed to. And now I have to go on a different diet and take a different drug. I don't understand."

"I understand your frustration," says Jessica. "You did do the right things. You took care of yourself and that baby. But you need to keep on doing it. You need to take care of yourself."

"It was so much easier to think about this when I was looking out for a baby. I don't know that I can do it with it just being me."

Jessica touches her arm. "Hey—you're worth it. You're worth all of this. Don't think for a minute that you're worth any less. You can do it for your boys if you want, but I think you should do it for yourself. You can make this happen."

"What if when they check me in six weeks I still have diabetes? What if I have to go on another diet and take more drugs on top of this diet and drug?" asks Susan.

"Then you'll keep doing what you did through your pregnancy. You'll eat the right foods, you'll exercise, and you'll take your medications," says Jessica. "You have a lot of control over this situation. You can make it worse, but you can also make it a million times better. That's pretty powerful, when you think about it."

"Powerful," says Susan. She feels like a cartoon supervillain.

"Yeah," says Jessica. "You are."

"If this is power, I'd say power isn't all it's cracked up to be."

The Newborn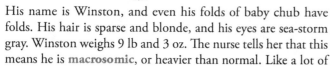

His name is Winston, and even his folds of baby chub have folds. His hair is sparse and blonde, and his eyes are sea-storm gray. Winston weighs 9 lb and 3 oz. The nurse tells her that this means he is **macrosomic**, or heavier than normal. Like a lot of

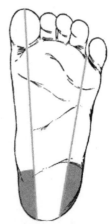

Figure 3.6. Infant heel-stick lancet and foot diagram. Preferred sites for heel blood sampling in infants (shaded areas). The limits of the calcaneus are defined by two lines, one drawn parallel to the lateral margin of the heel from the space between the fourth and fifth toes and the other drawn parallel to the medial margin of the heel from the center of the great toe. (Reprinted with permission from McMillan, J. A., Feigin, R. D., DeAngelis, C., & Jones, M. D. [Eds.]. [2006]. *Oski's solution* [4th ed., Fig. C.2]. Philadelphia, PA: Lippincott Williams & Wilkins.)

big babies, he is mellow and quiet, an early observer and not an instigator. It's a good thing, too, because he has had to go through a lot of heel sticks to check his blood glucose level, starting with one after his first bottle (Fig. 3.6 and Step-by-Step Skills 3.1).

It has taken a while for Susan to process the fact that her gestational diabetes has affected her baby. She remembers the conversation she had with her nurse, Betty, a few hours after delivery.

"But I was so careful," said Susan. "My sugars were really good, I stuck to my diet, I exercised, and I took my medication."

"I believe you," Betty said. "But Winston is a big baby. Between that and your diabetes, he's more likely to have a few days when he's producing extra insulin, and that can bring his blood sugar down to a dangerous level. With the little ones, we like to keep their blood sugar level above fifty, at least, for the first few days and above sixty after that."

"So you're not worried about his blood sugar being high like what I was worried about during the pregnancy—you're worried about it being low," said Susan.

 Step-by-Step Skills 3.1

Performing an Infant Heel Stick

1. Expose the infant's foot.
2. Select an area on either side of the heel that is away from bony prominences and nerves.
3. Wrap a heel warmer around the foot and leave in place for 5 min. This helps bring blood to the surface (optional).
4. Clean the area to be lanced with alcohol or an alternate cleanser.
5. Hold the foot securely in a dorsiflexed position with your thumb on the sole of the foot and your fingers around the calf.
6. Lance the preselected area.
7. Apply gentle pressure to express a drop of blood.
8. Wipe away the first drop of blood.
9. Collect blood for testing.

"Correct. If he was getting extra sugar from your blood during pregnancy, then his pancreas would have produced more insulin in response. And even now, after birth, his pancreas will continue to produce extra insulin because that's what it has been conditioned to do. It will take a while for his pancreas to catch up and realize he's not attached to your blood supply and that there isn't extra sugar," said Betty.

"What do we do if his blood sugar goes too low?" asked Susan.

"Well, it depends on how low. Two of the first things we do are put him up against you, skin to skin, and try to get him breastfeeding."

"Oh, I'm not breastfeeding," said Susan. "I can't. I can't stay home with him more than a few weeks before I go back to work. It was the same with my other little boy, Robbie. He came out okay."

Betty wrinkled her forehead. "Can you pump and give him the breast milk in a bottle? Breast milk is the perfect food for the little ones."

Susan shook her head. "I have nowhere to pump at work besides the store room, and people are in and out of it constantly. We have only one bathroom, and we share it with customers."

"You know with WIC you have the option of them giving you a pump. You wouldn't even have to buy it."

Susan was getting frustrated. "I know that, but that's not the issue. I don't have the time or place to pump. I don't want to feel bad about this. I'm doing my best. He'll do okay with formula just like millions of other babies do."

"Of course he will," said Betty. "You're absolutely right. And if his blood sugar goes too low, we'll do skin to skin and give him formula. That'll work perfectly."

Neither said anything more and the moment passed.

"How can I tell if he's getting low blood sugar? Is it just the heel stick?" Susan asked.

Box 3.10 Signs of Infant Hypoglycemia

- Jitteriness
- Irritability
- Poor feeding
- Weak, high-pitched cry
- Tachypnea (rapid breathing: >50 breaths per minute)
- Diaphoresis (sweating)
- Pallor (paleness)
- Lethargy
- Seizures
- Hypotonia (poor muscle tone)

Adapted from Committee on Fetus and Newborn from the American Academy of Pediatrics. (2011). Postnatal glucose homeostasis in late-preterm and term infants. *Pediatrics, 127*(3), 575–579.

Betty stroked the forehead of the sleeping baby, just below the cap. "He's a pretty mellow guy. If you see that he's getting jittery or fussy, you let me know" (Box 3.10).

"How often are you going to stick him?" asked Susan.

"We'd like to check him every three to six hours, just before he feeds, for the first few days," said Betty. "If he's having symptoms of low blood sugar, we'll check him then, as well."

Since that first day, baby Winston has done well. By the time of discharge, he is drinking enthusiastically from his bottle. Susan is doing well, too. She uses a cane to walk, but it is better than having to use the walker. She thinks she'll be able to walk by herself in time to go back to work in a few weeks. Robbie has met his baby brother and, with disappointment, notes that he is still too much of a baby to appreciate video games. Driving away from the hospital, Rob holds Susan's hand all the way home.

Think Critically

1. You are counseling a patient about DMPA. What do you tell her about this method of contraception?
2. Based on your reading of this chapter, what are some special considerations related to low income and pregnancy?
3. Describe the two strategies for diagnosing gestational diabetes. What are the advantages of each?
4. Why would oxytocin be given to a woman after a cesarean section?
5. You suspect your patient might have a deep vein thrombosis. Why would you want to examine both legs at the same time?
6. What risk factors did Susan have for gestational diabetes and pulmonary embolism?
7. What are the priority interventions for a suspected pulmonary embolism?
8. Describe the appearance of a newborn who is hypoglycemic.
9. Why do we perform regular glucose checks for macrosomic infants?

References

American Diabetes Association. (2015, October 19). *Create your plate.* Retrieved from http://www.diabetes.org/food-and-fitness/food/planning-meals/create-your-plate/

American Society of Anesthesiologists Task Force on Obstetric Anesthesia. (2016). Practice guidelines for obstetric anesthesia: An updated report by the American society of anesthesiologists task force on obstetric anesthesia and the society for obstetric anesthesia and perinatology. *Anesthesiology, 124,* 270–300.

Donovan, L., Hartling, L., Muise, M., Guthrie, A., Vandermeer, B., & Dryden, D. (2013). Screening tests for gestational diabetes: A systematic review for the US Preventive Services Task Force. *Annals of Internal Medicine, 159*(2), 115.

Elkins, D., & Taylor, J. S. (2013). Evidence-based strategies for managing gestational diabetes in women with obesity. *Nursing for Women's Health, 17*(5), 420–430.

Harrington, D. (2013). Preventing and recognizing venous thromboembolism after obstetric and gynecologic surgery. *Nursing for Women's Health, 17*(4), 325–329.

Lopez, L., Edelman, A., Chen, M., Otterness, C., Trussell, J., & Helmerhorst, F. (2013). Progestin-only contraceptives: Effects on weigh. *Cochrane Database Syst Rev, 7,* CD008815.

Paschall, S., & Kaunitz, A. (2008). Depo-Provera and skeletal health: A survey of Florida obstetrics and gynecologist physicians. *Contraception, 78*(5), 370.

Rowan, J., Hague, W., Gao, W., Battin, M., & Moore, M. (2008). Metformin versus insulin for the treatment of gestational diabetes. *New England Journal of Medicine, 328,* 2003–2015.

World Health Organization Department of Reproductive Health and Research and Johns Hopkins Bloomberg School of Public Health. (2008). *Family planning: A global handbook for providers.* Baltimore and Geneva: CCP and WHO.

Suggested Readings

American Diabetes Association. http://www.diabetes.org

Elkins, D., & Taylor, J. S. (2013). Evidence-based strategies for managing gestational diabetes in women with obesity. *Nursing for Women's Health, 17*(5), 420–430.

Harrington, D. (2013). Preventing and recognizing venous thromboembolism afterobstetric and gynecologic surgery. *Nursing for Women's Health, 17*(4), 325–329.

Women, Infants, and Children. http://www.fns.usda.gov/wic/women-infants-and-children-wic

4

Sophie Bloom:
Preeclampsia

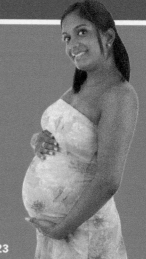

Sophie Bloom, age 23

1. Analyze the risk factors for preeclampsia.
2. Analyze the role of the nurses in the scenario.
3. Describe the impact of preeclampsia during pregnancy, labor and delivery, and the postpartum period.
4. Identify essential aspects of the management of preeclampsia.
5. List and explain psychosocial stressors common in unplanned pregnancies.

Key Terms

Beta-human chorionic gonadotropin (β-hCG)
Fundus
Group B streptococcus (GBS)
Last menstrual period (LMP)
Linea nigra

Nuchal translucency ultrasound
Preeclampsia
Variability
Vernix

Before Conception

Sophie, who is 23 years old, is the first person in her family to go to college and graduate. That's a big deal for her. It took her longer than she thought it would to get a job after she graduated, however, and she's not getting paid as much as she'd hoped, but she likes the small nonprofit organization she works for part time. She doesn't have any healthcare benefits through her employer and isn't eligible for Medicaid in the state where she resides. She's young and healthy and not that worried about getting sick or needing healthcare right now.

She's never been pregnant but also hasn't been very careful about using birth control. Because she's never been pregnant despite inconsistent use of birth control, she figures that she's likely not that fertile and doesn't worry about getting pregnant too much. After all, she has an older sister who has been trying to get pregnant for 2 years with no luck, so maybe it just runs in the family.

She was in a relationship with a guy for about 3 months, but they ended it 2 weeks ago, with no hard feelings. It was a pretty casual arrangement, and she thinks he was probably still seeing other people, anyway. They never talked whether the relationship was exclusive. He said he was clean and didn't have any sexually transmitted infections, and they usually used condoms, anyway.

Sophie once read that the average span for most women between the first day of one period (referred to clinically as last menstrual period, or LMP) and the next is 28 to 35 days. That's never been her experience. It's not unusual for Sophie to go up to a few months between periods, although as she's grown older her period has become more regular.

Sophie thinks her diet is pretty normal. She lives with a few roommates, but they rarely eat together because their schedules are so different. She eats most of her meals alone, and she knows she doesn't get as many fruits and vegetables as she should. She keeps gummy multivitamins at her desk. Sometimes she eats more than one serving, because they're completely delicious.

Sophie doesn't see any healthcare providers regularly and has no chronic conditions that she knows of (Box 4.1), but she did see a nurse practitioner at a women's health clinic a few years back

Box 4.1 Chronic Versus Acute Conditions

Chronic Condition

A chronic condition is one in which the course of the disease lasts 3 mo or more. More generally, it refers to conditions with a long-lasting duration or impact or both. Examples:

- Asthma
- Arthritis
- Diabetes

Acute Condition

An acute condition is one of short duration or rapid onset or both. Symptoms of an acute condition are typically sudden and may or may not be severe. Examples:

- Broken bone
- Acute leukemia
- Heart attack (myocardial infarction)

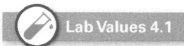

Lab Values 4.1

Beta-Human Chorionic Gonadotropin

β-hCG hormone can be detected in the blood and in the urine. Detection of this hormone in the blood or urine indicates pregnancy or a rare β-hCG–secreting tumor.

- Patients are often counseled not to take a pregnancy test until after the first missed period.
- A test is often positive as early as 3–4 d after implantation, or approximately 10 d after ovulation/conception and 4 d before the next period.
- Most laboratories report blood levels under 5 mIU/mL as negative.
- Most over-the-counter and in-clinic urine pregnancy tests indicate a positive finding when blood levels are between 10 and 20 mIU/mL.
- With a healthy pregnancy, β-hCG values usually double every 2 d for the first 4 wk.
- Doubling times lengthen after 4 wk, and at 6 wk the doubling time is about 3 d.
- β-hCG level peaks at 8–10 wk and then declines throughout the remainder of the pregnancy.

β-hCG, beta-human chorionic gonadotropin.

for her first Pap test at 21 years old. When her results came back, she was told there were no abnormalities and she wouldn't need another one for 3 years. She also tested negative for gonorrhea and chlamydia at that time. She had a finger-stick test for HIV at that visit, as well, and the results were negative. Nobody said anything about her blood pressure (BP), which she assumes was normal. She is 5 ft 4 in tall and weighs about 135 lb. She has a body mass index of 23, which is considered healthy and normal.

Pregnancy

First Trimester

One morning, Sophie wakes up feeling nauseous. She recalls that it's been about 2 months since her last period, so she decides to take a home pregnancy test, just in case, although she thinks she probably just ate something that didn't agree with her. One of her roommates, a nurse, recommends she take the test early in the morning, when her urine will be less diluted and contain more of the hormone **beta-human chorionic gonadotropin (β-hCG)**, which is the substance that is detected by the test (Lab Values 4.1). The friend warns her not to read her test after the time recommended or it might produce a false positive. Her test result, however, is a strong positive, and both the test and control lines show up long before the 3 minutes it's supposed to take to run the test (Fig. 4.1).

Sophie is shocked. She wasn't with her boyfriend for very long, and the relationship is over. They were pretty good about using condoms, but she can remember a few times when they didn't. She heard somewhere that women are fertile only for about 24 hours a month. She thinks it's just her luck that they didn't use a condom during those particular 24 hours. She has a decision to make.

Sophie decides to go ahead and tell her ex-boyfriend, Jeff, about the pregnancy. They haven't really spoken since the breakup, but

she wants him to know. Jeff says he really isn't interested in having a baby right now, but he'll respect Sophie's decision, whatever it is. She expected this response, but part of her wanted him to say that he wanted to make a family with her. Maybe next time he hooks up with someone he won't complain so much about using condoms (Patient Teaching 4.1).

After a lot of thought, Sophie decides to tell her mother but to beg her not to tell her father. She doesn't want him to know, but feels like she really needs her mother's good advice. Her mother lives 3 hours away in another state, so she calls her. She can hear the disappointment in her voice. They both cry over the phone. Her mother tells her that if she wants to keep the pregnancy she

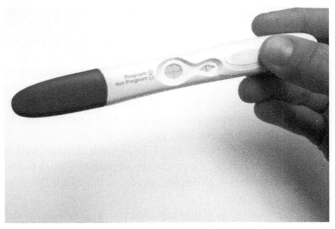

Figure 4.1. A positive home pregnancy test. Today's home pregnancy tests are highly accurate and very sensitive. One line means the test is working but is negative. Two lines indicate a positive pregnancy test.

Patient Teaching 4.1

Effective Condom Use

Effectiveness Rates

With *perfect* use, condoms are 95% effective for preventing pregnancy.

With *typical* use, condoms are 85% effective for preventing pregnancy.

Tips for Perfect Condom Use

- Use a new condom for every act of intercourse.
- If the penis is uncircumcised, pull the foreskin back before putting the condom on.
- Put the condom on after the penis is erect and before any contact is made between the penis and any part of the partner's body.
- If the condom does not have a reservoir tip, pinch the tip enough to leave a half-inch space for semen to collect.
- While pinching the half-inch tip, place the condom against the penis and unroll it all the way to the base.
- If a condom breaks during sex, stop immediately and pull out. Do not continue until a new condom is in place.
- After ejaculation and before the penis softens grip the rim of the condom and carefully withdraw from partner.
- To remove the condom from the penis, pull it off gently, being careful to not let semen spill out.

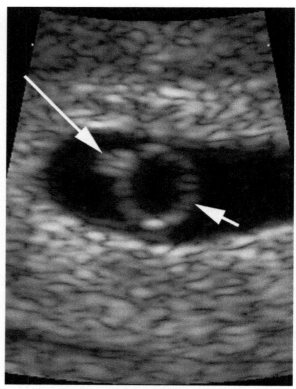

Figure 4.2. Ultrasound image of a gestational sac at 6 weeks. Shown are the embryo (long arrow) and yolk sac (short arrow). (Reprinted with permission from Doubilet, P. M., & Benson, C. B. [2011]. *Atlas of ultrasound in obstetrics and gynecology: A multimedia reference* [2nd ed., Fig. 1.6]. Philadelphia, PA: Lippincott Williams & Wilkins.)

could move home and her parents would help. Sophie thinks about the hard work to get through college and her struggle to work her way out of entry-level positions. She imagines all the good work she's been doing to build a future slipping away. She thinks about her sister, who has been trying so hard to get pregnant for 2 years now without any luck. According to Sophie's mother, who has learned a lot about infertility because of her daughter's problem conceiving, about 11% of women in the United States have impaired fertility (Centers for Disease Control and Prevention, National Center for Health Statistics, 2016). Sophie has not thought about this at all since a few months ago when her mother told her, but it now fills her with an irrational guilt.

Sophie decides she needs more information and schedules an ultrasound at a local reproductive health clinic to date the pregnancy. On ultrasound, a gestational sac, yolk sac, fetal pole, and heartbeat are seen. The nurse practitioner performing the ultrasound measures the fetal pole and tells her that she is 6 weeks and 3 days pregnant (Fig. 4.2). She tells her that because she can see a heartbeat, the pregnancy is much less likely to end in miscarriage (Box 4.2). Sophie asks for a copy of the image to take home with her.

Sophie makes a list of pros and cons and thinks about all she's done so far and what she wants to achieve. She thinks about how she doesn't have health insurance through her job and makes too much money to get on Medicaid. She knows how important it is to have good healthcare in pregnancy. If she quits her job

and moves in with her parents in the next state, which has more generous policies about healthcare coverage in pregnancy, she could have the costs of the pregnancy covered (Box 4.3). She'd have to leave the job she loves and worked so hard to get. What she'd do for work during pregnancy, and what she'd do afterward with a baby in tow, she's not sure, but she thinks she could figure it out. She starts to pack. She's going to continue the pregnancy.

Box 4.2 Uses for First Trimester Ultrasound

- Confirm pregnancy
- Confirm viability (is there a heartbeat?)
- Rule out ectopic pregnancy (a pregnancy occurring somewhere other than the uterus)
- Detect multiple pregnancies, such as twins and triplets
- Assess any vaginal bleeding
- Aid in chorionic villus sampling (a form of early prenatal testing for fetal congenital defects)
- Assess for a nuchal translucency (part of the first trimester screening)
- Assess for a maternal anatomical abnormality
- Estimate the age of the pregnancy

Box 4.3   The Approximate Financial Cost of Pregnancy for Medicaid Patients

Prenatal care: $2,406 for vaginal birth, $5,856 for cesarean birth
Uncomplicated childbirth: $6,117 for a vaginal birth, $7,983 for a cesarean birth
Infant healthcare for the first 3 mo: $558 for vaginal birth, $721 for cesarean birth
Total: $9,081–$14,560

Data from Truven Health Analytics. (2013). *The cost of having a baby in the United States.* Ann Arbor, MI: Author.

Box 4.5   Pregnancy Timing

Pregnancies are often calculated based on the last menstrual period, which typically occurs about 2 wk before ovulation and conception. This convention is used because women are more likely to know when they have had their period than when they have ovulated. Therefore, someone who is 8 wk pregnant is actually only about 6 wk past conception, and someone who is 40 wk pregnant is only about 38 wk past conception.

Sophie moves home. It's a tough transition. She hasn't lived at home since she left for college, and it makes her feel like a teenager again. She tries not to slide back into all the old fights she used to have with her parents then. She wants to be the adult she knows she needs to be for this baby, but that's hard when she feels like a kid herself, living in her parents' house and sleeping in her old bed.

Speaking of bed, she is so tired all of the time. She hasn't napped since she was a toddler, and now she always feels like sleeping. And coffee, which she's loved since high school, smells disgusting to her now and just adds to her morning sickness (which, by the way, isn't only happening in the morning). Her breasts are so sore she can't sleep on her stomach anymore. She's cranky, feels like she's peeing all of the time, and is so constipated she's started drinking her father's prune juice. She feels like she's gained at least 10 lb since yesterday. Not glamorous (Box 4.4).

Her mother makes an appointment for her with a nurse midwife at her obstetrician-gynecologist's office. Her name is Maria, and she seems nice enough. Sophie brings along a copy of her ultrasound image from the clinic, and the midwife says that this is helpful as they don't have an accurate LMP for Sophie (Box 4.5). Usually, if the mother is confident of this date, they can do a good job of figuring out how far along a pregnancy is. On the basis of the ultrasound, Maria determines the estimated date of delivery. She does warn her, however, that only about 5%

Box 4.4   Common Physical Changes in the First Trimester

- Fatigue
- Swollen, tender breasts
- Morning sickness
- Cravings or aversions to certain foods
- Moodiness
- Constipation
- More frequent urination
- Headache
- Heartburn
- Weight gain or loss

of women deliver on their due date. "Just think of your due date as more of an estimate than a promise," says Maria.

Maria talks with her about her current uncomfortable pregnancy symptoms and gives her some strategies for dealing with nausea. They talk over her pregnancy history and gynecologic history. Maria consults her health record and comments that she had a normal Pap smear 2 years ago and doesn't need another one until next year. Sophie confirms that, as far as she knows, she's never had a sexually transmitted infection. She says that she's never used any birth control besides condoms. She's healthy, has never had surgery, is looking for work, hasn't been to church since her grandmother died when she was 12, doesn't take any medications, is allergic to strawberries, doesn't do drugs, and hasn't had a drink since she found out she was pregnant. She doesn't smoke. She tries to fit protein and fruits or vegetables into every meal. She doesn't have an eating disorder, feels safe at home, is not in a relationship, and would rather not talk about the father right now, thanks anyway. All the questions are a little overwhelming. Well, what isn't right now, she thinks.

Maria conducts a physical exam and tells her, "everything seems just fine." She gives Sophie handouts on what she should and shouldn't do and what she should and shouldn't eat and a two-dollar off coupon for diapers (Table 4.1). The office nurse, Wendy, collects urine and blood samples from her for routine testing.

Sophie did this visit alone because she wants to be more independent, what with moving home and quitting her job. It felt terribly lonely, however. She's scared and excited and proud and disappointed and exhausted. She thinks next time she'll ask her mother if she wants to come with her. She doesn't know why, but she cries on the bus on the way home. Pregnancy hormones, she guesses.

By 11 weeks, Sophie feels like her morning sickness is starting to lift. Her pants are tight. When she mentions this at her second visit with Maria, she tells her it's not the fetus, which is only the size of a Brussels sprout, but rather because her uterus is growing and she's a little bloated. Plus, she's already gained 6 lb. Maria tells her that 6 lb is a little more than what is recommended for weight gain at this point in a healthy pregnancy, but that there's much variation in pregnancy weight gain (Box 4.6). She recommends that, going into the second and third trimesters, she increase her calorie intake to only about 300 above what she was eating before she became pregnant. It turns out that in reality, eating for two just means an extra apple and a container of yogurt.

Sophie's mother did come with her for this second visit, but warned her that because of her own job she won't be able to come

Table 4.1   What Not to Consume in Pregnancy and Why

Food	Reason for Avoiding
Raw or undercooked meat or eggs	Foodborne viruses, bacteria, and parasites
Hot dogs (fine if cooked to steaming hot)	Listeria (may cause miscarriage, stillbirth, or birth defects)
Lunch meat (fine if cooked to steaming hot)	Listeria (may cause miscarriage, stillbirth, or birth defects)
Unpasteurized dairy products, such as milk and cheese	Listeria (may cause miscarriage, stillbirth, or birth defects)
Large fish, such as shark and king mackerel	High mercury content (mercury is a neurotoxin and may impair brain and nervous system development)
Raw sprouts	Foodborne bacteria
Alcohol	There is no known safe level of alcohol, which is a teratogen and may cause permanent damage to the fetus.
Unpasteurized juice	Bacteria, especially *Escherichia coli*
Tap water that is high in lead	Linked with poor birth weight, preterm delivery, and developmental delays
Caffeine (avoid drinking more than 12 oz of coffee per day)	In greater amounts, may be associated with stillbirth, miscarriage, and reduced birth weight
Food or drink from vessels containing BPA	There is some conflicting evidence that BPA may have negative effects on the fetal brain.
Herbal teas or supplements	Consult a pregnancy care provider. Some may be associated with poor pregnancy outcomes, and none is regulated by the FDA.

BPA, bisphenol A; FDA, Food and Drug Administration.
Data from King, T. L., Brucker, M. C., Kriebs, J. M., Fahey, J. O., Gegor, C. L., & Varney, H. (2015). *Varney's midwifery* (5th ed.). Burlington, MA: Jones and Bartlett.

to all the visits. Her mom tells Maria that her daughter seems to be keeping her chin up. Her mom says she hopes that now that Sophie's morning sickness isn't as bad as it was, maybe she can think about getting a job. It's a lot having another person to support, her mom says, even though it has been a blessing to have Sophie in the house, and she does help with housework and cooking. But she is another mouth to feed, and a hungry one at that. Sophie just nods. She's imagining trying to work the grill at McDonald's while keeping her growing belly away from the heat. She'll look for a job with a desk.

Maria performs an abdominal exam and tells Sophie that her uterus is protruding just above her pubic bone. She then takes out a small white device that is attached to a little wand shaped like a wild mushroom. She calls it a Doppler and says that by this point in the pregnancy, 11 weeks, she'll probably be able to hear the fetal heart beat with it (Box 4.7 and Fig. 4.3). Sophie only saw a still picture when she had an ultrasound before. There was no sound. Maria applies some cold, blue gel to Sophie's abdomen, near her pelvic bone, and turns on the Doppler, which makes a sound like static on the radio. She applies the wand, which she calls a transducer, to the pool of gel and slowly rotates it and moves it all over the lower part of her abdomen. She stops, and then Sophie hears it: a little heart beating as fast as a rabbit's.

Box 4.6   Where Does the Pregnancy Weight Gain Go?

Fetus: 8 lb
Placenta: 2–3 lb
Amniotic fluid: 2–3 lb
Breast tissue: 2–3 lb
Blood supply: 4 lb
Stored fat for delivery and breastfeeding: 5–9 lb
Larger uterus: 2–5 lb
Total: 25–35 lb

Box 4.7   Fetal Heart Tones

A fetal heartbeat can typically be heard using a Doppler ultrasound (also called a Doptone, or just Doppler) by 10–12 wk.

A normal fetal heart rate through most of pregnancy is about 110–160 bpm.

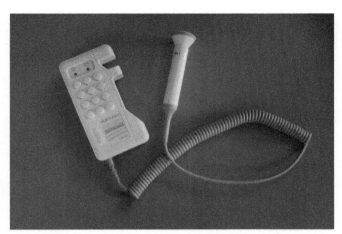

Figure 4.3. A Doppler ultrasound or "Doptone" device. Dopplers are used to auscultate fetal heart tones as early as 9 weeks' gestation. (Reprinted with permission from Evans, R. J., Brown, Y. M., & Evans, M. K. [2014]. *Canadian maternity, newborn, and women's health nursing* [2nd ed., unnumbered figure in Chapter 12]. Philadelphia, PA: Lippincott Williams & Wilkins.)

Maria offers her screening for Down syndrome, also called trisomy 21. She says the screening would also test for a much more rare mutation called Edwards syndrome, or trisomy 18. Human cells usually have 23 pairs of chromosomes. She explains that a trisomy is a genetic defect in which there are three of a particular chromosome instead of the pair you would expect (one from the mother and one from the father). The screening recommended involves a blood test and another ultrasound. This ultrasound would specifically measure the thickness of the skin at the back of the fetus's neck and is called a **nuchal translucency ultrasound** (see Table 1.1). Maria says the test is only for screening, which means a positive result would indicate that she has an increased chance of carrying a fetus with a trisomy. If the test indicates she is at higher risk, she'd need other tests to diagnose the problem definitively.

Sophie discusses it with her mother and decides to do the test. She has her blood drawn first and then has the ultrasound. This is the first prenatal ultrasound her mother has ever seen, and she says the fetus looks like an alien in a snowstorm, but a cute alien. The fetus is very active and Sophie is awed as she watches it stretch its legs and move its arms inside her. The person doing the ultrasound says everything looks perfect, and her blood tests come back just fine.

Maria says she'll see Sophie back in a month. At that time she will need to collect more blood samples for tests that will provide an even more accurate assessment of her risk of Down syndrome, as well as an assessment for neural tube defects. A neural tube defect, she explains, happens very early in pregnancy when the embryonic spinal column doesn't close completely. It often happens before a woman even knows she's pregnant. Maria will also order the fetal survey ultrasound at that time, and Sophie can learn the fetal sex if she wants to.

Second Trimester

Sophie has found an office job she likes. The pay is not very good, but it's part time. She's starting to get her energy back. She's 15 weeks pregnant now. She's hoping this employer will keep her on, even after she takes some time off to have the baby. She won't have been working there that long, however, and it's a small company. They won't have any legal obligation to hold her spot. She's trying not to worry about it. For the past week or so, when she has been sitting quietly at home, she's felt a "popcorn popping" sensation in her belly. She's not sure whether it is the baby moving or this wicked pregnancy gas she gets. Jeff hasn't called even once to check up on her. She wonders if he's even curious about the pregnancy, or if he's just as stubborn as she is.

She goes to her monthly visit with Maria and everything seems fine. She gets to hear the heartbeat again, trucking along at about 140 beats per minute (bpm). Maria finds her **fundus**, the top of her uterus, about midway between her pubic bone and her belly button, and tells her that's just where it should be (Fig. 4.4).

Sophie has now gained almost exactly 10 lb since the start of the pregnancy. She mentions that she now has a line of darker skin running from her belly button down to her pubic hair. Maria calls this the **linea nigra** and says that it occurs in about three-quarters of all pregnancies and that it usually disappears or at least fades quite a bit within a few months after the end of the pregnancy (Fig. 4.5). Maria asks her about cramping, and she says she's not having any, but sometimes she has pain near her groin when going up and down the stairs (Box 4.8). Maria says it's from the ligaments

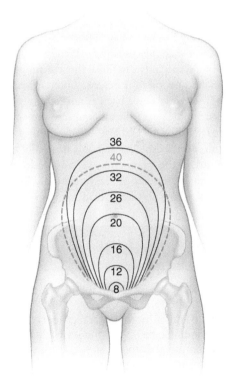

Figure 4.4. Fundal height according to weeks of gestation. In a normal singleton pregnancy in the vertex presentation, fundal height in centimeters roughly corresponds to gestational age from 16 to 36 weeks' gestation. (Reprinted with permission from Beckmann, C. R., Herbert, W., Laube, D., Ling, F., & Smith, R. [2013]. *Obstetrics and gynecology* [7th ed., Fig. 6.1]. Philadelphia, PA: Lippincott Williams & Wilkins.)

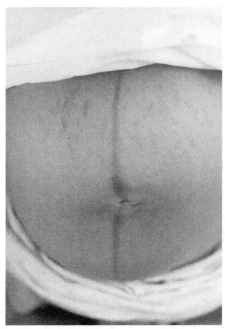

Figure 4.5. A linea nigra. This hyperpigmentation occurs in about three-quarters of pregnancies and is less common in women with pale skin. It typically resolves within several months after the birth. (Reprinted with permission from Hatfield, N. T. [2014]. *Introductory maternity and pediatric nursing* [3rd ed., Fig. 6-4]. Philadelphia, PA: Lippincott Williams & Wilkins.)

of her pelvis relaxing from pregnancy hormones, allowing those bones to move more than they usually do. Wendy, the nurse, draws another set of blood specimens to finish the screening for trisomy 21, trisomy 18, and neural tube defects. About a week later, the results of all of these tests come back as normal.

At 19 weeks, Sophie goes to another ultrasound appointment Maria set up for her (Box 4.9 and Fig. 4.6). She brings her mother to this one, too. Maria explains that this is usually the longest ultrasound exam of the pregnancy, as it includes evaluating and measuring many aspects of the fetus, including the face, skull, long bones, heart, abdomen, and many other parts. The

Box 4.8 Common Physical Changes in the Second Trimester

- Aches and pains, particularly in the pelvis, back, hips, and thighs
- Linea nigra: a line of more darkly pigmented skin running from the pubic hair up to the umbilicus, or even all the way up the abdomen; caused by estrogen and typically resolves after pregnancy
- Darkening of the nipples and areola
- Hyperpigmented patches of skin, particularly on the face
- Numbness or tingling of the hands and fingers
- Itchiness of the palms, soles of the feet, and abdomen
- Swelling of the face, feet, and hands (late second trimester)
- Heartburn

Box 4.9 Uses for Ultrasound in the Second and Third Trimesters

- Pregnancy dating (this becomes less and less accurate as pregnancy progresses)
- Evaluation of a fetal anomaly
- Evaluation of a pregnancy finding on exam that is different from expected
- Assessment of amniotic fluid
- Assessment of the placenta location
- In conjunction with procedures such as amniocentesis
- Assessment of fetal well-being
- Assessment of vaginal bleeding
- Evaluation of cervical length

ultrasonographer will also check the placenta, to make sure it's not too close to the cervix; the length of the cervix itself; the amount of amniotic fluid; and the number of blood vessels in the umbilical cord (there should be three). When the ultrasonographer asks if she wants to know if the baby is a boy or a girl, Sophie looks at her mother. Her mother nods. "Yes," Sophie says. On the way home she feels movement in her belly that she's sure for the first time isn't just gas.

At 24 weeks, Sophie is instructed go to the lab and take an oral glucose tolerance test to screen for gestational diabetes. It is explained that she will drink 50 g of glucose in a solution that tastes like flat orange soda. She will then have her blood glucose

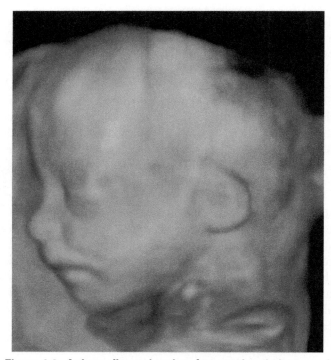

Figure 4.6. A three-dimensional surface-rendered ultrasound image of a 20-week fetal face. (Reprinted with permission from Doublet, P. M., & Benson, C. B. [2011]. *Atlas of ultrasound in obstetrics and gynecology: A multimedia reference* [2nd ed., Fig. 2.5]. Philadelphia, PA: Lippincott Williams & Wilkins.)

level checked an hour later. If her blood glucose level at the 1-hour mark is below 130 mg/dL, she does not have diabetes and will not require further testing for the condition. She's warned that the drink is so sweet it makes some people sick. She thinks it's absolutely delicious. Her blood glucose level is reported as 116 mg/dL, and she's almost disappointed that she won't get to drink another dose of that tasty medically sanctioned flat soda.

At her next visit, Maria again reviews danger signs and signs of preterm labor. She tells her that once she reaches 28 weeks or so, she should set aside some quiet time every day to be still and pay attention to fetal movement. Most pregnant women are able to count 10 fetal movements in an hour. If it takes more than 2 hours to feel 10 movements, she's to call Maria.

At 27 weeks she is given a Tdap vaccination, even though according to her records she had one a few years ago. Maria tells her that the vaccination is now recommended during each pregnancy to maximize her own protection against tetanus, diphtheria, and pertussis, but also to give the fetus some passive immunity to those diseases. Infants are at higher risk for acquiring these conditions because this vaccination is not administered until the age of 2 months and are more likely to have deadly complications if they do become ill (Centers for Disease Control and Prevention, 2016).

Sophie's starting to feel enormous, and her feet occasionally swell in the evening. She has heartburn and buys the big bottle of antacids. She can feel the top of her uterus, the fundus, well above her belly button. Maria says that's right where it should be, but she's wondering where else the fetus has to go as it grows. She tries calling Jeff, but he doesn't pick up and doesn't call back.

Third Trimester

By week 30 of the pregnancy, things are almost routine. The time when the baby becomes active each day is so regular that she can almost set her watch by it. Sometimes her abdomen moves so much it looks like a bag of cats. She usually works about 6 hours a day, 3 or 4 days a week. She buys at least one pack of diapers every week to stockpile them. She sees Maria every 2 weeks at this point.

Maria asks her how she wants to feed the baby after it's born: breast or bottle. Sophie knows that her mother bottle-fed her and she turned out okay, but the books and websites she's been reading all say that "breast is best." She does want the best for her little one, but the future seems so uncertain. What if she needs to work and can't be there to feed the baby? What if her work doesn't allow her the time and space to pump? What if she has no privacy to pump? When she thinks about having those cup things on her nipples sucking out milk, it makes her feel like Bessie the cow. On the other hand, formula feeding requires a lot of washing and sterilization and you have to remember to bring it with you. And formula is expensive. Maria gives her the contact information for Women, Infants, and Children, a program of the federal government that provides nutritional food in pregnancy and breastfeeding support or formula for low-income women. She says she's sorry she didn't think of it earlier in the pregnancy.

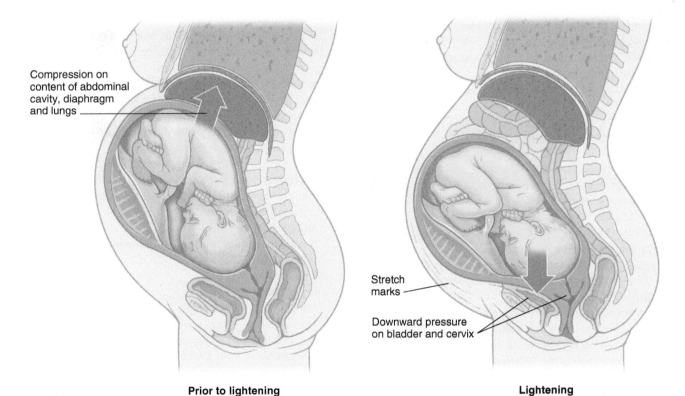

Compression on content of abdominal cavity, diaphragm and lungs

Stretch marks

Downward pressure on bladder and cervix

Prior to lightening

Lightening

Figure 4.7. A pregnant abdomen before (left) and after (right) the "drop" that often occurs prior to labor. (Right image: Reprinted with permission from Stager, L. [2008]. *Nurturing massage for pregnancy: A practical guide to bodywork for the perinatal cycle* [1st ed., Fig. 2.3]. Philadelphia, PA: Lippincott Williams & Wilkins.)

In her 36th week, Sophie stops wearing her rings because they've become tight and uncomfortable. Her shoes don't fit well, either, so she's begun wearing slippers and flip flops all the time. She feels like such a slob wearing them, but they're the only things that don't pinch.

On the plus side, she seems to be carrying the pregnancy a little lower than she was, and that's helped with her breathing (Fig. 4.7). On the minus side, her nausea has come back and that, on top of the continuing heartburn, is just a misery (Box 4.10). Her mother says that heartburn means the baby will be born with a lot of hair, and they both laugh because it seems so silly.

Sophie comes in for her week 36 visit. She knows this will be when the weekly visits start, and that makes it feel like the birth is coming up really soon. She's excited and nervous. She has been shopping for baby clothes on eBay and at a used clothing store in town. At this point she thinks she has enough cute outfits for two babies, not just one.

> ### Box 4.10 Common Physical Changes in the Third Trimester
>
> - Heartburn
> - Shortness of breath
> - Swelling of the ankles, feet, and face
> - Hemorrhoids
> - Breast tenderness
> - Colostrum (a yellow, sticky premilk) excretion from the nipples
> - Sleep disturbance
> - Contractions
> - Baby "dropping" (the descent of the baby into the lower abdomen, usually occurring 2–4 wk before birth in first pregnancies and often with labor in subsequent pregnancies; often improves the sensation of shortness of breath)

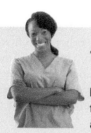

The Nurse's Point of View

Maria: At Sophie's next visit, she is instructed to leave a urine sample before being led to an exam room to have her vital signs taken. Teresa, the medical assistant who rooms her, comes to find me.

"Sophie's ready for you," says Teresa. "She's got some protein in her urine and her blood pressure (BP) is 146/92. She's up eight pounds since we saw her last two weeks ago."

"146/92?," I repeat, although none of what she's said is good news. "Yeesh. Did you recheck it."

"I did it twice," says Teresa. "Once on each arm. I got 144/94 the first time."

I'm not happy with anything Teresa has told me. I'm worried that Sophie may have developed preeclampsia. I knock on the door to Sophie's exam room and enter. Sophie is sitting on the table undressed from the waist down with a paper drape across her legs. Her mother is sitting in a chair next to the sink. I smile and nod to them both.

"Sophie," I say. "How are you today?"

"I'm alright," she says. "I gained more weight than I should have. My BP is high today."

"I know," I say. "Teresa told me. I'd like to do the usual check and a couple of other things. I'll tell you what I'm thinking after that."

I check Sophie's reflexes by hitting her knee with the reflex hammer and let her know that they're normal. This is a good thing as worsening preeclampsia can cause hyperreflexia. I listen to the fetus using the Doppler ultrasound and see that the heart rate is at a good 130 bpm. Sophie says the baby has been active, which is always reassuring.

"Today I'd like to take a sample from the opening of your vagina and anus with a swab," I tell her. "I'll be testing for group B streptococcus. That's a kind of really common bacteria that about a third of women are colonized with. It doesn't cause any issues day to day, but it can cause some serious issues for newborns who are exposed to it."

"What happens if she has it?" asks Sophie's mother. "Would she need antibiotics?"

"She would," I tell her. "But she'd have them IV during labor and delivery."

"I couldn't just take antibiotics before?" asks Sophie.

"Unfortunately no," I say. "It tends to recolonize quickly. If we give the antibiotics during labor and delivery, it treats you in the moment, but the fetus is also getting the antibiotic so is protected even if it is exposed. But let's worry about that if we come to it. How are you feeling otherwise?"

"Tired," says Sophie. "Kind of nauseous. Kind of like I did at the beginning. Is that normal?"

"I felt that way with both my kids," says Sophie's mother.

"For some women that's normal, yes," I say. "Do you have any pain? Any discomfort high up on your belly or under your ribs?"

Sophie shakes her head.

"Any headaches?"

"No, I'm mostly just tired and a little nauseous," says Sophie.

"Vision changes?"

Sophie shakes her head.

"Chest pain?"

"Are you kidding?" says Sophie's mother. "I promise you that if she has chest pain, I'm calling."

"Fair enough," I say. I turn back to Sophie. "Let me tell you what I'm thinking. Your BP being over 140/90 along with the protein in your urine makes me suspicious of preeclampsia."

"What's that?" Sophie asks.

"I had that with your sister," says her mother. "I told you about that."

"Well, that's good to know," I tell her. "Preeclampsia is a condition involving high BP that can be dangerous for you and the baby. It can lead to seizures and even death, in extreme cases. But as your mother can tell you, extreme cases are unusual. Most moms and babies come through just fine."

"You said extreme cases," says Sophie's mother, rattled. "Is this an extreme case?"

I shake my head. "Not that we know about, but it's important that we work this up thoroughly and keep a close eye on Sophie. Preeclampsia can often be managed with just close observation, but we need to act quickly if the situation changes."

I explain to them that Sophie will need to collect her urine for a 24-hour urine sample (Patient Teaching 4.2), return with it, and then have another BP check. We set up a non-stress test (see Fig. 1.11). We'll make a plan based on the results. I tell them not to be nervous and that we'll take good care of Sophie.

Sophie's mother is not so sure. "I'm not telling anyone how to do their job," she says, "but I remember almost dying with that first baby. Don't you think she should be taken care of in the hospital where people can keep an eye on her?"

"I understand your concern, I really do," I tell her. "But based on the exam today and the conversation we've just had, I don't see a call for hospitalization right now. I will be discussing the situation with the physicians I work with so everybody is on the same page, but right now we need to collect more information so we know how to best act."

"And we shouldn't be having that information collected in the hospital," says Sophie's mother, unconvinced.

"Not right now," I tell her firmly.

Patient Teaching 4.2

24-Hour Urine Collection

1. On day 1, urinate into the toilet when you get up in the morning.
2. After the first urination, collect all urine in a special container for the next 24 h.
3. On day 2, urinate into the container when you get up in the morning.
4. Close the container after each urination. Keep it in the refrigerator or a cool place during the collection period.
5. Label the container with your name, the date, and the time of completion, and return it as instructed.
6. Proteinuria is defined as 300 mg/dL or more protein in urine collected over 24 h.

She seems to accept that for the moment, but asks, "Is this my fault? Is this something I passed on to Sophie that's making this happen?"

I smile at her in a way that I hope is reassuring. "We know the risk factors of preeclampsia, and Sophie does have some of those, but a risk factor isn't the same thing as a diagnosis" (Box 4.11). "She might just as easily not have developed preeclampsia. It's not her fault, and it's not your fault. She's in good hands."

Box 4.11   Risk Factors for Preeclampsia

Maternal Risk Factors

- Age greater than 35 y
- Age less than 20 y
- African descent
- Low socioeconomic status
- Family history of preeclampsia
- Nulliparity (first pregnancy)
- Pregnancy with a new partner
- Preeclampsia in a previous pregnancy
- Urinary tract infection
- Gestational diabetes
- Type 1 diabetes
- Obesity
- Chronic hypertension (high BP that starts before 20 weeks' gestation; can accompany preeclampsia)
- Kidney disease
- Thrombophilia (an increased tendency to clot)

Pregnancy Risk Factors

- Chromosomal abnormalities of fetus, such as trisomies 18 and 21
- Hydatidiform mole (a disorder in which two sperm fertilize one egg or an egg without a nucleus is fertilized)
- Hydrops fetalis (the accumulation of fluid in the fetus, most common caused by maternal anemia, or low blood count)
- Multifetal pregnancy (such as twins or triplets)
- Donated eggs or sperm
- Structural congenital anomalies of the fetus

Data from King, T. L., Brucker, M. C., Kriebs, J. M., Fahey, J. O., Gegor, C. L., & Varney, H. (2015). *Varney's midwifery* (5th ed.). Burlington, MA: Jones and Bartlett; Lisonkova, S., & Joseph, K. (2013). Incidence of preeclampsia: Risk factors and outcomes associated with early- versus late-onset disease. *American Journal of Obstetrics & Gynecology, 209*(6), 544.e1–544.e12.

Box 4.12   Signs of Severe Preeclampsia

Any of the following:

- Hypertension: systolic BP >160 mm Hg or diastolic BP >110 mm Hg on two occasions at least 4 h apart while the patient is at rest (unless antihypertensive therapy is initiated before this time)
- Thrombocytopenia (platelet count < 100,000 platelets/μL)
- Impaired liver function (elevated blood levels of liver transaminases to twice the normal concentration), severe persistent right upper quadrant or epigastric pain unresponsive to medication and not accounted for by alternative diagnoses, or both
- New development of renal insufficiency (elevated serum creatinine level greater than 1.1 mg/dL or a doubling of serum creatinine level in the absence of kidney disease)
- Pulmonary edema (fluid in the lungs)
- New-onset cerebral or visual disturbances

Sophie returns after having collected her 24-hour urine sample and has her BP rechecked. It remains stubbornly at 146/92. Maria calls her later and tells her that there is protein in her urine and that she does have preeclampsia. She asks her about several different symptoms that she says would indicate that she has severe preeclampsia, but Sophie denies all of them (Box 4.12). Maria says that's reassuring, but that her supervising physician, Dr. Jennifer Riley, still wants her to be checked out in labor and delivery and monitored. Sophie turns to her mother, who is nodding.

"I'm glad that this Dr. Riley is taking the situation seriously," her mother says.

"I haven't even had a chance to pack my bag," says Sophie. She calls work and lets them know what's going on. She wonders if she'll ever get to go back.

The Hospital

When Sophie arrives on the labor and delivery floor, she is given a bed in triage and told that a nurse will regularly assess her. Her mother tells her stories about her childhood and tries to make her laugh. For her part, Sophie's mostly trying not to cry. She keeps on rubbing her belly like it's a genie's lamp. Her belly bumps back.

A nurse, Anne, tells Sophie that she's not to get out of bed except to use the bathroom, and that she should not eat or drink until her lab results come back. After a while, another nurse comes by and takes her blood. She tells her the orders are in to take blood to check her liver and something called a complete metabolic panel (Table 4.2).

Anne comes back a few minutes later and completes a head-to-toe exam. When she's done she reassures Sophie and her mother that everything looks fine but that she'd like to assess the baby now (Boxes 4.13 and 4.14). Anne places the tocodynamometer at the muscular top of her uterus, the fundus, and explains that this will detect any contractions she may have.

Sophie says, "I don't feel like I'm having any contractions."

Anne says, "That's fine, but sometimes women can have small contractions and not feel them. If you are having contractions, we need to see how the baby's heartbeat responds to them."

Lower down on her abdomen and off to one side, Anne places a second monitoring device that looks much like the first. She explains that this is for the fetal heart rate monitoring.

When everything is in place, Sophie, Anne, and Maria all look at the monitor. Maria explains that the image she's seeing on the screen is really two images. The top image is a line moving from left to right that indicates the fetal heart rate. The second line on the bottom matches the top line in terms of time, but is monitoring for contractions.

Because Sophie was not having contractions, Anne says the monitoring represents a nonstress test. Anne said that what she wanted to see was an acceleration of the fetal heart rate. If the heart rate went up, accelerated, twice in 20 minutes, the test would be referred to as reactive, which would be reassuring and would indicate that the baby is doing well (Fig. 4.8).

Table 4.2   Standing Orders for Sophie in Triage

Assessments	Blood pressure, heart rate, respiratory rate, and temperature every 15 min Deep tendon reflexes every hour Head-to-toe assessment every 4 h Breath sounds (lung auscultation) every 4 h Continuous pulse oximetry Fetal ultrasound for biophysical profile, including amniotic fluid volume One-hour fetal heart rate and uterine contraction monitoring three times daily
Precautions	Minimal outside stimuli
Laboratory tests	Comprehensive metabolic panel STAT Hepatic function panel (liver function tests) STAT Complete blood count with platelets
Medications	Promethazine 25 mg by mouth as needed for nausea Lactated Ringer's 500 mg IV bolus ×1 (for nonreassuring fetal heart pattern)

Box 4.13 Nursing Treatment for Sophie in Labor and Delivery Triage

1. Assess the patient history
2. Review orders
3. Wash hands
4. Introduce yourself
5. Identify the patient
6. Obtain fetal and maternal vital signs
7. Check the reflexes and clonus
8. Auscultate the heart and lungs
9. Obtain a blood sample
10. Obtain a fetal ultrasound
11. Continue with a focused maternal and fetal antepartum assessment
12. Initiate discharge instructions, including those related to bed rest and reduced environmental stimulation
13. Reassess maternal and fetal health status

Box 4.14 Assessment Guide

Assessment of Reflexes for Signs of Preeclampsia

- Preeclampsia can cause hyperstimulation of the central nervous system that can lead to seizure activity. Hyperactive reflexes and clonus may indicate worsening preeclampsia and impending seizure activity. Preeclampsia with seizure activity is called eclampsia.
- The patellar reflex is the one assessed most commonly in relation to preeclampsia.
- Preeclampsia is sometimes treated with an IV medication called magnesium sulfate. Magnesium sulfate can cause central nervous system suppression and hypoactive reflexes.

How to Check for Clonus

- Rapidly dorsiflex the patient's foot, stretching the gastrocnemius muscle.
- Beating of the foot three or more times indicates clonus, an abnormal finding.

Last of all, Sophie has another ultrasound, this one a specialized kind called a biophysical profile (BPP). The BPP, Anne explains to her, further assesses the well-being of the fetus by monitoring for breathing movements, fetal activity, fetal tone, and the volume of amniotic fluid (see Table 1.2).

Sophie and her mother are left alone for a time after the BPP. They try to watch some television. Sophie orders some food from the cafeteria and pushes it around her tray. After a time, Sophie's nurse, Anne, comes in to tell her that they'll be discharging her home. She tells her that the results from the lab tests they completed were all normal, the fetal heart rate is a healthy 132 bpm, and her BP has actually been a little lower while she's been here.

Anne tells her that Dr. Riley has advised she stay in bed until the delivery and try to minimize stress and stimulation. She

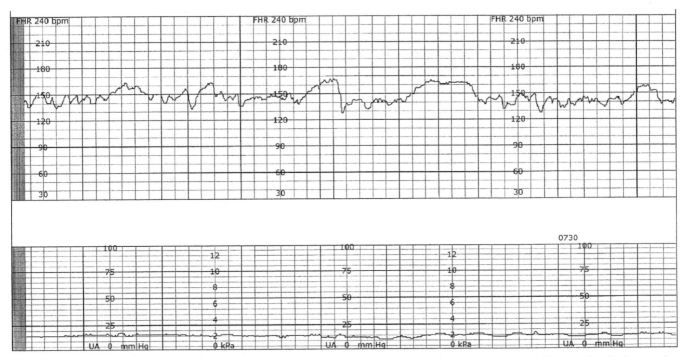

Figure 4.8. A reactive nonstress test. This nonstress test is reassuring, indicating fetal well-being. The top line indicates the fetal heart rate, whereas the bottom line indicates uterine contractions. Note the two areas where the fetal heart rate accelerates faster than baseline. Also note that no contractions register during the test. FHR, fetal heart rate. (Reprinted with permission from Gabrielli, A., Layon, A. J., & Yu, M. [2008]. *Civetta, Taylor, and Kirby's critical care* [4th ed., Fig. 101.4]. Philadelphia, PA: Lippincott Williams & Wilkins.)

tells her she is to eat a high-protein, low-sodium diet. She tells her that if she does not go into labor in the next week, she will likely be induced.

Sophie starts to cry, and Anne reassures her, saying, "Everything looks fine with your baby. There's no reason to think that it won't be born healthy."

Sophie replies, "That's not it. I really like my job, you see, and I need to work. I expected to be pregnant and working for another month. I don't think they'll hold my job for me if I'm out for that long—even if it is medical leave." She thinks about 4 years of student loans to pay off and starts crying even harder.

Anne looks thoughtful. "Let me have a talk with Dr. Riley," she says.

Anne returns after a few minutes. "I found Dr. Riley," she says. "I told her about your concerns. We agreed that although many providers, including Dr. Riley, still prescribe bed rest for preeclampsia, there's no good evidence that it results in better outcomes (Analyze the Evidence 4.1). There's also not any evidence to support a low-sodium diet, lowered stress, or reduced

stimulation. I'm telling you this so you can make choices about your own health. We're here to guide you, but you're still the boss of your own body. We can make recommendations but it's up to you to decide what you'd like to do." Anne goes on to tell her what management *is* supported by the evidence. "You're not a bad mother or a bad person for making the best decision based on your own judgment."

Sophie appreciates the nurse telling her about the evidence and the different options, but now she's more confused and stressed than ever. She has a new physician she hasn't met, she has this new diagnosis that people apparently can't decide what to do with, and as far as she knows, she's about to lose her job. She decides to go home and sleep on it. Surely everyone can agree that's a good idea, anyway.

Labor and Delivery

Sophie does sleep on it, and when she awakes, she feels rebellious. She has faced so many decisions this year and all of them tough.

 Analyze the Evidence 4.1 Bed Rest in Pregnancy

Routine bed rest is not advised in pregnancy for the treatment of preeclampsia.

Pro	Con
Some healthcare providers continue to prescribe bed rest for clients with preeclampsia. Some believe that avoiding the BP spike that may come with physical activity may improve outcomes, although this theory is not supported by the research.	The American Congress of Obstetricians and Gynecologists recommends against prescribing bed rest for clients with preeclampsia because of a lack of evidence (American College of Obstetricians and Gynecologists, Task Force on Hypertension in Pregnancy, 2013).

Adverse Effects of Bed Rest

Physical

- Weight loss
- Muscle wasting and weakness
- Bone demineralization and calcium loss
- Decreased plasma volume and cardiac output
- Increased risk of blood clots
- Cardiac deconditioning
- Alteration in bowel function
- Sleep disturbance and fatigue
- Prolonged postpartum recovery

Emotional

- Loss of control
- Dysphoria: anxiety, depression, hostility, and anger
- Guilt associated with difficulty in complying with activity restriction and the inability to meet role responsibilities
- Boredom and loneliness
- Emotional lability (mood swings)
- Financial strain associated with the loss of income and the cost of treatment

Effect on Caregivers

- Stress associated with increased responsibilities and disruption of family routines
- Financial strain associated with the loss of maternal income and the cost of treatment
- Fear and anxiety regarding the well-being of the mother and fetus

Keep the pregnancy or end it. Keep her job or move home. Call Jeff or stay stubborn. Go to work or stay in bed.

At first staying in bed sounds great. But then she starts to feel claustrophobic. And then she gets mad because it is yet another decision she has to make because of a lucky sperm. She decides to get up and go to work. She knows from what Anne told her at the hospital that she probably won't have more than a week before she has to go back to the hospital, anyway. At least this way maybe she can close out her time in a way that seems professional and responsible, and maybe someday they'll let her come back. Thank goodness she's been hoarding diapers.

Before she leaves for work, she calls her midwife, Maria, and tells her that she plans to go in to work for 2 or more days that week. She tells her she'll try to stop at a pharmacy to check her BP at the end of each day and will call with the results. Maria restates Dr. Riley's instructions but tells her that she can't be forced to rest and concedes that what Anne said about the evidence available is true. She lists the warning signs for worsening preeclampsia for her again and gives her strict instructions to call if the baby starts to move less or if she experiences any vision changes, increased swelling, pain under her ribs, worsening shortness of breath, or a headache (Box 4.15).

One night, a few days later, she is dreaming that she is in the water but can't remember how to swim, and then somehow she is out of the water and giving a presentation about the relative merits of each kind of diaper when suddenly she wets her own pants. She wakes up burning with embarrassment to realize two things. First, she has a nasty headache, and second, the bed is completely soaked with clear fluid. Well wouldn't you know it—it happened while she was in bed, anyway. She goes to her parents' room and shakes her mother awake. "It's time, Mom," she says, and goes back to her room to change her clothes. When she turns on the lights she realizes she's seeing spots.

Maria meets them in the triage area for labor and delivery and tells her that Dr. Riley is on her way, as well. A different nurse is on duty tonight, not Anne, and she tells them that the BP is much higher than it has been, 156/102. When Maria taps Sophie's knees with the reflex hammer, Sophie almost kicks her and apologizes.

"No apologies," says Maria, "but I think your preeclampsia is getting worse. We're going to check in on how the baby is doing and confirm that your water broke while you were sleeping."

Just like Anne did when she was in the hospital before, the new nurse, Fiona, puts the monitoring devices, which look like twin hockey pucks, on her abdomen, one close to her ribs, and one lower down her belly. Once the devices and elastic bands are in place, Fiona starts an intravenous (IV) line in the crook of her left elbow. Maria explains that Dr. Riley ordered magnesium sulfate to help prevent any seizures that might result from the preeclampsia and that she'd need to stay on it through the birth and for about a day after the baby was born. Sophie looks at the IV pole. There is a big bag of clear fluid dripping into the line, and a second bag running into the same line that has stickers all over it (The Pharmacy 4.1).

"Will this magnesium stuff hurt the baby?" Sophie asks.

Maria shakes her head. "You won't be on it for very long. Sometimes if mothers are on it for a long time before the birth

---

 The Pharmacy 4.1

Magnesium Sulfate Dosing and Toxicity Management

Common Magnesium Sulfate Dosing for Preeclampsia

- A loading dose of 4–6 g over 15–30 min
- 1–3 g/h from an IV piggyback (e.g., 40 g of magnesium sulfate in 1 L of Ringer's lactate)
- Therapeutic goal: a serum (blood) level of 4–7 mEq/L

Signs of Magnesium Toxicity

- Respiratory depression (under 12 breaths/min)
- Oliguria (low urine output)
- Absent reflexes
- Lethargy
- Slurred speech
- Muscle weakness
- Loss of consciousness

Nursing Interventions for Magnesium Toxicity

- Stop the magnesium sulfate infusion immediately.
- Notify the primary healthcare provider (i.e., the physician, nurse midwife, or nurse practitioner).
- Administer calcium gluconate if ordered.

Data from Brookfield, K., Su, F., Elkomy, M. H., Drover, D. R., Lyell, D., & Carvalho, B. (2016). Pharmacokinetics and placental transfer of magnesium sulfate in pregnant women. *American Journal of Obstetrics & Gynecology, 214*(6), 737.e1–737.e9; Institute for Safe Mediation Practices. (2005, October 20). Preventing magnesium toxicity in obstetrics. *Acute Care IMSP Medication Safety Alert.*

Box 4.15 Management of Mild Preeclampsia

- Delivery at 37 wk
- Assessment of maternal symptoms and fetal movement by the mother daily, particularly noting the following:
  - Reduced fetal movement
  - Vision change
  - Increased swelling
  - Epigastric pain
  - Shortness of breath
  - Headache
- Blood pressure checks twice weekly
- Weekly assessment of platelets and liver function tests

Data from the American College of Obstetricians and Gynecologists, Task Force on Hypertension in Pregnancy. (2013). *Hypertension in pregnancy.* Washington, DC: American College of Obstetricians and Gynecologists.

the baby can be a little floppy for a while, and it can make their bones thinner. But you won't be on it for that long."

"Don't I need some drugs to get my BP down?" Sophie asks.

"Not yet. If your BP gets above 160/110, I'm sure Dr. Riley will consider it."

While Fiona is setting up the IV and all the tubes, Maria is watching a monitor with the two different lines and the horizontal graphs. She reminds Sophie that the top line is the baby's heart rate and the bottom, the flat line, is monitoring contractions. She tells her that the baby's heart rate is still right where it needs to be, at about 140 bpm, with reassuring moderate **variability**. She tells her that variability refers to the sawtooth pattern she can see on the graph, which indicates that the fetal heart rate is going up and down.

Sophie is still not having any contractions. Maria explains that this is concerning because the longer she stays pregnant after her water breaks, the more likely she is to get an infection in her uterus. Because of this possibility, it is important to verify that her water broke.

"Breaking your water without having contractions for an hour," Maria explains, "is a condition called premature rupture of membranes."

Sophie laughs and then says, "Of course my water broke. I didn't wet my bed!" As she says this, though, she worries that she might be wrong. What if she came all this way and dragged everyone out of bed and all that happened was that she wetted the bed like a little kid?

Maria places a sterile speculum inside her vagina and explains that she is looking to see whether any fluid is pooling in her vagina, and that she would use Nitrazine paper to check the pH of the fluid. If the paper turns blue, it is highly likely that her membranes ruptured. The last test would be to look at the fluid under the microscope to see whether there is any ferning. Lastly, Maria takes out the speculum and reaches inside of her with a sterile-gloved hand.

"Your cervix is nice and ripe!" Maria says (see Analyze the Evidence 1.1). She confirms that fluid is pooling and that the paper has turned blue, and she says that she has collected some of the fluid to check under the microscope for ferning.

A few minutes after Maria leaves the room, a second woman comes in and introduces herself as Dr. Riley. "But you can call me Jen," she says. "We're going to be spending a lot of time together." She apologizes for not meeting earlier and confirms what Maria said earlier, that her water has broken.

"This baby is better out than in," she says. Jen explains that because Sophie is less than 37 weeks pregnant, her pregnancy just a little shy of term. She also explains, however, that the worsening preeclampsia and the premature rupture of membranes puts both her and the baby at risk for complications. She says that her nurse, Fiona, will be adding another bag to her IV, this time of something called oxytocin, which will make her contractions start.

Maria comes back in. Jen says to Sophie, "I'm leaving you in good hands. I'll be checking in with your team and I'll come see you after. You've got this."

"Sophie, my shift is done," says Maria. "Jen will be taking over your care and your nurse, Fiona, is excellent. We'll see each other soon. You've done a wonderful job so far."

Sophie nods and avoids catching Maria's eye or her mother's, because she's afraid if she does she will fall apart. Things just got real.

It's not until Fiona increases her oxytocin dose a half hour after starting the infusion that Sophie feels anything. Then she feels her uterus contract, and she thinks she can even see her big belly rise up a little under her hospital gown. Fiona is right there with her and shows her how the bottom line in the two-line stack goes up and down as the contraction comes and goes. Sophie tells Fiona that this isn't so bad. She can handle this. Fiona tells her to try to get some rest. Half an hour later, Fiona returns and increases the oxytocin dose a little more (see The Pharmacy 1.2).

After a few hours of contractions becoming stronger and more frequent and Fiona increasing the oxytocin dose every half hour or so, Sophie is starting to get anxious. "How bad does this get?" she asks. "Is this almost done?" Fiona tells her that she is in the first stage of labor (see Table 1.3). She says that the first stage has different phases and that Sophie might be moving into a later, more intense phase. Fiona asks her if she would like to talk about pain management. Sophie tells her she has no interest in talking about it but a lot of interest in getting an epidural.

Fiona explains to Sophie that the anesthesiologist on call would have to place the epidural and that it may take a few minutes for them to arrive. "But it will make the pain better and help me get through this, right?" Sophie asks.

Fiona nods. "Most women still feel pressure when the baby starts to come down, but you shouldn't have the contraction pain anymore."

"I can wait for the anesthesiologist," says Sophie.

Fiona smiles. "You'll have to wait for Jen, as well. We need to see how dilated your cervix is first."

As it turns out, Jen was already on her way in to check on her. She performs a pelvic exam and tells her that she is about 5 cm dilated. "About where we'd expect," Jen says. All Sophie can think is, five more to go.

A big man with a mustache comes in the room. "Hi. I'm Dr. Steve," he says. "I'll be the one to place your epidural" (Box 4.16). He explains that Sophie will have to stay very still while the epidural is being placed to avoid injury. He tells her that the most common side effects of the epidural are itchiness, an inability to urinate for a period of time, and nausea. He explains that the placement of an epidural is very safe, but rarely there can be more severe problems.

Another contraction is coming. Fiona asks if there is any more information she needs before she makes her decision, and Sophie shakes her head. She takes the consent form from Dr. Steve's hand and signs it.

Sophie elects to have the epidural inserted while she is sitting up, with her mother sitting in a chair in front of her holding her hands. During a contraction she can feel Dr. Steve cleaning her back, and he explains to her that he is going to numb the skin a little with a shot, just like the dentist does before filling a cavity. The contraction is intense, and when he numbs her she doesn't notice. She is vaguely aware of Fiona taking her BP again. She takes it a lot. When her contraction is over, Dr. Steve says he is starting the procedure. She thought she'd feel a pop or something, but all she feels is the catheter being taped up her back.

Box 4.16 Spinal and Epidural Anesthesia and Analgesia Options

Spinal Anesthesia

- Includes a local anesthetic, which may be combined with an opioid analgesic
- Is injected into the subarachnoid space to mix with the cerebrospinal fluid
- Is administered as a single dose of medication
- Lasts 1–3 h

Epidural Anesthesia or Analgesia

- Includes a local anesthetic or an opioid analgesic or both
- Is injected into the epidural space
- Preserves greater motor function than with spinal anesthesia
- Is administered by an indwelling catheter, which allows multiple doses or continuous dosing by a pump

Combined Spinal-Epidural Analgesia

- Includes a small amount of opioid, with or without a local anesthetic
- Is deposited into the subarachnoid space and then an epidural catheter is placed, as usual
- Allows superior motor ability than does epidural or spinal anesthesia/analgesia alone

Box 4.17 Maternal Hypotension After an Epidural

Sometimes an epidural can result in a 20% or more decrease in BP. This hypotension can result in less blood flow to the placenta, referred to as reduced placental perfusion, which can be dangerous for the fetus.

Signs

- A decrease in BP of 20% or more, or a systolic BP of 100 mm Hg or less
- A drop in the fetal heart rate below 120 bpm (fetal bradycardia)
- A reduction in fetal heart rate variability

Nursing Interventions

- Notify the patient's primary care provider or nurse midwife and/or the anesthesiologist or anesthetist.
- Position the patient on her side, if she is not already.
- Administer oxygen by a nonrebreather mask at 10–12 L/min.
- Administer a vasopressor intravenously per orders and institutional protocol.
- Elevate the patient's legs.
- Continue to monitor BP and fetal heart rate every 5 min until they are stable.

Fiona and her mother help position her so that she is lying on her side, and Fiona says this is to keep the baby off of major blood vessels to help with blood flow. Sophie has been hooked up to a machine since she arrived that automatically checks her pulse and BP every 15 minutes or so. Sophie notices that once Fiona has her lying on her side, she pushes a button that makes the machine check her pulse and BP yet again (Box 4.17). She notices her watching the fetal monitoring strip, as well. Another contraction starts, and Sophie feels just as much pain as she had before. "It didn't work," she tells Fiona.

"It will," says Fiona. "You'll start to notice about five minutes after it was placed. It may take about twenty minutes for full effect."

After another few contractions, the pain does dull, and Sophie notes that she and Fiona fall into a kind of routine of automated BP and pulse checks every 10 minutes and then every 15 minutes. At least hourly, Fiona asks about pain under the rib cage and whether those spots in front of her eyes are still there (they are, although her headache is better) and performs reflex checks. It begins to feel sort of normal. She is starting to understand why her room is equipped with a television. She even naps a little, she thinks. She knows that her mother does.

"Are you going to call that sperm donor of yours. What's his name? Jeff?" Sophie hears her mother say. Sophie thought her mother was asleep. In fact, her eyes are closed and she has her feet up in the industrial-style hospital recliner the room is furnished with.

"Some time," she says. "But I think I have enough going on just now." She gives up on the idea of napping.

"How about your sister, Leigh? We could call her." Leigh lives half way across the country and has been trying to get pregnant for years. She is also 10 years older than Sophie. They usually speak only on birthdays and major holidays.

"Are you bored, Mom? Is all of this not entertaining enough for you?" Sophie asks.

Sophie's mother sniffs. "I just thought it might be nice to reach out to family at a time like this."

Sophie looks at her mother shrewdly. The automatic BP cuff tightens around her arm again as she speaks. "We don't get a made-for-TV movie ending, Mom," she says. "This isn't the moment when I decide to give up this baby to my established older sister and head for the big city to make my fortune. This is just life. Not what I planned, but we'll be okay."

Sophie's mother starts to cry a little behind her hand. "I don't want things to be so hard for you," she says. "You're going to have to give up so much, to make so many compromises. I see the road you're traveling and it's just so hard."

Sophie reaches out her hand and her mother takes it. "Be happy for me, Mom. I'm happy for me." She makes a face and shifts in her bed as much as the epidural allows. "I'm feeling a lot of pressure. Can you find Fiona, Mom?"

Her mother returns with Fiona and Jen, who checks her cervix.

"Showtime," says Jen. "You are ten centimeter dilated and 100% effaced, and the head is at +2."

"That means," says Fiona, "that your cervix is all the way open and completely thinned out and that the baby's head is part way down the birth canal. We're going to get you pushing soon. You probably won't feel when your contractions are happening, so we'll tell you when you need to push. Got it?"

Sophie nods. "You tell me what to do."

Fiona nods back. "Try not to hold your breath while you push."

It takes less time than Sophie thought it would, maybe 45 minutes more, before Jen announces that the baby's head is crowning. Fiona brings around a mirror so Sophie can see her own vulva with the baby's head coming out of it. She is fascinated. It seems both hideous and beautiful, and she blesses the inventor of the epidural. When she reaches down, she can touch the dark, slimy curls on the baby's head, the face of which is looking down toward the floor. Fiona says this is normal—most babies come out face down.

Three more pushes and she is out: a slimy, bloody, gooey, spitting-mad, screaming baby girl. Jen puts her directly onto Sophie's abdomen, and Fiona rubs her with a warm baby blanket. Jen puts two clips on the umbilical cord and cuts between them. Fiona moves the baby from Sophie's abdomen to her chest and covers her with a fresh blanket. Sophie's hands go up automatically to steady the baby. She can hardly breathe, she is so relieved and scared at the same time.

"I can't believe it. I can't believe it," she says. And her placenta slips from her body and into Jen's hands without her even noticing. The automatic cuff inflates again, and Fiona removes the pink hockey pucks and elastic belts from her abdomen.

After Delivery

The baby is awake for almost an hour after the birth. Sophie and her mother watch as she seems to smell her little hands and scoot her way across Sophie's chest. At one point she seems to be eyeing Sophie's nipple but then just falls asleep, skin to skin with her mother. Fiona explains that most babies are very active in their first half hour of life, and then often have a nice long sleep of several hours (Box 4.18).

Box 4.18   Newborn Adaptation to Extrauterine Life

1. First period of reactivity
   a. Lasts up to 30 min after birth
   b. Heart rate of 160–180 bpm, decreasing to 100–120 bpm
   c. The newborn is alert and mobile.
2. Period of decreased responsiveness
   a. Lasts 60–100 min
   b. The newborn is less active and may sleep.
3. Second period of reactivity
   a. Lasts 10 min to several hours
   b. The first bowel movement (meconium) is likely to occur.

Data from Desmond, M., Rudolph, A., & Phitaksphaiwan, P. (1966). The transitional care nursery: A mechanism for preventative medicine in the newborn. *Pediatric Clinics of North America, 13*(3), 651–668.

By this time, Fiona and another nurse have Sophie all cleaned up and Jen has her stitched up. "You had just a little vaginal tear," she says. "It's not unusual." She still can't move or feel her legs very well.

After stopping the pump for Sophie's epidural, Fiona puts on a blue apron and pulls the tape from Sophie's back. She then puts on some gloves and pulls out the epidural catheter in one smooth movement. She cleans the area and puts on a fresh dressing.

Sophie calls and talks to her father for a few minutes after delivery, and her mother calls her sister. She texts Jeff to let him know that he has a daughter. He texts back a smiley face emoji. Jerk, she thinks.

An hour or so after the baby's birth, Fiona takes off the automatic BP cuff. She explains that she won't be checked as often now because she is stable, although they'll keep checking her reflexes and asking her questions about under-the-rib pain, vision changes, headache, shortness of breath, and increased swelling for another 24 hours or so.

Fiona then wheels Sophie next door to the postpartum floor, where she will likely spend the next few days. When she gets Sophie into her new room, Fiona reports off to another nurse, an older woman named Mary, who will be taking care of her for the remainder of her shift.

There is a recliner in this room just like in the labor and delivery room, and her mother sleeps in it, snoring a little bit. Sophie thought that sleep sounded like a great idea and that she would sleep while the baby did, but she finds instead that she is admiring perfect, tiny fingernails that look like little seashells on the tips of blue-tinged fingers and marveling at how soft babies' hair can be.

She looks at her IV pole. There is only one pump now that the epidural is gone. Another bag, the one for the oxytocin, is gone, as well. Just like Maria told her (it seemed like a million years ago), the magnesium sulfate is still there.

An hour after Sophie moves into her new room, Mary comes by and checks on her. She checks her BP, pulse, and breathing. She listens to her lungs. She checks her reflexes and, just like Fiona said she would, she asks about shortness of breath, pain under the ribs, vision changes, and headache. She tells Sophie that she'd like to check her bleeding and asks her to pull down the weird net hospital panties so she can look at her industrial-sized pad. While the pad is down, Mary starts to feel her belly, pushing particularly around where her belly button is.

"What are you checking for?" asks Sophie.

"I'm checking the size of your uterus and making sure it's nice and firm. I like to do it at the same time I check your bleeding, to see if we get any gushing."

Sophie just nods. It occurs to her that even 24 hours ago this would have been an embarrassing conversation.

"The top of your uterus is right where your belly button is, which is what we expect right now. It's nice and firm. Over the next few weeks your uterus will keep getting smaller and smaller until it's just about the size it was before the pregnancy."

"Do you have any swelling?" Mary asks.

"You tell me!" she says. "All I can see is swollen sausages where my toes used to be."

Mary laughs too and says it isn't at all unusual to have a lot of swelling in the legs for the first few days and that she is reassured that Sophie's legs appear to be equally swollen and that Sophie complains of no leg pain. Mary explains that when one leg is more swollen or painful than the other, it could indicate a blood clot. Mary also examines her legs and feels along the backs of her knees and calves, looking for warmth and hard areas and finding none. She explains that such signs could also indicate a blood clot.

Sophie had a catheter placed at some point (Mary says almost everyone who gets an epidural gets a catheter), and she is becoming increasingly aware of it, and not in a good way. She asks when she can have it taken out.

"We have to be sure you can make it to the bathroom and back safely before we remove it," Mary says. "We'll make two trips to the bathroom, and if all is well, we can take it out."

"I'm a little nervous about getting up," Sophie says, "but motivated. Between the cuffs on my legs and the catheter in my bladder, I'm feeling very cooperative right now."

Mary nods. "It's normal to be nervous, but I'll be right here. You've been lying down for a little while, however. I do want you to know that you may have a big rush of blood when you first stand up. It doesn't necessarily mean that you're bleeding that much, though."

Mary has her sit on the edge of the bed first and stay there for a few minutes. She lays some absorbent pads on the floor in case Sophie has the kind of bleeding she talked about. Slowly, then, and with some help from Mary on one side and her mother on the other, Sophie gets up and walks slowly to the bathroom. Truth be told, between the catheter and her jelly legs, it feels more like waddling. Mary carries with her the urine bag attached to the catheter, and her mother helps to push the IV pole next to her.

When she gets to the bathroom, she sits down on the toilet for a few minutes. Mary fills up a little squeeze bottle with warm water and shows her how to rinse off her vulva instead of using toilet paper to wipe. She explains that she'll likely be pretty sore there for a while, and that the water will be the most comfortable way to help keep clean. Sophie and the two other women then make the slow procession back to the bed. Mary clips the urine bag back to the side of the bed. About an hour later, Mary comes back and repeats the process. This time, however, she removes the catheter.

Sophie has been there for almost 24 hours, and she is eager to get the IV out of her arm and stop the magnesium sulfate. She thinks that it makes her feel dopey and tired. She and the baby have been practicing breastfeeding (it's harder than it looks, she's learning), and that makes her feel dopey, too. It is a bad combination. She has thinking to do and plans to make, and mostly she wants to nap.

Another nurse is on duty now, Kylie. She knocks softly on the door and asks if this would be a good time for an exam. She also tells her that the time is up for the magnesium sulfate. She stops the magnesium sulfate and reconfigures her tubes so that only the large bag is still active, with a line going through the pump. Then she detaches the tubes going from the pump to her arm until only a little stump remains attached to her.

"This is just a saline lock," Kylie explains. "If we need to get to a vein quickly, we can. We probably won't need it. I think everything's going to be just fine."

The Newborn

Her name is Gabrielle and she is beautiful. Well, truth be told, she looks a little bit like a hairy potato, but a really cute hairy potato. Her skin is a rich pinkish brown, and she has a white, cheese-like, creamy substance that Kylie says is called **vernix** in all of her many creases. Kylie handles Gabi with gloves until her first bath. She's 7 lb and 6 oz, which Sophie knows now is pretty standard. If you had asked her before the delivery, Sophie would have guessed that she weighed more like 10 lb. She was informed that she had an Apgar score of 8 at 1 minute and 9 at 5 minutes and that the only point she'd lost was for her blue fingers. Although Sophie isn't sure she'd say that she fell in love with her right away, she does immediately feel protective, like she wants to run for the hills and do anything she can to keep her little girl safe from harm.

After the first day, Gabi starts to spend more time awake, though for short periods. Sometimes she is just quietly alert, looking at her mother or participating (or not) as Sophie and Kylie work on getting her to latch to the breast. The contents of her first diaper are alarmingly black and tarry, but Kylie, who changes the diaper, assures her that this is normal and will last only a day or so. She calls the contents of the diaper "meconium." She advises that Sophie put a lot of petroleum jelly on Gabi's bottom at the end of each diaper change so that the meconium won't stick to her skin. It occurs to her then that she hasn't changed a diaper since she did some babysitting as a teenager. She'll have to watch carefully the next time Kylie does it.

Kylie has a different idea. She has Sophie change the next diaper and then has her watch while she bathes Gabi. Afterward, Kylie gives her another little squeeze bottle like the one she used on her vulva and a funny little sponge with a plastic brush on one side that Sophie can use at home to gently scrub Gabi's sparse hair. Kylie also teaches Sophie and her mother how to swaddle little Gabi.

Sophie and her mother decide that Gabi looks just like Sophie did when she was a baby and couldn't possibly look at all like Jeff. They think the shape of the baby's eyes is very similar to that of Sophie's father, and that she has her grandmother's chin. When her father comes to visit, he wiggles his eyebrows at his unimpressed granddaughter and calls her beautiful, and leaves a vase of sweet-smelling flowers for Sophie.

The following day a new nurse, Jeanine, takes Gabi to the newborn nursery to have her hearing checked and to have some blood taken from her heel for the newborn screening. She is also getting her first of a series of three hepatitis B vaccinations. Jeanine explains that the newborn screen has to be done at least 24 hours after birth because the baby has to eat something first. This is necessary because many of the genetic problems included in the newborn screen are associated with metabolism. For the test to be accurate, Gabi has to metabolize something first. Sophie will get the results when she takes Gabi to her first pediatrician visit in a few days.

While Gabi and Jeanine are in the nursery, Sophie packs. Her mother left a few hours before to get Sophie's room ready for the baby, and she and Sophie's father would be back with the car and a newly installed rear-facing car seat.

Sophie feels optimistic and she feels lucky. She knows she was fortunate to have the kind of support her parents could provide, and she knows that she won't need it forever. She feels smart and strong. Scared, too, but for Gabi's sake, she knows she can make things work. Because, really, what is the alternative?

Think Critically

1. What are four of the uses for ultrasound in early pregnancy?
2. Which common discomforts of pregnancy did Sophie experience each trimester?
3. What are Sophie's risk factors for preeclampsia?
4. Why does Sophie need to collect her urine for 24 hours?
5. What common findings during the third trimester of pregnancy might be confused with preeclampsia?
6. What dietary changes is Sophie encouraged to make because of her pregnancy and because of her preeclampsia, and why?

7. What constitutes a reactive nonstress test?
8. Why is magnesium sulfate used for patients with preeclampsia? What are some of the warning signs of magnesium toxicity?
9. If bed rest has not been found to improve outcomes but has numerous adverse effects, is it an acceptable recommendation? If not, what is the role of the nurse in this situation?
10. What is the goal range for oxytocin that would let a nurse know she does not need to further titrate the dose at this time? How is oxytocin titrated?

References

American College of Obstetricians and Gynecologists, Task Force on Hypertension in Pregnancy. (2013). *Hypertension in pregnancy.* Washington, DC: American College of Obstetricians and Gynecologists.

Centers for Disease Control and Prevention. (2016, January 25). *Pregnant? Get Tdap in your third trimester.* Retrieved from http://www.cdc.gov/features/tdap-in-pregnancy/

Centers for Disease Control and Prevention, National Center for Health Statistics. (2016, May 30). *Infertility.* Retrieved from http://www.cdc.gov/nchs/fastats/infertility.htm

Suggested Readings

Gray, J. B. (2015). "It Has Been a Long Journey From First Knowing": Narratives of unplanned pregnancy. *Journal of Health Communication: International Perspectives, 20*(6), 736–742.

Truven Health Analytics. (2013). *The cost of having a baby in the United States.* Ann Arbor, MI: Author.

Værland, I. E., Vevatne, K., & Brinchmann, B. S. (2016). An integrative review of mothers' experiences of preeclampsia. *Journal of Obstetric, Gynecologic, and Neonatal Nursing, 45*(3), 300–307.

Ybarra, N., & Laperouse, E. (2016). Postpartum preeclampsia. *Journal of Obstetric, Gynecologic, and Neonatal Nursing, 45*(3), S20.

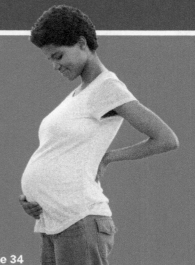

5 Letitia Richford: Cord Prolapse and Nonreassuring Fetal Status

Letitia Richford, age 34

Objectives

1. Calculate the most likely time in the menstrual cycle for conception to occur.
2. Differentiate between kinds of spontaneous abortion.
3. Explain the significance of the Rh-negative blood type in pregnancy and the priority assessments and interventions related to it.
4. Describe the signs of cord prolapse and nonreassuring fetal status and summarize the priority intervention.
5. Identify risks faced by late preterm infants and describe how to appropriately monitor them.
6. Define hyperbilirubinemia and describe how it is assessed for in the newborn.

Key Terms

Basal body thermometer
Cord prolapse
Corpus luteum
Engage
Fetal movement count
Folic acid
Follicular phase
Hyperbilirubinemia
Late preterm infant

Milia
Nasal flaring
Nonreassuring fetal status
Proliferative phase
Retractions
Secretory phase
Spinnbarkeit
Spontaneous abortion
Transcutaneous bilirubin monitoring

Before Conception

Letitia and her husband, Don, have been trying to get pregnant for nearly a year. She thought it would be easy. After spending half her life trying not to get pregnant, it never occurred to her that it might be difficult. She schedules an appointment with her gynecologist, Dr. Janachek, to see what she is doing wrong, because surely this isn't normal.

"This is normal," says Dr. Janachek. "If you're under thirty-five, we start to be concerned about your fertility when you have not conceived after a year of well-timed intercourse. If you're thirty-five or older, we start to look into it earlier simply because you have less time overall in which to conceive."

"What do you mean by well-timed intercourse?" Letitia asks.

"Women's ovaries typically release only one egg per month, and that egg can only be fertilized for about twenty-four hours after release. The challenge is figuring out when that twenty-four–hour time frame is. Most women ovulate about fourteen days before their period starts. If your cycle is regular, it is easy to find out when you're most fertile. If your cycle is irregular, it's not so easy."

"When you say 'cycle,' do you mean my period?"

"We consider your cycle to be the time from the first day of one period to the first day of the next period" (Fig. 5.1).

"Okay. Then I guess my cycle hasn't been that regular since I stopped my pill to get pregnant," says Letitia. "Some months it's

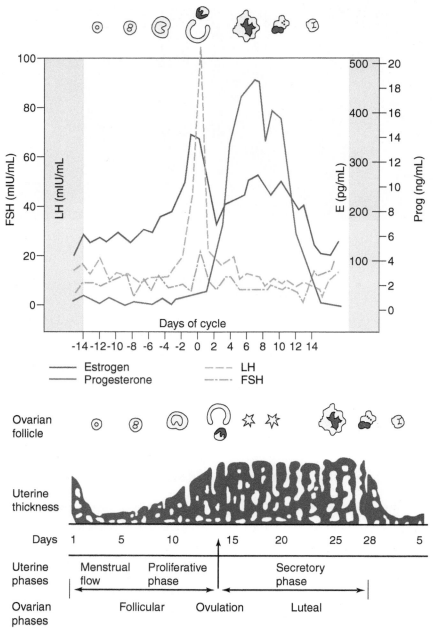

Figure 5.1. Changes during reproductive and menstrual cycles. (Top) Plasma hormone concentrations in the normal female reproductive cycle. **(Bottom)** Ovarian events and uterine changes during the menstrual cycle. FSH, follicle-stimulating hormone; LH, luteinizing hormone. (Reprinted with permission from LifeART © 2018 Lippincott Williams & Wilkins. All rights reserved.)

twenty-six days and other months it's a lot longer. I keep track of it on a calendar in my smartphone."

"That's a good start," says Dr. Janachek. "Let's discuss what else you can do."

Dr. Janachek removes a paper from the drawer and explains that Letitia should use it to keep track of her temperature throughout the month (Fig. 5.2).

"You'll need a special thermometer," says Dr. Janachek. "It's called a **basal body thermometer**, and it's a little more sensitive, a little more precise than regular thermometers. You may have to ask the pharmacist for it, and sometimes they have to specially order it."

"Is it expensive?"

"It's less than ten dollars, typically. The trick is how you use it. You need to take your temperature first thing in the morning, before you lift your head off the pillow, before you have water, before you have coffee."

"I can probably do that. So I take my temperature and I make a mark on this grid each day. What am I looking for?"

Dr. Janachek explains that she should look for a pattern in the temperatures rather than focus on individual measurements. She explains that in the first half of the cycle, which is the **follicular phase** in the ovarian cycle and

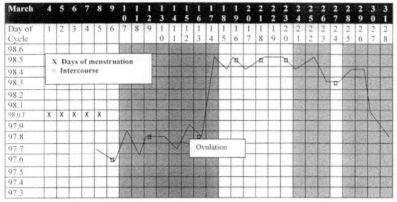

Figure 5.2. Menstrual cycle basal body temperature tracking chart.
(Reprinted with permission from Bienstock, J. L., Fox, H. E., Wallach, E. E.,
Johnson, C. T., & Hallock, J. T. [2015]. *Johns Hopkins manual of gynecology
and obstetrics* [5th ed., Fig. 35-1]. Philadelphia, PA: Lippincott Williams &
Wilkins.)

proliferative phases in the uterine cycle, her temperature
should remain fairly low.

"During this time the follicle that the egg will release from
on the ovary is forming, which is why we call it the follicular
phase of the ovarian cycle. After menses, the endometrial lining
starts to grow, or proliferate, again, which is why we call it the
proliferative phase of the uterine cycle."

If she ovulates, Letitia should expect to see a slight dip in
temperature one day followed by a sharp rise in temperature
the next day.

"Once you see the sharp rise, you're likely no longer fertile,"
Dr. Janachek explains. "That dip is your most fertile time, but
the dip can be subtle, and only obvious in retrospect."

The temperature, Dr. Janachek explains, would continue to
be elevated for the remainder of the cycle and then dip again just
prior to menstruation. This second part of the cycle, in which the
temperature is elevated, is the luteal phase of the ovarian cycle,
referring to the hormone-secreting corpus luteum on the ovary
that forms in the follicle from which the ovary was released. It
is also the secretory phase of the uterine cycle, referring to the
activity of the endometrium at this time.

"If this dip is so subtle, I'm not sure how helpful it will be,"
says Letitia. "I'm worried I'm going to miss it."

"There are two things to consider," says Dr. Janachek. "First,
look for trends over time. Many women get very good at predicting their cycles based on these charts. Second, check your
cervical mucus. Have you ever noticed how your discharge changes
throughout the month?"

"Sure," says Letitia. "It changes all the time when I'm not on
the pill. Sometimes I think I have a yeast infection, but it doesn't
itch. Sometimes it seems like there's a lot of it and sometimes it's
like there isn't any at all."

Dr. Janachek explains that after menses, vaginal discharge is
often thin and slippery, and then at the time nearing ovulation can
become thick and stringy like an egg white. This, she explains, is
when women are most fertile. Between the egg-white–like mucus,
also known as spinnbarkeit, and menses, the discharge can be

stickier, even curdy, and white. All of this, says Dr. Janachek,
is normal.

"So when should we have sex?" asks Letitia. "When I see the
egg-white mucus?"

"Sperm can live up to five days, we believe. In this practice,
we recommend having intercourse daily for the five days leading
up to the rise in temperature."

"But I don't know when that will be," says Letitia.

"That's why you need to look for trends in your chart. But in
the meantime, having sex when you see the change in mucus is
a great idea." Dr. Janachek says. "While I have you here, since
you are actively trying to get pregnant, I'd like you to fill out a
questionnaire about diet, exercise, and some risk factors that
can impact a healthy pregnancy. I'd also like to do some blood
work to determine whether you're a carrier for some of the more
common genetic variants that contribute to disease and some
routine blood work to assess for other health risks. That way we
can talk about any lifestyle changes now, and we'll have a better
idea of what your risks are for passing on certain conditions to
any offspring" (see Table 1.1; Boxes 1.2 and 5.1).

After reviewing her questionnaire, Dr. Janachek reminds Letitia
to take a daily prenatal vitamin. "Probably the most important
part of that vitamin is the folic acid," she says. "Women who have
too little folic acid are more likely to carry fetuses with neural
tube defects, such as spina bifida. Much of the benefit of taking
folic acid is only realized if you begin taking it before you even
know you're pregnant, so don't wait for a confirmed pregnancy
before you start taking your vitamin."

Miscarriage

For 3 months, Letitia continues to track her menstrual cycle
using an app on her smartphone, but now she is monitoring
her temperature and cervical secretions, as well. She comes to a
month in which the luteal phase of her ovarian cycle (the secretory
phase of her uterine cycle) lasts for 14 days and then 15 days
and then 16 days. Finally, on the 17th day, she decides to take

Box 5.1 Components of Preconception Care Questionnaire

Health Considerations

- Chronic disease and disease management (diabetes, polycystic ovary syndrome, endometriosis, asthma, depression, etc.)
- Medications, including prescription, over-the-counter, and herbal preparations
- Infectious diseases (hepatitis C, HIV, etc.)
- Vaccination history
- Reproductive history
  - Pregnancy history (including GTPAL; see Box 2.2)
  - Sexually transmitted infections
  - Surgical history
- Genetic conditions, self and family history (sickle cell anemia, cystic fibrosis, fragile X, thalassemia, etc.)

Behavioral Considerations

- Nutrition
  - Folic acid intake (supplements, green leafy vegetables, fortified baked products)
  - Diet, including daily intake of fruits, vegetables, protein
  - Exercise
- Current contraception
- Tobacco, alcohol, recreational drug use
- Current family structure, partner participation
- Intimate partner violence assessment
- Environmental exposures and other home or work hazards

a pregnancy test. She's a little crampy and her breasts are sore, just like she normally is right before her period, so she thinks she is probably wasting her money as she purchases the pregnancy tests (two for $9.99) at the pharmacy as well as her time and her hope as she unwraps the first test in a stall in the ladies' room at work and pees on the end of the paddle. She cries right there in the stall when the second pink line appears, her pants still down around her ankles.

After she has a good cry, blows her nose into a handful of scratchy toilet paper, and makes it back to her desk, she calls Don and gives him the good news. He's so excited that he starts laughing and yelling, and soon everyone in both his office and hers knows. Letitia then calls her mother, her best friend, and her sister. She spends the rest of her work day shopping for maternity clothes and daydreaming about the baby. She doesn't get much work done.

Two weeks later—and 8 weeks after the first day of her last period—Letitia's breasts are still sore, she's exhausted, and she nauseous. And this morning, she starts bleeding. It's not a lot of blood, just a little bit. It's dark on the toilet paper, and she's wearing an absorbent liner in her panties. It doesn't stop. She's had some cramping on and off like menstrual cramps for weeks now. Is the cramping more intense now? Is it happening more often? She just can't tell.

She makes an appointment to see Dr. Janachek. When she tells the office triage nurse why she needs an appointment, the nurse tells her to come in right away.

Dr. Janachek does an ultrasound right there in the office. When Dr. Janachek inserts the transducer into Letitia's vagina, it doesn't hurt, it just feels strange and mildly uncomfortable, like a too-big bite of food shoved to the side of the cheek.

Dr. Janachek rotates the transducer and moves the picture on the screen left to right. She wrinkles her forehead and freezes the image. She rotates the screen to show Letitia what she's seeing.

"You see this dark circle here? That's the gestational sac, where the pregnancy grows. This little circle right here is the yolk sac, which is producing red blood cells for the pregnancy right now."

Letitia looks at it for a second. "I think I'll have to take your word for it."

"This is what I'm concerned about," says Dr. Janachek. She indicates a darker gray streak that travels in a line from the black gestational sac. "This tells me that your cervix is opening. I'm sorry, Letitia. I don't think this pregnancy is viable."

"I don't understand."

"This line, the one that indicates that your cervix is opening, means that a **spontaneous abortion** is inevitable" (Table 5.1).

"What? What do you mean?" asks Letitia, alarmed. "I want this baby. I don't want an abortion."

"I'm sorry," says Dr. Janachek. "That was confusing. The technical term for a miscarriage is spontaneous abortion. I know how much you want this pregnancy."

"I don't understand why this is happening. Can't we stop it? What if I rest? Or is there some way we can just keep the cervix closed? Stitches? Something?"

Table 5.1 Types of Spontaneous Abortion (Miscarriage)

Type	Description
Inevitable abortion	The patient typically reports vaginal bleeding and cramping. The cervix is dilated.
Threatened abortion	Symptoms include vaginal bleeding without cervical dilation.
Missed abortion	The pregnancy is no longer developing and is not viable, but bleeding, cramping, and cervical dilation have not occurred.
Septic abortion	Any spontaneous abortion with intrauterine infection. Symptoms may include fever, chills, abdominal pain, bleeding, discharge, tachycardia, and tachypnea.
Incomplete abortion	Symptoms include vaginal bleeding, cramping, and cervical dilation. Some or all of the products of the conception remain in the cervix or uterus.

Dr. Janachek shakes her head and smiles sympathetically. "I'm sorry, but no. Most of the time we don't know what causes miscarriage, but we do know that as many as twenty to twenty-five percent of pregnancies end this way" (Hachem et al., 2017). "Some research suggests that as many as sixty percent of pregnancies end before a woman even knows she's pregnant" (Larsen, Christiansen, Kolte, & Macklon, 2013). "Many of these likely happen because something is genetically wrong with the pregnancy and the fetus cannot continue to survive" (Larsen et al., 2013).

"So this is happening," says Letitia. All of the joy and expectation she's been feeling about the pregnancy vanishes. She feels a lump forming in the back of her throat as she works not to cry. How will she tell Don? Her mother? Her sister? Everyone?

"I'm sorry. I know you very much want this pregnancy. At least now we know that you can get pregnant. We have no reason to think you can't get pregnant again and have a completely successful pregnancy. We should talk about what you want to do next, though."

"What do you mean?"

"Well, you have three options. We can wait and see whether you pass the pregnancy yourself in the next few days, which is likely. We could also give you a medication, misoprostol, which would encourage your body to pass the pregnancy. And lastly we could do an in-office procedure, a dilation and curettage, to remove the pregnancy from your uterus."

"I don't want to do the medication or a procedure," says Letitia. "I think I just want the wait and see option. Will it hurt?"

"It's different for everyone," says Dr. Janachek. "It may be like period cramps or it may be worse. It's very tiny, the pregnancy. You won't see anything that looks like a fetus. It will just look like period clots. It can take weeks for this process to be complete, though given your bleeding and your cervix opening, I suspect it won't take that long. If it hasn't happened in a month, however, we'll have to consider the medication or surgical option again. I'd like to schedule an appointment for you weekly until we're sure you're through this. And I'd like to see you earlier if anything changes."

"What kind of changes?" asks Letitia.

"Well, I'd like to see you if you pass any clots, bleed through more than two pads per hour for more than two hours, or have any signs of infection. Your pain and bleeding will likely be at their worst during the two to four hours it takes for you to pass the pregnancy. It's especially important for me to see you if the pain and heavy bleeding continue after you see the clots."

"If I change my mind and decide to do the medical or surgical option, can I just call?"

"Absolutely," says Dr. Janachek. She pauses for a moment and then says, "I know you may not want to think about this right now, but once you pass the pregnancy you can get pregnant again right away. If that's not something you want, you'll need to restart contraception. This pregnancy is very early, and your body won't need a recovery period. Keep in mind, however, that the hormone that we look for to detect a pregnancy, beta-human chorionic gonadotropin, or β-hCG, may be present for a time after the pregnancy ends. You might take a home pregnancy test in a few weeks and have it be positive. It doesn't mean that you're pregnant again, necessarily. It may still be positive from this pregnancy."

"I understand," says Letitia. "I think I'd like to give myself a few months before starting to try again, anyway. We'll just use condoms or something."

"You've been doing well tracking your cycle," says Dr. Janachek. "You could just reverse what you're doing. So instead of trying to have intercourse when you think you might be fertile, you'd avoid having sex during that time."

"Oh," says Leticia. "I guess that makes sense." "I'll think about it."

"That sounds wise. You do what makes the most sense for you," says Dr. Janachek. "One more thing—it appears we didn't check your blood type when you were here last. Do you know what it is?"

"I don't. I gave blood once but I lost the card."

"We just need to do a fingerstick to find out whether you're Rh negative or Rh positive. If you're Rh negative, we'll need to give you a shot before you leave" (Fig. 5.3).

"What's the shot for?" asks Letitia.

"When a woman is Rh negative, she may form antibodies to Rh-positive blood if exposed to it, which can occur when a fetus she carries is Rh positive and she has bleeding during pregnancy. In such cases we administer a shot of Rh_0 (D) immune globulin to the mother, which will stop her from developing the antibodies."

"What would happen if I developed antibodies to Rh-positive blood?" asks Letitia.

"If you were to become pregnant in the future with an Rh-positive fetus and you had antibodies against Rh-positive blood, your body would stage an immune reaction against the fetus that could end in fetal death."

No agglutination
(negative reaction)

Agglutination
(positive reaction)

Figure 5.3. Blood typing reactions. Letitia's Rh result is shown in the top circle, no agglutination. If she were Rh positive, her test would appear as in the lower circle, agglutination. (Reprinted with permission from Cohen, B. J., & DePetris, A. [2013]. *Medical terminology: An illustrated guide* [7th ed., Fig. 10-7B]. Philadelphia, PA: Lippincott Williams & Wilkins.)

"Well that's awful," says Letitia. "But that would happen only if the baby were Rh positive, right, not if the baby were Rh negative?"

"Correct."

Dr. Janachek tells Letitia she'll see her again in a week, if not sooner, and then leaves. A nurse arrives and introduces herself as Jeanine. She cleans the side of the tip of her middle finger with alcohol and pricks it with a spring-loaded lancet. She draws up the drop of blood in a little pipette and leaves the room, telling her she'll be back shortly (Step-by-Step Skills 5.1).

Jeanine returns within a few minutes. "You are Rh negative," she says. "I'll need to give you a shot of Rh_o (D) immune globulin before you go. Did Dr. Janachek explain to you why we're doing this already?" (The Pharmacy 5.1; Box 5.2).

"Yes, she did," Letitia says.

"Do you have any questions about it?"

"I don't think so."

Jeanine injects the medicine into the muscle of her left shoulder.

"I don't think you're going to bleed," Jeanine tells Letitia, "But I'll give you a bandage anyway."

The bandage is shaped like a blue crayon.

Three days later, just as Dr. Janachek predicted, she wakes up with intense cramping and heavy bleeding. The worst of it is over in an hour. She has been hoping that somehow Dr. Janachek was wrong, that the little flicker of life would somehow win the day. But it doesn't. She knows it. It is still a shock, even if it isn't a surprise. Dr. Janachek performs another ultrasound the next day and confirms that her uterus is just as unoccupied as it was before she ever thought to become a mother.

"You can try again anytime," Dr. Janachek says, gently patting her shoulder. "But you needn't rush it."

Letitia doesn't rush it. She and Don take a few months off from trying and grieve their loss.

Pregnancy

First Trimester

A few months later, not long after she and Don have started trying to get pregnant again, Letitia misses another period. And just like that, she's pregnant again. This time, she and Don don't tell anyone.

At 6.5 weeks after the start of her last period, the bleeding starts again, and she is glad they haven't told anyone about being pregnant. It's just spotting, though, and mild cramping. She asks Don to call Dr. Janachek's office to make the appointment.

"I can't make that call," she tells him. "I just can't."

That afternoon she goes in for her appointment. This time Don comes with her. She tells Dr. Janachek about her bleeding, which she describes as light, and her cramping, which she describes as very mild—similar to her normal premenstrual cramping. She tells her she hasn't passed any clots or tissue and doesn't feel ill or feverish, although maybe a little nauseous.

"I'd like to do another ultrasound," says Dr. Janachek. "Just like before, we'll look for the yolk sac and fetal pole and assess your cervix."

"I can't believe this is happening again," says Letitia. Don squeezes her hand.

"Well, hold on," says Dr. Janachek. "We don't really know what's happening yet. Bleeding in early pregnancy happens in up to forty percent of women. Sometimes it's just caused by how the pregnancy is implanted. It's not always bad news, but I know it's frightening."

Letitia and Don watch the ultrasound with Dr. Janachek. She points out the uterus, the black circle of the gestational sac, the yolk sac, and the pulsation at the center of the fetal pole, which is the heartbeat.

"This all looks beautiful," says Dr. Janachek. "All I see here is a very normal-looking early pregnancy, about six and a half weeks along. I don't see any opening of your cervix."

Letitia and Don both take a deep breath and smile at each other goofily with relief.

Dr. Janachek removes the ultrasound transducer, and Don helps Letitia into a sitting position.

"I think we should expect the best," says Dr. Janachek. "We did your genetic screening before your first pregnancy, and we know you're not a carrier for cystic fibrosis or sickle cell anemia, the two conditions you are most likely to have a predisposition for" (see Table 1.1). "Because of the bleeding, I'd like to see you in another week. If the bleeding has stopped completely, after that we'll see you again at twelve weeks" (Box 5.3).

In response to Dr. Janachek's questions, Letitia confirms that no changes have occurred in her health since her preconception

---

Step-by-Step Skills 5.1

Checking Rh Factor Using Point-of-Care Testing

1. Use an Anti D Eldon Card.
2. Obtain blood sample by finger stick.
3. Place a drop of water in the Control circle and the Anti D circle.
4. Place a drop of blood on the Control circle and stir for 10 s with EldonStick. Blood should fill the entire circle.
5. Dispose of EldonStick.
6. Place drop of blood on Anti D circle and stir with second EldonStick for 10 s. Blood should fill the entire circle.
7. Hold the card upright on end for 10 s.
8. Rotate the card an additional three times, holding it on end, for a total of 40 s.
9. While tilting the card, blood should not be allowed to run out of the circles.
10. After the 40 s of holding the card upright in four different directions, the card may be laid flat and read.
11. Look for evidence of agglutinate, or graininess, in the circles.
12. The control circle should show no evidence of agglutinate.
13. Agglutinate in the Anti D circle indicates Rh positive.
14. Absence of agglutinate in the Anti D circle indicates Rh negative.

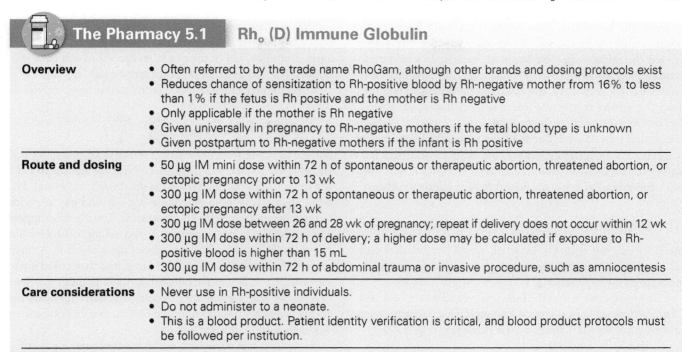

The Pharmacy 5.1 Rh₀ (D) Immune Globulin

Overview	• Often referred to by the trade name RhoGam, although other brands and dosing protocols exist • Reduces chance of sensitization to Rh-positive blood by Rh-negative mother from 16% to less than 1% if the fetus is Rh positive and the mother is Rh negative • Only applicable if the mother is Rh negative • Given universally in pregnancy to Rh-negative mothers if the fetal blood type is unknown • Given postpartum to Rh-negative mothers if the infant is Rh positive
Route and dosing	• 50 μg IM mini dose within 72 h of spontaneous or therapeutic abortion, threatened abortion, or ectopic pregnancy prior to 13 wk • 300 μg IM dose within 72 h of spontaneous or therapeutic abortion, threatened abortion, or ectopic pregnancy after 13 wk • 300 μg IM dose between 26 and 28 wk of pregnancy; repeat if delivery does not occur within 12 wk • 300 μg IM dose within 72 h of delivery; a higher dose may be calculated if exposure to Rh-positive blood is higher than 15 mL • 300 μg IM dose within 72 h of abdominal trauma or invasive procedure, such as amniocentesis
Care considerations	• Never use in Rh-positive individuals. • Do not administer to a neonate. • This is a blood product. Patient identity verification is critical, and blood product protocols must be followed per institution.
Warning signs	Monitor for anaphylaxis.

IM, intramuscular.

Box 5.2 Religious Convictions Regarding Blood Transfusions

Rh₀ (D) immune globulin is a blood product. Some people adhere to specific belief structures that prohibit the use of blood products. Some Jehovah's Witnesses and Christian Scientists, for example, may refuse Rh₀ (D) immune globulin for reasons of religious conviction. Such patients may be asked to sign a refusal indicating they have been educated about Rh₀ (D) immune globulin and understand the potential harm of refusing it.

---

visit and that she is taking a prenatal vitamin every morning. Dr. Janachek suggests moving her dose to the evening, as the vitamin makes some women nauseous and as pregnant women typically have less nausea in the evening.

Second Trimester

Dr. Janachek was right to be optimistic. The bleeding stops and does not return. Letitia completes her prenatal screening, as recommended (Box 5.3). She returns to the office for monthly visits with Dr. Janachek starting in week 12. At 20 weeks, she and Don watch the fetus by ultrasound. Letitia thinks it looks like a fish the way it swishes within the uterus. They give it the in utero name of Neptune. At 26 weeks, she gets another injection of Rh₀ (D) immune globulin. At 28 weeks, she starts coming in every other week for her visits.

With every test, particularly the early ones, Letitia tenses. She frets until the results come back showing that everything is

---

Box 5.3 Letitia's Schedule of Routine Prenatal Assessments

First Trimester

Screening for trisomies

Blood test 12 wk

- *Pregnancy-associated plasma protein:* low in abnormal test
- *Human chorionic gonadotropin:* high in abnormal test

Ultrasound between 12 wk

- *Nuchal Translucency (measurement by ultrasound of space at the back of the fetal neck):* Thick in abnormal test

Second Trimester

Integrated screening: Additional labs drawn at 16 wk (in addition to first trimester screening labs and ultrasound)

- *Maternal serum alpha-fetoprotein:* high levels associated with neural tube defects, low levels associated with Down syndrome
- *Human chorionic gonadotropin:* high levels associated with Down syndrome, low levels associated with trisomy 18
- *Unconjugated estriol:* low in Down syndrome and some neural tube defects
- *Inhibin-A:* high in Down syndrome

Fetal survey ultrasound (20 wk)

50 g one-hour glucose screen for diabetes (26 wk)

Third Trimester

Vaginal and rectal swab for Group B strep (36 wk)

normal. She knows that many miscarriages result from genetic anomalies of the pregnancy. She wonders whether this is what caused the miscarriage. She hopes so, because it would mean that nothing was wrong with her, that it was just a problem with that particular pregnancy, and that future pregnancies might be fine. She worries that maybe this pregnancy has similar defects, but that her quality control system just hasn't caught the problem the second time around. But all of the tests—the first trimester screening, the integrated screening, and Neptune's 20-week fetal survey ultrasound—all indicate that the pregnancy is fine. She's also relieved to learn that she doesn't have gestational diabetes.

Third Trimester

At 36 weeks, she visits Dr. Janachek again. Dr. Janachek feels all over her belly, explaining that she is trying to determine the position of the baby (see Fig. 1.7).

"The good news is that the little one is head down," she says. "I don't think the head is engaged, though. That basically means the baby has not deep down in your pelvis yet" (Fig. 5.4).

"Is that bad?" asks Letitia.

"It's not bad," says Dr. Janachek. "Babies typically engage at around thirty-eight weeks. Some don't even engage until labor. You still have plenty of time. We'll check again next week."

Dr. Janachek then has Letitia put her feet into the metal stirrups and slide her bottom down to the edge of the table. She swabs the rectum and the opening of the vagina, the introitus, for group B streptococcus. She adds some lubricant to her gloved fingers and reaches inside Letitia's vagina to feel her cervix. She frowns.

"You're dilated about three centimeters," she says. "That's fine, but I'd like it better if that fetal head was a little lower. We'll check again next week, but in the meantime, go ahead and pack your hospital bag and keep the office on speed dial."

Before the next scheduled check, Letitia starts to have contractions.

Labor and Delivery

She's been doing fetal movement counts since about week 30 (Analyze the Evidence 5.1; Box 5.4). Neptune has scared her a few times by not moving as often as she thought he should. Her usual approach is to lie quietly on her side and pay attention to the fetus until she feels 10 movements. Usually this happens within a half hour, but sometimes it takes as long as 2 hours. She called Dr. Janachek's office a couple of times about it. A nurse named Alicia called her back both times, and they talked about the normalcy of fetuses napping for up to 40 minutes at a time. And almost as if Neptune were listening, he moved his knees and elbows across her belly so it looked like she was carrying a litter of kittens instead of a single baby.

Sometimes this movement was so intense, particularly when the fetus stretched, that she thought it must be something like what a contraction feels like. But one morning, contractions begin and she quickly realizes that they are different. They are starting first thing in the morning, for one thing. This is unusual, because, like most third trimester fetuses, Neptune generally becomes more active throughout the day, and seems most active when Letitia is trying to sleep. And the contractions have a vise-like tightness, not a stretching tightness.

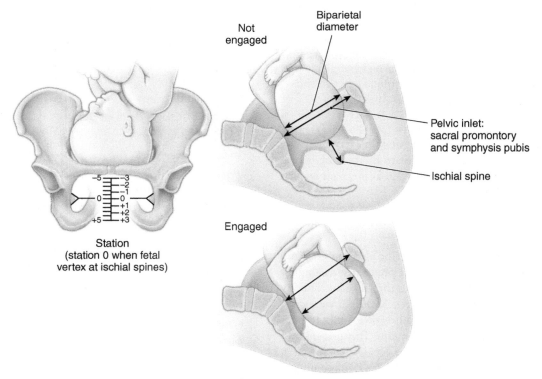

Figure 5.4. Fetal engagement. (Reprinted with permission from Beckmann, C. R., Herbert, W., Laube, D., Ling, F., & Smith, R. [2013]. *Obstetrics and gynecology* [7th ed., Fig. 8.4]. Philadelphia, PA: Lippincott Williams & Wilkins.)

Analyze the Evidence 5.1 Fetal Movement Count

Pro	Con
A large cohort study of 65,550 women found that maternal reporting of the following reduced the stillbirth rate from 4.2% to 2.4% (Tveit et al., 2009):	Although there is sound evidence that increased fetal movement is associated with positive fetal outcomes and decreased activity is associated with stillbirth, there is little consensus as to when women should be told to report reduced fetal movement and what evaluation and intervention is indicated (Flenady et al., 2009). To date, no robust studies exist to evaluate appropriate management strategies (Hofmeyr & Novikova, 2012).

1. Overall perception of reduced movement
2. Reporting reduced movement the same day it is perceived
3. Reporting if the fetus has moved less in a course of a single day or multiple days
4. Perception of fewer than 10 movements in 2 h during a typically active period

---

Box 5.4 Fetal Movement Count Methods

- Count to 10 method: At least 10 fetal movements over up to 2 h when pregnant woman is at rest
- At least 10 fetal movement during 12 h of normal maternal activity
- At least 4 fetal movements in an hour when the mother is at rest
- At least 10 fetal movements in 25 min for pregnancies 22–36 wk and 10 fetal movements in 35 min for pregnancies 37 or more weeks

Data from Heazell, A. E., & Froen, J. F. (2008). Methods of fetal movement counting and the detection of fetal compromise. *Journal of Obstetrics and Gynaecology, 28*(2), 147–154.

Box 5.5 Letitia's Hospital Bag

- Two changes of maternity clothes (she does not expect to fit into her regular clothes for some time)
- Tennis balls for Don to press into the small of her back in case of back labor
- A Bluetooth speaker for her phone to play music
- Mints
- A nursing bra
- Three pairs of socks
- A bag of travel toiletries
- A nightgown
- An extra phone charger
- Going home outfit for Neptune

Box 5.6 Letitia's Birth Plan

- My husband Don is my support person.
- I'd prefer my water to break on its own.
- I want to be able to get up and walk around.
- I prefer intermittent instead of continuous fetal monitoring.
- I would like to avoid all pain medications unless specifically requested.
- I'd like to be allowed to push according to instinct.
- I'd like to avoid an episiotomy.
- I would like to give birth in a squatting position.
- I would like to use a mirror to watch my baby being born.
- I would like the cord to stop pulsing before it is cut.
- Don would like to cut the umbilical cord.
- I would like to hold the baby skin to skin immediately after the birth.
- I would like to try to breastfeed the baby immediately after the birth.
- We would like to room with the baby and participate in all infant care.
- If the baby is a boy, we do not want him to be circumcised.

She wakes up Don and is impressed by how quickly he finds the stopwatch on his smartphone. Letitia recalls the mnemonic "411" that Dr. Janachek taught her to help her determine whether she is in active labor. It means that she should head to the birthing center when her contractions are 4 minutes apart or less, last for at least 1 minute each, and occur in this manner for at least 1 hour.

"Wait," says Don. "Is it four minutes from the end of one contraction until the beginning of the next?"

"No," says Letitia. She is lying on her side with her hand on her belly feeling Neptune churn. "It's four minutes from the start of one contraction until the start of the next one."

"Oh. Well, in that case, I think we have that."

"Just keep timing," says Letitia, as another contraction begins to swell. When it's over, she gets up from the bed, changes into maternity sweats, and retrieves the duffle bag packed with things for the hospital from the closet (Box 5.5). "Just in case," she tells Don, and adds two freshly printed copies of her birth plan to the bag (Box 5.6).

"I'm calling the office," says Don. "And then we're going." Letitia's contractions are 3 minutes apart and lasting over a minute each. Don has decided the third requirement of "411" can just be implied. He makes the call and rushes a newly dressed Letitia out

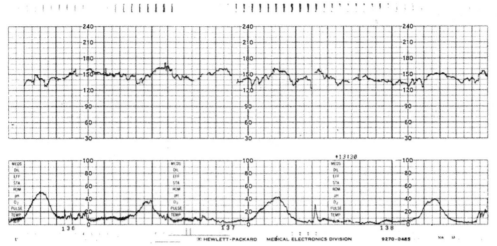

Figure 5.5. Fetal monitoring strip indicating reassuring fetal status. The top graph shows a reassuring fetal heart rate pattern, with good variability, no decelerations, and a heart rate of about 150 beats per minute. The bottom graph shows the mother's uterine contractions. (Reprinted with permission from Cabaniss, M. L., & Ross, M. G. [2009]. *Fetal monitoring interpretation* [2nd ed., Fig. 5.1]. Philadelphia, PA: Lippincott Williams & Wilkins.)

the door between contractions. Seconds later, he runs back into the house to retrieve his car keys from the hook inside the door.

The birthing center seems peaceful, almost eerily quiet when they arrive, and the nurse, Polly, who takes them to triage says that it's been a quiet night, with only one birth, which finished hours before. She confirms Letitia's health information, which was previously uploaded by staff at Dr. Janachek's office, and listens to Don's account about the timing of the contractions.

"The result from your group B strep test is back," says Polly. "It's negative, so you don't need an antibiotic right now."

Polly affixes the contraction monitor, which she calls a "toco," onto her belly below her rib cage and the fetal monitor on the lower part of the swell of her belly. She performs the Leopold's maneuvers on her belly, as Dr. Janachek did, to determine the position of baby Neptune. Satisfied with her exam, she moves the round pink fetal heart monitor over the lower right side of Letitia's belly.

"I think this little one is still high up in your belly," says Polly, before finding the sweet spot where she identifies a strong, reassuring fetal heart rate (Fig. 5.5).

"Is that bad?" asks Don, who didn't attend Letitia's most recent visit with Dr. Janachek.

"It's not bad, exactly," says Polly. "But we want to keep a careful eye on her. What we don't want is for the umbilical cord to slip between the baby and the mother's pelvis. That could compress the cord so that the baby isn't getting enough oxygen, a condition called **cord prolapse**."

"Well that sounds bad to me," says Don. He's holding Letitia's hand, and he looks at her apologetically.

"Cord prolapse is pretty rare," says Polly, "and harm to the baby is even more rare. We run drills here, so everyone on the team knows what to do if it happens. It's not likely to happen, but if it does, you have an excellent team to take care of it."

Remarkably, Letitia's amniotic sac breaks then, at the very moment that Dr. Janachek enters the room wearing blue scrubs.

In less than a minute, Dr. Janachek puts on a sterile glove and performs a vaginal examination. She looks at the fetal monitor (Fig. 5.6) and then at Polly.

"Prolapse protocol," she says calmly but firmly, and Polly hits a red button on the wall.

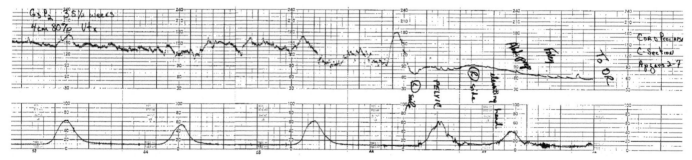

Figure 5.6. Fetal monitoring strip indicating nonreassuring fetal status, as may be seen with cord prolapse. Shown are fetal bradycardia, minimal or absent variability, and prolonged deceleration. (Reprinted with permission from Freeman, K. F., Garite, T. J., Nageotte, M. P., & Miller, L. A. [2012]. *Fetal heart rate monitoring* [4th ed., Fig. 6-25]. Philadelphia, PA: Lippincott Williams & Wilkins.)

Things move very quickly after that.

Polly puts a mask over Letitia's face, explaining that it may smell a little funny but that it's just oxygen.

Dr. Janachek's hand is still inside of Letitia.

"The cord is in your vagina ahead of the baby's head," says Dr. Janachek, who then instructs Polly to lower the head of the bed to Trendelenburg position.

"I was just telling her how this wouldn't happen," says Polly, to no one in particular. "I'm sorry."

"We need to relieve the pressure that the head is putting on the cord," explains Dr. Janachek. "A lack of oxygen to the baby can be dangerous and is causing an abnormal fetal heart rate and rhythm—what we call a **nonreassuring fetal status**. I know this is uncomfortable. I am manually lifting the head off the cord right now, but I can't do it for long. By lowering your head and keeping your bottom up, I'm hoping to get a little extra help. Polly has called the emergency delivery team. I'm sorry, but we need to perform a cesarean delivery right now."

It's all happening incredibly quickly. As she finishes talking, Dr. Janachek climbs onto Letitia's bed with her, her fingers still inside of her vagina, keeping the fetal head elevated and off the cord. There's a loud click as the brake is released from the bed and a team of two nurses, neither of them Polly, wheels the bed into a surgical suite at the end of the hall. Someone has covered the lower part of Leticia's body with a sheet for privacy.

In the surgical suite, a small woman in blue scrubs and a surgical mask appears at the head of the bed. She's wearing a cotton surgical cap covered with rainbow-colored lobsters.

"I'm Dr. Tripp," she says. "I will be administering the anesthesia. Have you ever had anesthesia before in the past?"

"No, I don't think so," says Letitia. She feels sick and breathless. The contractions are still coming, and the counterpressure Dr. Janachek is applying to keep the baby up off the cord feels tremendous. Don wipes away the tears that are streaming onto her forehead with his fingertips. She realizes that she is crying. "Am I getting an epidural?"

"I wouldn't recommend it," says Dr. Tripp. "An epidural would take too long. I'd strongly recommend general anesthetic. We'll bring you back up just as soon as we can. When did you last eat?"

"Last night," says Letitia. "I was tired. I think we ate around six and I went to bed soon after."

"Good," says Dr. Tripp.

Letitia doesn't ask why that is good. She holds closely to Don's hand, which is damp with her tears.

"She'll be okay," says Don, more a confirmation than a question.

"Yes," says Dr. Tripp.

Polly starts an intravenous (IV) line in Letitia's left wrist and gives her hand a squeeze with both of hers. "We've got this," she tells Letitia and Don. "You're in the very best place for this to happen."

Another masked person in a surgical cap comes into the room. He introduces himself as Dr. Needam, a pediatrician here on an "as needed basis." He seems inappropriately cheerful, almost jocular.

Polly asks Don to put on some scrubs, a hat, and a mask.

"I can stay?" he asks her.

"You can stay," she says. "Just make sure you stand where people tell you to."

Dr. Tripp says to Letitia, "I'm going to give you some medication by mask that's going to make you sleepy. Take deep, slow breaths."

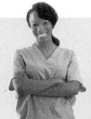

The Nurse's Point of View

Polly: As far as I'm concerned, umbilical cord prolapse is one of the scariest obstetric complications. Going through an entire pregnancy and then facing losing it at the very last moment is almost unimaginable. Fortunately, it's also pretty uncommon, occurring in less than one in five hundred births (Gibbons, O'Herlihy, & Murphy, 2014). That's why, even though I've worked on this floor for a while, I've never seen it happen until now. It's also why we run drills—so that if it does happen, we still know what to do.

I knew that Leticia was at risk for cord prolapse because the presenting part of the fetus, the head, wasn't engaged in the pelvis, giving the cord room to be washed out when her water breaks. Also, this baby is not quite term, and prematurity increases the risk, as well.

Right after Leticia's water breaks, I look at the screen right away. It's the single most important thing you can do after the water breaks, checking to see what the fetal heart rate is. What I see is a prolonged dip in the fetal heart rate, called bradycardia. The diagnosis of cord prolapse is confirmed when Dr. Janachek feels the cord inside of Letitia's vagina.

When Dr. Janachek says, "cord prolapse protocol," what she is asking for is notification of the nursing staff, an anesthetist, and the pediatric team, and the immediate preparation of an operating room. As do a lot of hospitals, we have an operating room right in the birthing center.

Dr. Janachek stays in position holding the fetus' head up off of the pelvis as much as possible to minimize compression of the cord. It's important to minimize manipulating the cord and to avoid exposing it to cold, which could happen if the cord prolapsed outside of the vagina, which is not the case here. Too much manipulation or cold exposure can lead to vasospasm of the cord, which can compromise fetal oxygenation just as cord compression can.

A prolapse can be overt or occult. With an occult prolapse, the cord is alongside the presenting part. With an overt prolapse, such as this one, the cord comes out ahead of the presenting part.

Delivery is a top priority with cord prolapse. Sometimes if the prolapse is occult, a vaginal delivery can be managed. Most of the time, however, an emergency cesarean section is needed. Leticia arrived just before everything started happening. I don't even know what her plans were for coping with pain. If a woman already has a neuraxial catheter in place for epidural or spinal anesthesia, sometimes this can be used for cesarean section anesthesia. As it is, starting something like that would take way more time than we have. That's why she will have to have general anesthesia.

Though the fetal heart rate is an important indication of fetal well-being, honestly, we hardly glance at it as we move Letitia to the operating room. An emergency cesarean section must occur either way.

Time is the important thing. The faster the baby is delivered, the less compromise there is to oxygenation. The longer the fetus stays in with a compressed cord, the more likely damage will occur because of poor oxygenation. That's why it's a good thing that Letitia arrived when she did. If this had happened at home, it would have taken much longer to deliver the baby. It might not have made it.

After Delivery

Letitia feels consciousness return to her in waves, like the ocean lapping the shore. It surges up a little, immersing her, and then falls back, a little more, and then rolls back in. She tries to open her eyes several times before she is successful, and it seems like sometimes her ears work and other times they don't. Her mouth feels strange, as though it has forgotten how to make saliva. She hears a baby cry, and then she doesn't.

"In retrospect," she says, her eyes still closed. "I'm not sure I should have spent as much time as I did working on that birth plan."

She hears a baby crying again.

Letitia feels strong, cool hands roll her onto her side. She vomits, and opens her eyes in time to see a pink, kidney-shaped emesis basin make its exit. The cool, strong hands return, and Letitia feels the blood pressure cuff on her arm being adjusted before it starts to inflate (Table 5.2).

"I feel better and kind of gross," she says to no one in particular. "I'm glad," says a male voice. It's Don. "We have a baby girl."

"A girl," says Letitia. "Neptune is a terrible name for a girl."

Letitia feels suddenly anxious and moves to sit up and then remembers, more or less, the events of the last few hours. "Is she okay? Am I okay? Why doesn't this hurt more? I thought I'd hurt more."

The person attached to the hands that held the emesis basin returns. The nurse introduces herself as Sheila. She explains that Letitia is receiving IV oxytocin for pain and will switch to oral oxycodone once her IV is discontinued.

Table 5.2 Letitia's Postoperative Cesarean Section Orders

Vital signs	• Every 15 min for the first hour • Every 30 min for the second hour • Every hour for the third and fourth hours • Every 4 h for next 8 h • Every 8 h after first 12 h **Report the following findings to the primary care provider:** • Systolic BP <90 or >150 mm Hg • Diastolic BP <50 or >100 mm Hg • Pulse <50 or >120 mm Hg • Temperature >38.0°F after the first 24 • Respiratory rate <10 or >20 breaths per minute
Exam	• Check the uterine fundus and lochia with every set of vital signs. • Using a numeric pain scale, assess pain with vital signs, prior to the administration of analgesics, and within an hour after administering analgesics.

Wound care	• Assess the incision dressing for bleeding, moisture, and odor every 4 h for 24 h.
	• After 24 h, remove the dressing, assess the wound, and change the dressing at every vital sign check. Assess for the following:
	  ◦ The wound edges should be well approximated.
	  ◦ The wound discharge should be scant.
	  ◦ No redness should be present around the incision site.

IV administration	• 30 units of oxytocin diluted in 500 mL of lactated Ringer's solution administered as follows:
	  ◦ 200 mL/h for the first hour
	  ◦ 135 mL/h for the second hour
	  ◦ 50 mL/h for next 4 h
	• If oral intake is <500 mL per shift, switch to dextrose 5% in 0.45% normal saline with 20 mEq KCl/L after oxytocin is finished.
	• Once oral intake is >500 mL per shift, switch to a saline lock.
	• The saline lock may be discontinued once oral intake is tolerated and oxytocin administration is complete.

Table 5.2	**Letitia's Postoperative Cesarean Section Orders (continued)**
Intake and output	• Monitor hourly for the first 2 h. • Monitor every 4 h for the next 8 h. • After the first 10 h, monitor every 8 h until both the IV and Foley urinary catheter are discontinued. • The Foley catheter may be discontinued when the patient is able to ambulate independently to the bathroom. **Report the following finding to the primary care provider:** • Output <30 mL/h
Analgesia	• Ibuprofen by mouth 600 mg every 6 h as needed • Acetaminophen by mouth 650 mg every 6 h as needed • Oxycodone immediate release by mouth 5–10 mg every 4 h as needed
Activity	• Early and frequent ambulation should be encouraged. • Sequential compression devices should remain in place on the lower legs until the patient is ambulating regularly. • Initial ambulation should be supervised. • The patient may shower after the removal of the initial incision dressing.
Serum testing and injection	• Kleihauer–Betke test on maternal blood to determine the volume of fetal blood transfer • Rh$_o$ (D) immune globulin injection based on Kleihauer–Betke test results (in the absence of significant transfer, the typical dose is 300 µg)

BP, blood pressure; IV, intravenous.

"You may find you don't need it long," says Sheila. "Most women recover well from a cesarean section."

Don folds back the blanket he's holding. A baby peers out, its eyes unfocused and face flushed. Letitia automatically reaches out her arms. What she feels isn't love exactly. It's more of an overwhelming maternal protectiveness. She feels like, if threatened, she could get up—despite having a catheter and IV and being in recovery from major abdominal surgery—and run with the baby to safety if she needed to. The baby looks toward her with dark gray eyes. Letitia looks up at Sheila.

"I'd like to breastfeed her," Letitia says. "I read that you're supposed to do that for the first time as soon as possible. Should I do it now? What about the oxytocin?"

"That's a great idea," says Sheila. "We don't believe that enough of the oxytocin gets into your milk to make a difference. Some women prefer to nurse their babies before they get their meds, however, just in case. I will warn you, however, that nursing causes your uterus to contract, and that can be painful for the first day or so. It can be helpful to be on your painkillers when you're getting started."

Letitia nods. "Well, the oxytocin is here now and she's awake. Let's do it."

Sheila helps Letitia unwrap the baby and places her tummy to tummy on top of her mother, skin to skin. She places a freshly warmed blanket over the pair of them. All three adults watch as the little one seems to scoot and shift her way toward Letitia's nipple, occasionally making small noises and seeming to sniff.

"I'm not sure what I should be doing," says Letitia. "Should I be getting her into position or something?"

"You could," says Sheila. "But babies can be smarter than we give them credit for. You have plenty of time to work on perfecting your breastfeeding technique. I think of this first feed as

a time for the two of you to get to know each other, you know, to get used to how you both smell and feel. She can find that nipple all by herself without any help. We have her in the right neighborhood. Just watch her go."

It takes a little time, but the baby does find her own way to the nipple, which she clamps onto with messy enthusiasm and, Letitia thinks, a small look of triumph. Letitia plays with the baby's hands and counts fingers and toes. She notes some little white bumps across the top of her nose. Milia, Sheila calls the bumps, explaining that they'd resolve within a few weeks and that they don't hurt (Fig. 5.7).

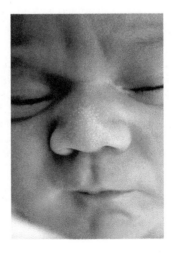

Figure 5.7. Milia. Very common on the faces of newborns, milia typically resolves within a few weeks without intervention. (Reprinted with permission from Jensen, S. [2015]. *Nursing health assessment* [2nd ed., unnumbered figure in Table 26.2, p. 829]. Philadelphia, PA: Lippincott Williams & Wilkins.)

Something wet falls onto the top of Letitia's head, once and then twice. She looks up and sees that Don is standing over her, watching his wife and daughter and crying tremendous tears behind his glasses and making no effort to wipe them away. She touches his face gently.

"I've never seen you cry," she says, and then realizes she's crying as well.

"I've never been so terrified," he says. "Just so, so terrified."

Recovery is easier than she expected, even with Sheila's reassurances. She walks the halls of the postpartum floor frequently, often pushing the baby in her little clear bassinet. She sees her incision after the initial bulky dressing is removed after 24 hours and is surprised to see such a little scar, a pale pink smile with interior stitches. Blood from the baby's umbilical cord is checked and found to be Rh positive. Letitia's blood is taken for a test called a Kleihauer–Betke, which she is informed would reveal whether more than 15 mL of fetal blood transferred to her own bloodstream, which would indicate she would need a larger dose of Rh$_o$ (D) immune globulin to avoid becoming sensitive to the baby's Rh-positive blood, which could harm a future pregnancy (as impossible as the idea of a future pregnancy seemed). The test comes back negative, and before the 72-hour mark, she receives a regular 300-µg dose of Rh$_o$ (D) immune globulin intramuscularly.

The Newborn

Earlier, soon after the birth, Don told Letitia that the baby's Apgar score at 1 minute was 6 but that it climbed to 8 by 5 minutes (see Table 1.4). She weighed 5 lb 5 oz. Her fingernails were perfect pink shells with only a suggestion of blue at the base of the nail beds. Letitia and Don decided to name her Salacia, after Neptune's wife, and call her Laci.

Debra, a neonatal nurse practitioner who works in the neonatal intensive care unit, informed them that because she was born between 34 and 36 weeks, 6 days gestation, Laci is considered a **late preterm infant**. Although most late preterm infants (about 6.8% of all births in the United States in 2015 [Hamilton, Martin, & Osterman, 2016]) are healthy and have an uneventful course after birth, Debra explained, they are at greater risk for some complications (Table 5.3).

Table 5.3   Increased Risks for Late Preterm Infants

Problem	Nursing Considerations
Hypoglycemia (low blood sugar)—the risk is approximately three times higher for late preterm infants than for term infants, likely because their immature system does not allow for an adequate metabolic response to premature removal from the maternal glucose supply. It's not uncommon for neonates to experience transient hypoglycemia as they transition to life outside the womb, but serum glucose levels typically do not drop below 40 mg/dL and numbers stabilize between 45 and 80 mg/dL at 6 h after birth.	Skin-to-skin contact and frequent feedings, breast or bottle, are good beginning strategies. Screen for hypoglycemia per institution protocols. A common protocol is screening prior to first feeding and then prior to feedings every 3–6 h for 24–48 h. *Symptoms of hypoglycemia* include jitteriness, poor feeding, poor muscle tone, changes in level of consciousness, rapid breathing, hypothermia, central cyanosis (blue skin color in areas besides hands and feet), bradycardia, apnea.
Hypothermia (body temperature below normal)—late preterm infants have less fat and less ability to maintain body heat.	Temperature should be maintained between 36.5°C and 37.4°C. Skin-to-skin contact with parents can be an excellent strategy. Temperature should be checked frequently until stable. No bath until temperature has been stable for at least an hour.
Hyperbilirubinemia (high bilirubin)—this is an excess of bilirubin that builds up in the blood and causes a yellowing of the skin and the sclera (whites of eyes). It is not uncommon for some yellowing (jaundice) to occur even in healthy infants, but when too much bilirubin accumulates, it can lead to serious acute and chronic neurologic problems.	Though an initial assessment of jaundice may be made visually, it should always be affirmed by testing. Many institutions have standing orders in place to assess for jaundice. A common screening test evaluates light reflecting from the skin's surface, and is known as a transcutaneous bilirubin. Hospital protocols may call for a single transcutaneous bilirubin assessment the evening prior to the day of discharge or may indicate more frequent screening as often as every 8–12 h while hospitalized. Abnormal results must always be confirmed and followed with serum bilirubin testing. • Feedings often aid in the excretion of bilirubin, and feedings are encouraged 8–12 times daily. • Confirmed high levels of bilirubin are typically successfully treated by light therapy. • Rarely, exchange transfusions of blood may be warranted.

Table 5.3 Increased Risks for Late Preterm Infants (continued)	
Problem	**Nursing Considerations**
Feeding problems—late preterm infants often have difficulty coordinating the suck, swallow, and breathing required for successful feeding.	• A lactation consultant should be a part of the care team. • Frequent assessment of latch and feeding efforts is indicated. • A nipple shield may be used to aid the infant in establishing a productive latch. • Infants may be weighed before and after feeding to determine intake. • Supplementation with pumped breast milk or formula is indicated for infants who lose more than 7% of their birth weight. • Mothers may be instructed to pump their breast milk immediately after nursing to encourage milk production and accumulate a supply of pumped milk should supplementation be indicated.
Respiratory problems—may be mild or life-threatening and include respiratory distress syndrome, transient tachypnea, and persistent pulmonary hypertension. All of these issues are likely related to immature organs development. • Transient tachypnea—caused by fluid not cleared from lungs during birth • Respiratory distress syndrome—insufficient surfactant in lung. Surfactant keeps the alveolar surfaces from sticking together, allowing the lungs to expand • Persistent pulmonary hypertension—a condition causing right-to-left shunting of deoxygenated blood through the foramen ovule causing hypoxemia	Nurses should always be vigilant for respiratory distress in neonates. Any changes should be immediately reported to the neonate's primary care provider. Signs include the following: • Nasal flaring • Tachypnea • Grunting • Cyanosis (blue skin tone) beyond hands and feet • Intercostal and subcostal retractions (the appearance that the spaces between the bones are being "sucked in" with breathing) • Seesaw breathing, in which the stomach rises as the chest falls and vice versa
Apnea—short pauses in breathing of 5–10 s is normal in neonates. When breathing ceases for 20 or more seconds, or when oxygen desaturation occurs, it is considered apnea. In premature infants it is thought to result from immature control of respiration.	Typically resolves spontaneously but intervention may be required. Episodes of apnea witnessed by nurse or neonate's family members should be reported to the primary care provider.

Data from Leone, A., Ersfeld, P., Adams, M., Schiffer, P. M., Bucher, H., & Arlettaz, R. (2011). Neonatal morbidity in singleton late preterm infants compared with full-term infants. *Acta Paediatrica, 101*(1), e6–e10; Stanley, C. A., Rozance, P. J., Thornton, P. S., Leon, D. D., Harris, D., Haymond, M. W., . . . Wolfsdorf, J. I. (2015). Re-evaluating "Transitional Neonatal Hypoglycemia": Mechanism and implications for management. *Journal of Pediatrics, 166*(6), 1520.e1–1525.e1; and Veit, L., Amberson, M., Freiberger, C., Montenegro, B., Mukhopadhyay, S., & Rhein, L. M. (2016). Diagnostic evaluation and home monitor use in late preterm to term infants with apnea, bradycardia, and desaturations. *Clinical Pediatrics, 55*, 1210–1218.

For example, Debra continued, she is more likely than a term baby to have hypoglycemia. Therefore, she would need to have her glucose checked regularly every 3 to 6 hours for 24 to 48 hours just prior to feeding (see Step-by-Step Skills 3.1 and Box 3.10) (Harris and Weston, 2012). She is also more likely to suffer from hypothermia. It is recommended that she be held skin to skin and kept warmly wrapped and that her temperature be checked frequently (Fig. 5.8).

She is at great risk for hyperbilirubinemia, too, a potentially dangerous condition in which her body does not sufficiently eliminate a product that results from the breakdown of red blood cells. She would need to be evaluated for this regularly by visual inspection as well as by transcutaneous bilirubin monitoring and a nomogram to interpret the level of risk associated with her serum level of bilirubin (Fig. 5.9). As with many late preterm babies, she is more likely to

have trouble coordinating the sucking, swallowing, and breathing required to feed and would require special evaluation from a lactation consultant. Her nurses and her parents would need to monitor her for signs of respiratory distress such as tachypnea, nasal flaring, and retractions (Fig. 5.10), as well as for cessation of breathing altogether for 20 seconds or more, a condition called apnea (Box 5.7).

"I don't understand," said Don. He was sitting in a chair next to Letitia's bed. Laci was in his arms, asleep. "She looks perfectly healthy, just a little tiny."

"She likely is perfectly healthy," said Debra. "But she is premature—late preterm, but still not term. The last few weeks of a term pregnancy, which Laci is experiencing outside the womb, aren't just about putting on weight. Many developmental changes occur during this time, especially in the central nervous system.

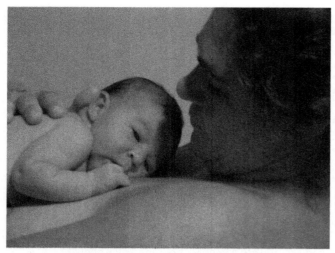

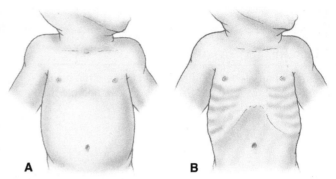

Figure 5.10. Infant intercostal retractions. (A) Normal inspiratory appearance of the chest during unobstructed breathing in the neonate. **(B)** Sternal and intercostal retractions during obstructed breathing in the neonate. This finding indicates respiratory distress of the infant and should be immediately reported and further evaluated. (Reprinted with permission from Porth, C. M. [2015]. *Essentials of pathophysiology: Concepts of altered health states* [4th ed., Fig. 22-11]. Philadelphia, PA: Lippincott Williams & Wilkins.)

Figure 5.8. Skin-to-skin contact, also called kangaroo care. Infants' temperatures are often best regulated by placing them in direct contact with their mothers' skin. (Reprinted with permission from Osborne, C. [2011]. *Pre- and perinatal massage therapy: A comprehensive guide to prenatal, labor, and postpartum practice* [2nd ed., Fig. 6-1]. Philadelphia, PA: Lippincott Williams & Wilkins.)

She's still laying down all the right wiring to coordinate things like breathing and eating, which her body really isn't programmed to do independently for a few more weeks. She'll likely catch up quickly, but we need to keep a careful eye on her in the meantime just to make sure she doesn't need extra help."

"It's funny," said Don. "I never really thought about it. I always thought that being a preemie just meant being a tiny kid. I never thought about the rest of it."

"If you're lucky," said Debra, "you will never truly have to."

"Breastfeeding isn't as straightforward as I thought it would be," said Don. He was watching Laci and Letitia work with a lactation consultant named Brenda. It was almost 24 hours since the birth.

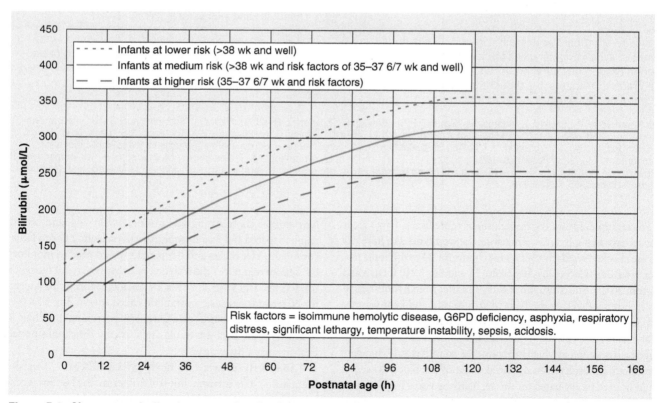

Figure 5.9. Nomogram indicating serum levels of bilirubin in the neonate. (Reprinted with permission from Chowdhury, S. H., Cozma, A. L., & Chowdhury, J. H. [2017]. *Essentials for the Canadian Medical Licensing Exam: Review and prep for MCCQE Part I* [2nd ed., Fig. 18-2]. Philadelphia, PA: Lippincott Williams & Wilkins.)

Box 5.7 Schedule of Nursing Evaluations and Interventions for Laci

Delivery Room Evaluations

- Assessment of muscle tone
- Assessment of crying and/or breathing
- Apgar scoring at 1 and 5 min (see Table 1.4)
  - Heart rate
  - Respiratory effort
  - Muscle tone
  - Reflexes
  - Color
- Vital signs (temperature, respiratory rate, heart rate)
- Measurements: length, weight, head circumference
- Sex determination, general survey for overt malformation

Delivery Room Interventions

- Routine erythromycin 0.5% ointment in eyes to prevent gonococcal ophthalmia
- Routine 1-mg vitamin K injection intramuscular to prevent bleeding due to vitamin K deficiency
- When Letitia is alert enough, breastfeeding should be attempted, preferably in first hour after birth
- Laci's blood glucose should be checked with sample obtained by heel stick within an hour of the birth after feeding
  - Hypoglycemic if *asymptomatic* with glucose <25 mg/dL
  - Hypoglycemic if *symptomatic* with glucose <50 mg/dL

Transitional Period (First 4–6 h) Evaluations: Every 30–60 min

- *Temperature* should stay between 36.5°C and 37.5°C. Infants with infections may have a temperature that is high or low. Hypothermia can lead to hypoglycemia or acidosis. Late preterm infants like Laci are more likely to experience hypothermia.
- *Heart rate* is anticipated to stay between 120 and 160 beats per minute, though it may drop below 100 in deep sleep and rise about 170 with crying. A sustained high or low heart rate is suspicious for cardiac disease. Heart rate should be counted for a full minute.
- *Color* of a neonate is typically pink, though hands and feet may be blue (acrocyanosis). Blue trunk, lips, and tongue are called central cyanosis and are concerning for heart or lung disease. Jaundice in this period of time (first 24 h) is unusual and would suggest a serious issue.
- *Tone* refers to flexion of the muscles. Most term infants preferentially stay in a curled position with arms and legs flexed. Hypotonia, poor tone, may indicate a neurologic issue, sepsis, a genetic syndrome, or exposure to maternal medications.
- *Respiratory rate* is expected to stay between 40 and 60 breaths per minute and should be counted for a full minute. In addition to rate, nasal flaring, retractions, and grunting should be evaluated.
- *Glucose* should be checked by heel stick every 3 to 6 h prior to being fed

- If symptomatic:
  - Hypoglycemia if glucose <50 mg/dL
- If asymptomatic:
  - Hypoglycemia if glucose <25 mg/dL within first 4 h
  - Hypoglycemic if glucose <35 mg/dL within 4–24 h

After Transition and Until Discharge

- *Routine vital signs* every 8 h (respirations, heart rate, temperature)
- *Full head to toe physical exam* within 24 h
- *Glucose* by heel stick every 3–6 h prior to being fed for at least 24 h
- If symptomatic:
  - Hypoglycemic if glucose <50 mg/dL within first 48 h
  - Hypoglycemic if glucose <60 mg/dL after first 48 h
- If asymptomatic:
  - Hypoglycemic if glucose <35 mg/dL in first 4–24 h
  - Hypoglycemic if glucose <50 mg/dL in 24–48 h
  - Hypoglycemic if glucose <60 mg/dL after 48 h
- Evaluation for *hyperbilirubinemia* (typically peaks at 72–96 h)
  - A visual assessment that may be followed by transcutaneous evaluation and /or serum testing
  - A serum bilirubin level above the 95th percentile for age is an indication for phototherapy.
- *Breastfeeding* assessment and intervention
  - Direct observation twice daily to assess for latch, swallow, and duration of feeding
    - Feeding challenges may indicate pumping after feeding to stimulate milk production and collect milk for supplementary feedings.
    - Infant weighing before and after feeding may be considered if poor intake is suspected.
    - Infant should not lose more than 7% of birth weight.
    - Breast shields may aid infant to form a productive latch.
- Assessment of *stooling* and *urination*
  - Anticipate one urinary void in first 24 h, two or three in second 24 h, five or six in each of the next 2 d, and six to eight thereafter.
  - First stool (meconium) should occur within the first 24 h. Anticipate at least three stools a day after 3 d.
  - Adequate urination and stooling is a good indication of breast milk intake.

Predischarge Evaluations

- Heel stick for newborn screening after 24 h (Fig. 5.12; Step-by-Step Skills 5.1)
- One-time pulse oximetry between 24 and 48 h
  - Check right hand and foot.
  - Anticipate value of 95% or higher with no more than 4% difference between numbers.
  - Abnormal values may indicate retesting in an hour or urgent referral for suspected cardiac disease.

(continued)

Box 5.7   Schedule of Nursing Evaluations and Interventions for Laci (continued)

- Observed minimum of two successful feeds
- Vital signs within normal range for at least 12 h
- Passage of urine and at least one stool
- Hearing test

Predischarge Interventions

- First in series of three hepatitis B vaccinations
- Follow-up visit with pediatrician scheduled within 48 h of discharge
- Car seat challenge test (Box 5.8)

Note: Specific institutional protocols may vary.
Data from Bhutani, V. K., Johnson, L., & Sivieri, E. M. (1999). Predictive ability of a predischarge hour-specific serum bilirubin for subsequent significant hyperbilirubinemia in healthy term and near-term newborns. *Pediatrics, 103*(1), 1520; Stanley, C. A., Rozance, P. J., Thornton, P. S., Leon, D. D., Harris, D., Haymond, M. W., . . . Wolfsdorf, J. I. (2015). Re-evaluating "Transitional Neonatal Hypoglycemia": Mechanism and implications for management. *Journal of Pediatrics, 166*(6), 1520.e1–1525.e1; and Committee on Fetus and Newborn. (2011). Postnatal glucose homeostasis in late-preterm and term infants. *Pediatrics, 127*(3), 575.

Box 5.8   Car Seat Challenge

A car seat challenge is indicated on discharge for preterm and low–birth weight infants and others who may be at a greater risk for oxygen desaturation, apnea, and bradycardia when placed in a car seat (Arya et al., 2016).

Criteria for Challenge

- Infants should be evaluated in the car seat that will be used to transport them home.
- The duration of the car seat challenge is 90–120 min or the amount of time anticipated to transport the infant.
- Heart and respiratory rates and oxygen saturation will be evaluated throughout the challenge.
- A "failure" is oxygen desaturation below 90% or 93% for more than 10 s according to institution protocol; apnea greater than or equal to 20 s; bradycardia equal to or less than 80 beats per minute.
- Infants failing the challenge may repeat it using a car bed. Discharge may be delayed and further evaluation of infant may be done for heart and respiratory problems.

Correct Car Seat Positioning

- Rear-facing car seat with less than 10 in from top of strap to seat bottom, and less than 5.5 in from crotch strap to seat back.
- Infant's back and buttocks should be placed flat against the back of the seat.
- For very small infants, inserts may be placed on either side between the infant and the sides of the seat to provide lateral support.
- The retainer clip, which holds the two straps together, should always be closed and located at the level of the infant's nipples.
- The car seat should always be located at the back seat of the car, rear facing.

"I hear that a lot," said Brenda. "People are amazed when I tell them that I needed one thousand hours total of clinical as well as coursework to be certified as a lactation consultant. Breastfeeding is not a simple thing. If it were, we wouldn't need lactation consultants."

Brenda was peering down at Laci, who had her lips wrapped around a plastic breast shield laid on top of Letitia's right nipple. Her eyes were open only by the smallest amount. As Letitia watched, Laci's hand started to move toward Laci's mouth and Brenda gently held it.

"Many a fine latch has been broken because the baby has tried to suck on a nipple at the same time as her fingers," Debra said. Still holding onto Laci's hand, she tickled her exposed feet. The baby began a rhythmic sucking motion.

"Is she doing it?" asked Letitia.

"She's doing it," said Brenda. "Do you hear that little click? That's a swallow."

"So she's getting milk?" asked Don.

"Right now she's getting colostrum, which is just right. She doesn't need anything more. Letitia's transitional milk will start coming in in about forty-eight hours." Brenda looked at the baby, who had stopped suckling again. She tickled the little feet again and was rewarded this time, with the baby coming off the nipple. She was asleep. "That's not bad for a little one in the first twenty-four hours," said Brenda. "I do want you to pump after each feeding, however, Letitia. It will help with your milk supply."

Letitia eyed the hospital-grade breast pump (Fig. 5.11) that was sitting next to the bed. "It makes me feel like a cow. I'm not saying I won't do it, I'm just saying that if there were a different way to magically transport the milk from my breasts to the bottle, I'd spend a lot of money to get it."

On the second day, after 24 hours had passed since the birth, the shift nurse, Bethany, came to retrieve Laci for a visit to the nursery for her newborn screening (Fig. 5.12, Step-by-Step Skills 5.2).

"What are you screening for?" asked Letitia. The baby had not left her side since shortly after she'd awoken from the anesthesia, and she felt a suspicious protectiveness of the baby that she knew was ridiculous but somehow felt normal and instinctive.

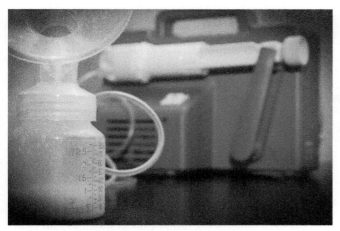

Figure 5.11. **Hospital-grade breast pump.**

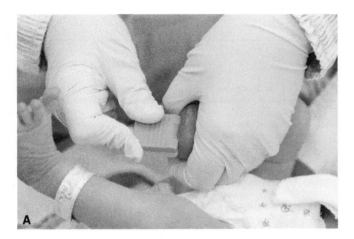

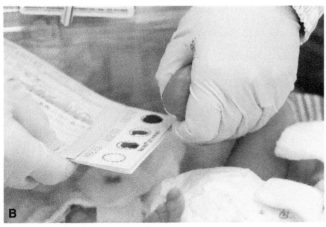

Figure 5.12. **Newborn screening card. (A)** The infant's heel receives a shallow cut for blood collection. **(B)** A nurse milks the infant's foot to obtain the blood needed to completely fill all the circles on the card. (Reprinted with permission from Ricci, S. S. [2013]. *Essentials of maternity, newborn, & women's health nursing* [3rd ed., Fig. 18.22]. Philadelphia, PA: Lippincott Williams & Wilkins.)

 Step-by-Step Skills 5.2

Newborn Screening

1. Collect blank newborn screening card (Fig. 5.12) and equipment for heel stick (see Step-by-Step Skills 3.1).
2. Fill out newborn screening card.
3. Perform infant heel stick (see Fig. 3.6 and Step-by-Step Skills 3.1).
4. Being careful not to touch the infant's heel to the card, fill all circles completely with blood.
5. Put card aside to dry and to be sent to lab for analysis.

"When you say a lot, how many tests do you mean and how much blood?" asked Don.

"In this state we routinely check for twenty-nine different conditions. We don't need much blood," said Bethany. "I'll stick her heel just like we do when checking her blood sugar. I'll have a piece of marked paper with five circles on it, each about an inch across. I need to saturate those five circles with blood. That's it. No vials or needles are involved."

Laci's blood sugar remained in the normal range for the first 24 hours and, besides a single check on the second day, no further screening was indicated for hypoglycemia. The color of her skin was evaluated frequently, first for central cyanosis and then for jaundice. She had a transcutaneous evaluation for jaundice daily, but her levels remained between the 50th and 65th percentiles, and no blood tests were indicated.

Also on the second day, Bethany performed a pulse oximetry. She recorded levels from Laci's right hand and right foot and compared them. Both levels were above the 95th percentile and were within a point of each other. No further evaluation was required for heart disease based on this screening.

By the third day, Letitia's milk came in vigorously. She woke to find her breasts firm and nearly painful. So engorged were they that Letitia feared Laci wouldn't be able to latch, and Letitia was forced to pump some of the milk before her daughter awoke to be fed. Every day Laci's suck and swallow became progressively more coordinated. Both Letitia and her care team were convinced by the plentiful wet diapers and the number of daily stools that she was well fed. She dipped 7% from her birth weight, but dropped no further.

On the morning of the fifth day since birth, the day they are to be discharged, Laci makes her last visit to the nursery. An audiologist tests her hearing (Don and Letitia are told that this would happen without waking the baby, which seems like nothing short of magic). A car seat challenge is done to ensure that Laci doesn't stop breathing when in a semireclining position and that her heart rate and oxygen saturation won't go down while in the car seat (Box 5.8).

Don brings the car seat up from the parking garage. Letitia spent weeks selecting just the right one. She went to every review website and looked at all the highway standards. She agonized between a rear-facing car seat and a convertible car seat that could start out as rear facing and then be switched to front facing. She considered multiple variations of car seat upholstery and padding. Now, Laci looks tiny in the seat that had appeared so small. They place rolled receiving blankets on either side of her to help prop up her head and neck and brace her body. She passes the car seat challenge. They are ready to go home.

Think Critically

1. You have a patient who is interested in preventing pregnancy by timing intercourse to avoid her most fertile times. Using the information you learned in this chapter about timing intercourse to achieve pregnancy, how could you educate the patient to avoid pregnancy?

2. Your patient wishes to optimize her chances of getting pregnant. How would you explain her cycle to her? What recommendations would you make?

3. You are caring for a patient who is identified in her chart as a Jehovah's Witness. She is Rh negative. Describe how you would explain the recommendation of Rh_o (D) immune globulin to her. What are your key considerations in this scenario?

4. Your patient is seeking information about performing fetal movement counts. How do you guide her?

5. What would make you suspect cord prolapse? How would you prioritize care?

6. What signs would make you suspect an infant in your care was experiencing respiratory distress?

7. You are taking care of a late preterm infant. What screening is indicated? How do you explain to the family the screening necessary for the infant in the first few days after the birth?

8. Describe to a new parent how and why a car seat challenge test is performed.

References

Arya, R., Williams, G., Kilonback, A., Toward, M., Griffin, M., Blair, P. S., & Fleming, P. (2016). Is the infant car seat challenge useful? A pilot study in a simulated moving vehicle. *Archives of Disease in Childhood—Fetal and Neonatal Edition*, F1–F6.

Flenady, V., MacPhail, J., Gardener, G., Chadha, Y., Mahomed, K., Heazell, A., . . . Frøen, F. (2009). Detection and management of decreased fetal movements in Australia and New Zealand: A survey of obstetric practice. *The Australian & New Zealand Journal of Obstetrics & Gynaecology, 49*(4), 358–363.

Gibbons, C., O'Herlihy, C., & Murphy, J. (2014). Umbilical cord prolapse—Changing patterns and improved outcomes: A retrospective cohort study. *BJOG, 121*(13), 1705–1708.

Hachem, H. E., Crepaux, V., May-Panloup, P., Descamps, P., Legendre, G., & Bouet, P.-E. (2017). Recurrent pregnancy loss: Current perspectives. *International Journal of Women's Health* (9), 331–345.

Hamilton, B. E., Martin, J. A., & Osterman, M. J. (2016). Births: Preliminary data for 2015. *National Vital Statistics Report, 65*(3), 1–15.

Harris, D., & Weston, P. H. (2012). Incidence of neonatal hypoglycemia in babies identified as at risk. *Journal of Pediatrics*, 161(5), 787-791.

Hofmeyr, G. J., & Novikova, N. (2012, April 18). Management of reported decreased fetal movements for improving pregnancy outcomes. *The Cochrane Library*, (4):CD009148.

Larsen, E. C., Christiansen, O. B., Kolte, A. M., & Macklon, N. (2013). New insights into mechanisms behind miscarriage. *BMC Medicine, 11*, 154.

Tveit, J. V., Eli Saastad, B. S. -P., Børdahl, P. E., Flenady, V., Fretts, R., & Frøen, J. F. (2009, July 22). Reduction of late stillbirth with the introduction of fetal movement information and guidelines—A clinical quality improvement. *BMC Pregnancy and Childbirth, 9*, 32.

Suggested Readings

Baker, B. (2015). Evidence-based practice to improve outcomes for late preterm infants. *Journal of Obstetric, Gynecologic, and Neonatal Nursing, 44*(1), 127–134.

Harris, J. (2015). A unique grief. *International Journal of Childbirth Education, 30*(1), 82.

How it Works. (n.d.). Retrieved from https://www.fertilityfriend.com/

Maher, M. D., & Heavey, E. (2015). When the cord comes first: Umbilical cord prolapse. *Nursing, 45*(7), 53–56.

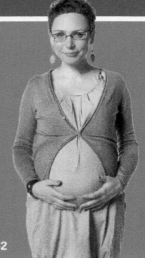

6 Rebecca Sweet: Placental Abruption and Fetal Loss

Rebecca Sweet, age 32

Objectives

1. Identify the potential causes of placental abruption and describe its effect.
2. Describe the characteristics of effective therapeutic communication and explain how caring can impact the experience of fetal loss.
3. Compare different kinds of decelerations and fetal heart rate variability.
4. Describe how you would prioritize assessments and interventions for a patient with suspected placental abruption.

Key Terms

Disseminated intravascular coagulation (DIC)
Fertility awareness–based contraception
Hemodynamic stability
Hypotension

Intrauterine device (IUD)
Placental abruption
Progestin-only pill
Vena cava

Before Conception

Rebecca Sweet is a careful person. As a child, she always reached for an adult's hand before crossing the street, even long after she could cross by herself. She was 10 before she agreed to ride her bike without training wheels.

She and her husband, Russ, are reference librarians at a university library, where they met a few years ago. Russ is also careful. In fact, it took him almost a year to build up the courage to have a conversation with her. She knew long before then, however, that he liked her, because he would often show up in her section for no good reason or send her emails about the most trivial things. She liked him, too. She liked that he was tall and husky, so much bigger than her. She liked it when he brought her coffee or some news article he thought she'd like. Most of all, though, she loved his gentle, compassionate nature. When he found her alone, crying in the reserve stacks after her dog died, and comforted her, she was hooked.

Before they were married, Rebecca carefully weighed all of her contraception options. Rebecca had a reliable 28-day cycle that she tracked meticulously (see Figs. 5.1 and 5.2). So, one of the options she considered was fertility awareness–based contraception, which involves abstaining from intercourse during fertile times of the cycle. In researching this method, however, she learned that it has a failure rate of approximately 24%, meaning that for every 100 people using it, 24 will be pregnant within a year (Centers for Disease Control and Prevention, 2014). For her meticulous nature, this degree of uncertainty was unacceptable.

She also considered an intrauterine device (IUD; see The Pharmacy 1.1), which provides years of contraception. But because she and Russ wanted to have children in a few years, this approach seemed like a poor return on investment. Rebecca was nothing if not frugal.

In college, she had tried the regular pill, a combination of the hormones estrogen and progestin, for a few months, but she hadn't liked how it made her feel (The Pharmacy 6.1). It had made her moody and stopped her period, which had made her nervous even though the nurse in the office had reassured her it was safe (Box 6.1).

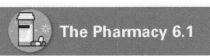

The Pharmacy 6.1   Combined Oral Contraceptives (the Pill) and the Progestin-Only Pill (the Minipill)

Combined Oral Contraceptives (the Pill)

Overview	• Contain a combination of estrogen and one of several different forms of progestin • Suppress ovulation and thicken cervical mucus so sperm cannot pass into the uterus from the vagina
Route and dosing	• Oral dose (containing 20–35 μg of estradiol, a kind of estrogen, plus a progestin) taken orally at the same time each day (to make remembering to take the pill simpler and to reduce the risk of break-through bleeding)
Care considerations	**Common side effects (many side effects improve within 2 mo of start)** • Nausea (better if taken at night with food) • Breast tenderness • Headache • Spotting, missed periods, and other bleeding irregularities • Mood changes • Changes in sex drive (libido) • Changes in vaginal discharge **Common contraindications** • Migraine headache with aura • Blood pressure > 130/90 mm Hg • A history of smoking and age over 34 y • Current pregnancy • History of blood clots • History of estrogen-dependent cancers
Warning signs	• *A*bdominal pain • *C*hest pain • *H*eadache (new onset, severe) • *E*yes: vision changes • *S*evere leg pain *All of these ACHES symptoms could be suspicious for a blood clot, a rare but serious side effect.*

Progestin-Only Pill (the Minipill)

Overview	• Contains only progestin and no estrogen • Is a good choice for women who cannot take estrogen because of migraine with aura, smoking after the age of 34 y, or a known history of blood clots
Route and dosing	• 0.35 mg of norethindrone, a kind of progestin, taken at the same time every day for effectiveness (a lower dose than that contained in combined oral contraceptives) • Must be taken within the same 3-h window every day • Contains no placebo pills; thus the patient must take a pill every day without a break
Care considerations	• A backup method of contraception is not necessary if started within first 5 d after menses. • If started after the first 5 d, a backup method should be used for 7 d. • Menstrual disruptions, including unscheduled bleeding and missed menses, are common.
Warning signs	• Though the risk of pregnancy is small, if it does occur it is more likely to be ectopic. • Unlike combined oral contraceptives, the minipill is not associated with increased clot risk.

She instead opted for the progestin-only pill, also known as the minipill, which her nurse practitioner told her did not contain any estrogen and only a third of the dose of progestin. She knew that it, too, was associated with bleeding irregularities but hoped that she might be less moody with it than she was with the regular combination pill (Patient Teaching 6.1; Fig. 6.1). Her nurse practitioner warned that she had to take it within the same 3-hour window every day, but for Rebecca, this made it almost more appealing. She liked the discipline it required.

Pregnancy

First Trimester

Now, almost 2 years later, Rebecca and Russ have decided they are ready to have a baby. In their typical way, they have planned out every aspect of the pregnancy. They bought a house the previous spring and spent months painting walls and arranging furniture until it looked and felt the way they wanted it to, like a home. They considered adopting a dog from an animal shelter for almost

Some women choose to skip the placebos in their pill pack to avoid having withdrawal bleeding. This is not a true period, and choosing not to have the withdrawal bleed will not have a negative impact on the woman's health. The first inventors of the pill in the 1960s thought that including a withdrawal bleed resembling a period might make the method more acceptable both to women and to the Catholic church. This modification, however, did not prove compelling to the Vatican, which continues to recommend that followers of the Catholic faith avoid all methods of artificial contraception, including the pill. Many women, however, do prefer to incorporate a withdrawal bleed, as they feel reassured that they are not pregnant.

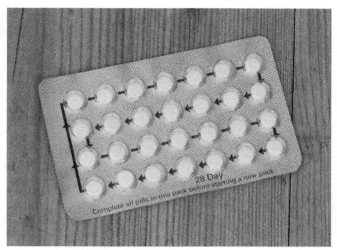

Figure 6.1. A pack of minipills.

a year before reluctantly deciding to wait until the children, not yet conceived, were 5 years old for safety, based on research that Russ had done in the library during breaks.

They agree on a birth control stop date that will allow the birth, assuming they successfully get pregnant within the first few months of trying, to coincide with summer vacation, the quietest time in both of their departments. On their second wedding anniversary, according to their plan, Rebecca stops taking her minipill. She takes her temperature and checks her cervical mucus. She uses an app to enter in her data and evaluate them online (see Figs. 5.1 and 5.2).

When she reaches the third month and still is not pregnant, she is frustrated. Concerned that the pregnancy will no longer occur according to the schedule she has so carefully planned out, she restarts her minipill. Her period does not arrive at the usual

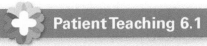

Patient Teaching 6.1

Progestin-Only Pill (Minipill)

- The pill must be taken within the same 3-h window every day to be effective.
- If a pill is taken outside of the 3-h window, a backup method, such as condoms or abstinence, must be used for a full week before again relying on the minipill for contraception.
- Unlike the combination pill, which has 3 wk of hormones and 1 wk of placebo pills, the progestin-only pill has no placebo week. Patients must take each pill all 4 wk.
- Missed periods, mistimed periods, and spotting are common with this method.
- The minipill, just like combined oral contraceptives, does not protect against sexually transmitted infections.

time, however, and when she is 2 weeks late, she takes a home pregnancy test. It is positive.

At her first prenatal visit, Dr. Walsh explains that there is a small increased chance of an ectopic pregnancy with progestin-only contraception methods because they slow the action of the cilia in the fallopian tube (Grimes, Lopez, O'Brien, & Raymond, 2013), causing the fertilized egg to implant in the tube instead of in the uterus (see Fig. 3.1). Rebecca is anxious, but Dr. Walsh reassures her that they will keep an eye on her and tells her how an ectopic pregnancy would present (see Box 3.2).

"Call me if you have any bleeding or cramping," Dr. Walsh tells her, "but an ectopic pregnancy would be a very rare complication of minipill use, and we have no reason at this point to expect anything other than a lovely, healthy pregnancy."

And it is a lovely, healthy pregnancy, or at least it is medically sound. Rebecca has wanted a child since she, herself, was a child and has dreamed of pregnancy and motherhood. She's been choosing names for her children since middle school. She's imagined what she'd wear in pregnancy and how cute her baby bump would be.

Then the morning sickness starts. Only it's not just in the morning. She has overwhelming, persistent vomiting that lasts all day. She has extra saliva in her mouth that no peppermint and no amount of tooth brushing can fix. She finds herself spitting, ladylike, into napkins she keeps in her pockets. Her breasts were so tender in that first week after she missed her period that she went and bought supportive bras on her lunch break one day. She develops nasal congestion, which at first she thinks is caused by allergies. At her next visit, however, Dr. Walsh tells her that it is a normal occurrence in pregnancy and that it might last through the birth (Table 6.1). At times fatigue overwhelms her and she naps at her desk while Russ goes and gets them soup and oyster crackers from a kiosk.

"How many times in your adult life do you have permission to be cute?" asks Russ, patting her belly.

Rebecca rolls her eyes. She doesn't feel cute. She is 12 weeks pregnant and has already gained 15 pounds because the only thing that made her feel better when she had morning sickness

Table 6.1   Common Complaints and Interventions of Early Pregnancy

Complaint	Care
Breast pain, tenderness, and tingling	• Typically most uncomfortable in the first several weeks • Wear a supportive bra
Nausea and vomiting (50%–75% of women)	• Most common in the first trimester • Avoid an over-full stomach and liquids with meals • Eat frequent small meals • Avoid fried and odorous foods • Fresh lemon smell, peppermint, ginger, acupressure, and B$_6$ may be helpful
Leukorrhea (increase in vaginal discharge)	• Not preventable • Wear a panty liner • Inform the provider of new-onset odor or itching (pruritus)
Ptyalism (excess salivation)	• May start in week 6 or 7 • Associated with nausea • Mouthwash and tooth brushing may have drying effects • Sucking hard candies and chewing gum may be helpful • Try the same interventions used for nausea and vomiting
Persistent nasal congestion	• Most likely to start in the second month • May persist for the duration of pregnancy • May be accompanied by epistaxis (nosebleed) • Saline nasal spray, use of a humidifier, exercise, and avoidance of irritants may be helpful

was eating. Saltines worked, but so did cookies—and sometimes ice cream and, yes, even pickles. In addition to the sometimes daily vomiting, nausea was a constant companion throughout the day for nearly 2 months. Now the nausea is gone, but the weight gain is here to stay (see Boxes 1.5 and 4.6; Fig. 6.2). She's already gained at least half of the weight recommended for someone with a normal body mass index, like the one she had before the start of the pregnancy.

"But the baby is the size of a lime!" says Russ (Table 6.2). "Isn't that cute?"

"I know limes, and limes are not cute," says Rebecca. "Plus, you'd need about a hundred limes to account for all of the weight I've gained."

"More of you to love."

"I hate that expression," says Rebecca, but leans into his kiss, anyway.

Second and Third Trimesters

As the pregnancy progresses without incident through the second and into the third trimesters, Rebecca takes careful notes at her visits with Dr. Walsh and keeps a list of reportable symptoms with her at all times (Table 6.3). Russ says she is compulsive, but Rebecca says she is just careful. With her body changing, she feels she is losing some measure of control. She goes with it as well as she can. She tries meditation. She wakes early every morning to do a prenatal yoga workout with a woman who looks too young to have ever conceived, let alone given birth to three children, which she says she did without any medications.

But it is her list she finds most helpful. Her list makes her feels as though she has distilled all possible complications into

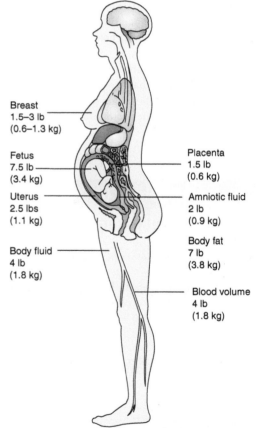

Breast
1.5–3 lb
(0.6–1.3 kg)

Fetus
7.5 lb
(3.4 kg)

Uterus
2.5 lbs
(1.1 kg)

Body fluid
4 lb
(1.8 kg)

Placenta
1.5 lb
(0.6 kg)

Amniotic fluid
2 lb
(0.9 kg)

Body fat
7 lb
(3.8 kg)

Blood volume
4 lb
(1.8 kg)

Figure 6.2. Weight distribution during pregnancy. (Reprinted with permission from Pillitteri, A. [2002]. *Maternal and child health nursing: Care of the childbearing and childrearing family* [4th ed., Fig. 12.1]. Philadelphia, PA: Lippincott Williams & Wilkins.)

Table 6.2 The Food Chart of Fetal Growth

Week of Gestation	Food of Comparable Size		Average Length and Weight of Embryo or Fetus*
Week 4	Poppy seed		Length: 0.13 cm (0.05 in) Weight: 0.11 g (0.004 oz)
Week 5	Sesame seed		Length: 0.23 cm (0.09 in) Weight: 0.09 g (0.007 oz)
Week 6	Lentil		Length: 0.38 cm (0.15 in) Weight: 0.28 g (0.01 oz)
Week 7	Blueberry		Length: 0.79 cm (0.31 in) Weight: 0.5 g (0.02 oz)
Week 8	Kidney bean		Length: 1.6 cm (0.63 in) Weight: 1 g (0.07 oz)
Week 9	Cherry		Length: 2.3 cm (0.09 in) Weight: 2 g (0.07 oz)
Week 10	Kumquat		Length: 3.1 cm (1.22 in) Weight: 4 g (0.14 oz)
Week 11	Brussels sprout		Length: 4.1 cm (1.61 in) Weight: 7 g (0.25 oz)
Week 12	Lime		Length: 5.4 cm (2.13 in) Weight: 14 g (0.49 oz)
Week 13	Pea pod		Length: 7.4 cm (2.91 in) Weight: 23 g (0.81 oz)
Week 14	Lemon		Length: 8.7 cm (3.42 in) Weight: 43 g (1.52 oz)

(continued)

Table 6.2 The Food Chart of Fetal Growth (continued)

Week of Gestation	Food of Comparable Size		Average Length and Weight of Embryo or Fetus*
Week 15	Macintosh apple		Length: 10.1 cm (3.98 oz) Weight: 70 g (2.47 oz)
Week 16	Avocado		Length: 11.6 cm (4.57 oz) Weight: 100 g (3.53 oz)
Week 17	Beet		Length: 13 cm (5.12 oz) Weight: 140 g (4.94 oz)
Week 18	Bell pepper		Length: 14.2 cm (5.59 in) Weight: 190 g (5.7 oz)
Week 19	Large tomato		Length: 15.3 cm (6.02 in) Weight: 240 g (8.47 oz)
Week 20	Artichoke		Length: 16.4 cm (6.46 in) Weight: 300 g (10.58 oz)
Week 21	Carrot length		Length: 26.7 cm (10.51 in) Weight: 360 g (12.7 oz)
Week 22	Papaya		Length: 27.8 cm (10.94 in) Weight: 430 g (15.17 oz)
Week 23	Eggplant		Length: 28.9 cm (11.38 in) Weight: 501 g (1.1 lb)
Week 24	Corn on the cob		Length: 30 cm (11.81 in) Weight: 600 g (1.32 lb)
Week 25	Acorn squash		Length: 34.6 cm (13.62 in) Weight: 660 g (1.46 lb)
Week 26	Zucchini		Length: 35.6 cm (14.02 in) Weight: 760 g (1.68 lb)

Table 6.2 The Food Chart of Fetal Growth (continued)

Week of Gestation	Food of Comparable Size		Average Length and Weight of Embryo or Fetus*
Week 27	Cauliflower		Length: 36.6 cm (14.41 in) Weight: 875 g (1.93 lb)
Week 28	Kabocha squash		Length: 37.6 cm (14.8 in) Weight: 1,005 g (2.22 lb)
Week 29	Butternut squash		Length: 38.6 cm (15.2 in) Weight: 1,153 g (2.54 lb)
Week 30	Cabbage		Length: 39.9 cm (15.71 in) Weight: 1,319 g (2.91 lb)
Week 31	Coconut		Length: 41.1 cm (16.18 in) Weight: 1,502 g (3.31 lb)
Week 32	Napa cabbage		Length: 42.4 cm (16.69 in) Weight: 1,702 g (3.75 lb)
Week 33	Pineapple		Length: 43.7 cm (17.2 in) Weight: 1,918 g (4.23 lb)
Week 34	Cantaloupe		Length: 45 cm (17.72 in) Weight: 2,146 g (4.73 lb)
Week 35	Honeydew melon		Length: 45.2 cm (18.19 in) Weight: 2,383 g (5.25 lb)
Week 36	Romaine lettuce		Length: 47.4 cm (18.66 in) Weight: 2,622 g (5.78 lb)

(continued)

Table 6.2 The Food Chart of Fetal Growth (continued)

Week of Gestation	Food of Comparable Size		Average Length and Weight of Embryo or Fetus*
Week 37	Long as Swiss chard		Length: 48.6 cm (19.13 in) Weight: 2,859 g (6.3 lb)
Week 38	Long as rhubarb		Length: 49.8 cm (19.61 in) Weight: 3,083 g (6.8 lb)
Week 39	Mini watermelon		Length: 50.7 cm (19.96 in) Weight: 3,288 g (7.25 lb)
Week 40	Small pumpkin		Length: 51.2 cm (20.16 in) Weight: 3,462 g (7.63 lb)

*Measurements are from crown to rump through 20 weeks and then from crown to heel.
Adapted from Doubilet, P., Benson, C., Nadel, A., & Ringer, S. (1997). Improved birth weight table for neonates developed from gestations dated by early ultrasonography. *Journal of Ultrasound Measurement, 16*(4), 241–249.

something she can fold up and put into her pocket. She thinks (and she knows it is foolish) that if she can visualize and imagine each of the potential complications, she can avoid them actually happening. She imagines that if she can predict any eventuality she can avoid having it sneak up and surprise her. She keeps it secret. She knows if she tells Russ he'll say that it is just magical thinking, and of course he would be right.

Labor and Delivery

One morning in her 38th week of pregnancy, Rebecca wakes feeling especially tired and decides to sleep a little more and go into work a couple of hours late. Russ has to be in early for a meeting, so they agree to drive separately. By the time Rebecca pulls out onto the highway, the dark storm clouds that have been looming overhead all morning finally break, and the rain begins to pour down. It's so heavy that Rebecca has trouble seeing the road. After fumbling with her windshield wipers and finally getting them on, she looks up and sees a red light ahead. Panicked, she slams on her brakes. Her car slips, hydroplaning, and crashes into a guardrail. The airbag explodes open and immediately begins to deflate. She sits there a moment in a cloud of airbag dust frightened and confused.

She feels tightness and pain all over her abdomen and in her lower back (Table 6.4). Is that a contraction? Her legs feel wet. She looks down and sees that her skirt is soaked with blood.

Moments later, she hears tapping on the driver's side window and turns to see a woman looking at her wide-eyed.

"Are you okay?" the woman yells through the glass.

Rebecca finds herself nodding mechanically.

"I called nine-one-one," the woman says. "I'll stay here with you until they come."

Rebecca nods. The pressure and pain in her abdomen are getting worse. This is not a contraction.

As she waits for the ambulance, she manages to retrieve her phone from her purse and calls Russ. She tells him about the accident.

"I'm so sorry. I'm just so sorry," she tells him. Her belly is tender and painful, the pressure on her back almost unbearable. "Please meet me at the hospital. And hurry."

"I'm pregnant" is the first thing she says as the ambulance crew arrives. She knows it's absurd as soon as she says it, because it's the most obvious thing about her. The paramedics move her to a stretcher and position her on her side. Her librarian's mind tries to distract her by recalling what Dr. Walsh said, that this side-lying position prevents the heavy uterus from resting on and

Table 6.3 Pregnancy Danger Signs and Concerns

Sign or Symptom	Associated Condition
Vaginal bleeding	• First trimester: miscarriage • Second and third trimesters: low-lying placenta (placenta previa), detaching placenta (placental abruption), or bloody show (the breakdown of the mucus plug that seals off the cervix)
Dysuria (painful urination) and urinary frequency and/or urgency	• Urinary tract infection (can cause pregnancy complications)
Fever	• Infection (although pregnant women are typically 0.4°F–0.6°F warmer than their baseline temperature)
Nonstop vomiting	• Hyperemesis gravidarum: nausea and vomiting, typically occurring in the first trimester that can result in weight loss, dehydration, nutritional and electrolyte imbalances, and even death, if untreated
Severe headache	• Preeclampsia: a dangerous hypertensive (high blood pressure) disorder exclusive to pregnancy that can start as early as 20 wk
Epigastric pain (pain in the upper, central abdomen)	• Preeclampsia
Fluid leakage from the vagina	• Premature rupture of membranes (rupture of membranes before contractions begin): may present as copious clear, odorless discharge • Infection (if accompanied by odor, itching, or irritation) • Note: It's normal to have an increase of milky, odorless discharge in pregnancy.
Uterine contractions, pelvic or abdominal pain or cramping, pelvic pressure, and lower backache	• Preterm labor

compressing her **vena cava** (Fig. 6.3), which can cause maternal **hypotension** and poor gas exchange between the placenta and fetus (Demma & Grace, 2015). A mask is put over her face for oxygen. Her vital signs are measured and measured again. The hospital is close and she is hopeful.

At the hospital, she bypasses the emergency room and is sent immediately to labor and delivery, where she is met by two nurses and the on-call physician, a man she's never met and whose name she doesn't catch. He skips the elastic straps entirely, and manually holds the toco over her uterus and the fetal heart monitor over her lower abdomen. He purses his lips and wrinkles his forehead.

"Will she be okay? Will they be okay?" Russ says. He has just arrived, and is at Rebecca's side, holding her hand.

Table 6.4 Symptoms of Placental Abruption

Class 0	Class 1 (40%)	Class 2 (45%)	Class 3 (15%)
• No symptoms • Diagnosis made postpartum with inspection of placenta	• No or mild vaginal bleeding • Normal vital signs • Back and/or abdominal pain • Uterus may be slightly tender • Normal fetal heart rate • No clotting issues (no DIC)	• No-to-moderate vaginal bleeding • Back and/or abdominal pain • Uterine tenderness • Possible tetanic contractions (uterus does not completely relax in between; reduces oxygen exchange with fetus) • Possible maternal tachycardia and hypotension • Fetal distress • DIC possible	• No-to-heavy vaginal bleeding • Back and/or abdominal pain • Painful tetanic contractions • Fetal distress • High risk for maternal shock • High risk for DIC

DIC, disseminated intravascular coagulation.
Data from Tikkanen, M. (2010). Etiology, clinical manifestations, and prediction of placental abruption. *Acta Obstetricia et Gynecologica Scandinavica, 89*(6), 732–740.

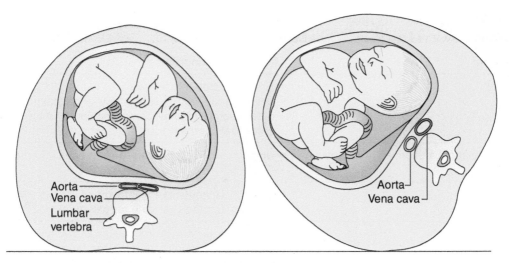

Figure 6.3. Compression of the vena cava by the uterus. As the uterus grows during pregnancy, it may compress the inferior vena cava when the pregnant woman lies in a supine position. This may cause hypotension and reduce perfusion of the uterus, placenta, and fetus. It is easily reversible by moving the woman into an upright or side-lying position. (Reprinted with permission from Pillitteri, A. [2002]. *Maternal and child health nursing: Care of the childbearing and childrearing family* [4th ed., Fig. 9.8]. Philadelphia, PA: Lippincott Williams & Wilkins.)

"I'm concerned that the placenta may have come partly away from the wall of the uterus," he says.

"Will you do an X-ray or something to find out?" asks Russ.

The physician shakes his head. "We don't see fifty percent of **placental abruptions** by ultrasound. Not seeing it wouldn't mean it wasn't there, and seeing it wouldn't change how we care for her at this point."

"**Placental abruption**? Is that what this is called?" asks Russ (Box 6.2).

"Yes," the physician says. "I'm worried about both the mother and the baby. Right now the priority is to deliver the baby."

"Do you mean a cesarean section?" asks Rebecca. She's sweating, and her abdomen *hurts*.

"Most likely, yes," he says. "I'm concerned about the fetal heart rate. It's a category two right now, which means we don't know

for sure that the baby is in trouble, but we're also not sure it's not in trouble. If it becomes a category three, then there is a high chance the baby is in trouble and we'll want to deliver immediately" (Table 6.5). "We also need to consider the possibility of a bleeding complication that can occur in the mother with placental abruption called **disseminated intravascular coagulation**, or DIC. If that happens, it will impact our thinking, as will the amount of blood loss. We need more information before we decide whether a vaginal birth would be safer. The nurses here are going to start some IVs, and we'll get some labs and see where we are shortly." He glances at one of the nurses. "STAT that" (Lab Values 6.1; Fig. 6.4).

"My name is Maryanne," says an older nurse as the physician leaves the room. Her voice is soft but no-nonsense, and her fingertips are chilly. "I'm going to start an IV in each arm, and then I'm going to place a catheter in your bladder so we can measure your urine more accurately. You're in good hands."

"Why two IVs?" asks Russ (Box 6.3). He seems completely collected. Rebecca knows him and recognizes that he's probably terrified.

"We want to make sure we have good access and can give her fluids quickly if we need to. Right now we're just going to run some fluid called Ringer lactate, but she may need blood later."

Rebecca nods. Russ holds her hand tightly.

"Why the catheter?" asks Russ.

"We need to measure her urine output, as well. If her kidneys aren't producing enough urine, it's probably because she has lost too much blood," says Maryanne.

"Does she need blood?" asks Russ.

"We're monitoring the status of her blood supply—what we call her **hemodynamic stability**—right now. We don't know whether she needs blood yet, but I promise you we'll keep you as informed as we possibly can."

Dr. Walsh, Rebecca's obstetrician, arrives.

Box 6.2   Risk Factors for Placental Abruption in Order of Significance

1. Previous placental abruption
2. Abdominal trauma
3. Cocaine or other illicit drug use
4. Eclampsia
5. Chronic hypertension
6. Polyhydramnios
7. Chorioamnionitis
8. Premature rupture of membranes
9. Hypertensive disorders of pregnancy (excluding eclampsia)
10. Preeclampsia in previous pregnancy
11. Small-for-gestational-age baby with previous pregnancy
12. Smoking in pregnancy

Table 6.5 Fetal Heart Rate Categories

Category and Status	Description	Appearance on Monitoring Strip
I: Reassuring, normal, not concerning	• No decelerations or early decelerations • With or without accelerations • Must have moderate variability (6–25 bpm) • Baseline heart rate 120–160 bpm	Early decelerations With an early deceleration, the FHR returns to baseline before the end of the contraction. The return to baseline is gradual, 30 s or less from onset to the slowest FHR (nadir).
II: Nonreassuring: indeterminate; further evaluation required and intervention may be indicated	• Any reading that is not Category I or III	

III: Nonreassuring: abnormal; expedited interventions required	• Sinusoidal pattern (smooth, undulating, and symmetric)
	• Absent variability (undetectable amplitude) and:
	  ◦ Recurrent late decelerations
	  ◦ Recurrent variable deceleration
	  ◦ Bradycardia (slow heart rate)
		Sinusoidal pattern
		
		Absent variability
		
		Late decelerations
		
		With a late deceleration, the FHR returns to baseline after the contraction ends. The return to baseline is gradual, 30 s or less from onset to the slowest FHR (nadir).

(continued)

Table 6.5 Fetal Heart Rate Categories (continued)

Category and Status	Description	Appearance on Monitoring Strip
		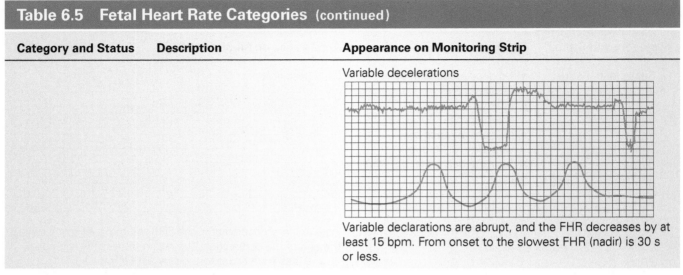Variable decelerations Variable declarations are abrupt, and the FHR decreases by at least 15 bpm. From onset to the slowest FHR (nadir) is 30 s or less.

FHR and bpm are relevant only if the patient is having contractions. Variability refers to changes in the amplitude range of the fetal heartbeats. bpm, beats per minute; FHR, fetal heart rate.
Figures adapted with permission from: (early, variable, and late decelerations) Stephenson, S. R. (2012). *Obstetrics and gynecology* (3rd ed., Fig. 25-7); (sinusoidal pattern) Menihan, C. A., & Kopel, E. (2014). *Point-of-care assessment in pregnancy and women's health* (Fig. 3-23); (absent variability) Gibbs, R. S., Karlan, B. Y., Haney, A. F., & Nygaard, I. (2008.) *Danforth's obstetrics and gynecology* (10th ed., Fig. 10-2A, p. 157), all published by Philadelphia, PA: Lippincott Williams & Wilkins.

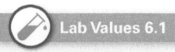

Lab Values 6.1

Evaluation for Disseminated Intravascular Coagulation

Disseminated intravascular coagulation is a condition in which there is widespread clotting throughout the body. Simultaneously, because the components of the blood used to stop bleeding are being used up, catastrophic bleeding can occur. It is always a complication of another condition. In Rebecca's case, it would be a complication of severe placental abruption.

- Fibrinogen: decreased
- Fibrin degradation products: elevated
- D-dimer: elevated (less reliable in pregnancy)

"Rebecca, your blood work results are back. The good news is I don't see any evidence of the clotting disorder, DIC. You urine output is sufficient for now, and your vital signs are stable. I'm advising an epidural and a cesarean section sooner rather than later. I have the anesthesiologist coming right now."

"So, the baby has a category three heart rate now?" asks Russ. He's been paying attention, collecting complicated jargon and storing it like the librarian he is.

"Yes—category three," confirms Dr. Walsh, looking surprised. "This baby needs to come out now. I'm afraid there's not enough placenta attached to the wall of your uterus for her to get the oxygen she needs from you. We can take better care of her out than in" (Fig. 6.5).

The IV bag of clear Ringer lactate empties into her arm through one of the two lines as Rebecca curls up her body around her abdomen for the epidural (see Boxes 4.16 and 4.17). She feels a

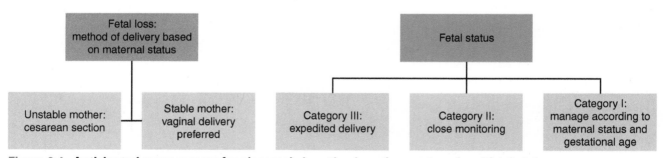

Figure 6.4. Anticipated management for placental abruption based on maternal and fetal status.

Box 6.3 Initial Monitoring and Interventions for Suspected Severe Placental Abruption

Monitoring for Hemodynamic Stability

- Heart rate, blood pressure (rapid heart rate and hypotension are concerning)
- Urine output (maintain >30 mL/h)
- Blood loss (weigh bloody materials and compare to identical nonsoiled materials)
- Continuous fetal heart rate monitoring

Interventions

- Administer a blood transfusion as ordered to maintain hemodynamic stability (typically for estimated blood loss over 500 mL or 1 L)
- Establish intravenous access with two wide-bore needles and administer lactated Ringer's

Laboratory Tests

- Blood type and cross (possibly cross-match for transfusion)
- Complete blood count
- Creatinine
- Liver function tests (if preeclamptic)
- Coagulation studies for disseminated intravascular coagulation evaluation (Lab Values 6.1)

Placental Abruption: Various Degrees of Separation of Normally Implanted Placenta

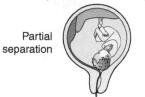

Partial separation

Marginal separation

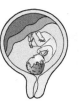
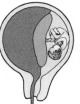

Complete separation with concealed hemorrhage

Complete separation with heavy vaginal bleeding

Figure 6.5. Degrees of placental abruption. (Reprinted with permission from Suresh, M. [2012]. *Shnider and Levinson's anesthesia for obstetrics* [5th ed., Fig. 21.1]. Philadelphia, PA: Lippincott Williams & Wilkins.)

pinch in her back and then little else as the anesthesia and analgesia of the epidural take effect (Fig. 6.6). The tightness and tenderness in her abdomen recede. The lack of pain is blissful, but her fear is still pervasive. Russ holds her hand, and the expression on his face reflects her emotions.

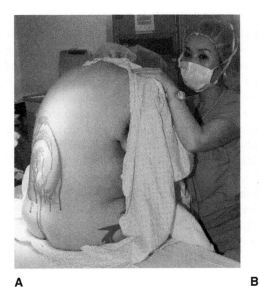
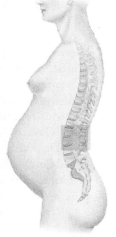
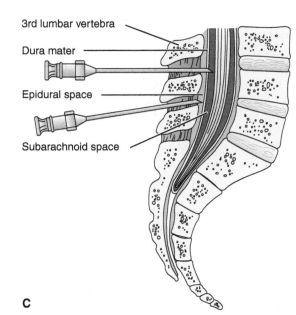

A **B** **C**

3rd lumbar vertebra

Dura mater

Epidural space

Subarachnoid space

Figure 6.6. Epidural placement. (A) The laboring woman is correctly positioned for epidural anesthesia. **(B)** The shaded area shows the location of epidural placement. **(C)** The different locations for an epidural and an intrathecal needle are shown. (Reprinted with permission from Hatfield, N. T., & Kincheloe, C. A. [2017]. *Introductory maternity and pediatric nursing* [4th ed., Fig. 9-5]. Philadelphia, PA: Lippincott Williams & Wilkins.)

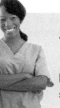

The Nurse's Point of View

Maryanne: I always try to imagine in circumstances like Rebecca's what it's like to be her, and to let that empathy guide my care as much as possible. We're worried about her. Very worried. We have quite a team assembled in the surgical suite. There's Dr. Walsh, an anesthesiologist, a resident, a medical student, a nursing student, two scrub nurses, Rebecca's husband, two pediatricians, and me. I identify the people by name and role to Rebecca and her husband, but it's just noise, something to say. They both look frightened, and I don't think they're listening. I don't think I would be, either.

Almost as soon as Rebecca arrived, we initiated our massive hemorrhage protocol. This protocol helps us to have the blood the patient needs on hand quickly and allows us to administer it safely. Typically we transfuse after an estimated blood loss of 500–1,000 mL. Contributing to the decision are signs of hemodynamic instability, such as a drop in blood pressure, a heart rate over 120 beats per minute (bpm), shortness of breath, or an altered level of consciousness. We have also checked her blood repeatedly for hematocrit, platelet count, and coagulation factors. We drew blood for a type and screen so that, in the event that she does need a transfusion, we'll be able to give her blood compatible with her own. We've been measuring blood loss as best we can, but she lost blood in the car and ambulance before she got here. There may be even more between her uterus and the placenta. We have blood on standby, but the call has not yet been made to use it.

Women with epidurals often have a sensation of tugging and pressure, but no pain. I hold Rebecca's hand and quietly tell her that this is expected and not to be alarmed if that's what she feels. Some television shows might have you think that the operating room is all people talking about golf and listening to Led Zeppelin. That hasn't been my experience. Conversation is limited to what needs to be said, and everyone is concentrating on what needs to be done.

I am concentrating on Rebecca. Her well-being is my responsibility right now as much as it is anyone's. There's a sheet between her face and her body, and she can't see what's happening. I can, however. The baby is out, and it's completely still. Dr. Walsh hands her off to the pediatric team.

"Your baby is born," I tell her. "The pediatricians have her now."

"I don't hear anything," Rebecca whispers. "I don't hear anything."

After Delivery

Rebecca can feel her legs again, now, and with it the incisional pain. It isn't bad. It's more distracting than anything else. Her mind is focused inward. Nurses come in and out of the room. She doesn't feel crowded, but she senses their presence and feels a little less alone. They say the right things: "What can I do to help? I'm so sorry; this must be hard for you." She must be saying the right things in response, though she's not really sure. Everyone looks at her kindly. They check her vital signs. They look at her incision. They hand her medications, which she swallows automatically. She has an IV for a while, and then she doesn't. The compression devices on her legs inflate and deflate to prevent her from developing clots (see Table 5.2). Russ spends most of his time in a chair next to her bed. At times he opens up the chair, transforming it into a narrow cot, and lies on it with his eyes open. He watches her. He watches the ceiling. They speak sometimes or hold hands. She cries so hard that she has to splint her abdominal incision with a pillow.

The Newborn

"I'm so sorry," Dr. Walsh had said after the delivery. "She didn't make it. The trauma was just too great."

Rebecca already knew it, somehow—maybe because of the silence following the birth or the somber mood of the staff—but the words still struck her like a sledgehammer, making her feel shattered into shards. She didn't scream or cry or wail. She felt like she couldn't breathe. She knew that she'd been holding onto just the smallest pocket of hope, which was now empty.

After a moment, she could manage only one word: "Why?" She wasn't looking at either Russ or Dr. Walsh. The question was rhetorical, but Dr. Walsh took it literally.

"The placenta is not elastic like the uterus," Dr. Walsh explained. "With trauma, the uterus may stretch but the placenta can't. It can be sheared partially or completely from the uterine wall and cause bleeding where it became detached. The less placenta that's attached to the uterus, the less nutrients and waste that can pass between the mother and the fetus. That's what happened here. After the accident, not enough placenta stayed attached to the uterus. Your baby just wasn't able to get enough oxygen."

"Oxygen," said Rebecca. "I couldn't give her enough oxygen."

Dr. Walsh touched her arm lightly. Rebecca flinched a little and Dr. Walsh drew back. "No one could have. It's natural and normal to blame yourself, but know that it was the trauma that caused the death. It wasn't anything you or anyone else did."

"Do you want to see her?" asks Dr. Walsh a little later. Russ is sitting upright in the chair. Rebecca has just swallowed some pills. The nurse told her what they were. She doesn't remember. "There's no one right answer to that question."

The question feels complex, almost cruel. Like being asked what kind of torture you'd prefer. Rebecca has no idea of how to respond.

"What would you recommend?" Russ asks Dr. Walsh, relieving Rebecca of the burden of responding. She is grateful.

"This is a very personal choice," Dr. Walsh replies. "If you decide that you want to spend some time with her, we can facilitate that.

Most studies tell us that viewing and holding the baby helps the mourning process. Some people want to spend a few minutes, some want to spend hours. Some people want pictures, some don't. Some people don't want to see the baby at all, and that's a completely acceptable choice, as well. Some studies suggest seeing the baby may contribute to depression and anxiety in the future" (Kingdon, Givens, O'Donnell, & Turner, 2015). "In any case, we'll do our best to respect and facilitate your choices."

"I'm frightened," says Rebecca. "I've never even seen a dead body, and to have that body be hers . . .'"

"Would it be helpful if I told you how she looks?"

Both Russ and Rebecca nod.

"A nurse named Melinda gave her a bath. She looks clean. She looks as though she's sleeping, but she's very pale—dusky."

"And cold," says Rebecca.

"Melinda has dressed and swaddled her in a blanket. She's wearing a knit cap. She doesn't look cold. Oh—and she has a lot of hair," Dr. Walsh says.

"What color?" asks Rebecca. Both she and Russ have straight blonde hair, and neither has much of it. She'd imagined a bald baby, or one with a puff of white fluff. She'd imagined blonde baby curls in ribbons as she grew older. She'd never considered one with a quantity of hair, or a child who would never have a chance to grow older.

"Dark," says Dr. Walsh. "Many babies are born with a lot of dark hair, though. It often falls out within a few months."

A lot of dark hair—imagine that. "I'd like to see her," says Rebecca. "Russ, can we see her?"

"You're sure?" he asks.

"I think I need to see her," Rebecca says. "I'm having a hard time making all of this seem real. I think I need to see her to be sure." She reaches her hand out to take his. "Please stay."

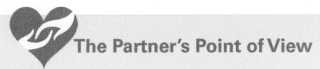

The Partner's Point of View

Russ: There is a sign on the door to Rebecca's room with a leaf and a drop of water. One of the nurses told me it's the universal sign for stillbirth. To me, it is a mark of tragedy; a warning to anyone who passes that beyond this door lies an all-consuming sadness; a plea for sensitivity; a cue to not ask unprompted questions. I've heard someone use the term "angel baby," and I wish I could believe in heaven. But I don't want to hear that the baby is in a better place or with God. This is the place Rebecca and I made for her. This is where she belongs.

When Rebecca tells me and Dr. Walsh that she wants to see the body of our stillborn baby, I feel an impulse to run away, to drive for miles, to find a space to hide. I'm terrified at the thought of seeing it . . . of seeing her. Nothing about this is natural or good. It is the most awful thing I've ever experienced, in fact.

But how could I refuse Rebecca? She was the one who carried the child for nine months in her body, after all. She was the one who had to go through the trauma of the car wreck with the baby. So if she has the courage to see the baby, I think I can, too.

Melinda comes in wheeling a clear bassinet, just as if it were any other baby, just as if the baby were alive and needed her own safe sleeping space and her own drawer full of diapers and wipes and extra blankets.

To Rebecca, looking into the bassinet feels like an act of courage. She feels heartbroken and frightened and even, she thinks, stupidly hopeful—as if she has an extra maternal instinct that will pick up a sign of life that everyone else has missed. Somehow, too, even with Russ and Melinda in the room, she feels profoundly alone.

Just as Dr. Walsh said, the baby is swaddled in a striped blanket and is wearing a pink cap knit by a hospital volunteer. A white T-shirt can be seen just above the blankets. She is clean and pale. The scene is still, like a photograph. Rebecca can see it now, though. The baby is unquestionably dead.

"Does she have a name?" asks Melinda.

"Heloise," says Rebecca. "She's named for my grandmother."

"Are we still using that name?" asks Russ.

"Of course," says Rebecca. "It's her name."

"Would you like me to pick Heloise up and hand her to you?" asks Melinda.

"I don't know," says Rebecca.

Russ moves closer and touches Heloise's cheek and her ear and the soft, dark hair peeking from underneath the cap. He lifts the cap. Dr. Walsh was right. There is a lot of hair.

"Some families like to keep a lock of hair," says Melinda. "We also have foot prints and hand prints, and a card with her height and weight."

Rebecca moves to sit on the edge of the bed. Melinda helps her remove the compression boots and eases her feet to the floor. Rebecca touches Heloise's face with the back of her hand and then tugs the swaddling loose and opens the baby's blanket.

It all looks so normal. There are the two arms and the 10 fingers with tiny fingernails. The rounded belly and the stump of an umbilical cord. Someone, probably Melinda, has put a diaper on the baby. This strikes Rebecca as a ridiculous kindness, to diaper a baby that will never need to be changed, but she is touched all the same.

"I'd like to hold her," she says.

In all, they stay together as a family of three for 2 hours. They take turns holding her and running a brush through the dark hair. They dab powder-scented lotion on Heloise's skin and sing to her. They soak her blanket with tears. Russ hands Melinda his smartphone and she takes dozens of pictures.

"I'm so sad for you," says Melinda as she leaves with the bassinet and the baby. "We're here for you. You just need to ask" (Box 6.4).

"I don't even know what I'd ask for," says Rebecca. "But you've been very kind. Everyone has been so kind."

Six weeks pass, and Rebecca's period returns. Her belly is still soft, with a pink scar above her pubic hair and slowing fading stretch marks. When she has gas in the night, for a brief and horrible moment each time she thinks to herself, "that's the baby moving."

She wrestles with guilt constantly. If only she hadn't slept in that morning. If only she'd gotten herself out of bed and ridden to work with Russ, like usual. If only it hadn't been raining or the traffic light had been green. If only she hadn't panicked and slammed on her brakes. Maybe if any one thing had happened

Box 6.4   Ways to Communicate Caring

- Open body language (arms open and lifted to the sides rather than crossed or behind the back, etc.)
- Eye contact, as culturally appropriate
- Gentle tone of voice (speak more quietly and slower)
- Unrushed presence
- Silence, as appropriate

Swanson's Middle Range Theory of Caring

- *Knowing:* striving to understand an event in the context of the person; using empathy
- *Being with:* a compassionate, responsive presence
- *Doing for:* acting on behalf of the person, as they would for themselves in different circumstances
- *Enabling:* providing a guide and means of reflection, validation, support, and perspective through the event
- *Maintaining belief:* retaining realistic hope

Data from: Cacciatore, J. (2010). Stillbirth: Patient-centered psychosocial care. *Clinical Obstetrics and Gynecology, 53*(3), 691–699; Swanson, K. (1991). Empirical development of a middle range theory of caring. *Nursing Research, 40*(3), 161–166.

differently at some point in her life she wouldn't have wrecked the car that day and killed her baby.

She and Russ have been seeing Virginia, a grief counselor with the hospital, regularly since the birth and death of the baby.

"When will I feel better?" asks Rebecca during a session. She looks at Russ, and then back at Virginia. "When will I stop feeling angry and guilty and sad?"

"Grief doesn't keep time," says Virginia. "I don't have an answer. Everyone copes differently. Some people feel guilty and sad and angry, like you do. Some people feel anxious and scared and like they want to find someone to blame. Some people will feel all these things at different times."

"Sometimes I feel like you're angry with me," says Russ. "Like you think I'm not sad enough."

Rebecca nods. "I am angry with you. I don't know why. I don't have a reason to be. I can't seem to shake it. I don't want to be angry. I want to be held. I want to feel better and I want you to be the person who holds me. I'm just having trouble working through all of this anger. I don't want to feel isolated but I do, and I know I'm doing it to myself."

"This can be a normal part of the grief reaction. Don't be too hard on yourselves," says Virginia. "But keep talking. Talk to each other, talk to me, talk to other people. There are excellent support groups locally and online I'd be happy to help you connect with. You will work through it."

"There's really no timeline?" asks Rebecca. "I don't want to mark my calendar, but I need some sort of light in this tunnel."

"I can tell you what some of the literature tells us," says Virginia. Rebecca smiles, just a little bit. "Most people who experience a loss like this will feel like they have some closure after six to twelve months. Were you to choose to try again, it's likely best to wait until you have this closure" (Kingdon et al., 2015).

"It's hard to imagine that," says Rebecca.

"To imagine what?" asks Russ. "Feeling closure or trying again? I'm having a hard time with both."

Rebecca moves her knee so it touches his, briefly. "We still have a lot in common, the two of us."

Think Critically

1. Draw early, late, and variable fetal heart rate decelerations.
2. How can trauma lead to placental abruption?
3. Why is placental abruption potentially dangerous for the fetus? Why is it dangerous to the pregnant woman?
4. What are the signs of hemodynamic instability? How is it treated?
5. What is DIC, and how do we monitor for it?
6. You are caring for a patient like Rebecca postpartum. Consider what actions you could take that might be therapeutic.

References

Centers for Disease Control and Prevention. (2014). *Appendix D: Contraceptive effectiveness*. Atlanta, GA: Author.

Demma, J. M., & Grace, K. T. (2015). Prenatal care. In T. L. King, M. C. Brucker, J. M. Kriebs, J. O. Fahey, C. L. Gegor, & H. Varney (Eds.). *Varney's midwifery* (pp. 657–722). Burlington, MA: Jones & Bartlett Learning.

Grimes, D., Lopez, L., O'Brien, P., & Raymond, E. (2013). Progestin-only pills for contraception. *Cochrane Database of Systematic Reviews*, (11), CD007541.

Kingdon, C., Givens, J. L., O'Donnell, E., & Turner, M. (2015). Seeing and holding baby: Systematic review of clinical management and parental outcomes after stillbirth. *Birth, 42*(3), 206–218.

Suggested Readings

Heavey, E., & Maher, M. D. (2015). Placental abruption: Are we going to lose them both? *Nursing, 45*(5), 54–59.

Hope After Loss. Retrieved from http://www.hopeafterloss.org/

Macones, G. A., Hankins, G. D., Spong, C. Y., Hauth, J., & Moore, T. (2008). The 2008 National Institute of Child Health and Human Development Workshop Report on electronic fetal monitoring: Update on definitions, interpretation, and research guidelines. *Journal of Obstetric, Gynecologic, & Neonatal Nursing, 37*(5), 510–515.

MISS Foundation. (2016). Retrieved from http://www.misschildren.org/

7 Hannah Wilder: Chorioamnionitis and Neonatal Sepsis

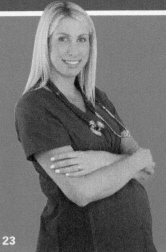

Hannah Wilder, age 23

Objectives

1. Identify and prioritize different kinds of testing for sexually transmitted infections.
2. Explain how to evaluate a woman with suspected premature rupture of membranes.
3. Describe the warning signs of chorioamnionitis.
4. Differentiate between the presentation of a healthy neonate and that of one with sepsis.
5. Explain the implications of a group B streptococcal infection during pregnancy and the intrapartum period.

Key Terms

Chorioamnionitis
Lamaze
Leukorrhea

Nitrazine dye
Sepsis

Before Conception

Hannah is a 23-year-old college student in a large 4-year nursing program. She works one shift a week at a community health center. She's a meticulous planner and tracks her work schedule and school assignments on a calendar app on her smartphone. She's been studying with one of the few men in the program, John, and their relationship has quickly become romantic.

"I want to be responsible," says Hannah, after kissing John for the first time.

"Hannah, you're the most responsible person I know," says John. "You make the rest of us look like disorganized losers."

"I'll take that as a compliment. What I was going to say is that I think we should get tested before we do anything, you know, sexual."

John teases her about being overly cautious but agrees to go in with her to be tested for sexually transmitted infections (STIs).

Hannah makes them back-to-back appointments at a local family planning clinic after assuring John it isn't just for women.

"This isn't really romantic," he says after they sign in and find seats in the waiting room.

"Neither is an STI," says Hannah quietly.

"I use condoms," he says.

"Every time?"

"Most of the time."

"That's like using a parachute *most* of the time when you jump out of an airplane," she says.

Hannah is called first. She produces a urine sample as instructed and waits in an examination room, perusing a binder containing information about STIs, birth control, and nutrition. After 15 minutes of reading about hepatitis C and trichomoniasis (Box 7.1), Hannah hears a knock on the door and a woman in a white coat enters the room. She introduces herself as Merit.

"Oh excellent," says Merit. "I see you've been browsing the menu. What questions do you have?"

Hannah shrugs. "I don't know. I just want to be tested."

Box 7.1   Common STIs at a Glance

Chlamydia

- *Cause:* The *Chlamydia trachomatis* bacterium
- *Who should be screened:* All sexually active women under 25 y of age, men and women in high-risk settings, pregnant women, men who have sex with men, and people with HIV
- *Incubation period:* 1–2 wk
- *Screening method:* Urine test or vaginal or rectal swab
- *Symptoms:* Usually none. Women may have dysuria, vaginal discharge, or pelvic pain; men may have dysuria, urethral discharge, or testicular pain.
- *Occurrence:* 456.1/100,000 people in the United States in 2014, up 2.3% since 2013
- *Treatment:* Antibiotics (curative)

Gonorrhea

- *Cause:* The *Neisseria gonorrhoeae* bacterium
- *Who should be screened:* All sexually active women under 25 y of age, men and women in high-risk settings, pregnant women, men who have sex with men, and people with HIV
- *Incubation period:* 2–7 d
- *Screening method:* Urine test or vaginal, rectal, and/or pharyngeal swabs
- *Symptoms:* Usually none. Women may have dysuria, vaginal discharge, or pelvic pain; men may have dysuria, urethral discharge, or testicular pain.
- *Occurrence:* 100.7/100,000 people in the United States in 2014, up 5.1% since 2013
- *Treatment:* Antibiotics are curative, but gonorrhea is increasingly resistant to the antibiotics available. Strains have been identified that do not respond to any antibiotics.

Syphilis

- *Cause:* The *Treponema pallidum* bacterium
- *Who should be screened:* Men who have sex with men; pregnant women, others identified as high risk.
- *Incubation period:* 10 d to 3 mo
- *Screening method:* Blood test. People with a suspicious lesion may be tested by culture.
- *Symptoms:* Varied based on the individual and the stage of disease. The patient may have no symptoms. Common initial presentation is a painless sore or multiple sores at the site of infection. Later symptoms may include a rash of the hands and feet, a disseminated reticular rash, alopecia, flu-like symptoms, and others.
- *Occurrence:* 6.3/100,000 people in the United States in 2014, up 15.1% since 2013; 11.6/100,000 live births (congenital syphilis), up 27.5% since 2013
- *Treatment:* Antibiotics (curative)

HPV (Genital Warts)

- *Cause:* The HPV. Strains 6 and 11 are responsible for 90% of genital warts.
- *Who should be screened:* No screening recommendation

- *Incubation period:* Varies widely
- *Screening method:* N/A; visual inspection for suspicious lesions
- *Symptoms:* Painless, cauliflower-like genital bumps
- *Occurrence:* 1.1%–4.9% in the United States in 2014
- *Treatment:* Genital warts can resolve spontaneously. They are commonly treated with liquid nitrogen or trichloroacetic acid application. They may also be treated with imiquimod, an immune response modifier, or podofilox. Vaccination is available and recommended for both men and women between the ages of 9 and 26 y.

Cervical, Anal, Rectal, Vulvar, and Vaginal Dysplasias and Cancers and Head and Neck Cancers

- *Cause:* High-risk forms of HPV, primarily strains 16 and 18, but other strains as well
- *Who should be screened:* Women 21 y and older should be screened every 3 y until the age of 30 y with Pap testing. Between the ages of 30 and 65 y, women should be screened every 5 y, with the addition of HPV screening with the Pap test. There are no screening recommendations for men at this time.
- *Screening method:* Pap test
- *Symptoms:* Usually no symptoms
- *Occurrence:* 34,788 new cancers in 2009
- *Treatment:* A combination of watchful waiting, lesion excision, and other treatment. Vaccination is available and recommended for both men and women between the ages of 9 and 26 y.

Genital Herpes Virus

- *Cause:* Herpes simplex virus I and herpes simplex virus II
- *Who should be screened:* No screening is indicated in the absence of symptoms.
- *Incubation period:* 2–12 d for symptoms; up to 3 mo for a positive blood test
- *Screening method:* Screening is not recommended. Patients with symptoms may undergo a swab of a fresh lesion or a blood test.
- *Symptoms:* Over 87% of people will have no or minor clinical manifestations. Symptoms may include flu-like symptoms with painful lesions primarily at the site of exposure.
- *Occurrence:* Approximately one in six people in the United States has genital herpes.
- *Treatment:* Antiviral medication, to treat and suppress outbreaks

Hepatitis B Virus

- *Cause:* Hepatitis B virus
- *Who should be screened:* People who may have been exposed to infected blood and other body fluids and have not been effectively vaccinated
- *Incubation period:* 6 wk to 6 mo
- *Screening method:* Blood test

Box 7.1   Common STIs at a Glance (continued)

- *Symptoms:* Often asymptomatic; may include fatigue, yellowing of the skin or whites of the eyes, abdominal pain, nausea, dark urine, and clay-colored stool
- *Occurrence:* 0.9/100,000 people in the United States in 2014. Approximately 5% of adults will go on to have a chronic infection, and 25%–90% of children under the age of 5 y may remain chronically infected.
- *Treatment:* Antiviral medications. A vaccination has been recommended for all infants since 1991.

Hepatitis C Virus

- *Cause:* Hepatitis C virus
- *Who should be screened:* People born between 1945 and 1965, people who are HIV positive, IV drug users, and others exposed to blood. Having multiple sex partners is considered a risk factor, although sexual transmission remains controversial.
- *Incubation period:* Up to 6 mo
- *Screening method:* Blood test
- *Symptoms:* Often asymptomatic; may include fatigue, yellowing of the skin or whites of the eyes, abdominal pain, nausea, dark urine, and clay-colored stool
- *Occurrence:* 0.7/100,000 people in the United States in 2014. Approximately 75%–85% develop a chronic infection.
- *Treatment:* Antiviral medications

HIV

- *Cause:* HIV
- *Who should be screened:* Everyone who is sexually active (at least once), pregnant women, people seeking screening and/or treatment for STIs
- *Incubation period:* 2–12 wk
- *Screening method:* Initial evaluation by saliva or finger stick; confirmatory testing by serum testing

- *Symptoms:* May have no symptoms. Later symptoms vary according to the course of the disease. Early symptoms may include a rash, joint pain, or flu-like symptoms.
- *Occurrence:* 44,073 people diagnosed in 2014, down 19% from 2005. Approximately 1.2 million people are estimated to be HIV positive in the United States.
- *Treatment:* Antiretroviral treatment

Pubic Lice (Crabs)

- *Cause:* Parasitic insects
- *Who should be screened:* No screening is indicated. Symptomatic people should be examined.
- *Incubation period:* 1–6 wk
- *Screening method:* Exam
- *Symptoms:* Possible rash; itching of hair-bearing genitals, which may be worse at night; and visible nits (eggs) or lice
- *Occurrence:* Reliable statistics are not available.
- *Treatment:* Topical over-the-counter and prescription treatments

Trichomoniasis

- *Cause:* The *Trichomonas vaginalis* parasitic protozoan
- *Who should be screened:* Patients who are HIV positive or high risk
- *Incubation period:* 4–20 d
- *Screening method:* Screening by urine test, vaginal swab; symptomatic patients may also be evaluated by microscopy of vaginal fluid, vaginal swab, or urine test.
- *Symptoms:* 70%–85% have no symptoms. Symptoms may include vaginal odor, itching, and discharge; penile discharge; and urethral irritation and dysuria.
- *Occurrence:* Most prevalent nonviral STI. Approximately 3.7 million people in the United States are infected.
- *Treatment:* Antibiotics

HPV, human papillomavirus; IV, intravenous; STIs, sexually transmitted infections.
Data from Centers for Disease Control and Prevention. (2015, September 24). *Genital herpes—CDC fact sheet (detailed)*. Retrieved from http://www.cdc.gov/std/herpes/stdfact-herpes-detailed.htm; Braxton, J., Carey, D., Davis, D., Flagg, E., Footman, A., Grier, L., . . . Weinstock, H. (2015). *Sexually transmitted disease surveillance 2014*. Atlanta, GA: U.S. Department of Health and Human Services; U.S. Preventive Services Task Force. (2016, June). *Final recommendation statement: Genital herpes: Screening*. Retrieved from http://www.uspreventiveservicestaskforce. org/Page/Document/RecommendationStatementFinal/genital-herpes-screening; Centers for Disease Control and Prevention. (2016a, August 4). Hepatitis B FAQs for health professionals. Retrieved from http://www.cdc.gov/hepatitis/hbv/hbvfaq.htm#overview; Centers for Disease Control and Prevention. (2016b, July 21). Hepatitis C FAQs for health professionals. Retrieved from http://www.cdc.gov/hepatitis/hcv/hcvfaq.htm#section1; Division of HIV/AIDS Prevention, National Center for HIV/AIDS, Viral Hepatitis, Sexual Transmitted Diseases and Tuberculosis Prevention, Centers for Disease Control and Prevention. (2016, June). *HIV in the United States: At a glance*. Retrieved from http://www.cdc.gov/hiv/statistics/overview/ ataglance.html; Division of STD Prevention, National Center for HIV/AIDS, Viral Hepatitis, STD, and TB Prevention, Centers for Disease Control and Prevention. (2015, June). *Human papillomavirus (HPV) infection*. Retrieved from http://www.cdc.gov/std/tg2015/hpv.htm; Workowski, K. A., & Bolan, G. A. (2015, June 5). Sexually transmitted diseases treatment guidelines, 2015. *MMWR Recommendations and Reports, 64*(3), 1–137.

"We can do that. Is there anything in particular you're concerned about—any symptoms you've experienced or rumors you've heard?"

"No. I broke up with my last boyfriend about six months ago. I heard later that he might have been cheating on me, but he denies it. Mostly I'm here because I have a new partner. We haven't done anything yet, but I want to get tested for everything to make sure I'm safe."

"I love to hear that," says Merit. "It's awesome when people come in at the start of the relationship. But let's go through the list of STIs and see which ones make the most sense to test for. Most people don't need to be tested for everything. You're twenty-three, correct?"

Hannah nods.

"Have you had a Pap test yet?"

"Yes. I think it was about two years ago. It was normal. I haven't had one since. Aren't you supposed to get them every year?"

Merit shakes her head. "The guidelines were changed a while ago. Now women should have their first Pap test at age twenty-one and then one every three years until age thirty" (see Patient Teaching 2.2). "We feel comfortable with this new guideline because the changes that happen to the cervix as a result of the human papilloma virus, or HPV, happen very slowly, and many of those changes regress over time. If we screened more often we'd be likely to overtreat you."

"Cervical cancer is usually caused by a virus," says Hannah. "Right. I totally forgot that."

"So that's one off of the list. If you had that two years ago, you don't need another until next year. Have you been screened for HIV?"

"I don't know. I don't think so. It's not like I'm using IV drugs. I'm not a gay man. Am I supposed to be screened?"

"The Centers for Disease Control recommends that you be tested at least once. A quarter of the people with HIV in this country are women, you know. And over eighty-five percent of them got it from having sex with a man who was positive" (Centers for Disease Control and Prevention, 2016).

"Really?"

"Really."

"Darn. Well, let's do that then. What else am I supposed to be screened for?"

"You're under twenty-five, so annual screening for gonorrhea and chlamydia is recommended. What about vaccinations? Given your age, you were likely vaccinated for the hepatitis B virus, unless your parents opted out of it."

"I definitely had that," says Hannah. "I'm a nursing student. I had to have a titer test to prove I'm immune. I think I had the three shots for that HPV vaccine, too. Do I even need to get a Pap test anymore?"

"You need to get your Pap tests," says Merit. "The vaccination covers only two, four, or nine of the strains of HPV, depending on which vaccine you got. There are around 40 strains of HPV that have been shown to cause the changes that can lead to cancer or genital warts. But I'm very glad you got the vaccination. It does protect against the strains of the virus that cause a vast majority of the harm."

"Well, what else should I get tested for? Hepatitis C? Herpes? Syphilis?"

"Hepatitis C virus is bloodborne. We don't believe that it transmits efficiently through sexual contact. It's more prevalent in IV drug users, and we routinely screen people born between 1945 and 1965, because three out of every four infected people we see are in that age range. Testing of the blood supply did not begin until 1992, so someone who had a transfusion or organ transplant before then would also be considered at risk."

"Okay. What about syphilis?"

"The main risk group for syphilis at this time is men who have sex with men."

"And herpes?"

"Have you ever had any symptoms associated with herpes?" Hannah shakes her head.

Merit shrugs. "Then no screening is recommended at this time" (U.S. Preventive Services Task Force, 2016).

"So that's it—HIV, chlamydia, and gonorrhea?"

"Unless there's something you haven't mentioned."

"I don't think so."

"Good. I'll send the medical assistant in shortly to do the finger stick for HIV screening" (Fig. 7.1). "We'll send your urine sample out to the lab for testing for gonorrhea and chlamydia, and we'll do the HIV test here. We'll use the new point-of-care test that takes about a minute to run. But first, tell me what you're planning on for birth control."

"Oh," says Hannah, not expecting the turn in conversation. "I don't know. Condoms?"

"Condoms are good. They do provide some protection against STIs. However, in terms of contraception, they're not the most reliable method. With typical use they're only about eighty-five percent effective in preventing conception" (see Patient Teaching 4.1).

"I know, but it's what I've always used and it's always worked fine for me before. I tried pills for a few weeks once, but I just didn't like them. They made me kind of nauseous."

"That's a really common side effect when you first start the pill," says Merit. "It usually goes away within a few months, though, and a lot of people find it helps to take the pill at night or with a little bit of food. But there are methods besides the pill. Some don't have any hormones, and some have low hormones. Some methods you'd only have to think about occasionally instead of every day. Would you like to hear about any of those?"

Hannah shakes her head. It's not something she wants to think about today. "I'm good for now. Just condoms."

Merit nods and nudges a large jar containing wrapped condoms in her direction. "You take as many as you want. I'm going to put in a prescription for emergency contraception, as well. You can come in and pick it up here if you need it."

"Isn't that the abortion pill?"

Merit shakes her head. "The evidence we have tells us that it stops fertilization, not implantation, and that it won't interfere with an established pregnancy. But it does need to be used within five days of unprotected intercourse, and the sooner the better" (Gemzell-Danielsson, Berger, & Lalitkumar, 2013).

"How effective is it?" asks Hannah.

"Somewhere between fifty-seven and ninety-five percent effective," says Merit. "There's a reason it's called Plan B and not Plan A" (Gemzell-Danielsson et al., 2013).

Pregnancy

First Trimester

Hannah and John use condoms, and they work out fine. She purchased a box of emergency contraception through the clinic for "just in case," but the box has remained at the bottom of her purse for a long time. It might have even expired. One day, she misses her otherwise predictable period.

"I always said that I was pro-choice but that it wasn't a choice I'd make for myself. But now that the choice is before me, I'm not so sure." says Hannah. She's holding a pregnancy test. It has two blue lines on it. She's pregnant.

HIV Type1/2 (Serum/Plasma) Test

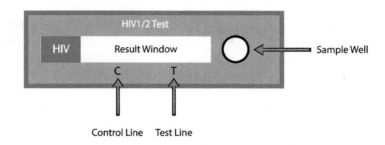

INTERPRETATION OF RESULTS

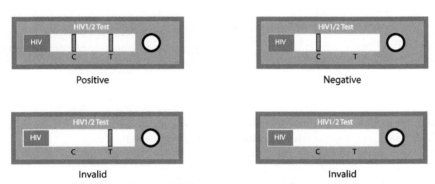

Figure 7.1. Point-of-care HIV test interpretation.

"You never know what you'll do in a situation until you're in it, I guess," says John. He's rereading the instructions for the test, as if somehow it was possible to screw it up. "You read it at three minutes, right? You didn't read it late?"

"It lit up like a Christmas tree in the first twenty seconds," says Hannah. She sits down next to him and puts her head on his shoulder. He puts his arm around her and gives her shoulder a vigorous rub. "I don't know what to do," she says.

"Well, I like to think I get a vote," says John. "But it's your body, so you get two votes."

"So then, what does the minority vote say?"

"I think you'd make a wonderful mother."

Hannah snorts. "A wonderful poor, single, unemployed mother with student debts that are breeding like rabbits."

"Well, let's think about it. By the time the baby comes we'll be graduated. Once we pass the NCLEX, we'll be employable. We'll be shift workers. Maybe we can arrange our schedules so we won't even need to use daycare."

"We?"

"Well, I was going to ask you to marry me after graduation. I've had it all planned out for months."

"You have not. You're just saying that," says Hannah.

"No, it's true! That's been the plan."

"Really? What now? You said you were planning to ask. Have you changed your mind?"

"No. I figured I'd just ask you now, instead."

"You reckon I'll say yes?"

A few weeks later, Hannah and John meet with a nurse midwife, Darla. Hannah's mother wanted her to see an obstetrician, but Hannah really enjoyed working with midwives during her maternity rotation in school. They seemed to spend more time with their patients and were more involved not just with the care but with the patients themselves than were physicians. The idea comforted her.

"What kind of birth would you like to have?" asks Darla.

"Short and painless," says John.

Hannah gives him a look. "I'd like a natural childbirth. I've read about epidurals and know all the facts and statistics, but the idea of a needle in my back still freaks me out."

"Are you serious?" asks John. "Why would you want to put yourself through this without an epidural? I mean, I read all the same sources you did for class, and there's no way I'd do that without some good pain killers."

"Well, then, it's a good thing I'm doing it and not you," says Hannah, lifting one eyebrow. "Think of it as a challenge, or a marathon. I want to prove to myself that I can do it. It's like a test, you know?"

"Yeah, well. I can't imagine wanting to run a marathon, either."

"Women have been giving birth without epidurals for most of our history. On the whole it seems to have worked out for the human race. I'm willing to try it."

"We'll respect your choice, whatever it is," says Darla. "Have you considered taking a childbirth preparation class?"

"Like Lamaze?"

"Sure, that's one option. Childbirth classes help prepare you for the birth. The best classes give you coping strategies. The breathing technique taught in Lamaze is one of those strategies."

John groans and says, "More classes?" Hannah playfully smacks him on his arm.

"One of the midwives in our practice offers a class, if you're interested. She teaches hypnosis, which many women find helpful."

"Hypnosis?" asks Hannah. "You mean I'll have to bark like a dog and cluck like a chicken?"

"It's a little different from that. Patients learn methods of relaxation, reframing, and visualization that help them through the contractions and the birth. For many people, it's a very natural, calm, peaceful method of birthing. There's very little barking and clucking, on the whole."

"What's the time commitment?" asks Hannah. "The class sounds great, but we're both still in school full time."

"I believe it's five sessions over about twelve hours. I'll give you the brochure. I think it costs a few hundred dollars. Fortunately, insurance often pays for it in our state, so that's worth looking into."

Second Trimester

Hannah's pregnancy proceeds normally in the second trimester, just the way her textbook described it. Her routine screenings are unremarkable (see Table 1.1), and the labs contain no surprises (see Lab Values 1.1). The ultrasound at the end of the first trimester is normal. She starts to feel the fetus move at 16 weeks, right on target. The fetal survey ultrasound at 20 weeks is also normal (see Box 1.8). Her blood pressure stays low and doesn't spike. She doesn't experience a urinary tract infection or even morning sickness. She doesn't develop gestational diabetes (see Lab Values 3.2), and after the belly measurements begin at 20 weeks, she is always within 2 cm of the measurements expected, based on her gestational age in weeks (see Fig. 2.8).

Third Trimester

Her third trimester goes well, too. By the end of it, she has gained exactly 24 lb (see Box 1.5). She feels lucky but also nervous, knowing that her luck could run out at any time. Sure enough, she gets some bad news shortly after her visit at 36 weeks.

"I knew things were going too well," says Hannah.

"This isn't so bad," says Darla. She's just told Hannah that her vaginal-rectal swab came back positive for group B streptococcus (GBS). "Think of it as a manageable concern. It's completely treatable. We'll start you on antibiotics when you get to the hospital and administer a new dose every four hours. You're not allergic to penicillin, so we can give you a medication that we know is most effective against GBS" (Box 7.2).

"What would happen if I did have an allergy to penicillin?"

"We'd still give you an antibiotic, but one that's safe for someone with a penicillin allergy. When using nonpenicillin antibiotics, however, there's a slightly higher risk of your passing the infection on to the newborn than when using penicillin or a related antibiotic. Remember, it's not really you we're worried

---

Box 7.2 Criteria for Treatment of GBS Infection During Labor and Delivery

Factors Indicating Treatment

- GBS disease in an infant of a previous pregnancy
- GBS found in the maternal urine during the current pregnancy
- A positive GBS rectal-vaginal swab of the mother between week 35 and 37 of pregnancy
- Unknown maternal GBS status plus any one of the following:
  - Membranes ruptured for 18 h or longer
  - Temperature of 100.4°F (38°C) or greater during labor and delivery
  - Positive GBS testing during labor and delivery
  - Preterm delivery (less than 37 weeks' gestation)

Factors Indicating That No Treatment Is Necessary

- A positive GBS rectal-vaginal swab (colonization) in a previous pregnancy but not in the current pregnancy
- GBS found in the maternal urine during a prior pregnancy
- A negative GBS rectal-vaginal swab in the current pregnancy
- A cesarean section prior to rupture of membranes

GBS, group B streptococcus.
Data from Verani, J. R., McGee, L., & Schrag, S. J. (2010a). *Prevention of Perinatal Group B Streptococcal Disease: Revised Guidelines from CDC, 2010.* Atlanta, GA: National Center for Immunization and Respiratory Diseases.

---

about with GBS; we're worried about passing the infection on to the baby, where it could cause complications. Many women are colonized with GBS, and it typically doesn't cause them any problems. We don't screen for it or worry about it unless someone is expected to give birth soon."

"Right, I know. It's fine," says Hannah. "It probably sounds dumb, but I had this whole fantasy of not being hooked up to anything, no IV, no monitors, nothing. I'm just disappointed I'll have to have an IV through the whole thing."

"I understand," says Darla. "It is possible we may be able to take you down to a saline lock between doses. But Hannah, one of the best things you can do for yourself going into labor is to decide to go with the flow. Don't get too attached to any one thing. Remember our goal is a healthy mama and a healthy baby."

"I know, I know," says Hannah.

Labor and Delivery

Hannah gets out of bed at 5:30 in the morning 3 days after her due date. She's been awake for much longer than that. The baby has been moving around and kicking her so hard when she is in her preferred comfortable position that she has finally given up. When she stands up, fluid gushes through her panties all the way to her socks. She walks quickly to the bathroom and wipes down her legs. She puts her contact lenses in her eyes. The baby moves one of its limbs and pushes it uncomfortably against the front of her abdomen. She gently pushes it back. She goes back into the bedroom, where John still sleeps on his back.

"Two things," she tells him after shaking him awake. "Thing one, we're out of contact lens fluid. Thing two, my water broke."

She and John get dressed and go to the hospital, as instructed by the triage nurse who returned their call to Darla's office. Another nurse, named Rochelle, meets them in the triage area of the labor and delivery floor.

"How are you feeling?" asks Rochelle as she attaches the automated cuff to Hannah's arm to get her blood pressure and pulse. She passes a temporal thermometer across her forehead to get her temperature.

"I feel fine," says Hannah. "I just feel kind of wet. It didn't hurt."

"Is the baby moving?"

"He never stops moving. I haven't noticed anything different."

"Good. Are you having any contractions?"

"I haven't noticed anything, but then I haven't noticed any Braxton Hicks contractions and my midwife says I'm definitely having those even if I can't feel them."

"Alright," says Rochelle. "I'm going to put these monitors on you to check the baby's heart rate and see if we pick up any small contractions you may not be feeling. I will also do a pelvic exam to confirm that your water broke" (Box 7.3).

"What else would it be besides her water breaking?" asks John.

"Sometimes it can be urine. Women also produce extra vaginal secretions during pregnancy. It's called **leukorrhea**. Sometimes if there's enough of that it can be confused with ruptured membranes."

"I know the difference between ruptured membranes and wetting myself," says Hannah. "I just graduated from nursing school. I can tell the difference. For one, it didn't smell like pee."

"You're probably right, but let's check it out anyway."

"I see no evidence that your water broke," says Rochelle about 15 minutes later. She has completed a sterile speculum exam, gathered samples, and checked them under the microscope and with cotton swabs impregnated with **nitrazine dye** (Step-by-Step Skills 7.1).

"Oh no, really?" says Hannah. "Are you telling me that I managed to graduate from nursing school without being able to tell the difference between amniotic fluid and urine?"

Box 7.3 Evaluation of a Woman Reporting Premature Rupture of Membranes

- Testing for rupture of membranes (Step-by-Step Skills 7.1)
- Nonstress test or biophysical profile
- Determination of fetal position
- Assessment of the pregnant woman
  - Contractions
  - Fever (suggests infection and chorioamnionitis)
  - Vital signs (tachycardia suggests infection and chorioamnionitis)
  - Uterine tenderness (suggests infection and chorioamnionitis)

Step-By-Step Skills 7.1

Testing for Rupture of Membranes

Note: It is usually helpful to verbally walk patients and support people through the procedures as you do them. Always explain the purpose of and approach to a procedure before performing it.

Procedure

1. Wash your hands and put on clean gloves.
2. Select a sterile speculum, being careful not to touch the blades or to allow the blades to touch nonsterile surfaces.
3. Insert the speculum and localize the cervix.
4. Observe for pooling of fluid in the vaginal vault. Pooling suggests amniotic fluid.
5. Ask the patient to cough, and observe for leakage of fluid from the cervix.
6. Nitrazine test: using nitrazine paper or cotton swabs impregnated with nitrazine dye, obtain a sample of pooled fluid, avoiding swabbing the cervix (see Fig. 1.12).
7. Ferning test: with a second sterile cotton swab not impregnated with nitrazine, obtain a second sample from the pooled fluids.
8. Remove the speculum and help the woman into a comfortable position. Explain that you will return after interpreting the results.
9. Wipe the second cotton swab on a slide and allow the fluid to dry. Dispose of the swab.
10. Examine the slide under low-power microscopy. Observe for ferning (arborization; see Fig. 1.13).
11. Wash your hands.

Interpretation

- Nitrazine test (see Fig 1.12)
  - Shades of yellow and green indicate that the membranes are likely intact.
  - Shades of blue-green to blue indicate that amniotic fluid is probably present.
  - Results may be compromised by semen, douching, insufficient amniotic fluid, bloody show, and vaginitis.
- Ferning test (see Fig. 1.13)
  - Ferning indicates that amniotic fluid is probably present. A false-positive finding is possible if the sample is compromised by cervical mucus.
  - Lack of ferning suggests that the reported fluid was urine or vaginal discharge.

Documentation

- The result of both the nitrazine test and the ferning test is typically reported as either positive or negative.
- Some institutions may further require the exact pH level to be reported.

"Embarrassing," says John, nodding.

"Yes," Hannah says.

With no signs of labor or membrane rupture, Hannah is discharged a little later and returns home with John.

The same thing happens the next morning. Still not having had a contraction, Hannah gets out of bed and feels the rush of fluid seep through her panties and into her socks. She shakes John awake.

"Call the office again, will you?" she asks. "I need to put my contact lenses in and then get checked again to see if I wet my pants."

"I'm going to break out those diapers early," he says, but he makes the call.

"Well this time you're right," says Darla. It's her day to be on call. She's in the hospital attending another birth and evaluated the fluid herself. "Your water broke."

"Well thank goodness for that," says Hannah. "I'm pretty sure they'll let me keep my RN license now."

Darla looks at the monitoring strip and then shows it to Hannah and John. "You're right about your uterus, too, Hannah. It is quiet. I'm not seeing any contractions. The baby looks lively, though. The baseline heart rate is sitting at about one hundred fifty beats per minute (bpm). There are no decelerations, but there are some nice accelerations. This is all reassuring."

"If there are no contractions, what now?" asks John. "Wait and see?"

"That is one option," says Darla (Analyze the Evidence 7.1). "But I wouldn't recommend it. There's a danger with premature rupture of membranes that an infection will start in the uterus that may be passed on to the fetus. We know you're GBS-positive, as well, which makes us even more concerned about infection. Whether we induce or not, I do want to get you started on some IV penicillin G" (Box 7.4).

"So I guess I'll have to be induced," says Hannah. "I hoped that my body would do it all on its own, that we would have that 'honey, it's time' moment."

"Think of it as just needing a jump start," says John.

"If we decided to just wait, what would happen?" asks Hannah.

"Well, if it wasn't for the GBS, I'd say you could go home and self-monitor for a while. We'd have you take your temperature every few hours and let us know if you got to 38°C or higher.

Box 7.4 Recommended Antibiotic Regimens for Treatment of Group B Streptococcal Infection During Labor and Delivery

General Treatment Guidelines

- Antibiotic dosing must start 4 or more hours prior to delivery to be considered adequate.
- Only treatment with penicillin G, ampicillin, or cefazolin is considered adequate; these antibiotics, however, are contraindicated in people with severe allergies to penicillin.

For Patients With No Penicillin Allergy

Either of the following:

- *Penicillin G:* first dose of 5 million U IV followed by IV doses of 2.5–3 million U every 4 h until delivery
- *Ampicillin:* first dose of 2 g IV followed by IV doses of 1 g every 4 h until delivery

For Patients With Penicillin Allergy NOT Including Anaphylaxis, Urticaria, Angioedema, or Respiratory Distress

- *Cefazolin:* first dose of 2 g IV followed by 1 g IV every 8 h until delivery

For Patients With Penicillin Allergy Including Anaphylaxis, Urticaria, Angioedema, or Respiratory Distress (High Risk for Anaphylaxis)

- *Clindamycin:* 900 mg IV every 8 h until delivery

For Patients at High Risk for Anaphylaxis From Penicillin but Having an Organism Not Susceptible to Clindamycin as Identified by Culture or if No Culture Is Available

- *Vancomycin:* 1,000 mg IV every 12 h until delivery

Note that the time between doses is counted from the beginning of one dose to the beginning of the next dose.

IV, intravenous.
Data from Verani, J. R., McGee, L., & Schrag, S. J. (2010a). *Prevention of Perinatal Group B Streptococcal Disease: Revised Guidelines from CDC, 2010.* Atlanta, GA: National Center for Immunization and Respiratory Diseases.

Analyze the Evidence 7.1 — Expedient Induction of Labor With Term or Near-Term Rupture of Membranes

Induction Within 24 h

- Pregnancies in group B streptococcus–positive women may benefit from induction rather than watchful waiting (Tajik et al., 2014).
- Induction of labor may reduce the incidence of neurodevelopmental delays at 2 y of age (Heyden et al., 2015).

Watchful Waiting as an Acceptable Alternative

- Induction of labor does not reduce the rate of neonatal sepsis or other neonatal outcomes and may slightly increase the risk for chorioamnionitis (Ham et al., 2012).
- Prolonged preterm rupture of membranes does not increase the risk of neonatal sepsis (Drassinower, Friedman, Običan, Levin, & Gyamfi-Bannerman, 2016).

We'd have you keep monitoring for fetal movement. We'd want you to come in if your discharge became foul smelling or colored" (Box 7.5).

"But you're not recommending that," says Hannah.

"I'm not. I'd like you to stay here and receive some antibiotics."

"And oxytocin?"

"Yes. In my professional opinion the risk of infection at this point is greater than any of the risks of induction."

"Do you think her water might have really broken yesterday?" asks John. "Do you think maybe the tests were wrong?"

"Anything is possible," says Darla. "But right now we have to go with what we know. We know her membranes are ruptured now and she's GBS-positive. We have to get some antibiotics started."

"What about my cervix?" asks Hannah. "I remember the Bishop score. Is my cervix ripe enough?" (see Analyze the Evidence 1.1).

"Right now your cervix is anterior and you're about two to three centimeters dilated and maybe fifty percent effaced. Your cervix is fairly soft, and thankfully the baby is at zero station, which is why we're not as worried about cord prolapse as we would be otherwise. I think you'll be fine without any further cervical ripening" (see Chapter 5).

"But if we did need to ripen the cervix we'd use misoprostol or prostaglandins, right?" asks John.

"That's right."

"Ha," says John, rolling his eyes dramatically at Hannah. "See? I totally studied."

Hannah is started on oxytocin. Soon afterward she feels her contractions begin. Gradually, the dose of oxytocin is increased, and gradually the contractions get stronger and closer together (see The Pharmacy 1.2). Hannah begins to lose track of time.

"She has a fever. It's 39°C," a nurse says (Box 7.6). Moments later the nurse hands her two tablets and a glass of water.

"It's acetaminophen," says the nurse.

"Is it for the pain?" Hannah asks. She is feeling frightened, and worries that she won't be able to manage the contractions much longer. She's been practicing the techniques she learned in birthing class and is able to relax deeply between contractions, but it skews her sense of time. She isn't sure how long it has been since the first dose of oxytocin. It might have been any amount of time.

"No, you have a fever. The medication is to help bring down your temperature."

"Why does she have a fever?" asks John. "What's going on? She's already on an antibiotic."

"We think she has an infection of the membranes surrounding the baby, a condition called **chorioamnionitis**," says Darla. "She has a fever and both her heart rate and the baby's are higher than we'd like to see. The acetaminophen should help, and we're going to switch from the penicillin G to broader-spectrum antibiotics, ampicillin and gentamicin" (Box 7.7).

"She's going to be okay? I mean, they're going to be okay?" asks John.

"This isn't uncommon and she's in the right place. You leaving the nursing stuff to us; it's our job today. You take care of her."

"I'm scared," says Hannah after the next contraction. "I'm scared and it hurts and I feel awful."

"Hannah, do you feel like your belly is tender in between contractions?" asks Darla. She gently pushes against Hannah's swollen abdomen. Hannah shrinks back a little.

"Yeah, it's tender," she says.

Box 7.5 Risk Factors for Chorioamnionitis

- Prolonged rupture of membranes
- PROM (may be a risk factor for chorioamnionitis or chorioamnionitis may be the cause of PROM)
- Long labor
- Vaginal exams after rupture of membranes (vaginal exams may be the consequence of long labor rather than the direct cause of chorioamnionitis)
- Nulliparity (no previous births)
- Previous chorioamnionitis
- Meconium-stained amniotic fluid (fetal stool in the fluid)
- Internal monitoring of the fetus and/or contractions
- Genital pathogens, including group B streptococcus and sexually transmitted infections
- Maternal smoking
- Maternal alcohol use

PROM, premature rupture of membranes; STI, sexually transmitted infection.
Data from Cohen-Cline, H. N., Kahn, T. R., & Hutter, C. M. (2012). A population-based study of the risk of repeat clinical chorioamnionitis in Washington State, 1989–2008. *American Journal of Obstetrics and Gynecology, 207*(6), 473.e1–473.e7; Soper, D. E., Mayhall, C. G., & Dalton, H. P. (1989). Risk factors for intraamniotic infection: A prospective epidemiologic study. *American Journal of Obstetrics and Gynecology, 161*(3), 562–568; Hunter, L. A. (2015). Complications during labor and delivery. In M. C. Bruker, T. L. King, J. M. Kriebs, J. O. Fahey, C. L. Gegor, & H. Varney (Eds.). *Varney's midwifery* (pp. 971–1030). Burlington, MA: Jones & Bartlett.

Box 7.6 Possible Causes of Intrapartum Fever

- Epidural anesthesia
- Chorioamnionitis
- Other infection (kidney, lung, etc.)
- Dehydration
- Overly warm room
- Use of prostaglandins to induce labor
- Extended water therapy (tub, shower, etc.)

Data from Hunter, L. A. (2015). Complications during labor and delivery. In M. C. Bruker, T. L. King, J. M. Kriebs, J. O. Fahey, C. L. Gegor, & H. Varney (Eds.). *Varney's midwifery* (pp. 971–1030). Burlington, MA: Jones & Bartlett; Higgins, R. D., Saade, G., Polin, R. A., Grobman, W. A., Buhimschi, I. A., Watterberg, K., Raju, T. N.; Chorioamnionitis Workshop Participants. (2016). Evaluation and management of women and newborns with a maternal diagnosis of chorioamnionitis: Summary of a workshop. *Obstetrics & Gynecology, 127*(3), 426–436.

Box 7.7 Criteria Required for the Clinical Diagnosis of Chorioamnionitis

Note: The definitive diagnosis of chorioamnionitis is made through a laboratory examination of the placenta and fetal membranes.

Must Be Present:

- Maternal oral temperature greater than 39°C (102°F) in a single reading or greater than 38°C (100.4°F) in two readings at least 30 min apart

Plus at Least One of Following:

- High maternal white blood cell count (>15,000/mm^3)
- Maternal tachycardia
- Fetal tachycardia (160 beats per minute or higher for 10 min or more)
- Cloudy or yellow discharge from the cervix

Data from Tita, A. T., & Andrews, W. W. (2010). Diagnosis and management of clinical chorioamnionitis. *Clinical Perinatology*, *37*(2), 339–354; Hunter, L. A. (2015). Complications during labor and delivery. In M. C. Bruker, T. L. King, J. M. Kriebs, J. O. Fahey, C. L. Gegor, & H. Varney (Eds.). *Varney's midwifery* (pp. 971–1030). Burlington, MA: Jones & Bartlett; Higgins, R. D., Saade, G., Polin, R. A., Grobman, W. A., Buhimschi, I. A., Watterberg, K., Raju, T. N.; Chorioamnionitis Workshop Participants. (2016). Evaluation and management of women and newborns with a maternal diagnosis of chorioamnionitis: Summary of a workshop. *Obstetrics & Gynecology, 127*(3), 426–436.

"Placenta abruption?" asks John. "That causes uterine tenderness, right? It's not that, is it?"

Darla shakes her head. "We don't have reason to think that," she says. "Her uterus feels relaxed between contractions even if it is tender. I'm not seeing excess bleeding. We know she has a fever and her membranes have been ruptured, maybe since yesterday. She's GBS-positive. No, the infection is a much more likely cause of the tenderness."

"I can't do it," says Hannah. "I'm sorry, I tried, but I need something to cut the pain, just a little."

Another contraction starts and she buries her head in her arm and tries to breathe normally. She tries to visualize a deer walking through an enchanted forest as she learned in birthing class. It doesn't work.

"Not an epidural. Just something," says Hannah. "John, I mean it. I know I told you to ignore me if I said I need something, but I need something."

"Alright," says Darla. "I'll give you some IV nalbuphine—that's Nubain. Just to warn you, it may make you groggy" (The Pharmacy 7.1).

"I don't care," says Hannah as another contraction starts. "I want it."

After taking the nalbuphine, Hannah feels like she is falling asleep between contractions and waking up to discover she's in labor.

"It's okay," John says. "Breathe, breathe."

"No, no, no," she moans. The contraction releases, like a car coasting to a halt, and she falls back to sleep. She wakes up again at the apex of the next contraction and falls back to sleep again, and again, and again, each time forgetting and waking up frightened.

"That baby's baseline heart rate is at one hundred seventy bpm and it's been at that rate for too long," says a new nurse, Phyllis. The shift changed an hour before, and Phyllis hasn't left the room since. "That baby needs to come out now."

"I don't know that she'll be ready to push. The last time I checked her, a few hours ago, before we gave her the nalbuphine and switched antibiotics, she was no more than four centimeters," says Darla. "Hannah, do you feel like you need to push?"

Hannah's face is buried in her pillow. The effects of the pain medication are waning, and she is starting to feel more present. "No, I don't think so."

"Hannah, I need to check your cervix to see if you're ready to push," says Darla.

"What if she's not?" asks John.

"We're not there yet. Ask me again if we get there."

The Pharmacy 7.1 — Nalbuphine (Nubain)

Overview	<ul><li>An opioid agonist–antagonist</li><li>Lower risk for respiratory depression and nausea than with an opioid agonist, such as fentanyl</li><li>Pregnancy category B</li></ul>
Route and dosing	<ul><li>10–20 mg/70 kg IV or IM every 3–6 h as needed in women with no history of opioid addiction</li><li>Predicted duration of action: 2–4 h IV and 4–6 h IM</li></ul>
Care considerations	<ul><li>Pain relief varies among patients.</li><li>Patients may be groggy. Neonates may also be groggy if the dose is administered 4 h or less before birth.</li><li>Laboring women may be sedated between contractions and have difficulty coping with the contractions themselves.</li><li>Encourage urination every 2 h and evaluate for bladder distention.</li></ul>
Warning signs	<ul><li>The medication may cause severe bradycardia in fetus. Bradycardia may be reversed with naloxone.</li><li>Newborns should be evaluated for bradycardia and respiratory depression.</li></ul>

IM, intramuscular; IV, intravenous.

With the next contraction, Darla inserts the fingers of her gloved hand into Hannah's vagina to feel the cervix.

Hannah moans. "It hurts," she says.

Darla removes her hand. "I'm sorry that hurts," she says to Hannah. "She's ten centimeters dilated. She's past ten centimeters," she says to Phyllis. "Hannah, it's time to start pushing. When you feel your next contraction, start pushing and keep pushing until the contraction is done."

"I'm scared," says Hannah. "I don't feel like I have to push. Why don't I feel like I have to push?"

"It may be the nalbuphine," says Darla. "I know you're scared. You can do this."

"It's the home stretch, sweetheart," says John. "Remember the stages. Stage two is the pushing stage. For a first birth, it averages a half hour to three hours" (see Table 1.3).

"You. Are. Not. Helping," says Hannah, and she pushes.

She feels burning and pressure—the hot, stretching feeling she learned about in class. She is surprised that pushing seems to help. When she pushes with the contraction, the pain gets better—much better than the previous pain of labor. She pushes with each contraction, resting as best she can against John's chest in between contractions.

"Oh, great work, Hannah!" says Phyllis after a half hour or so. "With that last push I could see a little fluffy head coming down. You can do this. Do you want to look in a mirror?"

Hannah shakes her head. As a student, Hannah thought of birth as almost a curiosity, an exhibition. Now that it is her own birth, she feels like she needs to focus on the task assigned, the pushing. Three more solid pushes is all it takes. The baby is crying about his rude eviction even before his shoulders clear the birth canal. He is passed into the waiting hands of a pediatric resident.

After Delivery

"You have a small laceration," says Darla (Fig. 7.2). "I'm going to suture it."

Hannah hardly cares. She is blissful over not having contractions. "What degree is it?" she asks. She feels like she's making polite conversation.

"It's just a first degree," says Darla. "There's no muscle involvement. A little lidocaine to numb you up and a few stitches to close it and you should be good to go."

"What about the placenta?" asks Hannah.

"You already passed it."

"Really?"

"Really."

"How did I not notice?"

"Well, in comparison it's pretty anticlimactic, and you're a little distracted. It's not unusual."

"We should take it home and make placenta smoothies," says John.

"No."

"We could grind it up and put it in gel caps. It's supposed to be great for milk production."

"No. And don't make me laugh. Darla's stitching my vulva. Do you want her to slip?"

"Alright. I'm all done," says Darla. "We're going to get you cleaned up and transfer you to the postpartum unit" (Box 7.8).

"The baby too, right?" asks John.

"Not just yet," says Darla. "We need to examine him first. We'll update you on his status as soon as we can."

The Newborn

After what seems like an eternity, a nurse who introduces herself as Julia arrives.

"A team is looking the baby over in the NICU, and he's wailing. He certainly doesn't seem ill. Because you had an infection during labor and delivery, Hannah, your baby is at risk for having one, too. The antibiotics we gave you also treated him, but there's a chance he'll need more antibiotics" (Box 7.9).

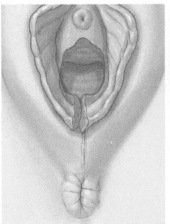
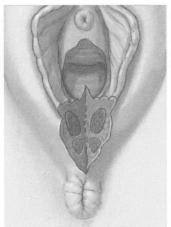
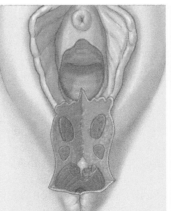
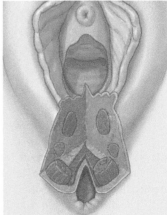

Figure 7.2. Degrees of perineal laceration. From left to right. First-degree laceration: injury to tissue of perineum and vagina, no injury to muscle; second-degree laceration: injury extends into fascia and muscle, anal sphincter intact; third-degree laceration: tearing extends into anal sphincter' fourth-degree laceration: injury extends through sphincter and rectal mucosa.

Box 7.8 Essential Information Required for Transfer From the Labor and Delivery Unit to the Postpartum Unit

- Patient name
- Allergies
- Duration of rupture of membranes
- Method of delivery
- Feeding method (breast or bottle)
- Course of labor
- Gestational age at delivery
- Gravidity and parity
- Time of birth
- Volume of blood loss
- Analgesia and anesthesia
- Preexisting medical conditions
- Medical conditions of pregnancy (gestational diabetes, preeclampsia, etc.)
- Names of support people
- Visitor restrictions
- Tubes: intravenous lines, urinary catheter, epidural, etc.
- Intake and output
- Bonding considerations
- Medications given during labor and delivery
- Scheduled medications
- Wounds: episiotomy or lacerations, cesarean incision

Box 7.9 Risks to Neonate of Chorioamnionitis

- Early-onset sepsis (within the first 3 d)
- Septic shock
- Pneumonia
- Meningitis
- Intraventricular hemorrhage (bleeding into the ventricles of the brain)
- Cerebral palsy
- Death

All of these risks are greater for preterm neonates than for term neonates.

Box 7.10 Management of a Newborn With a Group B Streptococcus–Positive Mother

Well-Appearing Infant

Adequate Maternal GBS Treatment (With Penicillin G, Ampicillin, or Cefazolin)

- Observation for 48 h
- Infants born at term may be released to home observation after 24 h

Inadequate Maternal GBS Treatment

- Infant born at term without PROM
  - In-hospital observation for 48 h
- Infant preterm or PROM
  - Limited diagnostic evaluation
    - CBC with differential and platelet count at birth and/or 6–12 h after birth
    - Blood culture at birth
- In-hospital observation for 48 h

Maternal Chorioamnionitis

- Limited diagnostic evaluation
  - CBC with differential and platelet count at birth and/or 6–12 h after birth and C-reactive protein
  - Blood culture at birth
- Antibiotics (empiric treatment for up to 48 h or until test result return)
  - Ampicillin dosing based on age, body weight, and the course of illness
  - Gentamycin dosing based on age, body weight, and the course of illness

Ill-Appearing Infant (Box 7.12)

Full Diagnostic Evaluation

- CBC with differential and platelet count
- Lumbar puncture
- Blood culture
- Chest radiograph

Antibiotics (May Be Adjusted Based on the Results of Diagnostic Testing)

- Ampicillin dosing based on age, body weight, and the course of illness
- Gentamycin dosing based on age, body weight, and the course of illness

CBC, complete blood count; GBS, group B streptococcus; PROM, premature rupture of membranes.
Data from Verani, McGee, and Schrag (2010); Polin, R. A. (2012a,b). Management of neonates with suspected or proven early-onset bacterial sepsis. *Pediatrics, 129*(5), 1006–1015.

"So do we just keep a closer eye on him for a few days?" asks John.

"We need to be more proactive than that," Julia says. "Right now they're doing a physical exam, but they'll also take blood samples to be cultured. The blood cultures may produce false-negative results, however, because of the antibiotics you've already had. So, they'll do a CBC and C-reactive protein and then repeat those at about the six-hour mark. If the CBC and C-reactive protein are off but the culture is fine, we'll probably still treat the baby with antibiotics for two to five days. In the meantime, we'll start him on some empiric antibiotics" (Polin, 2012; Box 7.10).

"Just in case?" asks Hannah.

"Just in case."

"Because he seems fine, right?" asks John.

"He sounds great," says Julia. "But don't take that as a diagnosis."

After the NICU team has finished examining baby Gaius, Julia wheels his bassinet into Hannah's room and then places him on his mother's chest.

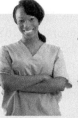

The Nurse's Point of View

Julia: My name is Julia and I'm a postpartum nurse, so I almost always take care of a couplet, both the mom and the baby. Depending on the day, I may also be taking care of partners, new grandparents, and siblings. But today I'm taking care of Hannah and baby Gaius. Hannah's fine. She had chorioamnionitis, but we gave her antibiotics both during and after the birth, and so far I don't have any reason to be concerned that she has a continuing infection. Her nurse during labor and delivery, Phyllis, said that the nalbuphine (Nubain) wore off around the same time that Hannah had to start pushing and that she was a champ at that.

Because she had chorioamnionitis and premature rupture of membranes, she is at greater risk for endometritis, an infection of her endometrial lining, which can produce a fever, tachycardia, and some uterine tenderness. Some women develop flu-like symptoms, as well. If this were to happen, one of my major concerns would be uterine subinvolution and atony, which could cause excessive bleeding. At the moment she's just on regular checks. So, unless something comes up, we don't need to take any further action now.

I'm more concerned about Gaius. Hannah had a fairly high fever, along with the chorioamnionitis, preterm rupture of membranes, and group B streptococcal (GBS) infection. According to Phyllis, there's also some question about whether her water had actually broken twenty-four hours before she was finally admitted for labor and delivery. I guess we'll never know, but either way we need to keep a more careful eye on Gaius to make sure he doesn't have **sepsis**, and treat him if he does. Sepsis in newborns with mothers who are GBS-positive is much less common than it used to be, but it definitely still happens, and the risk of it occurring in Gaius is higher because of the chorioamnionitis (Verani, McGee, & Schrag, 2010a). If it was just that Hannah was GBS-positive, we would most likely simply monitor Gaius for forty-eight hours and only do further testing and treatment if he developed symptoms. Because of the chorioamnionitis, however, we have to do more right from the outset.

Soon after his birth his blood was sent to be cultured. It usually takes about twenty-four to thirty-six hours to receive blood culture test results. Blood samples for a complete blood count (CBC) with differential and C-reactive protein (CRP) test were drawn then, as well, and an order is in to repeat those labs at

six to twelve hours. The blood culture is pretty straightforward to interpret most of the time: it's either positive or negative, and then there's a work-up to figure out which bacteria it is. The CBC and CRP are a little more challenging. In a neonate with an infection, the neutrophils can be either low or high, and many factors besides an infection can lead to a high count. A count that stays low is more suspicious for an infection than is a high count. An elevated ratio of immature to total neutrophils (the I/T ratio) can also suggest sepsis, but as many as half of infants without an infection can have this finding, as well. Like I said, it's not so straightforward.

The CRP isn't any easier to interpret. The CRP is increased with inflammatory conditions, and many factors can cause it to be elevated, including Hannah's fever. So a single measurement doesn't tell us much, but if we repeat it a few times and it stays high, that's more suspicious for sepsis. If it stays low, an infection is less likely.

Until we receive the culture test results, we'll keep Gaius on ampicillin and gentamicin. He gets the ampicillin every twelve hours and the gentamicin every twenty-four hours. If the blood culture test comes back positive and the bacterium involved is susceptible to penicillin, he may be switched to penicillin G every twelve hours for ten days. If the culture and lab test results are all negative for bacterial infection, we'll stop the ampicillin and gentamicin at forty-eight hours (Box 7.11).

> ### Box 7.11 Intravenous Therapy for Suspected Neonatal Group B Streptococcal Infection in Term Infant (excluding meningitis)
>
> **Empiric Antibiotics**
> Both of the following:
> - Ampicillin 150 mg/kg intravenously every 12 h
> - Gentamicin 4 mg/kg IV every 24 h
>
> **Typical Therapy After Confirmation of Diagnosis**
> - Penicillin G 50,000–100,000 U/kg/d in two doses for 10 d
>
> IV, intravenous.
> Data from Verani, McGee, and Schrag (2010a).

The nurses on the postpartum unit are keeping a close eye on Gaius. They check his temperature, pulse, and respirations every 4 hours and recruit Hannah and John to serve as eyes and ears monitoring the baby. Hannah packs her maternity nursing textbook in her hospital bag. For once, John doesn't make fun of her bookishness.

"There's a weird thing about baby fevers, right?" asks John.

"Yeah," says Hannah. "They can have either a high or a low temperature if they have an infection. I think preterm babies are more likely to have a low temperature than a high temperature."

"So we're worried about a high or low temperature," says John. "What else are we looking at?"

"Well, babies breathe super fast, so it's not considered tachypnea unless he's breathing over sixty bpm, and it's not bradypnea unless he's taking fewer than thirty bpm."

"And both are bad," says John.

"Both are bad. And tachycardia is over 160 bpm and bradycardia is under 100 bpm."

"Both bad."

"Both bad."

"So what are the two of us looking for?"

"Just changes, I think," says Hannah. "You know, if the baby seems listless, or doesn't feed. Seizures" (Box 7.12).

"You know, sometimes I think it's possible to know too much for your own sanity," says John.

Three days pass uneventfully, however. Three days of bonding with the baby, worrying over a possible infection, learning how to breastfeed, and dreaming about the future. Hannah and John take turns counting little Gaius' breaths and heartbeats.

The hospitalist pediatrician, Dr. Wittman, arrives.

"We've received Gaius' blood culture results, and they're positive for GBS," Dr. Wittman says.

"But he seems fine," says John. "He just seems like a baby. Do you think he looks sick?"

"I think he looks beautiful," says Dr. Wittman. "But I also think he has an infection. About eighty-five percent of these GBS infections are without focus, meaning that the infection is generalized and not specific to the lungs or the central nervous system or elsewhere. However, if his infection is focal, it will change how we care for him. We need to know. We need to evaluate his lungs and cerebral spinal fluid" (Verani, McGee, & Schrag, 2010b).

"So you're going to do a chest X-ray and a spinal tap on him?" asks Hannah. "Really?" She looks at her son, who is sleeping in her arms. She thinks about the needle she refused to have inserted into her own spine being inserted into his.

"That's our recommendation, yes," says Dr. Wittman. "Normally with this diagnosis we'd switch him to penicillin G at this point, but given that we had to switch you to a broader-spectrum antibiotic during labor, we're going to stick with the ampicillin and gentamicin he's currently on. We'd like to do the spinal tap and chest X-ray, and we'll do another blood culture in twenty-four to forty-eight hours, as well. We expect it to be negative at that point, but even if it is we'll continue the antibiotics for ten days. If the spinal tap comes back positive, we'll likely have to double the time he's on antibiotics."

"What happens if the blood culture is still positive after the next culture?" asks John.

"It shouldn't be," says Dr. Wittman. "But if it is we'll need to think about changing antibiotics."

Box 7.12   Select Signs of Neonatal Sepsis: What an Ill Infant Looks Like

Most Common Signs (>50% of Infants)

- Tachycardia (onset may be in utero)
- Hyperthermia (more common in term infants than preterm infants)
- Neonatal respiratory distress
  - Tachypnea or bradypnea (over 60 breaths per minute or under 30)
  - Seesaw respirations (the chest goes down while the abdomen goes up, and vice versa)
  - Nasal flaring
  - Grunting
  - Intercostal/subcostal retractions (pulling in of tissue between the ribs and under the rib cage with inhalation)
  - Pallor

Common Signs (25%–50% of Infants)

- Apnea
- Bradycardia
- Hypotension
- Lethargy
- Feeding difficulties
- Vomiting
- Jaundice
- Hepatomegaly (enlarged liver)

Least Common Signs (<25% of Infants)

- Irritability
- Seizures
- Central cyanosis
- Hypothermia (more common in preterm infants)
- Diarrhea
- Abdominal distension

Data from Nizet, V., & Klein, J. O. (2016). Bacterial sepsis and meningitis. In J. S. Remington, & J. O. Klein (Eds.). *Infectious diseases of the fetus and newborn infant* (pp. 217–271). Philadelphia, PA: Elsevier Saunders.

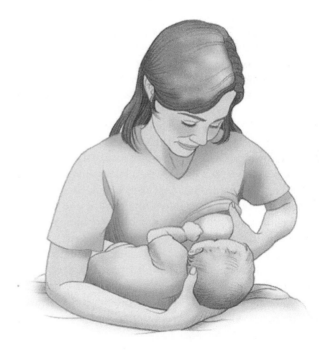

Figure 7.3. A proper breastfeeding latch. Note that Gaius has taken most of his mother's areola into his mouth. His lips are flanged out. Hannah holds her breast with her hand in a C shape. She supports his head at the occiput but is not pushing his head into her breast. Hannah and Gaius aren't skin-to-skin, but they are belly-to-belly, with Gaius's neck in a neutral position, not turned to either side. (Redrawn from the Office on Women's Health, U.S. Department of Health and Human Services. [2014]. Retrieved from http://www.womenshealth.gov/breastfeeding/learning-to-breastfeed.html)

"Can't he take these antibiotics at home?" asks Hannah. "I hate the idea of him staying here without us. We're trying to breastfeed, and it's hard to do that on demand if we're across town. Honestly, just talking about it is making me anxious."

"I wouldn't recommend caring for him at home at this point. I know you're both nurses, but that doesn't necessarily mean it's a good idea. We have a low census on the floor at this moment, however. You should be able to stay in this room until the treatment has ended. I'll let the charge nurse know we talked. You'll be discharged as a patient, Hannah, so you won't receive any more nursing care yourself, but you can stay."

"Really?" says Hannah. "That would be amazing."

Gaius does fine. His spinal tap is clear, as are his lungs. The second blood culture is clear. His temperature, heart rate, and respirations remain in the normal range. He eats like a champ.

"This kid needs to give eating lessons to the other babies," says Julia, the postpartum nurse, during the last feed before they pack to go home. "He has the best latch on the floor" (Fig. 7.3).

"I'm nervous about taking him home," says Hannah. "The upside of spending all this time in the hospital is having a community of people around helping to take care of Gaius."

"And the free diapers," says John. "Ten days of free diapers has been awesome."

Hannah glowers at him affectionately. "I'm a little nervous about doing it when it's just me and this dope."

"We're not going anywhere," says Julia. "If you think something's off, listen to yourself. Go to the ER, call the pediatrician. You're the eyes and ears now. Trust yourself if you think he seems lethargic or his breathing is weird. Get yourself a good thermometer. Keep your appointment with the pediatrician in a few days. You can do this."

"I can do this," says Hannah.

"Would it sound cornball if I said that we can do this?" asks John.

"Totally," Hannah says.

Think Critically

1. What risk factors does Hannah have for STIs? What STIs should she be screened for and why?
2. Write a brief dialogue illustrating how you would explain to a patient the procedure for evaluating for preterm rupture of membranes.
3. What clinical signs and symptoms would make you suspicious of chorioamnionitis in your patient?
4. Why are a CBC with differential and CRP not as reliable markers for infection for neonates as they are for adults?
5. Using Box 7.12, describe three different clinical presentations of neonates with sepsis, giving at least two different signs for each clinical presentation.
6. What are the care considerations for a patient postpartum with chorioamnionitis?

References

Centers for Disease Control and Prevention. (2016, March 16). *HIV among women*. Retrieved from http://www.cdc.gov/hiv/group/gender/women/index.html

Drassinower, D., Friedman, A. M., Običan, S. G., Levin, H., & Gyamfi-Bannerman, C. (2016). Prolonged latency of preterm premature rupture of membranes and risk of neonatal sepsis. *American Journal of Obstetrics and Gynecology, 214*(6), 743.e1–743.e6.

Gemzell-Danielsson, K., Berger, C., & Lalitkumar, P. (2013). Emergency contraception—mechanisms of action. *Contraception, 87*(3), 300–308.

Ham, D. P., Heyden, J. L., Opmeer, B. C., Mulder, A. L., Moonen, R. M., Beek, J., . . . Nijhuis, J. G. (2012). Management of late-preterm premature rupture of membranes: The PPROMEXIL-2 trial. *American Journal of Obstetrics and Gynecology, 207*(4), 276.e1–276.e10.

Heyden, J. L., Willekes, C., Baar, A. L., Wassenaer-Leemhuis, A. G., Pajkrt, E., Oudijk, M. A., . . . van der Ham, D. P. (2015). Behavioural and neurodevelopmental outcome of 2-year-old children after preterm premature rupture of membranes: Follow-up of a randomised clinical trial comparing induction of labour and expectant management. *European Journal of Obstetrics and Gynecology and Reproductive Biology, 194*, 17–23.

Polin, R. A. (2012). Management of neonates with suspected or proven early-onset bacterial sepsis. *Pediatrics, 129*(5), 1006–1015.

Tajik, P., Ham, D. P., Zafarmand, M., Hof, M., Morris, J., Franssen, M., . . . Mol, B. W. (2014). Using vaginal Group B Streptococcus colonisation in women with preterm premature rupture of membranes to guide the decision for immediate delivery: A secondary analysis of the PPROMEXIL trials. *BJOG: An International Journal of Obstetrics & Gynaecology, 121*(10), 1263–1272.

U.S. Preventive Services Task Force. (2016, June). *Final recommendation statement: Genital herpes: Screening*. Retrieved from http://www.uspreventiveservicestaskforce.org/Page/Document/RecommendationStatementFinal/genital-herpes-screening

Verani, J. R., McGee, L., & Schrag, S. J. (2010a). *Prevention of Perinatal Group B Streptococcal Disease: Revised Guidelines from CDC, 2010*. Atlanta, GA: National Center for Immunization and Respiratory Diseases.

Verani, J., McGee, L., & Schrag, S. (2010b). Prevention of perinatal group B streptococcal disease—revised guidelines from CDC, 2010. *Morbidity and Mortality Weekly Report, 59*(RR-10), 1–32.

Suggested Readings

Munro, M. L., Dulin, A. C., & Kuzma, E. (2015). History, policy and nursing practice implications of the plan b emergency contraceptive. *Nursing for Women's Health, 19*(2), 142–153.

Rubarth, L. B. (2003). The lived experience of nurses caring for newborns with sepsis. *Journal of Obstetric, Gynecologic, and Neonatal Nursing, 32*(3), 348–356.

Graciella Muñez:
8 Preterm Premature Rupture of Membranes and Neonatal Respiratory Distress Syndrome

Gracie Muñez, age 25

Objectives

1. Identify some initial nursing considerations for the assessment and treatment of a woman presenting with subfertility.
2. Identify signs of potential intimate partner violence and discuss proper nursing responses.
3. Distinguish between the risks and interventions related to preterm premature rupture of membranes (PPROM) and those related to premature rupture of membranes.
4. Describe the assessments commonly used with PPROM.
5. Identify signs of infant respiratory distress syndrome and describe appropriate nursing interventions to use in response to this condition.
6. Explain the potential risks of early postpartum discharge for a patient with PPROM.

Key Terms

Continuous positive airway pressure (CPAP)
Endometrial hyperplasia
Ferguson reflex
Leopold's maneuvers
Lochia alba
Lochia rubra

Lochia serosa
Luteinizing hormone
Neonatal respiratory distress syndrome
Oligomenorrhea
Preterm premature rupture of membranes (PPROM)

Before Conception

Graciella, known as Gracie by her friends and family, is a 25-year-old pharmacy technician who lives with her boyfriend, Freddie. They have been trying to get pregnant for the past year now, and Gracie is starting to worry that she may have fertility problems. She suspects that her weird menstrual cycle may be to blame.

Gracie was a late bloomer in many ways and had a difficult adolescence. She played with dolls until she was 14 years old, only stopping when her brother began teasing her about it. She didn't date much in high school. She was shy around boys and rarely spoke to anyone outside of her close group of friends. She was always plump. To lose weight, she ate hardly anything for breakfast or dinner and skipped lunch entirely, but then got so hungry that she overate late at night, after her family was asleep. She learned from the body mass index (BMI) chart in health class that she was overweight, but was relieved she wasn't obese—not quite (see Box 1.4). She got her first period when she was 15 years old and didn't have another for almost a whole year, at which point her mother became worried and took her to the pediatrician.

"Are you sexually active?" asked Dr. Munsch, after Gracie's mother told him what her concern was.

Gracie thought she'd die from embarrassment. She shook her head.

Dr. Munsch looked from Gracie to her mother. "Would you like to talk with your mother out of the room?"

Gracie thought it would be more humiliating to have to explain to her mother later why she wanted her to leave the room than it would be just to have her stay.

"No," Gracie managed. "I'm a virgin. I've never had sex."

"So, there's no chance you're pregnant," said Dr. Munsch. Gracie shook her head again. "No."

"It's not unusual for the timing of your period to be irregular when you're a teenager," said Dr. Munsch. "When the first day of one period is more than thirty-five days after the first day of your last period or you get fewer than nine periods a year, we call that oligomenorrhea. That's just a fancy way of saying you don't get a lot of periods. How's your skin? Do you have any acne?"

"Gracie has the most beautiful skin," said her mother. "She just washes with soap, and look how smooth her skin is—no pimples."

"Have you noticed any dark hair anywhere?" Dr. Munsch asked Gracie. "Have you seen any wiry hairs, maybe on your chin or your upper lip?"

Gracie blushed and shook her head.

"I think you're fine, Gracie," said Dr. Munsch. "This may well just be your body getting a period established. We've talked before about how you're overweight. You're not obese, but you are heavier than is healthy for someone of your height. Probably the best thing you could do for yourself is to lose weight. There's a chance that would help normalize your periods, as well."

"I try," said Gracie. "It's just hard."

"What do you see as the major obstacle to losing weight?" asked Dr. Munsch.

"I get hungry," said Gracie. "So I eat. When I get hungry I just grab anything."

"Have you tried keeping small, healthy snacks around that you can grab before you get too hungry?"

Gracie shrugged. Of course she had tried that. She felt like she'd tried everything. She didn't want to talk about it anymore. "I can try it," she said.

"Good," Dr. Munsch said. "I do want to run a few tests to make sure that there isn't anything else going on that is causing you to not get your period. While you're here I'd like to check your blood sugar and your cholesterol, as well. We haven't checked them in over a year, and, in light of your weight and the issue with your menses, I'd like to keep an eye on them. And I want to start you on a birth control pill to regulate your cycle" (Lab Values 8.1; see Patient Teaching 2.1).

Lab Values 8.1   Gracie's Labs for Oligomenorrhea

Lab Name	Rationale	Value
Labs to Rule Out Other Conditions		
Total testosterone	Assess for evidence of hyperandrogenism, which may indicate PCOS or a testosterone-producing tumor	For adult women, normal values are 40–60 mg/dL (1.4–2.1 nmol/L).
		Women with PCOS commonly have values between 20 and 150 ng/dL (1.0–5.2 nmol/L).
		Values over 200 ng/dL (6.9 nmol/L) suggest a testosterone-producing tumor.
TSH	Thyroid hormones may alter menstruation. Hypothyroidism (high TSH) may result in more menstrual bleeding than usual. Hyperthyroidism (low TSH) may cause amenorrhea or oligomenorrhea and lighter menstrual bleeding.	The normal range for TSH level is between 0.03 and 5.0 U/mL.
Prolactin	Prolactin is produced by the anterior pituitary. Some medications, as well as tumors of the pituitary, can cause elevated prolactin levels, which can lead to amenorrhea and oligomenorrhea.	A value of over 25 ng/mL suggests that a high prolactin level may be causing menstrual irregularities.
Labs to Monitor for Associated Conditions		
Fasting lipids	Women who are overweight with or without PCOS often also have elevated cholesterol.	• Desirable total cholesterol level is under 200 mg/dL. • Optimal LDL level is less than 100 mg/dL. • Optimal HDL level is greater than 59 mg/dL. • Normal triglycerides level is less than 150 mg/dL.

(continued)

Lab Values 8.1 — Gracie's Labs for Oligomenorrhea (continued)

Lab Name	Rationale	Value
Fasting glucose and hemo-globin A_{1c}	Insulin resistance and type 2 diabetes are common in women who are overweight with or without PCOS.	A fasting glucose level of 126 mg/dL (7 mmol/L) or higher on two different occasions indicates diabetes. Hemoglobin A_{1c}: • 4%–5.6%, normal • 5.7%–6.4%, increased risk for diabetes • 6.5% or higher, diabetes

HDL, high-density lipoprotein; LDL, low-density lipoprotein; PCOS, polycystic ovary syndrome; TSH, thyroid-stimulating hormone.

"Gracie is not having sex—she said so," said her mother. "Are you Gracie?"

Gracie shook her head vigorously, wanting to sink into the ground.

"I understand," said Dr. Munsch. "But there are other uses for the pill, and regulating your period is one of them. We'd like to see Gracie have a period at least once every three months so she doesn't develop a thickening of the lining of her uterus, a condition called **endometrial hyperplasia**. There are other ways to prevent this condition, but using an oral contraceptive is the most straightforward."

"Will it make me gain weight?" asked Gracie. "I don't want to take it if it means I'm going to gain weight."

"It is very unlikely that the birth control pill has any significant effect on weight," said Dr. Munsch. "I think this is a good choice for you" (Gallo et al., 2014).

So, Gracie began taking the pill every morning and went on with her life. She went to prom with a group of friends. She graduated from high school. And then she got a job as a pharmacy technician. That's where she met Freddie.

Freddie was almost 10 years older than her and worked as a deliveryman. Gracie had been working for the pharmacy for nearly 5 years and had seniority over the other techs she worked with. Freddie would drive up in his big truck and unload, and it was Gracie who handled the intake and paperwork.

Freddie was a talker. He'd chat about the weather and his route. He'd talk about other deliveries, what he'd had for lunch. He'd talk about the couple of kids he'd had with his ex-girlfriends. His teeth went in all directions and his breath always smelled like a combination of his lunch and the breath spray he kept in the front pocket of his uniform.

The first time they went out she didn't even know it was a date. It was a hot day and her pharmacy was the last stop for him. Her shift was ending and he said he was going next door for an ice cream and did she want to come. She said yes, mostly because she really did want an ice cream. She realized it was a date when he wiped her mouth with his own napkin.

They moved in together a few months after the first ice cream. Her mother thought it was too soon, and Gracie had her own reservations, which she shared with no one. But the allure of moving out of her mother's house and into the home of an older man who treated her kindly was enough to sway her.

"Why do you keep taking those pills?" he asked her one morning as she prepared to brush her teeth.

"They keep my period regular," she said.

"They keep you from having babies," he said. "Are you telling me you don't want to have a kid with me?"

"I don't know," she said. "I mean, maybe, someday. But we've only been together a little while. We're not even married. I just moved in."

"What do you want? Do you want me to say I'll marry you?"

"I don't know," said Gracie. She was confused by the turn of the conversation. "I don't know if I'm ready for that."

"I'm telling you I want to commit to you," said Freddie. "I don't want to see these pills anymore. I want you and me to make a family."

Gracie only nodded. She thought she loved him, but she wasn't sure she wanted to start a family, not yet. She was getting to know him better, though, and she knew the mood he was in. It was best just to agree with him. She decided to hide her pills at work and take them there. She didn't consider arguing the point. She didn't think she'd win.

It was harder to remember to take her pills at work because it was a change in habit and because she felt ashamed of it. It felt wrong that she and Freddie couldn't agree on when they wanted to start a family, that they couldn't even discuss it. She was ashamed that she didn't feel like she could just say no. She thought about talking with her mother about it but she knew her mother didn't like Freddie as it was. Her mother thought that Freddie didn't respect Gracie, but Gracie secretly thought she just hadn't done anything to earn that respect. And Gracie was sure her mother would never let a man tell her what to do with her body.

After a few months, she just stopped taking her pills entirely. Freddie was excited at first when she missed her period, but she knew this was normal for her. Her cycle wasn't regular without the pill and it might be months before she bled again. Freddie insisted week after week that she take pregnancy tests she bought discounted at the pharmacy, and week after week they came back negative.

"We know it's not me," said Freddie. "I got two kids. Maybe you can't get pregnant, you know?"

Gracie started wondering the same thing. After a few months she went from passively going along with the idea of getting pregnant to actively worrying that she couldn't get pregnant. What if she couldn't have children? What if Freddie left? She was already 24 years old and he was her first boyfriend in all these years. What if there was no one else for her?

And now, after a year of trying to get pregnant—of having only four periods and taking dozens of pregnancy tests—Gracie is anxious. Sex has become joyless and mechanical. Sometimes Freddie seems sympathetic and supportive, but other times he seems almost angry, as though she is intentionally avoiding getting pregnant. She tries to talk to him about it, but he just keeps telling her that it will happen, and his assurance just increases her anxiety. She needs advice.

She makes an appointment with a gynecologist for a month from now, the earliest time she can get in. She keeps a careful diary of her cycle during this month based on what she learns online. She tracks her temperature, which varies little from day to day, and her vaginal discharge, which always seems pretty much the same. She can't tell whether she's ovulated, at any rate (see Fig. 5.1; Fig. 8.1). Finally, the day of her appointment arrives.

"Our general rule is that we don't start evaluating and treating women younger than thirty-five years for infertility until a year of well-timed intercourse has passed without evidence of a pregnancy," says Dr. Jones. "About ninety percent of women get pregnant after a year of trying" (Slama et al., 2011). "The challenge here is the well-timed intercourse piece. Because your period is so irregular, we really don't know when you ovulate, so we don't know when to time intercourse."

Gracie nods. "That's what I thought. I was tested when I was a teenager for all kinds of things to figure out why I didn't get my period more regularly but the doctor didn't find anything. He thought it would help if I lost some weight, and he gave me the pill. That works when I'm taking it, but that's it."

"He was probably right about the weight loss," says Dr. Jones. "Did you lose weight?"

"I think I gained weight," says Gracie. Actually, she *knows* she's gained weight.

"That's one thing you can work on," says Dr. Jones. "Eat a lot of vegetables. Limit your caffeine and alcohol intake. Don't take drugs or smoke. Stay away from prepackaged foods, and eat lean proteins. I'd like to run some preliminary labs to look at what's going on with your irregular period, but we may come to the same conclusions as before."

"So what then?" asks Gracie. "Would we try in vitro fertilization?"

"That could be an option down the line," says Dr. Jones. "There are typically several steps before we get to that point, and a few health insurance policies cover infertility treatments. It can get expensive fast. In any case, you and your partner will have a lot of decisions to make."

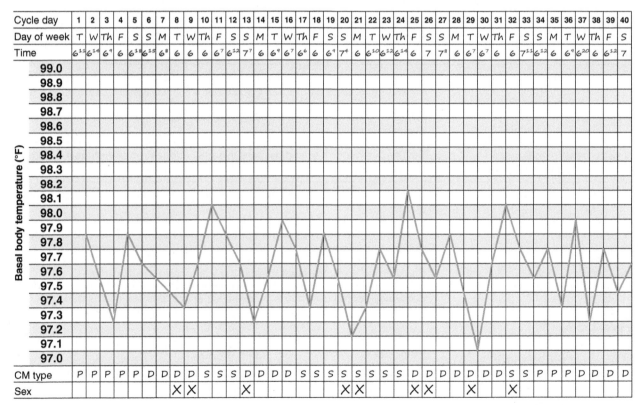

Figure 8.1. Anovulatory cycle chart. Note that with an ovulatory cycle, there is typically a small dip below the baseline temperature followed by an abrupt rise in the baseline temperature. In an ovulatory cycle that does not result in pregnancy, this baseline again drops with menstruation. In the case of an anovulatory cycle such as this one, there is no consistent baseline change or evidence of ovulation. CM, cervical mucus; P, period; D, dry; S, sticky rice.

"He's my fiancé," says Gracie. She's not sure why she feels the need to add this, but she does. "There's nothing wrong with him," she says. "He has two kids already."

"I see," says Dr. Jones. "That's good to know, though it doesn't necessarily rule out male factor infertility completely. Probably about twelve percent of men in this country have some kind of fertility issue" (Louis et al., 2013).

"I don't think he'd come in to get checked out," says Gracie. "He says this is my problem."

Dr. Jones is quiet for a minute. "Gracie, do you feel safe at home, safe with your fiancé?"

Gracie nods. "Yes, of course. He's just kind of old-fashioned, you know? But I don't feel like he's not safe to be around. We're fine."

"Are you scared of him?" asks Dr. Jones.

"Scared? No, I'm not scared," Gracie says.

Dr. Jones waits. Gracie plays with a pen she's holding.

"I feel like he'll leave me if I don't get pregnant, you know? Like I'm not even a woman to him anymore if I can't give him kids."

"That must be painful for you, thinking that," says Dr. Jones.

"It's just the way he thinks, the way he is," says Gracie. "I think maybe a lot of guys think that way, it's not just him."

"Maybe," says Dr. Jones. "But it doesn't make it right, Gracie. You have your own worth. Your ability to have children or wanting to have children is only one part of you. You're not just your ability to reproduce. You deserve someone who recognizes that."

"I know," says Gracie. "I'm probably making it sound way worse than it is. He loves me, I know it. And I love him. We just fight a lot about kids. You know, all the time when I take these pregnancy tests we get our hopes up and then nothing. It's hard on him. It's hard on us. It's not logical, but it's like a part of him thinks I'm not getting pregnant on purpose. He takes it personally."

"What about you, Gracie? Do you want to be pregnant?"

"Sure, I wouldn't be here otherwise, right?"

"Okay. I'm just checking because infertility workups and treatment can be emotionally grueling. They can be hard on individuals and couples. I want you to be comfortable with the decisions we make. Tell me if that stops being the case."

"I will," says Gracie. "What do we do first?"

Dr. Jones examines her (Table 8.1) and takes blood samples to send to the lab for tests, the same ones she had as a teenager when the oligomenorrhea was first identified. Dr. Jones also recommends gonorrhea and chlamydia screening just as a precaution and a Pap test because she was due for one (see Patient Teaching 2.2). The urine sample Gracie provided at check-in is negative for pregnancy, which is no surprise.

Table 8.1	Elements of Gracie's Infertility Health History and Exam
Element	**Rationale**
Health History	
Duration of infertility	Women younger than 35 y are typically evaluated only after a full year of well-timed intercourse. Women 35 y and older are generally evaluated after 6 mo.
Menstrual history	A regular cycle with molimina (breast tenderness and bloating) suggests ovulation.
Pain with menses and/or sex (dysmenorrhea and dyspareunia)	Severe dysmenorrhea and dyspareunia may suggest endometriosis, which can impair fertility.
History of STIs and PID	STIs and PID can cause scarring of the reproductive organs, which can impair fertility.
Obstetric history	A review of the patient's obstetric history may help identify events or conditions that lead to infertility.
Sexual history	Badly timed and infrequent intercourse can preclude pregnancy.
Lifestyle	Smoking, alcohol use, nutrition, exercise, and stress can all affect fertility.
Physical Exam	
BMI	Both high and low BMIs can impair fertility.
Acne and abnormal hair growth (hirsutism and male-pattern alopecia)	Acne and abnormal hair growth may indicate endocrine issues (PCOS, hypothyroidism, etc.) that may impair fertility.
Pelvic exam	An enlarged uterus, cervical or vaginal abnormalities, pain, masses, nodules, and inflammation may all suggest conditions that may impair fertility.

BMI, body mass index; PCOS, polycystic ovary syndrome; PID, pelvic inflammatory disorder; STI, sexually transmitted infection.

Her testosterone level is checked to rule out polycystic ovarian disease and any adrenal problems. Her blood levels of thyroid-stimulating hormone and prolactin are checked to rule out disorders of the thyroid and pituitary glands, respectively. Just as her pediatrician had, Dr. Jones checks her blood levels of cholesterol and glucose (the latter by way of a hemoglobin A_{1c} test) to rule out problems associated with being overweight.

"What if all these tests come back negative?" asks Gracie.

"Honestly," says Dr. Jones, "I expect they'll all be negative, except maybe the test for your blood sugar. In the meantime, there are two things I'd like to get started on. The first is weight loss. I'd like you to focus on diet and exercise, the old-fashioned way. As I said earlier, eat a lot of vegetables and lean protein and avoid simple carbs. Track everything you eat. Keep in mind that losing just five to ten percent of your body weight can make a tremendous difference to your fertility" (Best, Avenell, & Bhattacharya, 2017).

"I was worried you would say that," says Gracie. "I'm not saying I won't do it, but it's hard."

"I don't want you to think of weight loss as a short-term fix to your fertility problem. Any weight loss you achieve now, particularly weight loss you can sustain, will improve your overall health in the long term. Which brings me to part two. Have you noticed that your skin is different behind your neck and on your inner thighs around your groin?"

Gracie has noticed this and is self-conscious about it. She nods.

"That's a condition called acanthosis nigricans. It occurs in people who are insulin resistant" (Fig. 8.2).

"What does that mean?"

"Insulin resistance means that your cells require more stimulation by insulin before they'll take in the sugars that are circulating

in your bloodstream. It means that your pancreas has to work harder to make more insulin."

"Do you mean I'm diabetic?"

Dr. Jones shakes her head. "Not necessarily, not yet. We'll know more when we see the results of your blood work. But I do think you have a strong chance of developing type two diabetes over time, particularly if you don't lose weight and exercise. In addition to losing weight and exercising, I'd like you to start taking metformin. This may help with the acanthosis over time, and for some people, it also helps with weight loss and ovulation" (see The Pharmacy 3.2).

Gracie nods. She knows about metformin from the pharmacy. "So how long do you want me to work on the weight loss and take metformin?"

"Let's set a weight loss goal for you of twenty pounds over the next three months. If you still aren't menstruating more predictably, we can talk about trying clomiphene" (The Pharmacy 8.1). "That's a medication that stimulates ovulation and is associated with a really low rate of multiple pregnancies. It requires much less monitoring and has fewer side effects and complications than other fertility medications, so it's a good place to start. But keep in mind that your insurance will likely not cover the cost of clomiphene or other fertility drugs. You may have to pay for the medication and monitoring out of pocket."

"What do you mean by monitoring?" Gracie says.

"Patients take clomiphene for five days, starting on or around day five after their period starts. We estimate that if a woman is going to ovulate she'll do so about five to twelve days after stopping the clomiphene. If you don't, we can increase your dose. If you do but don't get pregnant, we can keep you on that same dose the following month if you decide to try again."

"How can you tell whether I've ovulated?"

"That's where the monitoring comes in. What I usually recommend for my patients is buying the urinary **luteinizing hormone**, or LH, strips. They're simple to read and tell you if you're having a surge in LH, the hormone that cues ovulation. You can get them from a pharmacy. Have you seen them?"

Seen them? She'd stocked them. Gracie nods.

"They're not expensive and you can use them to monitor at home and report back to us. That's what I recommend."

"I get an employee discount," says Gracie. "It's fifteen percent off."

"Good," says Dr. Jones. "I'd also like you to buy a prenatal vitamin now and start taking one every day."

"Should I do those LH monitoring strip things now even without taking the medicine?"

"You certainly could. If you do ovulate, you'll know about it, and if you get pregnant, we'll know exactly when it happened."

Now that she's trying to lose weight, Gracie realizes that her pharmacy is half candy store. Every season they stock new racks of seasonally packaged candy. Entire aisles are devoted to wine, chips, snacks, and nonseasonal candy. The freezers are stocked with ice cream and cheap frozen meals. She was in the habit of shopping for her food from the freezer and eating her lunch from the shelves.

"Why do you never have money anymore?" asks her coworker, Nina.

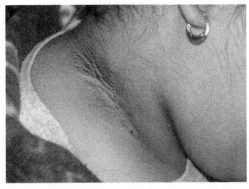

Figure 8.2. Acanthosis nigricans. This condition is present on the back of Gracie's neck and results in skin that is darkened and feels velvety. It typically occurs in folds, usually in the neck, groin, and axilla. It is closely associated with obesity, insulin resistance, and diabetes. In rare cases, it may be caused by a different endocrine problem, medications, some diseases, and cancer. (Reprinted with permission from Goodheart, H. P. [2003]. *Goodheart's photoguide of common skin disorders: Diagnosis and management* [2nd ed., Fig. 14.15]. Philadelphia, PA: Lippincott Williams & Wilkins.)

The Pharmacy 8.1   Clomiphene

Overview	• A selective estrogen receptor modulator used to stimulate ovulation
Route and dosing	• The first course is 50 mg by mouth daily for 5 d starting on or near day 5 of induced or spontaneous menses (if there is no recent or anticipated menses, it may be started at any time in the cycle). • Adjust the dose to 100 mg by mouth daily for 5 d for the next cycle if ovulation does not occur. • This medication may be used for up to six menstrual cycles.
Care considerations	• Side effects are rare and may include headache, hot flashes, and gastrointestinal symptoms. • Fertility treatment can be very stressful for women and families.
Warning signs	• Ovarian hyperstimulation syndrome is a rare but potentially serious complication. • Clinical manifestations include gastrointestinal distress, abdominal distension, respiratory distress, thromboembolism, oliguria, and others. • This condition is typically self-limiting but may require hospitalization.

"The doctor says I need to lose weight so I can get pregnant," Gracie says.

"If you're eating less, why does it cost more?"

"It costs more to eat healthy," says Gracie. "Vegetables and meat cost more than junk food."

"You're crazy."

"Yeah, well. You try going to a doctor and hearing you're too fat to have kids. It's embarrassing."

"Have you told that to Freddie?"

"No. I just told him we're eating better for when I get pregnant so our baby will grow and be healthy."

When Gracie returns to Dr. Jones' office to check-in at the 3-month mark, she weighs 20 lb less and has had two periods. The dark velvety patches of skin under her arms and along her inner thighs, the acanthosis, have faded a little, she thinks. She brings with her an LH test she took 2 weeks ago and a pregnancy test she bought that morning before her shift started. Both have two pink lines.

Pregnancy

First Trimester

"This is great," says Dr. Jones, "because you're pregnant, clearly, but also because we can do your first prenatal visit now."

"How often do I need to come in?" asks Gracie. "I need to let my manager at work know."

"Assuming there are no issues, we'll next see you around thirteen weeks, when the second trimester starts. Then we'll do monthly visits for three or four visits during the second trimester. In the third trimester, starting at twenty-eight weeks, we'll start seeing you every week."

"That's a lot of visits. I don't know if I can do all that. I have to work. I'm going to start buying diapers and stuff now and putting away some money. I'll have six weeks of leave when this baby comes, but I won't get any pay. I can't take time off now. I have to save up."

"I understand. However, it is important that you come to as many of the scheduled visits as possible. We can schedule you as the very first or very last visit of the day, if that would help."

"Maybe if I came in a half hour late to work I could stay later and make it up."

"Sure. Just let them know at the front desk what you decide," says Dr. Jones. "So the good news is we already took care of some of your labs. We'll draw blood today for some other routine assessments and then we'll see you again at about thirteen weeks" (Lab Values 8.2; see Table 1.1).

"Don't I need an ultrasound or something to see the pregnancy?"

"Not right now," says Dr. Jones. "We know when you ovulated and we know that you're pregnant. If we did an ultrasound this early, it might be too early to see anything at all. We'll order one at your next visit."

"So I'll get to see the baby at my next visit?"

"Yes," Dr. Jones says. She hands Gracie a sheet of paper. "This is our recommended schedule of testing" (Box 8.1).

"I hope you're keeping track of all this," says Gracie. "Because there's no way I can."

Second Trimester

For a while, things go pretty well. Freddie never comes with her to appointments because he has to work, but he gives her some money sometimes for expenses for the apartment and the car. He is taking more shifts out of town because they pay better, but he calls most nights when he is away. He jokes that he stays away at night so he won't have to eat all the vegetables she's cooking. She's started to cut costs by eating frozen instead of fresh vegetables.

Being pregnant is lonelier than she thought it would be. Her mother and stepfather left town shortly after she'd moved out for her stepfather's job. Her work friend, Nina, is single and likes to party. The last thing Nina wants is to spend all her time with a pregnant lady who always seems to be tired or nauseous or broke

Lab Values 8.2 Gracie's First Trimester Labs

Lab Name	Rationale	Value
Blood type and screen	To determine blood type, Rh factor, and any antibodies present in the blood from exposure to fetal blood. With certain maternal blood types, such as Rh negative, a fetus with the opposite blood type (in this case Rh positive) has the potential to promote maternal antibodies against that pregnancy.	A+
Complete blood count	To evaluate the blood for various kinds of anemia and infection	*RBC count:* 5.1 million cells/µL *WBC count:* 4,650 cells/µL *HCT:* 30% *HGB:* 13 g/dL *MCV:* 82 fL *MCH:* 27 pg/cell *MCHC:* 33 g/dL
Rubella blood test	To detect antibodies to the rubella virus in the blood, indicating immunity. Rubella is a virus that is routinely vaccinated for in childhood. A rubella infection in pregnancy can be highly damaging to a fetus (teratogenic). Because vaccinations don't always work and sometimes wear off, pregnant women are often screened in pregnancy to determine whether they're susceptible. The rubella vaccine is a live virus and cannot be given during pregnancy. It is often given in the hospital during the postpartum period.	11 IU/mL
HBV blood test	To detect antigens, antibodies, and DNA associated with HBV in the blood, indicating immunity or infection. Many people are now vaccinated for HBV. A person may also have an acute or chronic infection or no exposure. HBV is vertically transmitted, which means it can be passed from mother to fetus. HBV can lead to liver cancer.	*HBV antibodies:* positive (indicates Gracie is immune to HBV)
Syphilis blood test	To detect syphilis bacterium in the blood, indicating an infection. Syphilis infection is vertically transmitted from mother to fetus and is teratogenic.	Negative
HIV blood test	To detect antibodies, antigen, or the HIV virus in the blood, indicating an infection. HIV can be transmitted to a fetus vertically. With treatment of the mother in pregnancy, however, transmission is reduced to a less than 2% chance. The test can involve a finger stick, serum testing, or an oral swab.	Negative
Urine dipstick	To detect urinary tract infection, glucose in the urine (indicating high blood sugar), and protein in the urine (which may indicate kidney problems)	*Protein:* negative *Glucose:* negative *Ketones:* negative *Nitrites:* negative *Leukocytes:* negative *Blood:* negative

HBV, hepatitis B virus; HCT, hematocrit; HGB, hemoglobin; MCH, mean corpuscular hemoglobin; MCHC, mean corpuscular hemoglobin concentration; MCV, mean corpuscular volume; RBC, red blood cell; WBC, white blood cell.

or going to some appointment. Nina said at the beginning that she'd go to some appointments with Gracie if she wanted her to, but it never seems to work out because Nina usually covers at work for Gracie so she can go to her appointments.

She keeps up with her diet. Because her BMI is in the overweight range but not in the obese range, she is trying to keep her weight gain between 15 and 25 lb for the whole pregnancy (see Box 1.5). Some weeks are better than others, and during the first trimester, the only

Box 8.1   Gracie's Recommended Prenatal Screening

First Trimester

Screening Blood Tests at First Visit

- Cystic fibrosis (Gracie is determined based on family history and ethnic background to be a candidate for assessment for carrier status)

Blood Test at 12 wk for Trisomy Birth Defects

- Pregnancy-associated plasma protein: low in an abnormal test
- Human chorionic gonadotropin (hCG): high in an abnormal test

Ultrasound at 12 wk to Assess for Birth Defects

- Nuchal translucency (measurement by ultrasound of the space at the back of the fetal neck): thick in an abnormal test

Second Trimester

Integrated Screening: Additional Labs Drawn at 16 wk

- Blood tests for four markers:
  - Maternal serum alpha-fetoprotein screening
  - hCG
  - Unconjugated estriol
  - Inhibin A

These are interpreted in combination with the first trimester ultrasound and 12-wk labs.

Other Tests

- Fetal survey ultrasound to assess the fetus (20 wk; the sex may be assessed at this time)
- 50-g, 1-h glucose screen for diabetes (26 wk; Gracie's glucose level is 140 mg/dL, so she requires further testing with the 100-g, 3-h test, below)
- 100-g, 3-h glucose test (see Lab Values 3.2)

Third Trimester

- Vaginal and rectal swab for group B streptococcus (36 wk)

---

thing that made her nausea better was eating, so gained 10 lb. The weight gain slowed down after that, however, particularly once her fatigue wore off in the second trimester and she felt like she could walk more. She tries to walk to and from work most days, a round trip of 5 miles. At 24 weeks, her glucose level is elevated during her screening 1-hour glucose tolerance test, but her numbers are within the normal range for her diagnostic 3-hour glucose tolerance test (see Lab Values 3.2), ruling out gestational diabetes.

Third Trimester

It is a Thursday, and Freddie is home for the evening. Gracie is nearly 33 weeks pregnant. The baby has been its usual active self,

and they've been watching the movement of her belly as though it were live streaming television. She gets up to use the bathroom and feels a rush of fluid soak through her leggings.

Freddie laughs. "Did you pee yourself, girl?"

Gracie is confused. "No, I don't think so. I still have to pee, so this can't be pee."

Freddie stops smiling. "Your bag of waters broke, then?"

"I don't think so. I think it's too early, right? Isn't that what happens in the movies when the lady's water breaks and she's like, 'I'm having a baby! Take me to the hospital'?"

Freddie shrugs. "Maybe it's happening early?"

"I don't think it's supposed to," says Gracie. "Dr. Jones told me to call her with something like this."

She calls the office and a person working for an answering service tells Gracie he'll page the on-call provider. Gracie is relieved when it's Dr. Jones herself who calls back. She tells Gracie to head to labor and delivery for evaluation.

A half hour later, she and Freddie arrive in the triage area of labor and delivery.

"Are you having any contractions?" asks a nurse named Tiffany.

"I don't know," says Gracie. "I don't think so. There was just this fluid, and I think I'm still leaking."

"Do you think she peed herself?" Freddie asks.

"That can happen," says Tiffany. "The only way to be sure is to do an exam. I want to get a set of vital signs and a fetal heart rate to start with, and then we'll check."

A blood pressure (BP) cuff is wrapped around Gracie's arm and starts to inflate. Tiffany checks that baby's heart rate. The room fills with a strong, steady clip-clop noise, like the gallop of a miniature pony. It's the baby's heartbeat. Tiffany reads the display and tells Freddie and Gracie that the heart rate is 140 beats per minute (bpm).

"That seems fast," says Freddie.

"We expect the baseline heart rate for a fetus to be between about 110 and 160 bpm," says Tiffany. She turns back to Gracie. "I want to determine how your baby is positioned," she says. "I'm going to be feeling all over your belly doing something called **Leopold's maneuvers**. Do you want me to tell you what I'm feeling for?"

Gracie nods.

Tiffany places her palms on the fundus of Gracie's belly. "Right now I'm trying to find out if your baby is head down or butt down. What I'm feeling at the top of your uterus is soft and doesn't have a firm curve, which makes me think it's not the head but the butt up here. That's good. We want the baby to be head down right now."

Tiffany moves her hand down either side of Gracie's belly, still feeling with her palms and fingers. "I'd like to know how your baby is facing. One side is smooth, that's the back, but on the other side I'm feeling a lot of lumps and bumps—the hands, elbows, feet, and knees."

Gracie laughs. "I could have told you that's where the knees are," she says, thinking about the show the baby had been putting on before the wetness soaked through her leggings.

Using her right hand, Tiffany grasps the lower part of Gracie's abdomen and wiggles it. "The part down here is much firmer, so we've confirmed your baby is head down. It has some room to wiggle side to side, however, which tells us it's not deep in your pelvis. So, your baby is floating up above your pelvic bones instead of being engaged."

For the final maneuver, Tiffany shifts her body so her fingertips are facing toward Gracie's groin, one hand still on either side of her belly. She feels low on the side that is bumpy with knees and elbows. "I'm feeling for how the head is positioned. We know where it is, but I'd like to know whether the baby's head is tucked toward its chest or flexed back. Your little one seems tucked, which is good. Was any of this exam tender?" (see Fig. 1.7 and Box 7.3).

"Not really," says Gracie.

Tiffany then explains how she will check the fluid that Gracie reported (see Step-by-Step Skills 7.1). After performing the exam, she steps out to use the microscope and then returns. "I think your membranes did rupture," she says. "Your water broke."

"Does this mean the baby is coming now?" asks Gracie.

"We hope not," says Tiffany. "Gracie, it would be really early if your baby came now. We'd like it to stay in the womb a little longer to give it a better chance at being healthy. We've paged Dr. Jones' office, and someone should be here soon to discuss a plan with you."

"Early?" asks Freddie. "Like preemie? I thought that just meant a baby that's really tiny."

"Sometimes," says Tiffany. "But babies born early often haven't had enough time to completely develop important systems, like lungs. That can lead to some short- and long-term issues. The longer this pregnancy goes, the better off this baby is likely to be."

"If it's not the baby's time, I don't understand why this happened," says Gracie.

"Most of the time we don't know what causes preterm birth or **preterm premature rupture of membranes**—PPROM—which is what it's called when your water breaks before you're thirty-seven weeks pregnant and you have no contractions."

Dr. Jones arrives in time to see Gracie be moved from triage into a room.

"We're mainly concerned about two things," she says, "infection and prematurity. If you were a few weeks further along, we'd consider inducing labor to reduce the chance of infection, but you're early enough that this baby is better off in than out" (Box 8.2).

"What's she supposed to do?" asks Freddie. "Just keep her legs crossed or something?"

Dr. Jones smiles. "If that worked, no baby would ever be born preterm. Gracie, you were scheduled to be screened for group B streptococcus (GBS) at thirty-six weeks, but we're going to go ahead and test you for that now. We tested you at the beginning of the pregnancy for gonorrhea and chlamydia, but I'd like to check you for that again now, just to be safe."

"I don't have any disease," says Freddie.

"That's good," says Dr. Jones. "The test should come back negative. We're going to put you on some antibiotics, Gracie, and I'd like to keep you here for monitoring. We'll also be giving you a course of steroid shots to help your baby's lungs mature faster."

"So, what's the worst case scenario, Doc?" asks Freddie. "They'll both be okay if we do all that you were talking about, right?"

Box 8.2 Risks of Late-Term Premature Rupture of Membranes

- Infection (chorioamnionitis and others)
- Fetal malpresentation leading to cord prolapse
- Fetal malpresentation leading to cesarean delivery
- Placental abruption (risk increases with infection)
- Preterm birth
- Cord compression
- Oligohydramnios leading to malformations of limbs and lungs (rare after 23 wk of gestation)

"We hope so," says Dr. Jones. "We're concerned about infection and we're concerned about keeping the pregnancy going long enough for the lungs to mature a little longer, helped along by those steroid injections" (The Pharmacy 8.2). "We'll monitor the baby closely with nonstress tests that monitor the heart rate. If we have reason to think infection has set in or that the baby isn't doing well, we'll talk about ending the pregnancy early."

"So, how much longer is she supposed to be pregnant?" asks Freddie.

"We'd love it if we could get her to thirty-four weeks without an infection or problems with the baby. So, we'd like to delay the birth another week or maybe a little longer if everything looks safe."

"So you're telling me that if I get these shots my baby will be okay?" asks Gracie.

"We can't give you any guarantees," says Dr. Jones. "We know the steroid will help with lung maturity and may also reduce the risk of other complications we see sometimes with preterm babies, such as brain bleeds and severe damage to the intestines. This isn't a cure-all, however. You should be aware that there is still a risk for complications. We'll be keeping a close eye on your little one for a while after the birth, even if things go perfectly."

"Do I have an infection?" Gracie asks the nurse, Miriam, who has come to give her antibiotics a little while after the discussion with Dr. Jones. "Did the chlamydia test come back positive? Is that why I need an antibiotic?"

"I don't believe so," says Miriam. "I don't think that the tests we ordered have even made it to the lab yet. The purpose of the antibiotic I'm giving you right now is to treat any existing infection that may have caused the rupture of membranes and to prevent any new infection. If we can keep away infection, we might also keep labor and delivery at bay" (Box 8.3).

"Wait," says Gracie. "So, this can stop labor from happening?"

"That's what we hope," says Miriam. "Keep your eye on the prize. If we can get you through to 34 weeks, we have a much better shot at keeping your baby healthy."

"I hope so," says Gracie. "My boss said that if something like this happened I'd be using up my maternity leave time to be in the hospital. I can't afford to take more time than that, you know?"

Miriam nods sympathetically. "Yeah. I know."

The Pharmacy 8.2 — Betamethasone and Dexamethasone

	Betamethasone	Dexamethasone
Overview	• Administered to women at risk for preterm birth between gestational weeks 23 and 34 • Reduce the risks of neonatal death, as well as respiratory distress syndrome, necrotizing enterocolitis, and intraventricular hemorrhage	
Route and dosing	• Two doses of 12 mg IM 24 h apart	• Four doses of 6 mg 12 h apart
Care considerations	• Fetal heart rate changes (especially reduced variability) and fetal activity changes may be noted for 4–7 d after administration. • Some women may experience hyperglycemia starting at 12 h postpartum for up to 5 d. Closer monitoring of blood glucose is indicated in mothers with diabetes.	
Warning signs	• Rare anaphylaxis has occurred with the administration of corticosteroids. • Symptoms of anaphylaxis typically occur within a half hour of exposure and involve multiple systems. • Common symptoms are a pruritic rash, swelling of the throat and other body parts, breathing issues, gastrointestinal symptoms, and a feeling of impending doom.	

IM, intramuscular.

"So, how long am I taking all this medicine?"

"One week and we'll stop, even if you haven't gone into labor yet. But because you're so close to 34 weeks, expect that you'll be holding your baby soon after."

Gracie stays in the hospital for a week on antibiotics. Her vital signs, including her temperature, are taken every 4 hours. The fetus has its heart rate taken at the same time through her belly, and her nurses always ask if her abdomen is tender, which is a sign of infection, a nurse explained. Every evening, a nurse wheels in the fetal and contraction monitor for a nonstress test (see Box 3.6 and Fig. 4.8). By the middle of the week, Gracie can point right to the spot on her belly where the nurses can pick up the fetal heart tones. The tocodynamometer placed at the top of her uterus never picks up a contraction.

Box 8.3 — Sample Antibiotic Regimens for Preterm Premature Rupture of Membranes

Regimen #1
• Ampicillin 2 g intravenous (IV) every 6 h for 48 h
• *Followed by* amoxicillin 500 mg by mouth three times daily for 5 d
• *Plus* azithromycin, single dose, 1 g by mouth at the time of admission

Regimen #2
• Ampicillin 2 g every 6 h
• *And* erythromycin 250 mg every 6 h for 48 h
• *Followed by* amoxicillin 250 mg every 8 h
• *And* erythromycin 333 mg by mouth every 8 h for 5 d

Regimen #3 (for patients with a penicillin allergy but a low risk for anaphylaxis)
• Cefazolin 1 g IV every 8 h for 48 h
• *Followed by* cephalexin 500 mg by mouth four times daily for 5 d
• *Plus* azithromycin, single dose, 1 g by mouth at the time of admission

Regimen #4 (for patients with a penicillin allergy and a high risk for anaphylaxis)
• Clindamycin 900 mg IV every 8 h for 48 h
• *Plus* gentamicin 7 mg/kg ideal body weight for two doses 24 h apart
• *Followed by* clindamycin 300 mg by mouth every 8 h for 5 d
• *Plus* azithromycin, single dose, 1 g by mouth at the time of admission

Labor and Delivery

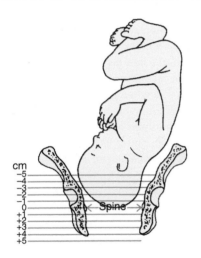

The Nurse's Point of View

Miriam: Gracie made it to thirty-four weeks without an infection. We're all relieved. Everyone on the floor is rooting for her. She's been really nice to work with in the week or so she's been here, but she's so quiet and seems lonely. There have been whole days when she doesn't get a phone call from her fiancé. Her mother came by once, and she has a friend from work who visits most days, but no one has been able to stay long. Everyone works, you know? She's scheduled to be induced in the morning because her obstetrician thinks the danger of prematurity at this point is less than the risk of infection, particularly since Gracie finished her course of corticosteroid injections. I sure hope her fiancé shows up for it.

It's 8:00 in the morning, and Gracie's fiancé Freddie still hasn't shown up. He was supposed to be here a half hour ago. Gracie said it was okay to go forward, so her obstetrician, Dr. Jones, did the cervix check. Her cervix is soft with an anterior orientation. She's about sixty percent effaced and two centimeters dilated. The fetal head is engaged at station 0 (Fig. 8.3), which is a change from when she was first admitted. She has a Bishop score of eight, which is favorable for delivery (see Analyze the Evidence 1.1). If she had a lower score, her team might have considered ripening her cervix with misoprostol

or prostaglandin E_2 before starting the oxytocin to increase the likelihood that her cervix will dilate sufficiently for a vaginal birth. As it is, she'll start with oxytocin and skip the ripening.

Freddie arrives at about 8:30, just as we're getting ready to start the oxytocin. Gracie seems happy to see him. He says he had an out-of-state route the night before and got home late and overslept. He does look pretty haggard. Gracie's IV is already started, so I attach the oxytocin to the most proximal port in her IV. I set the pump to administer one milliunit per minute. Depending on her response to the medication, I'll titrate that dose up by one or two milliunits every half hour or hour. My goal is that Gracie will have one contraction every two or three minutes that lasts about eighty to ninety seconds each. We want that to occur consistently, and the fetal monitoring strip, which also gives us a read on the contractions, is helpful for keeping track (Fig. 8.4).

Gracie says that she wants to try to go without any kind of pain relief. She does pretty well through the latent phase of the first stage, when the contractions are milder and do not last much longer than thirty seconds or so (see Table 1.3). As she moves into the active phase, though, I see a change in her. Her contractions get stronger, longer, and closer together, just like we want them to, but she appears to be frightened and in more pain. I hold her hand and rinse her face with a cool washcloth. I encourage Freddie to take my place, but he looks scared too. He watches from a chair on the other side of the bed. After a while, Gracie asks for an epidural, and we make the call to anesthesiology. Gracie seems really embarrassed, like somehow she's let everyone down, including herself and Freddie. I tell her it isn't like that, and besides, the important thing is that she is making the right decision for her.

Dr. Jones checks Gracie's cervix and reports that she's four centimeters dilated. I help Gracie to the bathroom to empty her bladder and then give her bolus of normal saline prior to the epidural placement to help prevent hypotension that could be dangerous to her baby after the epidural is placed. We'll encourage her to empty her bladder into a bedpan periodically so it doesn't hamper labor. If she can't do it spontaneously, we may have to do it for her with a straight catheter once or twice. Our hospital used to just do Foley catheters for everyone getting an epidural, so encouraging women to void spontaneously or just doing a straight catheter is a newer protocol for us (Suleiman et al., 2017).

Gracie sits on the edge of the bed while the anesthesiologist, Don, works behind her. I place a chair in front of Gracie and have Freddie sit in it so he can hold her hands. She makes a little noise when the numbing medication goes in, but that's it. I help Gracie lie on her side and reposition her toco and fetal monitor to make sure they're still in the optimal spots. So far everything looks good. We'll continue to monitor Gracie's

Figure 8.3.   Fetal stations. Note that Gracie's baby is in line with the ischial spines at 0 station. (Modified with permission from Weber, J. R. [2018]. *Nurses' handbook of health assessment* [9th ed., Fig. 24.8]. Philadelphia, PA: Lippincott Williams & Wilkins.)

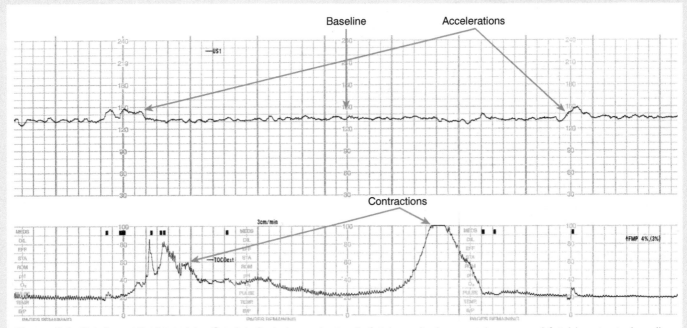

Figure 8.4. Fetal monitoring strip. Gracie's first-stage electronic fetal monitoring reveals a normal fetal heart rate baseline, moderate variability, presence of accelerations, and no decelerations. (Modified with permission from Freeman, R. K., Garite, T. J., Nageotte, M. P., & Miller, L. A. [2012]. *Fetal heart rate monitoring* [4th ed., Fig. 14.26]. Philadelphia, PA: Lippincott Williams & Wilkins.)

BP for hypotension and the baby for bradycardia and poor variability every five minutes until we're sure they're stable. If after twenty minutes of checking Gracie's vitals every five minutes everything is stable, we'll go down to checking every half hour. We'll keep the fetal monitor and toco on, however, so that we can observe changes in real time.

In all, Gracie's first stage of labor, the time until her cervix is fully dilated, takes almost twelve hours. That's normal, though it can seem like a long time. Thanks to the epidural, she's been able to rest a little bit through it. Her mother and friend both visit for a while and promise to come back when it's over. Gracie says she doesn't want anyone to see the birth who doesn't have to. She says she's worried it will be disgusting. She doesn't really even want Freddie here, I think. He left about an hour ago, anyway, saying he'd be back. He said he wanted some food and a smoke. We're lucky on this unit that we're only usually assigned one patient. Without a regular outside support person I think Gracie really needs me here. Sometimes just having another person in the room can make a difference.

Dr. Jones' on-call shift ends and her colleague Dr. Rheinhart comes in. I brief him on the progress so far. Gracie's cervix hasn't been checked for about four hours, and in the last half hour her contractions have been a little longer and her uterus has been firm to the touch while they're occurring. Dr. Rheinhart checks Gracie and finds that she is fully dilated and effaced.

He says that he wants her to labor down until she's at about +2 station. I explain to Gracie that laboring down means that you let the baby make its way down the birth canal without pushing, and that by doing that a woman can significantly shorten the amount of time she's pushing.

It takes Gracie almost an hour to labor down to +2. This is the time during the second stage (the second stage being the time between full dilation and effacement and the birth) when a lot of women will feel an urge to push. The urge is called the **Ferguson reflex**. It doesn't always happen, particularly if a woman has had an epidural, and it doesn't happen with Gracie. That means it's up to us to coach her as to when to start pushing and when to stop.

We start having her push with each contraction. I keep a hand on her abdomen so I can feel when each starts and ends. She's been pushing like this for nearly half an hour when Dr. Rheinhart says he can see the head and some curly hair peeking out. Gracie says she doesn't want to see, but she allows Dr. Rheinhart to guide her hand down so she can feel the baby's head. It takes about five more pushes before the head is out completely. A few more pushes later, the rest of the baby is born. Because he's so premature, he's handed off to the pediatric team immediately, and they work with him under a warmer (Fig. 8.5).

Gracie has a second-degree perineal laceration, a tear through skin and muscle that stops short of her anal sphincter

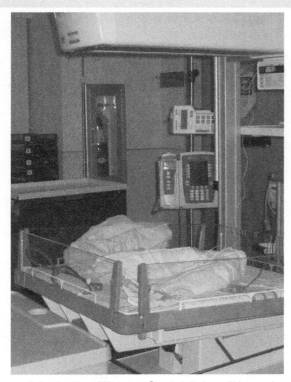

Figure 8.5. Radiant Warmer. Gracie's baby will be evaluated on this bed, which is heated by an element over the table. (Reprinted with permission from Tecklin, J. S. [2014]. *Pediatric physical therapy* [5th ed., Fig. 4-7]. Philadelphia, PA: Lippincott Williams & Wilkins.)

(see Fig. 7.2). I know from experience that the pressure of the head on the perineum often means that these aren't as painful as they look, but I'm still glad Gracie has an epidural, if for no other reason than she won't need any additional medication while Dr. Rheinhart sutures the injury. Tears like these are really common and usually heal very well.

As Dr. Rheinhart completes the sutures, Freddie enters the room. He looks well rested. He's carrying flowers and a silver balloon and at least has the decency to look sheepish. He tells Gracie he figured he'd just be in the way and that she did great, and he's proud of her.

The Newborn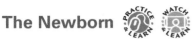

He doesn't cry when he's born. He's blue, not just his hands and feet but also his face. He flexes his arms and legs when his airways are suctioned, but he doesn't pull away. His heart rate is 150 bpm, and his limbs are flexed.

"Apgar one minute is five," says the pediatrician. "That's moderate depression" (see Table 1.4). A nurse enters it into the record.

The pediatrician suctions out the baby's mouth and then the nose using a tool attached to a panel on the wall. "This is to make sure the baby doesn't aspirate, or breathe in fluid," the nurse explains. The nurse attaches some kind of device to the baby's left wrist, which she explains is a pulse oximeter (Fig. 8.6).

"Apgar at five minutes is still five," the pediatrician says. Reading the pulse oximeter, he says, "Oxygen saturation is seventy percent" (Table 8.2). "He's tachypneic, with a respiratory rate of over sixty breaths per minute. Do you see that?" the pediatrician says to a nurse. "His nares are flaring and you can see intercostal and subcostal retractions when he inhales" (see Fig. 5.10). When the baby breathes out, he makes a small grunting noise that Gracie, listening closely, can hear from where she lies (Box 8.4).

"What's going on?" Gracie asks a nurse. "Is he okay?"

"They're working on him right now," the nurse tells her. "It's not uncommon for these little ones to have some breathing issues when they start out. That's why the pediatric team was brought in. We should know more soon. Your baby is in good hands."

"Alright," says the pediatrician from across the room. "Let's start a CPAP—**continuous positive airway pressure**—and get an umbilical line. We'll also need a chest X-ray" (Figs. 8.7–8.9).

"What is going on?" asks Gracie again, this time louder and with more force.

The pediatrician, who had been speaking earlier, nods to a second person in surgical scrubs, who takes his place.

"I'm Dr. Wallace," he says. "I work out of the neonatal intensive care unit (NICU). I think your baby has **neonatal respiratory distress syndrome**. It's not unusual in preterm babies."

"I thought I had those shots so he'd be okay," says Gracie.

"I'm sure the steroid shots helped," says Dr. Wallace, "but sometimes the little ones will have trouble anyway. This is usually very manageable. Right now we're using a CPAP device to deliver oxygen and help keep the lungs expanded. With respiratory distress syndrome, there's not enough of a substance called surfactant lining the inside surfaces of the lungs. Without it, the little air sacs in the lungs can collapse, and once they've done that, it's very difficult to open them back up. This CPAP should keep that from happening."

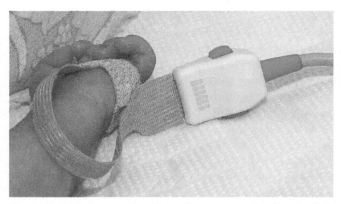

Figure 8.6. A neonatal pulse oximeter, attached to the left wrist/palm.

"Why doesn't he have enough of the stuff in his lungs?"

"Surfactant is one of the last things to develop in the baby prior to a term birth. If a baby is born early, there simply isn't enough time for the body to have produced enough surfactant. The steroids help speed up the process, which is why you got those last week. We do expect that within the next two or three days, however, he'll have produced enough that he'll be able to get by without the CPAP. We'll start trying to wean him of it then."

"Can't we just give him some of the lung stuff? Squirt it down his throat or something?"

"If he doesn't do well with the CPAP, our next step would be to intubate him—that means put a tube into his airway—and then add surfactant into that tube so it gets in the lungs. He's old enough now, however, and with the steroids you had I'd be surprised if it got to that point. We'll keep a close eye on his BP, as well, because that can sometimes become low, which would be concerning. That can happen sometimes with respiratory distress syndrome. We've ordered a chest X-ray to confirm the diagnosis, and we're starting a line where his umbilical cord was cut so we can keep an eye on the blood levels of oxygen and carbon dioxide every four to six hours or so."

Table 8.2 Target Spo$_2$ Levels at Sea Level for Term Infants

Time Postpartum (min)	Target Spo$_2$ Range (%)
1	60–65
2	65–70
3	70–75
4	75–80
5	80–85
10	85–95

Data from Wyckoff, M. H., Aziz, K., Escobedo, M. B., Kapadia, V. S., Kattwinkel, J., Perlman, J. M., et al. (2015). Part 13: Neonatal Resuscitation—2015 American Heart Association Guidelines update for cardiopulmonary resuscitation and emergency cardiovascular care. *Circulation, 132*(18 Suppl. 2), S543–S560.

Box 8.4   Clinical Manifestations of Respiratory Distress Syndrome

- Tachypnea (respirations over 60 breaths per minute)
- Nasal flaring
- Intercostal, subcostal, and subxiphoid retractions with inspiration
- Grunting on expiration
- Cyanosis
- Decreased breath sounds with auscultation
- Pallor
- Peripheral pulses diminished
- Oliguria (reduced urinary output)

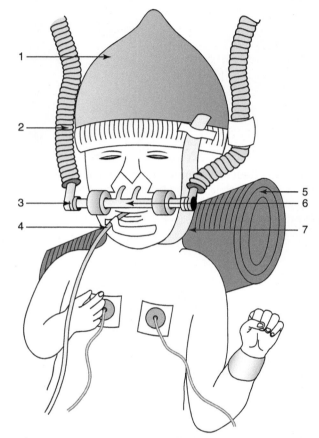

Figure 8.7. Nasal continuous positive airway pressure (CPAP). A CPAP machine may be used to deliver oxygen and help keep the lungs expanded in newborns with suspected respiratory distress. (1) Head cap (cap fit well on head covering down to eye brows, almost entire ears and back of head); (2) Breathing circuit tubes attached to side of hat while avoiding both eyes; (3) Three-way elbow on expiratory limb allows the attachment of pressure manometer or could be capped to preserve pressure within circuit; (4) Orogastric tube attached to lower lip and chin with Tegaderm; (5) Neck roll allowing slight neck extension (sniff position); (6) Nasal prongs applied to baby—prongs inserted into nares allowing a space between the transverse arm of the nasal prongs and nose to avoid damage to nasal columella; (7) Supporting chin strip. (Modified with permission from MacDonald, M. G., Ramasethu, J., Rais-Bahrami, K. [2012]. *Atlas of procedures in neonatology* [5th ed., Fig. 35-3]. Philadelphia, PA: Lippincott Williams & Wilkins.)

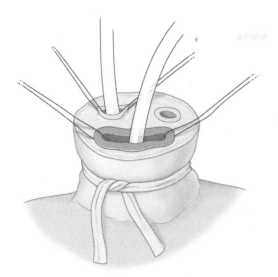

Figure 8.8. Umbilical line. A catheter may be inserted into the vein of a newborn's umbilical stump to monitor blood gases, in lieu of repeated intravenous punctures, to minimize the stress caused to the newborn.

"So, with having the thing in his umbilical cord, you don't have to stick him in his veins all the time?" asks Freddie, who has come to stand by the bed. "I'm the father."

"That's correct. We try to stress the infants as little as possible. We'll carefully regulate his temperature so he won't get cold stress. We want to make sure he has good nutrition, as well. For the short term, we'll plan to feed him by tube instead of by nipple."

"Like one of those nose tubes?" asks Freddie.

"We'll likely use an oral tube," says Dr. Wallace. He turns back to Gracie. "Are you planning to breastfeed?"

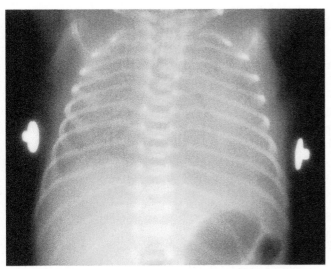

Figure 8.9. Chest X-ray of a neonate with respiratory distress syndrome. Note the granular appearance, sometimes referred to as "ground glass opacity," which is typical of this condition. (Reprinted with permission from Sabella, C., & Cunningham, R. J. [2017]. *The Cleveland Clinic intensive review of pediatrics* [5th ed., Fig. 21-3]. Philadelphia, PA: Lippincott Williams & Wilkins.)

"No," says Freddie. He snorts.

Gracie glances at Freddie. "We haven't really talked about it, but I don't think so. We were planning on formula."

"That's perfectly fine. I was going to have someone talk with you about pumping if that was something you were interested in."

"She's not interested," says Freddie. "How's the kid? Is he going to be okay?"

"I think he's going to be fine," says Dr. Wallace. "But he's going to need close care and monitoring for a while. We're going to keep him in the NICU for at least the next three days or so, probably more like a week, but we strongly encourage you to spend time with him there."

Gracie feels like she might cry, but stops herself. "His name is Edward," she says. "Can you make sure that everyone who takes care of him knows that's his name?"

"We're calling him Eddie," says Freddie.

After Delivery

Gracie is moved to the postpartum unit. Soon after arriving, she meets her postpartum nurse, Raven.

"I don't think I can pee," says Gracie. "I don't need to. I can wait."

"Sometimes after having a baby you have less of a sense that you need to pee," says Raven. "But it's still really important that you have an empty bladder. If your bladder is full, it might keep your uterus from firming up and shrinking, and that can make you bleed."

"But I'm all torn up down there," says Gracie. "I'm worried that if I pee it's going to really hurt."

"I understand," says Raven. "If you want, we can put a bowl of water in your toilet seat and you can urinate while sitting in it. It would dilute the urine and that might feel better."

"Then I'll have pee-water all over me," says Gracie.

"Well, how about this. I'll have you sit on the toilet normally, without the bowl of water, and as you pee I'll run some warm water over the area with a squeeze bottle."

"I don't think that will work," says Gracie.

"Women tell me it really does," Raven says. "We catheterize women who really, truly cannot urinate spontaneously, but I don't think you want that."

"Let's try using the squeeze bottle," says Gracie.

Gracie knows that her baby will be in the NICU for at least a week. She sleeps for almost 6 hours in the postpartum unit shortly after using the bathroom twice with Raven's assistance. Raven left off her compression boots after the second trip, which was a relief, and made sleep possible. She wakes before the change of shift in a room by herself. She sits on the edge of the bed for a minute considering the task of getting up to use the bathroom. She stands gingerly, and when she's not lightheaded, she goes into the bathroom to use the toilet. She doesn't hesitate or have any pain while urinating, which is a small triumph. She cleans herself off afterward with the peri bottle the way Raven showed her and then changes her pad and panties. She stands and looks in the mirror. There's a yellow florescent bulb in the overhead light fixture. She looks like herself, except maybe more tired, more rumpled. She still looks pregnant. A new nurse, Bethany, comes to take her vital signs and check her uterine fundus as she's getting back into bed. They introduce themselves, and Bethany takes a start-of-shift set of vital signs.

"I just peed," says Gracie. "It didn't hurt."

"Perfect," says Bethany. "Did you use the peri bottle?"

Gracie nods. "I used it after just to clean up."

"When you changed your pad, how was your bleeding?"

"Most of the pad was soaked with blood, but I hadn't changed it since before I went to sleep."

"Were there any clots?"

"Yes."

"How big were they?" asks Bethany.

"They were about the size of a grape."

"That sounds about right," says Bethany.

"How long am I going to bleed like this?" asks Gracie.

"Bleeding like this, with a lot of red blood, is **lochia rubra** and usually lasts about three days. After that, it starts to lighten up for another week or so. We call that type of bleeding **lochia serosa**. Then, you'll still have some discharge, but it will be more white than red. That's **lochia alba**."

"Alba? In Spanish that means dawn," says Gracie.

"Interesting," says Bethany. "I think it means white in Latin."

"So, how long does that last for?"

"Up to six weeks."

"Man," says Gracie. "It's a good thing I get a discount on maxi pads."

"True," says Bethany. "Where do you work?"

"I work as a pharm tech," says Gracie. "I wanted to ask about that. My baby, Eddie, is in the NICU, they think probably for a week or so. I want to spend time there with him but was thinking about maybe working some shifts before he comes home, so I have more time with him when he does come home, you know? I only get six weeks off from work to stay with him, and I already wasted one in here when my water broke early. If I take another whole week here before he comes home, I only get to be with him for a month and my daycare won't take him until he's six weeks old. Family and friends can probably watch him for maybe a week, but I don't know about two weeks."

"I can't tell you what to do," says Bethany. She sits in the armchair next to Gracie's bed. "But you're still recovering, too. You need time to heal."

"I feel okay," says Gracie. "It's not like I have to do a lot of running around at work. I can sit a lot. My work is not so far from here. I can still come see him a few times a day so he won't forget me, and I can answer questions and sign paperwork and stuff."

"Gracie, you've been through a lot lately, and you haven't even had time to process that you've had a baby. You're a mom now, Gracie. Will you think about staying out of work a little longer?"

Gracie nods. "I'll think about it, but I don't have a different idea about how to make everything work, you know? When do you think I can get discharged?" (Analyze the Evidence 8.1).

"Well, the law mandates that your health plan cover your hospitalization for at least 48 hours after a vaginal birth. In terms of how early you get discharged, it really depends on how you're doing."

"What if I'm doing fine?" asks Gracie. "Because I feel fine. Nothing hurts bad, and I can pee normally. I'm walking around. My bleeding's not bad. I'm a little sore down there and I still look kind of pregnant but besides that I'm fine."

"Your water did break early," says Bethany. "That makes you more likely to get an infection, which might go undetected if you leave early."

"What would the signs of that be?" asks Gracie.

"It's normal to have a slightly elevated temperature in the first twenty-four hours after the birth, but after that, it could mean you have an infection. Other signs of infection include soreness in your uterus, foul-smelling vaginal discharge, and bleeding that gets heavier. All of those things would make us concerned."

Gracie shrugs. "I never got an infection before he was born, and they gave me all of those antibiotics. And I know how to take my temperature and check my maxi pad."

"You have to do what you think is right," says Bethany. "But I want you to think about your heart and your head, too. This is a major time of adjustment for you. You need time to process all of this."

"But I can process at work, right?" says Gracie. "It doesn't have to be here."

"No, it doesn't have to be here; you just need to make sure you do it somewhere. Do you have someone you can talk to? Your partner, maybe?"

"I don't know. I guess I could talk to Freddie. Maybe I could talk to my mom, if I feel sad or something."

"Will you make that time for yourself?" asks Bethany.

Gracie snorts. "You think I'll have more time when I have a baby? No, I'm okay. I have some time right now, while other people are looking after Eddie. Thanks for being so nice to me, but I'm alright."

Analyze the Evidence 8.1   Early Discharge

Risks

- May be detrimental to the establishment of successful breast-feeding (James, Sweet, & Donnellan-Fernandez, 2017)
- May delay identification and treatment of problems in the mother and infant (Lain, Roberts, Bowen, & Nassar, 2015)

Benefits

- May be safe and cost-effective and encourage family bonding (Nilsson et al., 2015)

"Okay, well, I can tell Dr. Jones what you're thinking about. And Gracie—promise me that if you fill a maxi pad in fifteen minutes you won't ignore it, you'll go to Dr. Jones' office or you'll come here right away. That could be a sign that you're hemorrhaging."

"I will. It's not just me anymore. I have to be strong. I can't be a meek little mouse anymore," says Gracie. "I have this whole other person I have to think about now. I know going to work sounds crazy, but I can't raise a baby with no money.

And I don't know if his daddy is going to stick around. Now that he's been born, I feel like I see things more clearly. The baby and I are in this together; maybe there will be someone else with us and maybe there won't. It makes no sense for me to lie around here or at home while Eddie's in here. He doesn't need me here, he needs all you nurses and tubes and that doctor. He'll need me later, so that's what I have to get ready for."

"You're brave," says Bethany.

"No," says Gracie. "I'm just not rich."

Think Critically

1. Describe the challenges infertility poses to people seeking to expand their family.
2. Gracie was asked multiple times about her safety with her partner. What do you think prompted these questions? Would you be comfortable asking a patient questions about relationship safety? How do you think you'd approach a patient?
3. What are the major differences between Gracie's rupture of membranes and Hannah's in Chapter 7? Why was the management of the two women so different?
4. Draw an illustration that depicts the action of CPAP. Explain how this treatment would be helpful in Eddie's situation.
5. Imagine you have a patient, like Gracie, who wishes to be discharged early. What do you see as the nurse's role in this patient's decision?
6. Make a pro and con list. What are the advantages of early discharge? What are the disadvantages?

References

Best, D., Avenell, A., & Bhattacharya, S. (2017). How effective are weight-loss interventions for improving fertility in women and men who are overweight or obese? A systematic review and meta-analysis of the evidence. *Human Reproduction Update, 23*, 681–705.

Gallo, M. F., Lopez, L. M., Grimes, D. A., Carayon, F., Schulz, K. F., & Helmerhorst, F. M. (2014). Combination contraceptives: Effects on weight. *Cochrane Database of Systematic Reviews*, (1), CD003987.

James, L., Sweet, L., & Donnellan-Fernandez, R. (2017). Breastfeeding initiation and support: A literature review of what women value and the impact of early discharge. *Women and Birth, 30*(2), 87–99.

Lain, S. J., Roberts, C. L., Bowen, J. R., & Nassar, N. (2015). Early discharge of infants and risk of readmission for jaundice. *Pediatrics, 135*(2), 314–321.

Louis, J. F., Thoma, M. E., Sørensen, D. N., McLain, A. C., King, R. B., Sundaram, R., . . . Buck Louis, G. M. (2013). The prevalence of couple infertility in the United States from a male perspective: Evidence from a nationally representative sample. *Andrology, 1*(5), 741–748.

Nilsson, I., Danbjørg, D. B., Aagaard, H., Strandberg-Larsen, K., Clemensen, J., & Kronborg, H. (2015). Parental experiences of early postnatal discharge: A meta-synthesis. *Midwifery, 31*(10), 926–934.

Slama, R., Hansen, O., Ducot, B., Bohet, A., Sorensen, D., Bottagisi, S., . . . Bouyer, J. (2011). Estimation of the frequency of involuntary infertility on a nationwide basis. *Epidemiology, 22*(1), S122.

Suleiman, A., Mruwat-Rabah, S., Garmi, G., Dagilayske, D., Zelichover, T., & Salim, R. (2017). Effect of intermittent versus continuous bladder catheterization on duration of the second stage of labor among nulliparous women with an epidural: A randomized controlled trial. *International Urogynecology Journal*, 1–6.º

Suggested Readings

Allan, H. T. (2017). Shining a light into an unexplored area of nursing: Infertility and in vitro fertilisation. *Journal of Clinical Nursing, 26*, 887–890.

Flanagan, K. A. (2016). Noninvasive ventilation in premature neonates. *Advances in Neonatal Care, 16*(2), 91–98.

March of Dimes. (2016). Retrieved from www.marchofdimes.org

Stevenson, E. L., Hershberger, P. E., & Bergh, P. A. (2016). Evidence-based care for couples with infertility. *Journal of Obstetric, Gynecologic, and Neonatal Nursing, 45*(1), 100–110.

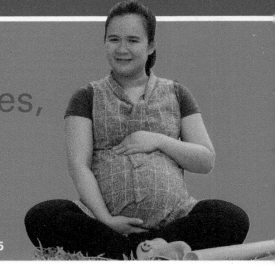

9

Nancy Ng:
Gestational Diabetes, Macrosomia, and Neonatal Cephalhematoma

Nancy Ng, age 25

Objectives

1. Identify special considerations associated with providing reproductive healthcare to a same-sex couple.
2. Discuss some implications of maternal obesity.
3. Identify strategies for resolving urinary retention postpartum.
4. Describe the care considerations for a patient diagnosed with gestational diabetes.
5. Compare the three different kinds of scalp injuries presented in the case.
6. Discuss the risks of macrosomia to the mother and the fetus or newborn.

Key Terms

Caput succedaneum
Cephalhematoma
Diabetogenic
Hemoglobin A$_{1c}$
Hypoxia
Intracervical insemination

Intrauterine insemination
McRoberts maneuver
Perineum
Periosteum
Polyhydramnios
Subgaleal hemorrhage

Before Conception

Nancy Ng is a third-generation American. If you ask her where her people are from, she'll tell you "Poughkeepsie." She and her wife, Missy, have a 1-year-old son, Teddy, who was conceived by artificial insemination and carried and delivered by Missy. Now, they would like for Nancy to be inseminated and to have their second child.

Nancy and Missy met at a party their junior year of college and started dating. They broke up once a few months later but soon got together again. Then, after graduation, they parted ways again. Missy moved to the city to start a production job for a multilingual online news organization, whereas Nancy stayed on at the college as an admissions counselor for a while. But Nancy couldn't stand being apart from Missy, and she bought a ticket on a cheap bus to the city.

"It always comes back around to you," said Nancy when Missy opened the door of her walk-up apartment. "Every conversation I have with a student about my time in college ends up being about you."

"We've done this twice, Nance. Why is now any different?"

"Miss, everything is better with you. Things smell and look and taste better. I like who I am when I'm with you. You make me a better version of me."

"My parents hate you."

"Your parents hate that you're with a girl—any girl. That's not going to change, Miss. You know that. It's nothing to do with me."

"They say you're big and loud."

"I am big and loud. I take up space, and why shouldn't I? Miss, if I were a man taking up this kind of space, do you think they'd complain?"

"Nan, I don't want to choose between you and them."

"I don't want that either, Miss. And if I thought that was the choice I'd walk out of here right now and leave you alone forever. But Miss, this is us we're talking about. We're a part of each other. You're not choosing between your parents and me. You're choosing

between your parents and us, between your parents and yourself. They'll come around, Miss. I promise."

"What if they don't?"

"Then we'll have one less set of people to keep happy at Thanksgiving."

They married 6 months later in a city park, attended by broad spreading trees, friends, and family, including Missy's parents, who implied that they continued to strongly hope for grandchildren.

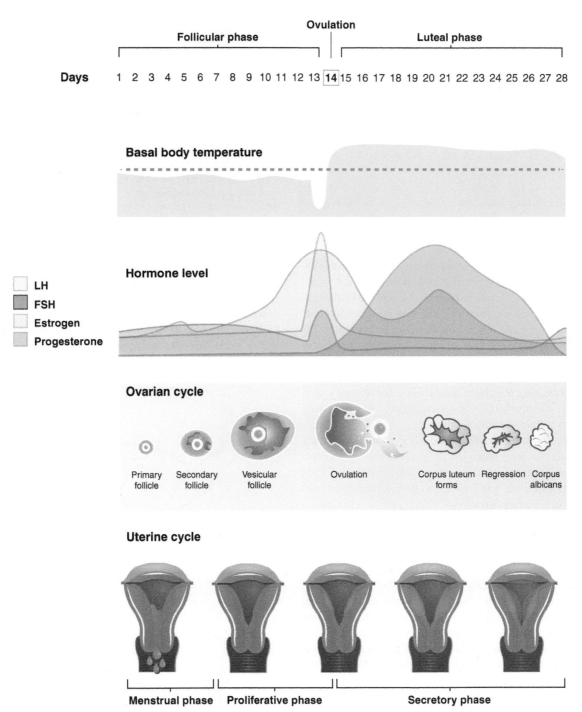

Figure 9.1 A simplified version of a cycle chart. Note that this chart applies to a 28-day menstrual cycle and that the timing of events varies by the duration of a woman's cycle. FSH, follicle-stimulating hormone; LH, luteinizing hormone.

They decided that Missy would go first.

"This is like buying shoes online," said Nancy.

They were looking through an online catalog of available donor sperm from a sperm bank on the other side of the country. They could narrow down the profiles by eye color, ethnicity, ancestry, availability, and previous successful pregnancies.

"I was hoping for one with more of a heel," said Nancy.

"Stop it," said Missy. "This is serious. This is the father of our future child."

"Perspective," said Nancy. "This is half the genetic material of our future child. We don't even have to buy this guy a drink."

Missy initially wanted the donor profile to match Nancy as closely as possible, but Nancy wanted to be able to use the same donor when her turn came, if possible.

"If we choose someone who seems like me now, when it's my turn the baby will be a little Nancy clone, and no one wants that."

In the end they chose someone whom they both thought they might be friends with, if ever they met. They reserved several vials of sperm, some for Missy and the rest for a second sibling pregnancy.

"You could just choose a friend to donate sperm," pointed out one of their old college classmates.

"We could," agreed Missy. "But then they have a claim to the child, and anything could happen. No sperm donor is going to claim parental rights. Plus, all of this sperm is cleaned and scrubbed and safe. No weirdness."

"Well, less weirdness," said Nancy. "In fairness."

An advantage of Missy going first was her extremely predictable 28-day menstrual cycle (Fig. 9.1). Each month of sperm, which would arrive in a container of liquid nitrogen, cost almost $1,000, all told, and the company estimated a 13% success rate with the at-home insemination method, which equated to a turkey baster. The method, also called **intracervical insemination**, required simply depositing the semen next to the cervix and hoping for the best. They'd learned in their reading that **intrauterine insemination** (Fig. 9.2), depositing the sperm directly into the uterus, would likely be more effective but also more expensive, and would need to be done by a trained medical provider.

"You're an absolute, amazing, disgusting show-off," Nancy told Missy affectionately when the pregnancy test returned two pink lines just 2 weeks after the first insemination attempt. "Truly you are. And I suppose you'll go on to have a boring, normal pregnancy and textbook birth."

Which she did; 40 weeks and 2 days later, she gave birth to a baby boy. They named him Theodore—Teddy for short.

Now, a year later, it's Nancy's turn. She begins with the at-home insemination approach that Missy used. They hope to have their second child about 2 years after Teddy's birth, but Nancy's menstrual cycle is unpredictable. As she begins, she takes her basal body temperature daily before she lifts her head from her pillow or has a drink of water. She evaluates her cervical mucus, assessing for the sticky spinnbarkeit (Fig. 9.3), which would indicate imminent ovulation. Sometimes she thinks she can predict when her ovulation will occur and other times not. The ease of Teddy's conception is almost intimidating. Nancy is worried her body will let her down somehow. She buys a large box of ovulation test strips to better determine when her predictive surge of luteinizing hormone will occur, cueing ovulation.

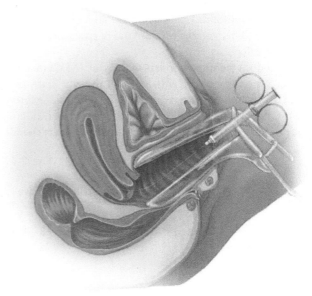

Figure 9.2 Intrauterine insemination. In this procedure, sperm that has been washed of the semen donor's white blood cells and prostaglandins, as well as dead sperm, is injected directly into the uterus via the cervical os through a narrow catheter. (Reprinted with permission from Ricci, S. S. [2013]. *Essentials of maternity, newborn, & women's health nursing* [3rd ed., Fig. 4. 2B]. Philadelphia, PA: Lippincott Williams & Wilkins.)

"We could go to a pro this time," suggests Missy, "If you're so worried about it. We could have someone do the intrauterine insemination."

"No, not unless we have to," says Nancy. "Most couples get to make babies at home without involving medical teams.

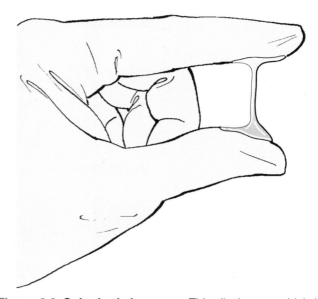

Figure 9.3 Spinnbarkeit mucus. This discharge, which is typical of ovulation, has the slippery, stretchy quality of egg whites and is usually colorless. (Reprinted with permission from Hatfield, N. T., & Kincheloe, C. A. [2017]. *Introductory maternity and pediatric nursing* [4th ed., Fig. 4-3]. Philadelphia, PA: Lippincott Williams & Wilkins.)

Obviously we need this outside sperm, but I'd rather not have other people involved."

"Well, we could order multiple vials each month," suggests Missy. "We could try it a few days in a row instead of having just one shot. It would be like having sex twice near ovulation."

"Double your chances, double your fun?" says Nancy. "Also double the cost. I don't want to end up having to raise Teddy on noodle soup because we're trying to give him a little brother or sister."

"So compromise. We'll try three times with a single vial for cycles, just us. If it doesn't work, we'll go for outside help," says Missy. She gives Nancy a shrewd look. "What's this really about? Do you not want to do it? Do you want me to do it again? Because I would. I loved being pregnant. I would definitely do it over again."

"No," says Nancy. "I do want to. It just feels weird, like a total change in identity. I'm not girly. I don't wear skirts, I don't wear make-up, and I get my hair cut by a barber. But part of me is all woman, and I don't know that part as well. It's daunting, but I want to get in touch with that part of me, too. This birth and pregnancy, growing a whole human—It's all so amazing."

"It is," says Missy. "But it's okay if you don't want to go through with it. There's no shame in wanting to bypass the experience."

"No," says Nancy again. "I want to. You're my family, both of you. Sometimes I feel like I just want to curl up with both of you and never go anywhere. But there's someone missing, you know? And that's this little person it's up to me to make."

Pregnancy

First Trimester

It takes a total of three inseminations 3 months in a row before Nancy has a positive pregnancy test, which is a relief and less than what they'd budgeted for. Based on some reading, they know that with sexual intercourse, there's a 30% chance of pregnancy with the first cycle and up to a nearly 59% chance of conception within the first 3 months of trying. They also know that the per-cycle success rate is much lower with donated sperm that have been processed, cleaned, frozen, shipped, and defrosted. So they had feared a longer wait. Seeing the results is like waking up to tulips in January. Nancy isn't ready for it. She sits in the bathroom for nearly 10 minutes, looking at the test and processing this monumental change and long-sought identity challenge.

"Oh thank goodness," says Missy. "I'm so excited! And you look like you just saw someone kick a puppy. What's going on?"

"No, I'm really happy," says Nancy. "It's just a big change. Remember how it was with Teddy? It's like working on a long, draining project, finishing it, and realizing that your reward is another long, draining project. I want to do it and I'm excited, but it's a lot to take in. This changes things—not bad changes, but changes, you know?"

Missy shakes her head no and smiles. "Yes, absolutely."

"Shush, you," says Nancy. "I have an OB appointment to make."

Nancy has never been small. She is nearly 6 feet tall and wears size 11 shoes and men's gloves because they fit better. She wears a lot of men's clothes in general because the sleeves and legs are longer, and she feels more like herself in them. She's never paid attention to a scale, but isn't surprised when

her obstetrician, a man who asks to be called Ron, tells her she's in the obese range.

"I've got big bones," Nancy tells Ron. "Look at these wrists, look at my hands. These bones are heavy!"

"Likely so," says Ron, "but you're still obese. Look at this chart with me. At five feet eleven inches, a normal weight for you is between 136 and 172 lb. Nancy, you're up here at 225" (Fig. 9.4).

"Big boned," says Nancy. "Besides, I'm muscular. Anyway, there's not much to do now but gain baby weight, right?"

"Nancy, I don't want you to be embarrassed," says Ron. "I'm not saying this to make you uncomfortable, but we need to think about how much weight you should be gaining in this pregnancy."

"My wife gained 26 lb for her pregnancy and you told her she was perfect," says Nancy.

"That may well have been perfect for Missy," says Ron, "but pregnancy isn't one size fits all. For someone with a normal body mass index, a weight gain between 25 and 35 lb is just right. For someone who is obese, weight gain should be 12 lb or less" (see Box 1.5).

"Seriously?"

"Seriously."

"I feel like I'm already eating that in saltines alone."

"Do you have nausea?"

"Yes, and it's awful. It's not just morning sickness, it's all-day sickness and in-the-middle-of-the-night sickness when I get up to pee."

"Well, no one seems to like me saying it, but nausea is a good sign. Women who have nausea, particularly severe nausea, are less likely to have a miscarriage" (Hinkle et al., 2016).

"So I just have to suffer through it?"

"If you like," says Ron. "Although I'd be happy to talk with you about some management strategies for the nausea. Tell me what you've tried."

"Saltines."

"That's it? What about real ginger tea, with ginger grated into it?"

"That sounds disgusting," says Nancy. "That sounds nausea-inducing."

"Well, some people think that the smell of fresh cut lemon is helpful, and peppermint. There's some evidence that a healthy dose of vitamin B$_6$ can help, as well."

"This sounds like hippy stuff, Ron," says Nancy. "What about meds?"

"There are some meds that can be helpful for some women," says Ron. "But we like to limit medications in pregnancy as much as we can, particularly in early pregnancy when the fetus is most vulnerable. We just don't know for sure that they don't do harm, so they're best avoided if we can do it."

"So I'll just suffer through it," says Nancy.

"Try the ginger tea. It's not bad if you add some lemon, and make it fresh so you can smell it, as well," says Ron. "When was the last time you visited your primary care provider?"

"For what?"

"For anything—a check-up, a Pap test—anything like that."

"College? Or maybe it was before, when I had to get my vaccination paperwork for school."

"So it's been a while."

"I haven't been sick," says Nancy. "Why go if I feel great?"

"It doesn't matter how good you feel. At your age, you still need a Pap every three years until you're thirty, and then every

Body Mass Index Table

	Normal						Overweight					Obese										Extreme Obesity														
BMI	19	20	21	22	23	24	25	26	27	28	29	30	31	32	33	34	35	36	37	38	39	40	41	42	43	44	45	46	47	48	49	50	51	52	53	54
Height (in)															Body Weight (lb)																					
58	91	96	100	105	110	115	119	124	129	134	138	143	148	153	158	162	167	172	177	181	186	191	196	201	205	210	215	220	224	229	234	239	244	248	253	258
59	94	99	104	109	114	119	124	128	133	138	143	148	153	158	163	168	173	178	183	188	193	198	203	208	212	217	222	227	232	237	242	247	252	257	262	267
60	97	102	107	112	118	123	128	133	138	143	148	153	158	163	168	174	179	184	189	194	199	204	209	215	220	225	230	235	240	245	250	255	261	266	271	276
61	100	106	111	116	122	127	132	137	143	148	153	158	164	169	174	180	185	190	195	201	206	211	217	222	227	232	238	243	248	254	259	264	269	275	280	285
62	104	109	115	120	126	131	136	142	147	153	158	164	169	175	180	186	191	196	202	207	213	218	224	229	235	240	246	251	256	262	267	273	278	284	289	295
63	107	113	118	124	130	135	141	146	152	158	163	169	175	180	186	191	197	203	208	214	220	225	231	237	242	248	254	259	265	270	278	282	287	293	299	304
64	110	116	122	128	134	140	145	151	157	163	169	174	180	186	192	197	204	209	215	221	227	232	238	244	250	256	262	267	273	279	285	291	296	302	308	314
65	114	120	126	132	138	144	150	156	162	168	174	180	186	192	198	204	210	216	222	228	234	240	246	252	258	264	270	276	282	288	294	300	306	312	318	324
66	118	124	130	136	142	148	155	161	167	173	179	186	192	198	204	210	216	223	229	235	241	247	253	260	266	272	278	284	291	297	303	309	315	322	328	334
67	121	127	134	140	146	153	159	166	172	178	185	191	198	204	211	217	223	230	236	242	249	255	261	268	274	280	287	293	299	306	312	319	325	331	338	344
68	125	131	138	144	151	158	164	171	177	184	190	197	203	210	216	223	230	236	243	249	256	262	269	276	282	289	295	302	308	315	322	328	335	341	348	354
69	128	135	142	149	155	162	169	176	182	189	196	203	209	216	223	230	236	243	250	257	263	270	277	284	291	297	304	311	318	324	331	338	345	351	358	365
70	132	139	146	153	160	167	174	181	188	195	202	209	216	222	229	236	243	250	257	264	271	278	285	292	299	306	313	320	327	334	341	348	355	362	369	376
71	136	143	150	157	165	172	179	186	193	200	208	215	222	229	236	243	250	257	265	272	279	286	293	301	308	315	322	329	338	343	351	358	365	372	379	386
72	140	147	154	162	169	177	184	191	199	206	213	221	228	235	242	250	258	265	272	279	287	294	302	309	316	324	331	338	346	353	361	368	375	383	390	397
73	144	151	159	166	174	182	189	197	204	212	219	227	235	242	250	257	265	272	280	288	295	302	310	318	325	333	340	348	355	363	371	378	386	393	401	408
74	148	155	163	171	179	186	194	202	210	218	225	233	241	249	256	264	272	280	287	295	303	311	319	326	334	342	350	358	365	373	381	389	396	404	412	420
75	152	160	168	176	184	192	200	208	216	224	232	240	248	256	264	272	279	287	295	303	311	319	327	335	343	351	359	367	375	383	391	399	407	415	423	431
76	156	164	172	180	189	197	205	213	221	230	238	246	254	263	271	279	287	295	304	312	320	328	336	344	353	361	369	377	385	394	402	410	418	426	435	443

Adapted from *Clinical Guidelines on the Identification, Evaluation, and Treatment of Overweight and Obesity in Adults: The Evidence Report.*

Figure 9.4 A body mass index (BMI) chart. BMI is an indicator of body composition that is calculated by dividing a person's weight in kilograms by height in meters. It does not reflect muscle or bone mass. (Adapted from The National Heart, Lung, and Blood Institute [NHLBI] of the National Institutes of Health. [2016]. *Aim for a healthy weight: Body mass index table.* Retrieved from www.nhlbi.nih.gov/health/educational/lose_wt/BMI/bmi_tbl.pdf)

five years" (see Patient Teaching 2.2). "We can do that for you today. I also want to check you for diabetes. If you're diabetic, we'll need to manage your pregnancy very differently."

"Who says I'm diabetic?" says Nancy, taken aback. "I'm not peeing all the time or downing water. I feel great."

"I know you do, and that's wonderful. But you're obese, and that can predispose you to having issues with your blood sugar levels and your insulin. We're going to screen you later in pregnancy because we screen everyone, but I also want to screen you today to make sure you don't already have diabetes."

"Is it just a blood test?"

"It's just a blood test. It just means we'll have to draw one more tube of blood in addition to the others we're drawing for other tests. I promise you'll never even miss it" (see Table 1.1).

"You're not diabetic," says Ron when he calls with test results a few days later. It's one of the reasons that Nancy and Missy like him, because he calls with his own test results. Most physicians don't.

"Great," says Nancy. "So I don't need to worry about it?"

"I won't say that," says Ron. "Nancy, the test I ran is something called a **hemoglobin A₁c**. It's like a snapshot of what your blood sugar has been like for the past two or three months. Normal is 4% to 5.6%. You can be diagnosed as diabetic at 6.5%. Your

hemoglobin A_{1c} was 5.7%, which means that you're not diabetic now, but you are at risk of developing diabetes during this pregnancy."

"Why would I be more likely to become diabetic during pregnancy?"

"Pregnancy is a **diabetogenic** state," Ron says, "particularly after the first trimester. That means the body demands progressively more insulin to do the job it can normally do with less. If your body is already having trouble keeping up with your insulin needs before pregnancy, it will likely keep up progressively less as you get into the second half of the pregnancy (Fig. 9.5). Now remember, the job of insulin is to get your cells to take in sugar, or glucose, from your blood. The more insulin you have circulating in your blood, the more glucose your cells will take in. If you don't have enough insulin, the cells won't take in the glucose, and you end up with too much glucose circulating in your bloodstream."

"So, too much glucose in the blood is bad," says Nancy.

"Yes," Ron says. "Too much sugar in the blood is definitely bad."

"What should do I do, then?" asks Nancy.

"I want you to start to live like you already have diabetes. First, I want you to exercise. It doesn't have to be strenuous. Start with

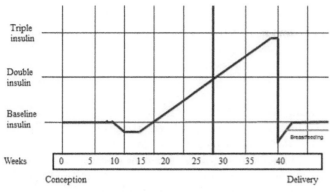

Figure 9.5 Insulin requirements during pregnancy. Baseline insulin needs are similar to what is required during the pre-pregnancy state. Note that insulin needs start to rise sharply after the first trimester of pregnancy and peak at the end of pregnancy. (Reprinted from California Department of Public Health. *California diabetes and pregnancy program.* Retrieved from https://www.cdph.ca.gov/programs/cdapp)

walking. Nothing is more effective at increasing cell sensitivity to insulin than exercise."

"Exercise," says Nancy, dully.

"Yes. And I want you to start eating like a diabetic. I'm going to give you some guidelines that you can take home and talk over with Missy. This is really a lifestyle change we're talking about, not a diet. You really need to embrace this" (Box 9.1).

"Okay, Doc," says Nancy. "What happens if I get diabetes anyway?"

"Well, then we'd treat you."

Box 9.1   Nutritional Recommendations for Nancy Ng

Caloric Intake

- BMI 18.5–29.9 (normal to overweight): 30 kcal/kg/d
- BMI ≥ 30 (obese): 22–25 kcal/kg/d
- Morbid obesity (BMI of 40 or higher or 30 or higher with health problems related to obesity): 12–14 kcal/kg/d

Nancy weighs 225 lb (102 kg) and has a BMI of 31.4. Ron suggests she consume between 2,224 and 2,550 kcal/d.

Nutrient Distribution

- 40% of calories from carbohydrates, primarily fruits and vegetables; avoidance of simple carbohydrates such as candy and baked goods
- 40% of calories from fat, avoidance of trans fats
- 20% of calories from protein

Timing of Calories

- Breakfast: 10% of calories
- Lunch: 30% of calories
- Dinner: 30% of calories
- Snacks: 30% of calories

BMI, body mass index.

"With what—medications and insulin?"

"Yes."

"Okay, so say I didn't take my medications. What's the worst that can happen?"

"Well, I would certainly recommend against that," says Ron. "Your baby could be very big and have some serious complications and you would be at significant risk for injuries at the time of birth." (See Chapter 4.)

"Diet and exercise," says Nancy.

"That's right," says Ron. "Besides the eating guidelines, I can also refer you to a nutritionist, if you'd like."

Nancy shakes her head. "I think we can figure it out. I'll let you know, though."

The results from Nancy's routine first trimester laboratory tests are normal, diminishing her concerns about fetal abnormalities (see Table 1.1).

Second Trimester

In the second trimester, starting in her 13th week of pregnancy, Nancy starts monthly visits with Ron. Her fetal survey ultrasound at 18 weeks is normal. After 20 weeks, each visit includes a fundal height measurement, with Ron measuring her uterus in centimeters from her pubic bone to the fundus (see Fig. 2.8).

"Is it normal?" Missy asks after the first measurement. She's come to as many visits with Nancy as her schedule has allowed.

"She's measuring about three centimeters larger than what I'd expect at this gestation," says Ron, "but the pattern is really more important than any isolated number. If she stays at this size over a series of measurements, that's fine. If the measurements become progressively larger than what I anticipate for the gestational age, we will be concerned."

"So we're good," says Nancy, sitting up with Ron's help and pulling her shirt back down.

"Nancy, we need to talk about your weight again," says Ron. "You're at almost 21 weeks, about halfway through the pregnancy, and you've gained 16 lb. Our goal was for you to gain 12 lb or less for the entire pregnancy."

"I can't help it," says Nancy. "I was nauseous until about a month ago, and the only thing that helped was food. I try not to eat much but my body is just gaining weight."

"I'd like you to think about seeing a nutritionist," says Ron. "Have you been exercising?"

"Not as much as she should," says Missy. "And I don't think having a nutritionist would help necessarily. I'm measuring out all of her meals, but she cheats."

"Missy!" says Nancy. "Tattle tale. I get hungry and I eat. I'm sorry."

"You're not sorry," says Missy.

"I don't think I've impressed on you the importance of diet and exercise at this time," says Ron.

"No, you have," says Nancy. "I'll get better. I promise. I'll go for walks every day and I won't sneak food. Much. I won't sneak much food."

"Nancy," says Missy.

"What? Fine. I'll be good. I'll be better than I have been."

"In a month, at 24 weeks, I want to test you for gestational diabetes," says Ron.

"Should we test for it earlier?" Missy asks.

"Studies have shown no value and no improvement in outcomes from earlier screening," says Ron, "but I like the way you're thinking" (Moyer, 2014).

"So she'll have the test where she drinks the orange soda and then has her blood taken an hour later?" asks Missy.

"Close," says Ron. "Nancy will have her blood taken first thing in the morning. Then she will drink the orange glucola and have her blood taken again one hour later and then two hours after she had the drink. It's a longer process than the standard test, but Nancy, you're so high risk I think you will have a positive result from the one-hour screening test and would have to have the three-hour test anyway. This saves us a step" (Box 9.2).

"Well," says a nurse named Tanisha shortly after taking Nancy's fasting blood sugar at twenty-four weeks. "Your fasting blood glucose is over one hundred five. Anything over ninety-two is diagnostic for diabetes."

"Are you kidding?" asks Nancy. "I haven't even had the drink yet and you're telling me I'm diabetic?"

"With this test you only need one elevated reading for a diagnosis, and you've got it."

"Well then," says Nancy. "As a consolation prize do I not have to do the drink or the other sticks?"

Tanisha shakes her head and hands her a bottle containing orange liquid. "Sorry. We need to measure your blood glucose level after sugar intake so we know how to adjust your insulin."

"Insulin?" says Nancy.

"Well, based on your chart, you've been working on diet and exercise since the beginning of the pregnancy. Ron typically starts women in your situation on insulin."

A few days after receiving the diagnosis of gestational diabetes, she and Missy are meeting with Ron.

"I have to take insulin?" asks Nancy. "I have to do finger sticks and get shots in the legs all day long? Really?"

"Insulin is our first-choice medication if diet and exercise fail, yes," says Ron. "Nancy, only one elevated level during a screening

is required for a diagnosis, and all three of yours were elevated. We need to take this seriously. You don't need to think about it every hour, but you do need to be diligent in testing your blood glucose level and injecting your insulin."

"I don't believe this," says Nancy. "That means months of jabs and shots, right?"

Ron nods. "Yes, for the duration of your pregnancy you will have gestational diabetes. It's certainly manageable, but you are correct that it will take no small effort on your part."

"Ron," says Missy, "could this still be managed with diet and exercise? She hasn't gained more weight and I think she's recently cut back on extra food, but she could walk more."

Ron shakes his head. "I wouldn't recommend that at this time. This is serious stuff, Nancy. This is about your health and your baby's health. I know both of these things are important to you."

"I know, I know," says Nancy. "I'm just in denial. So how does this go? What do I have to do?"

"I know this is challenging, Nancy. But you have good support from this office and at home. Tanisha will come in and explain our plan. I'd like to see you back in a week."

"I hate needles," Nancy mutters.

The nurse, Tanisha, enters and introduces herself again.

"Let's start with the finger sticks," says Tanisha. "At first, you'll do this six times a day so we can establish your general status and the effectiveness of the insulin."

"How long will I be doing that?" asks Nancy.

"We'll know more after we see the result logs for the first week," says Tanisha. "The machine will track the actual numbers, but during this time we encourage you to write down your results, times, food diary, and whether the level is fasting, before eating, or an hour after your first bite of food. This will give you an at-a-glance visual to see how you're doing."

Tanisha hands a little log book to Nancy, who flips through the empty pages (Fig. 9.6). Tanisha brings out a box containing a glucometer and a package of test strips (Fig. 9.7). She reviews with Nancy and Missy glucose targets and the technique for obtaining capillary blood from the side of the finger to test it (Step-by-Step Skills 9.1). It takes Nancy a couple of tries to stick her finger correctly. Her instinct is to pull her hand away as she triggers the lancet.

"Tough girl," Missy teases her. "You can do this."

"Six times a day," Nancy grumbles, milking a drop of blood from the middle finger of her left hand. "I hate this."

"It does get easier," Tanisha says. "Make sure not to use your fingertips. They'd hurt more because you use those more than the sides of your fingers."

"Fine," says Nancy. "I just need to do it. What about the insulin? I'll have to take another bunch of shots, right?"

"One," says Tanisha. "To start with."

"Why one?" asks Missy. "I'd think it would be after each meal."

"We generally start with two different kinds of insulin that are injected right before breakfast. One is rapid acting and kicks in within fifteen minutes and peaks between about a half hour and an hour and a half. The other one, called NPH, lasts four to ten hours. We'll start you on fifteen units of NPH and five units of the fast-acting type. And again, you'll take both of these before breakfast" (The Pharmacy 9.1).

Box 9.2 Single-Step Combined Screening and Diagnosis Testing

1. After an overnight fast, fasting glucose level is checked.
2. A solution containing 75 g of glucose is drunk.
3. Blood glucose is again checked after 1 and 2 h.
4. If one of the following values is elevated, gestational diabetes is diagnosed:
   - Fasting ≥ 92 mg/dL
   - One hour ≥ 180 mg/dL
   - Two hour ≥ 153 mg/dL

Data from Sacks, D. A., Hadden, D. R., Maresh, M., Deerochanawong, C., Dyer, A. R., Metzger, B. E., . . . Trimble, E. R. (2012). Frequency of gestational diabetes mellitus at collaborating centers based on IADPSG consensus panel–recommended criteria. *Diabetes Care, 35*(5), 526–528.

Name: Phone:

Month:

Day of the month	1	2	3	4	5	6	7	8	9	10	11	12	13	14	15
Before breakfast finger stick															
Breakfast foods															
Before lunch finger stick															
Lunch foods															
Finger stick 1 hour after first bite of lunch															
Finger stick before dinner															
Dinner foods															
Finger stick 1 hour after first bite of dinner															
Notes section for snacks and exercises															

Day of the month	16	17	18	19	20	21	22	23	24	25	26	27	28	29	30	31
Before breakfast finger stick																
Breakfast foods																
Before lunch finger stick																
Lunch foods																
Finger stick 1 hour after first bite of lunch																
Finger stick before dinner																
Dinner																
Finger stick 1 hour after first bite of dinner																
Notes section for snacks and exercises																

Figure 9.6 **A sample page from a blood glucose monitoring log.**

Tanisha coaches both Missy and Nancy on how to draw up the prescribed dose of insulin. She teaches them to draw up the rapid-acting insulin before the NPH. She has them practice using normal saline instead of insulin, first drawing it up and then injecting it into an orange using an ultrafine needle, only 6 mm long.

"Clear before cloudy, clear before cloudy," she makes Nancy and Missy repeat several times, a reference to the rapid-acting insulin appearing clear in the bottle, whereas the NPH appears cloudy.

"Remember this injection is subcutaneous, so the tip of the needle should end up between the skin and the muscle. Most people, including pregnant women, prefer to use the abdomen, but as this baby grows, you may find it easier to use a site along the sides of your belly instead of up front," says Tanisha.

Tanisha says that hypoglycemia, low blood glucose, is fairly unlikely with gestational diabetes, as long as no meals or snacks are skipped. If Nancy does feel like she's having a glucose low, Tanisha advises her to have a snack containing a mix of protein and carbohydrates.

"You don't want your blood glucose to drop below seventy, as a general rule," says Tanisha.

"So how will we know she's having low blood sugar?" asks Missy.

"I'll know," says Nancy. "I'll feel hungry, weak, irritable, and shaky."

"That's pretty close," says Tanisha, sliding yet another form across the table (Patient Teaching 9.1). "This sheet lists symptoms of hypoglycemia. If you experience any of these, have a small

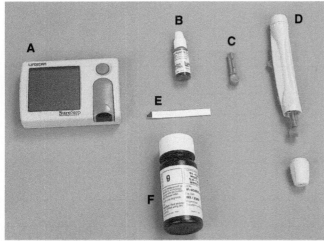

Figure 9.7 Equipment used to perform blood glucose testing. A glucometer **(A)**, control solution **(B)**, a lancet **(C)**, a lancet holder **(D)**, a test strip **(E)**, and a container of test strips **(F)**. The control solution contains a known amount of glucose and is used periodically to test the accuracy of the device. The lancet and lancet holders are used for the finger stick. (Photo by B. Proud.)

Step-by-Step Skills 9.1

Checking Blood Glucose Level

Target Glucose

- Fasting: <90 mg/dL
- Before lunch and the evening meal: <90 mg/dL
- One hour after the first bite of meals: <120 mg/dL

Nancy is informed that if all six daily readings are within normal range for a period of time, she may go down to twice daily readings.

How to Check Blood Glucose

1. Gather the monitor, test strips, lancet, and cotton.
2. Wash your hands (alcohol may be used if soap and water are unavailable).
3. Use the lancet on the side of the finger (note: some machines allow blood from other sites, such as the thigh or forearm; Nancy's does not).
4. Wipe the first drop of blood away with cotton.
5. Touch the test strip to the second drop of blood.
6. The result will appear on the readout of the machine.

Data from American Diabetes Association. (2017). Management of diabetes in pregnancy. *Diabetes Care,* 20(S1), S114–S119.

The Pharmacy 9.1 — Selected Categories of Insulin

Time Course	Agent	Onset	Peak	Duration	Indications
Rapid acting	Lispro (Humalog)	10–15 min	1 h	2–4 h	Used for rapid reduction of glucose level, to treat postprandial hyperglycemia, and/or to prevent nocturnal hypoglycemia
	Aspart (NovoLog)	5–15 min	40–50 min	2–4 h	
	Glulisine (Apidra)	5–15 min	30–60 min	2 h	
Short acting	Regular (Humulin R, Novolin R, Iletin II Regular)	30–60 min	2–3 h	4–6 h	Usually given 20–30 min before a meal; may be taken alone or in combination with longer-acting insulin
Intermediate acting	NPH (neutral protamine Hagedorn)	2–4 h	4–12 h	16–20 h	Usually taken after food
	(Humulin N, Iletin II Lente, Iletin II NPH, Novolin N [NPH])	3–4 h	4–12 h	16–20 h	
Very long acting	Glargine (Lantus)	1 h	Continuous (no peak)	24 h	Used for basal dose
	Detemir (Levemir)	6 h		24–36 h	
	Glargine (Toujeo)				
Rapid-acting inhaled insulin	Afrezza	<15 min	~50 min	2–3 h	Used as rapid-acting insulin

Reprinted with permission from Hinkle, J. L., and Cheever, K. H. (2018). *Brunner and Suddarth's Textbook of Medical-Surgical Nursing* (14th ed.; Table 51-3). Philadelphia, PA: Wolters Kluwer.

Patient Teaching 9.1

Signs of Hypoglycemia

- Hunger, gurgling in the abdomen (borborygmus)
- Shakiness, nervousness, weakness, anxiety
- Impaired judgment
- Dysphoria
- Irritability
- Nausea, vomiting
- Tachycardia
- Diaphoresis, subjective feeling of being hot
- Subjective feeling of being cold
- Paleness (pallor)
- Headache
- Dilation of pupils, vision changes
- Slurring of speech and poor coordination of movement
- Coma and seizures

snack if a meal is not imminent. Also, we'd prefer you verify your blood glucose first with a finger stick. Do your best."

"So I need to avoid ever being hungry but I need to restrict my diet as much as possible."

Tanisha nods sympathetically. "Try to hit the sweet spot."

Third Trimester

The sweet spot turns out to be a moving target. By the end of the pregnancy, she is up from one dose in the morning to three doses throughout the day. Each dose contains part NPH and part rapid-acting insulin. Her dosing schedule requires her to inject just prior to breakfast, lunch, and dinner.

"I don't understand," Nancy says to Ron. "We've been so much better about my diet and we're really good about the insulin and the finger sticks. Why does my dose keep going up?"

"Well remember, Nancy," says Ron, "Your peak insulin need doesn't come until the third trimester. When we started your insulin, you were just a month past the halfway mark. Since then your insulin needs have continued to climb. You'll go back to your baseline insulin needs very quickly after the birth. Having said that, I advise that we do another two-hour glucose tolerance test when you come back for your postpartum visit at six weeks to make sure this gestational diabetes hasn't become type two diabetes."

"That can happen?" asks Nancy.

"Oh yes. As many as half of the women who develop gestational diabetes go on to develop type two diabetes within ten years after the birth" (Damm et al., 2016). "However, should that occur, we likely would not keep you on insulin. Most people with type two diabetes are prescribed medications that are far easier to manage."

"Oh Ron, you're always a ray of sunshine," says Nancy.

"I try," says Ron. "Now look, I'd like to talk more about your care at this point."

"Please no more needles."

"No more needles. But you're in week 32 now and I'd like to start monitoring the baby more closely. There is an increased risk for stillbirth, and we want to make sure all is well" (Rosenstein et al., 2012).

"Increased risk from the diabetes?" asks Nancy.

"The gestational diabetes, yes, particularly as management with diet and exercise was unsuccessful," says Ron.

"What kind of monitoring? Ultrasound?"

"Part of it is ultrasound. We need to measure the pockets of amniotic fluid around the baby using an ultrasound machine and get a good look at the fetus, but we also will do something called a nonstress test, or NST."

"That's the one where you get hooked up with the thing on your belly to monitor the heart rate, right?" asks Nancy.

"That's correct. We use it twice a week to assess the variability in the fetal heart rate—the variation of the fetal heart rate within a discreet period of time—as well as heart rate accelerations" (see Box 3.6).

"Twice a week? That might be hard with my work schedule," says Nancy. "You do it here?"

"We do. We'd be happy to schedule you first thing in the morning, if that would be helpful. We open our doors at eight."

"What's the issue with the amniotic fluid?" asks Nancy.

"Sometimes with diabetes, not just gestational diabetes but also diabetes that predates the pregnancy, a condition called **polyhydramnios** can occur, which means extra amniotic fluid collects around the baby. It's associated with various complications, so if we suspect it's happening, we may elect to induce labor earlier" (Box 9.3).

"Okay, I'm worried. Is there anything else I need to know about?"

"I don't want you to worry. You have a good team, but we are taking your situation seriously. Now, as we've discussed before, babies of women with gestational diabetes are more likely to be very large, which can lead to myriad problems, including birth injuries. Although estimating fetal size in utero is challenging, I would like to get an ultrasound in the final month specifically to

Box 9.3 Complications Associated With Polyhydramnios

- Cord prolapse
- Preterm labor
- Premature rupture of membranes
- Fetal malpresentation
- Placental abruption with membrane rupture
- Prolonged second stage of labor
- Compromise of maternal respiration
- Uterine atony postpartum

Data from Samantha, L. Wiegand, C. J. (2016). Idiopathic polyhydramnios: Severity and perinatal morbidity. *The American Journal of Perinatology, 33*(7), 658–664; Karahanoglu, E., Ozdemirci, S., Esinler, D., Fadıloglu, E., Asiltürk, S., Kasapoglu, T., . . . Kandemir, N. O. (2016). Intrapartum, postpartum characteristics and early neonatal outcomes of idiopathic polyhydramnios. *Journal of Obstetrics and Gynecology, 36*(6), 710–714.

measure the baby. If the baby is likely to be very large, we may need to do a cesarean section."

"What do you mean by 'very large'?"

"If the baby is estimated to be four thousand five hundred grams or larger, I recommend a cesarean."

"What's that in pounds?"

"That's about nine pounds nine ounces."

"That's a big baby."

"A very big baby, yes," agrees Ron.

"I'm a pretty big lady myself," says Nancy.

"The size of the mother isn't always a good predictor of her ability to successfully give birth to a large newborn without interventions," says Ron. "Now, even if we don't think this baby is over 4,500 g, I recommend we induce your labor at 39 weeks, assuming labor hasn't started on its own."

"Why?"

"There is some indication that early induction can reduce the rate of complications and the risk for stillbirth (Rosenstein et al., 2012)."

Nancy feels a shiver of fear pass through her.

Labor and Delivery

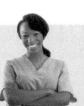

The Nurse's Point of View

Grace: Nancy has been admitted the night before she is scheduled to be induced to have her cervix ripened with twenty-five micrograms of misoprostol vaginally every four hours. The note in her chart says her Bishop score (Table 9.1) is four, so her admission

at this time makes sense. The induction is more likely to be successful this way.

The advantage of taking care of a patient who is being induced is that you have some time to review the chart before you meet her. For example, I know already that she has gestational diabetes that it is being managed with insulin, which explains the induction at thirty-nine weeks. Her physician, Ron, is most likely concerned that this baby will be particularly large. She

Table 9.1 Bishop Score

Component	Score				Further Explanation
	0	1	2	3	
Position	Posterior	Middle	Anterior	–	The cervix moves to "point" toward the woman's front at the very end of pregnancy.
Consistency	Firm	Medium	Soft	–	Prior to a birth, a cervix may feel firm, like a chin. Women who have given birth previously will have softer-feeling cervixes.
Effacement	0%–30%	40%–50%	60%–70%	≥80%	The cervix starts out about 3–4 cm thick. With full effacement, the cervix shortens to become part of the lower uterus.
Dilation	Closed	1–2 cm	3–4 cm	≥5 cm	Dilation refers to how open the cervix is.
Fetal station	–3	–2	–1, 0	+1, +2	Fetal station refers to the position of the fetus' head in relation to the distance from the ischial spines. These spines are part of the pelvis and are about 4 cm inside the vagina. In assessment of fetal station, negative numbers mean the fetus is above the spines, and positive numbers mean the fetus is below the spines.

Recommended Management

- Score of 5 or less: Labor is likely not imminent without induction.
- Score of 9 or higher: Spontaneous labor is likely.
- Score of 8 or higher: Induction is more likely to be successful.
- Score less than 8: Induction is less likely to be successful.

A successful induction is an uncomplicated vaginal delivery.

Data from Bishop, E. (1964). Pelvic scoring for elective induction. *Obstetrics and Gynecology, 24*(2), 266–268.

would also be at an increased risk for stillbirth if she were to carry the pregnancy through week forty. Her chart indicates that she's obese, which may also put her at greater risk for having a newborn who is large for gestational age, even without the diabetes. So far the ultrasounds have looked good, though, and they don't think the baby looks too big. These ultrasounds for size are notoriously inaccurate, however.

One aspect of care we'll have to prioritize is blood glucose monitoring. Because she's on insulin, she'll need to have a finger stick every two hours or so. This hospital's policy is to keep patients' blood glucose level below one hundred ten. Ron usually has a standing order in for intravenous (IV) insulin if blood glucose gets above one hundred twenty, so I expect that order to be added to her chart once she's admitted.

Nancy's wife Missy arrives just after 7:30 the morning of the induction (see The Pharmacy 1.2). I start the oxytocin infusion at one milliunit per minute and plan to titrate it up by one or two milliunit per minute every thirty to sixty minutes until Nancy's contractions are coming once every two to three minutes and lasting for about a minute and a half each. I've placed sensors on Nancy's abdomen that communicate with a monitor to track her uterine contractions and the fetal heart rate. So far, so good. The fetal baseline heart rate is one hundred fifty beats per minute, with moderate variability. Nancy looks pretty anxious, which is understandable. Missy holds her hand and talks about their son, Teddy, but she looks anxious, as well.

We consider four primary factors that affect the progress of labor, which are known as the "four Ps": passenger, passageway, powers, and position of the laboring woman. Because we're concerned this might be a big baby, the relationship between the passenger and the passageway is a major concern here. The powers are the uterine contractions, which we're stimulating with the oxytocin, and pushing, which will occur later. Again, if this does turn out to be a big baby, that third P is going to relate directly to the first two. The good news here about the fourth P, position, is that, for now at least, Nancy has opted not to get an epidural. This, along with the fact that she's on a wireless monitor, means that it will be much easier to get her on her feet and moving around the floor. By keeping her vertical and having her walk around, we're letting gravity assist in labor (Lawrence, Lewis, Hofmeyr, & Styles, 2013).

She's now been in the latent phase of the first stage of labor for nearly nine hours (see Table 1.3), and her cervix is only three centimeters dilated. Contractions during this phase are further apart and less intense, but that's still a long time to go with making so little progress, particularly with IV oxytocin.

Once she enters the active phase of her first stage, she progresses more quickly. Eight hours to go from three to seven centimeters. Seven hours into the active phase, Ron checks her cervix and decides to perform an amniotomy, or artificial rupture of the membranes. Sometimes this helps speed things along, but it can be done safely only if the fetus is head down and engaged in the pelvis to avoid the risk of cord prolapse (see Chapter 5). Of course, the cervix also has to be dilated sufficiently for the procedure to be performed.

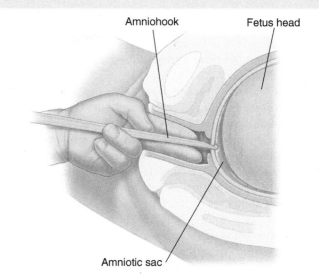

Figure 9.8 **Amniohook.**

"This isn't going to hurt," I tell Nancy and Missy, who look worried when they see the amniohook (Fig. 9.8). "Your amniotic sac doesn't have any nerve endings. You'll feel Ron's hands, but you won't feel the hook itself."

With the next contraction, Ron inserts two gloved fingers into Nancy's vagina along with the amniohook. Using his fingers as a guide, he nicks the amniotic sac overlying the baby's head. He keeps his fingers in place for a few moments to verify that the cord doesn't move down with the fluid and then removes his hand. The fluid now flowing out her vagina is clear with no evidence of fetal meconium, which would turn it greenish or brown. That's always a relief. If there had been meconium, we'd be concerned that the baby had hypoxia, although this finding can also be normal for some babies, particularly if they're past their due dates.

Labor progresses much more quickly after the amniotomy, and now, after seventeen hours of labor, she becomes really intense and focused. She's vocalizing much more and rests with her eyes closed between contractions. I'm pretty sure by her behavior that she's in the transition phase of the first stage, which occurs when the cervix is seven to ten centimeters dilated. Another clue is that her contractions are closer together, every two minutes, and they're lasting a full minute and a half. She doesn't get much rest between them.

She's entered the pushing stage, the second stage, and it's lasting a long time. The monitors indicate that the baby is doing fine, but Nancy is starting to get tired. I'm tired. I'm working a double, so I'm still here, but I'm just as eager for this little one to be born as anyone else is. Well, it's possible other people are more eager!

It's been almost two and half hours of pushing. I have Nancy empty her bladder into a bedpan, and I can see a little dab of scalp hair. Hopefully it won't be too long. After three hours, an arrest of labor can be diagnosed, and an operative delivery considered (American College of Obstetricians and Gynecologists, 2014). Maybe having her empty her bladder has given her a little more space, or maybe it's just the distraction she needs to get through. I have Nancy adjust her position so she's more upright. She's pretty tired and the temptation after pushing so long is to lie down, but we know an upright position can move the second stage of labor along faster (Gupta, Sood, Hofmeyr, & Vogel, 2017).

About fifteen minutes later and after more contractions, the baby's head emerges. There's a minute or so of further concern. Babies of mothers with diabetes tend to have larger shoulders and greater fat distribution in the upper part of the body, so there's a risk that the shoulders will get stuck even though the head is out, a condition called shoulder dystocia.

Ron tells Missy and me to help Nancy move her legs back toward her shoulders as much as she can, something called McRoberts maneuver (Fig. 9.9). This is supposed to change the configuration of the pelvis so the anterior shoulder of the baby can move out from under the pubic symphysis. It works, or maybe there wasn't a problem after all, because the little one slips out and Ron catches him. Missy cuts the cord. Sometimes Ron delays cutting the cord for a few minutes because there's evidence that it will increase the number of circulating red blood cells in the baby. Babies born to mothers with diabetes, however, are more likely to already have polycythemia, or too many blood cells, so delaying cord clamping could worsen that situation. Babies with polycythemia are more likely to have problems such as severe jaundice, so we don't delay clamping the cord this time.

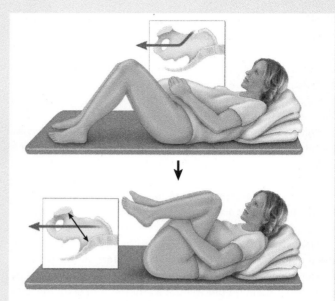

Figure 9.9 McRoberts maneuver. Hyperflexion and abduction of the hips cause cephalad rotation of the symphysis pubis and flattening of the lumbar lordosis that frees the impacted shoulder. (Reprinted with permission from Beckmann, C. R., Herbert, W., Laube, D., Ling, F., & Smith, R. [2013]. *Obstetrics and gynecology* [7th ed., Fig. 9.9A]. Philadelphia, PA: Lippincott Williams & Wilkins.)

The Newborn

After rubbing down baby boy Ng with warmed blankets, clearing his airways with a bulb syringe, and taking his first Apgar score at 1 minute (which is 8), Grace weighs the baby.

"Four thousand four hundred grams," she says to the room at large, and then turns to Nancy and Missy and says, "that's about nine pounds seven ounces."

She wraps the baby loosely in a blanket, places him on Nancy's chest, and then spreads a warm blanket over the pair. At 5 minutes she takes the second Apgar, and his score is 9. Another nurse comes in to relieve Grace, and Missy gives the original nurse a big, tired hug on her way out. The new nurse, Helena, admires the baby.

"He's huge," she says.

"He got a little stuck," says Nancy.

"Nancy," says Ron, "the good news is you're already anesthetized. The bad news is you have a fairly serious laceration of your vulva. I'm going to be making some repairs as well as delivering the placenta."

"How serious are they?" asks Missy.

"Well, she has what we refer to as a third-degree laceration, which is a tear into but not through the anal sphincter and that does not involve the rectal mucosa" (see Fig. 7.2).

"My God," says Nancy. "That sounds awful."

"No, no," says Ron cheerfully. "I'll put in some sutures and all will be well."

A few minutes later there's a sudden gush of blood from Nancy's vagina and an elongating of the umbilical cord that still protrudes from her vagina. There's a small shift as her uterus becomes more round and rises with the release of the placenta. Ron applies slight traction to the cord, and the placenta slides into a stainless steel bowl. Helena examines it to ensure it is intact, with no pieces left behind in Nancy's uterus that may cause atony or subinvolution and thus bleeding (see Fig. 1.2). Ron continues his repair work.

"This is a great time to get him started with breastfeeding," says Helena to Nancy. Helena has removed her gloves and washed her hands. "Big babies like this sometimes have a hard time keeping their blood glucose up for the first few days. One of the best things you can do is feed him."

"I'm not sure how," Nancy says. She watched Missy feed Teddy, of course, but doing it herself is something different. She feels like her arms are in the wrong place, or maybe she just doesn't have enough of them. The baby's little rosebud of a mouth suddenly seems like an impossible target. He has his own ideas of how to go about it, however, and makes his way to the nipple and mouths it. Nancy doubts that he actually manages to drink anything.

Within an hour of the birth, small drops of blood are obtained from the baby's heel to assess for polycythemia and for hypoglycemia, both of which are more common in babies who are large for gestational age (Boxes 9.4 and 9.5; see Fig. 1.16). Helena explains that his blood glucose level will be checked every 6 hours for the next 48 hours to make sure he doesn't become hypoglycemic.

"These blood checks are because of my gestational diabetes, right?" asks Nancy.

Helena nods. "Elevations in your blood glucose cause the baby to produce more insulin when he's inside you. After he's born, it may take his pancreas a little while to adapt to producing less

Box 9.4 Risks to Neonate of Large for Gestational Age

- Birth injury
- Respiratory distress
- Hypoglycemia
- Polycythemia
- Perinatal asphyxia (oxygen restriction)
- Congenital anomalies

Data from King, J., Korst, L., Miller, D., & Ouzounian, J. (2012). Increased composite maternal and neonatal morbidity associated with ultrasonographically suspected fetal macrosomia. *The Journal of Maternal-Fetal and Neonatal Medicine, 25*(10), 1953–1959.

Box 9.5 Assessment of Infant Size

- Small for gestational age (SGA): below 10th percentile
- Appropriate for gestational age (AGA): between 10th and 90th percentiles
- Large for gestational age (LGA): above 90th percentile

insulin. Until that happens, his blood glucose level will likely stay low. Usually we can fix it with feeding. Rarely, we need to provide dextrose through an IV. That's a kind of sugar."

"Besides the heel sticks, is there any way we can know whether his blood sugar is low?" asks Missy. "Is there something we should look for?"

"Some babies get kind of jittery," says Helena. "They may not feed so well, and their cry may seem off" (see Box 3.10). "We do extra blood checks as needed. In this hospital we ideally like to keep their blood glucose level above fifty for the first forty-eight hours and above sixty after that. If they're doing okay and are not having symptoms, we just encourage feeding. If they develop symptoms, we feed them more aggressively and possibly give them dextrose. It doesn't happen often" (Lab Values 9.1).

"What was the other test you did?" asks Missy.

Lab Values 9.1

Blood Glucose Parameters for Asymptomatic Neonates

- Within first 4 h of life, maintain plasma glucose levels >25 mg/dL (1.4 mmol/L).
- Between 4 and 24 h of life, maintain plasma glucose levels >35 mg/dL (1.9 mmol/L).
- Between 24 and 48 h of life, maintain plasma glucose levels >50 mg/dL (2.8 mmol/L).
- Greater than 48 h of life, maintain plasma glucose levels >60 mg/dL (3.3 mmol/L).

Data from Committee on Fetus and Newborn from the American Academy of Pediatrics. (2011). Postnatal glucose homeostasis in late-preterm and term infants. *Pediatrics, 127*(3), 575–579.

"That was for polycythemia," says Helena. "That means an overabundance of red blood cells. The test results show that he is fine. If his hematocrit had been over 65, though, we would have taken blood from somewhere other than his heel to make sure that the first reading was accurate. Even when polycythemia is verified in babies, we usually just observe them, feed them, and keep them hydrated, and they are fine."

"Speaking of which," says Nancy. "Not to complain, but I haven't eaten in about ten years. How do I get a turkey sandwich, in this place?"

A few days later, Nancy asks Missy, "Does his head look funny to you?". Nancy is lying on her bed with her knees up and the baby propped up against them, sleeping. She's carefully unwrapped him for inspection. She's removed his hat and is peering at his head. "Doesn't his head seem lopsided?"

Missy runs her hand over the baby's head. "I see what you mean. The left side of his scalp seems higher than the other."

A nurse who has been caring for the family, Rae, enters for her hourly check. Missy calls her over for another opinion.

"It looks like he has a **cephalhematoma**," says Rae (Fig. 9.10). "That's not uncommon. You had a long pushing stage."

"Is it dangerous?" asks Nancy.

"Not usually," says Rae. She gently runs her hand over the top of the baby's head. "It's a little collection of blood between the skull and the **periosteum**. That's a layer of connective tissue that covers the bone. See how the swelling stops right in the middle? That's where this bone of his skull stops and another one joins it, so we know that's where the swelling is. If this swelling didn't

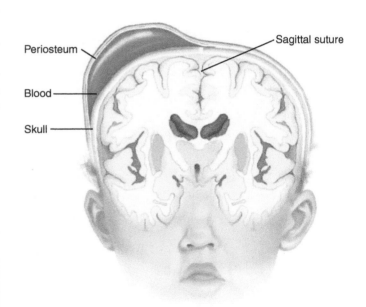

Figure 9.10 Cephalhematoma. With this condition, bleeding appears within the first 2 to 3 days after birth and does not cross the suture line. It may take weeks or even months to resolve completely, but typically does so without complications. (Reprinted with permission from Kyle, T., & Carman, S. [2016]. *Essentials of pediatric nursing* [3rd ed., Fig. 16.15B]. Philadelphia, PA: Lippincott Williams & Wilkins.)

stop midway at the suture line, we'd likely think it was something called **caput succedaneum**, which is just swelling under the skin of the scalp. That usually is obvious when the baby's born but resolves within a few days" (Fig. 9.11). "Or we might suspect a **subgaleal hemorrhage**, which is more rare. That can be much more serious, but because the swelling doesn't cross the suture line in this case, I'm reassured" (Fig. 9.12).

Missy and Nancy are silent for a moment. "Wait, are you sure?" Nancy asks. "It's the first thing and not the last thing?"

"I'm sure," says Rae, again indicating the lopsided nature of the swelling and the hard stop at the center of the scalp. "We'll monitor him for jaundice, which can occur with any kind of bleed, but we do that routinely, anyway. You lose enough sleep with a new baby. This isn't a reason to."

Nancy considers. "How do you monitor for jaundice?"

Rae lightly depresses the baby's right cheek. "The first thing is a visual inspection. When I press my finger down, the skin should be white when I take my finger away. Yellow would suggest there's extra bilirubin. It's ordinary for babies' faces to be a little yellow. We're more concerned when that color moves further down, onto the chest and belly. We also have a monitor that can estimate bilirubin levels through the skin" (see Fig. 5.9). "If we're concerned, we can use that or go straight to a blood test. We'll also check his bilirubin using the transcutaneous monitor before you're both discharged."

"So how does he look now?" asks Nancy.

"He looks beautiful," says Rae.

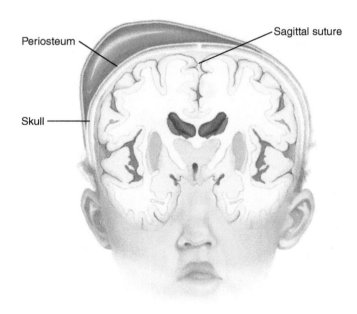

Figure 9.11 Caput succedaneum. With this condition, edema is noted at birth and crosses the suture line. It typically starts to resolve within a few days after birth. (Reprinted with permission from Kyle, T., & Carman, S. [2016]. *Essentials of pediatric nursing* [3rd ed., Fig. 16.15A]. Philadelphia, PA: Lippincott Williams & Wilkins.)

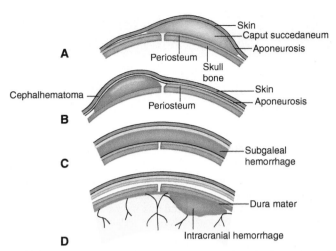

Figure 9.12 Neonatal scalp defects. (A) Caput succedaneum. **(B)** Cephalhematoma. **(C)** Subgaleal hemorrhage. **(D)** Intracranial hemorrhage. (Reprinted with permission from Bachur, R. G., & Shaw, K. N. [2016]. *Fleisher & Ludwig's textbook of pediatric emergency medicine* [7th ed., Fig. 14.24]. Philadelphia, PA: Lippincott Williams & Wilkins.)

After Delivery

"It's going to hurt," says Nancy. She hasn't had a bowel movement in 2 days and the pressure is building. "I think I can wait until tomorrow."

She's talking to a nurse named Robin. Missy is at home with Teddy and plans to bring him with her when she comes to pick up Nancy and the baby and bring them home.

"The stool will be very soft," says Robin. "You've been taking docusate, and it really does help the stool stay soft and your bowel movement more comfortable" (The Pharmacy 9.2).

Nancy has also had issues with urinating. It took her almost 12 hours to empty her bladder without the aid of a catheter. Her perineum (the area between her pubic symphysis and coccyx) was swollen from the duration of pushing and her anxiety about the pain was such that she had a hard time allowing her body to release. Her nurse at the time tried running water and putting her hand in water. Eventually, the nurse had to catheterize her—twice. She explained that it was important to keep her bladder empty because a full bladder could push against the uterus in such a way that it might stay soft and bleed. Nancy secretly thought this all sounded suspicious—after all, she didn't feel like she had to pee. Of course the nurse said that was normal, as well, just before she catheterized her (Box 9.6).

"Have you been walking?"

"Yes," says Nancy. "I've been walking up and down these halls pushing that bassinet. The baby likes the movement, and I like getting out of bed."

"That should help stimulate the movement of your bowels," says Robin. "Have you had any fiber or hot liquids?"

"Yes and yes. I even drank warm prune juice," says Nancy. "It tastes about as good as you would think."

"Have you tried peppermint tea?"

"Gallons," says Nancy. "Still, I'm worried this is going to hurt. I'm worried I'm going to tear through my stitches."

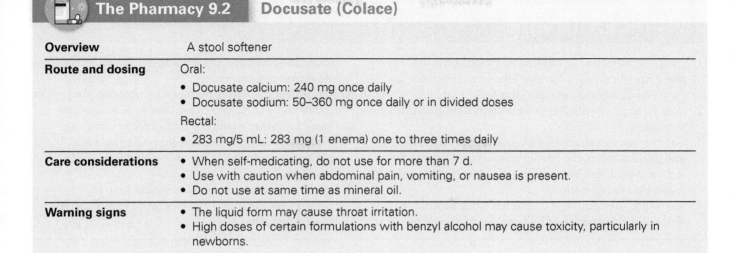

The Pharmacy 9.2 — Docusate (Colace)

Overview	A stool softener
Route and dosing	Oral: • Docusate calcium: 240 mg once daily • Docusate sodium: 50–360 mg once daily or in divided doses Rectal: • 283 mg/5 mL: 283 mg (1 enema) one to three times daily
Care considerations	• When self-medicating, do not use for more than 7 d. • Use with caution when abdominal pain, vomiting, or nausea is present. • Do not use at same time as mineral oil.
Warning signs	• The liquid form may cause throat irritation. • High doses of certain formulations with benzyl alcohol may cause toxicity, particularly in newborns.

"It might hurt," says Robin. "But you won't rip through your stitches. Take your time. Think about relaxing instead of pushing. Think about how much better your belly will feel afterward."

"Relaxing instead of pushing," Nancy repeats.

"You could try a laxative, if you like," says Robin. You have an order for one in your chart."

"I hate that stuff," says Nancy.

"Look, why don't you just go in there and sit on the toilet. I'll take the baby with me to the nursery. Run some water, bring a book, try to relax. If it doesn't work, you can try a laxative."

Later that afternoon, Missy returns with Teddy and the baby's car seat. Teddy is 3, now, with perfectly straight dark hair that always sticks out from his head as though by static electricity. He's watching the baby sleep in his clear plastic cot. He is on his best behavior with his hands jammed deep in his pockets, but he's bouncing lightly on his heels.

"He looks like a snap pea," he says. "And he smells weird."

"I guess he does look a little like a pea all wrapped up like that," says Nancy. "Do you want to touch him?"

Box 9.6 Ways to Stimulate Urination Postpartum

• Place your hand in warm water.
• Blow bubbles through a straw.
• Run warm water over the perineum.
• Listen to the sound of running water.
• Take a warm shower.
• Drink fluids.
• Ensure privacy while urinating.
• Void into a bed pan containing drops of peppermint oil.
• Place ice packs on the perineum prior to voiding.

Teddy considers. "No."

"The baby bought you a present, Teddy," says Missy. She brings out a flat, brightly wrapped package from her purse.

"It looks like a book," says Teddy. He turns away from Missy without taking the book and sits on the bed with Nancy, his shoulder against hers. Clearly the baby is lousy at choosing gifts. "Is he going to sleep in the bed with you now?"

"He's going to sleep in a little bed next to ours," says Nancy. "Babies wake up a lot in the night. They don't sleep all the way through like big boys."

"Like I do," says Teddy, who made a habit during Nancy's pregnancy of sleeping through the night not in his own bed but in his mothers'.

"Like you do."

"What's his name, anyway?"

"We thought you might like to name him," says Nancy.

"We thought you might like to *help* name him," says Missy. "Mommy and Mama have veto rights."

"Hmm," says Teddy. He makes a show of tapping his mouth with his finger and scrunching up his eyes. He sits up with one finger in the air. "Backhoe!"

"No," says Missy.

"Why not?"

"Because he's a baby, not a machine."

"John Deere?"

"Also a machine, but warmer," says Nancy.

"Bob?"

"Well," says Missy diplomatically. "Bob is a very fine name, but are you sure that it's *his* very fine name?"

Teddy considers this carefully. He looks at the baby again and pulls back his cap a little so that his hair, dark and straight like Teddy's, shows. Teddy is satisfied. "His name is Jonathan. Can I hold him?"

Think Critically

1. Using the resources you can find at www.diabetes.org, plan a day of eating for Nancy. Make sure to reference her particular dietary requirements (Box 9.1).
2. How do insulin needs change for women throughout pregnancy?
3. Consider the two screening protocols for the diagnosis of gestational diabetes, the 1-hour followed by 3-hour test and the 2-hour test. What do you see as the benefits and drawbacks of each method?
4. You suspect an infant in your care has cephalhematoma. Write a brief description of how you would explain to a patient the difference between this, a subgaleal hemorrhage, and caput succedaneum.
5. Your patient is suffering from urinary retention postpartum. How would you prioritize your intervention attempts?
6. Nancy and Missy would like more information about why baby Jonathan is more predisposed to jaundice than another baby might be. How would you explain it to them?
7. In your own words, explain why infants born to mothers with gestational diabetes have a higher risk for hypoglycemia after birth.

References

American College of Obstetricians and Gynecologists. (2014). Obstetric care consensus no. 1: Safe prevention of the primary cesarean delivery. *Obstetrics and Gynecology, 123*(3), 693.

Damm, P., Houshmand-Oeregaard, A., Kelstrup, L., Lauenborg, J., Mathiesen, E. R., & Clausen, T. D. (2016). Gestational diabetes mellitus and long-term consequences for mother and offspring: a view from Denmark. *Diabetologia, 59*(7), 1396–1399.

Gupta, J., Sood, A., Hofmeyr, G., & Vogel, J. (2017). Position in the second stage of labour for women without epidural anaesthesia. *Cochrane Database of Systematic Reviews,* (5), CD002006.

Hinkle, S. N., Mumford, S. L., Grantz, K. L., Silver, R. M., Mitchell, E. M., Sjaarda, L. A., . . . Schisterman, E. F. (2016, September 26). Association of nausea and vomiting during pregnancy with pregnancy loss. *JAMA Internal Medicine, 176*(11), 1621–1627.

Lawrence, A., Lewis, L., Hofmeyr, G., & Styles, C. (2013). Maternal positions and mobility during first stage labour. *Cochrane Database of Systematic Reviews,* (10), CD003934.

Moyer, V. A. (2014). Screening for gestational diabetes mellitus: U.S. Preventive Services Task Force recommendation statement. *Annals of Internal Medicine, 160*(6), 414–420.

Rosenstein, M. G., Cheng, Y. W., Snowden, J. M., Nicholson, J. M., Doss, A. E., & Caughey, A. B. (2012). The risk of stillbirth and infant death stratified by gestational age in women with gestational diabetes. *Obstetrics and Gynecology, 206*(4), 309.e1–309.e7.

Zuzelo, P. R. (2014). Improving nursing care for lesbian, bisexual, and transgender women. *Journal of Obstetric, Gynecologic, and Neonatal Nursing, 43*(4), 520–530.

Suggested Readings

American Diabetes Association. (2017). Retrieved from www.diabetes.org

Elkins, D., & Taylor, J. S. (2013). Evidence-based strategies for managing gestational diabetes in women with obesity. *Nursing for Women's Health, 17*(5), 420–430.

Lacker, C. (2012). Preventing maternal and neonatal harm during vacuum-assisted vaginal delivery. *The American Journal of Nursing, 112*(2), 65–69.

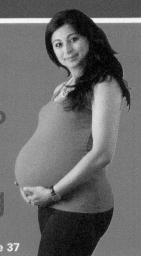

10

Lexi Cowslip:
Advanced Maternal Age, HELLP Syndrome, and Neonatal Necrotizing Enterocolitis

Lexi Cowslip, age 37

Objectives

1. Identify clinical manifestations of HELLP syndrome.
2. Describe the key complications of prematurity.
3. Identify key screening differences between a pregnancy designated low risk and one categorized as advanced maternal age.
4. Discuss potential stressors associated with the birth of a very preterm infant and their effect on the parents.
5. Describe the signs and symptoms of neonatal necrotizing enterocolitis and the appropriate nursing interventions to address this condition.
6. List and explain factors that contribute to the decision of whether a client should have a vaginal delivery or a cesarean delivery.
7. Explain the rationale for administering total parenteral nutrition to a premature neonate.
8. Define and discuss the benefits of skin-to-skin care for neonates.

Key Terms

Amniocentesis
Bronchopulmonary dysplasia
Cerebral palsy
Congenital
HELLP syndrome
Infiltrate
Intraventricular hemorrhage

Intubation
Necrotizing enterocolitis
Pneumatosis intestinalis
Surfactant
Total parenteral nutrition (TPN)
Vasectomy

Before Conception

Lexi Cowslip is 37 years old and would like just one more baby. She and her husband Joe have two boys, aged 9 and 3 years old. She has a copper intrauterine device (IUD; see The Pharmacy 1.1), which was placed immediately after the birth of her second son. Overall, the method has worked for her, but her periods are generally heavy and crampy and last for over a week. Joe has been talking about getting a **vasectomy**, a surgical procedure for male sterilization (Fig. 10.1), but Lexi is hesitant to agree.

"I'm willing to do it," says Joe. "Then you could have the IUD taken out and we wouldn't have to worry about another pregnancy."

"Well, technically," says Lexi, who likes to methodically research all of her options before making a decision, "after you have the procedure you are still considered fertile until a semen analysis is done three months later to confirm you've used up all the sperm in the tubes."

"Okay, fine. I have the vasectomy, I get my sperm analyzed, and then you get the IUD out and we don't need to worry about pregnancy."

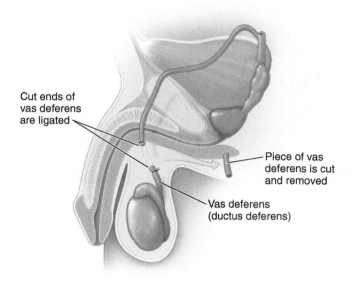

Cut ends of
vas deferens
are ligated

Piece of vas
deferens is cut
and removed

Vas deferens
(ductus deferens)

Figure 10.1. Vasectomy. In a vasectomy, a piece of the vas deferens is cut and removed, and the loose ends are ligated (tied). (Reprinted with permission from Nath, J. [2016]. *Stedman's medical terminology* [2nd ed., Fig. 14.15]. Philadelphia, PA: Lippincott Williams & Wilkins.)

"Yeah, I know," says Lexi. She plays with the sleeve of his sweater.

"What are you thinking, Lex?" asks Joe.

"I don't know. I love our boys, they're great boys. But I just feel like I'm not quite done, like maybe there's this one other kid out there who's supposed to be mine."

"Lex, you're the accountant. We talked about this. You made spreadsheets. We've figured out all of our expenses—college funds, car replacements—based on having two kids, not two or three kids, just two kids."

"I know, but this isn't a thinking thing. It's more of a feeling." Joe looks surprised. "A what?"

"Stop it."

"I'm just surprised is all," says Joe. "I'm usually the one making rash, emotional decisions and then thinking them through later."

"This isn't rash, Joe," says Lexi. "And I'm not saying I've made a decision. I'm just not sure I'm ready to not have any more children. A vasectomy is so final."

"Think about car seats," says Joe. "We're down to only one car seat. Remember how excited we were when Randy could start buckling his own seatbelt?"

"I know."

"And daycare. We're a year and a half away from Neil being in public school. That will save us hundreds of dollars every month. Remember how we were planning to use that extra money to pay down student debt?"

"I know," says Lexi. "But we'd only have a little bit of overlap with two of them in daycare and preschool, even if I got pregnant right away. That's not so bad."

"We donated all of the baby stuff. We don't have so much as a bouncy seat left."

"We always had way more than we needed for the boys. We can borrow from people and buy things used. We can budget and buy the things we really need in the months leading up to the birth."

"We have a three-bedroom house."

"Well," says Lexi. "The baby will sleep in our room for a year. I was reading the other day that having a baby sleep in the parents' room for a year reduces the risk of sudden death syndrome by half" (Moon, 2016). "And then maybe we could put the boys together in a room, or we could build an extension or move. We've been in this house almost ten years."

"What are we talking about here, Lexi? Because it sounds like you've made a decision, and I'm just wondering how long this has been in your head before you decided to tell me."

"It's not a decision. I'm just talking, just throwing out ideas, you know?" says Lexi.

"We've been married fifteen years. You never talk something out unless you've already made a decision inside your head."

"It took over a year to get pregnant with Neil," says Lexi. "And I'm older now. I may not even be able to get pregnant."

"But you want to try," says Joe.

"I could just have the IUD taken out and see what happens. We could leave it to the universe to decide."

"That's completely illogical," says Joe. "You barely let the boys pick out their own cereal and now you want the universe to decide if we're going to create another person?"

"I'm trying something new," says Lexi.

"Lex, you know I'd love to have another kid, but you seemed pretty sure it was a bad idea. Are you sure this isn't just an emotional reaction to the approach of menopause?"

"That's a lovely thought, husband, but no, I don't think so. One more baby, then I'm done."

Pregnancy

First Trimester

"You are thirty-seven years old now, Lexi," says Dr. Stone. He's older than her father and has a brusque if reassuring presence. "That means for the purposes of this pregnancy we consider you to be of advanced maternal age."

"Advanced maternal age?"

"Yes. It means a woman who is pregnant at or beyond the age of thirty-five years. You may have heard the term geriatric pregnancy."

"Are you kidding? No, I hadn't heard that term," says Lexi. "That's kind of awful."

Dr. Stone removed her IUD just 3 months ago. At the time, he advised her, in a businesslike way, that a woman's fertility diminishes sharply in her mid-30s and that she was at higher risk for subfertility, complications in pregnancy, and of having a fetus with a congenital defect (Box 10.1). He wrote her a prescription for a prenatal vitamin and told her that if she wasn't pregnant in 6 months she could consider evaluation for infertility.

"Normally we wait for a full year before we consider fertility assessment," he told her at the time. "But with clients who are over thirty-five, we start work at six months because the overall

Box 10.1 Increased Risks of an Advanced Maternal Age Pregnancy

- Ectopic pregnancy
- Spontaneous abortion
- Stillbirth
- Congenital defects, including Down syndrome
- Preeclampsia, eclampsia, gestational hypertension, and HELLP syndrome
- Gestational diabetes
- Placenta previa
- Placental abruption
- Preterm birth
- Low birth–weight infant
- Intrauterine grown restriction
- Cesarean delivery

Data from Mills, T., & Lavender, T. (2014). Advanced maternal age. *Obstetrics, Gynaecology and Reproductive Medicine, 24*(3), 85–90.

Box 10.2 Standard Schedule of Routine Early Fetal Assessments for Low-Risk Pregnancies

First Trimester

- Screening for trisomies
- Blood test at 12 wk
  - Pregnancy-associated plasma protein: low in an abnormal test
  - hCG: high in an abnormal test
- Ultrasound between 10 and 13 wk
  - Nuchal translucency (measurement by ultrasound of the space at the back of the fetal neck): thickening indicates an abnormal test.

Second Trimester

- Labs drawn at 16 wk (in addition to first trimester screening labs and ultrasound)
  - Maternal serum alpha-fetoprotein: high levels associated with neural tube defects; low levels associated with Down syndrome
  - hCG: high levels associated with Down syndrome; low levels associated with trisomy 18
  - Unconjugated estriol: low in Down syndrome and some neural tube defects
  - Inhibin-A: high in Down syndrome
- Fetal survey ultrasound at 20 wk

hCG, human chorionic gonadotropin.

time frame for a pregnancy is so much smaller. With clients who are forty years or older, we start right away."

With that kind of endorsement, Lexi felt less hopeful about a pregnancy and more anxious. She didn't tell Joe what Dr. Stone said and felt relieved when she got pregnant, as well as feeling the usual contrary tugs of excitement and anxiety she had with her previous pregnancies.

"It's wonderful you were able to get pregnant so quickly," Dr. Stone tells her during her visit today.

"Yes. After we met last time I was surprised."

"No two people are alike," says Dr. Stone. "But what we discussed at that time about a greater risk for complications in pregnancy and congenital defects of the fetus holds true still. You also have an increased risk for a cesarean delivery. I believe you've already had one. This is considered a high-risk pregnancy, even though your age is the only difference between this pregnancy and your previous ones."

"What do you mean by high risk? Do I have to do anything different?"

"Some of it's the same, but some of our monitoring of this pregnancy will be different. We'll do the routine blood and urine tests this visit that we did with your previous pregnancies (see Lab Values 1.1). We don't need to check your carrier status for genetic anomalies because we have your previous records. We do need to talk about the fetal evaluations we do for this pregnancy, however. Previously we've used blood tests and ultrasound to screen for abnormalities (Box 10.2). Your test results with previous pregnancies did not indicate a high probability of a problem. If they had, I would have recommended an **amniocentesis** for a definitive diagnosis. My recommendation with this pregnancy is that we bypass the blood tests and early ultrasound and go straight to the amniocentesis."

"Amniocentesis is when you stick the big needle in the belly," says Lexi.

"Yes. A needle is inserted into the amniotic sac through your abdomen with ultrasound guidance, and a small sample of the amniotic fluid is extracted. This fluid contains fetal cells that can then be definitively assessed for anomalies. We'll also be measuring the level of alpha-fetoprotein, which would alert us to a neural tube defect such as spina bifida" (Fig. 10.2).

"So no blood tests?"

"Not for congenital defects, no. If we were to do them and the results came back abnormal, I would recommend an amniocentesis," says Dr. Stone. "If they came back normal, I'd still recommend an amniocentesis."

"So our plan would be the same regardless of the blood test results."

"Correct."

"Is anything else different?"

"It has become routine for women in this country to have an ultrasound in the second trimester to survey the fetus regardless of medical indication," Dr. Stone says (Wax et al., 2014). "In your case, however, because of your age, I do think it is warranted to assess the health of the fetus."

"Is that it? Should I be looking for anything different?"

"No, the concerns are the same; it's just that the likelihood of complications is higher. So, you should notify this office immediately of any signs of a problem, such as bleeding. After twenty weeks, you should report abdominal pain or headaches immediately" (see Table 6.3).

"I really hoped to have a vaginal birth this time," says Lexi. "But you mentioned a cesarean is more likely."

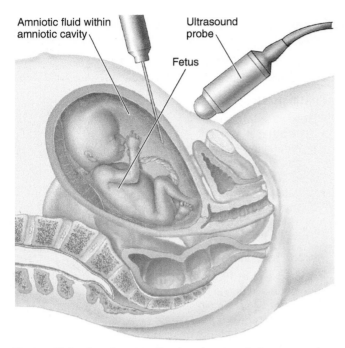

Figure 10.2. Amniocentesis. Amniocentesis is a procedure performed from 14 to 20 weeks of gestation in which a needle is inserted into the patient's abdomen under ultrasound surveillance, to make sure the fetus is not accidentally punctured, and a sample of amniotic fluid is withdrawn. DNA analysis of fetal cells floating in the fluid is then done to examine for genetic abnormalities. Alpha-fetoprotein levels are also often evaluated for neural tube defects. (Modified with permission from Anatomical Chart Company; reprinted with permission from Wingerd, B. [2013]. *The human body: Concepts of anatomy and physiology* [3rd ed., Fig. 18.14]. Philadelphia, PA: Lippincott Williams & Wilkins.)

"Your risk for a cesarean is higher than it would be for a younger woman, yes," says Dr. Stone. "And you've already had a cesarean section in the past."

"Yes, because the baby was having trouble. I did have my first vaginally, however. My physician mentioned he wouldn't do a vaginal birth after my cesarean section, were I to get pregnant again."

"That's not uncommon," says Dr. Stone. "There is increased risk. There is a small but real chance that your uterus could rupture during the delivery, which could have catastrophic consequences for both you and the baby. Many hospitals do not allow vaginal births after a cesarean section at all."

"What are the odds of that happening, a uterine rupture?" asks Lexi.

"Small," says Dr. Stone. "About one in two hundred" (Guise et al., 2010).

"Have you ever had anyone's uterus rupture?"

"Twice," says Dr. Stone. "But the circumstances were different each time. Before I can commit I need to verify your past surgical history. To go forward with a trial of labor for vaginal delivery, you need to have had a horizontal, or side-to-side, incision of your uterus in your previous cesarean birth. A uterus that has

undergone cesarean section in which a vertical incision was made is much more likely to rupture, and I would not attempt a vaginal delivery under that circumstance."

"My incision does go side to side," says Lexi.

"Yes, most women do have an incision of their skin that is transverse. What I'm referring to is the internal incision of your uterus, though most of the time this is also a transverse incision" (Fig. 10.3).

"Is there anything else we should be thinking about, or is it really just this incision?" asks Lexi.

"That's the most pertinent issue at the moment," says Dr. Stone. "Lexi, you're otherwise healthy and you'll be giving birth at a large, well-equipped hospital. Having your pregnancies close together can put you at greater risk for uterine rupture, but you've had three years since your last birth, which should be sufficient to mitigate that particular risk. Assuming this pregnancy goes to term and there are no other complications, I believe we can accommodate your request for a trial of labor. Keep in mind, though, that you may still need a cesarean section. If you do, it may be a decision that needs to be made quickly " (Analyze the Evidence 10.1).

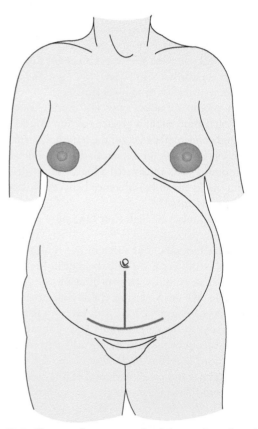

Figure 10.3. Types of cesarean incisions. Anterior view of a pregnant woman with the two types of cesarean incisions, classic (vertical pink line) and transverse (curved blue line), indicated. (Reprinted with permission from LifeART image, © 2018 Lippincott Williams & Wilkins. All rights reserved.)

Vaginal birth after cesarean (VBAC; also referred to as trial of labor after cesarean) may be an option for many women who have had a previous cesarean section. Both options have risks and benefits. Current guidelines suggest that resources and personnel should be immediately available to perform an emergency cesarean section in the case of uterine rupture.

VBAC Considerations	Repeat Cesarean Considerations
• Faster postpartum recovery and discharge than repeat cesarean • Reduced or absent risk of complications from anesthesia • Reduced or absent risk of surgical complications • Reduced risk of neonatal respiratory complications	• Risk of uterine rupture of approximately 1/200, which can pose a serious risk to mothers and newborns, including death • Small reduction in neonatal mortality • Increased risk of the placenta growing into the wall of the uterus (placenta accrete) in future pregnancies with repeat cesarean section

Data from Guise, J. M., Denman, M. A., Emeis, C., Marshall, N., Walker, M., Fu, R., . . . McDonagh, M. (2010). Vaginal birth after cesarean: New insights on maternal and neonatal outcomes. *Obstetrics and Gynecology, 115*(6), 1267–1278.

Second Trimester

At 15 weeks of gestation, Lexi presents for an amniocentesis to assess for neural tube defects and genetic disorders. Prior to the procedure, Lexi has to sign a form stating that she understands the risks of amniocentesis, including prolonged leakage of amniotic fluid, injury to the fetus, infection, and miscarriage.

"I think I'd like some perspective on this," says Lexi. "These are pretty scary risks. What are the chances of something bad happening from the amniocentesis, realistically?"

"Low," says Dr. Stone. "The risk of a miscarriage resulting from an amniocentesis is about one in three or five hundred" (ACOG, 2016).

"What's the chance of finding something with the amniocentesis that we need to worry about?" asks Joe.

"At Lexi's age, about one in one hundred, give or take," says Dr. Stone. "Which means the odds are still extremely good that this pregnancy is completely healthy. It's entirely your decision if you want to go forward with this. Some people feel like it wouldn't change their decision making about the pregnancy and they'd rather not introduce an extra risk. Other people feel like it may not change decision making, but they'd like to be prepared if there is a problem. Many people elect not to continue a pregnancy that has a significant issue. These are all very personal decisions. All we can do with the test is give you information."

Lexi nods. "Well, I appreciate the breakdown," she says. She looks at Joe. "I need to know."

"Me too," says Joe.

"Okay, so we'll do an ultrasound first," says Dr. Stone. "That way we can visualize the fetus, placenta, and amniotic fluid to make sure we're aiming for the right spot. After that I'll clean the injection site thoroughly and provide a little local anesthetic. Then I'll insert the needle under ultrasound guidance and draw out about an ounce of fluid to send off to the lab for analysis."

"Let's do it then," says Lexi, and she climbs onto the table indicated by Dr. Stone.

Lexi rolls down the waistband of her maternity pants, and Dr. Stone tucks a paper drape into the top of her pants. He covers her belly with cool, pale blue ultrasound jelly and moves an ultrasound transducer over it. Joe is by Lexi's bedside, and they glance at each other, and then at the screen, where they can make out a blurry assortment of white, black, and gray shapes.

"Can you tell anything just from the ultrasound?" asks Joe.

"We can get some general impressions, yes," says Dr. Stone. "But with this ultrasound we're really just focusing on getting a sample of the amniotic fluid. You'll have a fetal survey ultrasound in about a month when the fetus is more fully developed."

Dr. Stone thoroughly cleans a small spot on Lexi's belly. He picks up a syringe with a thin, short needle filled with clear fluid from a tray. "This is some local anesthetic. It's up to you if we use it or not. It feels a little like a bee sting when it first goes in. Some people think the procedure is actually more comfortable without it, but the choice is entirely yours."

"I think I'd like the anesthetic," says Lexi. She puts out her hand, and Joe holds it. Dr. Stone is right. It does feel like a bee sting.

Lexi closes her eyes when she sees the long amniocentesis needle. She feels only pressure as it is inserted through her abdominal wall and uterus and into the amniotic sac. Dr. Stone announces that he's drawing up the fluid, and then that he's removing the needle (Fig. 10.2).

"That's it," says Dr. Stone, "That's the whole show."

"That wasn't so bad," says Lexi.

"Good," says Dr. Stone. "A few things. You may have a little bit of cramping or vaginal bleeding, maybe some clear discharge from the vagina. That's all normal and should resolve quickly. Give us a call if the bleeding or discharge doesn't stop or if the cramping lasts for several hours. We want to know right away if you start running a fever."

"Okay," says Lexi. "Anything else? Do I just go about my day?"

"Maybe take it a little easy today," says Dr. Stone, "but that's it. We should have some results for you in one to two weeks."

A week later Dr. Stone calls to congratulate them on a perfectly normal pregnancy.

"Good," says Joe when Lexi tells him. "That sounds boring. I like boring in a pregnancy."

Third Trimester

It's a Thursday and Lexi is 29 weeks pregnant. She's been waking earlier and earlier as her pregnancy progresses, and when she wakes up this morning just after 4:30, she notices a pain in her right side under her ribs. It feels like a stitch in her side from exercising, yet not quite. Plus, she was sleeping, not exercising. She sits up holding her side. She feels a sudden surge of nausea, rushes to the bathroom, and vomits. She brushes her teeth and rinses her mouth. The pain is still there. She climbs back into bed. She's still nauseous. Her head hurts.

"You okay?" Joe asks.

"I think I have the stomach flu," says Lexi.

"Really? Is there something going around?"

"I don't know. But I just threw up and it hurts under my rib cage. It was just on the right side, but now it's in the middle, as well. And I have a headache. It's probably a virus."

Joe feels her head. "You feel warm, but you've been sleeping."

"I'm fine," says Lexi. "Maybe if I just go back to bed I can sleep it off."

"Maybe we should call the OB office."

"It's like five in the morning," says Lexi. "They're closed."

"I'm sure they have someone on call."

Lexi groans. "They open at eight. Just call them then. They're just going to say the same thing I just did."

Joe does call the office at 8:00, and by 8:30, Lexi has given a medical assistant a urine sample and is having her blood pressure (BP) taken while she waits for Dr. Stone to come in.

"I'm concerned about the pain and vomiting," says Dr. Stone as soon as he arrives a few minutes later. "I'm particularly concerned because your BP is one hundred forty-eight over ninety-eight and you have protein in your urine." As he says this he's inflating the BP cuff around her arm again to verify the reading the medical assistant got earlier. "It's still high," he says, but doesn't report the number.

"So I have high BP, a high protein level, pain, and vomiting," says Lexi. "You're not thinking it's a stomach bug, I take it."

"Did you have any BP issues or preeclampsia with your previous pregnancies?" asks Dr. Stone.

"Well no, not that I know of," says Lexi. "I'm sure it would say in my old chart."

"I want to draw some blood," says Dr. Stone. "Then I'll send the sample to the lab STAT. I want you back here by the end of day so we can check your BP and review the lab results" (Lab Values 10.1).

"You're making me nervous," says Lexi. "What are you thinking here?"

"I think at minimum you have preeclampsia, but I do want to verify your elevated BP in a second visit. The protein in your

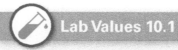

Lab Values 10.1

HELLP Diagnostic Labs

- Complete blood count with platelets: platelets ≤100,000 cells/μL indicates low platelets.
- Peripheral blood smear: appearance of schistocytes indicates hemolysis.
- Serum aspartate aminotransferase: a value greater than two times the limit of normal indicates liver damage and hemolysis.
- Total bilirubin: ≥1.2 mg/dL indicates hemolysis.

urine would also indicate preeclampsia, but I'm quite concerned that the headache, abdominal pain, and vomiting actually suggest a more serious condition called **HELLP syndrome**" (Box 10.3).

"Help? Seriously? That's what it's called?"

"It stands for hemolysis, elevated liver enzymes, and low platelets. It's quite dangerous for you and for your baby" (Boxes 10.4 and 10.5).

"Wait, this is nuts. What do you mean by dangerous? This is treatable, right? Like with bed rest or medications or something? We're going to be fine."

Dr. Stone furrows his brow and looks at her. "Lexi, if this is HELLP syndrome, this baby needs to be delivered within 48 hours. Usually we have some warning that this condition may happen because the woman develops preeclampsia first. You've had a very normal pregnancy, and so this is wholly unexpected.

Box 10.3 Prevalence of Symptoms in Patients With HELLP Syndrome

- Proteinuria (protein in the urine): 90%–95%
- Hypertension: 85%
- Right upper quadrant and/or epigastric pain: 60%–80%
- Nausea and vomiting: 40%
- Headache: up to 61%
- Visual changes: up to 20%
- Jaundice: 5%–10%

Data from Kirkpatrick, C. (2010). The HELLP syndrome. *Acta Clinica Belgica*, 65(1), 91.

Box 10.4 Definition of HELLP Syndrome

- *Hemolysis*
- *Elevated Liver enzymes*
- *Low Platelets*

Box 10.5 Prevalence of Maternal Complications in Patients With HELLP Syndrome

- Need for transfusion of blood or blood products: 55%
- Disseminated intravascular coagulation: 21%
- Placental abruption: 16%
- Renal failure: 8%
- Pulmonary edema: 6%
- Need for surgery for intraabdominal bleeding: 2%
- Liver hematoma: 1%
- Retinal detachment: 1%

Data from Sibai, B. M., Ramadan, M. K., Usta, I., Salama, M., Mercer, B. M., & Friedman, S. A. (1993). Maternal morbidity and mortality in 442 pregnancies with hemolysis, elevated liver enzymes, and low platelets (HELLP syndrome). *American Journal of Obstetrics and Gynecology, 169*(4), 1000–1006.

I'm sorry, but this isn't something I can break to you gently. We need to act on this quickly" (Box 10.6).

"I don't know," Lexi tells Joe on her cell phone. She's sitting in the waiting room. Dr. Stone told her he doesn't want her driving. "He just took my blood and said it could be serious and told me to come back this afternoon to have another BP check and come up with a plan."

"Well, what's serious?"

"*Serious* serious," says Lexi. "Like, I might not even be pregnant anymore by the end of the weekend." Lexi's voice catches at the last word. Saying it out loud makes it a real thing instead of an idea.

"I'll meet you there in a few minutes."

"No, I'm okay," says Lexi. "Really. I can hang just out here and wait for the results. I need to come back in later anyway. This will save a trip. You have a busy day. I'll be fine."

"Not likely. You don't have to be a hero, Lex. I'll come pick you up."

"Your BP has not improved," says Dr. Stone that afternoon. "And your labs confirm the diagnosis of HELLP syndrome."

"Really? It's called help syndrome?" asks Joe.

"It stands for hemolysis, elevated liver enzymes, and low platelets," says Lexi.

"Yes," says Dr. Stone. "Most women who develop it have preeclampsia first so we have a progression or warning. In a minority of cases HELLP presents symptomatically without a prior diagnosis."

"Well, are you sure?" asks Joe. "Could something have been missed before?"

Box 10.6 Risk Factors for HELLP Syndrome

- HELLP syndrome with a previous pregnancy
- A close relative with HELLP syndrome
- Preeclampsia (precedes HELLP syndrome in 80%–85% of women)

"I don't believe so," says Dr. Stone. "I reviewed her record thoroughly prior to this visit."

"Lex said the baby might have to be delivered early. Do you still think that?" asks Joe.

Dr. Stone nods. "I do. Lexi, I want you to be admitted. We're going to do a few things. I want to put you on intravenous magnesium sulfate. You're still early in the pregnancy, and this may provide some protection for the baby's brain" (Zeng, Xue, Tian, Sun, & An, 2016; see The Pharmacy 4.1). "The second thing we need to do is a course of two steroid injections. This will help hasten the development of some systems, including the lungs. It gives your baby a better shot" (see The Pharmacy 8.2).

"So, we aren't doing a vaginal delivery?" asks Lexi.

Dr. Stone shakes his head. "No, I'm sorry. I was willing to have you try under close observation, but it's just not possible now. After the course of steroids are done, your baby will be delivered by cesarean section."

"I wanted to try a vaginal delivery this time," says Lexi. She doesn't mean it as a challenge, just a statement.

"I would strongly recommend against that at this point. Very strongly."

"Mr. and Mrs. Cowslip?" says a man in a white coat standing in the doorway of Lexi's hospital room a few hours later.

"Yes," says Joe. "We're Joe and Lexi Cowslip. Are you from the NICU?"

The man enters the room and closes the door behind him. He shakes their hands. "I am. I'm Eric White. I'm a nurse practitioner in the NICU. I was hoping I could talk with you about some of what you might see over the next few weeks."

"This is happening so fast," says Lexi. "Two days ago I was worrying about staff coverage for my maternity leave and getting the car inspected. This morning I thought I'd just eaten something weird. And now all this. This just feels surreal."

"I completely understand that. But we're glad it was caught and we're glad you're here," says Eric. "You have a good team. We're going to work hard to get both you and the baby through this."

"We understand Lexi is getting steroid shots to try to head off complications, right?" asks Joe.

"That's correct. The steroids accelerate maturity in several systems that are underdeveloped in your baby at this point." Eric starts to tick points off on his fingers. "First thing is the lungs. The steroids help them to hurry up the production of something called **surfactant**, which keeps them from collapsing. Our hope is that the lungs will be mature enough that we can avoid invasive interventions, such as **intubation**, which have the potential to lead to other problems."

"Another complication we see in preterm infants is a kind of bleeding in the brain called an **intraventricular hemorrhage**. We can reduce this risk by about half with the steroids, so that's a very good thing" (Roberts, Brown, Medley, & Dalziel, 2017).

Eric pulls down another finger. "Third, we also reduce the risk of a serious gastrointestinal complication called **necrotizing enterocolitis** by about half. We also reduce the chance of a major infection in the first forty-eight hours to half, and we significantly improve the overall chances of infant survival" (Roberts et al., 2017).

Lexi looks up at Joe and then back to Eric. "We've heard this a couple of times, about the improved chances of survival. I guess, I don't know. I don't know if I want to ask."

"What are the survival rates for babies born this early?" Eric finishes for her. He says it gently, but both Joe and Lexi look away.

"Yes," says Lexi. "That's what I'm asking. I know every baby is different and there are no guarantees and all that. But I just want something. Some idea."

Eric nods. "You're right. Every baby is different. But overall, not accounting for your otherwise good health, Lexi, or any other variables, the overall mortality rate for infants born this early is about thirty-six percent" (Mathews, MacDorman, & Thoma, 2015).

"My God," says Joe. "That's really high."

"It does sound high," says Eric. "But remember you have things going for you. You're getting the steroids. You're getting the magnesium sulfate, which helps to protect the brain. Your pregnancy has been healthy and textbook perfect up to this point. I don't want to discount the real risk here, but I want you to know that we feel really hopeful about a good outcome."

"I want to do everything we can to help her," says Lexi. "Everything."

"I understand. Let's talk about the care your baby will be receiving." Eric hands them a laminated picture (Fig. 10.4). "The NICU is very open. It's not like an adult floor where everyone has a private room. Your baby will be in an enclosed bed like this one. An isolette. These little ones have a hard time maintaining their body temperature, so we regulate their ambient temperature as much as possible."

"Will we even be able to touch her?" asks Joe.

"Oh yes," says Eric. "It takes some coordination, but we strongly encourage skin-to-skin time with mom and dad. It's

not just about bonding, either, though that's important. It can also help to regulate temperature and blood sugar and is linked to better survival rates" (Boundy et al., 2016).

"Can other people come visit?" asks Lexi. "She has two little brothers."

Eric shakes his head. "No children visitors are allowed in the NICU, I'm afraid. These babies are very fragile, and even a mild infection could be dangerous. Although the two of you are welcome to visit anytime, other visitors will not be allowed. You can take lots and lots of pictures."

"Okay," says Lexi, who was expecting that anyway. "What else?"

"One of the first things we'll work on after she's born is breathing," says Eric. "Sometimes even the little ones like this can get by without help. Some need a mask, a CPAP, that provides constant pressure to keep their lungs from collapsing. And some babies need a tube to help them breathe and artificial surfactant to help keep their lungs from collapsing."

"Okay," says Joe. "So probably she'll need some sort help with breathing."

"Yes, I think that's fair to expect," says Eric. "She'll also have a feeding tube, either in her nose or in her mouth, depending on what sort of breathing support she has and what she tolerates."

"What will she be eating?" asks Lexi. "Formula?"

"Well, optimally we like to use expressed breast milk," says Eric. "We strongly encourage mothers of preterm babies to express their breast milk for their babies. We can also buy human milk from milk banks or use formula."

"Of course," says Lexi. "I thought I'd end up freezing milk to give her later, but this is better."

"In all likelihood you will end up freezing some milk," says Eric. "We start out giving these babies very small feeds and then gradually increase them in volume over time—a more gradual increase than for mature babies feeding from the breast on demand. We'd like first dibs of your milk, but you'll likely have leftovers to freeze for later."

"Can she get enough nutrition this way with just small amounts?" asks Lexi.

"Not at first," says Eric. "Shortly after birth something called a central line will be placed, likely into the vein of her umbilical cord. This allows for administration of something called **total parenteral nutrition**, or TPN, which is nutrition we deliver directly into the bloodstream. As the feedings directly into her belly through the feeding tube increase, though, we can start to back off on the TPN and eventually discontinue it all together."

"Why can't she just have all breast milk feeds?" says Joe.

"We believe that introducing feeds slowly and building them over time, along with the steroid shots, help prevent necrotizing enterocolitis."

"Alright," says Joe. "What else?"

"Expect stickers on her chest to monitor her heart rate and breathing with the cardiac apnea monitor. She'll have another sticker on her right hand or wrist to monitor her blood oxygen levels. She'll have another IV in an artery in her umbilical stump so we can monitor certain elements of her blood called arterial blood gasses."

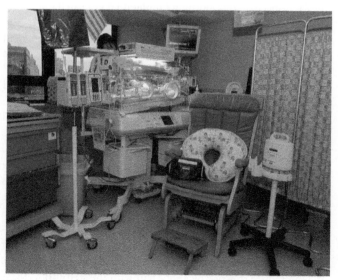

Figure 10.4. A breastfeeding-friendly neonatal intensive care unit environment. Note the presence of a comfortable chair, breastfeeding pillow, breast pump, human milk warmer, stool, portable screens, infant isolette, and pump array. (Reprinted with permission from MacDonald, M. G., & Seshia, M. M. K. [2016]. *Avery. Neonatología* [7th ed., Fig. 21.33]. Philadelphia, PA: Lippincott Williams & Wilkins.)

"Is that it?" asks Joe. He sounds like a combination of sarcastic and overwhelmed.

"Initially, yes," says Eric. "After a week or so the umbilical lines will be discontinued. Depending on what's going on, a central line may need to be placed in a different location. Other things, like the CPAP, may go on for a while or may be discontinued earlier depending on how things are going."

"It's a process," says Joe.

"Yes, it's a process," says Eric. "I don't want you to be afraid to ask questions through this process, of me, of your nurses, of the physicians. And I don't want you to be afraid to ask the same questions over and over. This kind of care can be complex and confusing and will change as she matures and the clinical picture changes. We want to keep you informed."

"What about long-term complications?" says Lexi.

"It's a really good question," says Eric. "I can tell you the risks but not give you any absolutes. There's a risk that she'll have damage to her vision; we'll screen her for that after a month. There is risk of brain damage from bleeding into the brain; we'll evaluate for that after a week and then around the original due date. Even in the absence of a brain bleed there is an increased risk of **cerebral palsy**, which can cause issues with movement. There's also an increased risk for learning and memory issues, and problems with attention. A lot of these kids end up being shorter and smaller than they might have been otherwise. Your baby may get sick more often than other kids. Or none of these things may happen. There's tremendous variation, but these are real risks" (Box 10.7). He pauses. "That was an overwhelming list, I know."

"This is it," says Lexi. "Do we really have no way of telling what her life will be like? She could be anything from a regular kid to a kid who needs round-the-clock support long term—like, forever long term."

Joe grabs her hand. "We can handle this. Whatever happens we can do this."

Lexi pulls her hand away. "We can? Maybe you can, but I don't personally feel like I'm handling right now."

"It's overwhelming," says Eric. "There's a tremendous amount of uncertainty. It's a lot to take in. I wish I could give you a more certain picture."

"I know you're doing your best," says Lexi. "It's just everything. In theory, when you sign up to be a parent, you sign up for whatever gets thrown your way. But in practice? I need time. I need to think about all this, but it's like a freight train coming at me whether I'm ready for it or not."

"Give yourself permission to be sad and to mourn. Even if everything turns out okay, this isn't the experience you've been anticipating. And for a while at least she won't be the healthy baby you've been planning for," says Eric.

"Is that what's going on?" says Lexi. "Maybe I am mourning. That sounds so awful."

"Everything you're feeling right now is normal. Even in this time of uncertainty there are things you can do and people you can talk with who may help you feel more prepared. We have wonderful hospital chaplains here we can call if you feel that spiritual support would be helpful. We have excellent social workers you can talk with who may offer a different perspective. I can see

Box 10.7 Potential Long-term Complications of Prematurity for the Child

- Increased hospitalizations in childhood
- Impairments of learning and memory
- Behavioral problems such as attention deficit hyperactivity disorder
- Cerebral palsy, resulting in problems of movement, balance, and coordination
- Sensory difficulties, including problems with vision and hearing
- Chronic kidney disease
- Respiratory disease, including asthma
- Impaired insulin regulation in adults
- Hypertension as adults
- Reduced reproductive capacity

Data from Stephens, A. S., Lain, S. J., Roberts, C. L., Bowen, J. R., & Nassar, N. (2016). Survival, hospitalization, and acute-care costs of very and moderate preterm infants in the first 6 years of life: A population-based study. *The Journal of Pediatrics, 169,* 61.e3–68.e3; Carmody, J. B., & Charlton, J. R. (2013). Short-term gestation, long-term risk: Prematurity and chronic kidney disease. *Pediatrics, 131*(6), 1168–1179; Saarenpää, H. K., Tikanmäki, M., Sipola-Leppänen, M., Hovi, P., Wehkalampi, K., Siltanen, M., . . . Kajantie, E. (2015). Lung function in very low birth weight adults. *Pediatrics, 136*(4), 642–650; Rotteveel, J., Weissenbruch, M. M., Twisk, J. W., & Delemarre-Van de Waal, H. A. (2008). Infant and childhood growth patterns, insulin sensitivity, and blood pressure in prematurely born young adults. *Pediatrics, 122*(1), 313–321; Swamy, G. K., Ostbye, T., & Skjaerven, R. (2008). Association of preterm birth with long-term survival, reproduction, and next-generation preterm birth. *Journal of the American Medical Association, 299*(12), 1429–1436.

that you have each other, but sometimes it helps to let someone else in so you don't always feel like you have to be the strong one."

"Yes, I think I'd like that," says Lexi. "The chaplain and the social worker. Anyone who's seen all this before."

"We're not really religious," says Joe.

"I don't care," says Lexi. She's crying silently, and dabbing at her cheeks with scratchy hospital tissues.

"You don't have to be religious for a chaplain to be helpful," says Eric. "We have all kinds of people with all sorts of beliefs who can find comfort."

"I'd rather not," says Joe.

"You," says Lexi, "don't have to."

"I want to be supportive," says Joe.

"I know you do, but you don't have to be everything right now," says Lexi. "Go home with the boys. They must be so frightened right now. I'll see if I can talk with the chaplain or maybe the social worker. If I can't I'll have my mom come by and stay. And honestly, some time alone to think wouldn't be awful."

"Divide and conquer," says Joe. He looks a little hurt, a little exasperated.

"I'm going to make some calls about the chaplain and social worker," says Eric, getting up from his chair. "Call me if you have any questions. We'll be apprising you of the situation as it develops. This is hard. I know it's hard—we all do. You're going to be scared and frustrated and angry. You're going to be getting a lot of advice, but here's mine. Take care of yourselves and take care of each other. Don't take those feelings out on each other."

The door makes a soft swish as he closes it behind him.

"Don't push me away," says Joe after Eric has left.

"I'm sorry, I know," says Lexi. "I'm just angry. Not with you or anyone. I just . . . I don't know. I'm just angry."

"I'm going to go home and see the boys," says Joe. "We'll call you later. Try to rest."

Labor and Delivery

"Help me understand why you're so resistant to a cesarean section," says Joe. "You heard Dr. Stone. He said he recommends a cesarean."

"Yes, I know, I heard," says Lexi. "And I didn't say I wouldn't agree to it, it's just that it sucks and I'm sad and I just need space to be disappointed about it.

I'm agreeing to the surgery. Okay?"

There's a light tap at the open door. "I'm Reggie Hampton," says a man in green scrubs. "Mr. and Mrs. Cowslip? I'm the anesthesiologist for your case. I was hoping I could review our plan and see if you have any questions."

"Come in," says Lexi. "I've had a few of these before, so I know what the epidural is like."

"Well, that's one reason why I wanted to come talk with you in person," says Reggie. "We've been watching your platelet levels. Dr. Stone feels comfortable performing your surgery with your count being where it is, but I have a lot of concerns about performing an epidural at this time. There is a risk that I could start a bleed in your spinal canal that we would not be able to stop."

"One thing. Can I have just one thing go right?" asks Lexi. She starts to cry, and Joe sits next to her and hands her the box of tissues.

"So what now?" asks Joe. "You can't do a cesarean section without anesthesia."

"You're absolutely right," says Reggie. "I'm proposing general anesthesia, meaning that we'll be putting you all the way under, Mrs. Cowslip" (Box 10.8).

"Call me Lexi." Lexi blows her nose. "So if I'm all the way under I won't see or hear anything? I'll just wake up and not be pregnant anymore?"

Reggie nods.

"I hate this," Lexi says. "Can't you just give me more platelets or something?"

"We may end up doing that before your surgery is planned tomorrow morning," says Reggie, "but from my perspective that's even more reason to not do the epidural. If your platelets are continuing to drop that means you could be increasingly more of a bleeding risk. I'm sorry, but it's my expert opinion that it's just too risky right now."

"What if we waited to see what my platelets do?"

"I'm not an expert in HELLP syndrome," says Reggie. "But I think Dr. Stone would strongly recommend against waiting, both for your health and for the baby's."

"I know," says Lexi. "It's not your fault. It's no one's fault. It just stinks."

The Newborn

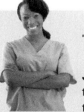

The Nurse's Point of View

Jack: It's the morning of the cesarean section to deliver baby Cowslip, and I'm part of a large team from the NICU assisting with the birth. Preterm babies often need to be resuscitated and require urgent support, which is why so many people are involved. Dr. Stone delivers the baby from the incision in her mother's abdomen and hands her off to me. I put her under a radiant warmer to help maintain her body temperature. Preterm babies have a harder time maintaining their body temperature than do term babies because they have less body fat, thinner skin, and a higher body surface-to-weight ratio and cannot curl up automatically. With really small babies, born under twenty-eight weeks, it's the policy of our institution to wrap the baby in a polyurethane bag to help maintain body temperature (Fig. 10.5). This baby is a little bigger and a little older, so we don't have to do that. I dry her and warm her as well as I can. In addition, all of our delivery rooms and our delivery operating rooms are kept at seventy-nine degree Fahrenheit. There's no need for warm-up jackets here.

I suction out her airways, nose first and then mouth, with a simple bulb syringe. She fusses when she's suctioned, and

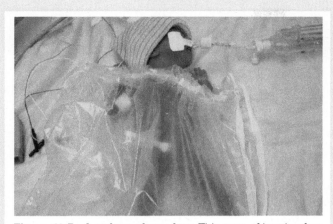

Figure 10.5. A polyurethane bag. This type of bag is often used to maintain the temperature of preterm infants, particularly those weighing less than 1,000 g. (Reprinted with permission from Bowden, V. R., & Greenberg, C. S. [2013]. *Children and their families: The continuum of nursing care* [3rd ed., Fig. 14.7]. Philadelphia, PA: Lippincott Williams & Wilkins.)

this is a good thing. We like fussy neonates. She's on her back with her neck in neutral position, meaning that her chin isn't rolled forward into her chest, which might make it a little harder to breath. Preemies don't need any more challenges with breathing than what they're born with, believe me.

The head of the team determines the Apgar scores at one and five minutes, just like we would for any baby (see Table 1.4). The scores don't tell us what care to provide, just whether things are moving in the right direction. An Apgar score of three or less is closely associated with the worst outcomes, including death and cerebral palsy (Iliodromiti, Mackay, Smith, Pell, & Nelson, 2014). All things considered, she is doing pretty well, with scores of six and seven at one and five minutes, respectively.

I place a pulse oximeter on her right wrist and auscultate her heart. It's fast but not too fast at one hundred fifty beats per minute (bpm). We'll need to keep an eye on that. I hook her up to an electrocardiogram (ECG) so we can have moment-to-moment monitoring. At one minute, her oxygen saturation as measured by pulse oximetry is just below where we want to see it, fifty-eight percent. We want to see it between sixty and sixty-five percent at one minute. She also has chest retractions and nasal flaring, which indicate respiratory distress syndrome, indicating she doesn't have enough surfactant in her lungs. We start with a nasal continuous positive airway pressure, or nCPAP, mask per protocol, with the fraction of inspired oxygen (FiO_2) set to 0.4. If we can keep her at or under 0.4, she won't need intubation or surfactant, which would be great. The less respiratory help we give her now, the less likely she is to develop bronchopulmonary dysplasia, which can have lasting effects. So far she's holding steady with an SpO_2 (blood oxygen saturation) of ninety-one percent with nCPAP. If she stays between ninety and ninety-five percent and her arterial blood gasses stay in the normal range, she shouldn't need anything more than the nCPAP.

We start an IV line in her umbilicus in case we need to rapidly give her medications. She'll also be getting a central venous line in her umbilical cord. The central line will allow us to give her TPN until she can get all of her nutritional needs met orally. We put another line into an umbilical artery (see Fig. 8.8). This will allow us to easily access arterial blood to assess arterial blood gasses.

She's looking stable for the moment. Her SpO_2 is holding steady at ninety-one percent, and the ECG reads a heart rate of one hundred eighteen bpm, which is not bad.

I see babies like this all day, every day, so I'm used to it, but for the parents I know it's scary, seeing their baby hooked to all sorts of tubes and stickers and monitors. I'll be spending a lot of time with this family. On my unit they try to keep us with the same kids and the same families. It's time to introduce myself, and introduce a dad to his little girl.

When I come in for my shift the next day, Baby Girl Cowslip has a name! The new tag on her warmer reads "Kylie" when I come in for my shift the next day. Her mom, Lexi, has been spending a lot of time up here, which we encourage. It's hard on families because we really need to limit visitors in the unit and there are lots of machines and tubes, and often alarms going off. The babies look, and often really are, very small. Each NICU nurse is usually assigned only one infant, but usually that means we have a whole family we're caring for. The saddest cases, which are fortunately pretty rare, are those where there isn't a family, just a really sick kiddo. It's tough whatever the case, though. I read that up to sixteen percent mothers with kids in the NICU meet the criteria for posttraumatic stress disorder (Feeley, Hayton, Golde, & Zelkowitz, 2017).

Kylie's feeding orders are pretty typical for a baby in her situation. Lexi has been expressing colostrum using a pump, and we swab out Kylie's mouth with it three times a day (Box 10.9). The thinking is that colostrum has great immune system benefits that we don't want Kylie to miss out on just because she's not ready to have a full-on feed yet. She's been getting parenteral feeds through a central line right into her bloodstream. We have to be careful to check the line every time we give a feeding because TPN can cause a lot of damage if it **infiltrates** (escapes from the tubing and into surrounding tissues). TPN is a vesicant, which

Box 10.9   Kylie's Feeding Protocol

- Swab the infant's mouth with the mother's colostrum every 3 h to benefit the immune system.
- Initiate parenteral feedings on day 1.
- Initiate oropharyngeal tube feedings on day 1 every 2 h, totaling 20 mL/kg/d, with expressed breast milk to prime the gastrointestinal tract.
- Titrate up enteral feedings by 15 mL/kg/d.
- Titrate down parenteral feedings as enteral feedings increase.
- Add fortifier to maternal milk once enteral feedings reach 80 mL/kg/d to increase caloric density.
- Discontinue parenteral feedings when enteral feedings reach 100 mL/kg/d.
- Target enteric intake of breast milk at 160 mL/kg/d.

Box 10.10 Assessments of the Baby's Feeding Tolerance

- Presence or absence of vomiting
- Presence or absence of abdominal distention, tenderness, and increased or diminished bowel sounds
- Gastric residual fluid (prior to each feeding): should be not greater than 2 mL/kg per feeding and/or less than half of the volume of the previous feeding
- Stool, for volume and the presence of blood

Box 10.11 Clinical Signs and Symptoms of Necrotizing Enterocolitis

Abdominal

- Gastric retention
- Vomiting
- Diarrhea
- Blood in the stool
- Abdominal tenderness
- Abdominal distention
- Bilious drainage
- Hypoactive bowel sounds

Systemic

- Lethargy
- Apnea
- Respiratory failure
- Hypotension (if severe)
- Poor feeding
- Temperature instability
- Reduced heart rate variability

Data from Gephart, S. M., Wetzel, C., & Krisman, B. (2014). Prevention and early recognition of necrotizing enterocolitis, a tale of two tools: eNEC and GutCheckNEC. *Advances in Neonatal Care, 14*(3), 201–210.

means it can cause tissue damage with infiltration. Infiltration of a vesicant like TPN is called extravasation.

She's also started feedings of expressed breast milk from Lexi through an oral tube every two hours. She weighs 1,432 g, or 1.4 kg, so she's getting a total of only twenty-eight grams in twelve divided doses this way. The plan is to titrate that up by fifteen milliliters per kilogram every day. As these oral feedings increase in volume, we'll be able to decrease her TPN feedings. When her total daily intake is up to one hundred milligrams per kilogram a day, we'll discontinue the TPN feedings altogether. Until feeding is established, we're also checking he blood glucose level prior to every feeding.

Before feeding, it's really critical to do some checks (Box 10.10). The first thing we do is to check for gastric residual. We do this by attaching an empty syringe to the feeding tube and pulling back to suction out any stomach contents. We anticipate that the total we withdraw should be less than half of the volume of the previous feed, or about two milliliters per kilogram.

It's also really important to assess the baby's belly before any feed. We're looking for distention and tenderness. We also auscultate bowel sounds to assess for hypo- or hyperactivity. We monitor for vomiting, stool volume, and bloody stool. Unfortunately, bloody stool, a tender distended belly, hypoactive bowel sounds, and a whole slew of other things that may at first seem unrelated (Box 10.11) can all indicate a condition called necrotizing enterocolitis, or NEC. It can be a devastating diagnosis. NEC is bowel ischemia that can lead to death of parts of the bowel. Up to thirty percent of kids diagnosed with NEC don't survive (Gephart, McGrath, Effken, & Halpern, 2012).

Kylie has been here for eleven days now. She's been steadily growing and thriving. I came on about an hour ago, though, and I'm starting to be concerned. Looking back in her chart, I see that her temperature has been a little low. Not very low, but it's unexpected when the room is always the exact same temperature and the baby is under a warmer.

I watch her breathing. I watch baby breathing a lot. The count at this point is automatic, I don't even think about it. Kylie has done well with just the nCPAP and hasn't had to be intubated or given a surfactant. Babies breathe really quickly and at irregular intervals. A rate of as many as sixty bpm is completely normal. They often do something called periodic breathing, which means that they'll cluster their breaths and then stop breathing for maybe ten seconds or so and then start again. Apnea, which

is really common in premature infants, occurs when they stop breathing for a full fifteen to twenty seconds before they start breathing again. It usually lasts for only two or three months. By itself, it's normally insignificant, but accompanied by other signs, it can be a cause for concern. Kylie has an alarm that will sound if she doesn't breathe for fifteen seconds or more. Since I've been here this shift, the alarm has sounded twice. The first time seems to have been a false alarm, and the second time she started breathing again right away when I touched her arm. So, it's pretty normal, but I'm keeping it in mind.

It's when I go to do Kylie's first enteric feeding of my shift that I really start to be concerned. The gastric residual is more than half of what's listed in her chart as her most recent feeding. That's bad. Gastric residual is often an early sign of NEC. Her abdomen, which has always been round, now appears distended. She becomes agitated when I feel it, which makes me think it's tender, as well. All of this is bad news. I auscultate her belly for fifteen seconds in each quadrant. Her bowels are certainly hypoactive, but not completely absent. I ask the charge nurse to get the neonatologist in charge.

Dr. Liz is on tonight, which is always good news. I like her and we work well together. The first thing Liz does is order abdominal radiography, to get a look at the bowel. What we see is bad, but it could be worse. The films show something called pneumatosis intestinalis (Fig. 10.6). It basically looks like bubbles inside the walls of the small intestine. It's diagnostic for NEC, which is bad, but like I said, it could be worse. If there was a lot of free air inside the abdomen, we would be concerned that the bowel had

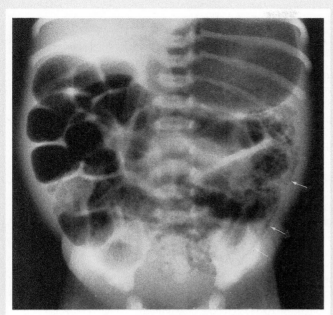

Figure 10.6. Necrotizing enterocolitis in a premature newborn. Pneumatosis intestinalis is shown on the left side (arrows). (Reprinted with permission from Daffner, R. H., & Hartman, M. S. [2013]. *Clinical radiology: The essentials* [4th ed., Fig. 7.27A]. Philadelphia, PA: Lippincott Williams & Wilkins.)

actually ruptured. We'll have to repeat imaging every six to twelve hours or so for at least a few days to track Kylie's condition. Liz requests a panel of tests, including complete blood count (CBC), blood urea nitrogen, creatinine, electrolyte, and pH. She puts in a standing order to repeat all these labs every twelve hours. We'll start checking her glucose level regularly again, as well. We will also culture Kylie's blood, because many babies with NEC are also septic. My charge nurse comes over and I describe the situation to her. She'll call Lexi and Joe and tell them what's going on.

Our first task will be to stabilize Kylie. We'll stop the feeds for the time being, and we'll regularly suction out her gut via her feeding tube to decompress it. She'll have to go back on TPN for a while. We'll continue to monitor her respiratory and cardiac status, and we may have to replace some fluid or even transfuse blood depending on the lab results. Disseminated intravascular coagulation can develop quickly in situations like this. Sometimes I feel like I need extra eyes in my head just to keep track of everything.

We start Kylie on three different antibiotics because it's important they be as broad-spectrum as possible, particularly because there's a chance the infection is in her blood as well. Liz chooses vancomycin, gentamicin, and piperacillin-tazobactam, which is a pretty standard cocktail for us. Depending on the results of the blood culture, we may change that combination. The results of that culture should come back within forty-eight hours. If it's positive, we'll adjust the antibiotics based on the results. If it's negative, Liz will likely discontinue the vancomycin and gentamicin and continue with just the piperacillin-tazobactam for ten to fourteen days total, depending on how things are looking.

Liz requests a surgical consult. Kylie doesn't necessarily need surgery, but if she does need it, she'll need it fast. If her bowel ruptures, surgery would definitely be indicated. Other findings that could indicate surgery include extensive bowel necrosis, overall clinical deterioration, or an abdominal mass. I hope Kylie won't need surgery, because it would mean her situation is really bad and because surgery has its own risks and complications. About half of the patients with NEC in this hospital do end up having surgery, so we'll have to see.

It's nearly two weeks later, and as these things go, Kylie has had a pretty easy course of it. Her platelet levels dropped at the beginning, which can be a sign that things are getting worse, but then they rebounded. Her pH level stayed stable, which is also a relief. Her blood glucose level has remained fairly stable. Those are the three lab values I consider most when assessing the status of the NEC. The presence of thrombocytopenia, hypoglycemia, and metabolic acidosis would indicate that the NEC is getting worse. We've gone from testing every twelve hours to every twenty four, and I think we may be getting toward the end of checking these labs so often.

The regular abdominal radiographs show that the NEC is regressing, so after one more confirmatory radiograph, we'll discontinue the imaging.

Overall, Kylie looks better, as well. One of the best things you can do for babies is give them skin-to-skin contact, especially with the mother. This can be challenging with preterm babies, particularly the sick ones, who may be hooked up to a lot of machines. Every now and then we get one who is so fragile that it's not a good idea, but that's rare. We have the caregiver get into a comfortable position and expose skin and then we put the baby right on top, with a warmed blanket over them both. We've been able to set up Kylie and her parents with skin-to-skin over the last few days, and it's been awesome. I think Joe in particular was nervous about it at first (though Lexi was not much better), but now he wears special button-down shirts when he comes to make it easier. One study reported a thirty-six percent reduction in neonatal mortality, reduced hypothermia and hypoglycemia, and a reduced rate of sepsis as a result of skin-to-skin contact (Boundy et al., 2016).

Another thing working in Kylie's favor right now is that she has no sepsis. So, we've been able to discontinue two of the three antibiotics. It goes a long way toward a more favorable prognosis. Kylie may have more battles ahead, but this one she almost certainly won. She's a fighter.

We'll start the enteric feedings again once Liz gives the go-ahead. We'll start them out slowly, just like we did at the start. Lexi has been pumping and freezing her breast milk, so we have a good supply to work from. Kylie has a few more hurdles to clear. Once she's four weeks old, an ophthalmologist will check her eyes for retinopathy of prematurity, which can cause blindness. In the next few days she'll have an ultrasound of her head to make sure she doesn't have bleeding into her brain, which is known as intraventricular hemorrhage. She'll have a similar exam around the time of her mother's original due date (Box 10.12).

Box 10.12 Common Complications and Their Prevalence in Infants With Very Low Birth Weight

- Respiratory distress (90%): increased work of breathing (tachypnea, retractions, grunting, etc.)
- Retinopathy of prematurity (60%): abnormal growth of blood vessels in the eye that can lead to retinal detachment and blindness
- Hyperbilirubinemia (59%): elevated levels of bilirubin that, when left untreated, can cause irreversible neurologic damage
- Patent ductus arteriosus (46%): a failure of closure of a fetal blood vessel that allows inappropriate shunting of blood from the left side of the heart back to the lungs
- Bronchopulmonary dysplasia (45%): a chronic lung disease caused by mechanical ventilation and long-term oxygen administration
- Early-onset sepsis (2%): a destructive immune response triggered by infection occurring in the first 3 d of life
- Late-onset sepsis (32%): a destructive immune response triggered by infection occurring 4–90 d after birth
- Hypoglycemia (15%): low blood glucose level
- Necrotizing enterocolitis (13%): tissue death of the bowel
- Severe intraventricular hemorrhage (5%–11%) bleeding into the ventricles of the brain.
- Periventricular leukomalacia (4%): necrosis of the white matter of the brain

Data from Altman, M., Vanpée, M., Cnattingius, S., & Norman, M. (2010). Neonatal morbidity in moderately preterm infants. A Swedish national population-based study. *The Journal of Pediatrics, 68*, 226–227; Stoll, B., Hansen, N., Bell, E., Walsh, M., Carlo, W., Shankaran, S., . . . Das, A. (2015). Trends in care practices, morbidity, and mortality of extremely preterm neonates, 1993-2012. *JAMA, 314*(10), 1039–1051.

We'll keep monitoring her as we have been. We'll start slowly feeding her again and slowly reducing her TPN. Once she's able to maintain her body temperature and is exclusively breastfeeding and gaining at least 20 g/kg/d, we can start talking about sending her home. Realistically, for most babies, that means about the time they would have been born anyway. So, we're getting there, slowly but surely. As I say, she's a little fighter.

After Delivery

Lexi's lab results actually got worse for the first 36 hours after birth before starting to improve. At one point, serious consideration was given to a platelet transfusion, but the next check showed that her platelet level had stabilized. Subsequent tests showed that her platelet level was rebounding. Because she had general anesthesia, she also had a course of oxytocin to keep her uterus firm to avoid hemorrhage.

"The cure for HELLP is delivery," says Dr. Stone. "But it's not unusual for lab results to actually worsen in the first forty-eight hours before they begin to improve, as yours are doing now. I expect your platelet count to normalize within a week. You are out of the woods, but anticipate staying in the hospital for the better part of the week for monitoring."

"I'll be closer to the baby that way, as well," says Lexi. She has been spending as much time as she can in the NICU, but has so far refused to hold the baby. Her fear of hurting her combined with an unreasoning and unreasonable sense of guilt inhibits her.

"I understand she's doing well," says Dr. Stone.

Lexi shrugs. "She's tiny and she's weak. I just feel so angry. It doesn't make sense and I don't even know who I'm angry with. Myself maybe. My body. My stupid idea for having another baby."

"Perhaps it's not helpful to hear," says Dr. Stone. "But this was not something that we could have predicted. When we first discussed a possible pregnancy for you a year ago, there was nothing besides your age that would have made you higher risk for this condition. This is a one in a thousand."

"I know, doc. Don't worry. I'm not mad at you. I'm just overwhelmed."

"You should sleep."

"I guess. I should take advantage of having a baby in the NICU, right?" Lexi hears herself. She sounds bitter. "You should go, Dr. Stone. I'm fine."

The next day, Lexi visits the NICU again.

"You can hold her, you know," says a nurse named Jack. He's with Kylie most days. Lexi feels a mix of gratitude to her daughter's caregiver as well as jealousy that someone else can provide the care to her daughter that she cannot.

"I don't know what to do," says Lexi. "I feel like a cow. I feel like the only thing I can meaningfully contribute is milk."

"I know it can feel that way," says Jack, "but I promise she needs you just like any other new baby does. It's important that she feels your touch and hears your voice."

"Everything feels weird and upside down right now," says Lexi. "I never prepared for anything but a healthy baby. And it's almost like being in mourning, you know? And then I feel guilty because she's right here in front of me and here I am being sad that she's not this perfect healthy newborn I was expecting. And that feels like I'm blaming her and I just feel like a jerk."

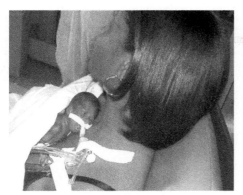

Figure 10.7. Transferring an infant on continuous positive airway pressure therapy to skin-to-skin care with the mother. (Reprinted with permission from Tecklin, J. S. [2014]. *Pediatric physical therapy* [5th ed., Fig. 4.26]. Philadelphia, PA: Lippincott Williams & Wilkins.)

"I've been doing this for a long time," says Jack. "And I can tell you that just about every mother I've ever met in your situation tells me the same thing you're telling me, or something really similar. It's normal to feel sad and angry and guilty. Don't hold that in. It takes a lot of energy to keep those feelings pent up. And you need that energy to help take care of yourself and your little girl."

"And the rest of my family," says Lexi. "I've seen my boys for maybe a half hour in the last three days. They're mostly with my husband and some family members. Add it to the list, I guess."

"Hey, I'm sure they understand, and you'll make it up to them. Don't beat yourself up. Don't add to your list," says Jack. "You know, the other thing about internalizing all that anger is that it has a way of jumping out and hurting people."

"Yeah," says Lexi. "I haven't been kind. My husband feels like I'm pushing him away."

"Talk to him," says Jack. "Is he coming in later?"

"Yes, this evening. My mom is coming over to watch the boys after she gets off work."

"Come up here with him. Show him how you can hold your daughter."

"But I can't," says Lexi. She feels her pulse quicken uncomfortably.

"You can," says Jack. He gestures to a padded chair next to Kylie's isolette, and Lexi sits.

"Because I'm going to help you" (Fig. 10.7).

Think Critically

1. What is the difference between a screening and a diagnostic test?
2. You are caring for a woman who has been diagnosed with HELLP syndrome. You take her BP and note petechiae where the cuff was. What could cause this? What would be your concern? What might you do next?
3. Why was Reggie Hampton unwilling to do an epidural for Lexi? What in particular made him cautious and why?
4. You are caring for an infant with irregular respirations. What signs shousld you look for that would indicate that the baby is exhibiting apnea? If these signs were present, what would you do next?
5. You are caring for an infant born at 29 weeks of gestation. What would make you suspicious that the infant had developed necrotizing enterocolitis?
6. What are some complications that are more common in pregnancies of women who are of advanced maternal age?
7. You are caring for an infant who is 10 weeks premature. Her mother has refused to hold her. How would you discuss skin-to-skin care with her?

References

ACOG. (2016). Practice Bulletin No. 162: Prenatal Diagnostic Testing for Genetic Disorders. *Obstetrics and Gynecology, 127*(5), e108.

Boundy, E. O., Dastjerdi, R., Spiegelman, D., Fawzi, W. W., Missmer, S. A., Lieberman, E., . . . Chan, G. J.. (2016). Kangaroo mother care and neonatal outcomes: A meta-analysis. *Pediatrics, 137*(1), e20152238.

Cooper, L., Morrill, A., Russell, R. B., Gooding, J. S., & Berns, S. (2014). Close to me: Enhancing Kangaroo care practice for NICU staff and parents. *Advances in Neonatal Care, 14*(6), 410–423.

Feeley, N., Hayton, B., Golde, I., & Zelkowitz, P. (2017). A comparative prospective cohort study of women following childbirth: Mothers of low birth-weight infants at risk for elevated PTSD symptoms. *Journal of Psychosomatic Research, 101,* 24–30.

Gephart, S. M., McGrath, J. M., Effken, J. A., & Halpern, M. D. (2012). Necrotizing enterocolitis risk: State of the science. *Advances in Neonatal Care, 12*(2), 77–89.

Guise, J. M., Denman, M. A., Emeis, C., Marshall, N., Walker, M., Fu, R., . . . McDonagh, M. (2010). Vaginal birth after cesarean: New insights on maternal and neonatal outcomes. *Obstetrics and Gynecology, 115*(6), 1267–1278.

Iliodromiti, S., Mackay, D. F., Smith, G. C., Pell, J. P., & Nelson, S. M. (2014). Apgar score and the risk of cause-specific infant mortality: A population-based cohort study. *The Lancet, 384*(9956), 1749–1755.

Mathews, T., MacDorman, M. F., & Thoma, M. E. (2015). Infant mortality statistics from the 2013 period linked birth/infant death data set. *National Vital Statistics Reports, 64*(9), 1–29.

Moon, R. Y. (2016). SIDS and other sleep-related infant deaths: Evidence base for 2016 updated recommendations for a safe infant sleeping environment. *Pediatrics, 138*(5), e20162940.

Roberts, D., Brown, J., Medley, N., & Dalziel, S. (2017). Antenatal corticosteroids for accelerating fetal lung maturation for women at risk of preterm birth. *Cochrane Database of Systematic Reviews,* (3), CD004454.

Stoll, B. J., Hansen, N. I., Bell, E. F., Shankaran, S., Laptook, A. R., Walsh, M. C., . . . Kennedy, K. A. (2010). Neonatal outcomes of extremely preterm infants from the NICHD neonatal research network. *Pediatrics, 126*(3), 443–456.

Wax, J., Minkoff, H., Johnson, A., Coleman, B., Levine, D., Helfgott, A., . . . Benson, C. (2014). Consensus report on the detailed fetal anatomic ultrasound examination indications, components, and qualifications. *Journal of Ultrasound in Medicine, 33*(2), 189–195.

Zeng, X., Xue, Y., Tian, Q., Sun, R., & An, R. (2016). Effects and safety of magnesium sulfate on neuroprotection: A meta-analysis based on PRISMA guidelines. *Medicine, 95*(1), e2451.

Suggested Readings

Busse, M., Stromgren, K., Thorngate, L., & Thomas, K. A. (2013). Parents' responses to stress in the neonatal intensive care unit. *Critical Care Nurse, 33*(4), 52–59.

Cooper, L., Morrill, A., Russell, R. B., Gooding, J. S., & Berns, S. (2014). Close to me: Enhancing Kangaroo care practice for NICU staff and parents. *Advances in Neonatal Care, 14*(6), 410–423.

March of Dimes Foundation. (2017). Your baby's NICU stay. Retrieved from http://www.marchofdimes.org/complications/becoming-a-parent-in-the-nicu.aspx

Preeclampsia Foundation. (2015). HELLP syndrome. Retrieved from http://www.preeclampsia.org/health-information/hellp-syndrome

11

Edie Wilson:
Migraine With Aura, Shoulder Dystocia, and Brachial Plexus Palsy

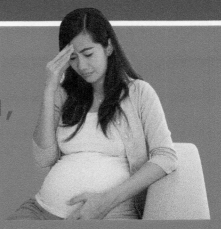

Edie Wilson, age 23

Objectives

1. Describe the features of a migraine headache, common triggers, and birth control considerations.
2. Identify the features of a precipitous birth.
3. Identify the signs of shoulder dystocia and common interventions.
4. List and discuss the risk factors and assessments for brachial plexus palsy.
5. Discuss the signs and symptoms of a hematoma of the perineum and interventions to address it.
6. Explain the importance of screening for depression.
7. Explain the importance of screening for intimate partner violence.

Key Terms

Aura
Brachial plexus
Diaphragm
Erb palsy
Hypoxic
McRoberts maneuver

Migraine headache
Precipitous birth
Prodrome
Shoulder dystocia
Vulvar hematoma

Before Conception

Edie Wilson is a 23-year-old secretary who regularly gets migraine headaches. She and her husband, Frank, live on the fringe of a large city in a 600-square-foot apartment in an older building. Edie commutes by train 45 minutes out of the city. Their neighborhood is more expensive to live in than the area where Edie's job is, but it's where they both grew up—only two blocks apart—and where they eventually want to raise a family, like their parents did. Frank has an associate degree and a job in information technology and works mostly from home, though he travels frequently by train to his company's headquarters in the next state.

Edie's migraine headaches, which she started having when she was 13 years old, tend to occur around the time of her period and

follow a predictable pattern. As the time of her period approaches, she starts to yawn more often and feels more irritable, which are early signs, or prodromes, that a headache is coming (Box 11.1). Then about a day later the headache starts, and with it an aura. The aura starts as a tiny area of bright light near the middle of her field of vision and then over 5 minutes or so progresses to zigzag lights and shapes and bright vision loss that expands to her peripheral vision. The aura always resolves within an hour, beginning with her central vision, but leaves behind the headache. The headache is always on one side and has a pulsing quality. Sometimes she vomits, and always she has photophobia (sensitivity to light) and phonophobia (sensitivity to sound), causing her to seek a dark, quiet room. The headaches last for 4 hours to 4 days and leave her exhausted.

Box 11.1   Sequence of a Migraine Headache

1. Prodrome depression, yawning, irritability, neck stiffness, constipation, euphoria, food cravings starting 24–48 h prior to headache (60% of migraine sufferers)
2. Aura visual, sensory, or language effects typically building for 5 min or longer and lasting for up to an hour prior to or in conjunction with headache (25% of migraine sufferers). May occur before and/or at beginning of headache
3. Headache usually unilateral with a pulsing quality. Can last 4 h to several days. Often involves photophobia and phonophobia and may include nausea and nausea and vomiting
4. Migraine postdrome common post-headache sensation of feeling exhausted or drained. May have recurrent pain at site of headache with sudden movement of head

Adapted from Laurell, K., Artto, V., Bendtsen, L., Hagen, K., Häggström, J., Linde, M., . . . Kallela, M. (2016). Premonitory symptoms in migraine: A cross-sectional study in 2714 persons. *Cephalalgia, 36*(10), 951–959; Headache Classification Committee of the International Headache Society. (2013). The international classification of headache disorders, 3rd edition. *Cephalalgia, 33*(9), 629–808; Charles, A. (2013). The evolution of a migraine attack—A review of recent evidence. *Headache, 53*(2), 413; Giffin, N., Lipton, R., Silberstein, S., Olesen, J., & Goadsby, P. (2016). The migraine postdrome: An electronic diary study. *Neurology, 87*(3), 309.

Box 11.2   Common Migraine Triggers

- Emotional distress
- Hormonal changes
- Eating infrequently
- Weather changes
- Sleep changes
- Trigger odors
- Neck pain
- Lighting
- Alcohol
- Smoke
- Heat
- Trigger foods
- Exercise
- Sex

Adapted from Lisicki, M., Ruiz-Romagnoli, E., Piedrabuena, R., Giobellina, R., Schoenen, J., & Magis, D. (2017). Migraine triggers and habituation of visual evoked potentials. *Cephalalgia*. doi:10.1177/0333102417720217

Frank witnessed one of Edie's migraines on their very first date, when Edie was 17 years old. She was yawning more than usual, though not tired, and feared that she might be getting a headache. She thought about canceling the date but really wanted to go out with him and was worried he'd think she wasn't interested or that he'd find someone else to ask out instead.

They'd planned to go to dinner at the diner down the street and maybe a movie, but before Edie's club sandwich came, the fuzzy ball of light appeared in her field of vision. She tried to will it away and ignore it as it grew. She covered her face with her hands, confusing Frank.

"What's going on?" he said.

"I'm getting a headache, I'm sorry."

"What kind of headache?" asked Frank. "Like a bad date headache or a real headache?"

"I feel sick," said Edie.

Frank left money on the table and explained to the waitress that they had to leave without eating. He guided Edie home and even held her hair as she retched into an alleyway. Despite her best efforts to hold it in, she cried because it hurt and because she was embarrassed. The sunlight and street noise made her headache worse. At home, Frank handed her off to her mother, who understood because she often had migraines as well, and left. Edie hid under her covers in a darkened room for the next 2 days. When she emerged headache-free, still fatigued but

relieved, she had three messages from Frank. In hindsight, the event has become an endearing memory and a joint experience that binds them together. When Frank tells the story, it is a comedy of errors.

As her mother had before her, Edie has learned to live with her migraine headaches. She knows that her main triggers are emotional stress and eating poorly (Box 11.2). She is careful to eat regularly and stay hydrated. She keeps her prescription antimigraine rescue medication with her at all times (The Pharmacy 11.1).

Edie's migraines have even affected her choice of contraceptive. After she and Frank had been together for nearly 6 months, she visited her nurse practitioner, Trish, to get a prescription for birth control.

"I just want the pill," she told Trish, "Or maybe the patch."

"Well, unfortunately the patch is out," said Trish. "There is an increased risk for stroke when we give estrogen to women who have migraines with aura" (Frieden, Jaffe, Cono, Richards, & Iademarco, 2016).

"I thought the pill has the same hormones at the patch does?"

"Most of them do," said Trish. "One kind, though, the progestin-only pill, doesn't have any estrogen. You do have to take it in the same three-hour window every day, however, or it won't be effective. It may also change the timing of your period and cause some spotting."

"I don't think I could keep track of that. I'm not that organized. What else? I don't want a shot and I don't want anything, you know, inserted."

"Well, there are the barrier methods. Besides abstinence, your best protection against sexually transmitted infections is condoms."

"We're both virgins."

"Still," said Trish. "Condoms are safe and effective, and using them gives your partner an active role in preventing pregnancy."

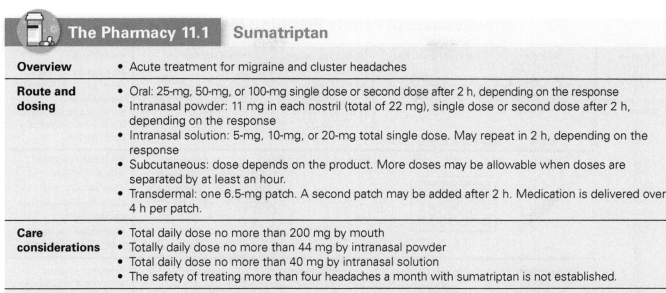

The Pharmacy 11.1 — Sumatriptan

Overview	• Acute treatment for migraine and cluster headaches
Route and dosing	• Oral: 25-mg, 50-mg, or 100-mg single dose or second dose after 2 h, depending on the response • Intranasal powder: 11 mg in each nostril (total of 22 mg), single dose or second dose after 2 h, depending on the response • Intranasal solution: 5-mg, 10-mg, or 20-mg total single dose. May repeat in 2 h, depending on the response • Subcutaneous: dose depends on the product. More doses may be allowable when doses are separated by at least an hour. • Transdermal: one 6.5-mg patch. A second patch may be added after 2 h. Medication is delivered over 4 h per patch.
Care considerations	• Total daily dose no more than 200 mg by mouth • Totally daily dose no more than 44 mg by intranasal powder • Total daily dose no more than 40 mg by intranasal solution • The safety of treating more than four headaches a month with sumatriptan is not established.
Warning signs	• Use is associated with cardiac events, stroke, elevated blood pressure, anaphylaxis, central nerve system depression, vasospasm, rare transient and permanent blindness, and serotonin syndrome

"My mom had a **diaphragm**," said Edie. "She said I should ask you about that."

"Old school!" said Trish. "It used to be that every married woman had a diaphragm in her nightstand. We don't see them much anymore. We have so many more effective, easy-to-use methods."

"But it works, right?"

"Yes, but let's do a comparison," said Trish, sliding a sheet of paper in front of Edie with a chart of different methods of birth control (Fig. 11.1). "If you look at the top of the chart, you can see that long-acting reversible methods such as intrauterine devices and implants are as effectives as sterilization or even more so. Pills are the next tier down. If you look at percentages, the diaphragm is not as reliable a method even as the pill."

"But it's not that much worse," said Edie, looking at the numbers.

"The thing to think about," said Trish, "is how you use each method. The pill can be a good choice if you take it every day. The diaphragm can be a good choice if you remember to use it prior to each time you have intercourse, and to use it correctly."

"Correctly?" asked Edie.

Trish pulled a sample diaphragm out of a box on the table (Fig. 11.2). "To use a diaphragm correctly you put about a teaspoon of spermicide into the cup and then a little more all around the edge of the diaphragm. You then fold it up and insert it into your vagina, angling it toward your backbone so that it completely covers your cervix. It's a good idea to then reach into your vagina and double-check the position. You'll also need to leave it in place for at least six hours after intercourse and insert new spermicide if you have sex multiple times while the diaphragm is in place" (Fig. 11.2).

"So I have to do this every time I want to have sex," said Edie. "Like, put my fingers inside myself? Tell me about the condoms again."

Edie went home with a white paper bag full of condoms in colorful round packets.

Now, 5 years later, Edie and Frank still use condoms as birth control but sometimes use the withdrawal method. They both know it can be a riskier form of birth control.

Pregnancy
First Trimester

When Edie does get pregnant, it's not really unexpected. They didn't plan to get pregnant, but they didn't try that hard to prevent it, either. They talked of wanting to be better established, to own a home, and to see a little of the world before having a baby. But it was just talk. They haven't even started saving money yet.

"I'm happy to be pregnant," Edie says to her mother. "I just thought I'd get to do some other things first, like visit Italy."

"Children are a blessing," says her mother, who is looking forward to her first grandchild.

"I know, mom; it's fine," says Edie. "Forget I said anything."

Edie decides to go to an obstetrics office closer to home rather than work because she expects to give birth at a hospital closer to home, so that it will be a briefer trip from home (assuming that she'll go into labor there) and so that it will be more convenient for friends and family to visit.

"I think my last period was a couple of months ago," Edie tells the receptionist when she calls to make her first appointment. "I put it in my calendar."

The receptionist asks Edie for an exact date of the first day of her last menstrual period, so Edie scrolls through the calendar on her phone, finds it, and tells it to the receptionist. The receptionist gives her an appointment that corresponded with 10 weeks past that day.

Effectiveness of Family Planning Methods

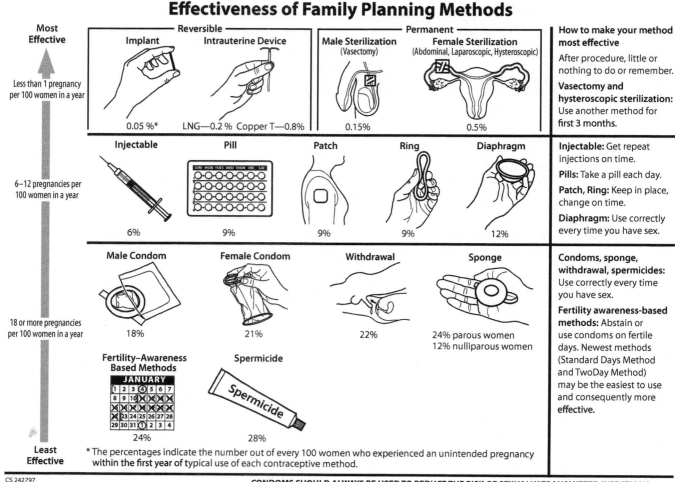

Figure 11.1. **Birth control methods.** (Reprinted from the Centers for Disease Control and Prevention. [2018]. US medical eligibility criteria [US MEC] for contraceptive use, 2016. Effectiveness of contraceptive methods chart. Retrieved from https://www.cdc.gov/reproductivehealth/contraception/mmwr/mec/summary.html)

Edie hangs up the phone. It all seems anticlimactic.

Frankie has begun kissing her belly when she comes home from work. "Kiss the baby," he says each time.

Edie swats him away. "Don't, I'm tired."

"What's wrong?" asks Frankie.

"I remember when it was my face you'd kiss when I got home," says Edie. "I'm not just an incubator."

"Are you feeling nauseous again, baby," Frank asks. He sounds sweetly concerned, which annoys Edie even more.

"Yes, but that doesn't make my feelings less important," says Edie. "It just means I have less patience."

"Do you feel safe at home and safe in your relationship?" asks Meredith, a nurse in Dr. Montgomery's office who is interviewing her during her first visit.

"I don't think anyone has ever asked me that before," says Edie. "I guess so. I'm not worried my husband would hurt me, if that's what you're asking."

"It is," says Meredith with a smile. "We've started asking all patients this question. We want them to know this is a safe space if they need help. All women are vulnerable to domestic violence, but pregnant women are particularly so because they may feel the pregnancy commits them more deeply to their situation."

"Oh," says Edie.

"And how are you feeling?" asks Meredith (see Table 6.1).

"Okay," says Edie. "I'm tired. I feel kind of nauseous, but I don't throw up. I'm congested, but I don't have a cold, I don't think."

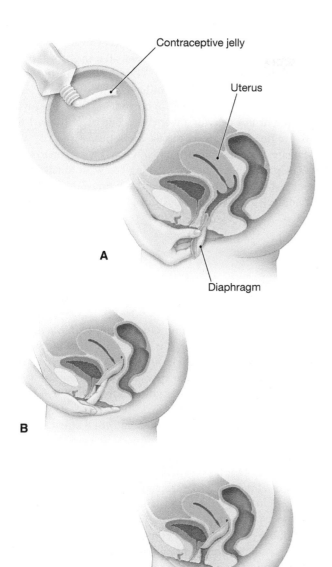

Figure 11.2. Diaphragm. (A) Insertion of the diaphragm. **(B)** Checking to ensure the diaphragm covers the cervix. **(C)** Diaphragm in place. (Reprinted with permission from Beckmann, C. R., Herbert, W., Laube, D., Ling, F., & Smith, R. [2013]. *Obstetrics and gynecology* [7th ed., Fig. 26.6]. Philadelphia, PA: Lippincott Williams & Wilkins.)

"That sounds normal," says Meredith. "I'm going to take your vital signs now and draw some blood for some routine labs. Then Dr. Montgomery will be in" (see Lab Values 1.1).

Dr. Montgomery asks more questions (see Box 1.2), including ones about her family history. "Given that your family came from Italy and Scotland, I recommend we include testing for cystic fibrosis and thalassemia today."

"I haven't heard of anyone in my family having either of those things," says Edie.

"That's good news," says Dr. Montgomery. "And being Italian and Scottish certainly doesn't mean you're a carrier for cystic fibrosis and thalassemia, it just makes it more likely. If you are a carrier,

we will test your husband. If he is positive, we'll recommend an amniocentesis to evaluate the fetus."

"What if we do all that and the results are positive?" asks Edie.

"We have much better treatments for cystic fibrosis now, but the truth is it is still at best a serious chronic condition and often a fatal one. As for the thalassemias, there are different kinds and different degrees of thalassemia, all determined by genetics. Some create little or no problem and others are not compatible with life."

"So we wait and see," says Edie. "So I shouldn't worry?"

"Worry is rarely productive," says Dr. Montgomery. "I don't think this is something you should lose sleep over. Before you leave, we'll also arrange for your first trimester lab work and ultrasound, which will screen for trisomies such as Down syndrome."

"Is that when we find out if we're having a boy or a girl?" asks Edie.

"That will be your second trimester fetal survey ultrasound," says Dr. Montgomery. "We will schedule that for around the eighteen-week mark. We will see each other before that, however" (see Box 2.6).

"What else do I need to think about now?"

"Enjoy this time," says Dr. Montgomery. He hands her a paper with food recommendations (see Table 4.1). "Take care of yourself. Eat well. Exercise moderately. You have big changes coming. Savor the time with your partner, your friends, and your family."

Edie's first trimester prenatal screening and fetal survey ultrasound results are normal (see Box 1.8 and Table 1.1).

Second Trimester

When the fundal height measurements begin with her visit at 22 weeks, they are consistently within the anticipated range, with nothing to suggest that her uterus or the pregnancy is growing too slowly or too rapidly. The fetal heart tones, picked up first at the time of her second prenatal visit after her uterus had risen out of her pelvis, stays consistently between 120 and 150 beats per minute (bpm). Because Edie has a body mass index of 23.2 (see Box 1.4) and has no other indications for early screening for diabetes (see Box 3.4), she is screened for gestational diabetes at 26 weeks with a simple 1-hour oral glucose tolerance test (see Lab Values 3.2). She passes the test with a blood glucose level of 90 mg/dL and so does not need to go on to the 3-hour glucose tolerance test.

Third Trimester

At 36 weeks, Edie undergoes a swab of the vaginal introitus and rectum; the results are negative for group B streptococcus (GBS).

"Are women usually really excited at this point?" Edie asks Margaret, the nurse in Dr. Montgomery's office. She's 38 weeks pregnant, and the fatigue of the first trimester, which had lifted in the second, has returned.

"Sometimes," says Margaret. "But often they're just eager to be done."

"I feel that way," says Edie. "When I was growing up, the idea of being pregnant was exciting. But actually being pregnant is not all that exciting. I don't really like it. And I feel bad that I don't like it."

"Don't feel bad," says Margaret. "It's normal. There's no right way to be pregnant. Some women love it and others don't. And every pregnancy is different, even in the same woman."

"I guess," says Edie.

"You sound sad," says Margaret, and then is quiet for a moment. "Do you feel like you might be depressed?"

Edie looks embarrassed and shakes her head. "No, I'm not depressed. Why would I be? I have a husband who loves me and I'll have a baby soon. I even get six weeks paid maternity leave from my job. Not everyone gets that, you know."

"Oh, I know," says Margaret. "But depression isn't necessarily linked to circumstances, Edie. And depression affects about ten percent of women in pregnancy. It can affect you and your baby and puts you at higher risk for depression after the baby is born" (Vigod, Wilson, & Howard, 2016). "There's no shame in talking about those feelings and asking for help."

Edie shakes her head again. "I'm not judging anyone or saying what's true or not true for anyone else, but it's not how I was raised. I'm fine. I don't want to talk about this."

Margaret hesitates and then nods. "Okay. I want you to know there's help available if that's something you want to talk about. We can just start with a conversation, any time."

"I appreciate that offer," says Edie. "But I'm not that kind of person."

Labor and Delivery

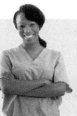

The Nurse's Point of View

Anna: We don't see women with precipitous labor all that often, but it's always exciting when we do. Labor is precipitous when it is three hours or less, from the beginning of regular contractions to birth. That's amazing when you think that for some women the second stage, the pushing stage, alone can take three hours. Women often think that's what they want, a brief labor. I've been doing this long enough, however, to know that the reality can be scary.

Most women ease into labor via the latent phase of the first stage. Contractions come every ten or twenty minutes, last only fifteen to twenty seconds, and are mild (see Table 1.3). They build from there, getting closer together and lasting longer. By the time the active phase of the first stage begins, they come every two to three minutes, last as long as a minute each, and are intense. When the transition phase begins, they come every two minutes or less, last a minute and a half, and are even more intense. Most women take a long time—hours—to build up to that point.

Every woman is different and every labor is different, but in general, women in precipitous labor quickly go from nothing to all-out, from zero to intense contractions every two minutes. They don't have time to get used to being in labor.

One thing I've heard a lot from women in labor over the years is that they're afraid that it will hurt so much that they'll lose control of themselves or the situation or be unable to cope. With a long labor or a labor of standard dilation, they work into it and find ways to get through it. Women with precipitous delivery, however, can *immediately* feel they've lost control of the situation and have no time to let go of the fear or ease into the idea of giving birth. It's just happening.

When Edie comes in, I have the sense of someone who has been preparing for this birth for a while with classes and books and such. We have no records preloaded in the system for her, which makes me think she was supposed to give birth in a different hospital than this one. Maybe she lives elsewhere, I don't know. She's still wearing a suit jacket, so maybe she's come straight from work.

She's doing great breathing but looks scared. Maybe not everyone can recognize that, but I've seen a lot of births, and most women are scared at least some of the time, so I'm familiar with that look. Now, Edie arrived by ambulance and was transferred here from the emergency room, which makes the whole experience even scarier.

This being a small regional hospital with a small birthing center, we don't have a physician or midwife here all the time, though one is always on call. We made the call while Edie was still in the ambulance, and the paramedics called ahead to tell us how close together the contractions were. Seeing her arrive here now, I'm glad a physician is expected to come in right behind her. All the same, I plan to stick to her like glue from now until the physician does come. The emergency medical technician said the contractions are two minutes apart. I ask the charge nurse to grab the emergency birth kit for me just in case (Box 11.3).

"How many weeks are you?" I ask Edie. My colleague Pat has returned with the birthing kit, and I indicate she should stay. If Edie does give birth shortly, there will be two patients, her and the baby, and it would be best for each to have a nurse.

"Thirty-nine, just," says Edie.

Box 11.3   Emergency Birth Kit Essentials

- A sterile drape for under the mother's buttocks
- Two sterile clamps for the umbilical cord (the cord is cut between these clamps)
- Sterile scissors to cut the cord
- A sterile clamp for the cord
- A bulb syringe for mucus clearance from the neonate's nares and mouth
- Blanket to wrap the neonate in
- Sterile gloves

That's good news. It means that though she's laboring fast, she's not premature. "Are there any issues with the pregnancy? Problems with the fetus?"

"No, nothing."

"Is this your first?"

Edie nods and screws her eyes up tight. Another contraction is coming, and I wait for it to pass before asking more questions.

"Do you have any pain under your ribs, or a headache?" I'm asking because I want to know if she might have preeclampsia.

Edie shakes her head again. I start to help her undress, starting with her pants.

"Have your waters broken?" I ask. She shakes her head again. "Are you GBS-positive?" I ask, though if she's laboring as quickly as I think she is, it won't matter. Even if we started antibiotics right now, she would likely give birth before they had time to make any difference. Edie shakes her head.

"Do you have any medication allergies?" I ask. She shakes her head.

"Do you feel like pushing?" I ask. She shakes her head no, which is a relief for as long as that lasts. Like many labor and delivery nurses, I've caught a baby or two in my time, but on the whole I'd rather not. "I'd like to take a look at your perineum," I tell her. "Your vulva, down below."

I really do just want a peak. I won't do a pelvic exam to check for cervical dilation. When I first started working in labor and delivery years ago, checking cervixes was a common practice for labor and delivery nurses. In the past several years, however, fewer and fewer of these sorts of exams are recommended, partly because they're uncomfortable for the patient and partly because the more exams that are done, the higher the risk for infection. At this point I'm not sure the exam would do much more than satisfy my curiosity, anyway. My prime concern is to see whether the top of a fetal head is visible or whether the perineum is bulging (Fig. 11.3), which would mean that birth is imminent. There's not much to see at this point, which buys us a bit of time, though I wouldn't like to guess how much.

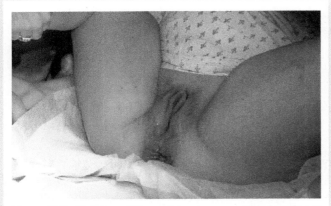

Figure 11.3. Bulging of the perineum, suggesting imminent birth. (Photo by B. Proud.)

I quickly take Edie's temperature and blood pressure (BP). Her temperature is normal, which is reassuring. I'm not really expecting her to have a fever, but it's still reassuring. Her BP is under 140/90, which is also reassuring. She didn't mention a diagnosis of preeclampsia and I already asked about some symptoms, but it can come on at any time—prior, during, or even immediately after a birth. I check the fetal heart rate with a Doppler ultrasound, and the heart rate is one hundred fifty bpm, which is fine, as I expect it to be anywhere from one hundred ten to one hundred sixty bpm. For the time being, unless I get other information, I'll be rechecking the fetal heart rate at least every fifteen minutes, assuming she's pregnant that long.

And then things start to change. "I need to push," she says, and I can see her bunching up to do it.

"I want you to breathe," I tell her. "Little puffy, panting breaths through the contractions, and then you can breathe normally in between."

My goal here with the little puffy breaths is to discourage her from pushing. I'm hoping to give the on-call provider a little more time to get here. The baby is coming out no matter what we do, but the slower it comes, the more likely we are to get a physician in the room and the less likely she is to have substantial tearing. There's a rush of, fortunately, clear fluid. The fetal membranes have ruptured. I listen to the fetal heart tones again, and everything seems fine. The heart rate is still one hundred fifty bpm.

Within just a few minutes, despite our best efforts, I can see her perineum bulge and catch a peek at some baby hair with the next contraction. I remind her about those little puffy breaths again and tell her she's doing just fine, which she is. It's just her body is a little speedy for my liking. I place a hand on top of the baby's head and apply pressure in the downward direction toward Edie's backbone. The baby is most likely face down at the moment, and I want it to stay in the flexed position with its chin (Fig. 11.4; Box 11.4). With my other hand, I support the perineum under the head.

Like many birthing centers, we have a transformer bed that breaks down so that the bottom half can be lowered so that it's easier for the provider to deliver the baby. I lower this bottom half of the bed a few inches but not all the way. No baby dropping on the floor today, thank you very much.

The head comes out with the next contraction. Even with all those little breaths and the downward pressure, I can tell the baby has come down too fast. Edie has a nasty laceration in her perineum (Box 11.5). We can't worry about it now; we'll take care of it later.

The baby's head rotates to the side; this is external rotation, which is just as it should be. I run my fingers along the back of the baby's head and neck to make sure there's not a loop of cord wrapped around it. There's not, but if there were, I would have pulled the loop over the baby's head. Something's not quite right, though. The little chin is stuck just inside, giving the baby a turtle-like appearance. Further pushing doesn't move the baby down more. Pat, bless her, hasn't left Edie's side. She's been coaching and soothing her. I think we're both full of adrenaline, but Pat looks cool, calm, and collected. I hope I

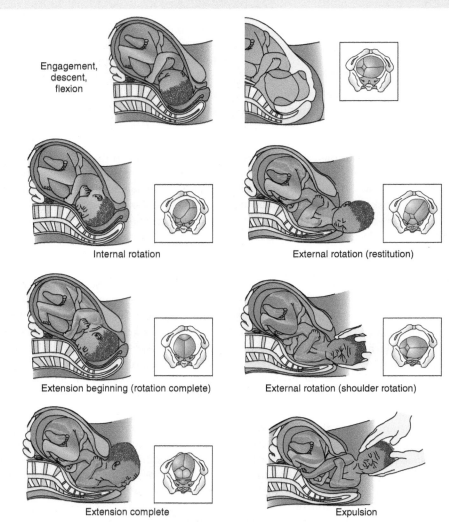

Figure 11.4. The cardinal movements of delivery. (Reprinted with permission from Nettina, S. M. [2014]. *Lippincott manual of nursing practice* [10th ed., Fig. 37. 4]. Philadelphia, PA: Lippincott Williams & Wilkins.)

Box 11.4   Cardinal Movements of Delivery

Movements 1 and 2: Engagement and Descent

The biparietal diameter (the largest measurement of the fetal head from side to side) enters the pelvic inlet, often prior to labor, particularly in nulliparous women; further descent into the pelvis

Movement 3: Flexion

The fetal head moves so that the chin touches the chest.

Movement 4: Internal Rotation

The widest part of the pelvis at the inlet is side to side, but the widest part of the outlet is anterior to posterior. The fetal head rotates to accommodate this difference.

Movement 5: Extension

The fetal chin comes off the chest and the neck arches as the head is born. At this point the pubic symphysis is located behind the fetal neck.

Movement 6: External Rotation (Restitution)

The fetal head, now born, rotates again to move the shoulders into position to fit through the pelvic outlet.

Movement 7: Expulsion

The body of the fetus is born.

Box 11.5 Potential Maternal Complications of Precipitous Labor

- Cervical tearing
- Grades 3 and 4 perineal lacerations
- Postpartum hemorrhage
- Placental retention
- Uterine rupture
- Hematomas of the vagina, perineum, and cervix

Adapted from Sheinera, E., Levyb, A., & Mazor, M. (2004). Precipitate labor: Higher rates of maternal complications. *European Journal of Obstetrics, Gynecology, and Reproductive Biology, 116*(1), 43–47.

Box 11.6 Risk Factors for Shoulder Dystocia

- Approximately 50% occur in the absence of known risk factors
- Infant > 4,000 g (8 lb 8 oz)
- Maternal diabetes
- Operative vaginal delivery (use of forceps or vacuum)
- Shoulder dystocia with previous pregnancy
- Precipitous second stage (pushing stage)
- Prolonged second stage
- Postterm pregnancy (42+ weeks of gestation)
- Male fetus
- Maternal obesity and excess weight gain in pregnancy
- African American
  Note that risk factors are cumulative.

Adapted from Øverland, E., Vatten, L., & Eskild, A. (2014). Pregnancy week at delivery and the risk of shoulder dystocia: A population study of 2,014,956 deliveries. *BJOG: An International Journal of Obstetrics and Gynaecology, 121*(1), 34–41; Kleitman, V., Feldman, R., Walfisch, A., Toledano, R., & Sheiner, E. (2016). Recurrent shoulder dystocia: Is it predictable? *Archives of Gynecology and Obstetrics, 294*(6), 1161; Kim, S. Y., Sharma, A. J., Sappenfield, W., Wilson, H. G., & Salihu, H. M. (2014). Association of maternal body mass index, excessive weight gain, and gestational diabetes mellitus with large-for-gestational-age births. *Obstetrics and Gynecology, 123*(4), 737–744; Laughon, S., Berghella, V., Reddy, U., Sundaram, R., Lu, Z., & Hoffman, M. (2014). Neonatal and maternal outcomes with prolonged second stage of labor. *Obstetrics and Gynecology, 124*(1), 57–67; Dall'Asta, A., Ghi, T., Pedrazzi, G., & Frusca, T. (2016). Does vacuum delivery carry a higher risk of shoulder dystocia? Review and meta-analysis of the literature. *European Journal of Obstetrics and Gynecology and Reproductive Biology, 204*, 62–68.

look half as reassuring. I look up to her as calmly as I can and say, "shoulder dystocia. Mark the clock. And hit the red button."

There is some good news. We've been doing some continuing education team walk-through simulations of scenarios just like this, situations in which the baby's shoulder gets stuck after the head is born. Now, when we've walked through this before, I've not had the role of the provider, but I'm familiar with the job description and I'm well aware of the stakes. In a normal birth it usually takes no more than about sixty seconds between the time the head is born and when the rest of the body slithers out. In situations like this one, though—shoulder dystocia—we're watching the clock. If a baby is stuck like this for more than five minutes, it is at increased risk of becoming hypoxic. So I told Pat to mark the clock because we have to be very clear on how much time we have. I told her to hit the button because we're going to need reinforcements.

So, Pat hits the emergency button and immediately starts to pull Edie's legs back as far as they will go while telling her to tuck her chin into a rolled position. She tells her she's doing great and she's in good hands.

"Don't push," I tell Edie. I'm hoping that this change in position with her legs back, called the McRoberts maneuver (Fig. 11.5; Table 11.1), will change the orientation of the pelvis in such a way that it will just slip easily over that anterior shoulder (that's the one on top).

I hear Cheryl's shoes in the hall before she opens the door. Cheryl's the charge nurse. "Shoulder dystocia," I tell her without looking up more than a second. "Time mark, Pat?"

"Fifteen seconds," says Pat.

"Fifteen seconds, McRoberts only," I tell her. I want to let her know how much time has passed and what we've done so far. Cheryl leaves the room to line up our resources. She'll be calling to make sure a surgeon, preferably an obstetrician, is available. She'll line up anesthesia, and she'll get a pediatrician down here. There is always an operating room prepped, but it will be Cheryl's job to double-check it.

"Suprapubic pressure between contractions," I tell Pat (Fig. 11.6). What I'm asking her to do is push down on Edie's lower abdomen just above the pubic symphysis while also pushing slightly laterally, in the direction the baby is facing. This will hopefully adduct the shoulder enough that the dimensions of the stuck parts will change to let the baby pass. It doesn't

work, though, and I'm wondering whether the baby just came down too fast to go through all the cardinal movements.

"Time?" I ask Pat. I'm worried now because I've done all that I know to do. I've certainly done McRoberts maneuver and suprapubic pressure before. I've seen other maneuvers used, but I've never had to do them myself.

"Minute thirty," says Pat.

The obstetrician, Maisie Reynolds, chooses that exact moment to come through the door. I've never been so glad to see anyone in my life. She's wearing pajama pants with suns and rainbows on them. I get up right away and let her have my stool.

"Minute thirty," I tell her. "McRoberts and suprapubic pressure."

"Nothing?" asks Maisie. I shake my head. Maisie takes a deep breath. "I'm going to deliver the posterior arm. What's her name?" she asks me as an aside. I tell her.

"Edie, I'm going to deliver your baby's arm. You're going to feel a lot of pressure," says Maisie.

No kidding. There's no time for anesthesia, and the anesthesiologist isn't here yet, anyway. At the head of the bed, Pat inserts two fingers into Edie's hand and tells her to squeeze as hard as she wants to. In come the pediatrician and the

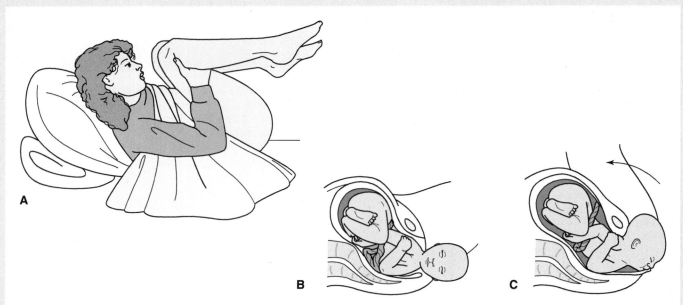

Figure 11.5. McRoberts maneuver. (A) Maternal position. **(B)** Normal position of the symphysis pubis and the sacrum. **(C)** The symphysis pubis rotates and the sacrum flattens. (Modified with permission from Kennedy, B. B., & Baird, S. M. [2017]. *Intrapartum management modules* [5th ed., Fig. 16. 5]. Philadelphia, PA: Lippincott Williams & Wilkins.)

Table 11.1   Maneuvers for Resolving Shoulder Dystocia

Maneuver	Description
General Maneuvers	
McRoberts maneuver	Hyperflexion of the hip to bring the knees back toward the laboring woman. Causes rotation of the pubic symphysis so that it may move over the anterior shoulder, releasing it. The woman should not push. Often used in conjunction with suprapubic pressure
Suprapubic pressure	Downward pressure just above the pubic bone. Pressure should be exerted at a slight angle toward the face of the fetus to attempt to rotate the anterior shoulder. Attempts should be made between contractions.
Rubin's maneuver	Fingers or hand are inserted into the vagina behind the fetal posterior shoulder. Pressure is put on the posterior shoulder to move it into a more oblique position. Pressure may alternately be placed on the anterior shoulder. The woman may push with this maneuver, and suprapubic pressure may be used simultaneously.
Delivery of posterior arm	Most infants are born with their anterior shoulder preceding their posterior shoulder. With this maneuver, a hand is reached into the posterior vagina, and an attempt is made to sweep the fetal arm across the chest and out of the vagina.
Gaskin maneuver	The woman is moved onto hands and knees.
Wood screw maneuver	Fingers or hand are inserted into the posterior vagina, and an attempt is made to rotate the fetus until the posterior shoulder becomes anterior while the fetus descends in a "screw-like" manner.
Fracture of the clavicle	May reduce the shoulder diameter. Usually done by moving the anterior clavicle forward
Rescue Maneuvers	
Zavanelli maneuver	Pushing back of the fetal head into the uterus and subsequent cesarean section
Abdominal rescue	An incision is made into the uterus, and the fetus is manually rotated into an oblique position for vaginal delivery.
Symphysiotomy	Incision made through the cartilage of the symphysis to allow separation of the pubic bones and passage of the fetus. Rarely used in high-resource settings where cesarean delivery is possible.

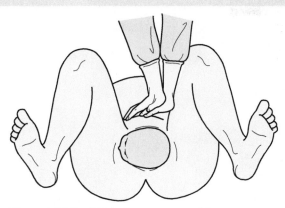

Figure 11.6. Applying suprapubic pressure.
(Modified with permission from Kennedy, B. B., & Baird, S. M. [2017]. *Intrapartum management modules* [5th ed., Fig. 16. 6]. Philadelphia, PA: Lippincott Williams & Wilkins.)

anesthesiologist. I see Maisie and the anesthesiologist lock eyes, and then Maisie shakes her head slightly and gets to work.

Maisie takes a deep breath and puts her entire hand into the posterior part of Edie's vagina. I watch as she sweeps her hand forward around to the baby's front like she's cleaning the inside of a cylinder with a damp cloth. She brings her hand out, firmly holding the baby's posterior arm. Out comes the arm and the posterior shoulder and then the rest of the baby. The baby makes an annoyed bubbly noise as Maisie deposits her onto Edie's belly, where she begins to cry in earnest.

Her mother is crying, too. In truth, she was screaming with the delivery of the posterior arm. She's whimpering now, and I can't imagine how she's feeling. I'm glad she has Pat with her. A **precipitous birth** can be traumatizing and so can a shoulder dystocia, not to mention the physical trauma of what looks to me like a grade four laceration (see Fig. 7.2). Maisie has a lot of work to do. At least Edie can be numbed up for the suturing.

The Newborn

Edie watches as a nurse vigorously rubs the baby off and quickly covers her with a warm blanket. The baby is crying, but the pediatrician suctions her nostrils anyway, which makes her sneeze. The baby's left arm is limp and hangs by her side rather than being flexed like her other arm and her legs. Edie might not have even noticed if the pediatrician hadn't asked the nurse to make note of this in the chart for later follow-up.

One of the physicians—she hears a nurse call her Maisie—puts clamps on the umbilical cord and asks Edie if she wants to cut it. Edie shakes her head, and the physician goes ahead and cuts between the clamps. She then applies a clamp to the end still attached to the baby about a ½ in from the baby's abdomen (Fig. 11.7).

"This clamp will be taken off in about twenty-four hours," Maisie tells Edie.

Edie just nods. She's watching the activity in the room through half-closed lids. She strokes the baby's cheek, and the baby turns toward her hand. Edie feels her uterus contract again and rise in her abdomen. She feels another rush of fluid between her legs.

"Am I bleeding a lot?" she asks, and even to herself she sounds detached from the situation. When she looks down, she sees that Maisie's forehead is furrowed.

"Your placenta detached," says Maisie. "That's the blood you felt that comes as that happens. The placenta is coming out now."

As she says it, the placenta slithers out and Maisie deposits it into a stainless steel vessel. A nurse takes it and inspects it; Edie doesn't catch her name.

"Edie, in her eagerness to be born, your daughter did some tearing of your vulva and vagina," says Maisie. "Don't worry, we can certainly repair, it but it's going to take a bit of time and some stitches."

About an hour later, Frank arrives, apologizing profusely. It wasn't his fault he missed the birth and Edie knows it, but she still feels sad about it, and Frank won't stop apologizing.

Later that day a new pediatrician arrives and introduces himself as Dr. Kellstrom.

After examining your daughter, we think "Your baby has sustained an injury to the **brachial plexus**, which is a fairly common complication with a delivery such as yours," Dr. Kellstrom says.

"The brachial what?" asks Frank.

"The brachial plexus. It's a network of nerves that occurs in the lateral aspects of the neck."

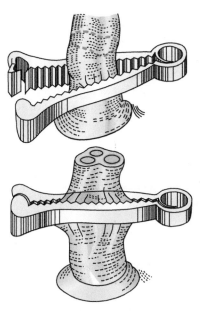

Figure 11.7. Cutting the umbilical cord. (Top) A plastic Hollister clamp is in position and open; the area to be cut is indicated by a dashed line. **(Bottom)** The clamp is closed, the cord has been cut, and three vessels are visible in the cord. (Reprinted with permission from LifeART image © 2018 Lippincott Williams & Wilkins. All rights reserved.)

Box 11.7 Complications of Shoulder Dystocia

Neonate Complications

- Occur in about 5% of cases of shoulder dystocia
- Temporary brachial plexus palsy
- Fracture of the clavicle
- Fracture of the humerus
- Permanent brachial plexus palsy
- Hypoxic brain injury
- Neonatal demise

Maternal Complications

- Postpartum hemorrhage
- Third- and fourth-degree lacerations

Adapted from Gachon, B., Desseauve, D., Fritel, X., & Pierre, F. (2016). Is fetal manipulation during shoulder dystocia management associated with severe maternal and neonatal morbidities? *Archives of Gynecology and Obstetrics, 294*(3), 505; Gauthaman, N., Walters, S., Tribe, I., Goldsmith, L., & Doumouchtsis, S. (2016). Shoulder dystocia and associated manoeuvres as risk factors for perineal trauma. *International Urogynecology Journal, 27*(4), 571.

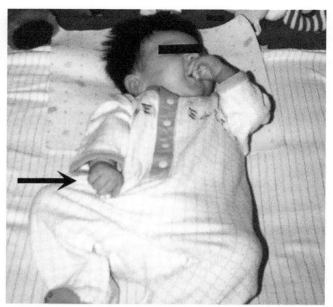

Figure 11.8. **Waiter's tip posture in Erb palsy, a brachial plexus injury of vertebrae C5 to C6.** (Reprinted with permission from Weinstein, S. L., & Flynn, J. M. [2014]. *Lovell and Winter's pediatric orthopaedics* [7th ed., Fig. 4. 23]. Philadelphia, PA: Lippincott Williams & Wilkins.)

"Lateral?" says Edie. "You mean off to the side?"

"Yes," says Dr. Kellstrom. "Bilaterally. Each side, though in most cases, including this one, only one side is injured. The type of injury in this case, a classic one, can cause a sort of paralysis called **Erb palsy**."

"Wait," says Frank. "Are you saying our baby is paralyzed? Can we fix this? Could you have broken that a little more gently?"

"I'm sorry," says Dr. Kellstrom. "I should explain that this is most often fully or partly reversible" (The American College of Obstetricians and Gynecologists, 2014). "You should know, however, that it can be permanent. I'm afraid only time will tell."

"Is this because of something that happened during the birth?" asks Edie (Box 11.7). "Is this because the doctor came so late?"

"It is true that these injuries are more common in cases of shoulder dystocia, though we see them with other births, as well," says Dr. Kellstrom. "It may be a product of the dystocia itself or of something else entirely" (American College of Obstetricians and Gynecologists' Task Force on Neonatal Brachial Plexus Palsy, 2014).

"So, I guess I don't completely understand what's going on," says Frank. "What exactly is Erb palsy?"

"It's an injury of the brachial plexus between C5 and C6 of the spine," says Dr. Kellstrom. "You'll notice your daughter keeps most of her limbs flexed, as is common to newborns. The left arm, however, remains straight and slightly adducted, meaning the shoulder is curving in slightly toward the front of the body" (Fig. 11.8).

"There's no possibility this is just how she's comfortable?" asks Edie. "Like, this is how she was positioned inside and it's how she likes it?"

Dr. Kellstrom shakes his head. "Babies have a variety of reflexes. Some of them persist into adulthood and others gradually fade as they develop. One, the Moro reflex (Fig. 11.9), is a startle reflex they exhibit when they have the sensation that they're falling. They're not actually falling when we test this reflex, of course, we just simulate the sensation. When they sense they are falling, they reach out their arms and then draw them back to their chest. In your daughter's case, however, she does this only with her right arm. Her left arm remains immobile."

"But this is temporary," says Frank. "This isn't a forever thing?"

"Most of the time, yes, it resolves spontaneously," says Dr. Kellstrom. "I advise that she start physical therapy in about a week, and after that it's just a matter of time. I would like to refer her to a pediatric neurologist for further assessment, but I believe she has an excellent chance of a full recovery" (Lagerkvist, Johansson, Johansson, Bager, & Uvebrant, 2010).

After Delivery

Edie feels confused. She's relieved the birth is over, traumatized by its speed, and mildly traumatized by its finale.

"It's not what I planned," she says to Frank.

"I'm sorry I wasn't here," he says. "You know I wouldn't have missed being here for you."

"I know," says Edie. "I'm not mad. And I'm really grateful that I'm going to be okay and it's over. I'm worried about her arm, but not super worried. I feel, I don't know, let down or something."

"Like, anticlimactic?"

"No. More like a little disappointed. I'm still a little freaked out. I know everything is fine now, but everything was so close to not being fine, and I was terrified there for about ten minutes."

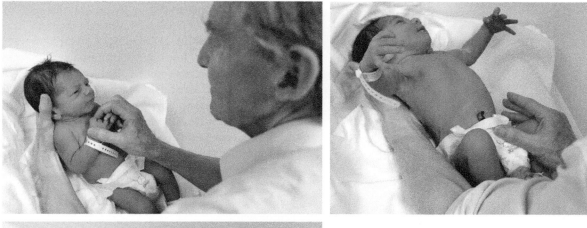

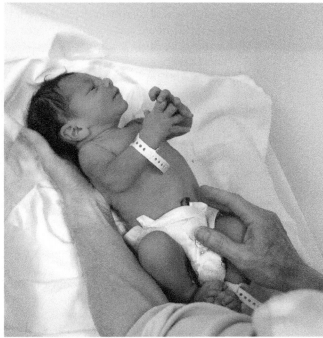

Figure 11.9. The Moro reflex. (A) In preparation for the Moro reflex, the head is supported and the hands are in the midline. **(B)** When support is removed and the head is allowed to fall backward, the arms abduct and extend. **(C)** After abduction, the arms then flex and adduct and the hands return to the midline. (Reprinted with permission from MacDonald, M. G., & Seshia, M. M. K. [2016]. *Avery's neonatology* [7th ed., Fig. 46.6A–C]. Philadelphia, PA: Lippincott Williams & Wilkins.)

Frank tries to lie down next to her on the barest sliver of the side of the bed. Edie winces as she shifts to make room. "Do you hurt?" he asks. "Should I get someone?"

"I don't know," says Edie, wincing. "I think maybe that anesthesia is wearing off down there. It's getting really uncomfortable."

"Do you want another ice pack?" Frank asks.

"No. I don't think so," says Edie. "Maybe I just need another ibuprofen. I just feel extremely sore and swollen."

"You did push a little lemonhead out your downstairs," says Frank.

"I pushed a watermelon out through my birth canal," says Edie, correcting him. She shifts uncomfortably again. "Yeah. Maybe I'll just push my call button."

A nurse they'd met at the beginning of the shift named Marnie answers the call.

"She's really uncomfortable," says Frank. "We were wondering if she could get some more ibuprofen or something?"

"I'll look in the chart and see what's scheduled, but why don't you tell me a little more about what's going on first," says Marnie.

"I don't know," says Edie. "It hurts down there. I tore up pretty good during the delivery, but it didn't hurt like this before. I thought maybe the numbing med they used when they were sewing me up has worn off."

"Maybe," says Marnie, "but I would have expected you to have felt the effects of that before. You delivered about six hours ago, right?"

Edie looks at Frank and then the clock. "I think so?"

"Yeah. Let me take a look at your perineum. You haven't been checked for a little while anyway. I can take a look at your bleeding while I'm at it."

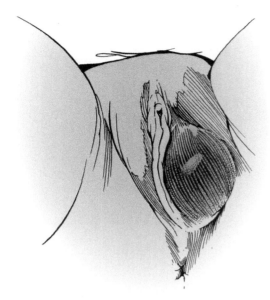

Figure 11.10. Hematoma of the vulva. (Modified with permission from Benrubi, G. I. [2010]. *Handbook of obstetric and gynecologic emergencies* [4th ed., Fig. 27.5]. Philadelphia, PA: Lippincott Williams & Wilkins.)

Edie adjusts herself slowly so she's positioned on her back. She feels uncomfortable in just about every way she can think of as she slides the net panties down her knees.

"Huh," says Marnie. She applies a small amount of pressure to Edie's perineum with a gloved finger and Edie sucks in her breath.

"That's really tender," she says.

"It looks tender," says Marnie. "Who is your provider?"

"You mean my OB? It's no one here. I was supposed to give birth in a different hospital, but there was no time. The baby came too fast. I called my OB afterward, but she said she doesn't have privileges to see patients in this hospital."

"That's too bad. Well, I'm going to contact the physician on call to come check you out. It looks like you have a collection of blood in your perineum that is stretching the skin and pulling on that laceration" (Fig. 11.10). "I want to take another set of vital signs before I do that and get an ice pack on that area" (Analyze the Evidence 11.1). "Do you feel different than you have been? Lethargic or light-headed? Anything like that?"

"No," says Edie. "Just really uncomfortable."

"When's the last time you emptied your bladder?"

"I don't know," says Edie. "Maybe an hour ago? Why?"

"Well, two reasons," says Marnie. "The first is that this kind of swelling can make it harder for you to pee, and the second is that if you're not peeing I'd be worried that you're bleeding quite a lot more than we're aware of. When you lose a lot of blood, you don't make much urine."

"I don't know," says Edie. "It wasn't hurting when I peed before. You think I could still be bleeding? Could this keep getting worse?"

"Well, that's why we need to get you checked out. If this just keeps on doing what it's doing and doesn't get bigger, you may get away with some ice and pain meds."

"Or else?" asks Frank.

"Let's not start looking for that trouble just yet."

Marnie leaves, only to return a few minutes later with the equipment for an intravenous (IV) procedure and oxycodone (The Pharmacy 11.2). She hands the oxycodone to Edie along with a cup of ice water from her bedside table (Box 11.8).

"This is for the pain," says Marnie. "It will take the edge off. The physician on call today is Dr. Brown, and he wants you to have this before he does an exam."

"Why, is it going to hurt more?" asks Edie.

"It might," says Marnie. "He also put through an order for an IV. We're just running normal saline for the time being, but if things change and we think you're bleeding more, we may have to start blood products as well."

"Seriously?" asks Edie. "After all this already, I might need a blood transfusion for a sore vagina?"

"I know it sounds strange, but sometimes when we see bleeding like this there can be bleeding into other places, like the abdomen. When that happens you can lose a lot of blood and we wouldn't even know about it until your vital signs were off or you felt weird or light-headed."

"I can't believe this," says Frank.

Analyze the Evidence 11.1   Do Cold Packs Help Postpartum Perineal Pain?

Yes	No
Study: The efficacy of cold-gel packing for relieving episiotomy pain—A quasirandomized control trial (Lu, Y. Y., Su, M. L., Gau, M. L., Lin, K. C., & Au, H. K. (2015). The efficacy of cold-gel packing for relieving episiotomy pain—a quasi-randomised control trial. *Contemporary Nurse, 50*(1), 26–35).	Study: Cryotherapy for the control of perineal pain following vaginal delivery: A randomized clinical trial (Neto, A. H. F., Amorim, M. M. R., Katz, L., Morais, I., Lemos, A., & Leal, N. V. (2015). Cryotherapy for the control of perineal pain following vaginal delivery: A randomized clinical trial. *Obstetrics and Gynecology, 125*, 64S–65S).
A study evaluating patient reports of pain relief. The study group used an ice pack and oral analgesics, whereas the control group used only oral analgesics. The study group reported better pain control, less intrusion of pain on daily activities, and better satisfaction with pain control.	A study evaluating the application of ice versus that of cold water found no difference in pain relief, edema, or the use of analgesia.

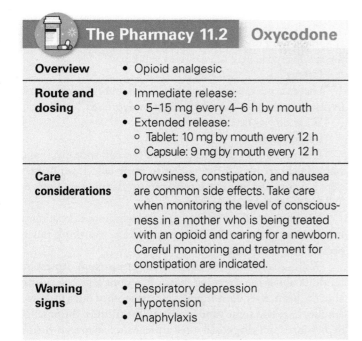

The Pharmacy 11.2 Oxycodone

Overview	• Opioid analgesic
Route and dosing	• Immediate release: ○ 5–15 mg every 4–6 h by mouth • Extended release: ○ Tablet: 10 mg by mouth every 12 h ○ Capsule: 9 mg by mouth every 12 h
Care considerations	• Drowsiness, constipation, and nausea are common side effects. Take care when monitoring the level of consciousness in a mother who is being treated with an opioid and caring for a newborn. Careful monitoring and treatment for constipation are indicated.
Warning signs	• Respiratory depression • Hypotension • Anaphylaxis

"I need to take some blood from you, as well," says Marnie. "For the time being, there's an order to get your blood every four hours to check for evidence of unusual bleeding."

Edie blows her cheeks out. "Sure. Great. Why not?"

Dr. Brown arrives soon afterward to perform an exam. "I'm sorry," he tells Edie. "This is no way to meet. I need to do a complete pelvic and abdominal exam to make sure this bleeding we can see is the only bleeding there is. And call me Mark."

"Mark. Okay. Marnie already told us there might be other bleeding. What happens if there is? Do you pop it?"

"I haven't heard it described like that. If we think you're still bleeding, especially into the abdomen, surgery is a distinct possibility. If we think this is stable, we'll likely monitor you for a while with blood work and vital signs and treat you with ice and pain medication."

Box 11.8 Initial Assessment and Orders for Marnie for Vulvar Hematoma

• Perform hourly vital signs to assess for hemodynamic stability.
• Establish a large-bore needle intravenous line with normal saline.
• Draw blood for complete blood count, fibrinogen level, prothrombin time, and partial thromboplastin time laboratory tests initially, to determine baseline, and then every 6 h.
• Hold 4 U of packed red blood cells, type and cross.
• Perform a complete examination of the abdomen, vulva, vagina, and perineum.
• Place a Foley catheter with initial examination.

"It's so much pressure," says Edie. "It feels like if you drained it, it would feel better, like a pimple, but about a zillion times worse."

"Well, let's see where we are," says Mark. "Generally speaking, any time we can avoid surgery we do. There's always risk for complications with surgery, including infection. I am ordering an anesthesia consult, however, just in case."

Mark does the exam and it is painful but tolerable. The abdominal exam doesn't feel much worse than the fundal checks she's been getting regularly, and the vaginal exam is mostly painful because it puts more pressure on the vulva.

"Edie, I want to insert a catheter into your bladder," says Mark (Step-by-Step Skills 11.1).

"Why?" asks Edie. "I peed just fine an hour ago."

"Well, my concern is that if this does get any larger it's going to make it hard to urinate and it will be that much harder to place a catheter. I also want to be able to more directly measure

Step-By-Step Skills 11.1

Instructions for Bladder Catheterization of a Female

1. Collect equipment, often a complete kit.
2. Wash your hands.
3. Prepare the kit and a sterile field.
4. Apply sterile gloves.
5. Verify that the catheter balloon is working.
6. Coat the insertion end of the catheter with sterile lubricant.
7. Using your nondominant hand, separate the labia and visualize the vaginal introitus and the urethra.
8. Using your dominant hand, clean the mucosa, one swipe per swab. Swab from the introitus outward, and from anterior to posterior.
9. Pick up the catheter with your dominant hand.
10. Locate the urinary meatus by observing how the cleaning fluid pools. It will be found just anterior to the vaginal introitus.
11. Gently insert the catheter. In females, the urethra is approximately 4 cm (1.5 in). Insert for about 2 in past where you begin to see urine inside the catheter, a total of 3–5 in.
12. Attach the provided syringe of sterile water or sterile saline to the balloon port and depress the syringe, inflating the balloon. For most catheters this will require 10 mL of liquid.
13. Apply gentle traction to the catheter until you feel that the balloon is snug against the bladder neck.
14. Attach the collection bag to the urine drainage port.
15. Place the drainage bag below the level of the bladder.
16. Secure the catheter to the thigh with straps, avoiding applying traction to the tubing.
17. Dispose of waste.
18. Remove the sterile gloves.
19. Wash your hands.
20. Document the procedure.

your urine output. Typically when someone is losing blood, urine production drops off. We could measure that by having you urinate into a hat in the toilet, but considering the risk that this swelling may constrict your urethra, I think this is the better choice."

"You know," says Edie. "This stinks."

"I know," says Mark. "I'm hoping this is going to be short term and that with a little ice and time the swelling will start to dissipate and that edema and blood will start to reabsorb and you can put this behind you. I'd like to do a series of ultrasounds of the area, however, to make sure this isn't growing."

"Ultrasound? Like when you were looking at the baby?"

"This will be of your vulva, of the labia where you have the collection of blood. Ultrasound does a good job of differentiating between the density of different tissues, so we will be able to see where the blood stops and where tissue starts. If we measure that several times over a period of time, we'll get a sense of whether it's growing, shrinking, or staying the same size."

"But you think it's going to go away all by itself, without surgery?" asks Frank.

"I do. I believe it's limited to the vulva. If it were extended into the vagina or another area within the pelvis, I'd be more concerned. We'll still keep an eye on her, however."

"I was hoping to go home soon," says Edie.

"We can revisit your discharge plan in a few days," says Mark. "But for now we need to keep a close eye on you."

Soon after Dr. Brown leaves, Marnie visits to check on her. "How are you?" she asks. Frank has gone to the cafeteria, and the baby is sleeping swaddled in Edie's arm, her limp arm curled up against her chest like the other one.

"This isn't what I planned, none of it," says Edie. She's been crying.

"That must be hard," says Marnie. She takes a seat in the soft chair next to the bed.

"I mean, forget even the things that have gone wrong. You know, giving birth at light speed and ripping and the baby getting stuck and her arm and this stupid blood thing. I couldn't even make it to the right hospital. It's not like I'm a big planner, but nothing went right."

"It sounds frightening," says Marnie.

"It all just feels so out of control, from the first contraction through to now. I've always been scared at the thought of my body doing things I had no control over."

"And now you feel like you were right?"

"I was so right. What if I hadn't even been able to make it here on time? She was stuck. We could have died."

"But you didn't. You knew things were going fast and you made it here on time to somewhere that you could be helped. You did great."

"Do you think she's going to be okay?" asks Edie, gesturing to her sleeping baby.

"Well, most babies recover from a brachial plexus injury with no lasting effects. But even if she doesn't, you and Frank are strong and she's strong. You will adapt if you need to."

"I wish I didn't have this blood thing down there."

"Does it still hurt?"

"The ice is helping, and the pain medication. I just want to be at home. I want my bed. I want my mom in the kitchen cooking for me. Everyone here is great, but, you know."

"I know."

"I haven't even talked to Frank about this, but I think the nurse in my doctor's office thought I might be depressed."

"What do you think?"

"I don't know."

"Do you want to talk about it? You can talk with me, if you want. Or I can ask a social worker to come talk. I can make a note in your chart and make sure your regular physician gets it. Tell me what makes sense for you."

"I don't know. There's a lot going on right now. I don't know if I want to deal with it," Edie pauses. "Do you think this is postpartum depression?"

"Well, usually when we think about postpartum depression we think about the screening that's often done a month or two after the birth, after the hormones have smoothed out a little and families have had some time to adjust. The truth is, the onset of depression that's diagnosed after a pregnancy may start before the baby is born and even before the pregnancy. Most of the time if the depression truly does start postpartum it starts in the first month after the birth, but it can start anytime in the first year. Ultimately it matters less what kind of depression it is. The important thing is that you get the help you need."

"I want to make a good start," says Edie. "I want this to be a good time for me and for everyone. I don't want to be sad, to be the one bringing everyone down. What would people think? What would Frank think?"

"Well," asks Marnie, "tell me what you're worried about people thinking."

"That I'm unhappy about how everything turned out," says Edie. "That maybe I don't love my baby. Maybe I don't love Frank or I wish . . . I don't know. Just something bad."

"Is that how you feel?" asks Marnie.

"No!" says Edie. "Well, not exactly. I don't know. I'm just overwhelmed by everything. I'm just sad. I feel kind of beaten down but like I don't even know why, like I shouldn't."

Marnie is silent for a minute. "I know when life is overwhelming like it is right now it can be easy to not take care of yourself and to beat yourself up. Promise me you won't let that happen."

"I won't," says Edie. "I'll be fine."

"Edie, do you ever have thoughts about wanting to hurt yourself?" asks Marnie.

"No!" says Edie. She starts to cry. "I wouldn't do that. I don't want to do that. I just want to feel better."

"Of course," says Marnie. "I had to ask. Edie, will you let me call a friend of mine to talk to you? She's a social worker here. I think she can help come up with a plan. You're going to be here for at least a few more days. She can come right to your room. You can work on feeling better mentally and physically all at the same time."

Edie thinks about it. "I don't want Frank to know. Not yet anyway."

"Tell me about that," says Marnie.

"I don't know if he'd approve. I think he'd take it personally, like it was about him," says Edie.

"But it's not about him," says Marnie. "It's about you."

"Yeah, I know. Maybe I'll talk with your friend, but maybe when Frank's not here."

"Do you feel safe with Frank?" asks Marnie.

"Why does everyone ask me that? Yeah, I feel safe. He's just old fashioned, you know?"

Marnie nods. "I'll see what I can do. Edie, your health is your health. You have no obligation to tell him anything you don't want him to know, and we won't share anything with him without you telling us to do so. This is a safe space for you. I want you to know that."

"Yeah," says Edie. "I'm fine."

Think Critically

1. Describe the features of migraine with aura.
2. Why should women who experience migraine headaches with aura not use contraception containing estrogen?
3. You have a patient who is considering using withdrawal as the primary means of contraception. How do you talk with this patient about this choice in a way that is factual and informative but nonjudgmental?
4. You are performing routine screening for intimate partner violence. Your patient is offended and asks what makes you think she is abused. How do you respond?
5. What constitutes a precipitous birth?
6. Why is it important to carefully monitor the time between the birth of the head and the birth of the remainder of the body?
7. Why is careful monitoring necessary for a woman diagnosed with a hematoma of the perineum?
8. Without referring to the chapter content, list three things you learned about brachial plexus injury.

References

American College of Obstetricians and Gynecologists. (2014). Patterns of neonatal brachial plexus palsy and outcomes. In *Neonatal brachial plexus palsy* (p. 65). Washington, DC: Author.

American College of Obstetricians and Gynecologists' Task Force on Neonatal Brachial Plexus Palsy. (2014). Executive summary: Neonatal brachial plexus palsy. *Obstetrics and Gynecology, 123*(4), 902–904.

Frieden, T. R., Jaffe, H. W., Cono, J., Richards, C. L., & Iademarco, M. F. (2016). *U.S. medical eligibility criteria for contraceptive use, 2016.* Atlanta, GA: U.S. Department of Health and Human Services.

Hansen, J., Lipton, R., Dodick, D., Silberstein, S., Saper, J., Aurora, S., . . . Charles, A. (2012). Migraine headache is present in the aura phase: A prospective study. *Neurology, 79*(20), 2044–2049.

Overland, E. A., Spydslaug, A., Nielsen, C. S., & Eskild, A. (2009). Risk of shoulder dystocia in second delivery: Does a history of shoulder dystocia matter? *American Journal of Obstetrics and Gynecology, 200*(5), 506.e1–506.e6.

Vigod, S. N., Wilson, C. A., & Howard, L. M. (2016). Depression in pregnancy. *BMJ: British Medical Journal, 352,* 492–495.

Suggested Readings

Beck, C. T. (2013). The obstetric nightmare of shoulder dystocia: A tale from two perspectives. *MCN: American Journal of Maternal/Child Nursing, 38*(1), 34–40.

Blake, C. (2012). "Did you just say... the baby's coming!!??": A nurse's guide to prepare for a safe precipitous delivery in the emergency department. *Journal of Emergency Nursing, 38*(3), 296–300.

Cox, E. Q., Raines, C., Kimmel, M., Richardson, E., Stuebe, A., & Meltzer-Brody, S. (2017). Comprehensive integrated care model to improve maternal mental health. *Journal of Obstetric, Gynecologic, and Neonatal Nursing, 46*(6), 923–930.

12

Loretta Hale:
Intimate Partner Violence, Formula Feeding, and Postpartum Depression

Loretta Hale, age 18

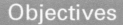

Before Conception

Loretta Hale is 18 years old, recently dropped out of high school, and lives with her boyfriend, Bryan. She is overweight, with a body mass index of 31 (see Box 1.4), and smokes and drinks alcohol. Bryan is older and sells marijuana out of their small apartment. He's out of high school and has a job and a car.

Loretta's earliest memory is of crying—not her own crying but that of her mother. In her memory, her mother lies next to her in the narrow bed Loretta slept in all throughout childhood. She doesn't have any other pieces of this memory that she can recall, but the memory of her mother crying next to her was reinforced numerous times throughout her childhood.

It was predictable, in its way. Her father was often effusive with her mother and with Loretta. He brought home small gifts and flowers. He told Loretta that she was pretty and sweet. He didn't drink. He kissed Loretta's mother on the cheek and sometimes full on the mouth right in front of Loretta. Loretta's mother laughed and said, "not in front of Loretta." These were the good times.

Her mother was better in those times as well. She acted happy and hopeful. She never told Loretta to shush.

Then there would be a shift. Little things started to bother her father that hadn't bothered him before. He brought home cases of beer. He criticized little things about how her mother looked or cleaned or cooked or took care of Loretta. He wasn't patient, and he didn't tell Loretta she was pretty or sweet. He got loud and yelled, and as he got louder, Loretta's mother got quieter. Loretta learned to be quieter, too.

And then came, predictably, in a pattern, the times when Loretta's mother came and lay in her bed. Before that there was usually more yelling and she heard her father say terrible things. Loretta covered her ears and hummed. She turned up the volume on the television. Once or twice Loretta's mother grabbed Loretta and left the house with her. Once they went to her grandmother's, and once they went to a shelter. Both times Loretta's mother explained she had nowhere else to go, and no money to get there. Her grandmother was strict and she had to be quiet all the time. The shelter was small and loud and shabby and her mother cried all the time.

Both times after they left, her father came for them, and they went with him. He said he was terribly sorry, that he'd stop drinking, and that he loved his family, loved Loretta's mother. Loretta's mother reassured him that it wasn't so bad, and that she would heal and that it was her fault, too, that they would heal as a family. Loretta's mother told her that he wasn't a bad man; he just had a lot of responsibilities, and sometimes he had a bad temper. In fact, he loved them both very much and would take care of them. Loretta was pleased to have her kinder father back. He told her that she was sweet and that she was pretty (Fig. 12.1). Later, though, true to pattern, he'd bring home beer instead of flowers, and she'd wake to find her mother crying in her bed.

High school was rough for Loretta. She skipped classes. She didn't go home any more than she had to. She avoided her parents.

She met Bryan when she was a junior. He was nicer to her than most people were. She was surprised that he even talked to

her. A lot of people were surprised by that. Boys weren't usually interested in her, and she was flattered by the attention. He gave her free joints, drank beer with her, and told her to come around whenever she wanted. When he wanted to have sex, it was not even a question. She would do anything for him, anything at all. She stopped going to class completely so she could spend more time with him. He told her she was pretty.

Then one day he called her a dumb pig. He'd had a bad day at work. He apologized but said that in fairness she could lose a few pounds. She did try to eat less. She starved herself for days and then got so hungry she binged on pies from the gas station across the street from his apartment. He was right; she knew he was right. He was just telling it like it is. She was lucky an older guy like him would go for someone as fat and stupid as she was. She asked him to use condoms so she wouldn't get pregnant, but he told her that he didn't like condoms, and if she didn't want to get pregnant, she was the one who would have to do something about it. She didn't get her period much

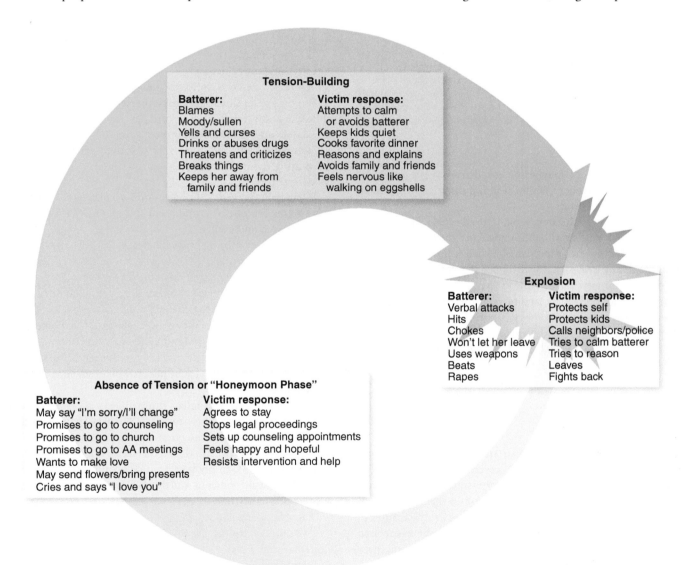

Figure 12.1. The cycle of violence. AA: Alcoholics anonymous. (Adapted with permission from Hatfield, N. T. [2013]. *Introductory maternity and pediatric nursing* [3rd ed., Fig. 16.3]. Philadelphia, PA: Lippincott Williams & Wilkins.)

Box 12.1 Risk Factors for IPV

- Personal history of prior victimization by IPV
- Female (though males can be victims, too)
- Under the age of 24 y
- High-risk behaviors with sex, alcohol, and drugs
- Witnessing IPV in childhood
- History of mental illness, including depression
- Poor education
- Poverty
- Income disparity between self and partner
- Male-dominated relationship
- Weak community support
- Strong traditional gender norms within community
- Underemployment, unemployment, and job insecurity

IPV, intimate partner violence.

Data from Tjaden, P., & Thoennes, N. (2000). *Full report of the prevalence, incidence, and consequences of violence against women: Findings from the National Violence Against Women Survey.* Atlanta, GA: Centers for Disease Control and Prevention; Gracia, E., López-Quílez, A., Marco, M., Lladosa, S., & Lila, M. (2015). The spatial epidemiology of intimate partner violence: Do neighborhoods matter? *American Journal of Epidemiology, 18*(6), 1456–1462; Khalifeh, H., Oram, S., Trevillion, K., Johnson, S., & Howard, L. M. (2015). Recent intimate partner violence among people with chronic mental illness: Findings from a national cross-sectional survey. *The British Journal of Psychiatry, 207*, 207–212.

anyway. She thought maybe she couldn't even get pregnant. Besides, there's nowhere within walking distance to get birth control, and she can't drive.

The hitting, when it came, was not unexpected and followed a pattern she was familiar with. The impatience and casual cruelty to Loretta seemed normal, expected. She knew from long experience at home that this was what love looked like for women like her mother and for girls like her. She looked forward to the times of gentleness and forgiveness, and savored them when they came. It was during one of these times when she left her parents' home for good and moved in with Bryan.

Now, she has no money, no job, and no high school diploma. Bryan says he'll take care of her (Box 12.1).

Pregnancy

First Trimester

Loretta does get a job, in a dollar store. There's no employee discount, but she can buy some groceries and other supplies without having to walk to the grocery store. She doesn't have a car, and there's no public transportation in their small town. She buys some off-brand tampons for a dollar in anticipation of her period. She realizes after a few months that she hasn't used them, and she buys a pregnancy test and uses it in the employee restroom. It comes up positive.

She thinks strategically. Bryan said that birth control was her job, but she didn't get it because there was no place within

walking distance that had it and no one to drive her. Bryan has a car, but he works during the times when the local clinic is open and she knew he wouldn't want to take time off to drive her; in fact, he'd probably get mad at her for even asking. She asked him to withdraw before ejaculation, but he refused. She took a risk in not using contraception, and now it looks like she'll have to face the consequences; but maybe it isn't a bad thing. Babies are all love and need, and a baby would bind them together.

She isn't sure how far along she is. Her period has always been irregular, anyway. She remembers having a very light period some months back but can't recall just when. She recalls that her breasts were tender like they are when she is expecting her period, but she can't remember having bled. She doesn't remember being particularly nauseous and knows she hasn't vomited. She's exhausted, but that's typical.

"I think I'm pregnant," she tells Bryan. She's made him his favorite dinner. The apartment is as clean as she can make it.

"Okay," he says.

Loretta waits. When it seems clear he doesn't plan to say more, she says, "I need to go to a doctor."

"I don't have money for that," he says.

"I have state insurance still," she says quickly. "It won't cost you anything. But I need to get there."

"I'll do it," he says. "But I'm coming in with you."

"To the appointment?" she asks, pleased he wants to be a part of it. She's been watching him carefully for anger and now she relaxes. He doesn't seem happy, exactly, but he's not mad either.

"I'm sorry," says the nurse who comes to get Loretta from the waiting room. "We need to see the patient by herself first. It's policy."

Bryan looks peeved. "But I want him to come back with me," says Loretta. She doesn't want him to be annoyed. She wants him to be involved and excited.

"It's only for a minute," says the nurse. "It's office policy."

Loretta hesitates and then goes with her reluctantly. She feels awkward and avoids looking the nurse in the eye.

When they reach the exam room, the nurse, who introduces herself as Julia, takes a set of vital signs and then asks, like it's just a normal conversation, like they've been talking about the weather, "Do you feel safe in your home and safe in your relationship?"

"I already answered that question in my paperwork," says Loretta. She filled out a stack of papers when they first checked in. "I'm fine."

"I know you did," says Julia. "But we like to ask twice. Sometimes people are more likely to tell us one way than the other, and when you answered the questionnaire, your boyfriend was sitting next to you. Do you think you can leave a urine sample?"

Loretta nods. "Can my boyfriend come in now?"

Dr. McDonald comes in shortly after Bryan and confirms the positive pregnancy test.

"How far along is she?" asks Bryan.

"We can't tell that just from the urine test," says Dr. McDonald. "Loretta, what was the first day of your last period?"

Loretta shrugs. "I don't know. It's been a while."

"What do you think? Has it been weeks? Months?"

Loretta shrugs again. "I don't know."

"Do you think it was in the spring or the summer?"

"Spring, maybe."

Dr. McDonald asks about first trimester symptoms such as breast tenderness, fatigue, and nausea (see Table 6.1), and Loretta confirms the fatigue but nothing else.

"I'd like to do an ultrasound to see if we can pin that date down a little bit for you," says Dr. McDonald.

"How much will that cost?" Bryan asks.

"You have insurance?" Dr. McDonald asks Loretta, who nods.

"State insurance," she says.

"That will cover it," says Dr. McDonald. "Have you thought about what you want to do with this pregnancy?"

"Do you mean if I want to keep it?"

"She wants to keep it," says Bryan. "That's my kid."

Dr. McDonald looks at him for a long moment and then looks back at Loretta. "Well, the first thing I want to do is confirm how far along this pregnancy is, and then we can make a plan. Have you ever had an ultrasound before?"

Loretta shakes her head.

"We'll start with the transvaginal ultrasound. In early pregnancy, we get a much better view this way. If you're further along, we'll need to switch to an abdominal ultrasound" (Fig. 12.2).

In the end Dr. McDonald does need to switch to the abdominal view.

"It's moving!" says Loretta as she watches the fetus kick and roll its spine.

"It looks like an alien," says Bryan.

"It's beautiful," says Loretta.

"You are sixteen weeks along, give or take," Dr. McDonald says. "Generally speaking, earlier ultrasounds give a more accurate date, but sixteen weeks should be pretty darn close" (Verburg et al., 2008).

"Sixteen weeks," says Loretta slowly. "That's almost half way."

"Almost," says Dr. McDonald. "You're just four weeks shy of half way, assuming you give birth at forty weeks."

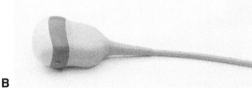
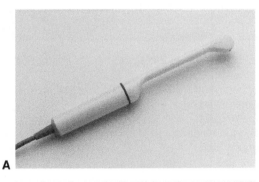

Figure 12.2. Ultrasound transducers. (A) Transvaginal. **(B)** Abdominal. (Reprinted with permission from Sanders, R. C. [2015]. *Clinical sonography: A practical guide* [5th ed., Figs. 2.12 and 2.14]. Philadelphia, PA: Lippincott Williams & Wilkins.)

"Can you tell what it is?" asks Bryan. "Like, boy or girl?"

"I can," says Dr. McDonald. "Loretta, would you like to know?"

"Yes," says Bryan, answering for her.

Dr. McDonald looks at Loretta, who nods. "It's a girl," she says.

"Oh," says Loretta. She isn't sure what to think. She's braced herself to be pregnant but not for details.

"I'd like to order a more thorough ultrasound," says Dr. McDonald, "One that will tell us a little more about the health of the pregnancy" (see Box 1.8).

"Can we do that today?" asks Bryan. "I can't keep taking all this time off of work for doctor's visits."

"It's important that Loretta be seen regularly," says Dr. McDonald (see Box 2.3). "Right now I'd like to see you monthly, Loretta, plus an appointment for the next ultrasound. We should schedule it for about a month from now, around the same time I'd like to see you next. You can schedule the appointments together, if you'd like."

Loretta glances at Bryan. "It depends on his schedule," she says, and looks away.

Dr. McDonald looks back and forth between Bryan and Loretta. "I understand the transportation difficulties. One option would be to arrange home visits with a maternity nurse. She may be able to help with transportation, as well."

"You mean having someone in the house?" asks Bryan. "I don't know about having someone in the house."

Dr. McDonald looks at him sternly. "This is about the health of the pregnancy and Loretta's health."

"I'll think about it," says Bryan.

Dr. McDonald looks back and forth at them again. "You should both think about it. In the meantime we should do some blood work today to screen for health issues and problems with the pregnancy" (Lab Values 12.1; see Table 1.1). "Then I need to ask you some more questions and conduct an exam" (see Boxes 1.2 and 1.3).

In the car on the way home, Loretta swallows hard and says in her softest voice, "So, if we got a home nurse, you maybe wouldn't have to drive me to visits so often. Maybe she could help with some other stuff, too. What do you think?"

"No. I'll take you," he says. There is a warning tone in his voice that dissuades her from pointing out the difficulties of the plan.

Instead, she stages a quiet action of rebellion. She calls Dr. McDonald's office and makes arrangements to have a visiting nurse come. Loretta is careful to arrange her work schedule and the visiting nurse schedule so there will be little chance Bryan will catch on, and she hopes the neighbors mind their own business. It feels exhilarating. It feels dangerous.

The nurse who comes is short and round. Loretta thinks she's probably her mother's age. She wears dark pants and a cardigan with an angled hem and looks nothing like what Loretta thinks a nurse should look like. She carries a backpack covered with pink flowers and introduces herself as Cara.

"It's not that I don't feel safe at home," Loretta tells Cara. "There are just times I feel like I have to be extra careful. He's got a temper, you know?" Loretta didn't mean to say anything to Cara. This was supposed to be a time to just get to know each other, but she likes Cara. She seems kind and she listens. And

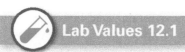

Lab Values 12.1

First-Visit Laboratory Tests for Loretta

Because Loretta presents in week 16 of pregnancy, she has some "catch up" screening to do.

Testing for Maternal Factors

- *Hemoglobin A$_{1c}$:* Elevated levels are associated with uncontrolled diabetes. Loretta is obese and at higher risk for diabetes and is thus screened for preexisting diabetes with her first visit.
- *Blood type and screen:* for Rh status (negative or positive)
- *CBC:* to evaluate for anemia
- *Rubella:* to screen for successful immunization. Vaccination indicated postpartum if not immune
- *HBV:* to evaluate for successful immunization for hepatitis or infection.
- *Syphilis:* to evaluate for infection
- *Gonorrhea and chlamydia:* to evaluate for infection
- *HIV:* to evaluate for infection
- *Urine dip:* one-time screening for UTI

Testing for Congenital Defects

- *Cystic fibrosis:* screen for carrier status. If positive, Bryan would be tested as well
- *Maternal serum alpha-fetoprotein:* High levels are associated with neural tube defects; low levels are associated with Down syndrome and trisomy 18.
- *Human chorionic gonadotropin:* High levels are associated with Down syndrome; low levels are associated with trisomy 18.
- *Unconjugated estriol:* Low levels are associated with Down syndrome and trisomy 18.
- *Inhibin-A:* High levels are associated with Down syndrome.

CBC, complete blood count; HBV, hepatitis B virus; HIV, human immunodeficiency virus; UTI, urinary tract infection.

Bryan has been in a difficult mood lately. He hasn't been talking and he seems coiled like a snake.

"Tell me about that, Loretta," says Cara. She's not taking notes. She's just like a friend having a conversation.

"He can be mean," says Loretta. "He can say hurtful things sometimes. Sometimes he'll swipe at me. Not very hard, but enough to let me know who's boss, you know?"

"Loretta, sometimes people say abusive things to other people to make them feel small. It can make them feel powerful, like they're in control."

"You think he's abusive?" asks Loretta, surprised. "He never beats me up. He's just not nice all the time. It's not like he's tossing me down the stairs or giving me black eyes."

"It doesn't have to leave a mark to be abusive," says Cara. "Every time he says something just to watch you hurt, that's abuse."

Loretta shifts in her seat. "I don't want to talk about this anymore. Bryan wouldn't like me talking about him like this.

He has a lot on his mind with taking care of me and thinking about the baby."

"We don't have to talk about it anymore. But, Loretta, thank you for trusting me with this information," says Cara. "I think that must have been a hard thing to do."

Loretta shrugs and looks away.

"Loretta, I'm going to tell Dr. McDonald what you told me. There are risks to the pregnancy from **intimate partner violence**" (Box 12.2).

Loretta looks up. "I didn't tell you so you'd tell other people," she says. "I told you only because you asked. I don't want to talk to anyone else about it."

"I'd like to help you," says Cara.

"I was just answering a question," says Loretta. "That's not the same as asking for help. Look, if Bryan knows I said something, who knows what he'd do. That's private. He wouldn't like it."

"It's alright," says Cara. "We don't have to do anything you don't want to do. Healthcare providers don't have to report the kinds of things you told me, not in this state, not if you don't want us to."

"I don't want you to," says Loretta. "This is private, like I said. I shouldn't have said anything."

"This is what I think, Loretta. I am a safe person for you. I really want you to believe that. I want you to know you can talk to me if that helps, or you can choose not to talk. If you want to talk to someone else, like a counselor or a social worker, I can help arrange that. If you want other help with shelter or safety or something else, you need only tell us."

"Don't take this wrong," says Loretta. "I'm not a trusting person. I don't feel like I can trust you. I trust him, but he hits me. What does that say about what I know about people?"

Box 12.2 Risks of Intimate Partner Violence in Pregnancy

- Two to three times increased risk for postpartum depression
- Pregnancy-induced hypertension
- Vaginal bleeding
- Hyperemesis
- Frequent urinary tract infection
- Preterm birth
- Small size for gestational age
- Placental abruption
- Perinatal injuries, including fracture, and death

Data from Parrish, J. W., Lanier, P., Newby-Kew, A., Arvidson, J., & Shanahan, M. (2015). Intimate partner violence victimization prior to and during pregnancy among women residing in 26 U.S. states: Associations with maternal and neonatal health. *Child Maltreatment, 21,* 26–36; Ludermir, A. B., Lewis, G., Valongueiro, S. A., Araújo, T. V., & Araya, R. (2010). Violence against women by their intimate partner during pregnancy and postnatal depression: A prospective cohort study. *The Lancet, 376*(9744), 903–910.

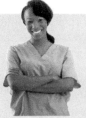

The Nurse's Point of View

Cara: It never does any good to judge anyone, or any person's situation. It would be easy for me to look at Loretta and say that she's foolish or weak or not worth my time. But the truth is much harder. Loretta has been taught by so many people in her life that she's not worth the trouble that she believes them. She doesn't trust because the people in her life don't have a track record of earning that trust.

Another thing, Loretta isn't weak, she just doesn't have power. Those are two different things. She doesn't feel she has a lot of control over her life because she believes that she shouldn't. She thinks it's the order of the world that someone else, in her case right now Bryan, makes the decisions. One of the most important, one of the kindest, things I can do for her right now is encourage her to make her own decisions. It would be wrong to tell her to leave, even if I truly believe that's what's best for her. If I tell Loretta what to do she might do it, and in the short term that might be a good choice, but it just continues the pattern of people telling her what to do and disempowering her. She needs to get strong. It's part of my job to help her become so.

It's so easy to think that you know what's best for someone, but the truth is, Loretta knows her situation best. She may not think she can afford to leave, and she may be right. She may think she has nowhere to go, and she's probably right about that. She may feel like she loves Bryan, and that if she leaves she risks never loving again. And she might be right about that, too. Part of earning trust is giving it. I need to trust that if I can help Loretta learn her strength, she'll make the decisions that are right for her.

Bryan surprises her. He does arrange his schedule so he can take her to visits, usually first thing in the morning or the last appointment of the day. He comes in with her to each of them from start to finish.

"I don't like it when they ask nosey questions about us, you know?" he says. "We're in this together. It's our relationship. No one else has any business here."

The results of Loretta's initial blood work are normal.

Second Trimester

A second, more thorough, ultrasound at 20 weeks confirms she is having a girl and that she appears healthy. The results of her initial blood work do not indicate preexisting diabetes, and those of her 1-hour glucose tolerance test at 26 weeks do not suggest the onset of gestational diabetes (see Lab Values 3.2). Loretta tries to keep her weight gain at 12 lb or less (see Box 1.5), as Dr. McDonald recommended, but it's hard. Food can be a friend when things are tough. She's still working at the dollar store, and it's where she buys most of her food. She knows she's supposed to be eating more fruits and vegetables, but she figures that the prenatal vitamin Dr. McDonald gave her for a prescription would fill in the chinks, along with the food she gets from WIC (see Box 3.1).

The next time Cara comes, Loretta has applied a thick layer of foundation to her face and turned off most of the lights in the apartment. Cara turns on the overhead lights without asking Loretta and then just looks at her for a moment. Loretta avoids her eyes.

"It's not like this all the time," Loretta says. "He can be loving and kind. He makes sure I get to all of these appointments because he cares about me and he cares about this baby. He's just sad. And sometimes I look at him and my heart just aches for him because he's so sweet. And he's damaged, just like me. For him it just comes out different, you know? He comes out swinging."

"He comes out swinging at you, Loretta," says Cara.

"I know. I'm just saying that's not all he does. He's loving and kind and he needs me," says Loretta. "Nobody else has ever needed me before."

"What about this baby?" Cara asks gently. "This baby needs you."

"This baby needs both of us," says Loretta. "A mom and a dad. A real family. Look, he mostly just says stuff. He usually hits only when he's been drinking a lot, and mostly he won't do that if I make sure not to say anything to make him mad. I've never had to go to the hospital. It's not that bad."

"What about your family," says Cara. "You're eighteen. You're still a teenager. Would they take you back in?"

Loretta makes a snorting noise. "Like it's so much better at home. Dad's just the same and I caused them plenty of trouble before I left. They said I can't do it, go it alone. But I can. I mean, I have to. I have nowhere else to go."

"There are places you can go," says Cara. "There are shelters and services and people who can keep you safe, you and the baby. I can help connect you with all of these. That's part of why I'm here."

Loretta is not sure whether to be exasperated with Cara or pity her. For a moment she feels like she's older than Cara. "Who would have me now if I left? I'm pregnant. I'm fat. I'm covered with stretch marks and my clothes are all stretched out and nasty. You think boys are lining up for me? Who's out there for me besides him? I don't want to be alone, not with the baby and not without the baby."

"You're not in this alone, Loretta. You have me to help. There are many people out there whose job it is to help people in your situation."

Loretta thinks for a long moment. When she looks up at Cara, she feels tears pricking her eyes. She wipes her nose with the back of her hand. "That's the loneliest thing you just said. That there's people out there who are paid to take care of people like me. Bryan and me, it's not perfect, but at least no one's paying us to take care of each other."

"Oh Loretta," says Cara, "I didn't mean . . ."

"I know you didn't," says Loretta. "But I'm taking my chances with what I've got. There's nothing I know about that says there's anything better out there."

At her next visit, Cara discusses infant care and feeding and asks Loretta whether she is planning to breastfeed the baby.

"The truth is, Bryan wouldn't like it," says Loretta. "He said my boobs are for him, not for some baby."

Cara raises her eyebrows. "It's your body, you know. And there are so many good things about breastfeeding, for you and for the baby. It's good for the baby's digestion, it's associated with lower rates of breast cancer, and it helps you bond with the baby" (Box 12.3).

"He wouldn't like it," repeats Loretta.

Cara sighs. "Don't you get mad?"

"Sure I do, I get mad all the time," says Loretta.

"What do you do when you're mad?"

"I don't know. I think about stuff. I go for a walk. I used to call a friend, you know, when I had a phone. I talked to my mom sometimes, but it's been a while since I've done that. I tried punching pillows once, but I just felt stupid."

"Have you ever hit anyone when you're mad?"

"No."

"Why not?" asks Cara.

"It's not my way, I guess," says Loretta. "I'm not the hitting kind."

"But Bryan is," says Cara.

"I guess."

"That's okay?"

"He's a man, you know," says Loretta. "They have more rage in them. Sometimes they have to hit and you might get in the way."

"Not all men hit, Loretta," says Cara.

Loretta is doubtful. "What kind of man doesn't get into fights? They have those hormones in them that make them tough and make them want to fight."

"A lot of men just talk through their problems," says Cara. "Or they do what you do. They go for a walk or talk it out. But they don't hit people, particularly not people who aren't as strong as they are and who can't protect themselves."

"I protect myself," says Loretta. "Sometimes I'm just not fast enough to do it all the way."

Cara decides to change the subject. "What happened to your phone?"

"Nothing really," says Loretta. "I just don't get much time. It's one of those where you pay for your minutes up front. Money's tight and Bryan says I can't get a new one until after the baby. I just need to be careful how much I use it."

"You know, Loretta, you're not alone," says Cara. "This isn't something that just happens every now and then to some women. I've read that one out of every five women is a victim of partner violence" (Breiding, Basile, Smith, Black, & Mahendra, 2015).

"It's pretty normal," says Loretta. This statement from Cara seems to confirm something she'd been thinking all along. "It's everybody."

"No," says Cara gently. "Not everybody. You're right that it's a normal part of the lives of a lot of people, but it doesn't have to be. It shouldn't be. Just because it's common doesn't mean it's right."

Loretta just shrugs. Cara sighs.

Box 12.3   Breastfeeding Benefits

Benefits to the Infant

- Improved gastrointestinal function
- Improved immunity to disease
- Reduced susceptibility to respiratory disease for the first year
- Reduced rate of otitis media, neonatal sepsis, and urinary tract infections
- Possible reduction in the occurrence of obesity
- Reduced rate of lymphoma and leukemia as well as other childhood cancers
- Improved dentition
- Reduced rate of type 1 diabetes
- Improved cognition
- Reduction in childhood behavioral issues

Benefits to the Mother

- Improved involution of the uterus
- Improved postpartum weight loss
- Reduced rates of breast and ovarian cancers
- Lower risk for heart disease
- Lower risk for type 2 diabetes

Economic Benefits

- Reduction in the cost of infant feeding
- Reduction in the cost of healthcare

Data from Victora, C. G., Bahl, R., Barros, A. J., França, G. V., Horton, P. S., Krasevec, J., . . . Rollins, N. C.; Lancet Breastfeeding Series Group. (2016). Breastfeeding in the 21st century: Epidemiology, mechanisms, and lifelong effect. *The Lancet, 387*(10017), 475–490; Horta, B. L., & Victora, C. G. (2015). *TI Optimal breastfeeding practices and infant and child mortality: A systematic review and meta-analysis.* Geneva, Switzerland: World Health Organization; Bowatte, G., Tham, R., Allen, K., Tan, D., Lau, M., Dai, X., & Lodge, C. (2015). Breastfeeding and childhood acute otitis media: A systematic review and meta-analysis. *Acta Paediatrica, 104*(S467), 85–95; Peres, K. G., Cascaes, A. M., Nascimento, G. G., & Victora, C. G. (2015). Effect of breastfeeding on malocclusions: A systematic review and meta-analysis. *Acta Paediatrica, 104*(S467), 54–61; Heikkilä, K., Sacker, A., Kelly, Y., Renfrew, M. J., & Quigley, M. A. (2011). Breast feeding and child behaviour in the Millennium Cohort Study. *Archives of Disease in Childhood, 96*(7), 635–642; Gunderson, E. P., Hurston, S. R., Ning, X., Lo, J. C., Crites, Y., Walton, D., . . . Quesenberry, C. P.; Study of Women, Infant Feeding and Type 2 Diabetes After GDM Pregnancy Investigators. (2015). Lactation and progression to type 2 diabetes mellitus after gestational diabetes mellitus: A prospective cohort study. *Annals of Internal Medicine, 163*(12), 889–898.

"The bottle-feeding isn't a problem. It's expensive, but WIC will help with that part. You'll think about what we've talked about though, won't you?"

Loretta nods but says nothing.

Third Trimester

Loretta is 34 weeks pregnant, and Cara stops in to talk more about infant care.

"I think you have the wrong idea about how it is with me and Bryan," says Loretta. "Most of the time he's normal, he's not hitting. He's just around, you know. He's not being violent. I mean, sometimes he says stuff, but that's not the same thing."

"What kind of stuff, Loretta?"

"Mean stuff—like that I'm fat or ugly or stupid. He doesn't mean it, he just says it to get to me, you know? I don't show him it hurts because it just eggs him on and it takes him longer then to get sweet. If I laugh along he gets better."

"Loretta, that's a kind of abuse as well," says Cara. "Making you feel small and worthless and frightened. That's psychological abuse."

"Maybe, but it's been that way nearly all along," says Loretta. "It started out kind of jokey, you know?"

"It's not unusual for abuse to start out just like that, with the psychological abuse, with getting inside your head first to make you feel badly about yourself. Then if he hits later you might even feel like you deserve it or that you don't deserve for someone to be kind to you. It's all part of what we call the cycle of violence (Fig. 12.1)."

Loretta is quiet for a minute. She inspects her fingernails. "Yeah, sometimes I feel like that. Like I'm so bad he can't help himself but to hit me. Like what's the point of leaving because I'd never find someone new the way I am and even if I did, what's to stop me from provoking them to hit me as well?"

"Abusers don't usually hit on the first date," says Cara. "They probably wouldn't get a second date if they did."

Loretta laughs a little. "No, I guess that's right."

They've agreed that Loretta will always call Cara, usually from work, to reduce the risk of Cara calling at an inopportune time.

When Loretta doesn't call for a full week, Cara stops by the dollar store and buys some tissues at Loretta's register. Loretta is pleased to see her.

"Are you spying on me?" she says and laughs.

"Loretta, I'm worried about you. You haven't called."

"We've been fighting," says Loretta, though it's not really an explanation for why she hasn't called. "He said he thought I was calling other men, but I told him he's stupid. What other men would be interested in me, with my belly hiding my shoes?"

"When's your break?" asks Cara. "Can I buy you lunch?"

An hour later they're sitting in Cara's car eating packaged sandwiches from a grocery store and drinking water out of plastic bottles that crinkle when they're squeezed.

"Loretta, tell me what you think his behavior is about," Cara says.

"He's correcting me," says Loretta. "I do something stupid or wrong and it just makes more trouble for him and it makes him mad. So things happen. I'm not saying I like how he does it, but it's at least partly my fault as well."

"A lot of people think about violence like this, not just the physical stuff but how he gets into your head as well, they think that's about control. What do you think about that?" asks Cara.

"Like he's wanting to control me?" asks Loretta. "I guess. We all want to feel like we're in control. And he can control me, so he does."

"Tell me about that."

"Well, some of it's just like life stuff. He's got the car so he controls when I go somewhere and where I go. He's the one with the money. He took my phone away completely. Not like I had much time left on it anyway."

"Could you tell a friend what's going on? That he took the phone away?"

Loretta shakes her head. "It's embarrassing. You're the first person I've ever even told about it. I left my parents' home because I didn't want to be treated like a child. Well, that and they kicked me out. But here I am with a man who's controlling my phone. It's childish. Besides, I haven't seen a friend in so long it would be weird to talk to them. They just sort of dropped off once Bryan and I started up. He didn't like them."

"Loretta, what would you do if you were at home alone without a phone and something happened? What if your water broke or you started having contractions?"

"I don't know," says Loretta. "I haven't thought about it. Maybe I could go across to the gas station and get them to call."

"Do you think you could talk with him about giving you your phone back, just for emergencies?"

"I'll have to think about it," says Loretta. "I don't want him to think I'm up to something. Maybe if I just had it so I could call in an emergency."

Loretta goes to her visit with Dr. McDonald at 36 weeks and has a swab taken from her introitus to test for group B streptococcus, which turns out to be negative. Dr. McDonald asks her about her plans for birth control after the pregnancy.

"I haven't thought about it," says Loretta.

"Can't you just give her a pill or something?" asks Bryan.

"We could. Several hormonal methods should be delayed until the milk supply is well established, however," says Dr. McDonald.

"I won't be breastfeeding," says Loretta quickly.

"I respect your choice," says Dr. McDonald, "but there are several benefits to breastfeeding over bottle-feeding. Would you like to go over any of that?"

Loretta shakes her head. "No. I'm fine. Lots of babies are bottle-fed. I was bottle-fed."

"Well, let's talk about birth control. We have many options we can talk about. We can place an intrauterine device or an implant in your arm even before you're discharged . . ."

"We'll think about it," says Bryan.

"Women can get pregnant shortly after giving birth, particularly if they're not breastfeeding," says Dr. McDonald, addressing Loretta. "Giving birth to children too close together is riskier for mom and baby. We recommend having a birth control plan on board even before you give birth."

Loretta opens her mouth to speak, but Bryan cuts her off. "I've got to get to work. Can't you just give her some pamphlets or something?"

During her next home visit, Cara says, "Loretta, you've told me before you didn't plan this pregnancy. Were you using birth control?"

"Well, I didn't plan it, but I didn't not plan it, either. It was too hard to get to the clinic and he said he didn't want to use condoms. I thought that maybe that meant he wanted me to have his baby. So I didn't try that hard to do anything honestly because I thought that was kind of sweet—like he wants the two of us to be linked forever. It made my heart melt a little bit. I still thought about getting birth control because I wasn't sure I wanted to have a baby yet, but I got pregnant before that happened, so here we are."

"Do you ever have sex with him when you don't want to?"

"Sometimes. He says he's paying for the cow so he wants the cream. Sometimes I say I don't want to, but he can get really mean, so I mostly don't try to stop him now. It's not worth it to me. I'd rather he just did it. And it's not all the time, you know? It's just sometimes. Other times he's really gentle and sweet and he makes me want to do it."

"You know what they call it when someone forces you to have sex when you don't want to, right?"

"It's not really rape," says Loretta quickly. "We live in the same place and we're having a baby. That's almost like being married, and you can't rape someone you're married to."

"That's not true. Any time someone forces sexual contact when you don't want it, that's sexual assault."

"I hadn't thought of it like that," says Loretta. "I'm not sure I want to think about it, to be honest. It's just how it is. It feels bad, but it's how we are, the two of us. I don't have to like it. I don't like a lot of things, but here we are."

"Does it bother you?" asks Cara.

"Well, sure," says Loretta. "But I've been raped before, when I was a teenager. It wasn't with a boyfriend or anything. It was just a guy. So I know what that is."

"I'm so sorry," says Cara. "Did you get help? Did you tell anyone?"

Loretta shakes her head. "No. I just wanted it to be done. I didn't want to go through the whole thing, with people thinking I was dirty or that I was asking for it. I never told Bryan, either. I told him I was a virgin when we first got together. I don't know if he believes it, but it's better than telling him and having him think I was being slutty with someone else."

"Being raped isn't being slutty," says Cara. "It's not that at all. It's an assault and it's wrong."

"I hear you saying it," says Loretta. "And in my heart I believe that, but there's all sorts of people who don't believe that. All the time you see it on the TV shows with people saying they're raped and other people saying they're asking for it. And here I am just a girl who had something happen to her and you think they're going to believe me? Nah."

When Loretta is almost 39 weeks pregnant, Bryan has taken to staying away for days at a time, and Loretta hasn't seen him since the day before. Cara arrives for a visit.

"Have you thought about leaving?" asks Cara.

"I think it must be hard for someone like you to understand why someone like me stays with someone like that," says Loretta.

"Tell me about that," says Cara. "Why do you say that?"

"Well, to you maybe it's obvious. Someone hits you and you leave because that's unkind," says Loretta.

"But you don't think like that," says Cara.

"I think like that a lot," says Loretta. "But it's not all I think about. I have no money. I'm not counting on my family to take me back, and I don't know that would be much better anyway. My friends are alright, but I've barely talked to them, and I'm not counting on any of them to try to help me out or get in his

way. He's known, you know? I'm not the only one he shows his temper to."

"There're other ways," says Cara. "We can leave right here and right now and take you to a shelter. There's not one but two organizations in this town whose sole purpose it to help women like you in situations like this."

"I know. And maybe one of these days that will be what I'm asking for, but this is what I'm talking about when I say that people like you can't understand people like me."

"Tell me. I want to understand," says Cara. "I want to help."

"I love him," says Loretta. "It's stupid and it's got me in a bad spot, but that's how it is. I've never felt this love for anyone like I have for him. What if I never feel anything like that for anyone again? You can say I'm stupid for letting him hurt me like this and maybe I am, but my heart says I'd be stupid to walk out on how he makes me feel when things are good."

"You're right that I can't understand it the same way you can," says Cara.

"You can't ever judge what's in someone's heart," says Loretta, "In someone's relationship. Everyone else is just looking in from the outside."

"Well, that's true," says Cara. "I can't understand it the way you do. But I've read about it, and I've talked to the people who can help. One thing they've talked to me about is a theory of **traumatic bonding** that says that when some people are threatened or hurt routinely while in a situation they can't easily escape, they bond with the person who is hurting them. It's a means of self-preservation."

"You think I'm crazy," says Loretta. "I tell you what's in my heart and you tell me I'm crazy."

"No," says Cara. "I truly don't think you're crazy. I think you have a brain that's trying to help you through a tough situation."

"I do feel trapped sometimes," says Loretta. "People think you can just walk out of the door, but it's not that easy."

"Tell me," says Cara. "Tell me how you feel trapped."

"Well, there's money for one," says Loretta. "That probably sounds stupid to anyone who has any money, but the only money I get is the little bit I make at work and that wouldn't feed a cat. I'd get a better job, but I don't even have my diploma. I don't have a car to get to a better job even if I could get one. And I love him. It's like a part of me would starve without him."

"I don't think you're crazy. Loretta, I want to tell you a story I heard from one of the advocates in the shelter near here. Back in the 1970s, there was a bank robbery in Sweden, in Stockholm. The robbers, I think there were two of them, took four hostages. They were in there for six days. That wasn't so weird. But what was interesting is that the hostages, despite being repeatedly threatened by their captors, took their side. They sympathized with them and befriended them. When the police came, they tried to fight them off."

"That's weird," says Loretta.

"It is weird," says Cara. "I have another weird story. This one happened a few years after what happened in Stockholm. There was a flight from Athens, Greece, with a final stop in the United States that was diverted by terrorists. Dozens of the passengers were held hostage. Some were beaten and threatened. One, a Navy

Box 12.4 The Link Between Intimate Partner Violence and Murder

In 2010, 13.4% of murders occurred as part of intimate partner violence (Stöckl et al., 2013). Many women are killed during the process of leaving and after they have left.

diver, was killed and his body thrown out onto the runway. This went on for weeks. Those passengers who survived also became sympathetic to their captors. They bonded with them."

"Why would they do that?" asks Loretta.

"I guess there's no easy answer to that, but it's a way our brains make sense of a bad situation. It helps us to cope and get through it. I've seen it called a lot of things. The most current term I think is traumatic bonding, like I mentioned before."

"He'd kill me if I left and he found me. No question," says Loretta.

Cara looks startled. "Why do you say that?" she asks.

"Because he told me so" (Box 12.4).

"Do you believe him?" asks Cara.

"I don't know," says Loretta. "He sounded like he meant it when he said it. It was a while ago, though. And the way he said it was kind of sweet, like if he couldn't have me no one else could either."

"Loretta, that's not sweet," says Cara. "That's a terrible thing to say to someone."

Loretta just shrugs.

"Why do you think he'd want to kill you?"

"Like I said, so no one else could have me. Plus, I think it would make him real mad. He'd take it like a rejection."

"You're telling me he'd get so mad about you leaving that you think he might kill you?"

"That's what he said. He's one to follow through, too."

"Loretta, I'm very worried that you're not safe here," says Cara.

"Listen to me," says Loretta. "I'm more worried I'll be unsafe if I leave. How am I supposed to do this on my own? My family won't help, and I can't count on my friends like that. How am I supposed to do anything for this baby? I can't take care of myself without him."

"There are people who can help and places you can go," says Cara patiently.

"You keep saying that," says Loretta. "But if you get people from the state involved, they'd take one look at me and decide I'm not a fit mother."

"Why would they think that?" says Cara.

"Well, look at me. I spent all this time with a man that hits. I have a job that pays nothing, no education, no prospects, no one to help me out."

"That's what they're there for. That's what I'm here for," says Cara. "To help you out."

"I hear what you're saying," says Loretta. "But I've heard the stories about kids being taken from their families. Better the devil you know than the devil you don't."

"Are you concerned he'll hurt the baby, or hurt you in front of the baby?"

"No," says Loretta quickly. "He wouldn't do that. I wouldn't let him. My dad never hurt mom in front of me."

"I want you to think about a few things. First, many abusers also abuse their children, if not physically then mentally. Second, even if you think you're hiding it and your child won't know how he treats you, children are affected by the abuse. It makes an impression."

"Well, that's true," says Loretta. "My mom thought she was hiding it pretty good, but I knew. He doesn't hit as much now, but my dad was wound pretty tight when I was a kid. He never hit me, but I knew he hit her. I used to think she was weak and stupid for letting him do it. I had no respect for her. I used to run wild."

"What do you think now?" asks Cara.

"I still think that way about her. It's just now I think it about me, too."

Labor and Delivery

Loretta is woken one night by an intense tightening in her belly. It feels kind of like menstrual cramps. Then she realizes that it is a contraction. Bryan is out. She waits for him. The contractions aren't strong at first, and, when she times them, none seems much longer than 30 seconds. At midnight she calls Bryan's phone and leaves a message on his voicemail. The contractions are now stronger and closer together and last a minute each. She can't remember whether Cara told her to time from the beginning of one contraction to the beginning of the next or from the end of one contraction to the end of the next. She calls Dr. McDonald's office and describes the situation, and the person on call tells her to go to the hospital for evaluation. She remembers as she gets up to change that she doesn't have transportation. She leaves another voicemail for Bryan.

When he finally comes in at two in the morning, Loretta is trying to blot up amniotic fluid from the bed. The towel she laid down just in case this were to happen is soaked.

"What's happening," asks Bryan. Loretta can see from his eyes that he's stoned. She's relieved. He's usually better stoned than drunk.

"Baby's coming," she says.

"You should have called," he says. He sits on the edge of the bed and seems to be preparing to take off his shoes.

"Bryan, we need to go," says Loretta. She feels her muscles bunching for another contraction. "We have to go now."

He squints at her and rubs his face with both hands. "Yeah. Let's do this thing."

Loretta is relieved once they reach the hospital, and she expects that her labor will progress quickly now. Her contractions do gradually become stronger and more frequent, but the whole thing is so much slower than she expected. She's known from the beginning that she wants an epidural and is disappointed to find that someone is not just waiting in the delivery room to make that happen. In reality, she has to wait for it almost a full hour while being poked and prodded and told to walk. She's glad Bryan is here, even if he spends a lot of time out of the room and watches television when he's in the room. He naps a bit, as well.

After spending 16 hours in active labor, she's told that it's time to push (see Table 1.3). At first, she has a hard time telling when she should push. Then, once she's got the pushing down, it seems like it will never end. She is glad of the epidural as she pushes and pushes without the emergence of a baby. She pushes for 3 hours.

"Do I need a cesarean section?" she asks her nurse, Rosalie. She started out with a different nurse, but the shift changed a while ago.

"Your baby is doing great," says Rosalie, gesturing to the little wiggly lines on the machine next to the head of the bed. "You're doing great. I know it's slow going."

"The baby's crowning," Rosalie says a little later. She brings in a mirror so Loretta can see the matted cap of dark hair emerging from the vaginal canal. Several pushes later the head is born, followed within a minute by the body. A nurse deposits the baby, already crying, on Loretta's abdomen and vigorously rubs it down and covers it with a fresh, warm blanket. Apgar scoring (see Table 1.4) is done at 1 and 5 minutes.

A few minutes later there is another rush of blood and the umbilical cord lengthens as the placenta detaches from the uterus and is delivered.

The newborn—in her mind Loretta has already named her Jacqueline, or Jackie for short—finds her exposed nipple with her mouth. Bryan leans down and gently kisses Loretta on the top of her head. Equally gently, he sweeps her nipple out of the baby's mouth.

"I'm proud of you babe," he says. "I'm going to have a smoke, and when I come back I'm going to fill up this whole room with flowers."

The Newborn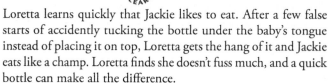

Loretta learns quickly that Jackie likes to eat. After a few false starts of accidently tucking the bottle under the baby's tongue instead of placing it on top, Loretta gets the hang of it and Jackie eats like a champ. Loretta finds she doesn't fuss much, and a quick bottle can make all the difference.

She also learns quickly the importance of a thorough burping during and after feeding. She initially tries to burp the air out of the baby's belly by holding her over her shoulder, but a single shower of warm, congealed formula down her back convinces her to burp Jackie in an upright, folded position on her lap. She also finds it easier to control the new baby's head on its floppy neck this way (Fig. 12.3).

"Let me try," says Bryan when it's time for Jackie's next feeding.

The family's nurse, Gretchen, seats him in a chair and hands him the baby, who appears alert if unfocused. She thrusts out her rolled tongue.

"She's hungry," says Gretchen. She quickly pulls a bottle of premixed formula out of the pocket of her scrubs along with a nipple and a ring to attach the nipple to the bottle. "Now when she's this little you want to use a low-flow nipple so she's not getting too much at one time. She probably won't have more than an ounce or two in one sitting right now" (Patient Teaching 12.1).

Gretchen helps Bryan to hold the bottle at a 45-degree angle. "It helps with gas bubbles in the tummy to hold it this way," she says. She points to bubbles rising from the nipple and up to the top of the liquid in the bottle. "These bubbles are a good sign. It means she's eating."

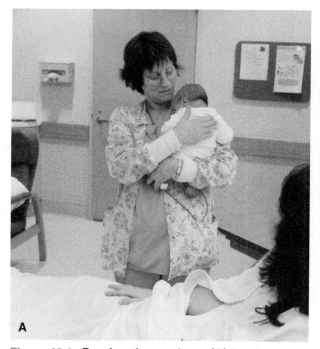
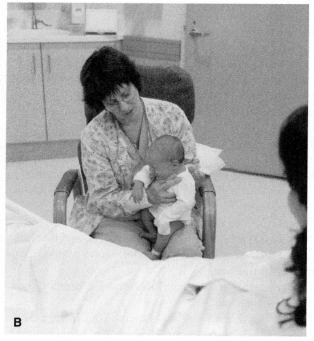

Figure 12.3. Burping the newborn. (A) Burping over the shoulder. **(B)** Burping with the newborn on the lap, while the nurse supports the head and neck. (Reprinted with permission from Evans, R. J., Brown, Y. M., & Evans, M. K. [2014]. *Canadian maternity, newborn, and women's health nursing* [2nd ed., Fig. 21.11]. Philadelphia, PA: Lippincott Williams & Wilkins.)

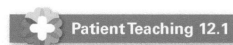

Patient Teaching 12.1

Formula Feeding Guidelines for Term Infants

Formula Types

- *Ready-to-feed, premixed:* the most expensive option; may be indicated for infants requiring sterile formula
- *Concentrated: must* be mixed with water before feeding, according to package instructions
- *Powdered:* the least expensive option, typically mixed with 60 mL (2 oz) of water. Mixing with too much or too little water may have serious health consequences for the infant.

Water Sources for Mixing

- Avoid natural mineral water, untested well water, and spring water.
- Use distilled water, tap water, or filtered tap water.
- If sterile water is indicated, keep the water at a rolling boil for 2 min and then cool it before using.
- If water without fluoride is indicated, as for infants under 6 mo of age, use distilled water or filtered tap water. If using water from the tap, use cold water and run it for a full minute before collecting.

Formula Preparation

1. Clean your hands, bottles, nipples, and other bottle supplies (this is essential).
2. Prepare only the volume required for one feeding.
3. If using concentrate, shake well before use.
4. If using powdered formula, use the scoop provided. Level off the scoop and do not pack it.
5. Do not add anything to the bottle besides formula and the recommended volume of water.
6. Do not allow fresh formula to sit at room temperature for longer than 2 h.
7. Warm the prepared formula in a bowl of warm water.

Formula Volume

- *First month:* 2–4 oz six to eight times daily
- *Second month:* 5–6 oz five to six times daily
- *Third through fifth months:* 6–7 oz six to seven times daily

Feeding

- Newborns require a slow-flow nipple. Older infants may graduate to medium- and high-flow nipples.
- Always hold the infant during feedings.
- Hold the bottle at a 45-degree angle.
- Bubbles rising in the bottle during feeding indicate effective sucking.
- Placement of the infant's tongue on the tip of the nipple rather than under it often results in ineffective feeding.
- Discard any milk that is left over in the bottle, because it is not safe.
- Burp the infant during and after feeding to avoid vomiting.

After an ounce, Gretchen has Bryan hold Jackie in his lap the same way Loretta has been taught to burp her. She shows him how to hold the lower part of her face to stabilize her head while he gently rubs and pats her back. She lets out an enormous belch. All three laugh.

After Delivery

Loretta calls to quit her job. She's known that she'd have to because she can't afford to pay anyone to look after Jackie while she works. It's not like she could keep a baby under the counter. She knows there is no other decision to make, but it feels like a door closing behind her, like a complete commitment to this man and this life (Boxes 12.5 and 12.6). Bryan's hours haven't changed. They are still long and he still sometimes spends nights away without calling. Loretta called her mother from the hospital, and she came to visit her new granddaughter before they went home, but Loretta's father didn't.

Box 12.5   Risk Factors for Postpartum Depression

- Past personal history of depression
- Past personal history of abuse
- Youth
- Unplanned pregnancy
- Lack of support
- Lack of a partner
- Unemployment
- Diabetes
- Bottle-feeding
- Family history of psychiatric illness
- Pregnancy loss

Adapted from Committee on Obstetric Practice. (2015). The American College of Obstetricians and Gynecologists Committee Opinion no. 630. Screening for perinatal depression. *Obstetrics and Gynecology, 125*(5), 1268–1271; O'Hara, M. W., & McCabe, J. E. (2013). Postpartum depression: Current status and future directions. *Clinical Psychology, 9,* 379–407; Norhayatia, M., Hazlina, N. H., Asrenee, A. R., & Emilind, W. W. (2015). Magnitude and risk factors for postpartum symptoms: A literature review. *Journal of Affective Disorders, 175,* 34–52; O'Hara, M. W., & Wisner, K. L. (2014). Perinatal mental illness: Definition, description and aetiology. *Best Practice and Research Clinical Obstetrics and Gynaecology, 28*(1), 3–12; Giri, R. K., Khati, R. B., Mishra, S. R., Khanal, V., Sharma, V. D., & Gartoula, R. P. (2015). Rates and risk factors associated with depressive symptoms during pregnancy and with postpartum onset. *BMC Research Notes, 8,* 111.

Box 12.6   Common Clinical Manifestations of Postpartum Depression

- Inability to sleep, even when the infant is sleeping
- Reduced appetite
- Reduced energy unrelated to lack of sleep
- Irritability
- A feeling of inadequacy related to infant care
- A sense of failure as a mother
- Anxiety and/or panic attacks
- "Scary thoughts" of harming self or the infant

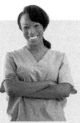

The Nurse's Point of View

Cara: This will be my last visit with Loretta as she and Jackie are at the end of the postpartum period. This is always a hard time. Sometimes I feel like I've helped as much as I can, and I'm frustrated I couldn't do more. Sometimes I feel like there's so much good left to do, if only I had more time. With Loretta, I feel something in between. I think maybe she's stronger than when I found her. I think she knows what resources are available. But at the same time, she's still in a tough situation, and it's hard to see how she'll make her way out. I don't have a wand, and I'm no kind of fairy godmother.

Postpartum depression is a common occurrence for women in situations like Loretta's. She's young, isolated, poor, and in a relationship with someone who abuses her. If I had to make up a recipe for depression, this is it. I'll do a formal assessment with her today and point her in the direction of help if it comes out the way I think it will. It will be down to Loretta to follow up, however. If she can.

I don't mean to say that Loretta's situation is hopeless; there's always hope. But she and Jackie have a long road ahead of them. I hope they find the right path for them. I hope their lives will be happy, and I hope they find safety. I think she's learned to trust a little, and that counts for something. I guess maybe I do know how I feel. I wish I could have done more.

"You look tired," says Cara when she visits. Cara has been coming twice a week since Jackie's birth. "Are you sleeping?"

"Not that much. I just can't. I'm up at all hours feeding Jackie. And when I'm not doing that, my brain starts spinning and that's it."

"What's making your brain spin?"

"Everything. I'm worried about how I can take care of Jackie when I'm barely taking care of myself," says Loretta. "I'm worried I'm already failing as a mother. I feel like I'm too young, too stupid to be a mother. I don't have the right food, I can't buy the baby anything."

"You're still using WIC, right?" asks Cara.

"Yeah, but then I eat something stupid like pie, and I feel like I'm going to have this baby fat forever," says Loretta.

"Loretta, do you ever think about hurting yourself?"

"Me? No. I've been thinking about death, like what it would be like and what the world would be like without me in it, but I'm not thinking about killing myself."

"I've had patients say that sometimes they think that if they didn't wake up in the morning, that wouldn't be such a bad thing," says Cara. "Do you ever have thoughts like that?"

"Yes," says Loretta. "That's it exactly. I don't want to hurt myself, but I think maybe it wouldn't be so bad to be dead. It's still scary, though, thinking like that, thinking about not being here and not existing anymore."

"What would you say if I told you I thought you might be depressed?"

"What, like postpartum depression? Isn't that when you're sad from not having enough time to take a shower and too much crying and stuff like that?"

"Well, I can see why you think that," says Cara. "Circumstances like not having a lot of support in the home and having a fussy baby can certainly contribute, and having a new baby can be a tremendous change in how you live and how you think about yourself. But there is likely a genetic component and a hormonal component and maybe other things contributing as well" (O'Hara & Wisner, 2014; Schiller, Meltzer-Brody, & Rubinow, 2015).

Loretta thinks for a moment. "I'm afraid that if I say I'm depressed you'll think I don't love Jackie—that I'm a bad mother."

"Oh Loretta, I don't think that at all," says Cara. "This has nothing to do with loving your baby. This is an illness, a sickness."

"So, do people take a medicine or something?"

"That's an option we can consider for you, but I'd like you to complete this questionnaire first. It's called the Edinburgh Depression Scale. It will give us a lot more information about where you stand and how best to help you."

"You do think I'm crazy," says Loretta. She's not angry, just matter of fact.

"I don't think you're crazy. I think you're feeling sad and you're in a tough spot in your life and that there are people, including me, who can help you."

"I just want a normal happy family," says Loretta, "With a nice husband and a couple of kids. Maybe I could even have a house and a dog someday, nice things like other people have. Other people don't even have to ask and they have everything and it makes me feel like I'm garbage, like I'm nothing. And I love my baby, honest I do, but I look at that lovely little thing and I think that every step I get closer to a nice, normal life is another step further away from her. Like, by having her, by having that part of it, it makes all the rest so much harder to make happen. Do you know what I mean?"

"I think so."

"I can't just put on my coat and walk out anymore. I can't just leave. Me and Bryan made this person, this baby, and it's my job to take care of her and it's his job to help. I used to think that was the way, that was the path, that if I could just hold on tight to him we'd come out on the other side of the birth with our nice life. But what if we're wrong? What if we come out on the other side and it's me and a baby who needs everything and a man who wants none of it?"

"How have things been since the birth?" asks Loretta. "Have you felt safe?"

"Alright," says Loretta, shrugging. "He's not here so much. I try to keep her quiet because he leaves if she cries too much, but he's not hitting. He curses some, but he's been alright."

"What do you want to do?" asks Cara.

"I want to start over, back at the beginning when I was as little as this one." Loretta gestures to the baby sleeping in Cara's arms.

"Will you take this test for me, the one about depression?"

Loretta shrugs. "If that's what you want. It doesn't make any difference."

"It might," says Cara. "There are people you can talk with, and medications. There are so many people out there who would like to help you—you and Jackie."

"You do think I'm crazy," says Loretta again. "You think I'm nuts to stay in this situation."

Cara thinks for a minute. "You know, Loretta, everyone always asks why, if it's so bad, do women stay. You know what they never ask? They never ask, if he's so unhappy with her, why doesn't he just leave?"

Think Critically

1. In this scenario, what risk factors does Loretta have for intimate partner violence? What risk factors does she have for postpartum depression? Do any of them overlap?

2. You are caring for a woman who is struggling with the cost of pregnancy and is worried about supporting her newborn. How do you discuss with her available supports in your community?

3. Imagine you have a patient who you suspect is being abused by her partner. How would you broach the topic?

4. Your patient asks you why someone would choose to breastfeed instead of bottle-feed. What are the top five reasons that you personally find compelling that you would share with the patient?

5. You overhear a fellow nursing student saying that he doesn't understand why someone would stay in an abusive relationship. What would you say?

6. You are educating a patient about how to correctly bottle-feed a baby at home. What critical points would you emphasize?

References

Breiding, M. J., Basile, K. C., Smith, S. G., Black, M. C., & Mahendra, R. (2015). *Intimate partner violence surveillance uniform definitions and recommended data elements version 2.0.* Atlanta, GA: Centers for Disease Control and Prevention, National Center for Injury Prevention and Control.

O'Hara, M. W., & Wisner, K. L. (2014). Perinatal mental illness: Definition, description and aetiology. *Best Practice and Research Clinical Obstetrics and Gynaecology, 28*(1), 3–12.

Schiller, C. E., Meltzer-Brody, S., & Rubinow, D. R. (2015). The role of reproductive hormones in postpartum depression. *CNS Spectrums, 20*(1), 48–59.

Stöckl, H., Devries, K., Rotstein, A., Abrahams, N., Campbell, J., Watts, C., & Moreno, C. G. (2013). The global prevalence of intimate partner homicide: A systematic review. *The Lancet, 382*(9895), 859–865.

Verburg, B. O., Steegers, E. A., Ridder, M. D., Snijders, R. J., Smith, E., Hofman, A., . . . Witteman, J. C. (2008). New charts for ultrasound dating of pregnancy and assessment of fetal growth: Longitudinal data from a population-based cohort study. *Obstetrics and Gynecology, 31*(4), 388–396.

Suggested Readings

Association of Women's Health, Obstetric and Neonatal Nurses. (2015). Intimate partner violence. *Journal of Obstetric, Gynecologic, and Neonatal Nursing, 44*(3), 405–408.

Centers for Disease Control and Prevention. (2016, May 3). *Intimate partner violence.* Retrieved from Injury Prevention & Control: Division of Violence Prevention: https://www.cdc.gov/violenceprevention/intimatepartnerviolence/

March of Dimes. (2015, June). *Depression during pregnancy.* Retrieved from March of Dimes: https://www.marchofdimes.org/complications/depression-during-pregnancy.aspx

Schwartz, M. R. (2012). When closeness breeds cruelty: Helping victims of intimate partner violence. *American Nurse Today, 7*(6).

13

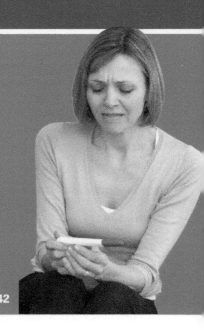

Tanya Green:
Gestational Trophoblastic Disease (Molar Pregnancy) and Advanced Maternal Age

Tanya Green, age 42

Objectives

1. Identify the characteristics and risk factors of molar pregnancies.
2. Differentiate between complete and partial molar pregnancies.
3. Describe the treatment options for molar pregnancies from the patient's perspective.
4. Identify the criteria for an advanced maternal age (AMA) pregnancy.
5. Explain why pregnancy may be more challenging for a woman of AMA.

Key Terms

Advanced maternal age
Cell-free DNA (cfDNA) screening
Choriocarcinoma
Complete molar pregnancy
Dilation and curettage (D&C)
Gestational trophoblastic disease (GTD)
Gestational trophoblastic neoplasm

Hyperemesis gravidarum
Hysterectomy
Invasive mole
Molar pregnancy
Partial molar pregnancy
Salpingoophorectomy
Theca lutein cyst

Before Conception

Tanya Green has two boys, twins who graduated from high school a year ago. She was divorced 2 years ago, after learning that her then-husband had been having an affair with a colleague, whom he subsequently married. Two years before the divorce, Tanya finished the coursework necessary to become a registered nurse. She passed her NCLEX exam on the second try. She now works as a visiting nurse. She likes the job because of its regular hours and because she rarely has to work evenings, nights, or weekends.

Tanya has had a few relationships since her divorce. One was with a fireman she met while on vacation in Jamaica. He moved in with her, but the relationship later soured. Then she dated a

much younger man, a friend of her son, for nearly 6 months before that relationship, too, failed.

"I'm not perfect," Tanya tells her friend Mandi, "But I am a heck of a lot of fun."

"You know, you can be picky and still be fun," says Mandi. "You're going to get yourself into bad trouble."

"I'm forty-two," says Tanya. "There's just so much trouble I can get into these days."

"Are you using birth control? Are you still having your period?"

"Condoms sometimes, and yes, I get my period."

"Girl, you won't just get into trouble, you are trouble," says Mandi. "It's people like you who think they can't get knocked up who end up shopping for maternity clothes. Just because you're old doesn't mean you can't get pregnant. And what about infections?"

"What? Like chlamydia? I'm clean."

"How do you know? Did you get tested?"

"No, but I feel fine."

"Look, I sat next to you during every class in nursing school. We both know that the reason people get screened for things like gonorrhea and chlamydia is that those infections don't typically cause symptoms. If you're going to go off and have fun fine, have a great time. But be smart about it. Protect yourself. Use condoms. Get screened for infections."

"You sound like an old married woman," says Tanya.

"I *am* an old married woman. And I'm boring. But I'm also your best friend. I know you have all this crazy divorcee empty nest stuff going on, but I want you to be safe."

"Okay," says Tanya, hugging her. "I'll be safe. For you."

"I don't want to be a godmother again," says Mandi.

"Come on," says Tanya. "At forty-two? What are the chances?"

She meets Mike at his mother's house. He's brought his mother her favorite flowers just because she likes them, which Tanya thinks is sweet of him. His mother needs regular nursing visits, and Tanya starts seeing a lot of Mike. She adjusts her schedule so she'll arrive at times he's likely to be there, and he brings her flowers when he brings them for his mother.

He's not wild and he's not particularly interesting. He works some sort of a desk job and he owns his house. He drives a sedan with an automatic transmission. When they go on their first date to a local restaurant with small tables, he holds the door open for her to walk through. She likes him well enough, and she's lonely.

"Are you protected?" he asks. "Are you taking the pill or something?"

"Don't worry about it," says Tanya. "We're fine."

Pregnancy

Tanya feels weird. She feels pregnant, but she also feels strange.

"It's probably because I'm so much older with this pregnancy," Tanya says to Mandi. "And it's been forever since I was pregnant. I probably just forgot what it feels like."

"I can't believe this," says Mandi. "Did you even try? Condoms? intrauterine device? Pill? Your God-given, natural common sense?"

"Thanks a lot," says Tanya.

"Well, what's the plan?" asks Mandi. "What does Mike say?"

"Not much," says Tanya.

"You didn't tell him."

"I did tell him," says Tanya. "He's not a big talker. He says he'll support me whatever I decide. He's an okay guy."

"Did he seem mad?" asks Mandi.

"Why would he be mad?" asks Tanya. "Things happen. I'm the one who got pregnant, not him."

"I can't believe you."

"I know it's a high-risk pregnancy automatically, just because of my age," says Tanya, ignoring her. "I'm classified as **advanced maternal age**. Can you believe that?" (Box 13.1).

"I don't even remember what that means," says Mandi.

Box 13.1 Risks Associated With an Advanced Maternal Age Pregnancy

- Reduced fertility and chance of conceiving
- Spontaneous abortion
  - 24.6% in women aged 35–39 y
  - 51% in women aged 40–44 y
  - 93.4% in women aged 45 y and older
- Ectopic pregnancy
- Hypertension
- Diabetes
- Placenta previa (low-lying placenta)
- Multiple (twins or more) pregnancy
- Cesarean section
- Congenital anomalies of the fetus
- Low birth weight and preterm birth
- Stillbirth

Data from Yogev, Y., Melamed, N., Bardin, R., Tenenbaum-Gavish, K., Ben-Shitrit, G., & Ben-Haroush, A. (2010). Pregnancy outcome at extremely advanced maternal age. *American Journal of Obstetrics and Gynecology, 203*(6), 558.e1–558.e7; Flenady, V., Koopmans, L., Middleton, P., Frøen, J. F., Smith, G. C., Gibbons, K., . . . Ezzati, M. (2011). Major risk factors for stillbirth in high-income countries: A systematic review and meta-analysis. *The Lancet, 377*(9774), 1331–1340; Richards, M. K., Flanagan, M. R., Littman, A. J., Burke, A. K., & Callegari, L. S. (2016). Primary cesarean section and adverse delivery outcomes among women of very advanced maternal age. *Journal of Perinatology, 36*, 272–277.

"Come on, you remember from school. It just means that something is more likely to go wrong, I think," says Tanya. "Like, I'm more likely to have a miscarriage or have complications."

"You are continuing the pregnancy, then."

"Well I haven't decided for sure. I have an appointment with my obstetrician next week."

"How is this all going to fit together?" Mandi asks. "I mean, if you wanted a baby maybe you could have talked with Mike about this and planned a little. This isn't like deciding what color to have your toes painted."

"Look, don't worry so much. Mike's good. I'm good. It'll work out. You'll see."

The following week, she goes to her obstetrician appointment. Dr. Wickham is petite and has soft gray curls that stick to her forehead. She delivered Tanya's sons by cesarean section almost 20 years ago.

"How are you feeling?" asks Dr. Wickham.

"Okay," says Tanya. "I'm feeling some pelvic pressure. I think that's normal. It's been a while. It's kind of a heavy feeling, you know?"

Dr. Wickham nods.

"I'm also having nausea. That's different for me. I didn't have any morning sickness with my boys, even though they were twins," says Tanya. "Maybe it means this one is a girl."

"Every pregnancy is different," says Dr. Wickham. "You never know. What are you doing for the nausea?"

"I have crackers in the morning before I get out of bed. It helps a little."

- Eating before rising in the morning
- Separating food and drink
- Smelling fresh lemon
- Having ginger tea
- Having ginger beer
- Drinking peppermint tea
- Consuming peppermint candies
- Taking vitamin B_6
- Receiving acupressure
- Eating small meals
- Drinking from covered cups
- Avoiding fragrant and fried foods
- Eating slowly

Dr. Wickham pulls a printed form from a drawer. "This is a list of some things you can do that will help with the nausea. Different things work for different people. Try a few and see what works for you" (Box 13.2).

"I'll need to get an amniocentesis, right? Because I'm older," asks Tanya. "Advanced maternal age and all that."

"You are more at risk for carrying a fetus with congenital anomalies because of your age," says Dr. Wickham. "Amniocentesis is a diagnostic test rather than a screening test, which means that it's confirmatory. If that testing comes back positive or negative, we don't require further testing to confirm those results. Because of your higher risk, we can skip the screening blood work, and ultrasound we typically do for lower-risk pregnancies and go straight for the diagnostic amniocentesis."

"Amniocentesis is when you put a giant needle in my abdomen," says Tanya. "I really hate needles" (see Fig. 10.2).

"It is a big needle," says Dr. Wickham, "but we do numb the area with some local anesthetic first. And we do use ultrasound to guide us to make sure that we're in the right spot for collecting amniotic fluid for testing and that we're not harming the fetus."

"Does that happen?" asks Tanya. "Hurting the fetus?"

"Rarely," says Dr. Wickham. "That happens as a result of only a tiny fraction of procedures. There is another option we can offer, however. We'd still have to stick you with needles, but it would just be for regular blood draws."

"Is it still diagnostic or just screening?"

"It's just screening. It's called cell-free DNA, or cfDNA, screening. It interprets fragments of fetal DNA, which we find in the maternal circulation in large-enough quantities to assess after about ten weeks of gestation. Although it's considered screening, it is much more accurate than the typical combined first trimester blood work and ultrasound we do. You'd still need more blood work in the second trimester, however, as it doesn't assess for neural tube defects."

"Like spina bifida?"

"Correct. The conditions that occur because of failure of the neural tube to close correctly."

"Okay," says Tanya. "So I could get this cfDNA testing done earlier than I'd normally get first trimester screening and it would

be more accurate, but either way you'd still recommend I get the amniocentesis."

"Correct," says Dr. Wickham. "Remember, though, that you always have the option of refusing any screening or diagnostic testing. You could elect to do the cfDNA screening and decide those results are all the information you want. You could decide to skip the cfDNA screening and go straight to amniocentesis. You could elect to do no screening. It's entirely up to you."

"Can I think about it?"

"Of course. You're eight weeks now. We couldn't even consider starting screening tests for at least another two weeks."

The next day Tanya starts bleeding. The blood is dark and thick and brown, like she sometimes gets at the end of her period. It's old blood, blood that has been sitting in her uterus for a while before coming out. The pelvic heaviness is still there. She throws up for the second time that morning and makes an appointment with Dr. Wickham for later in the day.

While performing the transvaginal ultrasound, Dr. Wickham's face is very still.

"That's not a happy face," says Tanya.

Dr. Wickham removes the ultrasound transducer from Tanya's vagina, pulls the protective sheath from it, wraps the sheath in her dirty glove, and throws it away in one motion. "You can sit up whenever you're ready," she says. Dr. Wickham moves the screen of the ultrasound machine so Tanya can see it. She indicates a mass of white speckled with black. "This is where I would expect to see a fetus."

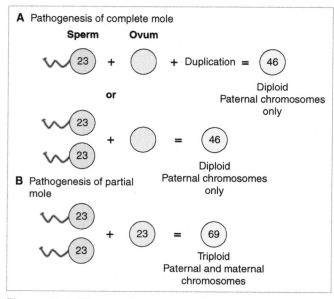

Figure 13.1. Molar pregnancy pathogenesis. Note that a complete molar pregnancy (**A**) can be caused by an egg empty of genetic material being fertilized by one or two sperm. The resulting product is diploid, having two sets of genetic material, both paternal. The partial molar pregnancy (**B**) is a normal egg with genetic material fertilized by two sperm. The resulting product is triploid, with one set of genetic material maternal and the other two sets paternal. (Reprinted with permission from Lewis, R. E., Saul, T., & Shah, K. H. [2012]. *Essential emergency imaging* [1st ed., Fig. 78.1]. Philadelphia, PA: Lippincott Williams & Wilkins.)

Box 13.3 Risk Factors for Molar Pregnancy

- Pregnancy over age 35 y
- Pregnancy under age 15 y
- Prior molar pregnancy
- History of two or more miscarriages
- Reduced consumption of dietary carotene

Data from Vargas, R., Barroilhet, L. M., Esselen, K., Diver, E., Bernstein, M., Goldstein, D. P., & Berkowitz, R. S. (2014). Subsequent pregnancy outcomes after complete and partial molar pregnancy, recurrent molar pregnancy, and gestational trophoblastic neoplasia: An update from the New England Trophoblastic Disease Center. *Journal of Reproductive Medicine, 59*(5–6), 188–194.

"I don't see anything," says Tanya.

"This is not a pregnancy that's meant to be," says Dr. Wickham. "I'm sorry. I'll have to have the diagnosis confirmed by pathology, but I'm confident this is a **molar pregnancy**. It's a form of **gestational trophoblastic disease (GTD)** and, from the looks of it, it's a **complete molar pregnancy**, which means that there is no fetus and no fetal parts."

"I don't understand," says Tanya. "I'm not pregnant?"

"Fertilization did occur," says Dr. Wickham, "and you certainly have detectable human chorionic gonadotropin, or hCG, in your bloodstream, so your body thinks you're pregnant. But what's developing in your uterus is a collection of cells that has no possibility of progressing to a normal pregnancy and birth. I'm sorry."

"Was there ever any possibility of a normal pregnancy?" asks Tanya. "Did I do something? Is it because I'm so old? I had wine before I knew I was pregnant. Was it the wine?" (Box 13.3).

"It wasn't the wine. It's not your fault or anyone's fault," says Dr. Wickham. "What happens with a molar pregnancy like this one, a complete molar pregnancy, is that an egg with no genetic material is fertilized by one or sometimes two sperm" (Fig. 13.1). "In any pregnancy, the maternal genetic material is more responsible for fetal growth, whereas the male genetic material is more responsible for placental growth. Without the maternal DNA, what you end up with is pathologic placental growth but no fetus."

"None at all?" asks Tanya. "Never?"

"In a **partial molar pregnancy**, in which two sperm fertilize one egg, fetal parts or even, very rarely, a viable fetus can develop. Also, a twin pregnancy can develop in which there is one viable fetus and one molar pregnancy. That's also very rare" (Table 13.1).

"But that's not what's happening in me," says Tanya.

"I'm sorry, no," says Dr. Wickham. "This is not a healthy pregnancy. There is no fetus."

"What do I do now? Do I just have to wait until it comes out or reabsorbs or something?"

"I wouldn't recommend that," says Dr. Wickham. "You have two options: evacuation of your uterus with a D&C or a **hysterectomy**."

"Back up," says Tanya. "Remind me what a D&C is?"

"It stands for **dilation and curettage**. It's a procedure we use to make sure that the molar pregnancy is removed from your uterus. Typically, we dilate the cervix and suction out the contents of the uterus."

"Wouldn't that option make more sense? If I have a hysterectomy I can't have any more children," says Tanya.

"That is true. But you are forty-two years old. Do you think you want to attempt another pregnancy?"

"I don't know, but I would like to have the option," says Tanya. "I didn't plan to get pregnant this time, but I didn't plan to not get pregnant. I didn't think I could get pregnant at my age, but when I did, I was excited about the idea of having another baby."

"I will tell you," says Dr. Wickham, "that even if you elect to not get a hysterectomy you will need to delay a further pregnancy. This kind of pregnancy, a molar pregnancy, can develop into a kind of neoplasm. One kind, an **invasive mole**, is less aggressive and doesn't usually metastasize, but the other, **choriocarcinoma**, does metastasize and can be dangerous if left untreated" (Table 13.2). "Both kinds are highly treatable, but we usually detect them by observing that the blood hCG levels rise or persist instead of

Table 13.1 A Comparison of Partial and Complete Molar Pregnancies

Characteristic	Type of Molar Pregnancy	
	Partial	**Complete**
Cause	Two sperm fertilize a single egg	One sperm fertilizes an egg without any of its own chromosomes.
Number of sets of chromosomes (ploidy)	Three (triploid): 69XXX, 69XXY, 69XYY	Two (diploid), from duplication of sperm genetics: 46XX; rarely, 46XY (if two sperm fertilize an egg that has no genetic material)
Fetus or fetal parts	Present	Not present
Risk of progression to gestational trophoblastic neoplasia	1%–5%	15%–20%

Table 13.2 A Comparison of Invasive Molar Pregnancy and Choriocarcinoma

Characteristic	Invasive Molar Pregnancy	Choriocarcinoma
Etiology	• Always arises from a molar pregnancy	• Arises from a molar pregnancy about 50% of the time • May arise from a normal precursor pregnancy • On rare occasions, may not be associated with pregnancy
Malignancy and metastasis	• Grows into and possibly through the uterus • May metastasize (4% of cases), most often to the lungs, vagina, and/or vulva	• More malignant than an invasive molar pregnancy • May metastasize to a variety of sites • May be more aggressive
Clinical features	• An increase or failure to decrease in blood hCG level after pregnancy • Possible bleeding or evidence of metastases	• An increase or failure to decrease in blood hCG level after pregnancy • Symptoms associated with location of metastases • May occur long after the pregnancy

hCG, human chorionic gonadotropin.

dropping after the end of the pregnancy. If you got pregnant again too soon, we'd have a much harder time identifying that this was occurring."

"But I'm forty-two," says Tanya. "If I delay I may not be able to get pregnant at all."

"I hear your concern," says Dr. Wickham. "But frankly, at your age, with a complete molar pregnancy, your chances of this becoming malignant are over fifty percent" (Elias, Shoni, Bernstein, Goldstein, & Berkowitz, 2012). "Even if we do a hysterectomy, there is about a four percent chance of that occurring" (Berkowitz & Goldstein, 2013). "If you decide to just do the D&C, I'm going to refer you to an oncologist for prophylactic chemotherapy. In fact, I may refer you anyway, even if you decide on a hysterectomy. We don't see these sorts of pregnancies much, and you may be better off with an oncologist. I know this is a lot to take in."

"So hold on. Until just a few minutes ago I was pregnant. And now I'm pregnant but not really pregnant because there's no baby. Not only that, but there's a good chance I could have cancer?"

"I'm sorry."

"It's not your fault, I just . . . my head is spinning. So my choice is between having a hysterectomy and never getting pregnant again but having a lower chance of getting cancer, or keeping my uterus, getting it suctioned out, having chemo just in case, and still maybe getting cancer?"

"Well, yes. Although I will say that your chances of developing a gestational trophoblastic neoplasm, either an invasive mole or a choriocarcinoma, are much lower with the hysterectomy than if you go with the other option and keep your uterus."

"So the mole thing and the chorio thing. Both of those are cancers?"

"The invasive mole is a less malignant neoplasm and is more localized, although it can spread, usually to the vagina and the lungs. The choriocarcinoma is more likely to metastisize and be more aggressive. We monitor for both and track them by observing your blood hCG levels, and they're both treated with chemo. Often we don't know which it is because we don't have tissue to biopsy for a definitive answer. They're both receptive to chemotherapy."

"Okay. So say I have the D&C and chemo and I get pregnant again. Am I likely to have another molar pregnancy?"

"Well, the first thing the oncologist would likely do after chemo is track your blood hCG level to make sure it gets to zero, and then for at least six months and up to a year after that point. Depending on how the oncologist assesses the risk, however, he or she may be willing to advise you to get pregnant sooner. If you were to do all that and get pregnant again, we'd want to do an ultrasound in the first trimester to make sure the pregnancy was normal. We'd also measure the blood hCG level six weeks after the birth to make sure there wasn't evidence of a neoplasm at that time."

"A neoplasm can happen that long after the molar pregnancy?"

Dr. Wickham nods. "You should also know that if you've had one molar pregnancy, you're more likely to have second."

"Really?"

"Really. It's not a huge risk, between one and two percent, but it is a risk" (Vargas et al., 2014).

"This is surreal," says Tanya. She's quiet for a moment "What else? I feel like there's more."

"Well, that's pretty much it in terms of a molar pregnancy," says Dr. Wickham. "But there are many other concerns about having a pregnancy at age forty-two, should you try for another one. There's a greater risk to you. There's a greater risk the fetus won't be healthy, and you have a greater than fifty-fifty chance of miscarriage with any given pregnancy. None of us is getting any younger, Tanya. You must not get pregnant while we're tracking your blood hCG levels. That means you'll be that little bit older when you start trying for another pregnancy, and the older you are, the worse your chances are for getting pregnant and having a healthy pregnancy."

"You think I should have the hysterectomy," says Tanya.

"I respect your choice, whatever you do. But from the perspective of your health, yes, I think a hysterectomy would be safer."

"Would they just take my uterus or would they take everything?"

"Usually, just the uterus is removed in a hysterectomy. Generally, we do not do a salpingoophorectomy for a molar pregnancy.

You get to keep your ovaries and your fallopian tubes. The surgery wouldn't initiate menopause like it would if your ovaries were removed, as well."

"So my choices are having a hysterectomy and definitely not getting pregnant or having any more babies ever again, or having a D&C and probably chemotherapy and trying again for a high-risk pregnancy maybe after six months."

"Probably longer than six months. It may be much longer, or it may be shorter. That's a discussion you'd have with your oncology team."

"My oncology team," says Tanya.

"Yes. This really is specialized care. Even if you do decide to have the hysterectomy, I'd like them on board to at least manage your initial care. You may be able to transfer back to this office at some point, but it really would be best to have a specialist at least initially. That goes double if you decide against the hysterectomy."

"What would happen if I just did nothing?"

"I would definitely not recommend that."

"But what would happen?"

"Well, we'll take your blood hCG level today. I expect it to be high. When hCG levels exceed 100,000 over a long period of time, the risk increases for hyperthyroidism, early preeclampsia in the second or even first trimester of pregnancy, and a kind of ovarian cyst called theca lutein cyst. We usually catch this kind of pregnancy so much earlier now, however, before those things can happen. It rarely gets to the point where we see this sort of effect. If you chose to put off your decision or let nature take its course, I suspect these are the sorts of complications we'd see" (Box 13.4).

Tanya thinks for a moment. "I thought I remembered something from school about getting lots of nausea and a giant uterus with a molar pregnancy."

"You're probably thinking about the classic symptoms of a molar pregnancy," says Dr. Wickham. "They include a uterus that's larger than you'd expect for gestation and hyperemesis gravidarum,

---

Box 13.4 Symptoms of Persistently Elevated (>100,000) Blood Human Chorionic Gonadotropin Level

- Hyperthyroidism
- Preeclampsia
- Ovarian theca lutein cysts
- Hyperemesis

---

which is a kind of nausea in pregnancy that is accompanied by vomiting, electrolyte imbalances, and weight loss."

"I guess," says Tanya. "I feel sick, but not that sick. I don't know about the size of my uterus."

"The classic symptoms of molar pregnancy aren't as relevant as they once were," says Dr. Wickham. "The uterus can be a little larger in early pregnancy for many reasons, not just in a molar pregnancy, and nausea in pregnancy is far from unusual. The real difference is that we now typically catch molar pregnancies so much earlier that it is too early for us to see these classic symptoms. Without the bleeding and ultrasound, your pregnancy looks totally normal, and even bleeding in early pregnancy is not uncommon, even in healthy pregnancies."

"So this is really happening."

"I'm afraid so."

"How much time do I have to think?" asks Tanya.

"The earlier you make the decision the better. Whatever you decide, I'd like to see it happen this week. I'll send the referral to oncology today, either way."

"If I were to book the hysterectomy today, could I change my mind later?"

"Yes, right up until the moment that the anesthesiologist puts you under."

"Alright. But I want to see pictures."

After Pregnancy

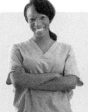

The Nurse's Point of View

Isabella: Tanya and I are going to be good friends for a while. I'm a nurse in a gynecologic oncology office who will be helping to monitor her care for the next 6 mo or more. It may be a lot longer, depending on how things go. Our usual protocol is to take blood for hCG levels weekly until the hormone is undetectable for 3 wk and then monthly for 6 mo to make sure it stays undetectable. If the levels plateau or go up, that's a bad thing (Lab Values 13.1).

Undergoing a hysterectomy can be tough emotionally on women and their families, and Tanya is no exception. I heard from the nurse in post op that she woke up crying after her hysterectomy last week. Of course, people wake up doing and saying all sorts of things after surgery. But my friend says that even with all the drugs wearing off, she was having a hard time pulling it together. She said only her friend was there for her. She has no husband or boyfriend. She hasn't mentioned the father of the pregnancy to me, and it's not my business to ask.

I know she was at higher risk for developing a neoplasia, mostly because of her age. Usually, when a molar pregnancy goes bad, it's an invasive mole, which can grow through the uterus and beyond, or a choriocarcinoma, which is worse. Sometimes it's a kind of placental site tumor, although that's rarer. I've been in gynecologic oncology for 10 y now, and I've helped care only for one woman with a placental site tumor. Tanya, however, is older, has had a complete molar pregnancy, and had blood hCG levels of over 100,000 before her surgery.

Lab Values 13.1

Assessment of Blood hCG Level After a Molar Pregnancy

Monitoring

- Weekly until hCG is not detectable in the blood
- Monthly for an additional 6 mo
- Note: Pregnancy should be prevented until hCG monitoring is complete.

Diagnostic Criteria for Gestational Trophoblastic Neoplasm

- hCG levels plateau over a 3-wk period.
- hCG levels increase more than 10% over 2 wk.
- hCG is present 6 mo after the end of pregnancy in the absence of a new pregnancy.

hCG, human chorionic gonadotropin.
Data from Soper, J. T., Mutch, D. G., & Schink, J. C. (2004). Diagnosis and treatment of gestational trophoblastic disease: ACOG Practice Bulletin No. 53. *Gynecologic Oncology, 93*(2), 575–585.

Box 13.5   Risk Factors for Developing Gestational Trophoblastic Neoplasm After a Molar Pregnancy

- Complete molar pregnancy
- Multiple molar pregnancies
- Maternal age of 35 y or older
- Uterine size in pregnancy greater than expected for gestational age
- Blood human chorionic gonadotropin level >100,000 mIU/mL
- Ovarian theca lutein cysts with a diameter >6 cm

Data from Berkowitz, R. S., & Goldstein, D. P. (2009). Molar pregnancy. *New England Journal of Medicine, 360*, 1639–1645.

That certainly puts her in a higher-risk category, even with the hysterectomy (Box 13.5).

The good news is that even if she develops a choriocarcinoma, which is less likely because she had the hysterectomy, it is a highly treatable condition. Most women can be cured with a short dose of a single chemotherapeutic agent, although some women may need additional treatment (The Pharmacy 13.1). She'll be okay. Her heart will heal over time, as well. I'm sure of it.

The Pharmacy 13.1   Methotrexate

Overview	A chemotherapeutic agent used primarily to treat neoplastic disease, but also for psoriasis, rheumatoid arthritis, and other off-label uses
Route and dosing	For gestational trophoblastic neoplasia: • IM or IV, dosed weekly, every other day, or on consecutive days repeated over several weeks • Dose of 0.3–0.5 mg/kg or 30–50 mg/m² standard
Care considerations	• Contraindicated in pregnancy • Toxic to liver • People with reduced kidney function are at greater risk for toxicity. • May cause bone marrow suppression • May induce lung disease • May cause gastrointestinal distress, bleeding, and even perforation and hemorrhage • Patients may be prone to opportunistic infections. • Gloves must be worn when handling this product.
Warning signs	• Monitor for signs of hypersensitivity (anaphylaxis), including shortness of breath, swelling of the tongue or throat, vomiting, itchy rash, low blood pressure, and lightheadedness • Monitor renal function, complete blood count, and liver function tests • Monitor for gastrointestinal distress and bleeding • Monitor for signs of infection • Monitor for pulmonary symptoms, especially a dry, nonproductive cough

IM, intramuscular; IV, intravenous.

Think Critically

1. You have a 43-year-old patient who is considering a pregnancy next year. What should you discuss with her in terms of pregnancy timing and risks?

2. You are caring for a newly pregnant patient who is considering cell-free DNA testing instead of amniocentesis. What points should you be careful to discuss when talking about the advantages and disadvantages to this approach?

3. You have a patient who has received no prenatal care and is presenting in the second trimester with hyperemesis gravidarum. She is diagnosed with a complete molar pregnancy. What additional complications do you know she is at risk for as a result of this diagnosis?

4. Your patient has just been diagnosed with a complete molar pregnancy. How do you describe to her the differences between a complete and partial molar pregnancy?

5. You have a patient who is trying to decide between a dilation and curettage and a hysterectomy with a molar pregnancy. How can you as the nurse help facilitate her decision-making?

6. Your patient was diagnosed with a molar pregnancy and treated with a dilation and curettage. She has had three assessments of her blood hCG level in a row, and the levels have been subclinical every time. When do you expect her next blood hCG test to be scheduled?

References

Berkowitz, R. S., & Goldstein, D. P. (2013). Current advances in the management of gestational trophoblastic disease. *Gynecologic Oncology, 128*(1), 3–5.

Elias, K., Shoni, M., Bernstein, M., Goldstein, D., & Berkowitz, R. (2012). Complete hydatidiform mole in women aged 40 to 49 years. *Journal of Reproductive Medicine, 57*(5–6), 254–258.

Soper, J. T., Mutch, D. G., & Schink, J. C. (2004). Diagnosis and treatment of gestational trophoblastic disease: ACOG Practice Bulletin No. 53. *Gynecologic Oncology, 93*(2), 575–585.

Vargas, R., Barroilhet, L. M., Esselen, K., Diver, E., Bernstein, M., Goldstein, D. P., & Berkowitz, R. S. (2014). Subsequent pregnancy outcomes after complete and partial molar pregnancy, recurrent molar pregnancy, and gestational trophoblastic neoplasia: An update from the New England Trophoblastic Disease Center. *Journal of Reproductive Medicine, 59*(5–6), 188–194.

Suggested Readings

American Cancer Society Medical and Editorial Content Team. (2016). *About gestational trophoblastic disease*. Retrieved from http://www.cancer.org/cancer/gestationaltrophoblasticdisease/detailedguide/gestational-trophoblastic-disease-what-is-g-t-d

March of Dimes. (2016). *Pregnancy after age 35*. Retrieved from http://www.marchofdimes.org/complications/pregnancy-after-age-35.aspx#

Monchek, R., & Wiedaseck, S. (2012). Gestational trophoblastic disease: An overview. *Journal of Midwifery and Women's Health, 57*(3), 255–259.

O'Connor, A., Doris, F., & Skirton, H. (2014). Midwifery care in the UK for older mothers. *British Journal of Midwifery, 22*(8), 568–577.

Unit 2
Maternity and Newborn Nursing for Uncomplicated Pregnancies

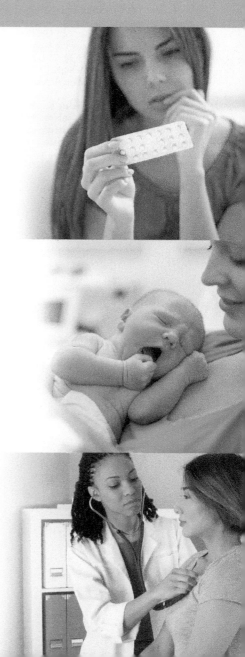

14 Before Conception

225

Objectives

1. Discuss cultural considerations when working with a patient and how to provide culturally competent care.
2. Describe different family structures.
3. Explain how maternity healthcare is funded.
4. Explain how a client's preconception age, health history, and health status can affect pregnancy and birth.
5. Identify the components of a health history.
6. Identify and explain the function of key female reproductive hormones.
7. List and discuss the phases and processes of the reproductive cycle.
8. Identify the steps of gametogenesis and fertilization.
9. Identify the different ways of confirming a pregnancy.

Key Terms

Acrosome
Amenorrhea
Ampulla
Arthralgia
Autosomes
Biochemical pregnancy
Capacitation
Chadwick's sign
Cohabitating-parent family
Conception
Corona radiata
Corpus luteum
Cortical reaction
Diploid
Endometrial
Extended family
Fertilization
Follicle-stimulating hormone (FSH)
Gametogenesis
Gonadotropin-releasing hormone (GnRH)

Goodell's sign
Graafian follicle
Haploid
Hegar's sign
Hook effect
Hypothalamic–pituitary–ovarian (HPO) axis
Infundibulum
Luteinizing hormone (LH)
Menstrual cycle
Microcephaly
Nuclear family
Oocyte
Oogenesis
Organogenesis
Ovarian cycle
Periodontal disease
Postnatally
Spermatogenesis
Teratogen
Zona pellucida

Cultural Context

Culturally competent care does not, as many students worry, require understanding all of the nuances of an individual's culture. Instead, cultural competence is about recognizing and respecting a person's culture and integrating the aspects important to that individual into their care (Fig. 14.1). Culture does not simply mean that a person comes from another country or practices a religion not typical to the region. Culture may also include variations of profession, age, gender identity, disability, income level, sexual orientation, and education.

You'll recall from Chapter 9 that Nancy is married to Missy, a woman. Sexual orientation is a facet of Nancy's culture. Does the gender of Nancy's partner change care considerations? If so, how?

Key to cultural competence is good communication and an open mind. A nurse cannot assume that an aspect of a culture is important to a patient simply because they identify with that culture. For example, a patient may identify with a religion that prohibits blood donation, but the patient is receptive to such a donation. Another patient may carefully follow the diet prescribed by a particular belief system but choose not to participate in the ceremonial aspects of the religion. It is not essential that nurses understand all aspects of a culture but rather that the nurse respects a patient's cultural context and takes the individual patient's preferences and beliefs into consideration when providing care.

Another aspect of cultural competence is the importance of respecting the value a patient may place on a belief or tradition that may impact their care or the delivery of that care. Culture can include food, religion, language, beliefs, values, and the nature of various relationships, but it can also color how a patient views illness and what care is appropriate and acceptable. These culturally based expectations may at times contradict or compete with prescribed care. It is a job of the nurse to help the patient understand the recommendations of the healthcare team while also striving to understand, respect, and integrate the patient's perspective. Ultimately, all decisions are the patient's.

You'll recall from Chapter 12 that Loretta is poor and young. Although we often think of culture in terms of ethnicity or place of origin, factors such as age and socioeconomic status also contribute to an individual's culture. Loretta is in a relationship with Bryan, a man who is abusive. It is clear to Cara, a home health nurse visiting Loretta, that her relationship with Bryan is detrimental to her mental and physical health. For Loretta, however, the relationship is acceptable and in some ways desirable within the confines of her own cultural context, which includes multigenerational intimate partner violence.

Contrasts with our healthcare system and a patient's culture may be overt, as in members of immigrant or refugee populations who may maintain traditions and beliefs customary to a particular culture, or they may be more subtle. The decision by many patients to pursue traditional and alternate means of healthcare, such as acupuncture, acupressure, naturopathy, and herbalism, must also be respected as cultural variations. Failure to acknowledge the part that different traditions and beliefs play in the life of the individual can be polarizing and distressing for both the patient and the nurse and is the antithesis of holistic care. It would not be appropriate, for example, to dismiss a patient's trust in herbal medicine. It would be appropriate, however, to determine the specifics of that care, as certain herbs or supplements may conflict with Western medications or be dangerous in the context of the patient's overall health.

Family Context

Many people often think of the family structure of a husband, wife, and children as being a typical family structure. In fact in 2014, 40% of babies born in the United States were born to women who are not married and were either single or in a partner relationship but unmarried (Hamilton, Martin, Osterman, Curtin, & Mathews, 2015). As of 2013, approximately 27% of female same-sex couples and 11% of same-sex male couples in the United States were raising children (Gates, 2013). An additional 22% of children in the United States are being raised in a blended married family (Pew Research Center, 2015). The remaining

CULTURAL DESTRUCTIVENESS	CULTURAL BLINDNESS	CULTURAL AWARENESS	CULTURAL SENSITIVITY	CULTURAL COMPETENCE	CULTURAL HUMILITY
Making everyone fit the same cultural pattern and excluding those who don't fit—forced assimilation. Emphasis on differences as barriers.	Do not see or believe there are cultural differences among people. Everyone is the same.	Being aware that we all live and function within a culture of our own and that our identity is shaped by it.	Understanding and accepting different cultural values, attitudes, and behaviors.	The capacity to work effectively and with people, integrating elements of their culture—vocabulary, values, attitudes, rules, and norms. Translation of knowledge into action.	The lifelong process of self-reflection and self-critique that begins, not with an assessment of a client's belief but rather an assessment of your own.

Figure 14.1. Cultural competence continuum. (Reprinted with permission from Silbert-Flagg, J., & Pillitteri, A. [2018]. *Maternal and child health nursing: Care of the childbearing and childrearing family* [8th ed., Fig. 2.3]. Philadelphia, PA: Lippincott Williams & Wilkins.)

children, approximately 4% to 5%, were being raised without parents (Pew Research Center, 2015). The context of a family includes its support systems. Family structure is not necessarily indicative of available support. A woman who is married may have a spouse who is not supportive, whereas a woman without a partner may have a committed and supportive **extended family**.

Nuclear Family

A traditional **nuclear family** is conceptualized as a married mother, father, and their biologic or adopted children. Less than half of children in the United States today are being raised in such a family (Blackwell, 2010). Of our case studies, 7 of the 13, (Bess Gaskell in Chapter 1, Tatiana Bennett in Chapter 2, Letitia Richford in Chapter 5, Rebecca Sweet in Chapter 6, Graciella Munez in Chapter 8, Lexi Cowslip in Chapter 10, and Edie Wilson in Chapter 11) are all married.

Same-Sex Parents

In June of 2015, the United States Supreme Court made same-sex marriage a legal right nationwide. Although this victory was remarkable, families headed by couples of the same sex, such as Nancy and Missy from Chapter 9, are far from unusual. The United States Census from 2014 showed that 17.3% of same-sex households included children. Same-sex couples are approximately four times as likely to be raising an adopted child and they are six times more likely than heterosexual parents to be raising foster children (Gates, 2013).

Depending on individual circumstances and communities, women who are pregnant and identify as lesbian and men who are expecting the birth of a child by surrogacy may feel judged or marginalized. Adoptive parents may feel equally unsupported. It is important to remember to follow the lead of these parents and acknowledge any same-sex partner of a pregnancy just as you would the father of a heterosexual pregnancy (Fig. 14.2).

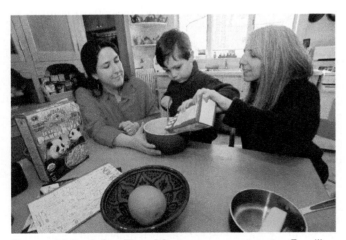

Figure 14.2. A family with same-sex parents. Families with same-sex parents are composed of parents of the same sex—married, in a civil union, or otherwise committed to parenting together—and their biologic, adopted, or foster children. (Reprinted with permission from Kyle, T., & Carman, S. [2016]. *Essentials of pediatric nursing* [3rd ed., Fig. 2.3C]. Philadelphia, PA: Lippincott Williams & Wilkins.)

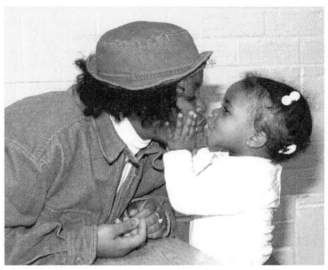

Figure 14.3. Single-parent family. More than a fourth of children in the United States are raised in single-parent families, most often by their mothers. (Reprinted with permission from Allender, J. A., Rector, C., & Warner, K. D. [2014]. *Community and public health nursing: Promoting the public's health* [8th ed., unnumbered figure in Chapter 28]. Philadelphia, PA: Lippincott Williams & Wilkins.)

Nancy and Missy each experience pregnancy and give birth to healthy baby boys. Although both women chose to grow their families with the help of donor sperm, other same-sex couples may choose to adopt, care for foster children, or employ a gestational carrier. Some may also bring into their current relationship children from a prior relationship.

Single-Parent Family

In 1960, only 9% of children lived in single-parent families. Today, 26% of children live with only one parent, who is six times more likely to be a mother rather than a father (Pew Research Center, 2015; Blackwell, 2010). In our case studies, only Sophie Bloom of Chapter 4 was without a partner. Single mothers, regardless of whether they became single prior to, during, or after a pregnancy, may experience more financial insecurity. In fact, in the United States, 35% of single-mother families live in poverty (Misraa, Mollerb, Stradera, & Wemlinger, 2012). In addition, these mothers may report an increased susceptibility to illness and to stress and reduced social support (Rousou, Kouta, Middleton, & Karanikola, 2013). These additional stressors will likely impact decisions as diverse as whether or not to continue a pregnancy, and how to fill out a birth certificate (Fig. 14.3).

You'll recall from Chapter 4 that Sophie is a single mother. Sophie was aware when she made the choice to parent that the decision came with compromises to her finances, career, and living situation.

Blended Family

Approximately 16% of children are living in a family with a stepsibling, half-sibling, and/or stepparent (Pew Research Center, 2015). Children may move between multiple blended families if both parents have started new relationships. The parent may have remarried or may be cohabitating without marriage. When a family is blended in the absence of a new marriage, it may be referred to as a **cohabitating-parent family**.

Financial Context

According to a 2013 report, the average charges for pregnancy care that includes a vaginal birth are $32,093. The average cost for similar pregnancy care inclusive of a cesarean section is $50,373. Commercial insurers will generally negotiate the fees down to a little over half this cost. Medicaid will reimburse the hospital by an average of $9,131 for a vaginal birth and $13,590 for a cesarean section. Care of the newborn during the initial hospitalization and 3 months of care was paid at an average rate of $5,809 for a vaginal birth and $11,193 for a cesarean birth by commercial payers, and $3,014 and $5,607, respectively, by Medicaid (Truven Health Analytics, 2013).

For Sophie in Chapter 4, the cost of healthcare was a significant part of her early decision-making about her pregnancy that spurred her to leave her job and move back into her parents' home in a state with superior Medicaid provisions related to pregnancy and birth.

In the United States, healthcare may be paid for in cash by individuals or by private insurance such as BlueCross BlueShield, Cigna, or MVP purchased by the individual or employer. Healthcare may also be paid for using state and federal money via Medicaid, Medicare, Title X funding, and other public funding. In the United States in 2015, 49% of people were insured through an employer, 7% of people bought insurance policies as individuals, 20% of people were insured by Medicaid, 14% were insured by Medicare, 2% took advantage of other public funding, and 9% remained uninsured (The Henry J. Kaiser Family Foundation, n.d.).

The Cost of Healthcare

Healthcare costs in the United States were equivalent to 17.1% of the gross domestic product (GDP) of this country in 2014. This means that of every $100 made in the United States in 2014, $17.10 was spent on healthcare. For context, the world healthcare costs are equivalent to 9.9% of the world GDP, and the European Union healthcare costs are equivalent to 10% (The World Bank, n.d.). Per capita healthcare spending in the United States in 2013 was $9,086. In the same year, Canada spent $4,569 per person, and Australia spent $4,115 per person. Cost drivers in the United States include a heavier reliance on expensive imaging

technology, comparatively low investment in social services that may mitigate health outcomes, and the higher overall cost of healthcare (Squires & Anderson, 2015).

Higher costs are not associated with superior outcomes. In 2015, the infant mortality rate was 6 out of every 1,000 births in the United States, 4 out of every 1,000 births in the European Union, 3 out of every 1,000 births in Australia, and 4 out of every 1,000 births in Canada (United Nations Children's Fund, 2015). The maternal mortality rate is 14 out of every 100,000 live births in the United States, 7 out of every 100,000 live births in Canada, 6 out of every 100,000 live births in Australia, and 8 out of every 100,000 live births in the European Union (World Health Organization, United Nations Children's Fund, United Nations Population Fund, World Bank Group, & the United Nations Population Division, 2015). Life expectancy in the United States in 2013 was 78.8 years, when compared with 82.2 years in Australia and 81.5 years in Canada (Organization for Economic Cooperation and Development, 2015).

Medicaid

Medicaid is healthcare coverage funded by a combination of state and federal funds. Eligibility for Medicaid is decided at the state level with the enforcement of minimal federal requirements. The Patient Protection and Affordable Care Act (ACA) gave states the option of extending Medicaid eligibility to people living at or below 133% of the federal poverty level, although some states may elect to provide coverage to people with a higher income level. For example, in Vermont, adults with household incomes at or above 138% of the federal poverty level are eligible, but children and pregnant women are eligible with household incomes up to 317% of the federal poverty level (Vermont Health Connect, 2015). Eligibility for Medicaid in pregnancy depends on income, household and, in some states, the trimester of pregnancy. Services covered in pregnancy may be comprehensive or narrower, depending on the pregnant woman's state of residence. Women are covered through the month in which their 60-day postpartum period ends (Singh, 2013).

Susan has Medicaid coverage for her pregnancy in Chapter 3 (as do Sophie in Chapter 4 and Loretta in Chapter 12). Nationwide, approximately half of pregnancies and births are covered by Medicaid.

Additionally, several states have Medicaid-funded waiver programs that provide contraception and other family planning services to low-income individuals who do not otherwise qualify for Medicaid. An example of one such program in California is estimated to have prevented 200,041 unintended pregnancies in 2009. Each averted adult pregnancy is estimated to save $5,469 in public funding in social services, including healthcare and welfare. Each averted adolescent pregnancy is estimated to save $11,077, for a total savings of $4.08 billion (Bixby Center for Global Reproductive Health, 2012). The Hyde Amendment, a rider first attached to an appropriations bill in 1976 and renewed annually and routinely since, prohibits spending federal spending on abortion, although individual states may elect to use state dollars to fund abortions for Medicaid patients.

Title X

The Title X appropriation for 2016 distributed among 4,400 family planning clinics was $286 million (The Henry J. Kaiser Family Foundation, 2015; National Family Planning & Reproductive Health Association, n.d.). In 2013, the funds provided services to 4.6 million patients and prevented an estimated 1 million unplanned pregnancies and 345,000 abortions (Hasstedt, 2015). The program was first enacted under the Nixon administration to provide comprehensive family planning services to low-income individuals. Approximately 92% of Title X beneficiaries are women. The funding allows clinics to provide family planning and reproductive health services free of charge for people at or below 100% of the federal poverty level and to provide the same services to higher-income individuals on a sliding scale (The Henry J. Kaiser Family Foundation, 2015). Abortion services are not covered by Title X funds in keeping with the Hyde Amendment. Title X funds may be administered as an entirely separate program or as a subprogram of Medicaid.

Medicare

People aged 65 and over who are eligible to collect social security are also eligible for Medicare (Table 14.1). People with certain disabilities or end-stage kidney disease may also be eligible for coverage. Medicare is broken into four categories: A, B, C, and D. Medicare Part A is hospital insurance, Medicare Part B is medical insurance, Medicare Part C refers to a system of private insurance providing the Medicare Part A and Part B coverage, and Medicare Part D is prescription drug coverage. Parts B and D are partially funded by fees paid by subscribers and Part A also includes a deductible and co-pays. Medicare does cover pregnancy services and screening for sexually transmitted infections (STIs) and cervical cancer. There is no federal requirement that Medicare covers contraception, although as of 2015, 920,000 women of reproductive age received insurance coverage from Medicare (The Henry J. Kaiser Family Foundation, 2015).

Private Insurers

Before the ACA came into being, a 25-year-old woman could pay 81% more for health insurance than a similarly aged man did for a policy that did not include maternity coverage. Of the policies sold prior to the ACA, 62% did not cover maternity care. Since the ACA, however, insurance companies may no longer charge women more for coverage, and they are required to cover maternity and newborn care. Insurers are also obligated to pay for contraceptive counseling and methods for women without a co-pay, even if a woman has not met her insurance deductible. Employers may opt out of the contraception rule for reasons of religious conviction. Employers may elect to provide abortion coverage as part of their policies for employees, although the law does not require it. Policies purchased prior to the passage of the ACA are not subject to these rules (U.S. Department of Health and Human Services, 2015).

Health Context

The first few weeks of a pregnancy can be the most critical, yet only 31% of women in the United States report receiving preconception care (Oza-Frank, Gilson, Keim, Lynch, & Klebanoff, 2014). **Organogenesis**, the formation of fetal organs, occurs primarily between weeks 3 and 10 of gestation, thus potentially making early education and interventions critical to a healthy pregnancy, mother, and neonate (Fig. 14.4). Compounding the problem is that approximately 50% of pregnancies are unplanned, suggesting that all women of reproductive age should have regular access to some form of preconception counseling regardless of their immediate or long-term reproductive intentions. Opportunities for providing preconception counseling include office visits for contraception, vaginitis, STIs, and periodic wellness visits. The three overarching goals of preconception care are risk identification, patient education, and interventions to mitigate identified risk.

In Chapter 5, Letitia's preconception counseling was extensive as she sought care after not becoming pregnant after nearly a year of trying. When Bess and Jake decided to try for another child, Bess had her intrauterine system removed and received brief preconception counseling regarding prenatal vitamins (Chapter 1). Lexi had a similar experience (Chapter 10).

Table 14.1 A Comparison of Medicaid and Medicare

Characteristic	Medicaid	Medicare
Description	A joint state and federal program of healthcare insurance	A federal program of healthcare insurance
Source of funding	State and federal funds	Federal funds
Eligibility requirements	Determined at the federal level, but individual states may opt to extend coverage to people outside of the mandated federal minimum.	Determined by age (65 y and over). People with certain disabilities who are not yet age 65 y are also covered, as are people with end-stage kidney disease.

Fetal Development Chart

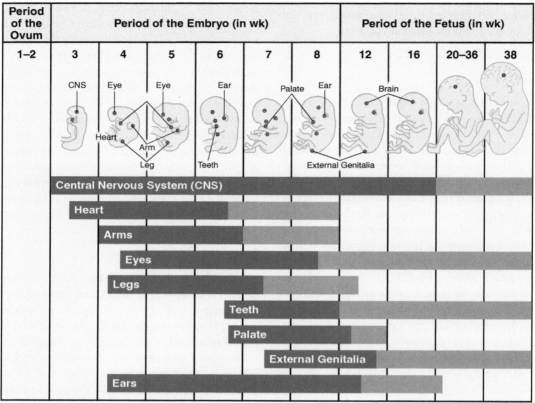

● Most common site of birth defects

Figure 14.4. Organogenesis. Critical periods of fetal development. Dark blue denotes highly sensitive periods. (Adapted from the National Organization on Fetal Alcohol Syndrome. Reprinted with permission from Morton, P. G., & Fontaine, D. K. [2013]. *Critical care nursing: A holistic approach* [10th ed., Fig. 11.1]. Philadelphia, PA: Lippincott Williams & Wilkins.)

Multiple factors comprise risk. In pregnancy, age, medical history, environmental exposures, and information gained from a physical exam or laboratory test may all be pertinent to risk identification.

Age

In the United States, the average maternal age at the time of the first birth is 26.3 years (Centers for Disease Control and Prevention, 2016). Based on age alone, pregnancies between the ages of 20 and 34 are not considered high risk. Pregnancies after age 34 years, such as Lexi Cowslip's in Chapter 10 and Tanya Green's in Chapter 13, are considered high risk because of advanced maternal age and largely because of the higher potential for diminished egg quality and an increased risk for pregnancy-related complications as well as the greater likelihood of preexisting health conditions. Adolescent pregnancies under the age of 20 years, such as Loretta Hale's in Chapter 12, are considered high risk primarily because of socioeconomic considerations.

Adolescence

Approximately 10% of young women between the ages of 15 and 19, like Loretta Hale in Chapter 12, become pregnant annually, and these pregnancies are less likely to be planned

(Finer & Zolna, 2016). Of the adolescent pregnancies that end in a birth, approximately 20% are to young women who already have at least one child (Centers for Disease Control and Prevention, 2013). Pregnant adolescents often seek care later in pregnancy (Fig. 14.5). Teens are often abandoned by their partner in pregnancy and may struggle to complete their education. Both single parenting and diminished education limit opportunities going forward, and adverse pregnancy outcomes are more common (Oringanje, Meremikwu, Eko, Esu, Meremikwu, & Ehiri, 2016).

Loretta was 18 years old when she became pregnant for the first time. The pregnancy was unintended. Women 18 to 24 years old are at particularly high risk for an unintended pregnancy. Other risk factors Loretta had for unintended pregnancy included poverty, cohabitating with her partner, and lack of a high school diploma. These disadvantages made Loretta's unintended pregnancy more likely, whereas, in turn, the pregnancy and birth of baby Jackie made it less likely that Loretta would complete her education or gain financial security (Finer & Zolna, 2016).

The major developmental task of adolescence is the formation of the sense of self, which may be at odds with the developmental

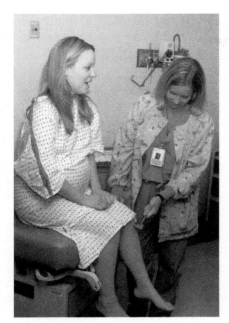

Figure 14.5. Adolescent mother. Adolescents often delay accessing care and may have social and economic disadvantages more routinely than do older mothers. (Reprinted with permission from Bowden, V. R., & Greenberg, C. S. [2013]. *Children and their families: The continuum of nursing care* [3rd ed., Fig. 7.10]. Philadelphia, PA: Lippincott Williams & Wilkins.)

tasks of pregnancy and becoming a new parent. A lower level of maternal competence may be achieved when compared with an older mother. Teens with high levels of support and self-esteem may demonstrate superior competence and improved adaptation to their new situation. Strong family support and social programs for pregnant teens and new mothers in the home, community, and schools improve outcomes (Angley, Divney, Magriples, & Kershaw, 2015; Barkana et al., 2014).

Nurses should be aware that the laws regarding disclosure of adolescent healthcare information to parents or guardians vary from state to state. Some states protect the privacy of teens regarding issues pertaining to sexual behavior, including contraception, STIs, and abortion. Others require consent from or notification of a parent or guardian for some or all of these services. It is important, however, even in states that do not require disclosure of information, that adolescents are encouraged to discuss their healthcare decisions with parents or guardians (American Medical Association, 2014). Nurses also have a legal duty to report abuse of teens and other minors according to individual state laws.

Advanced Maternal Age

Between 1973 and 2012, the rate of first births to women between the ages of 35 and 39 went from 1.7 out of every 1,000 births to 11 out of every 1,000 births. The rate of first births for women between the ages of 40 and 44 went from 0.5 out of every 1,000 births in 1985 to 2.3 out of every 1,000 births in 2012 (Mathews & Hamilton, 2014). The overall mean age of firsttime mothers rose from 21.4 to 26.3 between 1970 and 2014 (Mathews & Hamilton, 2014; Centers for Disease Control and Prevention, 2016). It is

important that women considering a pregnancy know that their likelihood of getting pregnant spontaneously (fecundity) begins to reduce at the age of 32 years (American College of Obstetricians and Gynecologists, 2014). Equally, it is important that women not rely on their diminishing fertility as a method of contraception. Women are still considered to have the potential for pregnancy until they are deemed menopausal a year after their last period. Although less likely to become pregnant, pregnancies in women age 35 and over are more likely to end in abortion than in any other age group (Finer & Henshaw, 2006).

As discussed in Chapters 10 and 13 with Lexi Cowslip and Tanya Green, a pregnancy is considered advanced maternal age at age 35 and very advanced maternal age at 45, although variations exist. In many cases pregnancies for women over 35, and even women over 50, have excellent outcomes. There is a higher risk of complications, however, including higher risks for fetal abnormalities, spontaneous abortion, hypertension, neonatal morbidity, and complications in labor and delivery (see Box 13.1).

Tanya's pregnancy at the age of 42 years in Chapter 13 was unintended although not unwelcome. Her pregnancy was a molar pregnancy, however, which is not viable. Although this is a rare pregnancy complication, molar pregnancies are more common in women of advanced maternal age, as well as among adolescents.

Health History

A health history is a series of questions that help a healthcare provider learn about a patient. Although people often think of a health history as limited to physical ailments, important aspects of a health history include a sexual history, questions about self-care and health promotion, a review of systems, biographic data, allergies, diet, sleep patterns, immunizations, workplace and environmental hazards, eating habits, and a family history.

The nurse typically need not memorize all of the information to be collected because prompts are provided by the electronic health record or by a form filled out in advance by the patient. It is, however, important that the nurse know *how* to ask the questions.

The nurse should conduct the interview in private. Partners, friends, and other families may be present, but only after the nurse has asked the patient privately if this is what she wishes. If a patient declines to have others present during any point of her visit, her wishes must be respected.

The nurse should provide a comfortable seat for the patient and refer to her by her name or title (such as Dr. Munez, or Mrs. Smith) unless the patient invites the nurse to address her by her first name. The use of open body language is important to gain trust. The nurse should make sure she's facing the patient and not a computer screen. Arms should be uncrossed. Leaning toward the patient indicates interest. The nurse should reassure patients that all aspects of the conversation are confidential, unless she wishes the information to be shared, and that all questions are relevant. Trust is a critical component of the nurse–patient relationship. In some cases, the nurse must earn this trust over several visits.

Often, open-ended questions are best for guiding the conversation while allowing the patient to provide important information. Direct questions may limit the person answering to the scope of the question, such as, "What did you eat for dinner?," as opposed to, "Tell me about the food you eat." The first question gives you a focused snapshot that may not reflect the person's typical intake. The second question allows the person answering to provide a broader answer that may yield more pertinent information. Direct questions may, however, be important when specifics are required. If you need to know the day of a woman's last period, "Tell me about your period," is a less helpful question than, "When was the first day of your last period?"

A health interview is not a one-sided conversation. Nurses are the facilitators of the conversation, and it is the responsibility of the nurse to ask questions and encourage answers. Different techniques that may be appropriate to use during the course of a patient interview include the following:

- Interpretation: This is the summarizing of a patient's narrative as a means of clarification. For example, "What I'm hearing you say is that you're mostly feeling pain in your right abdomen, but sometimes it's on both sides or in the middle."
- Reflection: Reflection, unlike interpretation, is repeating a patient's own words or phrases. For example, "Okay, so 'more achy than painful.'"
- Confrontation: This is the process of pointing out an inconsistency in what a patient is expressing or how she is behaving. For example, "You're telling me that you feel confident about when your last period was, but you'd like a dating ultrasound. Tell me what you're hoping to learn from this ultrasound today."
- Clarification: This technique is requesting clarification of what a patient has said. For example, "When you say that you don't feel well, what do you mean by that?"
- Empathy: This technique involves making statements that acknowledge a patient's feelings. For example, "That must have been frustrating for you."
- Facilitation: This technique involves encouraging the patient to continue the narrative by the use of words or body language, such as nodding. For example, "Tell me more about that."

Family Planning

Approximately 50% of pregnancies in the United States are unplanned (Centers for Disease Control and Prevention, 2015). Reducing this number is the priority of a number of governmental and nonprofit organizations, including the Centers for Disease Control, Healthy People 2020 (Box 14.1), Planned Parenthood, and the Oregon Foundation for Reproductive Health.

In 2012, the Oregon Foundation for Reproductive Health launched the One Key Question© initiative. The initiative recommends asking all women aged 18 to 44 if they would like to be pregnant in the next year. Women answering "yes" may be

provided with preconception counseling, including advice about lifestyle modification. Patients answering "no" will be provided with contraceptive counseling and access (Oregon Foundation for Reproductive Health, 2012). Similarly, in 2014, the Centers for Disease Control recommended a set of three routine questions to help guide clinicians in supporting women's reproductive health choices (Step-by-Step Skills 14.1).

Reproductive History

We record a woman's pregnancy history in one of two ways: G0P0 or G0T0P0A0L0. In both systems, the G stands for "gravidity," or the number of pregnancies. With the first system, the P stands for "parity," or the number of births. The GP (Gravidity and Parity)

Step-by-Step Skills 14.1

Centers for Disease Control and Prevention Quality Family Planning Recommendations

Ask the following three questions to every woman of a fertile age to determine the need for contraception or preconception counseling:

1. Do you have any children now?
2. Do you want to have (more) children?
3. How many (more) children would you like to have and when?

Data from Gavin, L., Moskosky, S., Carter, M., Curtis, K., Glass, E., Godfrey, E., . . . Zapata L; Centers for Disease Control and Prevention. (2014). Providing quality family planning services: Recommendations of CDC and the U.S. office of population affairs. *Morbidity and Mortality Weekly Report, 63*(RR04), 1–29.

Box 14.2 GTPAL and GP

GTPAL

G: The number of pregnancies a woman has had in her lifetime

T: The number of pregnancies that have ended at term (37 wk plus)

P: The number of pregnancies that have ended preterm (20–37 wk)

A: The number of pregnancies that end by spontaneous or elective abortion before 20 wk. This information may also be reported as two separate numbers, with the first representing spontaneous abortions and the second elective abortions. A patient with a pregnancy history including one spontaneous abortion and one elective abortion might have "1/1" following the A or "2," depending on the system used.

L: The number of living children

GP

G: The number of pregnancies a woman has had in her lifetime

P: The number of pregnancies carried to viable gestational age (variously defined as 20–24 wk gestation)

GTPAL, Gravidity, Term, Preterm, Abortion, Living children; GP, Gravidity and Parity.

and GTPAL (Gravidity, Term, Preterm, Abortion, Living children) systems were reviewed earlier in Chapter 2 during Tatiana's pregnancy and can also be found in Box 14.2.

Reproductive Notation System: GTPAL

Although the GTPAL reproductive notation system seems simple on first review, it has some variations that can be challenging, which are discussed below.

- *Gravidity:* This term refers to any pregnancy, regardless of how it ended. Pregnancies that ended in a birth, miscarriage, and abortion should all be accounted for.
- *Term:* The T stands for term, indicating all pregnancies that ended at or beyond 37 weeks. It is important to count the number of pregnancies and not the number of infants born.

Box 14.3 American Congress of Obstetricians and Gynecologists Recommendations for Further Delineating Term Pregnancies in Documentation

- *Early term:* 37 0/7 wk through 38 6/7 wk
- *Full term:* 39 0/7 wk through 40 6/7 wk
- *Late term:* 41 0/7 wk through 41 6/7 wk
- *Postterm:* 42 0/7 wk and beyond

Data from The American College of Obstetricians and Gynecologists Committee on Obstetric Practice Society for Maternal-Fetal Practice. (2015). *Definition of term pregnancy.* Washington, DC: ACOG.

A twin pregnancy is still counted as one. It should be noted that a more current recommendation calls for further dividing term into early term, full term, late term, and postterm (The American College of Obstetricians and Gynecologists Committee on Obstetric Practice Society for Maternal-Fetal Practice, 2015) (Box 14.3). Outcomes and risk factors for a neonate and mother vary widely in the 5 or more weeks accounted for in this category, and this modification is an effort to systematically capture this variation.

- *Preterm:* A pregnancy should be counted as preterm if it ends between 20 and 36 weeks 6 days. As with term, a twin pregnancy would still be counted as one, not two.
- *Abortion:* Any pregnancy ending prior to 20 weeks should be accounted for as an abortion, regardless of the number of fetuses included in a pregnancy. A twin pregnancy ending prior to 20 weeks would still be counted as one. This category may also be split into spontaneous abortions and elective abortions. If a woman had one spontaneous abortion and one elective abortion, it may be accounted for as 1/1.
- *Living Children:* This category accounts for children alive at the time of the recording (Table 14.2).

Obstetric History

Although GTPAL and GP give us a helpful shorthand for understanding the number of pregnancies a woman has had and

Table 14.2 A Sample Obstetric History Using GTPAL and GP

	G	T	P	A	L	G/P
The client is pregnant for the first time.	1	0	0	0/0	0	1/0
The client's pregnancy ends in an elective abortion.	1	0	0	0/1	0	1/0
The client is pregnant again, but has a spontaneous abortion.	2	0	0	1/1	0	2/0
The client is pregnant for a third time with twins and delivers at 30 wk.	3	0	1	1/1	2	3/1
The client is pregnant again and delivers a stillborn infant at 38 wk.	4	1	1	1/1	2	4/2
The client is pregnant for the final time. She delivers a viable infant at 40 wk.	5	2	1	1/1	3	5/3

GTPAL, Gravidity, Term, Preterm, Abortion, Living children; GP, Gravidity and Parity.

the overall outcomes of those pregnancies, this is not the sum of our data collection. Other information may help us better predict considerations and complications that can help guide care (Table 14.3).

Gynecologic History

Although most women of reproductive age will not have a complicated gynecologic history, it is important to identify those who do. A current or past history of gynecologic problems may create risk for the woman going forward regardless of whether or not she attempts a pregnancy. They may also impede her chances for pregnancy (Table 14.4).

Medications

A complete medication list is a critical part of preconception planning and should be inclusive of over-the-counter medications, prescriptions written for people other than the patient, herbal preparations, and other supplements. A **teratogen** is any substance a woman may be exposed to that causes damage to pregnancy, leading to physical or functional birth defects. A medication may be a teratogen, and an estimated 94% of

women will take a medication while pregnant or breastfeeding, and 70% of women will take a medication during the critical first trimester of pregnancy when the pregnancy is particularly vulnerable (Temming, Cahill, & Riley, 2016). Some medications that may be used routinely in otherwise healthy women who are not pregnant without a reasonable expectation of undue harm may be strongly contraindicated in pregnancy.

In the United States, the Food and Drug Administration (FDA) requires specific labeling of medications to reflect risk in pregnancy (Table 14.5). This designation has long been a pregnancy category (A, B, C, D, or X) that informs as to the broad nature of the risk of the medication to the pregnancy. A rule change of 2014 has revised the reporting of the impact of medications in pregnancy to make it more specific and informative (Department of Health and Human Services Food and Drug Administration, 2014). Unfortunately, the risk of teratogenicity is ill-defined for a majority of prescription medications. Of the prescription medications approved by the FDA between 1980 and 2011, the teratogenic risk has been determined for fewer than 2% (Adam, Polifka, & Friedman, 2011).

Table 14.3 Obstetric History

Information Collected	Rationale
Dates of prior deliveries	A distant history of past delivery may help us understand a woman's current knowledge base. A very recent past delivery within the prior year may increase her chance of pregnancy complications, including preterm birth.
Gestational age at deliveries	A significant risk for preterm birth is a prior preterm birth. A woman who delivers postterm is more likely to subsequently deliver postterm.
Mode of delivery	A past cesarean section may preclude a future vaginal birth or make a future cesarean section more likely. A past vaginal surgical birth may indicate the need for one in the future or the preemptive intervention of a cesarean section.
Type of anesthesia	Prior use of anesthesia and any complications associated with it should be carefully recorded.
Location of delivery	Delivery may be planned to occur at home, in a hospital, or in a birthing center. In some cases, as in the case of a delivery planned to occur in the home but transferred to a hospital by necessity or in the case of a very precipitous birth, the venue may not be the one preferred by the patient prior to the birth.
Outcome	Although the GTPAL notation provides us with a general outline for the outcome, it does not capture variations such as ectopic pregnancies, stillbirths, gestational age at the time of abortion, or precise gestational age at the time of birth.
Sex of the child	The sex of existing children may inform how a family views the preferred sex of future children. A sex-linked chromosomal defect may also be revealed.
Birth weight and percentile according to gestational age	Past small-for-gestational-age or large-for-gestational-age infants may highlight complications of past pregnancy such as malnutrition, hypertension, or gestational diabetes.
Length of labor	The length of past labors may indicate the length of future labors and thus assist in planning.
Complications	Complications of past pregnancies, including maternal complications such as preeclampsia, fetal complications such as intrauterine growth restriction, and neonatal complications such as respiratory distress syndrome, should be carefully recorded.

GTPAL, Gravidity, Term, Preterm, Abortion, Living children.

Table 14.4 Gynecologic History

Age at menarche (first menses)	Both early and late menarche may be associated with certain physical conditions as well as socioeconomic correlations.
Date of LMP	The first day of the most recent menses is referred to as the LMP. This date helps us predict when a woman may be most likely to conceive.
Cycle length and regularity	The length of a woman's cycle from the beginning of one menses to the beginning of the next menses can help predict when she has ovulated and will be most fertile. The regularity of her cycle (i.e., consistency of length of cycles) is helpful for determining how accurately we can determine ovulation based on cycle length alone. A short cycle, particularly in older women, may indicate reduced fecundity (see Menstrual Cycle below).
STIs	Patients seeking pregnancy should be screened for STIs (see Assessments below). Past STIs may have a negative impact on a pregnancy. Gonorrhea and chlamydia may cause permanent mechanical damage to the fallopian tubes, impairing fertility. Patients testing positive for HIV must be treated during pregnancy to prevent transmission to the newborn. Patients with genital herpes must be treated immediately before and during delivery to prevent transmission. If a mother tests positive for hepatitis B, measures will need to be taken after birth to prevent the neonate from contracting the disease; if a woman is not vaccinated at the time of preconception care, vaccination is recommended. A woman with hepatitis C may pass the infection onto her child.
Gynecologic surgeries	Certain surgeries may make pregnancy or labor more challenging or even dangerous. For example, surgery on the cervix may make it less likely to dilate, whereas surgery on the uterus may make it more likely to rupture during labor. Surgery for a woman with endometriosis may improve her chances of getting pregnant.
Gynecologic conditions	Gynecologic conditions such as endometriosis can make it more difficult to get pregnant, whereas a malformed uterus may make it less likely that a pregnancy can be successfully carried to term.

LMP, last menstrual period; STIs, sexually transmitted infections.

Table 14.5 Food and Drug Administration Pregnancy Risk Categories

Category	Description
Current categories	Older medications still use these current categories but are gradually transitioning to the updated criteria, listed below.
A	Human studies have demonstrated fetal safety in the first trimester, and there is no evidence of harm in later trimesters.
B	Either animal studies have not demonstrated harm but there are not sufficient human studies OR animal studies have shown harm but human studies have not.
C	Animal studies demonstrate harm and there are not sufficient human studies, but benefit may outweigh risk, OR sufficient studies are not available.
D	There is evidence of harm in humans, but therapeutic benefits may outweigh this harm.
X	There is evidence of fetal harm, and the risk clearly outweighs benefits in pregnant women.
Updated criteria	New labels will contain specific information and guidance pertinent to the specific medications within the following three categories instead of providing the general lettered categories of the current criteria.
Pregnancy	This section includes information about pregnancy and registries that women taking medications during pregnancy may participate in to further knowledge. It also includes information pertinent to labor and delivery.
Lactation	This section includes information on the potential impact of a complication on a breastfeeding infant.
Females and males of reproductive potential	This section includes information on pregnancy testing and contraception considerations, as well as the potential for infertility.

Adapted from the Department of Health and Human Services Food and Drug Administration. (2014). *Content and format of labeling for human prescription drug and biological products; requirements for pregnancy and lactation labeling.* Silver Spring, MD: Author.

Because we have such limited information about the teratogenicity of medications, use is often minimized as much as possible in preconception and pregnancy to avoid harm to the pregnancy or potential pregnancy. Older drugs with better known safety data may replace newer drugs with less well-established information for some patients. If no replacement medication is available, dosing may be minimized to continue treating the mother while reducing fetal exposure.

Chronic Diseases

Optimization of the treatment and control of chronic diseases is important to the health of both the mother and the pregnancy. Examples of chronic diseases that are relatively common in women of reproductive age include diabetes, hypothyroidism, hypertension, and lupus. A poorly controlled diabetic is at higher risk for a pregnancy with congenital defects. Optimal replacement of the thyroid hormone is important because uncontrolled hypothyroidism can compromise neurologic development in the fetus. Some medications used to control hypertension, such as angiotensin-converting enzyme inhibitors and angiotensin receptor blockers, are not recommended in pregnancy. Women treated for conditions such as lupus will often need to work closely with their prescribing provider to adjust medications to minimize exposure of the pregnancy to teratogens, and lupus-related comorbidities may complicate the pregnancy (see Chapter 19 for more about preexisting conditions).

Although Susan in Chapter 3 and Nancy in Chapter 9 were screened early in pregnancy for preexisting diabetes, in Chapter 8, Gracie worked hard in advance of becoming pregnant to minimize her chances of becoming diabetic while improving her chances of becoming pregnant.

Substance Use

Substance use includes street drugs such as heroin, cocaine, crack, methamphetamines, and marijuana, but also refers to alcohol use, smoking, and medications prescribed for someone else. There is no known safe amount of alcohol consumption in pregnancy and no known safe point in the pregnancy to drink (Centers for Disease Control and Prevention, 2016). Because of this, many healthcare providers will recommend that a woman seeking to conceive abstain from alcohol completely, or at least during the last 14 days of their menstrual cycle when a pregnancy may have begun but is not yet detectable. Street drugs in pregnancy can also cause serious health issues before, during, and after a pregnancy and all illicit drug use is ideally addressed prior to a pregnancy. Approximately 5% of women will take illicit drugs in pregnancy (March of Dimes, 2016). Medications prescribed for someone other than the patient, just as medications prescribed for the patient, may be contraindicated during pregnancy. Similarly, smoking cessation should be strongly encouraged prior to attempting conception (see Chapter 19).

Vaccinations

Although inert vaccines such as influenza and the tetanus, diphtheria, and pertussis (Tdap) may be given in pregnancy, vaccinations containing live virus are contraindicated because of a theoretical chance of fetal harm. Titers may be drawn for measles, mumps, and rubella and vaccinations administered prior to conception if the patient is not immune (Box 14.4).

Weight and Nutrition

Weight loss in pregnancy is generally not advised, and the amount of recommended weight gain is dictated by the patient's body mass index (BMI) (see Fig. 9.4) before conception. Patients are strongly encouraged to reach and maintain a goal weight between the BMIs of 18.5 and 30 prior to seeking pregnancy. Obesity in pregnancy is associated with birth defects, infertility, gestational diabetes, and other complications. A maternal BMI below 18.5 is correlated with low birth weight and preterm birth (Tabet, Flick, Tuuli, Macones, & Chang, 2015).

All patients of a reproductive age should be encouraged to take a supplement including at least 400 to 800 µg of folic acid daily in advance of conception and through pregnancy, although patients with certain medical conditions may be advised to take more. The neural tube closes between 18 and 26 days post conception; thus, waiting to start folic acid until after a pregnancy has been confirmed may well be too late. Adequate folic acid intake could eliminate approximately 70% of neural tube defects such as spina bifida (Cavalli, 2008). In the United States, however, food products have been supplemented with folic acid since 1998 without evidence of a reduction in neural tube defects, although studies done before 1998 predicted benefit (Viswanathan, Treiman, & Kish-Doto, 2017). A balanced diet including lean protein, fruits, vegetables, and a minimum of processed foods and simple sugars should be encouraged for all patients, including women seeking pregnancy.

Box 14.4 Vaccinations in the Preconception Period and Pregnancy

Vaccinations That May Be Administered During Pregnancy

- Annual influenza vaccine
- Tdap during each pregnancy (27–36 wk)
- Hepatitis B virus

Vaccines That Should Be Administered Preconception or Postpartum if Indicated

- Measles, mumps, and rubella virus
- Varicella virus
- Hepatitis A virus
- Pneumococcal virus
- Polio virus
- Human papillomavirus

Environmental Exposures and Infections

Environmental toxins may also be teratogens and cause birth defects, childhood cancer, impaired brain development, miscarriage, and stillbirth. The American Congress of Obstetricians and Gynecologists advise that, beginning prior to pregnancy, women limit their exposure to large fish with high mercury content, pesticides, solvents, dietary animal fat, BPA-containing plastics, processed foods, and fruits and vegetables that have not been thoroughly washed (American Congress of Obstetricians and Gynecologists, n.d.; Renzo, et al., 2015). Many toxins pass the placenta to impact the fetus, and toxins may also be found in breast milk.

Infectious diseases are another form of environmental exposure. The Zika virus became an emergent health concern in 2016 (World Health Organization, 2016). Zika is transmitted by mosquito and, in 20% of people infected, will result in a mild fever, rash, arthralgia (joint pain), or conjunctivitis. It can also be transmitted sexually. A very small number of adults infected will develop neurologic symptoms. It is not believed at this time that children infected postnatally (occurring after birth) have different manifestations of the infection than adults do, or that there are long-term consequences of an infection (Karwowski, et al., 2016).

For an infant born to a woman who has contracted Zika, however, the infection can be devastating. The current rate of complications resulting from maternal infection is unknown, but in one small study, 29% of pregnancies to infected women resulted in fetal abnormalities including microcephaly (Vouga & Baud, 2016). Infection may also result in spontaneous abortion, stillbirth, fetal growth restrictions, and other complications.

Couples seeking pregnancy and pregnant women are advised to avoid traveling to active Zika areas (http://www.cdc.gov/zika/geo/index.html). Women with confirmed exposure should wait for at least 8 weeks after the onset of symptoms or last possible exposure to attempt to conceive. Men should avoid attempting conception with their partner for at least 6 months since the onset of symptoms or most recent possible exposure (Petersen et al., 2016).

Social Situation

All patients presenting for preconception care should be evaluated for financial and food insecurity, as well as support systems and intimate partner violence (IPV), and nurses should not wait for the patient to introduce the topics. Some issues, such as IPV, may require long-term trust building before the problem can be meaningfully addressed with the patient, whereas others, such as financial and food insecurity, may best be mitigated by helping connect patients with federal, state, and community resources. Interprofessional help from a social worker can be critical to this process.

Current Health Status

Physical Examination

A physical exam by a nurse practitioner, nurse midwife, physician assistant, or physician may be done as part of preconception care. It would be highly unusual for a registered nurse to be responsible for such an examination. A physical examination, if indicated, would be a part of routine preventative care. There are no examination elements that are specific to preconception in a well woman. For example, a Pap test should be done only at the time of a preconception visit if a woman was due for one per the standard screening or follow-up schedule. A woman with a preexisting health condition may, however, require specific examination elements as determined by her care team.

Besides a blood pressure and BMI assessment, exam elements may include auscultation of heart and lungs, a thyroid exam, an abdominal and genital exam, and an exam of the mouth. The oral exam is important because periodontal disease (oral disease) has been associated with poor pregnancy outcomes, including preterm birth. Conversely, pregnancy can also have a negative impact on periodontal health (Armitage, 2013). Depending on the state of residence, some Medicaid patients may have access to dental coverage. Other Medicaid patients may have access to dental coverage only during pregnancy, making it an optimal time to seek dental care that may have been deferred because of cost (Medicaid.gov, n.d.). Optimally, patients will receive dental care prior to pregnancy, although pregnancy is not a contraindication to dental care.

Laboratory Studies

Laboratory studies are individualized to the patient. All patients regardless of risk are tested for human immunodeficiency virus (HIV) on an opt-out basis, meaning that they are screened unless they decline. Screening for other STIs including gonorrhea, chlamydia, hepatitis B, hepatitis C, and syphilis will be based on risk, although opt-out screening is common as the presence of STIs may cause subfertility, pregnancy complications, and vertical transmission (infection passed from a pregnant woman to the fetus). Other lab studies are also based on risk (Table 14.6).

Preconception Anatomy and Physiology

The female reproductive cycle can be described in the context of the ovarian cycle or the menstrual (uterine or endometrial) cycle. The ovarian cycle refers to the activity of the follicles within the ovaries, and the menstrual cycle refers to the endometrial changes within the uterus. Both are hormonally regulated (Fig. 14.6).

The female reproductive system consists of internal and external structures (Fig. 14.7). Students are encouraged to review the anatomy and physiology of the reproductive system presented in previous courses. A brief overview is provided here.

External Genitalia

The overarching term for the external female genitalia is vulva. This term includes all of the following structures:

- Bartholin's glands: Glands on either side of the vaginal vestibule that secrete mucus for vaginal lubrication
- Clitoris glans: The visible portion of the clitoris and the most sensitive erogenous zone of the female body
- Fourchette: The skin at the posterior of the vulva

- Hymen: A membrane partially covering the opening of the vagina
- Labia majora: The exterior skin folds, which are hair-bearing in mature females and extend from the mons pubis to the perineum
- Labia minora: The inner mucosal skin folds, which extend from the mons pubis to the perineum
- Mons pubis: A rounded area, padded with fat, that is anterior to the pubic symphysis; hair-bearing in mature females
- Urethra meatus: The opening to the urethra
- Perineum: The area between the vulva and the anus
- Skene's glands: Glands at the anterior of the vulva that drain into the urethra
- Vaginal vestibule: The opening into the vagina. When referred to as the vulvar vestibule, the term includes the urethral meatus.
- Introitus: The vaginal orifice

Table 14.6 Preconception Lab Work

Test	Rationale
Rubella	Documentation of vaccination is sufficient. If no documentation exists, a titer should be drawn. Lack of rubella immunity is an indication for preconception vaccination.
Genetic carrier testing	If a woman or her partner has a personal or family history of a heritable disease or if ethnicity indicates risk, she may elect to seek genetic carrier testing prior to seeking pregnancy. Testing may inform decisions related to planning a pregnancy, sperm or oocyte donation, preimplantation genetic evaluation, early prenatal testing, or avoidance of pregnancy, surrogacy, or adoption. Testing may be done in collaboration with a genetic counselor for the following: • Cystic fibrosis • Thalassemia • Fragile X syndrome • Sickle cell trait • Spinal muscular atrophy Screening more common for the Ashkenazi Jewish population: • Tay-Sachs disease • Canavan disease • Familial dysautonomia • Mucolipidosis IV • Niemann Pick disease type A • Fanconi anemia group C • Bloom syndrome • Gaucher disease
Hemoglobin A_{1c}	Patients with a diagnosis of diabetes type 1 or 2 or patients at risk for diabetes should be screened preconception. Optimized glucose control prior to conception and through pregnancy diminishes the chance of diabetes-related complications, including pregnancy loss and birth defects. The hemoglobin A_{1c} allows for assessment of glucose control over the prior 2 or 3 mo.
Tuberculin skin test	Women who have a family member with active pulmonary tuberculosis or who have had limited contact with a person with a highly active form of the disease should be screened. Women who have traveled to areas with a high prevalence of the disease should also be screened. The concern in this case is not so much the disease injuring the pregnancy but rather that the treatment is potentially teratogenic and will optimally be completed prior to pregnancy.
Lead	High lead levels can have a negative impact on the mother and the fetus. Of particular concern are women living in homes built prior to 1978 and women who may be exposed by work or a hobby to certain art paints, car repair, plumbing, soldering, pottery glaze, guns, glass working, plastic manufacturing, battery manufacturing, rubber manufacturing, printing, lead working, and some hair dyes and cosmetics. Levels that are safe for adults may be toxic to a pregnancy, leading to pregnancy loss, preterm birth, and low birth weight (Agency for Toxic Substances and Disease Registry, 2016).
Serum phenylalanine	Phenylketonuria is generally diagnosed shortly after birth during routine newborn screening. A woman who has not been assessed previously and is suspected to have phenylketonuria should be screened. Dietary management of the disorder in pregnancy will help protect the fetus.

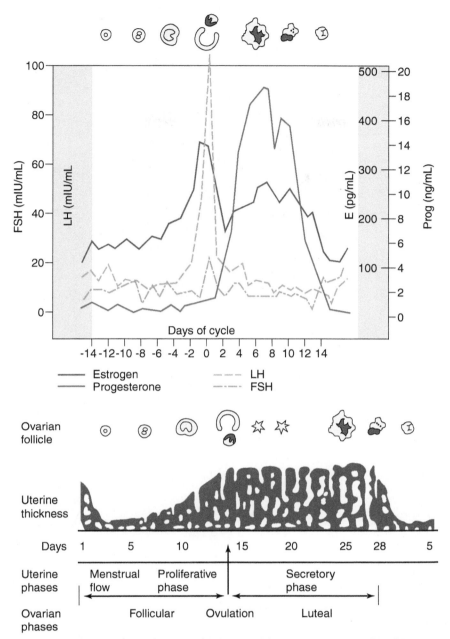

Figure 14.6. Changes during reproductive and menstrual cycles. (Top) Plasma hormone concentrations in the normal female reproductive cycle. **(Bottom)** Ovarian events and uterine changes during the menstrual cycle. LH, luteinizing hormone; FSH, follicle-stimulating hormone. (Reprinted with permission from LifeART image copyright © 2018 Lippincott Williams & Wilkins. All rights reserved.)

Internal Genitalia

The major structures of the internal female genitalia include the ovaries, fallopian tubes, vagina, and uterus, of which the cervix is a part. Structures of the internal genitalia are briefly detailed here.

- Ovaries: Paired reproductive organs that produce ova, estrogen, testosterone, and progesterone and are approximately the size and shape of walnuts
- Uterus: Also called the "womb"; the site of implantation of fetal growth and development. The innermost layer of the uterus, the endometrium, sheds with menstruation. When a pregnancy implants in the endometrium, the

endometrium is referred to as the decidua. The middle layer, the myometrium, is primarily smooth muscle. The outer layer is called the serosa or perimetrium. A nonpregnant uterus is approximately the size and shape of an upside-down pear.

- Fundus: The uppermost, rounded part of the uterus, which contains the greatest volume of smooth muscle
- Corpus: The main body of the uterus, located between the isthmus and the fallopian tubes
- Isthmus: The area of the uterus between the cervix and the corpus, which has thinner, more narrow musculature

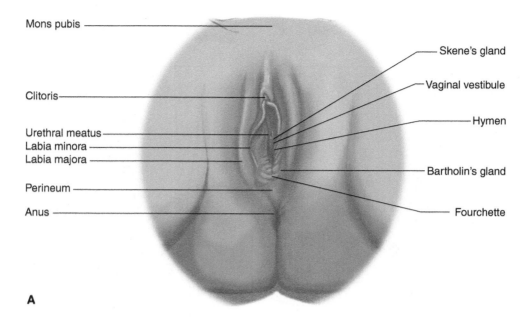

Mons pubis

Clitoris

Urethral meatus
Labia minora
Labia majora

Perineum

Anus

Skene's gland

Vaginal vestibule

Hymen

Bartholin's gland

Fourchette

A

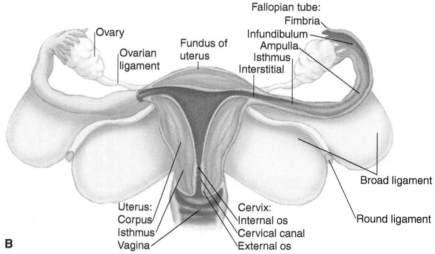

Ovary

Ovarian
ligament

Fundus of
uterus

Fallopian tube:
Fimbria
Infundibulum
Ampulla
Isthmus
Interstitial

Broad ligament

Round ligament

Uterus:
Corpus
Isthmus
Vagina

Cervix:
Internal os
Cervical canal
External os

B

Figure 14.7. Female reproductive system. (A) External genitalia. **(B)** Internal genitalia. (Reprinted with permission from Craven, R. F., Hirnle, C. J., & Jensen, S. [2013]. *Fundamentals of nursing* [7th ed., Fig. 41.2]. Philadelphia, PA: Lippincott Williams & Wilkins.)

- Vagina: A muscular tube that extends from the vestibule to the cervix and that accommodates penetrative sex and childbirth
- Cervix: The lowest portion of the uterus, which extends into the vagina. It is approximately an inch in diameter and has a small opening at its center called the os.
  - Internal os: The opening between the cervix and the body of the uterus
  - Cervical canal: The canal between the internal os and outer os
  - Outer os: The opening between the cervix and the vagina
- Fallopian tubes: A pair of cilia-lined tubes between the uterus and the ovaries, also referred to as uterine tubes
  - Interstitial: The portion of the tube that travels through the musculature of the uterus
  - Isthmus: The portion of the tube between the interstitial and the **ampulla**

- Ampulla: The distal portion of the tube, located between the isthmus and the **infundibulum**, where **fertilization** most often occurs
- Infundibulum: The funnel-shaped part of the tube, located between the fimbriae and the ampulla
- Fimbriae: A fringe of tissue at the end of the fallopian tube, not attached to the ovary, that gently draws the ovum into the fallopian tube with a sweeping motion
- Ovarian ligaments: A pair of ligaments attaching the ovaries to the uterus
- Round ligaments: A pair of ligaments starting where the fallopian tubes join the uterus (the "uterine horns") and ending deep in the pelvis. Stretching of these ligaments in pregnancy can cause pain.
- Broad ligaments: A wide ligament connecting the uterus to the pelvis

Female Reproductive Hormones

Interactions between the ovaries, anterior pituitary, and hypothalamus (the **hypothalamic–pituitary–ovarian [HPO] axis**) regulate the female reproductive cycle (Fig. 14.8). The hypothalamus, a region of the forebrain, releases **gonadotropin-releasing hormone (GnRH)**. In response, the anterior pituitary secretes **luteinizing hormone (LH)** and **follicle-stimulating hormone (FSH)**. FSH is the primary hormone responsible for maturation of the follicles of the ovary that will subsequently release eggs for fertilization. LH is responsible for the final maturation and release of the egg from the follicle. Levels of LH peak approximately 12 to 24 hours prior to follicle rupture (ovulation).

After follicle rupture, LH stimulates the ruptured follicle, free of its ovum, in a process called luteinization. The follicle, now called the **corpus luteum**, produces large amounts of progesterone and a smaller amount of estrogen, which was the dominant hormone prior to ovulation. The progesterone is responsible for the secretory phase of the endometrial cycle, during which the lining of the uterus is nourished and maintained in the event of a fertilized embryo and implantation.

The corpus luteum begins to lose its secretory function approximately a week after ovulation, lowering levels of both progesterone and estrogen. This lowering of progesterone and estrogen stimulates the hypothalamus to produce GnRH, thus cueing the anterior pituitary to produce FSH and LH, thus restarting

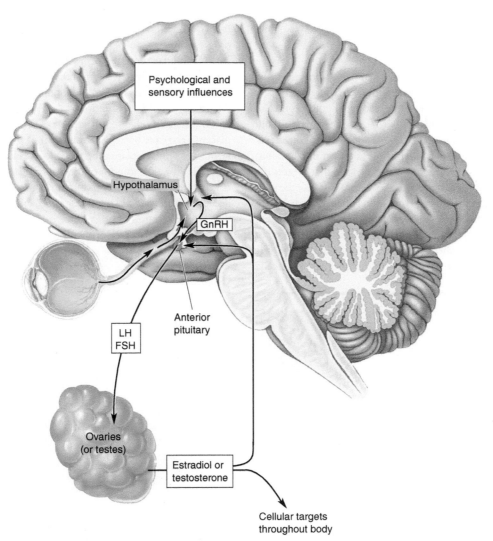

Figure 14.8. Bidirectional interactions between the brain and the gonads. The hypothalamus is influenced by both psychological factors and sensory information, such as light hitting the retina. GnRH from the hypothalamus regulates gonadotropin (luteinizing and FSH) release from the anterior pituitary. The testes secrete testosterone and the ovaries secrete estradiol, as directed by the gonadotropins. The sex hormones have diverse effects on the body and also send feedback to the pituitary and hypothalamus glands. GnRH, gonadotropin-releasing hormone; LH, luteinizing hormone; FSH, follicle-stimulating hormone. (Reprinted with permission from Bear, M. F., Connors, B. W., & Paradiso, M. A. [2015]. *Neuroscience* [4th ed., Fig. 17.7]. Philadelphia, PA: Lippincott Williams & Wilkins.)

the cycle. If conception occurs, however, the pregnancy cues the continuation of the corpus luteum and the maintenance of the endometrium (called the decidua in pregnancy) by producing human chorionic gonadotropin (hCG), thus inhibiting GnRH and the response of the anterior pituitary.

Estrogen

Estrogen is secreted by the ovaries and, to a smaller degree, by the corpus luteum after ovulation. Small amounts of estrogen are also secreted from the renal cortex and from fat cells. Estrogen is the hormone primarily responsible for female patterns of fat distribution, including the development of breasts. Estrogen is the dominant hormone in the first half of the menstrual cycle prior to ovulation and causes proliferation (growth) of the endometrial lining after menstruation as well as the contributing to the maturation of the ovarian follicles.

Progesterone

Progesterone is produced by the corpus luteum after rupture of the ovarian follicle. In pregnancy, progesterone production is eventually taken over from the corpus luteum by the placenta. In the second half of the menstrual cycle after ovulation, progesterone helps maintain the uterine lining as well as relaxing the smooth muscle of the uterus and causing vasodilation, all of which would support implantation of a pregnancy. Progesterone is also the hormone that creates the small rise in body temperature (about 0.3°C to 0.6°C) we see after ovulation. This rise is helpful when tracking the menstrual cycle using body temperature because it lets us know that ovulation has occurred. A subsequent dip approximately 2 weeks later tells us that fertilization did not occur, whereas a stabilized rise in temperature after the expected time of menstruation tells us that pregnancy is likely.

When Letitia was checking her temperature every morning when trying to become pregnant (Chapter 5), she was monitoring for the rise in temperature caused by progesterone in the second half of pregnancy, indicating that ovulation had occurred.

Reproductive Cycle

Ovarian Cycle

The ovarian cycle is broken into two phases, the follicular phase prior to ovulation and the luteal phase after ovulation. The luteal phase is 12 to 14 days for most of a woman's reproductive life. As a woman approaches menopause, the luteal phase shortens, making successful implantation and maintenance of a pregnancy less likely. Variation in the length of a woman's menstrual cycle (the time between the first day of one menses and the first day of the next menses) is typically due to variations in the follicular phase and not in the luteal phase. The follicular phase may be as short as 8 days, but may also be considerably longer, with the average follicular phase lasting 14 to 21 days. As the name implies, during the ovarian cycle, the follicular phase concerns maturation of the follicles and the associated **oocytes**.

At the end of the follicular phase, the now mature follicle is called the **graafian follicle** and measures about 5 to 10 mm, about the size of a pencil eraser or a dime. The cells lining the follicle are the granulosa cells, which will produce the progesterone after ovulation when the empty follicle becomes the corpus luteum.

The enlarging of the graafian follicle containing the ovum brings it closer to the capsule, the outside, of the ovary. The tissue between the follicle and the outside of the ovary thins and finally ruptures, expelling the ovum. The cilia of the fimbriae of the fallopian tube sweep the ovum into the fallopian tube where may be fertilized. The cilia within the fallopian tubes will help move the egg toward the uterus, where it will arrive approximately 72 to 96 hours after ovulation.

With ovulation begins the luteal phase of the ovarian cycle. The luteal phase refers to the activity of the corpus luteum that results from the ruptured graafian follicle under the influence of the LH from the anterior pituitary gland. The corpus luteum produces the progesterone that creates a hospitable environment within the uterus for a fertilized ovum. The corpus luteum begins to disintegrate after a week unless the ovum is fertilized within a 6-to-24 hour window and successfully implants into the endometrium of the uterus. Should fertilization and implantation occur, the pregnancy will secrete hCG, which stimulates maintenance of the corpus luteum until the placenta can take over the production of progesterone. Failure of fertilization and implantation will cue increased production of LH and FSH from the anterior pituitary as the corpus luteum begins to degenerate. When the corpus luteum is no longer functional, either because fertilization did not occur or because the placenta has taken over the production of progesterone, it becomes a connective scar tissue, referred to as the corpus albicans (Fig. 14.9).

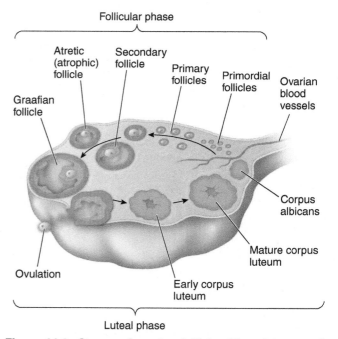

Figure 14.9. Stages of ovarian follicles. The origin, growth, and rupture of an ovarian follicle and the formation and retrogression of a corpus luteum. (Reprinted with permission from Braun, C. A., & Anderson, C. M. [2011]. *Pathophysiology* [2nd ed., Fig. 12.5]. Philadelphia, PA: Lippincott Williams & Wilkins.)

Menstrual Cycle

The menstrual cycle (also called the uterine cycle) refers to the period of time between the start of one menses to the start of the next. The duration of the entire cycle is usually 21 to 35 days, with a majority of the variation stemming from the variation of the length of time between the start of menstruation and ovulation and not the time between ovulation and the next menses. The menstrual cycle can be broken down into four phases: menstrual, proliferative, secretory, and ischemic.

- Menstrual: Menstruation occurs when an ovum is not fertilized and the lining of the endometrium is no longer maintained by progesterone released by the corpus luteum. Menstruation typically begins 12 to 14 days after ovulation. Many women find factors such as illness and stress cause the timing of their menses to vary, whereas others find that their menstrual cycle remains consistent regardless of circumstances. Although the loss of blood may seem significant, the menstrual flow consists of blood, vaginal, and cervical secretions, bacteria, and other cellular debris. The loss of actual blood is only 10 to 80 mL over 2 to 7 days. Menses may be red to brown depending on the duration of time the blood has pooled in the uterus. Older blood is brown, whereas newer blood is redder.
- Proliferative: During the proliferative phase, the endometrial glands enlarge and the endometrium thickens in response to estrogen produced by the ovaries. Close to ovulation, the cervical mucus becomes particularly elastic with a consistency akin to egg white.
- Secretory phase: After ovulation, the endometrium is maintained by progesterone. Increased blood and secretions to the endometrium, as well as reduced contractility of the uterine, smooth muscles and create a hospitable environment for implantation. If fertilization occurs, this process continues. If it does not occur, the final phase of the menstrual cycle, the ischemic phase, begins.

- Ischemic phase: The ischemic phase begins as the corpus luteum begins to disintegrate, eliminating the source of progesterone. Vascular changes lead to necrosis and the breakdown of the endometrial lining, which sheds during menstruation, leaving behind the tips of the glands from which a new endometrium will grow.

Conception

Gametogenesis, or the creation of gametes (ova and sperm), occurs by a process called meiosis. Unlike mitosis, which creates two daughter cells identical to the parent cell, meiosis creates four cells, each with half of the chromosomes of the parent cell creating cells that are haploid (one set of chromosomes) rather than diploid (two sets of chromosomes [Table 14.7; Fig. 14.10]).

Oogenesis

Females are born with a complement of approximately 1 to 2 million oocytes in their ovaries. This diminishes to approximately 200,000 to 400,000 by puberty. During the 30 to 40 years of a woman's reproductive life span, one ovum that may be fertile for up to 24 hours is typically released every month in the absence of pregnancy, lactation, or hormonal suppression of ovulation. This accounts for the release of approximately 400 to 500 ova in a lifetime. The remaining ova will reabsorb so that, by the time of menopause, the store is depleted.

Meiosis requires two divisions of an oocyte. The primary oocyte has 46 chromosomes. Meiosis I of the oocyte splits and extrudes a polar body and half of its chromosomes, leaving a secondary oocyte and one polar body, each with 23 chromosomes. These oocytes begin this process of meiosis I when a female is still in utero, and then the process pauses until puberty. After puberty, this process continues, oocyte by oocyte, once a month, as part of a female's reproductive cycle. Immediately after meiosis I, meiosis II begins and then pauses. The secondary oocyte

Table 14.7	Meiosis Versus Mitosis	
Characteristic	**Meiosis**	**Mitosis**
Processes	Production of reproductive cells only	Growth, tissue repair, and cell replacement
Reduction of chromosome number	From diploid (46 chromosomes; two sets) to haploid (23 chromosomes; one set)	None
Number of stages of cell division	Two	One
Number of daughter cells	Four: two from each stage of division, each having half the complement of chromosomes (i.e., 23)	Two: each identical to the parent cell and with 46 chromosomes
Types of division, by sex	*Oogenesis (female):* One ovum and three polar bodies are produced. *Spermatogenesis (male):* Four spermatozoa are produced.	N/A

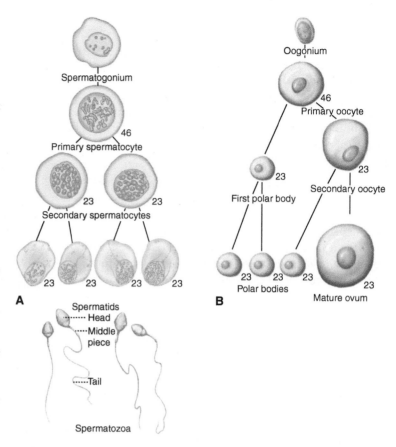

Figure 14.10. The formation of gametes by the process of meiosis (gametogenesis). (A) Spermatogenesis. One spermatogonium gives rise to four spermatozoa. **(B)** Oogenesis. From each oocyte, one mature ovum and three polar bodies are produced. The chromosomes are reduced to one half the number characteristic for the general body cells of the species. In humans, the number in the body cells is 46 and that in the mature spermatozoon and ovum is 23. (Reprinted with permission from Ricci, S. S. [2017]. *Essentials of maternity, newborn, & women's health nursing* [4th ed., Fig. 10.1]. Philadelphia, PA: Lippincott Williams & Wilkins.)

completes meiosis II only if fertilization occurs. In this second meiosis, the ovum will retain a majority of the cytoplasm of the original cell, while retaining only 23 chromosomes. A polar body is also produced in meiosis II, and the polar body from meiosis I may also divide, for a total of one viable ovum and two to three polar bodies, which disintegrate. If the secondary oocyte is not fertilized, meiosis II does not complete. Of the 23 chromosomes contained in each ovum, one is an X chromosome and the other 22 are **autosomes** (an autosome is a chromosome that is not a sex chromosome).

Spermatogenesis

Unlike gametogenesis in females, **spermatogenesis** does not begin until puberty in males. The first cell in this case is the diploid (two sets of chromosomes) spermatogonium. The spermatogonium undergoes meiosis I, producing two secondary spermatocytes, each of which has 23 chromosomes. During meiosis II, the two secondary spermatocytes split, creating four daughter cells called spermatids, each of which has 23 chromosomes. Two of these spermatids will have an X chromosome in addition to the 22 autosomes, and two will have a Y chromosome and 22 autosomes. These four daughter cells then undergo a process by which they become sperm. The nucleus of the spermatid is enclosed in the head of the sperm, which is covered by a cap called the **acrosome**, which is then covered by a plasma membrane. A tail is also produced to propel the sperm. In total, four gametes are produced in spermatogenesis to the one gamete produced in **oogenesis**.

Fertilization

Ova may be viable for fertilization for as few as 6 hours and as many as 24, whereas sperm may be capable of fertilizing an egg for as few as 24 hours and as long as 5 days. Fertilization most often occurs in the ampulla, the distal third of the fallopian tube (Fig. 14.11). As many as 500 million sperm are produced in a single ejaculation, but only a small fraction of these will make it to the ovum. Sperm are propelled by the movement of their tails but are also helped by an action of the cilia that moves the ovum down the fallopian tube toward the sperm but also move the sperm toward the ovum.

Through the removal of the plasma membrane overlying the acrosome cap on the head of the sperm by an action of uterine enzymes, the sperm undergo the process of **capacitation**. Hundreds of sperm that have undergone capacitation then surround the ovum and may undergo a collective acrosomal reaction that helps release enzymes to break down the outer layer of the ovum, the **corona radiata**, in advance of the action of the single sperm that will fertilize the egg. The acrosome of this single fertilizing sperm binds with a glycoprotein of the **zona pellucida**, allowing passage into the ovum (Fig. 14.12). Immediately after this binding, the zona pellucida undergoes a process by which it blocks any additional sperm that attempt penetration. This is called the **cortical reaction**.

In addition to blocking the penetration of other sperm, the ovum completes meiosis II immediately after fertilization, thus ejecting half of its chromosomes as another polar body. The

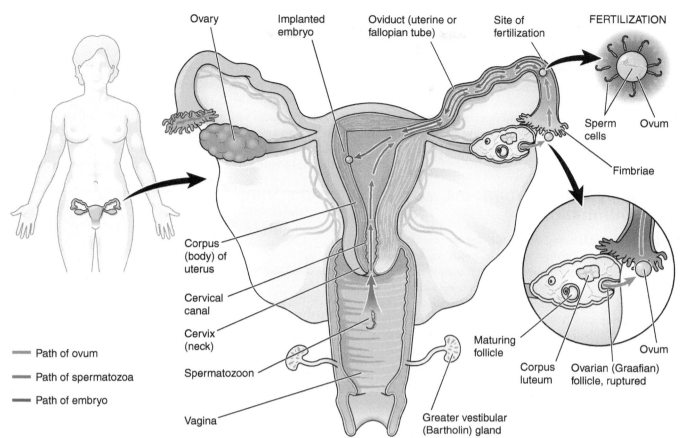

Figure 14.11. The process of conception. Conception occurs as a result of multiple coordinated events illustrated here. Arrows show the pathways of the sperm and the ovum, fertilization of the ovum, and implantation of the blastocyst. (Reprinted with permission from Stephenson, S. R., & Dmitrieva, J. [2017]. *Obstetrics and gynecology* [4th ed., Fig. 12.2]. Philadelphia, PA: Lippincott Williams & Wilkins.)

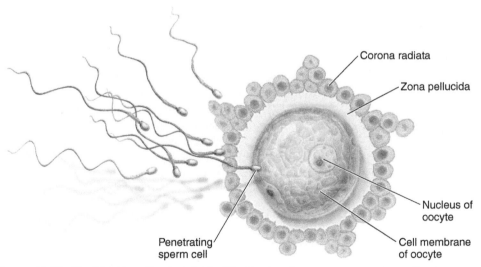

Figure 14.12. Fertilization. Successful fertilization involves an acrosomal reaction to overcome the corona radiata, followed by a single sperm cell penetrating the zona pellucida. (Modified with permission from Anatomical Chart Company. Reprinted with permission from Wingerd, B. [2013]. *The human body: Concepts of anatomy and physiology* [3rd ed., Fig. 18.1]. Philadelphia, PA: Lippincott Williams & Wilkins.)

23 chromosomes of the sperm unite with the 23 remaining chromosomes of the ovum, creating a diploid zygote with 46 chromosomes. Because half of the chromosomes came from the mother and half from the father, this cell is unique. In addition to the unique genetic complement formed at this moment, the sex of the pregnancy is determined. The ovum can only ever contribute an X chromosome. The sperm may contribute a Y chromosome or an X chromosome. A zygote that is XX is female. A zygote that is XY is male.

Pregnancy Signs, Symptoms, and Confirmation

For the purposes of learning, the signs and symptoms of pregnancy are typically broken into presumptive, probable, and positive. Although positive signs are considered confirmatory of pregnancy, presumptive and probable signs and symptoms warrant further investigation. It may be helpful here to differentiate between a sign and a symptom. A sign is objective and may be witnessed by an observer. Blood pressure would be an example of a sign. A symptom is subjective and reported by the patient. An example of a symptom would be a patient report of a headache.

Presumptive Symptoms

Many women who present for assessment of pregnancy come because they are having symptoms they believe are consistent with pregnancy. Often they did not get their menses when they anticipated it, or their menses was of a different quality or quantity than what is typical for the patient. **Amenorrhea** (lack of menses) may have several causes, however, including stress, intense exercise, and endocrine problems.

You may recall that Tatiana Bennett in Chapter 2 first became suspicious of pregnancy when she missed her period.

The patient may complain of breast tenderness, common in early pregnancy, but also common prior to and with menstruation. Many women will complain of fatigue, which is a finding common to the late first trimester of pregnancy, but is also common to anemia, poor sleep, stress, illness, and other physical or emotional reasons.

Bess Gaskell, who was pregnant for the third time (Chapter 1), anticipated fatigue as a normal part of early pregnancy.

Other women will have nausea they feel is unexplained by food poisoning, a virus, or other reasons. A patient may complain of breast enlargement, which, like breast tenderness, may result

from pregnancy, but may also have its roots in upcoming menses or in the use of estrogen-containing contraception. Urinary frequency is common in women who are 6 to 12 weeks pregnant, but may also occur in women with urinary tract infections, stress, pelvic organ dysfunction, or change in the level of hydration. Gas moving through the gastrointestinal tract may feel similar to fetal movement, which is typically first felt between weeks 16 and 20 of pregnancy. Darkening of the pigment of the skin, which may happen after week 16 of pregnancy, can also happen with the use of estrogen-containing contraception and sun exposure.

In Chapter 9, Nancy Ng's physician, Ron, referred to nausea as a good sign indicating a healthy pregnancy.

Probable Signs

Because these are signs, we know they're objective, and thus observable to others. The exception to this is Braxton Hicks contractions. Braxton Hicks contractions may be reported between 16 and 28 weeks of pregnancy, but may or may not be observable by a clinician. Conversely, Braxton Hicks contractions may be obvious to an experienced observer although not felt by the patient.

In Chapter 7, Hannah Wilder could not feel her Braxton Hicks contractions. Her midwife, Darla, informed her that they were occurring, even if she did not feel them.

The most common probable sign is a positive pregnancy test. Because of the high sensitivity of home urine pregnancy tests now, many women know they are pregnant before they miss their first menses. Home hCG tests are sensitive, starting at a urine concentration of 20 to 50 mIU/mL, depending on the test. hCG doubles in early pregnancy approximately every 48 to 72 hours, and is produced starting at the time of implantation. Caution should be exercised, however, as some brands of tests may have a disappointing degree of accuracy, well below the 99% many advertised (Johnson et al., 2014; Greenea et al., 2013). If the woman has a negative pregnancy test but a pregnancy is still suspected, the test should be repeated at a later date, preferably between 3 and 7 days. Samples that are more concentrated with a higher concentration of hCG are more likely to produce accurate results (Fig. 14.13).

False positive pregnancy tests are usually caused by user error, particularly reading the test late. A false positive may also be caused by a pregnancy that ends shortly after implantation, sometimes called a **biochemical pregnancy**. hCG is often used as part of fertility treatments and may cause a false positive, as may a tumor secreting hCG. The pituitary gland may also secrete hCG in women who are perimenopausal, thus creating a false positive hCG. A recent pregnancy loss may cause a false positive

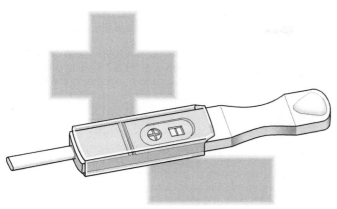

Figure 14.13. A urine pregnancy test. (Reprinted with permission from LifeART image copyright © 2018 Lippincott Williams & Wilkins. All rights reserved.)

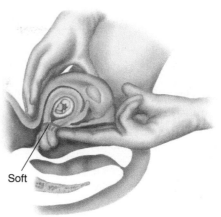

Soft

Figure 14.14. Heger's sign. (Reprinted with permission from Bickley, L. S., & Szilagyi, P. [2003]. *Bates' guide to physical examination and history taking* [8th ed., unnumbered figure in Chapter 12]. Philadelphia, PA: Lippincott Williams & Wilkins.)

because it may take several weeks for hCG to completely leave the system after a pregnancy.

In Chapter 13, Tanya's molar pregnancy produced high levels of hCG despite the pregnancy not being viable. With a molar pregnancy, regular hCG levels are assessed to monitor for possible postmolar gestational trophoblastic neoplasia.

The most common reason for a false negative pregnancy test is running a test too soon after conception. A false negative may also be read if the hCG is 500,000 mIU/mL or higher as in a molar pregnancy. This is called the **hook effect**.

Although some women, particularly those who have already had one or more prior pregnancies, will have abdominal enlargement in the first trimester, abdominal enlargement happens for almost all women by week 14 of pregnancy and is considered a probable sign of pregnancy, particularly in combination with other signs. **Goodell's sign** is a softening of the cervix and may be felt as early as 5 weeks into the pregnancy. Similarly, **Hegar's sign** (Fig. 14.14), a softening of the isthmus (lower portion) of the uterus, may be felt between 6 and 12 weeks. **Chadwick's sign**, a slight bluing of the female genitalia, including the labia and the cervix, may be seen as early as 6 weeks into the pregnancy.

Positive Signs

Visualization of the pregnancy by ultrasound is a positive sign of pregnancy. A pregnancy and its location in the uterus can usually be confirmed by 5 weeks, and the fetal heartbeat can typically be seen by 6 weeks. Fetal movement can usually be confirmed by the clinician by abdominal palpation by 20 weeks. Fetal heart tones may be heard as early as 9 weeks using a Doppler ultrasound fetal monitor, and almost certainly by 12 weeks. All positive signs are considered confirmatory of a pregnancy.

Think Critically

1. You are caring for a patient who is of an ethnicity unusual in your community. Write a brief dialogue that exemplifies culturally competent care.
2. You are caring for a patient without a partner. How might care considerations differ?
3. Medicaid and Medicare often compensate healthcare providers at a lower rate than do private insurers. Can you imagine this impacting care? How?
4. Consider the preconception Healthy People 2020 goals provided in the chapter. Write briefly about their significance to the health of a future pregnancy.
5. Women at the very beginning and at the very end of their reproductive lives are considered high risk. How do their specific risks differ?
6. From memory, list 10 suggested components of the health history. Go back and check your work.
7. When are estrogen, progesterone, LH, and FSH most prominent in the reproductive cycle?
8. Draw a diagram to illustrate the hormones of the female reproductive cycle.
9. List three ways that oogenesis differs from spermatogenesis.
10. List one presumptive, one probable, and one positive sign of pregnancy. Why is a positive pregnancy test considered only probable and not positive?

Unfolding Patient Stories: Fatime Sanago • Part 1

Fatime Sanogo, a 23-year-old, is being seen by the nurse in the prenatal clinic. The nurse learns that this is her first pregnancy, she is Muslim, and she recently moved to the United States from Mali, West Africa with her husband. What cultural factors are important for the nurse to assess that guide culturally competent care during her pregnancy and preparation for delivery? (Fatime Sanogo's story continues in Unit 3.)

Care for Fatime and other patients in a realistic virtual environment: **v*Sim* for Nursing** (thepoint.lww.com/vSimMaternity). Practice documenting these patients' care in DocuCare (thepoint.lww.com/DocuCareEHR).

Unfolding Patient Stories: Carla Hernandez • Part 1

Carla Hernandez is a 32-year-old gravida 2 para 1. She is at 39 5/7 weeks' gestation when her husband brings her to the hospital. How does the nurse determine that she is in active labor? If she is in active labor, how will the nurse monitor the progress of labor? What nursing assessments are done to identify the signs of potential complications during labor? What questions would the nurse ask Carla to identify symptoms of potential complications of labor? What nursing interventions can assist the couple's ability to cope with pain and stress experienced during labor? (Carla Hernandez's story continues in Unit 4.)

Care for Carla and other patients in a realistic virtual environment: **v*Sim* for Nursing** (thepoint.lww.com/vSimMaternity). Practice documenting these patients' care in DocuCare (thepoint.lww.com/DocuCareEHR).

References

Adam, M. P., Polifka, J. E., & Friedman, J. (2011). Evolving knowledge of the teratogenicity of medications in human pregnancy. *American Journal of Medical Genetics Part C: Seminars in Medical Genetics, 157*(3), 175–182.

Agency for Toxic Substances and Disease Registry. (2016, August 25). *Lead toxicity: Who is at risk of lead exposure?* Retrieved from Environmental Health and Medicine Education: https://www.atsdr.cdc.gov/csem/csem.asp?csem=34&po=7

American College of Obstetricians and Gynecologists. (2014). Female age-related fertility decline. Committee opinion no. 589. *Obstetrics and Gynecology, 123*(3), 719.

American Congress of Obstetricians and Gynecologists. (n.d.). *Toxic environmental agents.* Retrieved from https://www.acog.org/About-ACOG/ACOG-Departments/Public-Health-and-Social-Issues/Toxic-Environmental-Agents

American Medical Association. (2014). AMA code of medical ethics' opinion on adolescent care. *AMA Journal of Ethics, 16*(11), 901–902.

Angley, M., Divney, A., Magriples, U., & Kershaw, T. (2015). Social support, family functioning and parenting competence in adolescent parents. *Maternal and Child Health Journal, 19*, 67.

Armitage, G. C. (2013). Bi-directional relationship between pregnancy and periodontal disease. *Periodontology 2000, 61*(1), 160–176.

Barkana, S. E., Salazarb, A. M., Estepa, K., Mattosa, L. M., Eichenlauba, C., & Haggerty, K. P. (2014). Adapting an evidence-based parenting program for child welfare involved teens and their caregivers. *Children and Youth Services Review, 41*, 53–61.

Bixby Center for Global Reproductive Health. (2012). *Cost benefits from the provision of specific methods of contraception.* San Francisco, CA: University of California.

Blackwell, D. (2010). *Family structure and children's health in the United States: Findings from the National Health Interview Survey, 2001–2007.* Hyattsville, MD: National Center for Health Statistics.

Cavalli, P. (2008). Prevention of neural tube defects and proper folate periconceptional supplementation. *Journal of Prenatal Medicine, 2*(4), 40–41.

Centers for Disease Control and Prevention. (2013). Vital signs: Repeat births among teens—United States, 2007–2010. *Morbidity and Mortality Weekly Report, 62*(13), 249–255.

Centers for Disease Control and Prevention. (2015, January 22). *Unintended pregnancy prevention.* Retrieved from https://www.cdc.gov/reproductivehealth/unintendedpregnancy/

Centers for Disease Control and Prevention. (2016, June 21). *Alcohol use in pregnancy.* Retrieved from Fetal Alcohol Spectrum Disorders (FASDs): https://www.cdc.gov/ncbddd/fasd/alcohol-use.html

Centers for Disease Control and Prevention. (2016, October 7). *Births and natality.* Retrieved from http://www.cdc.gov/nchs/fastats/births.htm

Department of Health and Human Services Food and Drug Administration. (2014). *Content and format of labeling for human prescription drug and biological products; requirements for pregnancy and lactation labeling.* Silver Spring, MD: Author.

Finer, L., & Henshaw, S. (2006). Disparities in rates of unintended pregnancy in the United States, 1994 and 2001. *Perspective on Sexual and Reproductive Health, 38*(2), 90–96.

Finer, L. B., & Zolna, M. R. (2016). Declines in unintended pregnancy in the United States. *New England Journal of Medicine, 374*, 843–852.

Gates, G. J. (2013). *LGBT parenting in the United States.* Los Angeles, CA: The Williams Institute, UCLA School of Law.

Greenea, D. N., Schmidtb, R. L., Kamer, S. M., Grenacheb, D. G., Hokea, C., & Lorey, T. S. (2013). Limitations in qualitative point of care hCG tests for detecting early pregnancy. *Clinica Chimica Acta, 415*(16), 317–321.

Hamilton, B. E., Martin, J. A., Osterman, M. J., Curtin, S. C., & Mathews, T. (2015). Births: Final data for 2014. *National Vital Statistics Reports, 64*(12), 1–64.

Hasstedt, K. (2015, August). *Title X: The lynchpin of publicly funded family planning in the United States.* Retrieved from Guttmacher Institute: https://www.guttmacher.org/article/2015/08/title-x-lynchpin-publicly-funded-family-planning-united-states

Healthy People. (2016, December 20). *Healthy people.* Retrieved from healthypeople.gov: https://www.healthypeople.gov/

Johnson, S., Cushion, M., Bond, S., et al. (2014). Comparison of analytical sensitivity and women's interpretation of home pregnancy tests. *Clinical Chemistry and Laboratory Medicine (CCLM), 53*(3), pp. 391–402. Retrieved 10 May. 2018, from doi:10.1515/cclm-2014-0643.

Karwowski, M. P., Nelson, J. M., Staples, J. E., Fischer, M., Fleming-Dutra, K. E., Villanueva, J., . . . Rasmussen, S. A. (2016). Zika virus disease: A CDC update for pediatric health care providers. *Pediatrics, 137*(5), e20160621.

March of Dimes. (2016, November). *Street drugs and pregnancy.* Retrieved from http://www.marchofdimes.org/pregnancy/street-drugs-and-pregnancy.aspx

Mathews, T., & Hamilton, A. B. (2014). *First births to older women continue to rise.* Hyattsville, MD: National Center for Health Statistics.

Medicaid.gov. (n.d.). *Dental care.* Retrieved from https://www.medicaid.gov/medicaid/benefits/dental/index.html

Misraa, J., Mollerb, S., Stradera, E., & Wemlinger, E. (2012). Family policies, employment and poverty among partnered and single mothers. *Research in Social Stratification and Mobility, 30*(1), 113–128.

National Family Planning & Reproductive Health Association. (n.d.). *Title X.* Retrieved from http://www.nationalfamilyplanning.org/title-x_budget-appropriations

Oregon Foundation for Reproductive Health. (2012). Retrieved from One Key Question: http://www.onekeyquestion.org/

Organization for Economic Cooperation and Development. (2015). *OECD health data 2015.* Paris, France: Author.

Oringanje, C., Meremikwu, M. M., Eko, H., Esu, E., Meremikwu, A., & Ehiri, J. E. (2016). Interventions for preventing unintended pregnancies among adolescents. *The Cochrane Library, (2),* CD005215.

Oza-Frank, R., Gilson, E., Keim, S. A., Lynch, C. D., & Klebanoff, M. A. (2014). Trends and factors associated with self-reported receipt of preconception care: PRAMS, 2004–2010. *Birth, 41*(4), 367–373.

Petersen, E. E., Meaney-Delman, D., Neblett-Fanfair, R., Havers, F., Oduyebo, T., Hills, S. L., . . . Brooks, J. T. (2016). Update: Interim guidance for preconception counseling and prevention of sexual transmission of Zika virus for persons with possible Zika virus exposure—United States, September 2016. *Morbidity and Mortality Weekly Report, 65*(39), 1077–1081.

Pew Research Center. (2015, December 17). *The American family today.* Retrieved from http://www.pewsocialtrends.org/2015/12/17/1-the-american-family-today/

Renzo, G. C., Conry, J. A., Blake, J., DeFrancesco, M. S., DeNicola, N., Martin, J. N., Jr, . . . Giudice, L. C. (2015). International Federation of Gynecology and Obstetrics opinion on reproductive health impacts of exposure to toxic environmental chemicals. *International Journal of Gynecology and Obstetrics, 131*(3), 219–225.

Rousou, E., Kouta, C., Middleton, N., & Karanikola, M. (2013). Single mothers' self-assessment of health: A systematic exploration of the literature. *International Nursing Review, 60*(4), 425–434.

Singh, D. (2013, November 8). *Q&A on pregnant women's coverage under Medicaid and the ACA.* Retrieved from National Health Law Program: http://www.healthlaw.org/publications/browse-all-publications/QA-Pregnant-Women-Coverage-Medicaid-and-ACA#.WFJyoKIrLdQ

Squires, D., & Anderson, C. (2015). U.S. health care from a global perspective: Spending, use of services, prices, and health in 13 countries. *The Commonwealth Fund.* Retrieved from: http://www.commonwealthfund.org/publications/issue-briefs/2015/oct/us-health-care-from-a-global-perspective

Tabet, M., Flick, L. H., Tuuli, M. G., Macones, G. A., & Chang J. J. (2015). Prepregnancy body mass index in a first uncomplicated pregnancy and outcomes of a second pregnancy. *American Journal of Obstetrics and Gynecology, 213*(4), 548.e1–548.e7.

Temming, L. A., Cahill, A. G., & Riley, L. E. (2016). Clinical management of medications in pregnancy and lactation. *American Journal of Obstetrics and Gynecology, 214*(6), 698–702.

The American College of Obstetricians and Gynecologists Committee on Obstetric Practice Society for Maternal-Fetal Practice. (2015). *Definition of term pregnancy.* Washington, DC: ACOG.

The Henry J. Kaiser Family Foundation. (n.d.). *Health insurance coverage of the total population.* Retrieved from http://kff.org/other/state-indicator/total-population/?currentTimeframe=0

The Henry J. Kaiser Family Foundation. (2015, July 10). *Private and public coverage of contraceptive services and supplies in the United States.* Retrieved from http://kff.org/womens-health-policy/fact-sheet/private-and-public-coverage-of-contraceptive-services-and-supplies-in-the-united-states/

The World Bank. (n.d.). *Health expenditure, total (% of GDP).* Retrieved from http://data.worldbank.org/indicator/SH.XPD.TOTL.ZS?year_high_desc=true

Truven Health Analytics. (2013). *The cost of having a baby in the United States.* Retrieved from: http://transform.childbirthconnection.org/wp-content/uploads/2013/01/Cost-of-Having-a-Baby1.pdf

United Nations Children's Fund. (2015). *Child mortality estimates.* Retrieved from http://www.childmortality.org/index.php?r=site/compare

United States Census Bureau. (2014). *American community survey data on same sex couples.* Retrieved from https://www.census.gov/topics/families/same-sex-couples/data/tables.html

U.S. Department of Health and Human Services. (2015, May 13). *HHS.gov.* Retrieved from The Affordable Care Act and Maternity Care: https://www.hhs.gov/healthcare/facts-and-features/fact-sheets/aca-and-maternity-care/index.html

Vermont Health Connect. (2015). Retrieved from https://portal.healthconnect.vermont.gov/VTHBELand/welcome.action

Viswanathan, M., Treiman, K. A., & Kish-Doto, J. (2017). Folic acid supplementation for the prevention of neural tube defects: An updated evidence report and systematic review for the US preventive services task force. *JAMA, 317*(2), 190–203.

Vouga, M., & Baud, D. (2016). Imaging of congenital Zika virus infection: The route to identification of prognostic factors. *Prenatal Diagnosis, 36*(9), 799–811.

World Health Organization. (2016, February 1). *WHO Director-General summarizes the outcome of the Emergency Committee regarding clusters of microcephaly and Guillain-Barré syndrome.* Retrieved from http://www.who.int/mediacentre/news/statements/2016/emergency-committee-zika-microcephaly/en/

World Health Organization, United Nations Children's Fund, United Nations Population Fund, World Bank Group, & the United Nations Population Division. (2015). *Trends in maternal mortality: 1990 to 2015.* Geneva, Switzerland: World Health Organization.

Suggested Readings

Centers for Disease Control and Prevention. (2015, July 31). *Preconception health and health care.* Retrieved from https://www.cdc.gov/preconception/hcp/index.html

Whitworth, M., & Dowswell, T. (2009). Routine pre-pregnancy health promotion for improving pregnancy outcomes. *The Cochrane Database of Systematic Reviews,* (4), CD007536.

15 Pregnancy

Objectives

1. Identify the three stages of intrauterine development and describe the key events that occur in each.
2. Describe the development and functions of the placenta and the umbilical cord.
3. List the key anatomic and physiologic changes that occur in each body system during pregnancy.
4. Identify the normal discomforts of pregnancy and explain their relation to the anatomic and physiologic changes of pregnancy.
5. Discuss the self-care measures patients can take to address the normal discomforts of pregnancy.
6. Compare the various types of obstetric care providers and the care they provide.
7. Describe the elements and timing of prenatal care in each trimester.

Key Terms

Amnion
Blastocoel
Blastocyst
Blastomere
Chloasma
Chorion
Decidua basalis
Diastasis recti
Dirty Duncan
Dizygotic
Ductus arteriosus
Ductus venosus
Ectoderm
Embryoblast
Endoderm
Epulis
Fetal pole
Fetus
Foramen ovale
Human chorionic somatomammotropin

Hyperplasia
Hypertrophy
Mesoderm
Monozygotic
Morula
Multizygotic
Operculum
Palmar erythema
Pica
Placenta
Ptyalism
Relaxin
Shiny Schultze
Striae gravidarum
Syncytiotrophoblast
Tidal volume
Wharton's jelly
Zygote

Pregnancy Development

Prenatal development is commonly divided into three stages: preembryonic, embryonic, and fetal (Arey & Sapunar, 2017). These stages, along with the development of the **placenta** and umbilical cord, are discussed below.

Preembryonic Stage

The preembryonic stage of pregnancy development begins with conception and ends about 2 weeks later, with the establishment of the fetal membranes. After fertilization, which is described in Chapter 14, the fertilized ovum—now diploid, with half of its chromosomes from the mother and half from the father—is referred to as a **zygote**.

Mitosis

The zygote then begins to divide and generate new cells via the process of mitosis, also called cleavage, as it travels down the fallopian tube toward the uterus. By approximately 3 days after fertilization and while it is still in the fallopian tube, the preembryonic mass has developed into a collection of approximately 12 to 32 very small cells referred to as **blastomeres**. These cells are so small that, despite their number, they are combined not

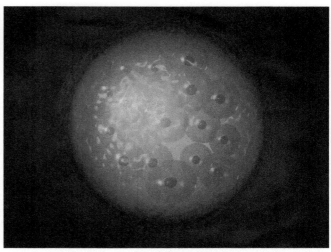

Figure 15.1. Morula. (Reprinted with permission from LifeART image © 2018 Lippincott Williams & Wilkins. All rights reserved.)

much larger that the ovum was at fertilization. This structure is referred to as the **morula** (Fig. 15.1; Table 15.1). These cells all remain within the bounds of the zona pellucida layer of the ovum until this structure disappears at the time of implantation in the uterus.

Table 15.1	Stages of Pregnancy by Developmental Age and Cell Division Status			
Stage	**Age Span (Time Since Fertilization)**	**No. of Cells**	**Notes**	**Image**
Morula	From day 3 to day 4	12–32	Cells (called blastomeres) are each hardly larger than the original fertilized ovum.	Reprinted with permission from LifeART image © 2018 Lippincott Williams & Wilkins. All rights reserved.
Blastocyst	From day 5 to day 9 (ending with implantation)	200–300	Differentiation begins. The outer cells, the trophoblast, become the placenta. The inner cell mass becomes the embryo.	Reprinted with permission from LifeART image © 2018 Lippincott Williams & Wilkins. All rights reserved.

Table 15.1 Stages of Pregnancy by Developmental Age and Cell Division Status (continued)

Stage	Age Span (Time Since Fertilization)	No. of Cells	Notes	Image
Embryo	From day 10 (implantation) to week 8	Many	Differentiation is completed. The inner cells of the former blastocyst differentiate into the germ layers: ectoderm, mesoderm, and endoderm. From these layers originate all organs and other structures.	An embryo at 4 wk. Reprinted with permission from Klossner, N. J. (2005). *Introductory maternity nursing* (1st ed., Fig. 5.3B). Philadelphia, PA: Lippincott Williams & Wilkins.
Fetus	From week 9 until the end of pregnancy	Many	Significant growth and development occur.	A fetus at 10 wk (shown in 3D ultrasound). Reprinted with permission from Doubilet, P. M., & Benson, C. B. (2011). *Atlas of ultrasound in obstetrics and gynecology: A multimedia reference* (2nd ed., Fig. 1.5B). Philadelphia, PA: Lippincott Williams & Wilkins.

Formation of the Blastocyst

As the morula enters the uterus, a cavity is created inside, separating the morula into different types of cells: an outer layer within the zona pellucida called a trophoblast and an inner cell mass adherent to the trophoblastic ring called an **embryoblast**. The fluid-filled cavity within the trophoblastic layer is called the **blastocoel**. With this change, the structure becomes known as a **blastocyst**. The trophoblast then "hatches" from the zona pellucida, allowing for implantation to proceed.

Implantation

Implantation of the blastocyst into the wall of the uterus occurs between day 6 and day 10 after fertilization. This stage of development occurs in the secretory phase of the endometrial cycle when, progesterone stimulates the endometrium of the uterus to become more vascular and glands to secrete nutrients, thus facilitating implantation. When the blastocyst reaches the endometrium, the trophoblast releases enzymes that further prepare the endometrium for implantation. The blastocyst then burrows down into the endometrium, typically in the posterior wall of the upper uterus, until it is completely enveloped. At this point, the endometrium is referred to as the decidua. The portion of the decidua underneath the implantation is called the **decidua basalis**, which will form the maternal part of the placenta. The embryoblast develops into the embryonic disk.

Formation of the Germ Layers, Embryonic Membranes, and Yolk Sac

Approximately 15 to 16 days after fertilization, the embryonic disk develops into the three germ layers: the **ectoderm** (outer layer), the **mesoderm** (middle layer), and the **endoderm** (inner layer). Each

Table 15.2 Body Structures Derived From Germ Cell Layers

Layer	Structures
Ectoderm (outer)	• Epithelium: anterior two thirds of the tongue, buccal surfaces, hard palate, external auditory meatus, lower anal canal, distal penile urethra, hair, nails, epidermis, nasal cavity, sinuses, tooth enamel, cornea, and lens of the eye • Glands: sweat and sebaceous glands, mammary glands, and pituitary gland • Peripheral and central nervous systems
Mesoderm (middle)	• Dermis • Skeleton and cartilage • Smooth, striated, and skeletal muscles • Circulatory system: bone marrow, blood, heart, spleen, and lymphatic tissue • Other organs: kidneys, adrenal cortex, and genitourinary systems
Endoderm (inner)	• Mucosa: lining of the gastrointestinal and respiratory systems • Endocrine organs: pancreas, liver, thyroid, and parathyroid • Other organs: gastrointestinal system and urinary bladder

of these layers goes on to develop into specific tissue types, body systems, and organs, as shown in Table 15.2 (Sadler, Chapter 5: Third Week of Development: Trilaminar Germ Disc, 2014).

The two embryonic membranes also develop and differentiate at this time: the **amnion** and the **chorion**. The inner layer, the amnion, arises from the ectoderm and is smooth. The space between the amnion and the embryo is known as the amniotic cavity, and the fluid inside the cavity is the amniotic fluid. Once the amnion is formed by day 10 or 12, the blastocyst is then considered an embryo.

The outer layer, the chorion, derives from the trophoblast cells, which made up the outer circle of the blastocyst inside the zona pellucida. As the chorion forms, it creates finger-like projections called chorionic villi. Over time these degenerate, except for those underlying the embryo, which will form the fetal portion of the placenta. Initially, the chorion is much larger than the amnion. Later in pregnancy the amnion expands more quickly than the chorion until the two meet and fuse, creating the amniotic sac.

At the same time that the amnion and chorion are developing, a cavity known as the yolk sac is also developing (Fig. 15.2). It is the first structure that can be visualized within the gestational sac with early ultrasound (about 5 weeks of gestation) (Brown, Stages of Development of the Fetus, 2017). Although in birds the yolk sac contains yolk to sustain the pregnancy, in mammals, very little nutrition is contained (Arey & Sapunar, 2017).

Embryonic Stage

The embryonic stage of pregnancy development begins once the amnion is formed, about 10 to 12 days after fertilization and lasts through the eighth week after fertilization or when the embryo measures 3 cm from crown (the top of the head) to rump (the posterior end) (Fig. 15.3) (Brown, Stages of Development of the Fetus, 2017). A **fetal pole**, the earliest form of the embryo that may be visualized by ultrasound, may be seen at 3 to 4 weeks after fertilization (5 to 6 weeks of pregnancy).

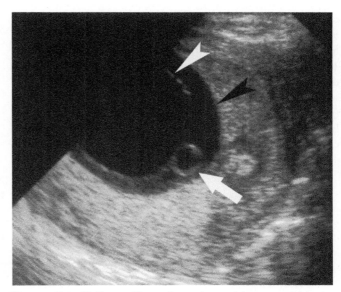

Figure 15.2. Yolk sac. The yolk sac (*arrow*) is seen within the gestational sac by transvaginal ultrasound. The normal yolk sac is less than 6 mm in diameter, spherical, filled with fluid, and has a thin wall. The yolk sac is in the fluid space between the thin membrane of the amnion (*white arrowhead*) and the chorion (*black arrowhead*). (Reprinted with permission from Brant, W. E., & Helms, C. A. [2006]. *The Brant and Helms solution: Fundamentals of diagnostic radiology* [3rd ed., Fig. 38.3]. Philadelphia, PA: Lippincott Williams & Wilkins.)

The critical task of the embryonic stage is the formation and development of the organs, a process known as organogenesis. During this stage, the pregnancy is most vulnerable to teratogens and spontaneous abortion is common, often because of chromosomal errors.

Developmental Versus Gestational Age

When discussing the development of an embryo or **fetus**, one can say that the age is based on the time since conception, not the

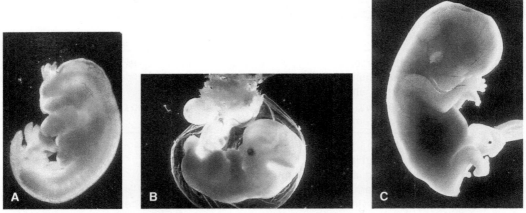

Figure 15.3. Embryos at various developmental ages (time since fertilization). (A) 4 weeks. **(B)** 5 weeks. **(C)** 6 weeks. (Reprinted with permission from Rosdahl, C. B., & Kowalski, M. T. [2016]. *Textbook of basic nursing* [11th ed., Fig. 65.4]. Philadelphia, PA: Lippincott Williams & Wilkins.)

time since the first day of the last menstrual period (LMP; as when calculating gestational age and estimating the due date). For the purpose of pregnancy dating, the presumed length of a menstrual cycle is 28 days. The luteal phase between ovulation and menses is 14 days if fertilization does not occur. With a 28-day cycle, the follicular phase between the first day of menses and ovulation is also 14 days. By this calculation, ovulation and fertilization occur 14 days after the first day of the LMP, so the embryonic or fetal age is 2 weeks less than gestational age. Thus, if a woman is 6 weeks pregnant (gestational age), her embryo is 4 weeks old, and when she reaches her estimated date of delivery (EDD) at 40 weeks of gestation, she carries a fetus with a postconception age of 38 weeks (Fig. 15.4).

Development of the Cardiovascular System

The cardiovascular system is the first functional system to develop in the embryo. The circulation required to support an embryo and later the fetus is considerably different from that observed in humans after birth, requiring a dramatic shift at the time of birth.

The key function of the cardiovascular system in the embryo is the same as that after birth, to supply the body's tissues with oxygen and nutrients and to remove waste products. However, because the lungs have no exposure to air in utero, the embryonic circulatory system is also exclusively responsible for gas exchange at the level of the placenta.

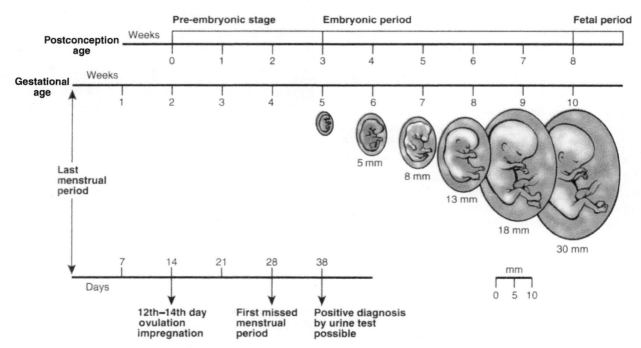

Figure 15.4 Stages of in utero development: preembryonic, embryonic, and fetal. The fetal period continues until the birth of the neonate, normally at approximately gestational week 40. (Reprinted with permission from Evans, R. J., Brown, Y. M., & Evans, M. K. [2014]. *Canadian maternity, newborn, and women's health nursing* [2nd ed., Fig. 6.1]. Philadelphia, PA: Lippincott Williams & Wilkins.)

By the end of the third week after fertilization (fifth week of gestation), a primitive tubular heart has begun to beat and may be visualized when the fetal pole measures 5 mm (Brown, Physiology of Pregnancy, 2016). Connected to the **chorion** (outer membrane) and the yolk sac, it pumps primitive red blood cells produced by the yolk sac through early blood vessels. This early tubular heart differentiates into the familiar four-chambered heart by the end of the fifth week (seventh week of gestation). By week 8 of the pregnancy, the liver and bone marrow take over the function of producing red blood cells in place of the yolk sac (Sadler, Chapter 13: Cardiovascular System, 2014).

In the embryonic (and later the fetal) circulation, oxygenated blood moves from the umbilical vein to the inferior vena cava via the **ductus venosus**, where it mixes with deoxygenated blood from the abdomen and lower extremities. This mix of oxygenated and deoxygenated blood enters the right atrium of the heart (unlike after birth, when only deoxygenated blood enters the right atrium). It may then go directly through the **foramen ovale** (an opening in the heart wall that is anatomically normal in the embryo and fetus but abnormal after birth) into the left atrium or, via the route typical of mature circulation, through the tricuspid valve into the right ventricle. From the right ventricle, blood is then pumped through the pulmonary valve and into the pulmonary artery. Here, however, the prenatal circulation differs again from mature circulation. Between the pulmonary artery and the descending artery is the embryonic and fetal structure of the **ductus arteriosus**. This structure allows for blood to be shunted directly between the pulmonary artery and the descending aorta, bypassing the lungs. Oxygen-poor blood leaves the fetal/embryonic circulation via the umbilical arteries, which pick up blood from the internal iliac arteries and return it to the placenta (Fig. 15.5).

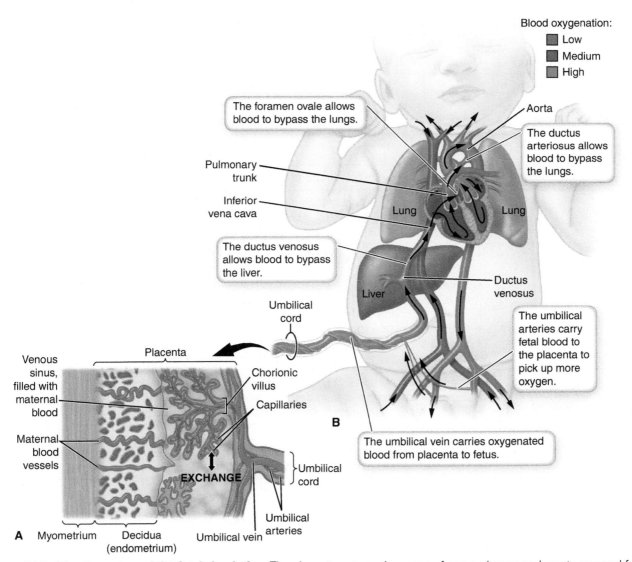

Figure 15.5. The placenta and the fetal circulation. The placenta acts as the organ of gas exchange and waste removal for the fetus. **(A)** The placenta. The placenta is formed by the maternal endometrium and fetal chorion. Exchanges between fetal and maternal blood occur through the capillaries of the chorionic villi. **(B)** Fetal circulation. During fetal life, specialized vessels and openings shunt blood away from nonfunctioning lungs and toward the placenta. The different colors show the relative oxygen content of the blood. (Reprinted with permission from Cohen, B. J., & Hull, K. [2014]. *Memmler's the human body in health and disease* [13th ed., Fig. 24.2]. Philadelphia, PA: Lippincott Williams & Wilkins.)

Fetal Stage

The fetal stage of pregnancy development begins in the ninth week after fertilization (11th week of gestation) and ends with birth. During this stage, it is referred to as a fetus. Vulnerability to teratogens declines significantly in most structures during this stage, although the central nervous system remains most vulnerable because it continues to change and develop dramatically throughout the pregnancy. The fetal stage involves rapid growth but also refinement of the organs and structures created in the embryonic stage. For the major developmental tasks of the embryonic and fetal stages, see Table 15.3. Table 15.4 shows the chances an infant has of surviving birth at different gestational ages.

A multiple pregnancy is one that involves more than one fetus: twins, triplets, or more. In 2015, the Centers for Disease Control and Prevention (CDC) reported that one out of every 30 births in the United States resulted in twins, up from one out of every 53 births in 1980. This rise is likely due to two factors: increased availability and use of fertility treatments and increased prevalence of births among women of older maternal age (CDC, 2015).

A multiple pregnancy may occur as a result of the fertilization of just one ovum (**monozygotic**), two ova (**dizygotic**), or more than two ova (**multizygotic**). In a monozygotic multiple pregnancy, a single zygote divides into two or, rarely, more zygotes within the first 2 weeks of fertilization. These twins or other multiples are of the same sex and identical and may share a placenta and amniotic sac. The propensity to have monozygotic twins does not run in families.

Dizygotic and multizygotic pregnancies are not identical, and each embryo/fetus has its own placenta and amniotic sac.

Table 15.3   Developmental Events of Pregnancy by Stage and Time Since Fertilization

Time Since Fertilization	Developmental Event
Preembryonic Stage	
Week 1	• Fertilization occurs approximately 2 wk before the first day of menses is anticipated and typically occurs in the ampulla of the fallopian tube. • The fertilized ovum will become a morula and then a blastocyst before entering the uterus.
Embryonic Stage	
Week 2	• Implantation occurs by the end of this week.
Week 3	• The embryonic disk that arose from the blastocoel of the blastocyst differentiates into the three germ layers: ectoderm, mesoderm, and endoderm. • The neural tube fuses at its center and the tubular heart begins to beat.
Week 4	• Fetal blood type is determined at the moment of conception but becomes manifest at 6 wk. • Maternal sensitivity to Rh-positive blood by an Rh-negative mother is possible after this time. • The head and the tail fold inward, and the embryo takes on the shape of a C. • Neural tube fusion concludes. • Respiratory and digestive tracks begin to form, as do the eyes and internal ears, the thyroid gland, the epidermis, and muscle and bone tissue.
Week 5	• The four-chambered heart begins to arise from the tubular heart. • Upper limb buds appear with notches between where fingers form. • Lower limb buds begin to form, as do the kidneys and pancreas.
Week 6	• The heart gains its final form. • The extremities, eyes, and face continue to develop. • The outer ear and nasal pits, which will define the nose, begin to develop.
Week 7	• Sex differentiation begins, along with testosterone secretion in males. • Two layers of the epidermis are present. • The face continues to develop and eyelids begin to grow. • Gastrointestinal development progresses faster than abdominal growth, and much of the intestines is housed in the umbilical cord.
Week 8	• Hematopoiesis (formation of blood) starts in the embryonic liver, spleen, and lymph nodes. • The first brain waves are detectable, and nerve fibers form. • The embryonic thyroid begins to secrete thyroxine.

Table 15.3   Developmental Events of Pregnancy by Stage and Time Since Fertilization (continued)

Time Since Fertilization	Developmental Event
Fetal Stage	
Week 9–12	• Fetal movement begins, and the head is about half the total length of the fetus. • Rapid growth begins. • The portions of the intestines in the umbilical cord move to the abdomen, and the digestive tract is fully formed from mouth to anus. • Blood production, which is primarily in the liver during week 9, moves to the spleen by week 11, and glycogen storage also begins in the liver. • Bile begins to form. Eyelids fuse, fingernails begin to grow, and lanugo appears on the upper lip and eyebrows. • The kidneys begin to function, and the islets of Langerhans of the pancreas, which will produce insulin, form. • Respiratory movements begin, the genitalia are fully differentiated, and heart tones can be picked up by Doptone.
Week 13–16	• The head becomes proportionately smaller, and the eyes face forward. • Ridges that will form in the finger, hand, foot, and toe prints are present. • Women may feel fetal movement for the first time. • Oogenesis is established in females. • The trachea, bronchi, and larynx form; the lungs begin to form. • Blood vessels are visible under the skin.
Week 17–20	• Lanugo is present over the entire body, which is also covered with cheesy vernix caseosa. • Fetal swallowing of amniotic fluid begins in month 5, as does the first response to taste. • Insulin production begins from the islets of Langerhans of the pancreas.
Week 21–24	• The lungs begin to produce surfactant, which is critical to preventing the collapse of the alveoli after birth. • The skin appears thin and red with little subcutaneous fat. • The first response to sound occurs.
Week 25–28	• Rods and cones present in eyes, and testes descend in males. • Scalp hair appears and eyelids are open. • The fetus often moves into a head-down position at this time because of a combination of the relative weight of the fetal head and the inverted pear shape of the uterus. • Blood production shifts to the bone marrow.
Week 29–34	• Subcutaneous fat deposits begin, and the skin is pigmented according to genetic inheritance. • Fingernails reach the fingertips, and fetal heartbeat variability is more pronounced due to greater central nervous system maturity.
Week 33–38	• Toenails reach the ends of the toes, and fingernails grow beyond the fingertips. • Visual acuity is 20/600. • Ovaries contain about 1 million follicles, and the testes have descended into the scrotum. • Vernix caseosa occurs only in skin creases and lanugo only on the upper back and shoulders. • The lungs and the central nervous system mature, and growth and weight gain are the major tasks of this period.

Dizygotic or fraternal twins may be the same sex or different sexes, as they each have a unique set of chromosomes. For more on multiple pregnancies, see Chapter 20.

Placenta

The placenta is a temporary organ of pregnancy that acts as a circulatory interface between the mother and embryo or fetus and serves several other functions essential to the pregnancy. Below, we will consider its formation, structure, and functions.

Formation

The placenta grows from the site where the blastocyst implants on the wall of the uterus and is composed of tissues that derive from both the blastocyst and the uterus. It begins to form when

Table 15.4   Chance of an Infant Surviving Birth at Various Gestational Ages

Gestational Age (wk)	Chance of Survival (%)	Chance of Survival Without Moderate or Severe Lifelong Impairment (%)
22	5.1	2
23	23.6	–
24	54.9	–
25	72	44
26	81.4	58.5
29	90	–

Data from Rysavy, M. A., Li, L., Bell, E. F., Das, A., Hintz, S. R., Stoll, B. J., . . . Higgins, R. D.; Eunice Kennedy Shriver National Institute of Child Health and Human Development Neonatal Research Network. (2015). Between-hospital variation in treatment and outcomes in extremely preterm infants. *The New England Journal of Medicine, 372*, 1801–1811 and Platt, M. J. (2014). Outcomes in preterm infants. *Public Health, 128*(5), 399–403.

the finger-like projections known as the chorionic villi arise from the trophoblast of the blastocyst and burrow into the decidua basalis of the uterus. Thus, the fetal side of the placenta is formed by the chorionic villa and lined by the amnion. The maternal side is formed by the decidua basalis. The placenta expands over the inner surface of the uterus until about 20 weeks of gestation. After this point, it will continue to grow thicker but will no longer expand outward (Brown, Physiology of Pregnancy, 2016).

Structure

Once fully developed, the placenta is approximately 2.5 to 3 cm thick and 38 to 51 cm in diameter. The outer surface, arising from the amnion, is smooth and translucent and is therefore often referred to as **shiny Schultze**. The side that joins with the decidua has a red, meaty appearance and is therefore often called the **dirty Duncan** (see Fig. 1.2). The functional part of the placenta, the **syncytiotrophoblast**, sits between the maternal and fetal blood supply (Brown, Physiology of Pregnancy, 2016; Sadler, Chapter 8: Third Month to Birth: The Fetus and Placenta, 2014).

Function

The placenta serves three primary functions: circulation, protection, and hormone production.

Circulation

As the circulatory interface between the mother and the embryo or fetus, the placenta is responsible for delivering oxygen and nutrients from the mother's bloodstream to that of the embryo or fetus and removing carbon dioxide and cellular waste products from fetal circulation. While performing this function, remarkably the maternal and the fetal blood do not mix. This is important because incompatibilities between elements of the maternal blood and fetal blood, such as ABO and Rh blood types, could compromise the pregnancy, as maternal antibodies would attack the fetal blood. A dose of Rh_o (D) immune globulin (RhoGAM) is

recommended for women who are Rh negative in the 28th week of pregnancy. This is done because there is a small potential for circulatory interface that can lead to alloimmunization and fetal compromise, particularly in cases of maternal abdominal trauma and vaginal bleeding when the exact source of bleeding cannot be determined.

In Chapter 5, Letitia required a Rh_o (D) immune globulin injection during her 28th week of pregnancy because her blood was Rh negative. Dr. Janachek explained that this would prevent her from developing antibodies that would attack the blood of an Rh-positive fetus.

The degree of gas and nutrient exchange varies throughout pregnancy, because the permeability of the syncytiotrophoblast varies with gestational age. It is less permeable at the beginning of the pregnancy and becomes more permeable around month 5, as the membrane, the syncytiotrophoblast, begins to thin. It again becomes less permeable in the final month of pregnancy (Sadler, Chapter 8: Third Month to Birth: The Fetus and Placenta, 2014).

Additionally, some necessary nutrients are stored in the placenta, such as vitamins, minerals, carbohydrates, and protein, and are passed into the fetal circulation according to need.

Protection

Also of critical importance is the role of the placenta in providing protection to the embryo or fetus. First, it transfers the mother's immunoglobulins that will provide passive immunity to the embryo or fetus, giving the neonate temporary protection from certain pathogens during early infancy. Second, it prevents some viruses and medications present in the maternal circulation from entering the embryonic or fetal circulation (Sadler, Chapter 8: Third Month to Birth: The Fetus and Placenta, 2014).

However, this protection is not universal. Some viruses, such as rubella, can pass through the placenta, as can many medications and other potential teratogens, such as nicotine, alcohol, and cocaine. Moreover, bacterial infections, such as syphilis, and parasitic infections, such as toxoplasmosis, may infect both the placenta and the fetus, compromising both (Sadler, Chapter 8: Third Month to Birth: The Fetus and Placenta, 2014).

Hormone Production

Finally, the placenta serves as a temporary endocrine gland, producing hormones that help establish and sustain the pregnancy and prepare the body for birth (Fig. 15.6). On implantation, the placenta begins to excrete human chorionic gonadotropin (hCG). This hormone signals the corpus luteum of the follicle abandoned by the ovum to continue excreting progesterone and estrogen, which are required to cue the endometrium and uterine musculature to maintain an environment conducive to pregnancy (Sadler, Chapter 8: Third Month to Birth: The Fetus and Placenta, 2014).

hCG rises predictably in early pregnancy, doubling about every 48 to 72 hours in a healthy pregnancy. When hCG levels fail to rise at this rate or drop, the probability of a miscarriage or an ectopic pregnancy increases. Later in the embryotic period, the rate of doubling slows to every 96 hours. After that, hCG levels plateau and then drop between weeks 8 and 11. At 25 weeks, it is approximately 75% lower than it was at peak (Rhoades & Bell, 2017).

hCG levels vary greatly between pregnancies. A pregnancy at 6 weeks of gestation may have an hCG level anywhere from 1,100 to 56,000 mIU/mL. Thus, interpretation of the meaning of hCG levels requires evaluation of the pattern of the rise (or fall) of hCG. Importantly, an hCG level of 2,000 mIU/mL or

higher typically indicates a pregnancy that may be visualized in the uterus on ultrasound. An hCG level 2,000 mIU/mL or higher without evidence of pregnancy by ultrasound is concerning for a possible ectopic pregnancy (Dulay, 2017).

A second hormone exclusively produced by the placenta is **human chorionic somatomammotropin** (hCS; sometimes referred to as human placental lactogen, or hPL). Unlike hCG, which peaks in the first trimester and then levels off and drops, hCS appears later in pregnancy and continues to rise. hCS acts directly on the mother's metabolism, increasing the insulin resistance of her cells, and thereby increasing her circulating glucose. The passage of this surplus glucose across the placenta to the pregnancy is also facilitated by hCS. This hormone also cues the breasts to prepare for lactation (Sadler, Chapter 8: Third Month to Birth: The Fetus and Placenta, 2014).

A third hormone produced by the placenta is progesterone, which also encourages breast development and changes in the mother's metabolism. Although the corpus luteum, cued by placental hCG, continues to produce progesterone in early pregnancy, this production is taken over by the placenta by the fourth month of pregnancy (Sadler, Chapter 8: Third Month to Birth: The Fetus and Placenta, 2014).

A fourth hormone produced by the placenta is estrogen, which, like progesterone, is initially produced by the corpus luteum. Like progesterone and hCS, estrogen promotes the development of the mother's breasts in preparation for future lactation. Unlike progesterone, which relaxes the muscles of the uterus, estrogen promotes contraction of the myometrium, the muscular layer of the uterus. It also promotes uterine growth and blood flow to the uterus and the attached placenta (Sadler, Chapter 8: Third Month to Birth: The Fetus and Placenta, 2014).

A fifth hormone produced by the placenta is **relaxin**. The corpus luteum initially produces relaxin in both nonpregnant and pregnant females. In the event of a pregnancy, this activity is eventually taken over by the placenta, decidua, and fetal membranes. Relaxin levels are highest in the first trimester and at the time of delivery. Relaxin appears to have several functions, including preparation of the endometrium for implantation at the beginning of pregnancy and softening of the cervix at the end of pregnancy. It also plays a part in the joint laxity that allows the mother's pelvic joints to move, while, unfortunately, also making all joints less stable and more prone to injury. Relaxin also helps optimize the circulatory system during pregnancy. Too much relaxin may trigger preterm birth because of the inappropriate softening of the cervix, whereas too little may disrupt maternal glucose metabolism (Marshall, Senadheera, Parry, & Girling, 2017).

Umbilical Cord

The umbilical cord, which arises from the fetal side of the placenta, serves as the conduit for blood traveling to and from the embryo or fetus. At the time of birth, it is 55 cm long and 2 cm in diameter, on average. It normally contains one large vein and two smaller arteries. A slippery substance called **Wharton's jelly** surrounds these blood vessels, which helps the cord slide back and forth between the fetus and the wall of the amniotic sac, thereby

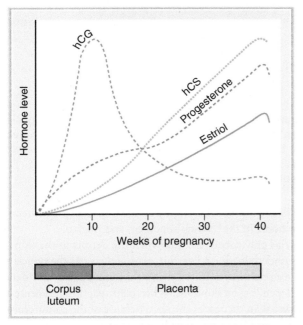

Figure 15.6. Hormone levels during pregnancy. hCG, human chorionic gonadotropin; hCS, human chorionic somatomammotropin. (Reprinted with permission from Costanzo, L. S. [2011]. *BRS physiology* [5th ed., Fig. 7.20]. Philadelphia, PA: Lippincott Williams & Wilkins.)

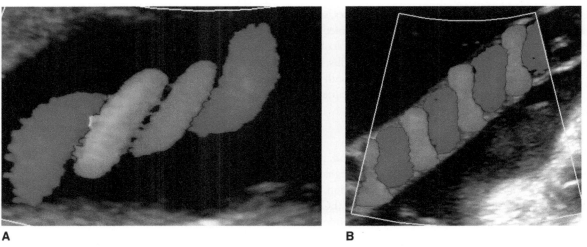

A **B**

Figure 15.7. Umbilical cords with different numbers of vessels, shown by color Doppler ultrasound, sagittal view. (A) Three-vessel umbilical cord: two arteries and one vein, with appropriate cord coiling. **(B)** Two-vessel umbilical cord: one artery and one vein. (Reprinted with permission from Stephenson, S. R. [2015]. *Obstetrics and gynecology* [3rd ed., Fig. 18.29]. Philadelphia, PA: Lippincott Williams & Wilkins.)

preventing compression of the cord. Approximately one out of every 200 cords has only two blood vessels: one artery and one vein. Although these pregnancies may be otherwise normal, this cord variation is associated with a higher rate of congenital abnormalities (Sadler, Chapter 8: Third Month to Birth: The Fetus and Placenta, 2014). In most pregnancies, the umbilical cord inserts into the center of the placenta. The umbilical cord often appears as a spiral, most likely from fetal movement (Fig. 15.7).

Maternal Anatomy and Physiology in Pregnancy

A woman's body changes throughout her pregnancy, sometimes in ways that she's witnessed in others and expects, such as an expanding belly and weight gain, and sometimes in ways she may not have anticipated. Some changes may be uncomfortable or confusing, and the nurse should discuss with the patient the broad range of expected changes.

Integumentary System

The integumentary system includes the skin, hair, and nails. Hormonal fluctuations can cause various changes in all of these structures. These changes may vary from woman to woman but also from pregnancy to pregnancy in the same woman.

Skin

Common skin changes during pregnancy include **striae gravidarum** and changes in pigmentation and vasculature.

Striae Gravidarum

One of the most familiar changes in the skin during pregnancy is stretch marks (Fig. 15.8), also called striae gravidarum. Many women already have some on their breasts and hips from rapid

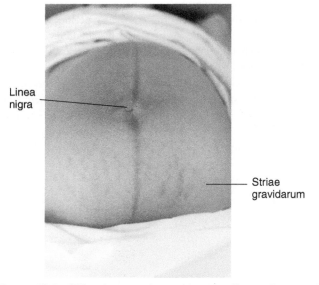

Linea nigra

Striae gravidarum

Figure 15.8. Skin changes in pregnancy: linea nigra and striae gravidarum. (Reprinted with permission from Evans, R. J., Brown, Y. M., & Evans, M. K. [2014]. *Canadian maternity, newborn, and women's health nursing* [2nd ed., Fig. 12.5]. Philadelphia, PA: Lippincott Williams & Wilkins.)

growth and hormonal changes during puberty. In pregnancy, they often occur in the breasts, abdomen, and thighs.

Striae gravidarum develop when the dermis of the skin, the layer underlying the epidermis, tears and creates the typical scar of the stretch mark. Initially, stretch marks appear very dark or red, depending on skin tone. When palpated, they feel depressed, or lower than the rest of the skin, because of the compromise of the dermis. Over time, they become paler and, on lighter skin, develop a silvery appearance.

Laser and light therapies may be effective for reducing the appearance of stretch marks in some. Topical treatments, however, have not been shown to be effective (Al-Himdani, Ud-Din, Gilmore,

& Bayat, 2014). Many women believe that keeping their skin well moisturized with products such as cocoa butter and vitamin E helps prevent stretch marks. Although its effectiveness has not been substantiated by research, this practice is also unlikely to cause harm (Yamaguchi, Suganuma, & Ohashi, 2014).

Pigmentation Changes

A classic pigmentation change in pregnancy, the linea nigra, occurs more commonly in women with darker skin. It starts at the pubic symphysis and varies in length, in some women going all the way to the top (the fundus) of the uterus. As with other pregnancy-related hyperpigmentation conditions, such as the darkening of existing nevi (moles) and macules (freckles) and of the areolae of the breasts, the linea nigra generally disappears after pregnancy as estrogen, progesterone, and melanocyte-stimulating hormone decrease to their normal, prepregnancy levels (McNulty-Brown & Vaughan-Jones, 2016).

Chloasma of pregnancy is another hyperpigmentation change more common in women with darker pigmented skin (Fig. 15.9). Chloasma manifests as a collection of brownish patches over the face and is often referred to as "melasma" or "the mask of pregnancy," although it may also occur with the use of estrogen-containing birth control methods, such as the pill, the patch, and the ring. Exposure to sun tends to darken chloasma, and the use of sunscreen may prevent this. As with linea nigra, chloasma typically resolves spontaneously after pregnancy, but may persist for many months or even years in some women (McNulty-Brown & Vaughan-Jones, 2016).

Vascular Changes

Superficial blood vessels often become more prominent in early pregnancy, especially in women with pale skin, as blood vessels dilate and proliferate because of increases in estrogen level. Redness of the soles of the feet and palms of the hands, called **palmar erythema**, is another common change caused by increased blood flow and is harmless and painless. Small vascular changes, such as telangiectasias and spider angiomas (Fig. 15.10), may occur

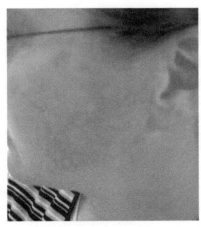

Figure 15.9. Chloasma. Also called melasma or "the mask of pregnancy." (Reprinted with permission from Jensen, S. [2014]. *Nursing health assessment: A best practice approach* [2nd ed., Fig. 25.5]. Philadelphia, PA: Lippincott Williams & Wilkins.)

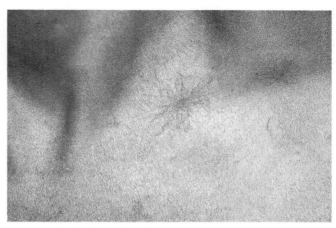

Figure 15.10. Spider angioma. (Reprinted with permission from Weber, J. R., & Kelley, J. H. [2014]. *Health assessment in nursing* [5th ed., unnumbered figure in Chapter 14]. Philadelphia, PA: Lippincott Williams & Wilkins.)

and, unlike other vascular changes, may not resolve completely after pregnancy (McNulty-Brown & Vaughan-Jones, 2016).

Hair and Nails

Thicker and more abundant scalp hair is another common change in pregnancy, and one that many women welcome. Hair grows in cycles. At any given time, 10% to 15% of scalp hair follicles are in the telogen phase, during which the hair does not grow, and the rest are in the anagen phase, during which the hair does grow. When a follicle reaches the end of the telogen phase and is about to enter the anagen phase, it drops its hair to make room for a new one. Most people lose about 100 hairs a day this way (Abraham, Chu, & Elder, 2014). In pregnancy, however, estrogen stimulates the hair follicles, causing both phases to last longer and resulting in more hair growth and less hair loss. Hair growth generally returns to normal within the first 4 months postpartum, creating actual excessive hair loss or the impression of excessive hair loss, which may be concerning to the patient. In some cases, scalp hair may be permanently thinned after pregnancy. Some women may alternately experience an increase in hair loss during pregnancy. This may be a result of poor nutrition or illness or may be normal for this pregnancy (McNulty-Brown & Vaughan-Jones, 2016).

Body hair, both fine vellus and course, also tends to become more abundant during pregnancy. Vellus hair tends to shed after birth, but new growth of coarse hair, often on the abdomen, chest, and face, persists. Changes in nails are diverse, as they may become softer, harder, or more brittle (McNulty-Brown & Vaughan-Jones, 2016).

Endocrine System

The roles of hCG, hCS, progesterone, estrogen, luteinizing hormone, and follicle-stimulating hormone in pregnancy are discussed above and in Chapter 14. Other hormones critical in pregnancy include those secreted by the thyroid gland (tri-iodothyronine and thyroxine), pancreas (insulin), adrenal glands (cortisol and aldosterone), and pituitary glands (prolactin and oxytocin).

Thyroid Gland

Because the fetus cannot produce its own thyroid hormones until the 12th week of pregnancy, the mother must supply them in early pregnancy. Adequate amounts of the thyroid hormones tri-iodothyronine and thyroxine are critical to fetal neurologic development. In addition, maternal hypothyroidism has been associated with miscarriage, preeclampsia, gestational diabetes, preterm birth, placental abruption, cesarean section, and induction of labor. Hyperthyroidism has also been linked with preeclampsia and cesarean section (Männistö, Mendola, Grewal, Xie, Chen, & Laughon, 2013).

During pregnancy, production of thyroid hormones may be cued by thyroid-stimulating hormone from the pituitary gland, as normal, as well as by estrogen and hCG. As a result, blood levels of thyroid hormones are often increased in pregnancy, which can make it difficult to distinguish between a normal adaptation of pregnancy and a thyroid disorder.

Pancreas

Insulin needs in pregnancy initially are the same as they are previous to pregnancy and then drop slightly in the late first trimester and early second trimester, after which they increase steadily until the end of pregnancy (see Fig. 9.5). These changes in the demands on the islets of Langerhans of the pancreas are largely due to the reduction in the responsiveness of the cells of the mother's body to insulin. This reduced responsiveness can be overcome by a greater production of insulin. Women whose pancreases cannot keep up with the cellular demand for increased insulin develop gestational diabetes.

Adrenal Glands

During pregnancy, the adrenal glands—which sit atop the kidneys—increase the production of both cortisol and aldosterone. Cortisol levels begin to climb in the second trimester and peak at the end of the third trimester of pregnancy. This late surge may help promote both lung and neurologic development of the fetus. Aldosterone helps retain sodium that would otherwise be excreted from the kidneys. This retention of sodium helps swell blood volume over the course of the pregnancy (Rhoades & Bell, 2017).

Pituitary Gland

Like luteinizing hormone and follicle-stimulating hormone (Chapter 14), prolactin is produced primarily by the anterior pituitary. Prolactin is active in milk production. Oxytocin, produced by the posterior pituitary, also has a role in lactation; it stimulates milk ejection. Oxytocin also acts on the uterus to produce contractions prior to labor and during childbirth. It further works to keep the uterus contracted postpartum to prevent atony and excessive uterine bleeding (Rhoades & Bell, 2017).

Respiratory System

Oxygen consumption increases approximately 15% to 20% in pregnancy. Several adaptations are necessary to make this change possible. The first is an increase of 40% to 50% in tidal volume, the amount of air that goes in and out of the lungs during quiet breathing (Costantine, 2015). During tidal breathing, very little of the total lung capacity is actually used. The average tidal volume of a nonpregnant adult is about 0.5 L/breath, and the average lung capacity of a nonpregnant female is 4.2 L/breath. Respiratory rate does not change from prepregnancy rates; instead, each breath taken is approximately 30% to 50% greater in volume than that before pregnancy (Costantine, 2015). In other words, if a woman's tidal volume is typically 0.5 L/breath, in pregnancy her tidal volume may be closer to 0.75 L/breath.

This mild hyperventilation causes the pregnant woman to "blow off" more CO_2 than she normally would, allowing for CO_2 in the fetal circulation to diffuse into the maternal bloodstream, and O_2 to diffuse from the mother to the fetus, thus improving oxygenation of the fetus. This is a state of physiologic respiratory alkalosis, meaning that the pH of the blood is slightly higher than it would be in the nonpregnant woman as a result of an increase in respiration volume and that this is a normal finding at this time.

As the uterus grows during pregnancy, the diaphragm is elevated approximately 5 cm, effectively shortening the thoracic cavity. To accommodate this change, the ribs expand and the subcostal angle at the middle of the chest between the left and right rib cages grows from approximately 68.5° prior to pregnancy to 103.5° at term (Fig. 15.11). As a result of this remodeling, respiratory capacity is not reduced, although many women may experience dyspnea (shortness of breath) throughout pregnancy, starting as early as the first trimester. This sense of dyspnea may result more from the reflex that leads to respiratory alkalosis or changes in the maternal metabolism than it does from the actual mass of the pregnancy displacing or compressing the lungs (LoMauro & Aliverti, 2015).

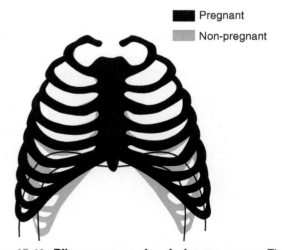

Figure 15.11. Rib cage expansion during pregnancy. The rib cage in pregnancy (black) expands laterally, which increases the subcostal angle and chest diameter, when compared with the nonpregnant state (blue). (Reprinted with permission from Irion, J. M., & Irion, G. L. [2009]. *Women's health in physical therapy* [1st ed., Fig. 11.9]. Philadelphia, PA: Lippincott Williams & Wilkins.)

Increased estrogen levels in pregnancy cause congestion of the mucous membranes because these tissues become more vascular. For some women, this congestion can cause problems. For example, swelling of the pharynx, trachea, and larynx may cause temporary deepening of the voice. Swelling of the sinuses may cause nasal congestion that can be chronic throughout the pregnancy. Engorged capillaries may cause frequent nose bleeds (epistaxis).

Cardiovascular System

Pregnancy places increased demands on the cardiovascular system, which results in significant changes in cardiac output, total blood volume, white blood cell count, blood pressure, and heart sounds.

Cardiac Output

Overall cardiac output (the volume of blood pumped by the heart each minute) increases by as much as 50% in pregnancy, peaking between 25 and 30 weeks' gestation. This output is made possible by a heart rate increase of 15 to 20 beats per minute (bpm), as well as an increase of 25% to 30% in stroke volume (the amount of blood pumped by the left ventricle of the heart per beat). This increased work may cause a minor hypertrophy (enlarging) of the heart (Sharma, Kumar, & Aneja, 2016).

Total Blood Volume

Total blood volume increases by 40% to 45% above prepregnancy levels. The volume of plasma, the portion of the blood that suspends the blood cells, increases by 40% to 50% in pregnancy, whereas the red blood cell count increases by 30% (de Haas, Ghossein-Doha, van Kuijk, van Drongelen, & Spaanderman, 2017). Because the volume of red blood cells is considered in proportion to the total blood volume, the relative increased volume of plasma over the red blood cell count results in hemoglobin and hematocrit values in pregnancy that would suggest anemia in a woman who was not pregnant. In fact, this is a physiologic anemia, also referred to as a pseudoanemia. For context, the normal hematocrit range is 37 to 47 for a nonpregnant woman and 33 to 39 for a pregnant woman. The normal hemoglobin range is 12 to 16 for a nonpregnant woman and 11 to 13 for a pregnant woman (CDC, 1989).

White Blood Cell Count

White blood cell production also increases in pregnancy, and therefore an elevated white blood cell count should not necessarily be considered a sign of infection. The normal white blood cell count range is 4.5 to 11 in nonpregnant women and 9 to 15 in pregnant women. The white blood cell count typically drops to prepregnancy rates by 1 week postpartum. Platelet counts in pregnancy do not vary considerably from nonpregnant values, although fibrinogen levels, as well as those of other clotting factors, may rise considerably, particularly in late pregnancy and the postpartum period. This rise is believed to help prevent excessive postpartum bleeding, but it also puts women at a higher risk for a dangerous blood clot that could lead to a pulmonary embolism or stroke.

Blood Pressure

Despite the increased blood volume and stroke volume, maternal blood pressure typically decreases, particularly in early pregnancy, and then returns to prepregnancy values at the end of pregnancy. This decrease in blood pressure is due to hormones acting on blood vessels to reduce peripheral vascular resistance.

Heart Sounds

All of these changes—reduced peripheral vascular resistance, heart hypertrophy, and increased cardiac output—commonly cause temporary changes in heart sounds that start after the first trimester and should resolve in the first week postpartum. Variations in heart sounds include an S1 split in most pregnant women, a systolic murmur (90% of women), a third heart sound (80% of women), and a diastolic (S2) murmur (20% of women). All of these heart sounds changes are considered benign (Sanghavi & Rutherford, 2014).

Urinary System

The kidneys function to eliminate waste, regulate fluid and electrolyte balance, stimulate red blood cell production, and regulate blood pressure. The kidneys must adapt all of these roles to the hormonal and physical changes of pregnancy.

The renal pelves and the proximal portions of the ureters that attach to the renal pelves dilate by the end of the first trimester of pregnancy. Because of the position of the ureters between the kidneys and bladder and the continuous growth of the uterus, the ureters must also stretch and grow and will retain a larger volume of urine at any given time. The kidneys themselves are larger due to the retention of fluid (Cheung & Lafayette, 2014).

Blood flow to and through the kidneys increases by 80% during pregnancy because of the combination of increased blood volume, particularly plasma volume, and increased cardiac output. Because of the increased volume, there is also about a 50% increase in the glomerular filtration rate, which is the rate at which blood plasma filters through the kidneys. Because of changes in the tubular function, which shunts nutrients back into the bloodstream while disposing of waste into the renal pelves and ureters, it is not uncommon for women to spill glucose and protein into the urine. In a nonpregnant person, this condition might signal diabetes or kidney disease, but, like the anemia common to pregnancy, it is considered physiologic in small amounts. It should be noted, however, that new glucose in the urine may signal gestational diabetes, and new protein in the urine may cue evaluation for preeclampsia, especially after the 20th week gestation (Cheung & Lafayette, 2014).

In pregnancy, the threshold of hydration at which thirst is cued and the release of antidiuretic hormone is lower than it is for women who are not pregnant. Dehydration could lead to lower plasma volume and decreased placental perfusion, thus compromising the pregnancy. Although more salt is re-absorbed during pregnancy, more water is also preferentially absorbed, leading to lower serum sodium proportion but an overall sodium gain of between 900 and 1,000 mEq. Overall water gain is approximately 1.6 L. Because of the action of progesterone, potassium levels also increase in pregnancy, as the tubular reabsorption of potassium is prioritized (Cheung & Lafayette, 2014).

Reproductive System

The changes to the reproductive system are the most overt, the most obvious during the course of a pregnancy. **Hyperplasia** (growth caused by production of new cells) and **hypertrophy** (growth caused by increase in the size of existing cells) are clearly observable, but many more subtle changes also contribute to the success of a pregnancy.

Breasts

For some women, the first symptom of pregnancy is a change in breast sensation that may range from mildly heightened sensitivity to pain. Exposed to high levels of estrogen and progesterone, the internal structures of the breast—the ducts, lobes, lobules, and alveoli—grow and the breasts become fuller (Fig. 15.12). In some women, this combination of growth and

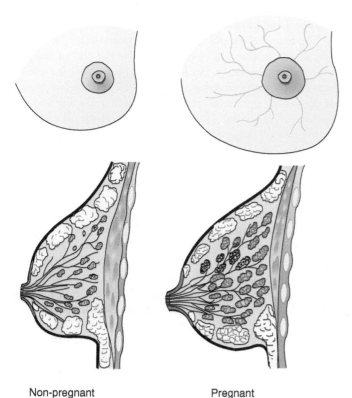

Figure 15.12. Comparison of nonpregnant and pregnant breasts. (Reprinted with permission from Pillitteri, A. [2002]. *Maternal and child health nursing: Care of the childbearing and childrearing family* [4th ed., Fig. 9-5]. Philadelphia, PA: Lippincott Williams & Wilkins.)

Non-pregnant   Pregnant

hormonal stimulation may lead to stretch marks similar to those common over the abdomen, as mentioned previously. The vascular expansion to the breasts is particularly obvious over the breasts of women with a pale skin tone. Nipples and areolae darken, more so in women with a darker skin tone. Montgomery tubercles (also called Montgomery glands') sebaceous glands that cover the areolae and moisturize the nipples, also hypertrophy.

In Chapter 3, one of the first early discomforts of pregnancy Susan reported was breast tenderness, along with nausea, fatigue, and an aversion to the smell of coffee.

Colostrum, a yellowish, early form of milk, starts being produced midway through the pregnancy or earlier. Some women may spontaneously leak colostrum, whereas others may produce colostrum in response to nipple stimulation. Pregnancies that end as early as the second trimester may cue limited lactation in some women.

Ovaries

On implantation, the placenta begins secreting hCG, which cues the corpus luteum of the ovary to persist in producing progesterone as well as smaller amounts of estrogen and relaxin, as reviewed previously in this chapter. The corpus luteum, a temporary structure, begins to regress in the second half of the first trimester. The combination of high levels of estrogen and high levels of progesterone during pregnancy suppresses the release of the luteinizing hormone and the follicle-stimulating hormone from the pituitary gland during pregnancy, preventing follicle recruitment and ovulation during pregnancy (Sadler, Chapter 3: First Week of Development: Ovulation to Implantation, 2014).

Uterus

The uterus grows from approximately the size of an egg to the size of a grapefruit from the start of pregnancy to the beginning of the second trimester because of hypertrophy and hyperplasia of the organ. After the first trimester, the growing fetus primarily accounts for growth. The pattern and rate of growth are predictable in a normal pregnancy (see Fig. 4.4). Between 16 and 36 weeks of gestation, the size of the uterus in centimeters, when measured from the pubic symphysis to the fundus, should equal the number of weeks of gestation. For example, the uterus in a 34-week pregnancy should measure approximately 34 cm.

Braxton Hicks contractions are contractions of the uterus that do not lead to progressive cervical changes, as contractions of labor do. They can first be detected clinically as early as 6 weeks' gestation, but are unlikely to be felt by the mother or a clinician until well into the second trimester. These contractions are irregular and painless and typically resolve with hydration or rest.

Just as with true labor contractions, Braxton Hicks contractions alter blood flow to the placenta, but this is not believed to harm the pregnancy (Sindinga et al., 2016). The blood flow to the uterus increases 20-fold during pregnancy, with most of this blood traveling through the intervillous space of the placenta so the exchange of nutrients and oxygen from the mother and waste from the fetus can occur (Browne et al., 2015). In very early pregnancy, this increased vascularity of the uterus causes Hegar's sign, a softening of the lower portion of the uterus that can cause the entire uterus to flex forward in early pregnancy (anteflexion). This exaggerated flexion may put extra pressure on the bladder and contribute to uncomfortable symptoms, such as urinary frequency.

Cervix

Early in pregnancy, the same vascularization that causes Hegar's signs also causes Goodell's sign, a softening of the cervix. The glandular cells of the cervix hypertrophy in pregnancy, creating an irregular network of mucus-producing cells and an overall enlargement of the cervix. The mucus produced by these cells form a mucus plug inside the cervical canal, which is called the **operculum**. This operculum creates a barrier against outside pathogens during pregnancy. As the cervix opens in late pregnancy just prior to or during labor, the operculum passes. The appearance of this blood-streaked mucus is often referred to as bloody show.

Vagina and Vulva

Increased vascularity of the sexual organs causes various changes. An early clinically observable change is Chadwick's sign, which is a bluing of the vulva, vagina, and cervix that is observable by the eighth week of gestation, 6 weeks after fertilization. Increased vascularity can also lead to heightened sexual interest and response, although it may cause vulvar varicosities and perineal edema. Sex in pregnancy is generally considered safe in the absence of bleeding or membrane rupture. However, sexual response may vary throughout pregnancy because of both physiological and psychological factors, such as how a woman feels about her changing body, the pregnancy, and her partner.

Normal vaginal discharge also changes in pregnancy. Leukorrhea of pregnancy is a discharge that is white and relatively thick and may be copious. Leukorrhea may have a musty odor but should not smell foul or fishy. There should be no blood in normal discharge. Although there may be minor vulvar irritation due to increased moisture, there should not be any pruritus. The pH of the vagina is slightly more acidic in pregnancy, which generally protects against some bacterial pathogens, although women may be more prone to *Candida* (yeast) infections. The *Candida* organisms that cause yeast are not adverse to an acidic environment and do particularly well with the slight elevation in body temperature typical of pregnancy, as well as the glycogen-rich vaginal environment caused by the changes in glucose and insulin metabolism (Aguin & Sobel, 2015).

In Chapter 7, Hannah thought her water had broken, but this impression was not confirmed by further evaluation. Rochelle, the nurse caring for her, told her the fluid she noticed was likely either urine leakage or leukorrhea of pregnancy.

Musculoskeletal System

Common changes that occur in the musculoskeletal system during pregnancy include those related to posture, ligaments and joints, abdominal muscles, and calcium stores in bone.

Posture

As her abdomen grows during pregnancy, the mother experiences postural changes, including a more exaggerated curve to her lumbar spine, called lordosis, which may contribute to back pain and other discomforts. This shift in posture, along with uterine growth and reduced tone of the abdominal muscles, causes a shift in the mother's center of gravity and puts her at a higher risk for falls.

Ligaments and Joints

This increased fall risk may be exacerbated by changes to the joints caused by the hormones relaxin and progesterone that make them less stable, while also increasing the mobility of the pelvis in preparation for delivery. This softening of the joints also accounts for the classic "waddle" often seen in pregnant women. As the pelvic ligaments relax, many women also experience sharp pain at the level of the mons pubis from hypermobility of the symphysis pubis in the latter part of pregnancy. This pain is most common with activities such as walking and climbing stairs. This condition, referred to as symphysis pubis dysfunction, typically resolves spontaneously after delivery (Mackenzie, Murray, & Lusher, 2018).

Musculature overlying the abdominal cavity and the round ligaments of the uterus within the abdominal cavity are also subject to alterations in pregnancy. The two round ligaments of the uterus attach to the uterus at the level of the fallopian tubes, travel through the inguinal canal, and attach at the level of the groin. These ligaments work to position and stabilize the uterus. During pregnancy, both hormonal factors and the mechanical force of the growing uterus cause these ligaments to stretch and spasm. Pregnant women often identify round ligament pain as sharp, brief, and unilateral. It may also present as a dull, persistent, unilateral pain, particularly after a long period of physical activity.

Abdominal Muscles

The abdominal muscles stretch over the growing uterus and lose tone, but gradually recover after delivery. Abdominal muscles may also ultimately separate at the midline. When this separation, referred to as **diastasis recti**, occurs, the muscle no longer overlies the central portion of the abdominal wall (Fig. 15.13). Diastasis recti occurs more commonly in women who have

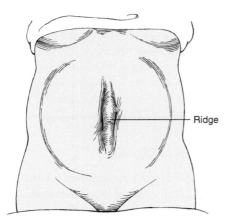

Figure 15.13. Diastasis recti. This condition occurs when the two rectus abdominis muscles separate and a section of the bowel protrudes through the separation, appearing as a midline ridge. The bulge may appear only when a supine client raises her head or coughs. (Reprinted with permission from Weber, J. R., & Kelley, J. H. [2003]. *Health assessment in nursing with case studies on bonus CD-ROM* [2nd ed., Fig. 18.6]. Philadelphia, PA: Lippincott Williams & Wilkins.)

carried multiple pregnancies. This condition is benign but is not reversible without surgical intervention, although physical therapy may also be helpful (Benjamin, Water, & Peiris, 2014).

Calcium Stores in Bone

Increased levels of parathyroid hormone in pregnancy increase renal reabsorption of calcium. The parathyroid hormone also leaches a small amount of calcium from bones for redistribution to the fetus. Although this amount of reabsorption is not typically clinically significant and is usually completely reversible after pregnancy, it may negatively affect the health of women who live in low-resource areas of the world, who have poor maternal access to nutrition and contraception, and who have large numbers of closely spaced pregnancies. These negative health impacts can include osteoporosis and bone fractures.

Gastrointestinal System

Reduced peristalsis (movement) of the gastrointestinal tract causes a delay in stomach emptying starting in the first trimester. Reduced peristalsis may also contribute to slowed emptying of bile from the gallbladder and/or liver. These physiologic changes can result in several common complaints of pregnancy, such as heartburn, constipation and gallstones, which are discussed in greater detail below.

Metabolism is another aspect of the gastrointestinal system that undergoes changes during pregnancy. Over the course of the pregnancy, because of increased needs of the fetus and the mother, the maternal basal metabolic rate increases by approximately 10% to 20%. To meet these increased metabolic needs, the mother must consume about 350 additional dietary calories per day in the second trimester of pregnancy and 450 additional calories in the third trimester of pregnancy (Academy of Nutrition and Dietetics, 2014). Weight gain is expected and desirable in most pregnancies

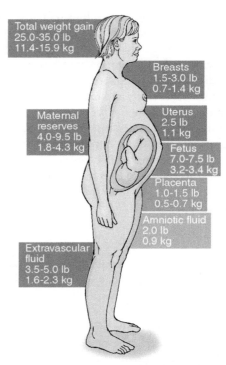

Figure 15.14. Distribution of weight gain during pregnancy. (Reprinted with permission from Weber, J. R. [2018]. *Nurses' handbook of health assessment* [9th ed., Fig. 24.1]. Philadelphia, PA: Lippincott Williams & Wilkins.)

(see Boxes 1.5 and 4.6; Fig. 15.14). Too little weight gain may result in a small-for-gestational age infant, whereas too much may increase the risk for complications such as pregnancy-induced hypertension and a greater risk for surgical delivery.

Normal Discomforts of Pregnancy and Self-Care

The myriad changes that occur as part of a normal pregnancy may cause various uncomfortable symptoms, discussed below. Some problems may simply require the nurse to reassure the client, whereas others call for more directed self-care.

Many of the discomforts of pregnancy, such as constipation, back pain, and leg cramps, may be relieved or even prevented by regular exercise. There are very few contraindications to exercise in pregnancy, and all women should be encouraged to participate in both aerobic and strength training activities unless instructed not to by her physician, nurse practitioner, or midwife. Scuba diving and activities that may result in trauma to the abdomen should be avoided. Some activities may need to be modified because of the changes of pregnancy, but it is generally considered safe to continue activities initiated prior to pregnancy and to start new programs of exercise (Artal, 2016).

Fatigue

Fatigue is particularly common in pregnancy, especially in early and late stages. Encourage women to rest or even nap when possible. Reassure the client that fatigue is common and will not persist, and give her "permission" to prioritize her own rest and well-being and to enlist help.

In Chapter 8, Gracie's weight gain peaked in the first trimester when she felt too fatigued to exercise. Her weight gain slowed once she regained some energy and started exercising regularly.

Respiratory Discomforts

Some women experience dyspnea, or difficulty breathing, in pregnancy because of hormonal and anatomic changes. Reassure the client that this experience is common in pregnancy, and show her the results of her routine pulse oximetry to affirm that her O_2 saturation is normal (assuming that it is). Teach the client strategies for improving her posture during pregnancy, particularly if she has adopted a slumped shoulder stance, because this position limits lung expansion. Provide instruction on stretching, controlled breathing exercises, and light exercise, which may help alleviate the sensation of breathlessness. Women experiencing chronic nasal congestion or epistaxis in pregnancy may benefit from saline nasal sprays or humidifiers, although the use of over-the-counter medications such as decongestants should be discouraged, because they present a small increased risk for birth defects (Yau, Mitchell, Lin, Werler, & Hernández-Díaz, 2013).

Cardiovascular Discomforts

Common discomforts of pregnancy associated with the cardiovascular system include postural hypotension, edema, and varicosities.

Postural Hypotension

Lightheadedness is common in early pregnancy and is often attributed to low blood pressure and orthostatic hypotension. It is most common when a woman is standing and is relieved by lying down. Lightheadedness that does not resolve with lying down or that occurs with an abnormality of heart rate or rhythm requires further evaluation.

Women who experience lightheadedness when rising to an upright position (a sign of orthostatic hypotension) should be instructed to avoid sitting up or standing abruptly. Orthostatic hypotension can be confirmed by taking two blood pressure measurements: one after a patient has been lying supine for at least 5 minutes and a second within 2 to 5 minutes after standing. A fall in systolic pressure of at least 20 mm Hg or a fall in diastolic pressure of at least 10 mm Hg when standing confirms the diagnosis.

Many women also experience supine hypotension, which is a temporary state caused by compression of the inferior vena cava (a large vein carrying blood from the lower body back to the heart) by the pregnant uterus when the woman lies on her back (see Fig. 6.3). This condition typically first occurs midway

through pregnancy and may recur at any point until after delivery. Symptoms of supine hypotension include nausea, dizziness, and lightheadedness. This condition can be alleviated by the woman shifting to her side or into an upright position such that her uterus is no longer compressing the inferior vena cava.

In Chapter 6, Rebecca was told to lie on her side to sleep to avoid compression of the vena cava and diminished oxygen exchange between the placenta and the fetus. She remembered this advice when the paramedics placed her on the stretcher in a side-lying position after her accident.

Moreover, emerging evidence suggests a correlation between sleeping in a supine position and stillbirth, as this position also contributes to reduced placental perfusion. Therefore, even women who do not become light-headed, diaphoretic, anxious, or nauseous while lying supine should lie on their sides (Gordon et al., 2015; O'Brien & Warland, 2014; Rådestad, Sormunen, Rudenhed, & Pettersson, 2015).

Edema

Swelling of the extremities, particularly the feet and ankles but also the hands, and face is a normal part of pregnancy and happens for a few different reasons. The increased volume of fluid in the blood vessels causes a change in the colloid osmotic pressure, meaning that the protein concentration is higher in the interstitial space (outside the blood vessels) than in the intravascular space (inside the blood vessels). This pressure causes passage of extra fluid from the intravascular space into the interstitial space to dilute the protein in the interstitial space, so that it equalizes with that of the intravascular space. Later in pregnancy, this process is compounded by the weight of the gravid uterus on the veins of the pelvis. This extra weight partially occludes these veins, delaying vascular return and forcing fluid from the veins into the interstitial space. A side-lying position is recommended to remove the pressure from the pelvic veins and allow for normal vascular return. Edema that arises suddenly, particularly with other symptoms, such as blurred vision, epigastric pain, or headache, is concerning and suggests preeclampsia, particularly in the presence of hypertension.

Approximately 10% to 15% of women develop nondependent edema in pregnancy in areas such as the face or hands. This kind of swelling may indicate preeclampsia, but it is not considered a specific or particularly sensitive sign (Task Force on Hypertension in Pregnancy, 2013). Edema that is present in only one leg or that is more pronounced in one leg than the other is suggestive of a deep vein thrombosis.

Dependent edema of the legs and feet can be an uncomfortable feature of late pregnancy. Advise clients that light exercise, avoidance of prolonged periods of sitting and standing, elevation of the legs, and sleeping in the left side-lying position promote optimal venous return from the lower extremities and thus may help alleviate edema.

Varicosities

The pressure of the pregnancy on the pelvic vasculature also contributes to an increased incidence of varicosities (distended veins) in later pregnancy, which may present as varicose veins, vulvar varicosities, or hemorrhoids. Although many varicosities may present only cosmetic concerns, some—particularly vulvar varicosities and hemorrhoids—may cause much discomfort. Varicosities may resolve spontaneously after pregnancy or persist.

Advise patients that they can reduce the incidence and frequency of hemorrhoids in late pregnancy by avoiding constipation, as bearing down may contribute to their formation. Self-care measures that are effective in relieving symptoms temporarily include application of topical witch hazel or ice to the affected area and sitz baths. Inform your patient that lying down, particularly with elevated hips, improves venous return and may help resolve the hemorrhoids, but is unlikely to provide relief to the immediate pain and itching they can cause. Steroid cream treatment is likely safe in pregnancy, although treatment should be limited to a week or less. Refer clients with severe hemorrhoids to a gastroenterologist (Zielinski, Searing, & Deibel, 2015).

As with dependent edema, light exercise, avoidance of prolonged periods of sitting and standing, and sleeping in the left side-lying position may relieve some of the discomforts of varicosities. Compression stockings, however, do not appear to help symptoms. Small studies have indicated some symptom relief from reflexology and water immersion if both varicosities and edema are present (Smyth, Aflaifel, & Bamigboye, 2015).

Neurologic Discomforts

Neurologic changes in pregnancy typically occur secondary to pregnancy-related edema, postural changes, and vascular alterations and not as a direct effect of the hormonal changes of pregnancy.

Carpal Tunnel Syndrome

A temporary form of carpal tunnel syndrome may occur in pregnancy because of edema around the nerves of the wrist. Carpal tunnel syndrome, which causes paresthesia (changes of sensation, including tingling) of the affected hand, is caused by compression of the median nerve of the wrist. In pregnancy, edema often causes this compression; thus, resolution of the edema also resolves the symptoms. Similar symptoms may also be caused by the common stooped-shoulder stance of pregnancy causing traction on the brachial plexus, which emphasizes the importance of good pregnancy posture. Similarly, compression of the pelvic nerves may cause sensory changes in the legs.

Headaches

Headaches are common in pregnancy and may be caused by stress, hormones, vascular changes such as those that cause vasodilation of the sinuses, or vision changes. Postural changes may also contribute to headache. Rest may help with headaches, as well as cool compresses, massage, stress reduction, and avoiding headache triggers. Ibuprofen should not be used to treat headache symptoms after 24 weeks of gestation because of concerns about premature closure of the fetal ductus arteriosus. Acetaminophen is generally believed to be safe in pregnancy, although newer evidence suggests a correlation between use of this medication in pregnancy and behavioral problems in offspring (Stergiakouli, Thapar, & Davey Smith, 2016).

A headache after 20 weeks of pregnancy is concerning for preeclampsia and requires further evaluation. Other headache danger signs requiring follow-up are the sudden onset of a severe headache, a change in mental status, a headache that wakes the sufferer from sleep, a headache that does not respond to pain medications, a change in pattern from the woman's usual headache, vision changes, neck stiffness, and a headache in a woman with a suppressed immune system.

Vision Changes

Some women may also experience slightly worsened vision, blurred vision, or dry eyes as a result of hormonal changes and edema. Such changes are generally minor and temporary and reverse in the first several months postpartum. Some women, however, may find they need a change in their prescription for glasses or contact lenses. Contact lens wearers may be unable to comfortably wear their lenses during pregnancy because of the irritation of dry eyes. Moisturizing eye drops may help increase comfort and are not contraindicated in pregnancy. The nurse should instruct women to report reduced or distorted vision and blind spots, however, as these can be symptoms of a rare complication of pregnancy called central serous chorioretinopathy (Errera, Kohl, & Cruz, 2013).

Reproductive Discomforts

Some common discomforts of the reproductive system during pregnancy include breast tenderness and leaking, Braxton Hicks contractions, and vaginal discharge.

Breast Tenderness and Leaking

Acutely tender and enlarged breasts are one of the earliest discomforts of pregnancy for many women. Reassure women who experience this discomfort that it usually resolves by the end of the first trimester, and encourage use of a supportive, well-fitting bra to provide relief. Advise women with large breasts who experience breast tenderness in pregnancy to consider wearing a soft sleep bra at night.

In Chapter 2, one of the earliest discomforts of pregnancy for Tatiana was breast tenderness.

From the middle of pregnancy on, women may leak small amounts of yellow colostrum. Reassure such women that this is normal, and advise them to wear breast pads inside of their clothing to avoid staining and leakage.

Braxton Hicks Contractions

Although some women won't notice Braxton Hicks contractions of the uterus in pregnancy, others may find them uncomfortable or concerning. Reassure clients that these are normal, but also teach them how to distinguish these contractions from true contractions (see Patient Teaching 2.3). True contractions are regular, progressively grow stronger, do not resolve with rest and relaxation, and become more intense with ambulation. Braxton Hicks contractions may have periods of regularity but are not regular overall. They often resolve with rest, hydration, and ambulation. Although Braxton Hicks contractions are typically felt only over the abdomen, true contractions are also felt as back and pelvic pressure.

In Chapter 2, Tatiana began to notice Braxton Hicks contractions after 20 weeks of pregnancy. She was told to rest and hydrate when they occurred and to evaluate for labor if they continued. Nina, a nurse practitioner, told her about the 411 of labor: having contractions at least every 4 minutes lasting for at least 1 minute for 1 hour suggests labor.

Vaginal Discharge

Leukorrhea, a condition of increased vaginal discharge that is common in pregnancy, may be troubling for some women. Reassure clients that this discharge is normal in the absence of a foul odor, pruritus, color change, or bleeding. Advise clients to wear a panty liner, preferably unscented, and to cleanse their genitals with plain water. Strongly discourage douching and cleaning the genitals with soap, because these practices may disrupt the normal vaginal flora, which can contribute to vaginitis and vaginosis.

Urinary Discomforts

Urinary frequency and urgency are a common complaint starting in early pregnancy, even in the absence of a urinary tract infection. In early pregnancy, such symptoms are more likely to be caused by hormonal changes, uterine changes, and increased blood flow through the kidneys. In late pregnancy, urinary frequency and urgency, along with nocturia (the need to urinate at night) and bladder irritability, are more likely to be caused by compression of the bladder by the uterus.

Urinary incontinence is another common complaint of pregnancy and may be caused by either bladder irritability (urge incontinence) or actions, such as sneezing or laughing, that overcome the urinary sphincters and cause involuntary loss of urine (stress incontinence).

Approximately three quarters of women experience some stress incontinence during pregnancy, and over 80% report urinary frequency and nocturia (Nigam, Ahmad, Gaur, Elahi, & Batra, 2016). Reassure clients that these conditions are normal responses to pregnancy and do not necessarily indicate urinary tract infection

(although having the additional symptom of blood in the urine or pain with urination would be concerning). Also, inform clients that these symptoms usually resolve after pregnancy without further intervention. Kegel pelvic floor exercises can be helpful for alleviating stress incontinence. However, many women find that the changes of pregnancy make it difficult or impossible to perform these exercises while pregnant. Kegels are ideally started prior to pregnancy and can be beneficial for regaining pelvic tone after pregnancy (Patient Teaching 15.1).

Nurses should also be aware that urinary tract infections occur at approximately the same rate for women who are pregnant as for women who are not pregnant, although the spread of infection to the kidneys, leading to pyelonephritis (a kidney infection), is more common. Asymptomatic bacteriuria (bacteria in the urine) is more common in pregnant women (Smaill & Vazquez, 2015). Common teachings to avoid urinary tract infections include urinating before and after sex, wiping from front to back after using the toilet, and excellent oral hydration.

Gastrointestinal Discomforts

Pregnancy produces many familiar discomforts related to the gastrointestinal system, including nausea and vomiting, food cravings, bleeding gums, salivation, heartburn, constipation, and gallstones.

Nausea and Vomiting

Nausea and vomiting is a common feature of early pregnancy and is likely caused by increased hCG levels and metabolic alterations. Nausea is more common in pregnancies involving more than one fetus, and pregnancies that include nausea are less likely to result in spontaneous abortion (Koren, Madjunkova, & Maltepe, 2014). Approximately two thirds of women experience pregnancy-related nausea, and about 1% have a severe form called hyperemesis gravidarum (Almonda, Edlundb, Joffec, & Palmed, 2016). Nausea may begin as soon as week 4 of pregnancy and typically stops by the end of the first trimester. It is rarely dangerous for the mother or the pregnancy.

In Chapter 9, Nancy experienced nausea in early pregnancy and was offered supportive measures to help with symptoms. (Tanya, too, in Chapter 13 experienced nausea in her pregnancy, which she had not had with previous pregnancies.)

Nausea in pregnancy, although self-limiting, can be very distressing, particularly if coupled with fatigue. Although most women are aware that nausea in pregnancy is normal and generally resolves with the end of the first trimester, reassurance may still be comforting. Nausea that is coupled with dehydration and weight loss is particularly concerning, as it may indicate hyperemesis gravidarum (O'Donnell et al., 2016). See Chapter 20 for additional information about hyperemesis gravidarum. Women may try various strategies to cope with nausea and may sometimes be prescribed an antiemetic, particularly if they are vomiting frequently (see Box 13.2).

Food Cravings, Bleeding Gums, and Salivation

Women in pregnancy may experience both food aversions and cravings and may report changes in how foods taste or smell. Pica, a craving for nonfood items such as starch and ice, is thought to be associated with nutritional or mineral deficits. Report any cases of pica to the woman's obstetric provider and warn the client not to consume any nonnutritive substances, as they may be dangerous for the mother or the pregnancy.

The increased vascularity of the gums that occurs normally in pregnancy may cause them to bleed easily, particularly with the development of an epulis (Fig. 15.15). An epulis is a friable (bleeding easily) nodule that typically appears late in the first trimester, grows progressively, and resolves spontaneously after pregnancy. Women with gums that are tender and bleed easily should continue to engage in careful oral hygiene using a soft toothbrush twice daily and flossing. Dental care should be continued throughout pregnancy as recommended.

Many women may complain of ptyalism (increased saliva). This may be due to either increased salivation or decreased swallowing due to nausea. For some women, ptyalism may compel them to regularly spit rather than swallow their saliva to avoid provoking nausea. Women who experience ptyalism, with or without nausea, may find that sucking on hard candies or use of an astringent mouthwash helps alleviate the symptoms of this condition. Reassure clients that these symptoms typically resolve at the end of the first trimester.

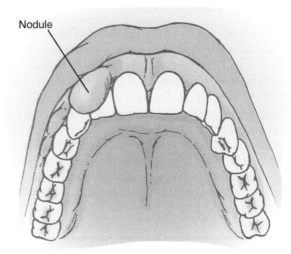

Nodule

Figure 15.15. Epulis. (Reprinted with permission from Weber, J. R., & Kelley, J. H. [2018]. *Health assessment in nursing* [6th ed., Fig. 29-6, p. 707]. Philadelphia, PA: Wolters Kluwer.)

Heartburn

Heartburn, also known as acid reflux, is another common complaint of pregnancy and is provoked by both mechanical and hormonal factors. Reduced peristalsis (movement) of the gastrointestinal tract causes a delay in stomach emptying starting in the first trimester, which contributes to reflux of stomach acid through the lower esophageal sphincter (between the esophagus and stomach) and into the esophagus. Later in pregnancy, pressure within the abdominal cavity may also cause a hiatal hernia, a condition in which part of the stomach, which normally sits below the diaphragm, pushes up through the diaphragm. The hiatal hernia also contributes to increased reflux of stomach contents into the esophagus and thus to heartburn. Hiatal hernia is more common in obesity and in pregnancies including two or more fetuses. Curiously, women who experience heartburn in pregnancy are more likely to give birth to infants with an abundance of hair, possibly because of a shared hormonal cause (Baumgardner, 2017).

Advise clients with heartburn to avoid fatty foods and consuming liquids with meals. Recommend, too, that they avoid lying down after eating and, if heartburn occurs during sleeping hours, not eat for at least 3 hours prior to sleep. As with nausea, smaller and more frequent meals may help prevent symptoms.

In Chapter 4, Sophie started to experience heartburn in the second trimester, which continued through to the end of the pregnancy. Her mother told her this meant the baby would be born with a lot of hair.

Constipation

Constipation is a familiar discomfort of pregnancy. Many factors contribute to constipation, including reduced peristalsis, increased water absorption by the colon due to the influence of estrogen and progesterone, increased iron intake from prenatal vitamins or supplements, and compression of the intestines by the gravid uterus. As in nonpregnant individuals, low-bulk dietary choices and a sedentary lifestyle can also contribute to constipation. Reduced peristalsis may also contribute to the sensation of bloating.

To help prevent constipation, encourage clients to take a fiber supplement throughout pregnancy to increase the bulk of stool. Promote the benefits of good hydration and exercise in alleviating the impact of pregnancy on the bowel. Stool softeners such as docusate sodium may also be advised, but laxatives should not be recommended without provider supervision because of a theoretical risk for electrolyte imbalance (Zielinski et al., 2015). Such measures may also help mitigate the additional flatulence that is common throughout pregnancy. Avoidance of gaseous foods such as beans may be helpful but can be impractical.

Gallstones

Reduced peristalsis in pregnancy may also contribute to slowed emptying of bile from the gallbladder or liver. Impaired bile flow from the gallbladder can contribute to the formation of gallstones. Women with suspected gallbladder disease in pregnancy will be instructed to eat a low fat diet, and medications or even surgery may be prescribed to control the condition, which may be ongoing after the birth.

Musculoskeletal Discomforts

Pregnancy discomforts of the musculoskeletal system include low back pain, ligament pain, and leg cramps.

Low Back Pain

Low back pain is a common complaint of pregnancy due to changes in the alignment of the body and the mobility of joints. To help your client avoid injury and alleviate low back pain, demonstrate to her good body mechanics and posture. Some evidence indicates that exercise, such as pelvic rocking (Fig. 15.16) and pelvic

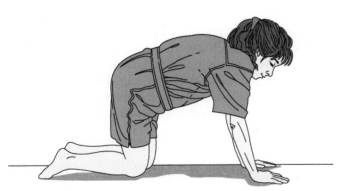

Figure 15.16. Pelvic rocking. This exercise is helpful for relieving backache during pregnancy and labor. To do it, the woman first hollows her back and then arches it. (Reprinted with permission from Pillitteri, A. [2014]. *Maternal and child health nursing: Care of the childbearing and childrearing family* [7th ed., Fig. 14-4]. Philadelphia, PA: Lippincott Williams & Wilkins.)

tilts, may offer some short-term relief and strengthen postural muscles. A specially designed pregnancy pillow may provide for a more comfortable sleeping position (Pennick & Liddle, 2013).

Ligament Pain and Leg Cramps

Round ligament pain may be felt anytime from the middle of pregnancy onward. It is usually noted on one side of the abdomen but may also present as sharp, brief hip, or groin pain that resolves quickly. Pain that persists or worsens should be evaluated. Flexing toward the side that is painful allows the muscle spasm to relax, as does moving into the flexed knees-to-abdomen position. Also, bending forward when anticipating laughing, sneezing, or other activities that trigger the pain may help prevent it.

Leg cramps may happen at any time in pregnancy, but are most common in the final trimester. They are likely related to nerve compression and vascular congestion and may be exacerbated by fatigue and plantar flexion of the feet while stretching (pointing the toes). Dorsiflexion of the toes or the entire foot, massaging the leg, or standing on a cold surface may help alleviate leg cramps.

Integumentary Discomforts

Pregnancy discomforts of the integumentary system include acne, pigmentation changes, and dry skin.

Acne and Pigmentation Changes

Because of the hormone changes of pregnancy, some women are more prone to acne in pregnancy, whereas others notice that acne improves. Women are most likely to note acne in the first two trimesters. Advise women with acne to use gentle cleansers and lotions designed for facial use and to avoid using retinoids and products containing salicylic acid, which can be harmful to the pregnancy. Antibiotics that are often used to control acne are also contraindicated in pregnancy. Women who choose to use moisturizers or makeup should be instructed to use products that are oil free. Women experiencing the hyperpigmentation of melasma can minimize its appearance by avoiding exposure to the sun and using sunscreen.

Dry Skin

Dry skin and resulting pruritus in later pregnancy is common as a result of the hormonal changes in pregnancy. To help prevent dry skin, advise clients to use mild, moisturizing soaps and emollients and to avoid hot water when taking a shower or bath, as it tends to be more drying than tepid water. Good oral hydration may be helpful.

Prenatal Care

Care in the prenatal period involves evaluation of the patient, screenings, identification of complications, and interventions, but it is also a crucial time for educating women about self-care, nutrition, danger signs, and planning. It is a time of guided transition that can be used to optimize the health and well-being of the mother and the pregnancy. For a woman with an uncomplicated pregnancy, prenatal care is preventative care that may focus more on developmental transition and support than on medical tasks. Improved early access to adequate prenatal care is a Healthy People 2020 goal. In 2007, fewer than 71% of pregnant women received this level of care in pregnancy (Office of Disease Prevention and Health Promotion, n.d.).

Schedule of Care

The traditional recommended schedule of prenatal care consists of one-on-one visits with an obstetric care provider. The first visit is scheduled for the first trimester, and then subsequent visits are scheduled to occur monthly until week 28 of gestation, every 2 weeks until week 36 of gestation, and then weekly until the end of pregnancy (see Box 2.3). The average visit takes fewer than 10 minutes. Given an average of 12 to 16 prenatal visits, the client is likely to receive a total of approximately 2 hours of direct prenatal care for each pregnancy (Carter et al., 2016). Although the actual direct care time is relatively small, clients face many barriers to accessing this care, including the following: transit time, time away from work, transportation difficulties, and care of existing children.

An alternate program of prenatal care delivery called CenteringPregnancy is gaining popularity. CenteringPregnancy involves 2-hour long group sessions every 2 to 4 weeks with an obstetric provider, a cofacilitator, and 5 to 12 pregnant women. The program is designed to empower women and to promote health behaviors, as well as providing considerably more time to allow for coverage of a greater breadth of information. Women may also benefit from the shared experience with other women in a similar life stage. Although some studies have found that this approach improves breastfeeding rates, reduces neonatal intensive care unit admissions, increases infant weights, and improves the uptake of contraception postpartum, among other positive impacts, others have found no difference in outcomes between the traditional schedule of care and CenteringPregnancy (Carter et al., 2016).

Obstetric Care Providers

Rapport building is an important task of any healthcare relationship but particularly in the case of providers of obstetric care, which includes developmental tasks for the pregnant woman and family. Pregnancy is a time of profound change: physical, mental, emotional, and social. It is a time in which women are more likely to make decisions and implement changes that will have a positive impact on their health and the health of their family (Artal, 2016). It is a critical time in which to discuss productive changes such as smoking cessation, alcohol and drug use, exercise, nutrition, weight management, and, particularly in the case of intimate partner violence, personal safety. Although brief interventions have been shown to be effective in inspiring various changes (Joseph & Basu, 2017), the repeated contacts

with healthcare providers should be viewed as a period of valuable therapeutic opportunity that may be unique in the life of the patient. This work starts with the very first visit.

One of the first pregnancy-related decisions a woman makes is who her pregnancy care provider will be. Different kinds of providers are appropriate for different sorts of patients. Different providers also attend births in different settings. For example, a family medicine physician or obstetrician is most likely to attend a birth in a hospital or birthing center, whereas a nurse midwife is more likely to incorporate home births into her practice, in addition to attending hospital or birthing center births. A lay midwife typically attends only home births. Some specially trained nurse practitioners, particularly family nurse practitioners and women's health nurse practitioners, may provide prenatal and postpartum care but not attend births. Typically, they work in collaboration with midwives or physicians who do attend births. Physician assistants may also provide routine prenatal and postpartum care in collaboration with other team members but not attend births.

Midwives

There are two different kinds of midwives: nurse midwives and lay midwives. Nurse midwives are registered nurses with advanced training that allows them to supervise and manage their own patients, either with our without collaboration with a physician. In many countries, such as the United Kingdom, nurse midwives are the primary providers of obstetric care and physicians are typically involved only in high-risk situations, such as surgical births. In the United States in 2014, nurse midwives attended just over 8% of all births (American College of Nurse Midwives, 2016). Nurse midwives may attend births in hospitals, birthing centers, or in the patient's home.

Nurse Midwives are generally provided more holistic care and spend more time with patients during prenatal care and birth. They do not perform cesarean sections or complex repairs to maternal birth injuries. Women with complex medical conditions or high-risk pregnancies may not be appropriate candidates for care managed exclusively by a midwife. Nurse midwives may work in collaboration with a team that includes a physician in such circumstances, however. In general, births attended by nurse midwives include fewer interventions such as instrumental birth and cesarean section (Wong, Browne, Ferguson, Taylor, & Davis, 2015).

Lay midwives attend a small percentage of births in the United States, primarily caring for women in their homes. They may be trained formally or apprenticed and may require a license in some states.

In Chapter 7, Hannah's mother wanted her to choose a physician as her obstetric care provider, but Hannah chose a nurse midwife named Darla. It was Hannah's impression during her time in nursing school that the nurse midwives spent more time with their patients than did the physicians, and she found this reassuring.

Physicians

Obstetricians oversee most births in the United States, although family practice physicians are also qualified to attend deliveries. Most physician-attended births occur in hospitals. Obstetricians may be generalists or may specialize in high-risk patients. Women with high-risk pregnancies or certain medical conditions may be more appropriately cared for by an obstetrician. Obstetricians may perform cesarean sections, operative vaginal births, and complex repairs. Although midwives are often thought of as the holistic obstetric care providers, some physicians may approach patient care in this manner. Physicians generally attend births in the hospital setting.

Doulas

Doulas attend births as support people. They are not responsible for the delivery itself but for anticipating and responding to a family's nonmedical needs during birth. They provide emotional and physical, but also informational, support. Although most doulas serve as labor support people, some also care for families in the postpartum period. Abortion doulas offer support to women electing to terminate a pregnancy.

First Trimester: Initial Prenatal Visit

The highlight of prenatal care in the first trimester is the initial visit, during which some critical screenings and assessments, laboratory tests, patient education, and care planning occur. The tasks of the first prenatal visit are typically similar to those of a preconception visit, as described in Chapter 14. Below are unique considerations of the initial prenatal visit.

Interview

The interview, including information about the health history, occupation, and lifestyle, are similar (see Boxes 1.2, 5.1, Table 14.4). Variations in approach from that of the preconception visit may include asking questions about pregnancy symptoms, such as nausea and breast tenderness, and feelings about the pregnancy. Women, even those who have been actively working to achieve pregnancy, may have complicated feelings about their pregnancy that they would like to discuss. It may be helpful to discuss past experiences with pregnancy and hopes and expectations for this pregnancy.

The nurse should ask women about any cramping or bleeding they may be experiencing, as well as timing of the pregnancy. LMP is important to know when dating a pregnancy, and it is helpful if the patient has been tracking her cycles or can report that her cycles are regular. Information about the timing of intercourse, the nature of the last menses, and any diagnosed or suspected spontaneous abortions may help direct care and facilitate dating of the pregnancy.

A discussion about any medications or supplements a patient may be taking, either prescription or over the counter, is important, because some may be generally safe but contraindicated in pregnancy. The nurse must educate patients to avoid street drugs, tobacco, and alcohol and to limit caffeine intake to two cups or less daily.

The nurse should encourage patients to view the nurse as a safe person and the office as a safe space. Disclosures about issues such as the use of opioids and intimate partner violence are essential information for a nurse striving to facilitate a safe and successful pregnancy.

Maternal Psychological Responses

Early pregnancy is a time of uncertainty. Many women may suspect they are pregnant, hope they are pregnant, or dread they might be pregnant before a pregnancy test can reasonably be expected to be accurate. Women may doubt the accuracy of their home test and seek confirmation from a healthcare provider in the way of a urine test, blood test, or even pelvic ultrasound.

Early pregnancy is often a time of ambivalence. Approximately half of pregnancies are unplanned, in which case the woman's ambivalence may be expected, but many pregnancies may also be mistimed. Even women who wanted and planned for their pregnancies may grow ambivalent because pregnancy and the life changes it brings become real.

Early pregnancy provides little in the way of proof of itself beyond a woman's often uncomfortable symptoms. There is no overtly growing abdomen, fetal movement, or regularly auscultated heartbeat to confirm the fetus. The birth and newborn, which are anticipated to arrive months later, may seem a distant reality. The first trimester of pregnancy can bring some rapid changes, however, and a woman may focus more on these physical and often emotional changes she is feeling associated with the pregnancy. These changes may disrupt a woman's relationship with herself as well as with her partner, family, friends, and associates.

In Chapter 9, Nancy found the psychological transitions of early pregnancy challenging.

Patient Education

A critical aspect of the initial prenatal visit is patient education. The nurse should take time to teach the client the pregnancy-related implications of nutrition, food safety, exercise, work, sexuality, substance use and abuse, exposure to environmental hazards, general safety, and travel safety. Patients should be advised of warning signs and symptoms that warrant follow-up and should be assessed for these clinical signs with each visit (see Table 6.3).

Nutrition

The nurse should provide essential nutrition guidance at the first prenatal visit. A 24-hour food recall is a helpful tool for evaluating a patient's diet, but should be supplemented by assessing the impact to her normal diet she perceives as resulting from the nausea, cravings, and food aversions of pregnancy. Weight gain is an expected part of pregnancy, but this does not give the client permission to eat indiscriminately. The additional daily calories recommended in the second half of pregnancy is equivalent to about two small containers of plain, full-fat yogurt. Recommended weight gain is based on body mass index (BMI) (see Boxes 1.4 and 1.5; see Fig. 9.4). Women who are particularly anxious about the idea of weight gain may find information about the typical distribution of the extra weight reassuring (see Box 4.6).

Many women may find it helpful to review appropriate portion sizes. The nurse should recommend whole foods instead of processed foods when economically and logistically possible. Women may generate a personalized eating plan from the MyPlate website (https://www.choosemyplate.gov/MyPlate-Daily-Checklist-input) that will help guide them to make healthy food choices and build habits that may extend beyond pregnancy. Low-income women may be referred to the Special Supplemental Nutrition Program for Women, Infants, and Children at this time for access to nutrition support (see Box 3.1).

Fluid intake adequate to quench thirst should be encouraged. Women may restrict fluids because of the urinary frequency associated with pregnancy. This practice may further predispose them to urinary tract infections and may trigger Braxton Hicks contractions and induce constipation.

Use of caffeine in pregnancy has been correlated with pregnancy loss, particularly at higher doses (Chen, Wu, Neelakantan, & Chong, 2015). The March of Dimes (2015) and other organizations recommend limiting caffeine intake to 200 mg, the equivalent of 12 oz of coffee or less. Women should be aware that chocolate, black and green teas, energy drinks, and many soft drinks also contain caffeine.

Women who are not already taking a prenatal vitamin should be instructed to do so. Women experiencing nausea may find it helpful to take the supplement at night and with food. Some women may instead opt for a chewable vitamin. A supplement of the essential fatty acid docosahexaenoic acid (DHA) may also be recommended and is associated with improved birth outcomes, including longer gestation and increased birth weight (Makrides, 2016). It is also essential to healthy neurologic development of the fetus. Optimally, DHA is obtained from foods sources in which it naturally occurs, fish being particularly rich in this nutrient; however, it may also be obtained from foods that are fortified with it. It is recommended that women consume fish three times a week, but many do not because of concern about mercury exposure or preference (Box 15.1).

Food Safety

Thorough washing of the hands as well as vegetables and fruits, particularly those that will be eaten raw, is important to reduce the risk of harmful pathogens, including *Escherichia coli*. Similarly, meat, including fish and poultry, should be cooked thoroughly, as should eggs. Raw eggs and undercooked poultry may contain *Salmonella*, and undercooked beef may contain *E. coli* or *Toxoplasmosis*. All food surfaces and cooking tools should be thoroughly cleaned before and after preparation of eggs and meats. Although all of these foods may be eaten provided that safe food handling is observed, some foods and beverages should not be

---

Box 15.1 Guidelines for Fish Consumption in Pregnancy

- Eat 8–12 oz of fish weekly.
- Choose fish that contain low levels of mercury, such as the following:
  - Catfish
  - Cod
  - Light canned tuna
  - Pollock
  - Salmon
  - Shrimp
  - Tilapia
- Limit intake of albacore tuna to 6 oz a week.
- Limit intake of fish from streams, rivers, and lakes to 6 oz a week, or according to the local fish advisories.
- Avoid fish that contain high levels of mercury, such as the following:
  - King mackerel
  - Shark
  - Swordfish
  - Tilefish from the Gulf of Mexico

Data from U.S. Food and Drug Administration. (2015, February 24). *Fish: What pregnant women and parents should know.* Retrieved from http://www.fda.gov/Food/FoodborneIllnessContaminants/Metals/ucm393070.htm

---

consumed in pregnancy because of the risk for *Listeria*, which may cause pregnancy loss, preterm birth, low birth weight, and birth defects (Box 15.2; see Table 4.1). In addition, raw sprouts such as alfalfa sprouts should be avoided because of the risk for *E. coli*. No amount of alcohol is known to be safe in pregnancy, and even small amounts, 1 to 2 units per week (a unit is 12 oz of beer, 4 oz of wine, or 1 oz of spirits), is associated with preterm birth and low birth weight (Mamluk et al., 2016). Alcohol is a known teratogen that may cause damage to the fetus that will have a long-term, potentially devastating, impact (Fig. 15.17).

Exercise

Women should be encouraged to continue to exercise as tolerated, both aerobic and strength training. As with people who are not pregnant, exercise improves cardiorespiratory function and

---

Box 15.2 Foods to Avoid in Pregnancy That Are Common Sources of Listeria

- Soft cheeses made with unpasteurized milk (such as brie, feta, camembert, and queso fresco)
- Refrigerated meat spreads such as pâtés (canned is fine)
- Refrigerated smoked seafood (except in cooked dishes; okay if canned or shelf-stable)
- Cold cuts, or lunch meats, not heated to steaming
- Hot dogs not heated to steaming
- Raw or unpasteurized milk or milk products

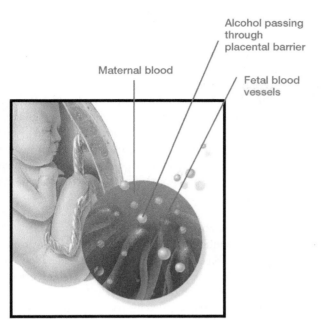

Figure 15.17. **A fetus with fetal alcohol syndrome**. Excessive alcohol consumption may cause impotence and damage to sperm in men. For women, alcohol use may cause interruptions in menstruation and damage to eggs. Alcohol may also cause serious problems for the developing fetus that can affect its entire life. The baby can be born with fetal alcohol syndrome, be underweight, grow more slowly, and have birth defects, as well as have a smaller brain and a lower intelligence quotient, or mental retardation. Alcohol may also be passed to a baby through breast milk. (Reprinted with permission from Anatomical Chart Company.)

psychological and physical well-being. Pregnancy is an excellent time to make positive lifestyle changes, including starting and increasing physical activity. In pregnancy, exercise can help avoid excess weight gain, back and pelvic girdle pain, and urinary incontinence. Infants born to women who exercise regularly are less likely to be macrosomic. Research also suggests a possible reduced risk for preeclampsia, gestational diabetes, and cesarean section, as well as a shorter first stage of labor (Aune, Saugstad, Henriksen, & Tonstad, 2014; Owe, Nystad, Stigum, & Vangen, 2016; Perales et al., 2016; Wiebe, Boulé, Chari, & Davenport, 2015).

There are contraindications to aerobic exercise in pregnancy, however. Absolute contraindications include significant heart disease, some forms of lung disease, a diagnosis of an incompetent cervix or a cerclage, a multiple gestation pregnancy with a risk of preterm delivery, persistent vaginal bleeding in the second or third trimesters, placenta previa after 26 weeks gestation, premature labor with this pregnancy, ruptured membranes, pregnancy-induced hypertension or preeclampsia, or severe anemia. Relative contraindications include heavy smoking, poorly controlled seizure disorder, poorly controlled hyperthyroidism, orthopedic limitations, poorly controlled hypertension, intrauterine growth restriction with the current pregnancy, extreme morbid obesity, extreme underweight, poorly controlled type 1 diabetes, chronic bronchitis, unevaluated maternal cardiac arrhythmia, and anemia (American College of Obstetricians and Gynecologists [ACOG], 2015b).

A commonly prescribed exercise program includes 5 to 10 minutes of warm-ups and stretching, 30 minutes of aerobic exercise or weight lifting, and a cool down lasting 5 to 10 minutes. Exercise is recommended at least 5 days a week (ACOG, 2015b).

Women who are starting a new exercise program should start slow and increase intensity and duration of activity over time. Women are often asked to base their activity intensity on the "talk test." For an activity to pass the "talk test," women must be able to carry on a normal conversation. If she cannot, she should reduce the intensity of exercise. Women who wish to work to a particular heart rate, particularly those coming into pregnancy very fit, may be instructed to aim for 145 to 160 bpm if aged between 20 and 29, and 140 to 156 bpm if aged between 30 and 39 (Bø et al., 2016).

Exercises that are considered safe include Kegel floor exercises, strength training, racquet sports, running or jogging, pilates (modified as needed for changing body), yoga (again, modified as necessary), low-impact aerobics, stationary biking, swimming, and walking. Activities to be avoided include contact sports, scuba diving, sky diving, hot yoga, and activities with a high risk of falling (skiing, surfing, gymnastics, etc.) (ACOG, 2015b).

Women should stop exercising if they experience regular painful contractions, leakage of copious clear fluid from the vagina, vaginal bleeding, dizziness, headache, impaired balance, calf pain or swelling, or chest pain. Women should not exercise with new shortness of breath prior to exercise but should rather be evaluated urgently (ACOG, 2015b).

In Chapter 2, Tati, an experienced marathon runner, wished to continue running throughout her pregnancy. Alice, a nurse practitioner, told her that she could continue running, but that she should listen to her body and slow down if she got too tired or was breathing so hard that she couldn't talk.

Work

Approximately two thirds of women pregnant with their first child work, and over 80% of them will work until within a month of the birth (Pew Research Center, 2015). Standard working conditions, such as shift work, lifting, standing, and physical labor present little risk to the health of a woman or her pregnancy if uncomplicated (Palmer, Bonzini, & Bonde, 2013).

Certain substances should be minimized in pregnancy and may warrant leaving a job if exposure cannot be limited. These substances include some pharmaceuticals, battery acid, benzene, manufacturing dyes, formaldehyde, heavy metals, solvents, pesticides, inks used for printing, wood preservatives, radiation, and some products used in manufacturing, such as lead and mercury (Katz, 2012). Women who encounter potential chemical hazards at work should be advised to consult the Occupational Safety and Health Administration manual that is mandated by law to be accessible on site to all workers. They may also check www.osha.gov for information about specific substances.

Workplace discrimination based on pregnancy and childbirth is prohibited for employers with 15 or more employees. Pregnant workers must have access to the same temporary disability benefits as any other disabled employee, including sick leave, work accommodations, and reinstatement privileges. Pregnant women must be allowed to work as long as they can do their jobs, and alternate work must be provided as necessary. Employers cannot mandate leave for a pregnant employee who is capable of fulfilling the obligations of her job. Pregnancy may not be used to discriminate against a woman during the hiring process (U.S. Equal Employment Opportunity Commission, n.d.).

Women experiencing nausea and vomiting in pregnancy may be triggered by certain odors at work and can be encouraging to manage symptoms with snacks, hydration, and possibly medication. In severe cases, a medical accommodation may be requested to adjust a work schedule to a time when the woman is less nauseous or even a temporary medical leave. Physical discomfort and fatigue may also limit a woman's ability to complete certain tasks. Accommodations may be required to minimize fatigue, prolonged standing, lifting, and bending.

Sexuality

Sex is not contraindicated in pregnancy in the absence of bleeding, ruptured membranes, or evidence of preterm labor. Pregnant women should be careful to protect themselves from sexually transmitted infections with the use of condoms, dental dams, abstinence, or alternate sexual activities such as intimate caressing because sexually transmitted infections can lead to pregnancy complications. Although orgasms and the prostaglandins in semen can theoretically stimulate labor, they are unlikely to provoke preterm labor.

Women should be educated about the changes in their bodies, such as vulvar and breast swelling, breast tenderness, and leukorrhea of pregnancy. Although all are normal, they may change how sex feels and how a woman and her partner feel about sex. Open communication about sex is optimal in any sexual relationship, but particularly in one that includes numerous physical, emotional, and role changes. Some women and their partners find sex more pleasurable during pregnancy, whereas others do not. The libidos of patients and their partners may also vary in response to the pregnancy.

Women should tell their partner if sex is uncomfortable at any point, and alternate positions or activities should be sought. Women and partners should be reassured that sex will not harm the pregnancy. Although cunnilingus for the pregnant woman is generally safe, it should be avoided if the woman's partner has a cold sore. A dental dam may be used if there is a concern for the transmission of HSV (Herpes simplex virus) or a different sexually transmitted infection that may be passed via the oral–genital route, as chlamydia.

Substance Use and Abuse

Smoking cessation is strongly encouraged in pregnancy. The safety of nicotine replacement strategies in pregnancy is not well established, and they may be no better than a placebo for facilitating smoking cessation (Coleman, Chamberlain, Davey, Cooper, & Leonardi-Bee, 2015). Resources such as http://women.smokefree.gov/ may be helpful to women seeking support and strategies to stop smoking.

Although illicit drug use and the use of medications prescribed for other people is strongly discouraged, pregnant patients using opioids such as heroin or oxycodone or medications that are used to manage opioid addiction, such as buprenorphine, buprenorphine/naloxone, or methadone, should not be instructed to stop use. Abrupt withdrawal of these substances may lead to pregnancy loss. These patients are instead managed medically throughout pregnancy and carefully monitored, often by specialized high-risk obstetric providers.

Exposure to Environmental Hazards

Home and work conditions may impact the health of a pregnancy. Women should be asked about their exposure to lead, radon, and second-hand smoke as well as the presence of smoke detectors and carbon monoxide detectors in their homes (CDC, 2014).

Many women may be aware that the parasite toxoplasmosis can be acquired from contact with cat feces and that exposure to the parasite can result in damage to the brain, hearing, and vision of the fetus. However, of the 400 to 4,000 new cases of toxoplasmosis in pregnancy that occur annually, approximately 50% actually result from exposure to untreated water or undercooked or mishandled meat (U.S. Food and Drug Administration, 2015). Women may also be exposed to this parasite when gardening. The infection is transmitted by the fecal–oral route: the fecal material gets on a woman's hands, which transport the parasite to her mouth, where it is ingested. Toxoplasmosis does not travel through the skin directly and is not airborne. Although it is preferable to have another person take care of a cat litter box, a pregnant woman may safely keep a cat providing she follows common-sense precautions to avoid ingesting the parasite (Box 15.3).

Box 15.3 Tips for Avoiding Transmission of Toxoplasmosis From Household Cats During Pregnancy

- Have someone else manage the cat litter box, if possible.
- If you must take care of the litter box, be sure to do the following:
  - Wear disposable gloves.
  - Carefully wash your hands with soap and water afterward.
  - Change the litter daily, because the parasite becomes infectious 1–5 d after it is shed in feces
- Do not feed the cat raw meat, only commercial cat food.
- Keep indoor cats indoors.
- Do not obtain a new cat, especially a stray, during pregnancy.

Data from U.S. Food and Drug Administration. (2015, February 24). *Fish: What pregnant women and parents should know.* Retrieved from http://www.fda.gov/Food/FoodborneIllnessContaminants/Metals/ucm393070.htm

Bathing

Women should take special precautions when bathing during pregnancy. Providing the water temperature remains below 102°F and she soaks for fewer than 10 minutes, warm baths are not believed to pose a health risk for the pregnancy. Pregnant women should be cautious, however, particularly in early pregnancy, to monitor themselves for lightheadedness when getting out of a warm tub, as the warmth in combination with orthostatic hypotension may make her more prone to syncope. Women may also be reassured that there is no risk of the bath water coming in contact with the fetus, because the cervix is blocked by the mucus plug and the fetus is inside the amniotic sac.

Travel Safety

Travel is generally considered safe in pregnancy. Women should be made aware, however, that their blood is more subject to clotting during pregnancy and that they should get up and walk at least hourly to avoid stasis. Seat belts should continue to be worn throughout pregnancy. As her uterus grows, the woman needs to adjust the seat belt to ensure it overlies her hips and not her abdomen. Pregnancy complications are most common in the first and last trimesters, making the second trimester the better time to travel. Airlines may choose to prohibit a woman from traveling in late pregnancy. As of this writing, the CDC recommends pregnant women not travel to areas with active Zika virus transmission.

Physical Examination

The initial prenatal physical exam should include a blood pressure, height, and weight. The blood pressure is a baseline measurement that will provide a context for measurements later in pregnancy. A high blood pressure during this visit would be consistent with preexisting hypertension, but not with pregnancy-induced hypertension or preeclampsia, which manifest later in pregnancy. The height and weight is used to calculate the BMI, which is used to counsel the patient about optimal weight gain (see Boxes 1.4 and 1.5).

A complete physical exam is usually done, which includes a pelvic exam. The size of the uterus can be assessed during this exam for consistency of size with the dates provided. The adnexa can be palpated to assess for a mass that may suggest an ectopic pregnancy or ovarian or fallopian tube abnormality.

A uterine size not consistent with dates is an indication for ultrasound to assess for a multiple pregnancy, uterine fibroids, or incorrect dating. A uterus that is difficult to assess, as can be the case with a patient who is obese or with a uterus that is retroverted (angled toward the back rather than the front), may also be an indication for having an ultrasound. Women complaining of pelvic pain or vaginal bleeding may have an ultrasound to assess for ectopic pregnancy, as well as serial hCG measurements, as described earlier in this chapter.

Cardiac activity may be viewed by 6 weeks gestation by transvaginal ultrasound. Fetal cardiac activity can be auscultated through the abdominal wall using a Doppler ultrasound by 12 weeks gestation.

Laboratory Testing and Imaging

If the pregnant woman is due for a Pap test, it is done at this time (see Patient Teaching 2.2). If a woman is uncertain of the first day of her LMP or has an irregular cycle, an ultrasound may be ordered to determine her EDD, in addition to the pelvic examination described in the last section (see Box 4.2). If the woman has a regular cycle and a known LMP and her dates are consistent with her pelvic examination, her EDD can be determined using Naegele's Rule (see Box 1.1). Tools such as a pregnancy wheel (see Fig. 2.4), online calculators, and electronic health records also rely on this simple calculation.

Some lab studies, such as those testing for Rh(D) factor or for genetic predisposition to certain congenital traits such as sickle cell anemia and Tay Sachs, may not be done if they were already completed at the time of a preconception visit or during a previous pregnancy (see Table 14.6). Congenital traits, such as Rh(D) factor, do not change during the course of a lifetime and thus do not need to be repeated.

If the mother is found to be Rh(D) negative, an antibody screen is warranted because the mother may already be sensitized to Rh(D)-positive blood. In the case of a woman who is Rh(D) negative and has antibodies indicating she is sensitized to Rh(D)-positive blood, the fetus will be monitored closely for anemia and may require either early delivery or blood transfusion via the umbilical cord while in utero (ACOG, 2013).

Screening for human immunodeficiency virus (HIV) is offered on an opt-out basis, meaning that the test will be run unless the woman declines it. The use of some screening, such as that for tuberculosis and syphilis, is based on the individual patient's risk factors. Screening for gonorrhea and chlamydia is done routinely.

Second Trimester

After the initial prenatal visit, the traditional visit schedule calls for a return visit every month until the 28th week of gestation (through the end of the second trimester). Depending on when the first visit occurred, a woman may have an additional visit in the first trimester or no further visits until the second trimester. These subsequent visits usually include the following:

- Review of the patient's chart and history taking about the time between visits
- An interval history, including questions about nutrition, exercise, and possible complications (Box 15.4) and typical discomforts
- Vital signs assessment
- Fetal heart rate (normal is between 110 and 160 bpm) assessment
- Weight assessment
- Fundal height measurement after 16 weeks of gestation (see Fig. 2.8)
- Maternal assessment of fetal activity

Box 15.4 Problems Requiring Urgent Assessment During Pregnancy

- Leakage of fluid from the vagina
- Vaginal bleeding
- Reduced fetal activity
- Headache that does not improve with acetaminophen
- Right upper quadrant pain
- Vision changes
- Persistent contractions
- New-onset lower back pain
- Sensation of pelvic pressure
- Menstrual-like cramps
- Dysuria

Routine Laboratory Tests

Routine laboratory tests in the second trimester include urinalysis, diabetes screening, and Rh(D) factor screening, as well as screening for fetal anomalies.

Urinalysis

A urinalysis may be done periodically as part of a routine visit, although this is not a universal recommendation. Protein in the urine may indicate preeclampsia, but spillage of protein into the urine is common and is found to be pathologic and associated with preeclampsia only 2% to 11% of the time. Additionally, false-positive results are common. Thus, routine screening for protein is not indicated without corroborating evidence, such as hypertension, in which case more accurate screening with 24-hour urine collection or a random protein:creatinine ratio is indicated (Henderson, Thompson, Burda, & Cantor, 2017). Equally, spilling of glucose into the urine during pregnancy is not unusual or diagnostic for diabetes. Routine glucose tolerance testing between 24 and 28 weeks of gestation is more specific and diagnostic (see Lab Values 3.2). The United States Preventative Services Task Force recommends that all pregnant women be screened for asymptomatic bacteria with a urine culture between weeks 12 and 16 of pregnancy, with no repeat screening indicated in low-risk women with a negative result (Lin & Fajardo, 2008).

Diabetes Screening

In the United States, universal screening of pregnant women is recommended between weeks 24 and 28 of pregnancy using either the one-step or two-step oral glucose tolerance test (see Lab Values 3.2). Women who are considered higher risk may have been tested with the first prenatal visit or at a visit before conception for nongestational diabetes. Earlier screening and treatment in pregnancy for gestational diabetes has not been associated with better outcomes and is not generally recommended.

Rh(D) Factor Screening

Women are routinely screened for Rh(D) factor during their first prenatal visit. Women who are Rh(D) negative are further tested to evaluate for antibodies to Rh(D)-positive blood that may have developed because of prior exposure to Rh(D)-positive blood, such as may occur during a pregnancy with an Rh(D)-positive fetus. Women who are Rh(D) negative and also negative for antibodies with the first prenatal visit are retested for antibodies prior to the administration of Rh(D) immune globulin at 28 weeks of gestation (see The Pharmacy 5.1).

Fetal Anomaly Screening

There is no one prenatal screening protocol for fetal anomalies. A common approach includes blood work at the very end of the first trimester and an ultrasound of the back of the fetus' neck between 11 and 13 weeks of gestation (Box 15.5; see Fig. 1.5). Results of the blood tests combined with those of the ultrasound, if in the normal range, are reassuring that congenital anomalies such as Down syndrome are unlikely. The woman may elect to have a second set of blood work tests a few weeks later. This blood work provides information about the possibility of congenital anomalies but also includes screening for neural tube defects. A fetal survey ultrasound typically occurs between 18 and 23 weeks of gestation and provides information about the fetus' anatomic development (see Box 1.8).

Box 15.5 Standard Schedule of Routine Fetal Assessments for Low-Risk Pregnancies

First Trimester

- Screening for trisomies
  - Blood tests (12 wk)
    - Pregnancy-associated plasma protein: Low in an abnormal test
    - hCG: High in an abnormal test
  - Ultrasound (11–13 wk)
    - Nuchal translucency (measurement by ultrasound of the space at the back of the fetal neck): Thick in an abnormal test

Second Trimester

- Integrated screening: Laboratory tests (14–16 wk) conducted in addition to the first trimester screening tests and ultrasound
  - Maternal serum alpha-fetoprotein: High levels are associated with neural tube defects; low levels are associated with Down syndrome.
  - hCG: High levels are associated with Down syndrome; low levels are associated with trisomy 18.
  - Unconjugated estriol: Low levels are associated with Down syndrome and some neural tube defects.
  - inhibin-A: High levels are associated with Down syndrome.
  - Fetal survey ultrasound (usually 18–23 wk)

hCG, Human chorionic gonadotropin.

A newer approach to screening uses cell-free DNA (cfDNA) from the fetus that is found in the maternal circulation. Analysis of cfDNA is up to 99% accurate for the diagnosis of Down syndrome and trisomies 13 and 18 as well as abnormalities in the number of sex chromosomes. The fetal sex may also be discovered with this testing. Although it is highly accurate, it is still not as accurate as the more invasive chorionic villi sampling or amniocentesis and is thus considered screening rather than diagnostic. A cfDNA test suggesting a fetal abnormality will be followed by one of these diagnostic tests. cfDNA may be offered instead of the more traditional first and second trimester screening or it may be offered in the event of abnormalities in traditional screening. Testing may be as early as 9 weeks, but it is typically performed after 10 weeks (ACOG, 2015a).

Diagnostic Tests

Although screening tests such as first trimester screening and cfDNA testing provide information that may strongly suggest fetal anomalies, diagnostic testing confirms the diagnosis. Both amniocentesis and chorionic villi sampling are considered diagnostic tests.

Amniocentesis

Amniocentesis is offered to women who carry pregnancies deemed to be at high risk for fetal anomalies. Amniocentesis is offered routinely to women who will be 35 years or older at the time of delivery because of the increased risk for fetal anomalies in fetuses of women in this age bracket. The procedure, the ultrasound guided removal of amniotic fluid using a needle introduced through the abdomen, is most frequently done between 15 and 17 weeks gestation, but may be done as early as 11 weeks (see Fig. 10.2).

In addition to analysis for fetal genetic abnormalities, amniocentesis may be used to evaluate for fetal lung maturity in late pregnancy or to assess for intrauterine infection, fetal blood type, hemolytic anemia, and neural tube defects. It may also be used to remove excess amniotic fluid in the case of polyhydramnios. There is a small risk for leakage of the amniotic fluid, injury to the fetus, and fetal loss with the procedure.

Chorionic Villus Sampling

Like amniocentesis, chorionic villus sampling (CVS) is considered diagnostic (Fig. 15.18). Although amniocentesis requires the removal of a small amount of amniotic fluid for assessment, CVS involves the removal and assessment of a small portion of the chorionic villi of the placenta. The sample may be obtained using ultrasound guidance via a needle inserted in the abdomen or a catheter introduced through the cervix. The decision about the approach, abdominal or cervical, is guided by the position of the placenta and provider preference. Like amniocentesis, it is offered to women who are at higher risk for carrying pregnancies with genetic anomalies. CVS may be performed as early as 10 weeks gestation. Potential complications include fetal loss and maternal bleeding. CVS performed prior to 10 weeks is associated with fetal limb reduction.

Maternal Psychological Responses

A woman's physical changes begin in earnest in the second trimester, when a growing abdomen, weight gain, and enlarging

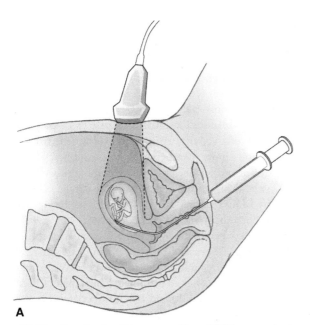
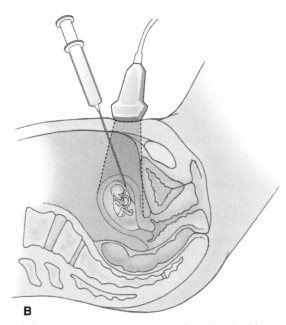

Figure 15.18. Chorionic villus sampling. (A) Transvaginal sampling. **(B)** Transabdominal sampling. (Reprinted with permission from Evans, R. J., Brown, Y. M., & Evans, M. K. [2014]. *Canadian maternity, newborn, and women's health nursing* [2nd ed., Fig. 11.25]. Philadelphia, PA: Lippincott Williams & Wilkins.)

breasts signal that she is really pregnant. These changes, along with changes in skin pigmentation and, later in pregnancy, striae, can alter a woman's body image. Women who have particularly focused on their physical form prior to pregnancy as a source of their sexuality, attractiveness, and worth may particularly struggle with these changes.

These physical changes, as well as the visual proof of ultrasounds, the regular audio proof of the fetal heartbeat, and the tactile evidence of fetal movement, make the fetus seem much more real. Often, the woman's focus at this time switches from her experience of being pregnant to a greater awareness of the fetus as a separate but entirely dependent entity. This awareness creates a prime time to help women initiate positive changes such as good nutrition and smoking cessation.

Third Trimester

In the third trimester, the woman sees her obstetric care provider every 2 weeks until week 36 of gestation and then weekly until the end of the pregnancy. Just as in the second trimester, each visit includes a review of her chart and an interval health history. She has her vital signs taken and is asked questions about fetal movement (see Analyze the Evidence 5.1). The fetal heart rate is assessed and the fundal height is measured when the woman's bladder is empty.

The fundal height, which is the distance from the pubic symphysis to the fundus of the uterus, should measure within a few centimeters of the number of weeks of gestation. For example, a woman who is 22 weeks pregnant is anticipated to have a fundal height of 20 to 24 cm. The purpose of the fundal height measurement is to detect abnormal fetal growth, either large or small for gestational age. Although this is routine care, a recent meta-analysis found little evidence to either support or change this common assessment (Japaraj, Ho, Valliapan, & Sivasangari, 2015). Leopold's maneuvers may be done several times in the last trimester to confirm that the fetus is head down and has not moved from this position (see Fig. 1.9).

Routine Laboratory Tests

Routine laboratory tests in the third trimester include those for hemoglobin or hematocrit, sexually transmitted infections, and group B streptococcus.

Hemoglobin or Hematocrit

Hemoglobin or hematocrit should be checked early in the third trimester. As mentioned previously, a form of physiologic anemia is typical during pregnancy. In the first and third trimesters of pregnancy, anemia is defined as a hemoglobin level of less than 11 g/dL (hematocrit under 33%). In the second trimester of pregnancy, hemoglobin and hematocrit values reach their lowest point, and a hemoglobin level of less than 10.5 g/dL (hematocrit below 32%) is considered diagnostic. Note that a hemoglobin

level that is as much as 0.8 g/dL lower than what is acceptable in people of other ethnicities is considered normal in those of African descent (CDC, 1989; Institute of Medicine, 1993). Women who are diagnosed with anemia may be treated with iron supplementation and should be rescreened 4 to 6 weeks after diagnosis.

Sexually Transmitted Infections

The CDC recommends rescreening for chlamydia for pregnant women 25 years and younger between weeks 28 and 36 of pregnancy. In addition, women who were diagnosed with a sexually transmitted infection earlier in pregnancy or who have a new sexual partner or other risk factor should be rescreened for chlamydia, gonorrhea, syphilis, HIV, and other infections based on risk (Workowski & Bolan, 2015).

Group B Streptococcus Screening

A swab is done of the rectum and the introitus of the vagina between 35 and 37 weeks of gestation. The presence of group B streptococcus is an indication for prophylactic treatment with intravenous antibiotics during labor and delivery (see Box 7.2).

In Chapter 2, Tatiana tested positive for group B streptococcus in late pregnancy and required prophylactic intravenous antibiotics during labor and delivery. Tatiana had hoped that she would not need an intravenous line during labor and delivery, and was disappointed by this news.

Maternal Psychological Responses

In the third trimester of pregnancy, women often feel progressively more vulnerable and more dependent on their partners. They may become anxious about the possibility of late fetal loss even in the absence of risk factors and complications. Many pregnant women feel reassured by fetal movement, although it may be uncomfortable at times. Sleep is often compromised by positional limitations, the discomforts of pregnancy, and nocturnal fetal activity. Positive reinforcement from partners, friends, and family members may be reassuring. Women in the third trimester often become fixated on the approaching due date and birth, although only approximately 4% of babies are born on their EDD (Moore, 2015). Women may become distressed if labor does not start by a particular date.

At the very end of pregnancy, many women elect to take time off from work because of physical discomfort, renewed fatigue, or to complete preparations for the newborn. Many take time at this point in pregnancy to formulate a birth plan. Often, time is devoted to reading books and watching programing about birth and newborn care.

Think Critically

1. From memory, write the steps of development from fertilization until week nine of development. Go back and check your work.
2. What are the major functions of the placenta?
3. Why is it important that the blood of the mother and of the embryo/fetus do not mix?
4. Why is Wharton's jelly important?
5. Review the changes and discomforts of pregnancy. Draw a map for yourself to illustrate what changes contribute to which discomforts.
6. You are working as a triage nurse in a midwifery office. A patient calls complaining of contractions. What important questions should you ask?
7. From memory, describe the traditional schedule for prenatal visits. What drawbacks do you see to this model? What advantages?
8. Summarize in a check list the nutritional considerations of pregnancy.
9. What are the danger signs of pregnancy, and what makes each concerning?
10. A patient's partner calls concerned that his wife seems "clingy" and emotional. Write a script of your conversation with the husband. Explain to a classmate or friend Rh(D) factor testing, implications, follow-up, and interventions.

References

Abraham, R. M., Chu, E. Y., & Elder, D. E. (2014). The skin. In D. S. Strayer, E. Rubin, J. E. Saffitz, & A. L. Schiller (Eds.), *Rubin's pathology: Clinicopathologic foundations of medicine* (7th ed.). Bethesda, MD: Wolters Kluwer.

Academy of Nutrition and Dietetics. (2014). *Practice paper of the Academy of Nutrition and Dietetics Abstract: Nutrition and lifestyle for a healthy pregnancy outcome 2014.* Retrieved from https://www.eatrightpro.org/practice/position-and-practice-papers/position-papers/nutrition-and-lifestyle-for-a-healthy-pregnancy-outcome

Aguin, T., & Sobel, J. (2015). Vulvovaginal candidiasis in pregnancy. *Current Infectious Disease Reports, 17*(6), 462.

Al-Himdani, S., Ud-Din, S., Gilmore, S., & Bayat, A. (2014). Striae distensae: A comprehensive review and evidence-based evaluation of prophylaxis and treatment. *British Journal of Dermatology, 170*(3), 527–547.

Almonda, D., Edlundb, L., Joffec, M., & Palmed, M. (2016). An adaptive significance of morning sickness? Trivers–Willard and Hyperemesis Gravidarum. *Economics and Human Development, 21,* 167–171.

American College of Nurse Midwives. (2016, February). *Midwives & birth in the United States.* Retrieved from http://www.midwife.org/Essential-Facts-about-Midwives

Arey, L. B., & Sapunar, D. (2017, March 21). *Prenatal development.* Retrieved from https://www.britannica.com/science/prenatal-development

Artal, R. (2016). Exercise in pregnancy. *Clinical Obstetrics and Gynecology, 59*(3), 639–644.

Aune, D., Saugstad, O., Henriksen, T., & Tonstad, S. (2014). Physical activity and the risk of preeclampsia: A systematic review and meta-analysis. *Epidemiology, 25*(3), 331–343.

Baumgardner, D. J. (2017). The value in verifying medical folklore. *Journal of Patient-Centered Research and Reviews, 4*(3), 101–103.

Benjamin, D., Water, A. V., & Peiris, C. (2014). Effects of exercise on diastasis of the rectus abdominis muscle in the antenatal and postnatal periods: A systematic review. *Physiotherapy, 100*(1), 1–8.

Bø, K., Artal, R., Barakat, R., Brown, W., Davies, G., Dooley, M., . . . Khan, K. M. (2016). Exercise and pregnancy in recreational and elite athletes: 2016 Evidence Summary from the IOC Expert Group Meeting, Lausanne. Part 1—Exercise in women planning pregnancy and those who are pregnant. *British Journal of Sports Medicine, 50*(10), 571–589.

Brown, H. L. (2016, October). *Physiology of pregnancy.* Retrieved from http://www.merckmanuals.com/professional/gynecology-and-obstetrics/approach-to-the-pregnant-woman-and-prenatal-care/physiology-of-pregnancy

Brown, H. L. (2017). *Stages of development of the fetus.* Retrieved from http://www.merckmanuals.com/home/women-s-health-issues/normal-pregnancy/stages-of-development-of-the-fetus

Browne, V. A., Julian, C. G., Toledo-Jaldin, L., Cioffi-Ragan, D., Vargas, E., & Moore, L. G. (2015). Uterine artery blood flow, fetal hypoxia and fetal growth. *Philosophical Transactions of the Royal Society B, 370*(1663).

Carter, E. B., Temming, L. A., Akin, J., Fowler, S., Macones, G. A., Colditz, G. A., & Tuuli, M. G. (2016). Group prenatal care compared with traditional prenatal care: A systematic review and meta-analysis. *Obstetrics and Gynecology, 128*(3), 551–561.

Centers for Disease Control and Prevention. (1989). Current trends CDC criteria for anemia in children and childbearing-aged women. *Morbidity and Mortality Weekly Report, 38*(22), 400–404.

Centers for Disease Control and Prevention. (2014, September 2). *Preconception health and health care.* Retrieved from https://www.cdc.gov/preconception/careforwomen/exposures.html

Centers for Disease Control and Prevention. (2015, November 6). *Three decades of twin births in the United States, 1980–2009.* Retrieved from https://www.cdc.gov/nchs/products/databriefs/db80.htm

Chen, L.-W., Wu, Y., Neelakantan, N., & Chong, M. F. (2015). Maternal caffeine intake during pregnancy and risk of pregnancy loss: A categorical and dose–response meta-analysis of prospective studies. *Public Health Nutrition, 19*(7), 1233–1244.

Cheung, K. L., & Lafayette, R. A. (2014). Renal physiology of pregnancy. *Advances in Chronic Kidney Disease, 20*(3), 209–214.

Coleman, T., Chamberlain, C., Davey, M., Cooper, S., & Leonardi-Bee, J. (2015). Pharmacological interventions for promoting smoking cessation during pregnancy (Review). *The Cochrane Database of Systematic Reviews,* (12), CD010078.

Costantine, M. M. (2015). Physiologic and pharmacokinetic changes in pregnancy. *Frontiers in Pharmacology, 5*(65).

de Haas, S., Ghossein-Doha, C., van Kuijk, S., van Drongelen, J., & Spaanderman, M. (2017). Physiological adaptation of maternal plasma volume during pregnancy: A systematic review and meta-analysis. *Ultrasound in Obstetrics and Gynecology, 49*(2), 177–187.

Dulay, A. T. (2017, October). *Ectopic pregnancy.* Retrieved from http://www.merckmanuals.com/professional/gynecology-and-obstetrics/abnormalities-of-pregnancy/ectopic-pregnancy

Errera, M. H., Kohl, R. P., & Cruz, L. (2013). Pregnancy-associated retinal diseases and their management. *Survey of Ophthalmology, 58*(2), 127–142.

Gordon, A., Raynes-Greenow, C., Bond, D., Morris, J., Rawlinson, W., & Jeffery, H. (2015). Sleep position, fetal growth restriction, and late-pregnancy stillbirth: The Sydney stillbirth study. *Obstetrics and Gynecology, 125*(2), 347–355.

Henderson, J., Thompson, J., Burda, B., & Cantor, A. (2017). Preeclampsia screening: Evidence report and systematic review for the US Preventive Services Task Force. *JAMA, 317*(16), 1668.

Institute of Medicine. (1993). *Iron deficiency anemia: Recommended guidelines for the prevention, detection, and management among U.S. Children and Women of Childbearing Age.* Washington, DC: National Academy Press.

Japaraj, R. P., Ho, J. J., Valliapan, J., & Sivasangari, S. (2015). Symphysial fundal height (SFH) measurement in pregnancy for detecting abnormal fetal growth. *The Cochrane Database of Systematic Reviews*, (9), CD008136.

Joseph, J., & Basu, D. (2017). Efficacy of brief interventions in reducing hazardous or harmful alcohol use in middle-income countries: Systematic review of randomized controlled trials. *Alcohol and Alcoholism, 52*(1), 56–64.

Katz, V. (2012). Work and work-related stress in pregnancy. *Clinical Obstetrics and Gynecology, 55*(3), 765–773.

Koren, G., Madjunkova, S., & Maltepe, C. (2014). The protective effects of nausea and vomiting of pregnancy against adverse fetal outcome—A systematic review. *Reproductive Toxicology, 47*, 77–80.

Lin, K., & Fajardo, K. (2008). Screening for asymptomatic bacteriuria in adults: Evidence for the U.S. Preventive Services Task Force reaffirmation recommendation statement. *Annals of Internal Medicine, 149*(1), W20.

LoMauro, A., & Aliverti, A. (2015). Respiratory physiology of pregnancy. *Breathe, 11*(4), 297–301.

Mackenzie, J., Murray, E., & Lusher, J. (2018). Women's experiences of pregnancy related pelvic girdle pain: A systematic review. *Midwifery, 56*, 102–111.

Makrides, M. (2016). Understanding the effects of docosahexaenoic acid (DHA) supplementation during pregnancy on multiple outcomes from the DOMInO trial. *Oilseeds and Fats, Crops and Lipids, 23*(1), D105.

Mamluk, L., Edwards, H. B., Savović, J., Leach, V., Jones, T., Moore, T. H., . . . Zuccolo, L. (2016). Effects of low alcohol consumption on pregnancy and childhood outcomes: A systematic review and meta-analysis. *The Lancet, 388*(Suppl. 2), S14.

Männistö, T., Mendola, P., Grewal, J., Xie, Y., Chen, Z., & Laughon, S. K. (2013). Thyroid diseases and adverse pregnancy outcomes in a contemporary US cohort. *The Journal of Clinical Endocrinology and Metabolism, 28*(7), 2725–2733.

March of Dimes. (2015, October). *Caffeine in pregnancy.* Retrieved from http://www.marchofdimes.org/pregnancy/caffeine-in-pregnancy.aspx

Marshall, S. A., Senadheera, S. N., Parry, L. J., & Girling, J. E. (2017). The role of relaxin in normal and abnormal uterine function during the menstrual cycle and early pregnancy. *Reproductive Sciences, 24*(3), 342–354.

McNulty-Brown, E., & Vaughan-Jones, S. (2016). An overview of pregnancy dermatoses. *Dermatological Nursing, 15*(1), 24–30.

Moore, K. (2015, February 3). Keith Moore. *BBC News Magazine.* Retrieved from: http://www.bbc.com/news/magazine-31046144

Nigam, A., Ahmad, A., Gaur, D., Elahi, A. A., & Batra, S. (2016). Prevalence and risk factors for urinary incontinence in pregnant women during late third trimester. *International Journal of Reproduction, Contraception, Obstetrics and Gynecology, 5*(7), 2187–2191.

O'Brien, L. M., & Warland, J. (2014). *Typical sleep positions in pregnant women. Early Human Development, 90*(6), 315–317.

O'Donnell, A., McParlin, C., Robson, S. C., Beyer, F., Moloney, E., Bryant, A., . . . Vale, L. (2016). Treatments for hyperemesis gravidarum and nausea and vomiting in pregnancy: A systematic review and economic assessment. *20*(74), 1–268. doi:10.3310/hta20740

Office of Disease Prevention and Health Promotion. (n.d.). *Maternal, infant, and child health: Objectives.* Retrieved from https://www.healthypeople.gov/2020/topics-objectives/topic/maternal-infant-and-child-health/objectives

Owe, K., Nystad, W., Stigum, H., & Vangen, S. (2016). Exercise during pregnancy and risk of cesarean delivery in nulliparous women: A large population-based cohort study. *American Journal of Obstetrics and Gynecology, 215*(6), 791.e1–791.e13.

Palmer, K., Bonzini, M., & Bonde, J. (2013). Pregnancy: Occupational aspects of management: Concise guidance. *Clinical Medicine (London, England), 13*(1), 75.

Pennick, V., & Liddle, S. (2013). Interventions for preventing and treating pelvic and back pain in pregnancy (Review). *The Cochrane Database of Systematic Reviews*, (8), CD001139.

Perales, M., Santos-Lozano, A., Sanchis-Gomar, F., Luaces, M., Pareja-Galeano, H., Garatachea, N., . . . Lucia A. (2016). Maternal cardiac adaptations to a physical exercise program during pregnancy. *Medicine and Science in Sports and Exercise, 48*(5), 896–906.

Pew Research Center. (2015). *Working while pregnant is much more common than it used to be.* Retrieved from http://www.pewresearch.org/fact-tank/2015/03/31/working-while-pregnant-is-much-more-common-than-it-used-to-be

Rådestad, I., Sormunen, T., Rudenhed, L., & Pettersson, K. (2015). Sleeping patterns of Swedish women experiencing a stillbirth between 2000–2014—An observational study. *BMC Pregnancy and Childbirth, 16*(1), 193.

Rhoades, R., & Bell, D. (2017). Chapter 38: Fertilization, Pregnancy, and Fetal Development. In R. Rhoades, & D. Bell (Eds.), *Medical physiology: Principles for clinical medicine* (5th ed.). Bethesda, MD: Wolter Kluwer Health.

Sadler, T. (2014). Chapter 13: Cardiovascular system. In T. Sadler (Ed.), *Langman's medical embryology.* Bethesda, MD: Wolters Kluwer Health.

Sadler, T. (2014). First week of development: Ovulation to implantation. In T. Sadler (Ed.), *Langman's medical embryology* (13th ed.). Bethesda, MD: Wolter Kluwer Health.

Sadler, T. (2014). Third week of development: Trilaminar germ disc. In T. Sadler (Ed.), *Langman's medical embryology* (13th ed.). Bethesda, MD: Wolters Kluwer Health.

Sadler, T. (2014). Third month to birth: The fetus and placenta. In T. Sadler (Ed.), *Langman's medical embryology.* Bethesda, MD: Wolter Kluwer Health.

Sanghavi, M., & Rutherford, J. D. (2014). Cardiovascular physiology of pregnancy. *Circulation, 130*(12), 1003–1008.

Sharma, R., Kumar, A., & Aneja, G. (2016). Serial changes in pulmonary hemodynamics during pregnancy: A non-invasive study using Doppler echocardiography. *Cardiology Research, 7*(1), 25.

Sindinga, M., Peters, D. A., Frøkjærc, J. B., Christiansena, O. B., Uldbjerge, N., & Sørensen, A. (2016). Reduced placental oxygenation during subclinical uterine contractions as assessed by BOLD MRI. *Placenta, 39*, 16–20.

Smaill, F., & Vazquez, J. (2015). Antibiotics for asymptomatic bacteriuria in pregnancy. *The Cochrane Database of Systematic Reviews*, (8), CD000490.

Smyth, R., Aflaifel, N., & Bamigboye, A. (2015). Interventions for varicose veins and leg oedema in pregnancy (Review). *The Cochrane Database of Systematic Reviews*, (10), CD001066.

Stergiakouli, E., Thapar, A., & Davey Smith, G. (2016). Association of acetaminophen use during pregnancy with behavioral problems in childhood: Evidence against confounding. *JAMA Pediatrics, 170*(10), 964.

Task Force on Hypertension in Pregnancy. (2013). *Hypertension in pregnancy.* Washington, DC: American College of Obstetricians and Gynecologists.

The American College of Obstetricians and Gynecologists. (2013, September). *The Rh factor: How it can affect your pregnancy.* Retrieved from http://www.acog.org/Patients/FAQs/The-Rh-Factor-How-It-Can-Affect-Your-Pregnancy#positive

The American College of Obstetricians and Gynecologists. (2015a). Committee Opinion No. 640: Cell-free DNA screening for fetal aneuploidy. *Obstetrics and Gynecology, 126*(3), e31–e37. doi:10.1097/AOG.0000000000001051

The American College of Obstetricians and Gynecologists. (2015b). ACOG Committee Opinion No. 650: Physical activity and exercise during pregnancy and the postpartum period. *Obstetrics and Gynecology, 126*(6), e135.

U.S. Equal Employment Opportunity Commission. (n.d.). *Pregnancy discrimination.* Retrieved from https://www.eeoc.gov/laws/types/pregnancy.cfm

U.S. Food and Drug Administration. (2015, February 24). *Fish: What pregnant women and parents should know.* Retrieved from http://www.fda.gov/Food/FoodborneIllnessContaminants/Metals/ucm393070.htm

Wiebe, H., Boulé, N., Chari, R., & Davenport, M. (2015). The effect of supervised prenatal exercise on fetal growth: A meta-analysis. *Obstetrics and Gynecology, 125*(5), 1185.

Wong, N., Browne, J., Ferguson, S., Taylor, J., & Davis, D. (2015). Getting the first birth right: A retrospective study of outcomes for low-risk primiparous women receiving standard care versus midwifery model of care in the same tertiary hospital. *Women and Birth, 28*(4), 279–284.

Workowski, K., & Bolan, G. (2015). Sexually transmitted diseases treatment guidelines, 2015. *Morbidity and Mortality Weekly Report, 64*, 1–137.

Yamaguchi, K., Suganuma, N., & Ohashi, K. (2014). Prevention of striae gravidarum and quality of life among pregnant Japanese women. *Midwifery, 30*(6), 595–599.

Yau, W., Mitchell, A., Lin, K., Werler, M., & Hernández-Díaz, S. (2013). Use of decongestants during pregnancy and the risk of birth defects. *American Journal of Epidemiology, 178*(2), 198–208.

Zielinski, R., Searing, K., & Deibel, M. (2015). Gastrointestinal distress in pregnancy: Prevalence, assessment, and treatment of 5 common minor discomforts. *The Journal of Perinatal and Neonatal Nursing, 29*(1), 23–31.

Suggested Readings

Clark, A. R., & Kruger, J. A. (2017). Mathematical modeling of the female reproductive system: From oocyte to delivery. *Wiley Interdisciplinary Reviews: Systems Biology and Medicine, 9*(1), e1353.

Nazik, E., & Eryilmaz, G. (2014). Incidence of pregnancy-related discomforts and management approaches to relieve them among pregnant women. *Journal of Clinical Nursing, 23*(11–12), 1736–1750.

Office on Women's Health. (2017, June 12). *Prenatal care.* Retrieved from https://www.womenshealth.gov/a-z-topics/prenatal-care

U.S. Food and Drug Administration. (2016, January 4). *Food safety for moms-to-be.* Retrieved from http://www.fda.gov/food/resourcesforyou/healtheducators/ucm081785.htm

16 Labor and Delivery

Objectives

1. Discuss delivery venue options and the advantages and disadvantages of each.
2. Identify the five Ps of labor and explain how each affects the process of labor.
3. Describe the potential mechanisms behind the onset of labor and the signs of impending labor.
4. Identify the four stages of labor and the three phases of the first stage, and describe the key characteristics of each.
5. Discuss the important nursing assessments and care interventions required in each stage and phase of labor.
6. Describe the types of fetal monitoring and discuss common fetal heart rate changes and their significance.
7. Describe how pain and discomfort manifest throughout the stages of labor and identify common pharmacologic and nonpharmacologic methods for managing them.

Key Terms

Acme
Decrement
Dilation
Duration
Effacement
Engagement
Ferguson reflex
Fetal attitude
Fetal lie
Fetal position

Fetal presentation
Frequency
Increment
Intensity
Intrauterine resuscitation
Nuchal cord
Open glottis pushing
Pelvimetry
Station

Labor and delivery is also referred to as childbirth or the intrapartum period. It starts with the regular contractions that dilate the cervix and ends with the delivery of the placenta. Contractions that do not cause cervical changes are not considered true labor, and often cease with hydration and rest.

Delivery Venue

In the United States, most women deliver their newborns in a traditional hospital setting. Usually, hospital births are attended by physicians, although approximately 8.3% of births are attended by midwives (Martin, Hamilton, Osterman, Curtin, & Mathews, 2015). In 2012, 1.36% of births occurred outside of a hospital, up from 1.26% in 2011. Of these 53,635 nonhospital births, 35,184 occurred at home and 15,577 occurred in birthing centers (MacDorman, Mathews, & Declercq, 2014).

Hospital

In the United States, 98.6% of births in 2012 occurred in hospitals (Martin et al., 2015). Labor and delivery nurses often take care of only one patient at a time and are responsible for a broad range of tasks, including starting intravenous (IV) lines, scrubbing in to assist during cesarean sections, fetal monitoring, medication administration, patient support and advocacy, and immediate newborn care.

Some hospitals keep a maternity patient in one room for labor, delivery, and recovery and then move her to another for postpartum care. Other hospitals offer a single room for a family's entire stay, where labor, delivery, recovery, and postpartum care all occur. Although rooming the infant with the mother is the current standard of care, most hospitals still offer a newborn nursery, in which the neonate may receive temporary care, interventions, screening, and monitoring. A hospital birth has the advantage of ready access to key personnel, equipment, and care in the case of an obstetric emergency, as well as access to a broader range of interventions and pain control options. Some women, however, prefer a less clinical setting for a birth anticipated to be uncomplicated.

Home

Approximately 88% of home births are intentional; the remaining 12% are precipitous or to mothers who are belatedly aware of the extent of their labor progress (MacDorman et al., 2014). Women may choose home births because of negative prior hospital experiences or perceptions of the hospital birthing experience or because they feel more empowered and in control or comfortable in the home environment (Zielinski, Ackerson, & Low, 2015). Although home births remain rare in the United States, other countries, such as the Netherlands, report that 20% of infants are born at home (Zielinski et al., 2015).

An advantage of home births is that they are far less likely to include medical interventions such as episiotomy, surgical birth, or invasive monitoring. However, home births in the United States are twice as likely to result in perinatal death (demise of a fetus or neonate near the time of birth) and three times as likely to involve a seizure or neurologic damage to the neonate (Wax & Barth, 2016). These statistics are not universally discovered, however, and other studies on the subject have found little to no difference in outcomes between planned home births and hospital births (Zielinski et al., 2015). Variations in statistics and outcomes are at least partly due to infrastructure differences between countries and regions: places such as the Netherlands, with a strong tradition of home births, also have robust systems for hospital transport and emergency consultations, whereas the United States does not.

Birth Center

Approximately 0.3% of births occur in independent birth centers, most of which are freestanding and not located in a hospital (Martin et al., 2015). Midwives attend most of these births. Birth centers are designed to be more home-like and comfortable and cater to women with low-risk pregnancies. Approximately 85% of women who are pregnant are eligible to deliver in a birth center rather than a hospital. Birth centers have standing transfer agreements with hospitals, and approximately 16% of women, 82% of whom are primigravidas (Box 16.1), or infants

> ### Box 16.1 Terms Describing Current and Past Pregnancy Status
>
> - *Gravida:* A pregnant woman
> - *Multigravida:* A woman who has had more than one pregnancy
> - *Multipara:* A woman who has carried a pregnancy past the 20th week of gestation or delivered an infant weighing more than 500 g more than once
> - *Nullipara:* A woman who has never carried a pregnancy beyond the 20th week of gestation or carried a fetus weighing more than 500 g
> - *Para:* The number of pregnancies carried to the 20th week of gestation or deliveries of an infant weighing more than 500 g, regardless of the outcome
> - *Primigravida:* A woman who is pregnant for the first time
> - *Primipara:* A woman who has been or is currently pregnant for the first time past the 20th week of gestation

are transferred to the hospital from the birthing center before, during, or after the birth (Stapleton, Osborne, & Illuzzi, 2013). Birth centers focus on pregnancy as a state of wellness and on women and families as a whole. The rate of cesarean delivery for women choosing to deliver in a birth center is approximately one-fifth that of women who deliver in hospitals, and neonate morbidity and mortality rates are equivalent to those of low-risk deliveries in hospitals (Stapleton et al., 2013).

Components of Labor: The Five Ps

Labor consists of five components, referred to as the five Ps. Dysfunction in any of these domains can cause complications that may require intervention to preserve the health and well-being of the mother, fetus, or both.

Power

Power in labor may be either primary or secondary. The primary powers of labor are the involuntary uterine contractions and **Ferguson reflex** (the reflex to push). The secondary power is the voluntary action of pushing itself.

Primary Powers

Involuntary uterine contractions occur in the muscular upper two thirds of the uterus and apply pressure to the fetus, which in turn applies pressure to the amniotic fluid, the lower portion of the uterus, and the cervix. In response, the cervix, in the lower portion of the uterus, dilates and effaces, allowing for passage of the products of conception (fetus, placenta, amniotic fluid, membranes, etc.).

Dilation of the cervix is the drawing up and opening of the cervix from fully closed or only a few centimeters in diameter at the onset of labor to 10 cm in diameter when fully open at the end of the first stage of labor. When the cervix is fully dilated, it can no longer be palpated. In first pregnancies, dilation typically progresses more slowly than effacement, whereas in subsequent pregnancies, effacement and dilation happen more or less simultaneously. Dilation is expressed in centimeters.

In Chapter 2, Tatiana was 2 cm dilated at 39 weeks of gestation. Her physician, Joy, told her this was a common finding at this point in pregnancy.

Effacement is the thinning and shortening of the cervix from about 2 to 3 cm long and 1 cm thick to effectively absent, with the exception of a small lip, as it is drawn up. Effacement is expressed as a percentage (Figs. 16.1 and 1.15).

During a contraction, blood flow to the placenta is decreased. Thus, it is critical that each contraction also has a resting phase, which allows for the perfusion of the placenta by the maternal blood and, in turn, the fetus. The contraction has three phases: increment, acme, and decrement (Fig. 16.2):

- *Increment:* The buildup phase of the contraction. As the uterus contracts, the sensation becomes more acute. This is the longest phase of a contraction.
- *Acme:* The peak and shortest but most acute phase of the contraction. Some laboring women may find it helpful

to remember that after the acme the contraction releases rapidly.
- *Decrement:* The relaxation of the uterine muscle and the second shortest phase.

In Chapter 2, Tatiana thought of her contractions as a hill she needed to run up and then come back down. The uphill was the increment, the top of the hill was the acme, and the downhill was the decrement.

While increment, acme, and decrement describe the actions of individual contractions, frequency, duration, and intensity describe the overall pattern of contractions. All of these factors are considered in monitoring the progress of labor.

In Chapter 5, Letitia learned about the 411 from Dr. Janachek. The 4 refers to contractions occurring 4 minutes a part or less (frequency), the first 1 refers to contractions lasting 1 minute or longer (duration), and the second 1 refers to the previous two criteria having occurred for at least 1 hour.

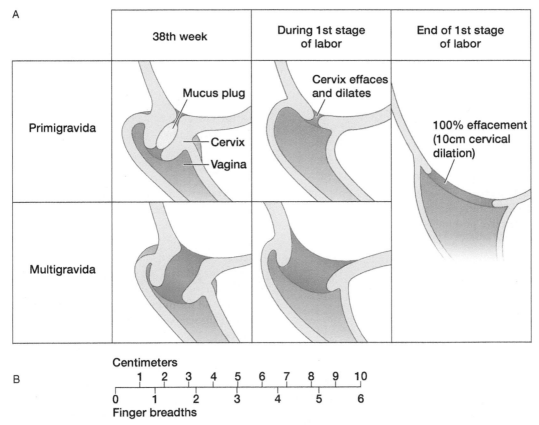

Figure 16.1. Stages and measurement of cervical dilation. (A) Stages of cervical dilation. **(B)** Measurement of cervical dilation. (Reprinted with permission from Irion, J. M., & Irion, G. L. [2009]. *Women's health in physical therapy* [1st ed., Fig. 15.3]. Philadelphia, PA: Lippincott Williams & Wilkins.)

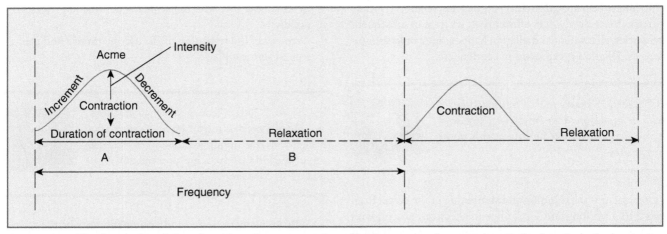

Figure 16.2. The interval and duration of uterine contractions. The frequency of contractions is the time from the beginning of one contraction to the beginning of the next contraction. It consists of two parts: (*A*) The duration of the contraction and (*B*) The period of relaxation. The broken line indicates an indeterminate period because the relaxation time (*B*) is usually of longer duration than the actual contraction (*A*). (Reprinted with permission from Pillitteri, A. [2002]. *Maternal and child health nursing: Care of the childbearing and childrearing family* [4th ed., Fig. 18-10]. Philadelphia, PA: Lippincott Williams & Wilkins.)

- *Frequency:* The frequency of contractions is the time from the beginning of one contraction to the beginning of the next contraction. In other words, the frequency of contractions is the time from the beginning of one increment phase to the beginning of the next increment phase. A woman who is having contractions every 3 minutes is actually starting a new contraction every 3 minutes.
- *Duration:* The duration of a contraction is different from the frequency of contractions. Although frequency includes the active and resting phases combined, duration refers only to the active, contracting phase of the contraction. A woman may have, for example, a contraction frequency of 3 minutes and a contraction duration of 60 seconds. In this example, she is contracting for 1 minute but not contracting (resting phase) for 2 minutes.
- *Intensity:* In low-risk pregnancies, the intensity, or strength, of a contraction is measured by uterine indentability. To evaluate intensity, a nurse presses her fingertips into the abdomen. The degree of intensity is determined by the firmness of the uterus.
  - Mild: feels like pushing the tip of your nose
  - Moderate: feels like pushing your chin
  - Strong: feels like pushing your forehead

Although the primary power of contractions is present through all stages of labor, the primary power of the bearing down reflex, called the Ferguson reflex, comes into play during the second stage of labor. The second stage is the time from complete dilation of the cervix (10 cm) to the birth of the fetus. The Ferguson reflex is cued when the presenting part of the fetus (usually the head) reaches the pelvic floor.

In Chapter 8, the nurse caring for Gracie during labor recognized that Gracie did not have a Ferguson reflex. She speculated it was likely because Gracie had an epidural in place.

Secondary Powers

Secondary powers are voluntary, meaning that they are controlled by the laboring woman. The secondary powers are the bearing-down movements of the abdomen and diaphragm, which help push out the fetus. These pushing efforts do not have a direct effect on the uterus but rather increase intraabdominal pressure such that the contractions of the uterus are potentiated. Secondary powers must not be enlisted prior to full dilation, as they do not contribute to effacement and dilation and may cause the cervix to become edematous and to open more slowly.

Passageway

The passageway refers to the anatomy of the bony pelvis and the soft tissue of the pelvic floor muscles, introitus (opening to the vagina), and vaginal canal.

Bony Pelvis

The bony pelvis can be divided into two parts, the false pelvis and the true pelvis. The false pelvis is the winged portion consisting of the ilia and iliac crest. The front is open and the ilia are joined at the back by the sacrum. The false pelvis serves to support the internal structures of the abdomen but typically has little to no obstetrical significance.

The true pelvis is the lower portion of the pelvis between the proximal pelvic inlet and the distal pelvic outlet. The area between the inlet and the outlet is called the midpelvis. The joints of the pelvis are the symphysis pubis and the right and left sacroiliac joints (Fig. 16.3). These joints become mobile in pregnancy because of the effects of increased estrogen and relaxin levels, allowing the pelvis to conform to the fetal passage. There are four generally recognized shapes for the true pelvis, along with many variations that combine the four types: gynecoid, android, anthropoid, and platypelloid (Fig. 16.4). Although traditionally gynecoid is acknowledged as the optimal configuration for a vaginal birth, newer research suggests that dimensions of the true pelvis have

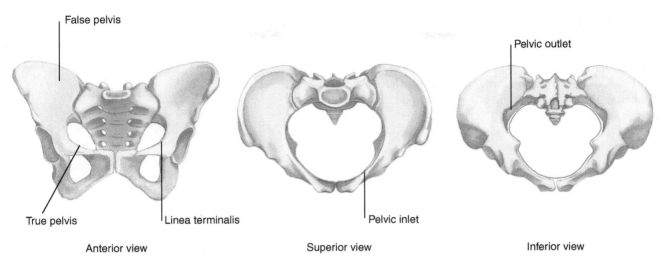

False pelvis

True pelvis

Linea terminalis

Anterior view

Pelvic inlet

Superior view

Pelvic outlet

Inferior view

Figure 16.3. The bony pelvis. (Reprinted with permission from Ricci, S. S. [2017]. *Essentials of maternity, newborn, & women's health nursing* [4th ed., Fig. 13.1]. Philadelphia, PA: Lippincott Williams & Wilkins.)

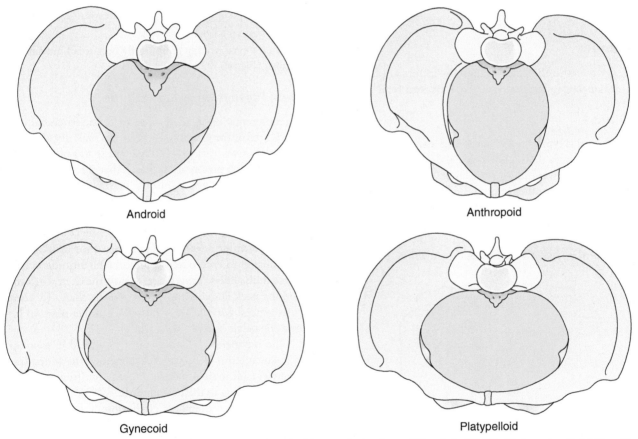

Android

Anthropoid

Gynecoid

Platypelloid

Figure 16.4. The four types of true pelves. (Reprinted with permission from Pillitteri, A. [2002]. *Maternal and child health nursing: Care of the childbearing and childrearing family* [4th ed., Fig. 10-9]. Philadelphia, PA: Lippincott Williams & Wilkins.)

little bearing on the potential success of a vaginal, as opposed to a cesarean, birth (Korhonen & Heinonen, 2014).

Although **pelvimetry** (assessment and measurement of the bony pelvis) is still done in many settings, it is not well supported by the evidence available as it is not well standardized and poorly predicts the course of labor. Unfavorable pelvimetry measurements do not preclude a trial of labor to attempt a vaginal birth

(Korhonen, Taipale, & Heinonen, 2013; Pattinson, Cuthbert, & Vannevel, 2017). The dimensions and size of the pelvis are less important than the size of the pelvis in relation to the size of the fetal head, which is not something that can be ascertained using only traditional pelvimetry (Korhonen & Heinonen, 2014).

The ischial spines of the true pelvis are located inside the midpelvis about midway between the inlet and the outlet.

This is the narrowest part of the interior of the true pelvis. When describing the descent of the presenting part through the true pelvis, we use the ischial spines as the reference. The level of the ischial spines is referred to as zero **station**. When a fetus is described as engaged, that means the presenting part has reached zero station. When the presenting part moves beyond the ischial spines, it is described as +1 through +5 station, with +5 indicating crowning (the presenting part visible at the introitus). Negative numbers indicate that the presenting part is still "floating" above station 0 and is not engaged (Fig. 16.5).

Soft Tissue

The soft tissue is rarely an impediment to fetal passage. On occasion, such as in the case of surgery to remove cancerous cells from the cervix, scarring may inhibit effacement and dilation. In general, however, tissues soften and dilate to allow fetal descent. The muscles of the pelvic floor help turn and orient the fetus through the cardinal movements of delivery (see Box 11.4 and Fig. 11.5).

Passenger

Passenger refers to the fetus. Important factors are fetal head, fetal presentation, fetal attitude, fetal lie, and fetal position.

Fetal Head

The fetal head is typically the largest and least malleable part of the fetus. Although the shoulders are wider, they are also more easily collapsed inward toward the chest, and the chest itself is also malleable. The sutures joining the fetal head are not immobile as they will be later in life, however. Molding is the process by which the sutures and the fontanels (nonbony intersections of the sutures) move such that the shape of the head changes in reference to the birth canal (Fig. 16.6). At times, bones of the

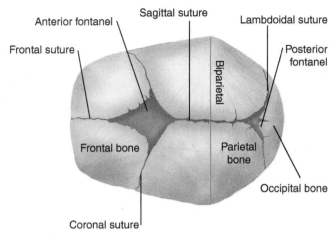

Figure 16.6. Fetal skull. (Reprinted with permission from Ricci, S. S. [2013]. *Essentials of maternity, newborn, & women's health nursing* [3rd ed., Fig. 13.3]. Philadelphia, PA: Lippincott Williams & Wilkins.)

skull may even overlap temporarily because of movement of the sutures (Fig. 16.7).

Fetal Presentation and Attitude

Fetal presentation refers to the part of the fetus that enters the pelvis first, or the presenting part. A vast majority of infants enter the pelvis head first, which is referred to as a cephalic presentation. A breech presentation means that the infant's buttocks or feet are descending first into the pelvis (Fig. 16.8). A shoulder presentation, wherein the shoulder is entering the true pelvis first, is not compatible with a vaginal delivery without correction and occurs in fewer than 1% of women presenting for delivery at term.

Fetal attitude refers to the position of the fetal body parts in relationship to each other. A typical fetal attitude includes legs flexed at the knees, arms flexed against the chest, back rounded, and the neck flexed with the chin on the chest. This is referred to as general flexion. This is also the optimal position for entry into the pelvic inlet.

The biparietal diameter of the fetal head is approximately 9.25 cm at term. The biparietal diameter is the widest transverse diameter (side to side). The anteroposterior (front to back) length varies according to the flexion of the fetal neck. This dimension is smallest with the fetal neck in flexion. If the neck is less flexed, with the chin off the chest, the anteroposterior diameter increases and the fetus may not be able to pass into the true pelvis. This variation in fetal attitude causes variations in the cephalic presentation (Fig. 16.9).

- Vertex presentation: In this, the most common presentation, the fetal attitude is general flexion with the fetal chin on the chest. The largest diameter entering the true pelvis is the biparietal diameter.
- Sinciput presentation: The fetal chin is off the chest, and the neck is straight. This is often called the military attitude. The anteroposterior diameter is wider than the biparietal diameter.

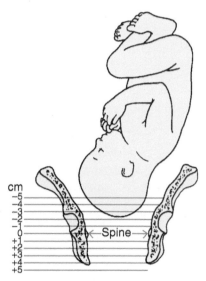

Figure 16.5. Fetal station. (Reprinted with permission from Weber, J. R. [2018]. *Nurses' handbook of health assessment* [9th ed., Fig. 24.8]. Philadelphia, PA: Lippincott Williams & Wilkins.)

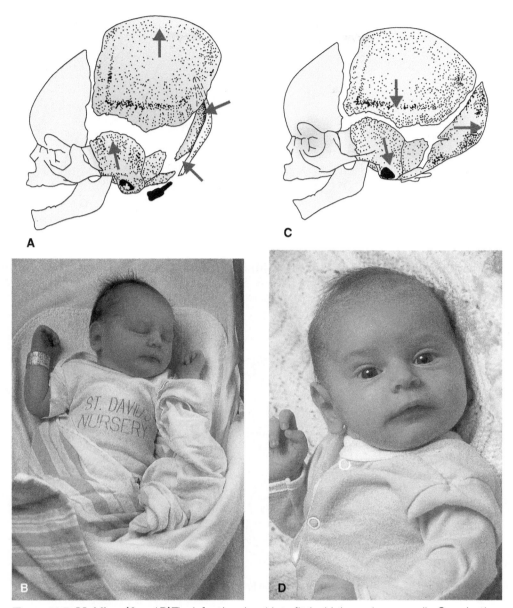

Figure 16.7. Molding. (A and **B)** The infant head molds to fit the birth canal more easily. On palpation, the skull sutures are felt to be overriding. **(C** and **D)** The head shape returns to normal within 1 week. (Reprinted with permission from Pillitteri, A. [2014]. *Maternal and child health nursing: Care of the childbearing and childrearing family* [7th ed., Fig. 18-18]. Philadelphia, PA: Lippincott Williams & Wilkins.)

- Brow presentation: The fetal chin is off the chest, and the neck is extended. The fetal brow enters the true pelvis first. The anteroposterior diameter is wider than the biparietal diameter.
- Facial presentation: The fetal chin is off the chest, and the neck is sharply extended. The fetal face enters the true pelvis first. The anteroposterior diameter is wider than the biparietal diameter.

Fetal Lie

Fetal lie is similar to fetal presentation. Unlike fetal presentation, which has three primary variations (cephalic, breech, and shoulder), lie has only two primary variations, longitudinal (or vertical) and transverse (or horizontal). The longitudinal lie is either a cephalic or breech presentation, and the transverse lie is a shoulder presentation. Fetuses in an oblique lie that is neither cephalic nor transverse typically convert during labor to one of the two primary lies (Fig. 16.10). Although the fetal lie may only be longitudinal or transverse (or, more rarely, oblique) and refers only to the relation of the fetal spine to the maternal spine, the fetal presentation refers to the specific fetal part.

Fetal Position

Fetal position is the relationship of the presenting part to the maternal pelvis. In the case of the most common presentation, the vertex presentation, the occiput of the fetal skull is the reference part, meaning that it is the relationship of the occiput to the

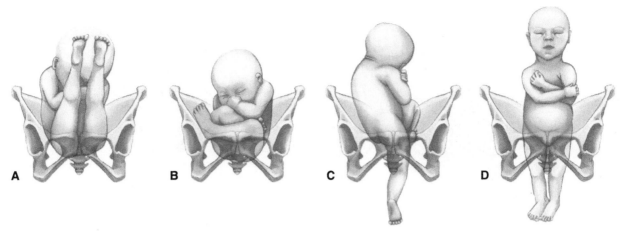

Figure 16.8. Breech presentations. (A) Frank breech. **(B)** Complete breech. **(C)** Single footling breech. **(D)** Double footling breech. (Reprinted with permission from Ricci, S. S. [2013]. *Essentials of maternity, newborn, & women's health nursing* [3rd ed., Fig. 13.8]. Philadelphia, PA: Lippincott Williams & Wilkins.)

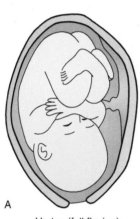

A   Vertex (full flexion)

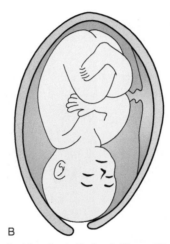

B   Sinciput (moderate flexion [military attitude])

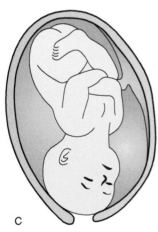

C   Brow (partial extension)

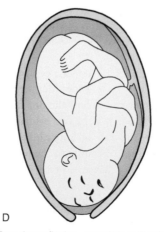

D   Face (poor flexion, complete extension)

Figure 16.9. Fetal attitude. (A) The fetus in full flexion presents the smallest anteroposterior diameter (suboccipitobregmatic) of the skull to the inlet in this good attitude (vertex presentation). **(B)** The fetus is not as well flexed (military attitude) and presents the occipitofrontal diameter to the inlet (sinciput presentation). **(C)** The fetus is in partial extension (brow presentation). **(D)** The fetus in complete extension presents a wide (occipitomental) diameter (face presentation). (Reprinted with permission from Pillitteri, A. [2014]. *Maternal and child health nursing: Care of the childbearing and childrearing family* [7th ed., Fig. 15-4]. Philadelphia, PA: Lippincott Williams & Wilkins.)

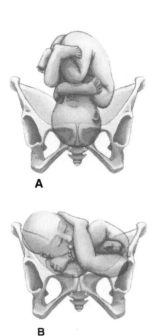

A

B

Figure 16.10. Fetal lie. Fetal lie is the relationship of the long axis of the fetus to the long axis of the mother. **(A)** Longitudinal lie occurs when the long axis of the fetus is parallel to that of the mother (fetal spine to maternal spine side by side). **(B)** Transverse lie occurs when the long axis of the fetus is perpendicular to the long axis of the mother (fetal spine lies across the maternal abdomen and crosses her spine). Note that although this longitudinal lie shows a cephalic presentation, a breech presentation is also a longitudinal lie. (Reprinted with permission from Cox-Davenport, R. [2016]. *Lippincott fast facts for NCLEX-RN* [2nd ed., Fig. 2-2]. Philadelphia, PA: Lippincott Williams & Wilkins.)

pelvis that is evaluated. Because the occiput is at the back of the head, fetal position in the case of vertex presentation is indicated from the orientation of facing the fetus's back. In other words, the fetal position is not the direction in which the fetus is facing, but rather the position of the back of the head.

Fetal position is described by a series of three letters. The first letter describes left (L) or right (R). The second letter describes the presenting part: occiput (O); mentum (M), for a brow or face presentation; scapula (Sc), for a transverse lie; and sacrum (S), for a breech presentation. The final letter describes the position of the presenting part as posterior (P), anterior (A), or transverse (T). The position of a fetus entering the true pelvis head down (cephalic) with chin tucked (vertex) and facing the mother's right buttock would thus be LOA, left occiput anterior, because the occiput is located in the left anterior quadrant of the pelvis. The position of a fetus entering the true pelvis buttocks first (breech, sacrum) and facing the mother's left abdomen would be RSP, right sacrum posterior, because the sacrum is positioned in the right posterior portion of the pelvis. The position of a fetus entering the true pelvis face first (mentum) with the chin oriented neither posterior nor anterior but to the right of the pelvis would be RMT, right mentum transverse (Fig. 16.11).

Psyche

A woman's state of mind; her feelings about herself, her pregnancy, and her surroundings; and her psychological health can all impact her experience of labor and delivery. These factors may also impact the process of labor. For example, anxiety, stress, and fear can reduce pain tolerance and delay the progress of labor (Stark, Remynse, & Zwelling, 2016). Conversely, relaxation may augment labor.

Childbirth education courses such as Lamaze, Hypnobirthing, Birthing from Within, and others seek to teach women and birthing partners strategies for coping with the psychological pressures of the intrapartum period. Strategies include a thorough education about normal birth processes, breathing exercises, visualization, hypnosis, and mindfulness. Approximately one-third of all women participate in childbirth education courses, including 59% of primiparas (Declercq, Sakala, Corry, Applebaum, & Herrlich, 2013). A woman's trust in her birthing support person or people, her care providers, and herself can also have a significant impact on her perception of labor and delivery, her use of analgesia, and whether she has a cesarean delivery or vaginal birth. On average, labor is shorter for women who have continuous support (Hodnett, Gates, Hofmeyr, & Sakala, 2013).

In Chapter 7, Hannah, encouraged by her midwife Darla, elected to take a birthing class that included hypnosis intended to promote relaxation and productive visualization. Although Hannah found these techniques initially helpful, she eventually elected to have IV nalbuphine to manage pain.

Position

The final of the five Ps refers to maternal position. Gravity can assist in successful labor and delivery. Contractions are more acute and productive for a woman who is upright and ambulating. The angle of the pelvis is more conducive to the passage of a fetus when a woman's hips are sharply flexed, as when squatting. In addition, perfusion of the uterus and placenta is superior if a woman is not flat on her back in the lithotomy position, which has become standard practice in Western cultures.

Furthermore, encouraging women to move into a position they feel is more comfortable, particularly upright or lateral, has been associated with improved outcomes. These improvements include a reduced rate of cesarean section and surgical vaginal birth, a reduction of episiotomies and spontaneous perineal lacerations, an increased sense of maternal comfort and control, and shorter first and second stages of labor (Gizzo, et al., 2014; Cox & King, 2015) (Fig. 16.12).

The preference for the lithotomy position may have evolved for the ease of the provider attending the birth or out of concern that women would exhaust themselves by remaining in an upright position. The medicalization of birth, during which it moved from

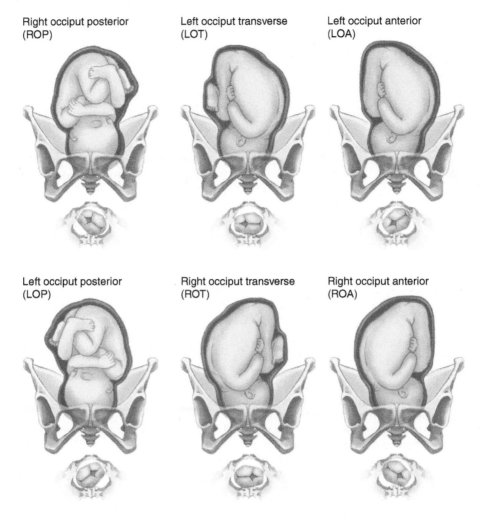

Figure 16.11. Examples of fetal positions in a vertex presentation. The lie is longitudinal for each illustration. The attitude is one of flexion. Notice that the view of the top illustration is seen when facing the pregnant woman. The bottom view is that seen with the woman in a dorsal recumbent position (i.e., the maternal sacrum is at the bottom of the image). (Reprinted with permission from Ricci, S. S. [2009]. *Essentials of maternity, newborn, & women's health nursing* [2nd ed., Fig. 13.9]. Philadelphia, PA: Lippincott Williams & Wilkins.)

the home to the hospital, where people are generally unwell and recumbent, may also be a factor. Monitoring of the patient and the fetus may be perceived as more convenient if the woman is sedentary and in bed.

Onset of Labor

Although the mechanisms that initiate labor remain unclear, many physical signs indicate that labor is impending occur. One familiar sign, the spontaneous rupture of membranes (SROM), actually occurs in only a minority of women. True labor is marked by contractions with dilation of the cervix.

Mechanisms of Onset

Many factors are involved in triggering labor, including a combination of maternal factors and fetal factors that initiate the beginning of

regular contractions and cervical dilation and effacement. Expansion of the uterus is likely involved and may cue hormonal processes that ultimately trigger productive contractions. Additionally, newer research suggests that a cue from fetal proteins in the lungs may play a significant part in the initiation of labor (Gao et al., 2015; Menon, Bonney, Condon, Mesiano, & Taylor, 2016).

Signs of Impending Labor

Women are often anxious for true labor to start, and the frequent contractions and monitoring for signs of labor may be stressful. Educating women about how to distinguish true labor from false labor is helpful for the patient and may result in fewer unnecessary visits with the obstetric provider for labor assessment (see Patient Teaching 2.3). Labor is not confirmed unless contractions are continuous and progressive and result in dilation and effacement of the cervix.

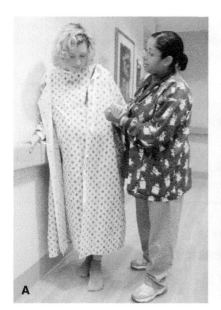
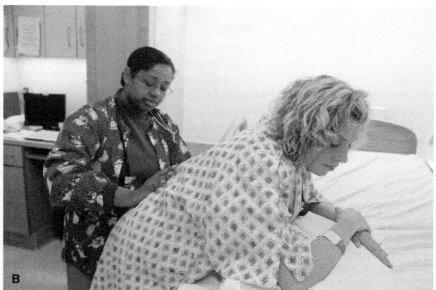
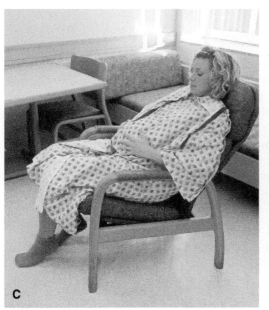
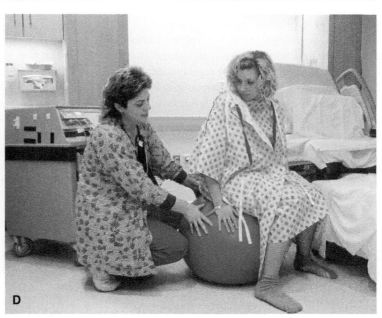

Figure 16.12. Positions for labor. (A) Ambulation. **(B)** Leaning forward. **(C)** Sitting in a chair. **(D)** Using a birthing ball. (Reprinted with permission from Ricci, S. S. [2013]. *Essentials of maternity, newborn, & women's health nursing* [3rd ed., Fig. 14.9]. Philadelphia, PA: Lippincott Williams & Wilkins.)

In Chapter 2, Tatiana was evaluated by a labor and delivery nurse, Judy, who determined she was having Braxton Hicks contractions and was not in labor. Judy sent Tatiana and Caleb home to relax. Two days later, true labor started.

The 411 rule is a memory device that women can use when deciding whether they should present for an assessment of labor. According to the 411 rule, assessment is warranted if the woman is experiencing the start of a new contraction at least once every 4 minutes that lasts for 1 minute, and if such contractions have been occurring for at least 1 hour. Some providers may want women to be evaluated when the contractions are less frequent, perhaps every 5 or 6 minutes apart, particularly if the woman lives far away from the birthing venue or has given birth previously. A woman should contact her obstetric provider immediately if she experiences intense pain—particularly if constant—rupture of membranes, or bleeding.

Although not reliable indicators of the onset of true labor, the following are signs that labor may be impending:

- Braxton Hicks contractions: These contractions are typically felt from midway through the pregnancy onward. Some women may never feel these contractions, although it is believed that all women have them. As labor approaches, they may become more coordinated, with periods of regularity, and it can become more difficult to discern Braxton Hicks contractions from true labor.

- Bloody show: Bloody show is mucus streaked with blood from the operculum as the cervix begins to open and change in the approach to labor. However, if the cervix has been manipulated prior to the appearance of bloody show, it cannot be considered a reliable sign of impending labor.
- Lightening: This term refers to the descent of the fetal head into the pelvis. This typically occurs with labor for a multigravida and about 2 weeks prior to the onset of labor for a primigravida.
- Nesting: Some women may experience an urge to put everything in order and clean as labor approaches. However, this surge of energy may result more from wishful thinking than any physical change, as a woman anticipates the nesting urge as proof of impending labor.
- Cervical changes: Labor is marked by regular contractions that contribute to cervical changes, but changes to the cervix happen prior to the onset of regular contractions at the end of pregnancy, as well. Women may be partially effaced and as many as 4 cm dilated for days or even weeks prior to the start of regular contractions.
- Gastrointestinal symptoms: Some women may have gastrointestinal distress around the time of delivery in the form of diarrhea, heartburn, or nausea.
- Weight loss: Some women lose 1 to 3 lb just prior to the onset of labor.

Assessment for Rupture of Membranes

Despite depictions in popular culture, SROM occurs prior to labor only 8% of the time and typically happens instead when labor is well established (Wojcieszek, Stock, & Flenady, 2014). Late in pregnancy the breakdown of the operculum may present as an increase in vaginal fluid. Additionally, leukorrhea or urinary incontinence may be mistaken for SROM.

If a woman presents with suspected SROM with regular contractions or rupture of membranes without contractions (premature rupture of membranes), she will need an exam to discover whether the fluid is amniotic fluid, urine, part of her mucus plug, or vaginal discharge (see Step-by-Step Skills 7.1). Assessment of the fetal heart beat is also critical, because there is an increased risk for prolapse of the cord between the fetus and the maternal pelvis with rupture of membranes, particularly if the fetus is not yet engaged in the pelvis. Further assessment of the fluid itself is needed to detect other complications. Normal amniotic fluid is clear, whereas fluid that is cloudy or has a foul odor may indicate an intrauterine infection. Fluid stained with meconium may be normal, particularly in postterm pregnancies, but it may also indicate fetal hypoxia in utero. Obstetric providers may elect for watchful waiting or induction of labor. Although watchful waiting may involve a small risk for infection, labor induction also carries risks, including a higher rate of cesarean delivery (see Analyze the Evidence 7.1).

In Chapter 8, Gracie's membranes ruptured prior to the onset of contractions, prior to term. Gracie's team decided not to induce, and she was given antibiotics to treat and prevent infection. (In Chapter 7, Hannah's membranes ruptured prior to the onset of contractions and labor was induced.)

Stages of Labor and Nursing Interventions

There are four stages of labor, each of which has its particular parameters and tasks (see Table 1.3 and Fig. 16.13).

First Stage

The first stage of labor is the longest, lasting an average of 12 hours for primigravidas and 8 hours for multigravidas, although the length of labor varies tremendously. The first stage begins with the start of regular contractions that cause progressive changes to the cervix and ends when the cervix is dilated 10 cm. During this stage, the membranes of pregnancy typically rupture spontaneously but may instead be ruptured by the obstetric provider. Maternal cardiac output and pulse increase, whereas peristalsis of the gut and gastric emptying decrease.

Phases

The first stage of labor is divided into three phases: latent, active, and transition.

Latent Phase

The latent phase of the first stage of labor is the period during which the cervix progressively dilates from 0 to 3 cm. During this phase, contractions are mild to palpation, enough so that women can typically talk through them. For some women, the latent phase is a period of excitement because the long-anticipated birth is finally immanent, whereas for others it may be a period of anxiety. Contractions last approximately 30 to 40 seconds in this phase, and may be as close together as every 3 minutes or as far apart as every 30 minutes. Contractions may feel like menstrual cramps and may be accompanied by a low backache.

Active Phase

The active phase of the first stage of labor is the period during which the cervix progressively dilates from 3 to 7 cm. It lasts about 5 hours in a primiparous patient and 2 to 3 hours in a multiparous patient. In the active phase, contractions are

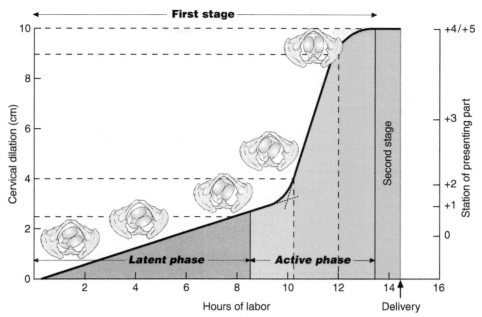

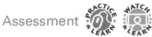

Figure 16.13. Progress of the successive stages of labor. Note the relationship between changes in cervical dilation and phases of labor as well as fetal descent (station). Also note the rotation of the fetal head in a right occiput-anterior presentation in the successive stages of labor. (Reprinted with permission from Callahan, T. L., & Caughey, A. B. [2018]. *Blueprints obstetrics & gynecology* [7th ed., Fig. 4.11]. Philadelphia, PA: Lippincott Williams & Wilkins.)

moderately strong to palpation and last 30 to 45 seconds. Contractions are more frequent in this phase, coming every 3 to 5 minutes. During the active phase, women may be more focused than they were during the latent phase and may at times become anxious and restless.

Transition Phase

The transition phase is the final period of cervical dilation and typically lasts less than 2 hours. Contractions are strong and close together, a new one starting every 1 to 2 minutes and lasting 40 to 60 seconds each. Women may feel out of control, irritable, uncooperative, exhausted, or dependent. Some women experience nausea and vomiting, and perspiration may be noted on the upper lip and forehead. An increase in bloody vaginal discharge is also typical of this phase. Delivery preparation begins at this time. If the woman's membranes have not already ruptured by this point, the provider will likely perform an amniotomy, or artificial rupture of the membranes.

In Chapter 9, the nurse, Grace, noticed that Nancy had become more focused and intense, and that she was vocalizing more. She deduced from these changes in behavior that Nancy was most likely in the transition phase of the first stage of labor.

Admission to the Delivery Venue

Most admissions occur in the first stage of labor, after the cervix has dilated to at least 3 cm and regular contractions are well established. Evidence of cervical changes, rupture of membranes, and maternal or fetal distress are other reasons for admission. Most women who have not given birth previously present for admission earlier than those who have previously given birth. Women may call the venue or the office of their obstetric provider prior to presenting for evaluation. Women receiving prenatal care typically have records on site at the birthing venue that were previously forwarded by the obstetric provider.

Assessment

Patient assessment by interview and physical exam is the first priority when the woman presents for assessment of labor. Pertinent information is collected about the duration and frequency of contractions and how long she has been aware of them. She is asked about vaginal discharge and the nature of that discharge (watery, bloody, etc.). A pain assessment is performed. The woman is asked to describe the intensity of her contractions and to identify any other discomfort. Persistent uterine pain that continues between contractions would be concerning. The nurse asks about the woman's last food and drink and notes this in the chart.

A physical assessment is done that includes the mother's vital signs and the fetal heart rate (FHR). Contractions are monitored at the same time as the FHR to obtain information not just about the contractions but also about how well the fetus is tolerating them (see Fig. 1.8). A sterile speculum exam may be done by a nurse to evaluate for pooling of fluids suggestive of rupture of membranes as well as for bleeding. A sterile vaginal exam is done to assess for cervical dilation and effacement and fetal station, presentation, and position (Step-by-Step Skills 16.1). If the fetal position cannot be discerned by vaginal exam, Leopold's maneuvers may be done (see Fig. 1.10).

When Gracie presented to labor and delivery in Chapter 8, Tiffany, a nurse, performed her evaluation. She was careful throughout to tell Gracie what she was doing and what she was learning from the examination.

Step-by-Step Skills 16.1

Sterile Vaginal Exams

1. Place a dollop of sterile water-based lubricant on a sterile drape.
2. Don sterile gloves.
3. With your nondominant hand, separate the labia.
4. Lubricate the first two fingers of your dominant hand and insert them into the vagina to locate the cervix.
5. Note: Straightening your arm at the wrist may allow for better access to the cervix.
6. Check the following:
   - Cervical dilation: Sweep your finger from one side of the cervical opening to the other to estimate the distance between the two in centimeters.
   - Cervical effacement: Estimate the length of the cervix. Two centimeters long is 0% effaced, and paper thin is 100% effaced. A cervix that is 1 cm long is 50% effaced.
   - Cervical position: A posterior cervix is oriented so that it "points" toward the pregnant woman's back, whereas an anterior cervix is oriented with its opening toward the vaginal introitus. A mid-position cervix is between these two orientations. A posterior cervix suggests an "unripe" cervix and indicates that labor is unlikely.
   - Station: The station refers to the level of the presenting part in relation to the ischial spines of the pelvis. Station zero means that the presenting part is at the level of the ischial spines and generally means that the fetus is engaged.
   - Presentation: Presentation refers to part of the fetus that is presenting to the maternal pelvis: head (cephalic), buttocks and/or feet (breech), or shoulder.
   - Fetal position: Fetal position refers to the relation of the presenting fetal part to the maternal pelvis (right occiput posterior, for example).

Chart Review

If the woman's chart is not already on the unit, a copy is ordered as soon as she presents to the unit. This prenatal record includes all visit information, including laboratory studies, ultrasounds, and pertinent information about each visit. Patient medications, allergies, prior obstetric history, and the estimated date of delivery are carefully reviewed. Particular note is made of conditions such as preeclampsia, diabetes, known cardiac conditions, and other health issues that may complicate labor, delivery, or the postpartum period. For patients known to be group B streptococcus positive, antibiotics are started when labor is confirmed per orders (see The Pharmacy 2.1 and Box 7.2). Maternal Rh status is also noted.

The woman's birth plan is reviewed with her nurse at this time. A birth plan is a wish list, and the nurse is clear about what requests can and can't be accommodated as well as hospital policies that may preclude implementation of aspects of the plan. The nurse may ask the patient to prioritize requests so the nurse will know what is most important to the patient.

Care

After this evaluation, the nurse should orient the patient and her birthing partner, if present, to the unit.

Depending on the policies of a particular birthing venue, the orders of the obstetric provider, and the wishes of the patient, the nurse may start an IV line, draw blood for laboratory work, and collect urine for assessment. During the first stage of labor, the nurse should take vital signs every hour unless the obstetric provider puts in a different order. If continuous fetal monitoring has not been ordered, the nurse is likely to receive orders to periodically monitor the fetus and contractions every 30 minutes initially and then every 15 minutes as labor progresses into the transition phase at the end of the first stage.

The nurse should encourage the laboring woman to void at least every 2 hours and should assess her bladder periodically, particularly in the late first stage, because a distended bladder may preclude fetal descent. Although frequent vaginal examinations to assess labor progress were once common, nurses now perform fewer such examinations because of the discomfort to the patient, the increased risk of infection, and the limited value of the examination itself. According to the policies of the individual institution, nurses often no longer perform vaginal examinations to assess labor progress at all, this responsibility instead falling exclusively to the obstetric provider.

The nurse should encourage the patient to participate in activities and positions that make her comfortable during labor. Walking has been shown in several small studies to reduce the duration of the first stage of labor by an hour and a half while decreasing the rate of the cesarean section and epidural use (Lawrence, Lewis, Hofmeyr, & Styles, 2013). Women often do best when ambulating with a partner or the nurse present for reassurance and companionship. When the patient is not ambulating, the nurse should remind her to not lie flat on her back to avoid supine hypotension from compression of the vena cava.

In Chapter 9, Nancy was encouraged to walk frequently during labor, particularly during the latent phase of the first stage. To facilitate this, Nancy's monitoring device was wireless so she was not restricted to her bed.

The nurse should update the patient regularly regarding her status and the status of her fetus as the information is available. The nurse should encourage the patient and partner or family members present to ask questions and should accommodate their requests as is feasible and appropriate. The nurse should pay particular attention to any cultural beliefs or needs a patient expresses. When determining appropriate communication methods and priorities, the nurse should assess the patient's maturity, knowledge level, and experience.

To provide support as contractions progress, the nurse should speak in a soothing voice, offer positive affirmations, and reassure the patient of the normality of the birthing experience and the control the patient has over her experience. In transition particularly, the nurse should encourage the patient to breathe deeply during contractions and to rest in between contractions. Some women may relax so deeply between contractions that they develop a sort of amnesia concerning the time between contractions. Other women may find it useful to count their breaths during contractions and to notice at what number the contraction peaks and then starts to release. Some women find it helpful to vocalize during this time; others do not.

The nurse should take care to include the patient's birthing partner, if present, in supporting the patient as much as is feasible and in keeping with the patient's wishes. The nurse should encourage the partner to stay with the patient when possible and include the partner in teaching. The nurse should review with the partner breathing exercises and comfort measures that the partner can do independently to support the laboring woman and prompt the partner to follow the lead of the laboring woman.

As transition ends, the nurse should prepare the room, the patient, and the partner for delivery. At this time, the patient is likely to have limited ability to assimilate new information or instructions, so the nurse should keep communication very focused. Also during this time, the nurse should no longer leave the room without a replacement present, because the patient's status may change quickly.

Second Stage

Childbirth reaches the second stage when the cervix is fully dilated to 10 cm. The second stage ends with the birth of the infant. Early in this stage, the woman experiences a lull between the end of dilation and the beginning of the urge to push known as the latency period. Delaying pushing until the patient feels the urge to push (known as the Ferguson reflex, a primary power) may reduce maternal fatigue. The Ferguson reflex typically starts when the presenting part is at station +1. Neither delayed pushing nor passive descent (waiting for the Ferguson reflex) is associated with increased rates of cesarean section, perineal injury to the mother, or other negative outcomes for mother or neonate. The woman should push according to her preferences and the recommendations of her obstetric provider in accordance with the clinical situation (Lemos, Amorim, de Souza, Cabral Filho, & Correia, 2015) (Fig. 16.14). The second stage may last as little as 20 minutes for some women who have given birth before or may last for hours for a subset of women who are giving birth for the first time. Some obstetric providers limit the time a woman may push before initiating a surgical intervention, whereas others base the decision on the woman's preference and the clinical situation.

Cardinal Movements of Labor

As the fetus descends, it rotates so that the orientation of the head in relation to the mother's pelvis is optimal for delivery. These movements are called the cardinal movements of labor (see Box 11.4 and Fig. 11.4).

- **Engagement.** The fetal head reaches the level of the ischial spines of the pelvis, typically at station 0, which may occur prior to labor or in early labor.
- Descent. The fetus moves past station 0 during the first and second stages of labor. The patient typically first feels the Ferguson reflex when the fetus is at station +1.
- Flexion. The fetal head moves so that the chin touches the chest in response to the resistance of maternal tissues, typically in the first stage. This flexion causes the biparietal diameter to be the widest dimension of the presenting part.
- Internal rotation. The fetal head rotates to align its widest part with the widest part of the pelvis through which it is passing at any given point, which at the pelvic *inlet* is lateral but at the pelvic *outlet* is anterior to posterior. This rotation occurs primarily in the second stage.
- Extension. The fetal chin comes off the chest as the maternal tissue is no longer pushing down on the head, and the neck arches as the head is born. At this point the pubic symphysis of the mother is located behind the fetal neck if the fetus is in an occiput-anterior position (Fig. 16.15). This occurs toward the very end of the second stage.
- External rotation (restitution). The fetal head, now born, rotates again as the shoulders move into position to fit through the pelvic outlet (remembering that the broadest dimension of the pelvic outlet is anterior to posterior).
- Expulsion. The body of the fetus is born.

Care

The nurse typically checks the FHR every 5 to 15 minutes in the second stage, depending on the protocols of the institution, the clinical situation, and the obstetric provider preferences. Alternatively, the nurse may assess the FHR after each contraction. The nurse should continue to check the mother's vital signs hourly or according to orders or protocols. The nurse should position the woman for labor according to the woman's preference, as

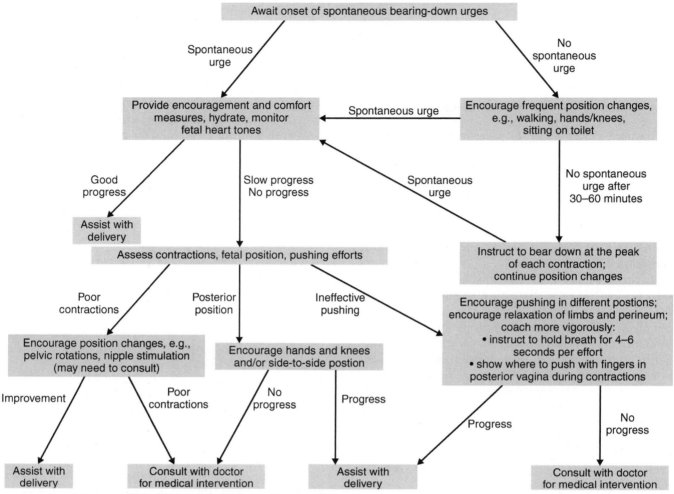

Figure 16.14. Suggested algorithm for the second stage of labor. FHR, fetal heart rate. (Adapted with permission from Cosner, K. R. , & deJong, E. (1993). Physiologic second-stage labor. MCN: The American Journal of Maternal Child Nursing, 18(1), 38–43.)

much as possible, and should help her assume and maintain the position, as an advocate for her choice. Nurses provide support and encouragement and, if the situation warrants it, coaching to push. **Open glottis pushing**, which is pushing without the breath being held, is encouraged because it has a positive impact on fetal oxygenation. The nurse may give the patient sips of water and ice chips, as the patient desires. If the woman passes stool when pushing, which is not uncommon, the nurse should discreetly dispose of it.

In some cases, the obstetric provider performs an episiotomy, which is an incision of the perineum to widen the introitus and thus facilitate delivery. An episiotomy may be cut midline between the introitus and the rectum or mediolateral (Fig. 16.16). A mediolateral incision starts at the same point in the posterior introitus but is cut at a 45-degree angle. Episiotomies are no longer done routinely in the United States because naturally occurring perineal lacerations heal more successfully. Lacerations may be first, second, third, or fourth degree depending on the depth of the extension of the tear (see Fig. 7.2).

In Chapter 7, Hannah had a first-degree laceration. Her midwife, Darla, explained that this designation indicated there was no tearing of the musculature of the perineum.

After the fetal head clears the introitus, the obstetric provider checks the neck for a **nuchal cord**. A nuchal cord is an umbilical cord that is wrapped around the neck of the fetus. In about half of the births in which a nuchal cord occurs, the cord can be easily slipped over the fetus's head and no harm is done to the fetus. This procedure is referred to as "reducing a nuchal cord." After the birth of the head and reduction of the nuchal cord, if present, the obstetric provider may apply gentle pressure to encourage the birth of the anterior shoulder. The provider then may apply pressure in the opposite direction to facilitate delivery of the posterior shoulder and the rest of the body.

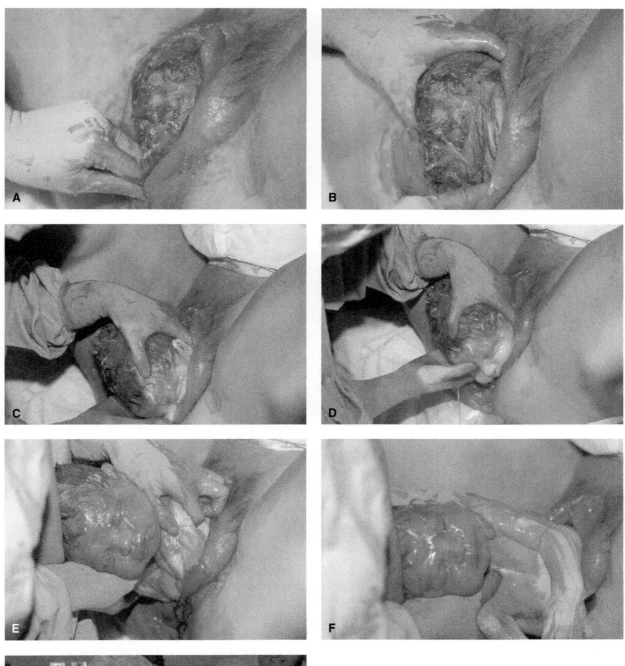

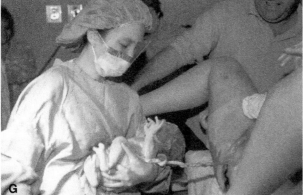

Figure 16.15. **Birth sequence, from crowning through the birth of the newborn. (A)** Early crowning of the fetal head. Notice the bulging of the perineum. **(B)** Late crowning. Notice that the fetal head is appearing face down. This is the normal occiput-anterior position. **(C)** As the head extends, the occiput is to the mother's right side—right occiput-anterior position. **(D)** The cardinal movement of extension. **(E)** The shoulders are born. Notice how the head has turned to line up with the shoulders—the cardinal movement of external rotation. **(F)** The body easily follows the shoulders. **(G)** The newborn is held for the first time. (Photos by B. Proud.)

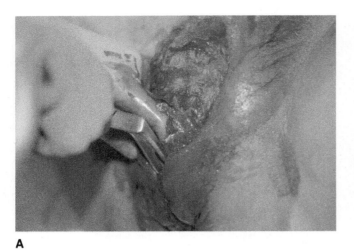
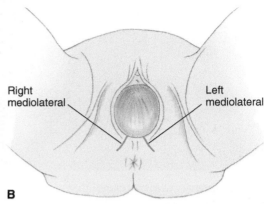

A

B

Figure 16.16. Episiotomy locations. (A) Midline episiotomy. **(B)** Right and left mediolateral episiotomies. (Reprinted with permission from Ricci, S. S. [2009]. *Essentials of maternity, newborn, & women's health nursing* [2nd ed., Fig. 14.14]. Philadelphia, PA: Lippincott Williams & Wilkins.)

Third Stage

The third stage of labor starts when the neonate is born and ends with the birth of the placenta. After the birth of the neonate, the patient's uterus contracts, diminishing the overall surface area of the decidua and the size of the decidua basalis (the area of the decidua underlying the placenta). This causes the placenta to detach in approximately 5 to 30 minutes. The uterus continues to contract, and "pinches" closed the open blood vessels in the decidua to prevent maternal hemorrhage. Failure of the uterus to contract, a condition known as uterine atony, is the primary cause for maternal postpartum hemorrhage.

In Chapter 2, Tatiana was diagnosed with late postpartum hemorrhage (postpartum hemorrhage occurring 24 hours to 12 weeks after the birth) due to uterine atony.

After delivery, the nurse may place the neonate on the mother's abdomen to initiate skin-to-skin contact or under a warmer, if the neonate requires special evaluation and care by nurses and other healthcare providers, such as neonatologists (pediatricians who care only for newborns). The obstetric provider may clamp the cord immediately or after a few minutes, depending on the clinical situation and the preferences of the parents and the obstetric provider (Analyze the Evidence 16.1). The obstetric provider clamps the cord in two places and then cuts it between the two clamps (see Fig. 11.7). Alternatively, if desired, the patient's birthing partner or the patient herself may cut the cord. If cord blood is being collected for banking, the nurse usually collects it at this time, although the nurse may also collect it after delivery of the placenta. Cord blood contains a kind of stem cell that is useful in the treatment of many diseases.

Signs of separation of the placenta from the uterus and its impending delivery include a change of the uterus to a more globular, round form. A rush of bright red blood that quickly slows is also typical, as is a sudden lengthening of the umbilical cord as the placenta detaches from the uterus and moves toward the introitus.

Delivery of the placenta may be active or passive. Active interventions include the use of an uterotonic, such as oxytocin (see The Pharmacy 1.2), early cord clamping, and gentle traction (pulling) on the cord. Passive delivery occurs without intervention. Although active management reduces the amount of blood loss over what is normal for a vaginal birth (500 mL, on average), it significantly increases the risk of afterpains, the use of analgesia, postpartum vomiting, and return to the hospital after discharge due to bleeding (Begley, Gyte, Devane, McGuire, & Weeks, 2015).

Nursing care during this stage includes taking vital signs every 15 minutes and, if necessary, coaching the mother to breathe with contractions. Not all women are aware of having contractions in the third stage and thus may not need this support. If the newborn is stable and with the mother, the nurse may facilitate family interactions, including skin-to-skin contact and breastfeeding according to the preferences of the mother (Fig. 16.17). If the partner is present, the nurse should encourage and facilitate the partner's bonding with the neonate, as well.

When the placenta was born in Chapter 7, Hannah was surprised that she didn't notice it. Darla told her this was not unusual, and John suggested they make smoothies from the placenta.

Fourth Stage

The fourth stage of labor begins with the birth of the placenta and ends after 4 hours or when the mother becomes clinically stable. The nurse should carefully examine the maternal portion

Analyze the Evidence 16.1 Timing of Cord Clamping

Immediate cord clamping (within the first minute)	Delayed cord clamping (after the first minute)
• Lower rate of neonatal jaundice	• Higher birth weight • Higher hemoglobin • Higher iron stores, lower iron deficiency • Possible increased cardiovascular stability • Possible reduction in necrotizing enterocolitis and intraventricular hemorrhage

No difference
- Apgar scoring
- Neonatal intensive care unit admissions
- Maternal postpartum hemorrhage
- Maternal hemoglobin
- Use of uterotonics for uterine atony

Adapted from The American College of Obstetricians and Gynecologists. (2016, December 21). *ACOG recommends delayed umbilical cord clamping for all healthy infants.* Retrieved from https://www.acog.org/About-ACOG/News-Room/News-Releases/2016/Delayed-Umbilical-Cord-Clamping-for-All-Healthy-Infants; Argyridis, S. (2017). Delayed cord clamping. *Obstetrics, Gynaecology & Reproductive Medicine, 27*(11), 352–353; McDonald, S. J., Middleton, P., Dowswell, T., & Morris, P. S. (2013). Effect of timing of umbilical cord clamping of term infants on maternal and neonatal outcomes. *Cochrane Database of Systematic Reviews,* (7), CD004074.

of the placenta (Fig. 1.2). If parts of the placenta remain attached to the decidua, the uterus will fail to contract completely, which significantly increases the risk of postpartum bleeding. At this time, the obstetric provider repairs any lacerations or episiotomies and the nurse administers any uterotonics and analgesics, per orders.

Because uterine atony can lead to postpartum hemorrhage, the nurse must frequently assess the woman's uterine fundus for tone, position, and location. Within an hour after the birth, the fundus should involute to the level of the umbilicus. For each day postpartum, it should descend by approximately one fingerbreadth, or 1 cm (Fig. 16.18). Similarly, the nurse should frequently check the woman's lochia. During the fourth stage

and the first few days postpartum, red lochia, called lochia rubra, is the norm and may include clots. Normal blood loss from a vaginal birth is approximately 500 mL.

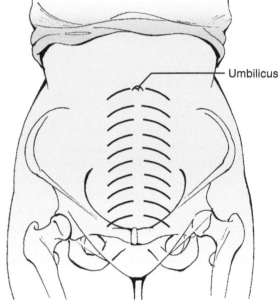

Figure 16.18. Normal uterine involution occurs at a predictable rate. One hour after childbirth, the fundus is at the level of the umbilicus. On the first postpartum day, the fundus is approximately 1 fingerbreadth or 1 cm below the level of the umbilicus. Thereafter, it descends downward at the rate of 1 fingerbreadth per day until it becomes a pelvic organ again on the 10th day postpartum. (Reprinted with permission from Klossner, N. J. [2005]. *Introductory maternity nursing* [1st ed., Fig. 12.1]. Philadelphia, PA: Lippincott Williams & Wilkins.)

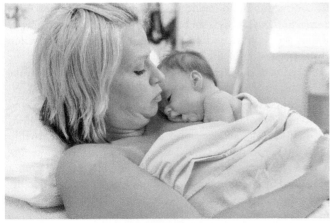

Figure 16.17. Implementation of skin-to-skin contact in the delivery room. (Reprinted with permission from Lippincott's Professional Development Programs, May 2013 release.)

In Chapter 1, Bess experienced early postpartum hemorrhage (postpartum hemorrhage within 24 hours after the birth) immediately after the birth of her son due to uterine atony.

The nurse may apply ice packs to the patient's perineum as tolerated, although this practice is not universally soothing and some women may find it uncomfortable. After the provider has made necessary repairs to the perineum, the nurse should monitor it for unusual swelling, which may suggest a growing hematoma. The nurse should also assess the patient's bladder function and assist the patient in using the bathroom. The nurse should assist a woman who is catheterized, such as for a spinal or epidural, to the bathroom successfully prior to removing the catheter.

In Chapter 11, Edie developed a vulvar hematoma after sustaining a grade 4 laceration to her perineum. In her case, watchful waiting with the use of serial ultrasounds was prescribed.

Fetal Monitoring

Fetal monitoring is the assessment of the FHR for patterns that may indicate fetal compromise. A normal pattern (often called reassuring) is associated with positive outcomes for the neonate. Abnormal patterns (often called nonreassuring) are associated with hypoxemia (low oxygen) of the fetus that may lead to fetal hypoxia. Hypoxia indicates that the low oxygen levels have caused inadequate oxygenation of the fetus at a cellular level, resulting in metabolic acidosis from disproportionately high levels of carbon dioxide in relation to oxygen.

Although continuous electronic fetal monitoring is not recommended for routine, low-risk pregnancies and deliveries, it is still used routinely for women who deliver in a hospital setting. Continuous electronic fetal monitoring does not reduce the risk of cerebral palsy or perinatal mortality, as is often thought. It may reduce the rate of neonatal seizures that do not appear to have long-term implications and is well documented to increase the rate of operative deliveries and intervention-related complications (Alfirevic, Devane, Gyte, & Cuthbert, 2017; Alfirevic, Devane, & Gyte, 2013; "ACOG Practice Bulletin No. 106," 2009; American Academy of Nursing, 2015). Intermittent monitoring, in which the fetus is periodically assessed, should be considered first for low-risk pregnancies and deliveries. However, consistent intermittent monitoring requires one-on-one nursing care, which may not be possible in a given facility.

Types of Fetal Monitoring

Fetal monitoring may be either intermittent or continuous.

Intermittent Fetal Monitoring

Intermittent fetal monitoring is the checking of the FHR at predetermined intervals and as otherwise indicated. There is no proven optimal frequency of monitoring, and different recommended guidelines are used according to the judgment of individual obstetric providers and the policies of birthing venues. Generally, the nurse should auscultate the FHR every 15 to 30 minutes during the active phase of the first stage and every 5 to 15 minutes in the second stage (American Academy of Nursing, 2015). The nurse may monitor the FHR with various devices, including a fetoscope, a Doppler ultrasound device, or a Pinard stethoscope (Fig. 16.19).

Letitia had included in her birth plan a wish for intermittent rather than continuous monitoring. However, Letitia's labor quickly changed as the umbilical cord prolapsed, and she required delivery by emergency cesarean section.

The first step in auscultating a fetal heart is to locate the fetal back, over which the fetal heart is best heard. An experienced nurse can initially assess this location by performing Leopold's maneuvers (see Fig. 1.7). It may still take time to identify the fetal heartbeat, however, and the nurse should reassure patients that he or she is trying to find "the best spot" or "the loudest spot" if this is taking longer than expected and the patient or her support person appears anxious. A bedside ultrasound may be ordered if the heartbeat cannot be located.

If a Doppler ultrasound is being used, the nurse should place ultrasound gel on the abdomen in the most likely spot for auscultation prior to the use of the transducer. To ensure proper placement, the nurse should find the maternal pulse at the same time as auscultation of the FHR so that the two heart rates, the fetal and the maternal, are not confused.

The nurse should also auscultate the FHR in conjunction with palpation of the abdomen for contractions. The nurse should palpate for an entire contraction cycle, noting the intensity of the contraction (mild, moderate, or strong), the duration of the contraction in seconds from beginning to end, and the frequency of contractions in seconds from the beginning of one contraction to the beginning of the next. The nurse should also note the resting tone of the uterus, soft or hard, between the end of one contraction and the beginning of the next.

The nurse typically auscultates the FHR before, during, and for 30 to 60 seconds after a contraction to note the baseline heart rate (Table 16.1), accelerations, and decelerations. The rhythm of the fetal heart may be noted as regular or irregular. Note that variability is assessed visually and not by auscultation and cannot be assessed by intermittent auscultation. Assessment of variability can be done only using electronic fetal monitoring. Careful documentation is important with all assessments and interventions, but particularly with intermittent auscultation because, unlike with continuous monitoring, there is no printed record that can be reviewed retrospectively.

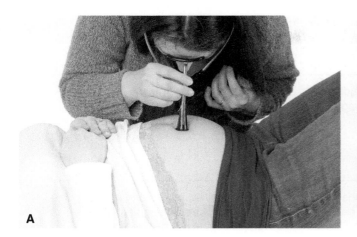

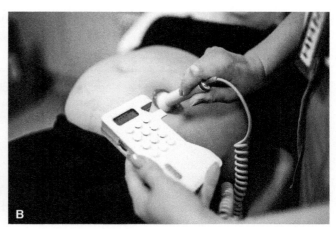

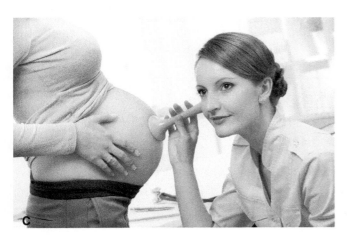

Figure 16.19. Methods of assessing fetal heart rate. (A) Auscultation of the fetal heartbeat using a fetoscope (photo by Beth Van Trees/Shutterstock.com). **(B)** A Doppler ultrasound device can be used to monitor fetal heart rate intermittently in low-risk labor (photo by COLLATERAL/Shutterstock.com). **(C)** A nurse-midwife using a Pinard stethoscope (photo by Capifrutta/Shutterstock.com). (Reprinted with permission from Silbert-Flagg, J., & Pillitteri, A. [2018]. *Maternal and child health nursing: Care of the childbearing and childrearing family* [8th ed., Fig. 15.15]. Philadelphia, PA: Lippincott Williams & Wilkins.)

Continuous Electronic Fetal Monitoring

It is common practice in the United States to monitor uterine contractions and FHR continuously for 20 to 30 minutes at the time of admission. In a majority of laboring women, this monitoring continues throughout labor. With a low-risk labor, nurses review the results of the monitoring approximately every half hour during the active phase of the first stage and every 15 minutes during the second stage. Women deemed higher risk may have their monitoring strips reviewed more frequently, often every 15 minutes in the active phase and every 5 minutes in the second stage.

External Fetal Monitoring

Continuous electronic fetal monitoring is most commonly done externally, with a tocotransducer placed at the fundus of the uterus to detect contractions and an ultrasound transducer placed so as to best detect the FHR. This approach is noninvasive, but may limit the patient's mobility. Wireless monitoring may be available for mothers who wish to ambulate. The ultrasound transducer may need to be adjusted periodically to account for maternal or fetal movement. Although the external tocotransducer is useful for monitoring the frequency and duration of contractions, it cannot detect the strength of the contraction. Contraction strength must still be monitored by abdominal palpation. Both the tocotransducer and the ultrasound transducer are kept in place with soft elastic bands that wrap around the mother's abdomen. The nurse should place the ultrasound transducer atop conductive gel, the same gel used with a Doppler ultrasound or an ultrasound used to visually monitor a pregnancy. The tocotransducer does not require conductive gel. Both the tocotransducer and ultrasound transducer may be less sensitive if the mother is obese.

Internal Fetal Monitoring

Internal fetal monitoring is more accurate because fetal or maternal movement or maternal obesity it is not impacted by. In addition, unlike external monitoring, internal monitoring allows contractions to be assessed for intensity as well as frequency and duration. Although it is more accurate, internal monitoring is also invasive. It can be performed only if membranes are ruptured and the cervix is dilated at least a few centimeters.

During internal fetal monitoring, the FHR is monitored via a small spiral electrode that is attached to the presenting part, usually the scalp. Contractions are monitored with a catheter introduced into the uterus via the vagina (Fig. 16.20). Contractions compress the pressure-sensitive tip of the catheter, which then converts the reading into millimeters of mercury (mm Hg). Montevideo units (MVUs) may be calculated using this pressure: The pressure of the resting uterus is subtracted from the peak pressure of the contractions, and the result is then multiplied by the number of contractions that occur in 10 minutes.

Table 16.1   Components of FHR Monitoring and Their Implications

Characteristic of FHR Monitoring	Implications
Baseline heart rate: The FHR between contractions, not including accelerations or decelerations. Baseline heart rate is an average within a 10-min increment for at least 2 min. • Normal baseline: 110–160 bpm • Tachycardia: >160 bpm • Bradycardia: <110 bpm	• Tachycardia can be an early sign of fetal hypoxemia. • A FHR <80 bpm or >200 bpm is an emergency. • Persistent bradycardia may cause fetal hypoxia.
Variability: The sawtooth, irregular pattern of fluctuations in the baseline heart rate, also assessed over a 10-min period and excluding accelerations and decelerations. Assessment is based on amplitude: the difference between the peak and trough of the FHR in bpm. • Absent: No amplitude • Minimal: Amplitude is ≤5 bpm • Moderate: Amplitude is 6–25 bpm • Marked: Amplitude is >25 bpm	Absent or minimal variability may: • Be caused by fetal sleep or age <32 wk • Indicate supine hypotension, uterine tachysystole, or cord compression • Result from medications
Acceleration: An increase in the FHR from baseline. The change is abrupt, with the increase of bpm peaking in ≤30 s. Return to baseline heart rate is the end of an acceleration. • Before 32 wk of gestation, the acceleration is an increase of ≥10 bpm above baseline lasting ≥10 s but <2 min. • After 32 wk of gestation, the criteria for an acceleration is an increase of ≥15 bpm above baseline lasting ≥15 s but <2 min. • A prolonged acceleration lasts 2–10 min. • An acceleration lasting >10 min is a new baseline heart rate.	Normal pattern

Deceleration: A decrease in the FHR from baseline.
• Early deceleration: A benign change, occurring because of pressure on top of the fetal head. It appears as a decrease in FHR simultaneous with a contraction that returns to baseline FHR with the end of the contraction. The nadir (lowest point) of the FHR typically happens at the same time as the apex (peak) of the contraction. Onset to nadir is ≥30 s.
• Variable deceleration: An abrupt drop in FHR, with the nadir reached in <30 s. The decrease is by ≥15 bpm for 15 s to 2 min. May or may not be linked with contractions. Associated with compression of the cord
• Late deceleration: A deceleration with a nadir occurring after the peak of the contraction. Gradual onset of >30 s to nadir. Caused by poor placental function
• Prolonged deceleration: A decrease in the FHR of ≥15 bpm lasting 2–10 min.
	• Early deceleration: No intervention required
	• Variable deceleration:
	  ○ Change maternal position
	  ○ Notify obstetric provider
	  ○ Discontinue any oxytocin infusion
	  ○ Administer 8–10 L/min of oxygen via a nonrebreather mask
	  ○ Assist with examination for cord prolapse
	  ○ Assist with amnioinfusion, if ordered
	  ○ Assist with birth, if the pattern remains uncorrected
	• Late deceleration:
	  ○ Move the woman to lateral position
	  ○ If hypotensive, elevate legs and increase the IV rate to expand circulating blood volume
	  ○ Stop oxytocin if infusing, and palpate the abdomen for tachysystole
	  ○ Inform the obstetric provider
	  ○ Administer 8–10 L/min of oxygen via a non rebreather mask
	  ○ Assist with birth, if the pattern remains uncorrected
	  ○ Consider internal monitoring

Sinusoidal pattern: A regular, smooth, undulating FHR pattern persisting for ≥20 min.	Associated with profound fetal anemia

bpm, beats per minute; FHR, fetal heart rate; IV, intravenous.

Adapted from American Congress of Obstetricians and Gynecologists. (2009). ACOG Practice Bulletin No. 106: Intrapartum fetal heart rate monitoring: Nomenclature, interpretation, and general management principles. *Obstetrics and Gynecology, 114*(1), 192–202.

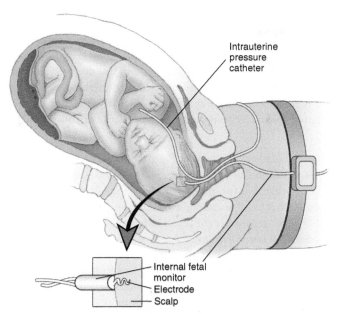

Figure 16.20. **Internal monitoring of fetal heart rate and contractions.** (Reprinted with permission from Lippincott's Nursing Procedures and Skills, 2007.)

For example, if the amplitude of a contraction is 50 mm Hg (the pressure of the resting uterus subtracted from the peak pressure of the contraction) and four contractions occur in 10 minutes, the MVUs would be 200. Decisions about oxytocin titration may be made based on MVUs.

Evaluation of FHR

Monitoring paper is split into a top portion and a bottom portion. Tracings in the top section represent the FHR, and those in the bottom section represent contractions (Fig. 16.21). The information is recorded on the paper from left to right. Each boxed vertical column represents 10 seconds, and every block of six columns represents 1 minute. Note that the pressure (mm Hg) in the bottom contraction section is pertinent only with internal monitoring. With external monitoring, the movement of the line representing contractions can be interpreted only for contraction frequency and duration, not for intensity.

Baseline

The first step in evaluating a FHR is determining the baseline. The baseline is determined over 2 minutes in a 10-minute monitoring

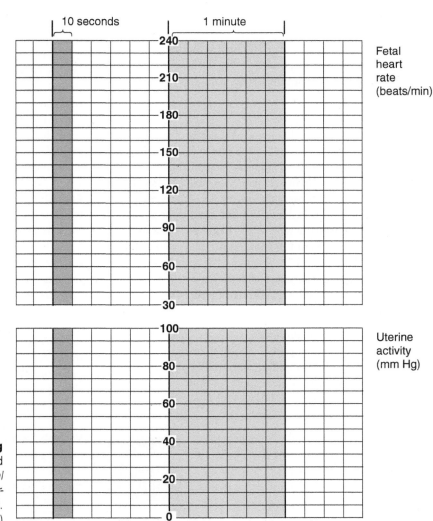

Figure 16.21. **A paper strip for recording electronic fetal monitoring data.** (Reprinted with permission from Pillitteri, A. [2014]. *Maternal and child health nursing: Care of the childbearing and childrearing family* [7th ed., Fig. 15-17]. Philadelphia, PA: Lippincott Williams & Wilkins.)

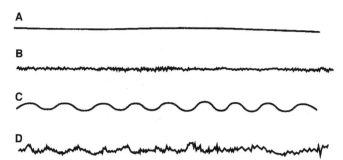

Figure 16.22. Fetal heart rate variability. (A) Short-term variability absent, long-term variability absent—abnormal. **(B)** Short-term variability present, long-term variability absent—abnormal. **(C)** Short-term variability absent, long-term variability present—abnormal. **(D)** Short-term variability present, long-term variability present—normal. (Reprinted with permission from Gibbs, R. S., Karlan, B. Y., Haney, A. F., & Nygaard, I. E. [2008]. *Danforth's obstetrics and gynecology* [10th ed., Fig. 10-2]. Philadelphia, PA: Lippincott Williams & Wilkins.)

strip. The 2 minutes do not need to be consecutive but must occur when there are no accelerations or decelerations or marked variability. The baseline heart rate is rounded to the nearest 5 beats per minute (bpm). If the baseline heart rate ranges from 130 to 140 (an amplitude of 10) bpm, the baseline heart rate is reported as 135 bpm. The normal heart rate for a fetus at term is 110 to 160 bpm. A FHR over 160 bpm indicates tachycardia and below 110 bpm indicates bradycardia. The baseline heart rate should be reevaluated each time a strip is interpreted.

Variability

Variability, or baseline variability, refers to the degree of fluctuation in the baseline heart rate. As with the baseline heart rate, accelerations and decelerations are not considered when assessing variability. Although baseline heart rate is assessed over 2 minutes, variability is assessed over 1 minute. The difference between the lowest point of the baseline heart rate (the trough) and the highest point (the peak) is the amplitude and determines the degree of variability. For example, a baseline heart rate that ranges from 130 to 140 bpm over 1 minute would have an amplitude of 10 bpm (Fig. 16.22). A sinusoidal pattern is a rare, regular, undulating FHR pattern associated with fetal anemia (Fig. 16.23).

The degree of variability is indicated by the size of the amplitude, as follows:

- Absent variability: no amplitude
- Minimal variability: amplitude of 5 bpm or less
- Moderate variability: amplitude of 6 to 25 bpm
- Marked variability: amplitude above 25 bpm

In Chapter 4, Maria, a midwife, explained to Sophie that the FHR was showing moderate variability. She described variability as the sawtooth pattern seen on the monitor that reflects the FHR going up and down.

Episodic and Periodic Changes

Episodic changes are accelerations and decelerations that do not occur regularly in conjunction with contractions. Periodic changes are accelerations, early decelerations, and late decelerations that occur regularly in relation to contractions. Variable decelerations are defined by their abrupt change from baseline, not by their relation to contractions, and may be periodic or episodic.

Accelerations

An acceleration is a rise in the FHR from baseline of at least 15 bpm that lasts for more than 15 seconds. In fetuses younger than 32 weeks of gestation, a rise in heart rate by 10 bpm for 10 or more seconds is considered an acceleration. A prolonged acceleration is one that lasts for 2 to 10 minutes. An acceleration that lasts for longer than 10 minutes is considered a change in baseline. Accelerations are reassuring and suggest that the fetus is well oxygenated. The absence of accelerations, however, is not a reliable predictor of fetal compromise. They often occur in conjunction with fetal activity and require no intervention. An acceleration of 20 bpm or more for less than 20 seconds that comes before or after a deceleration is a "shoulder" and is a compensatory response to hypoxemia.

Decelerations

A deceleration is a decrease in FHR below the baseline that lasts for less than 10 minutes. A deceleration lasting for 10 minutes or more is a change in baseline. Decelerations are classified according to timing in relation to contractions, shape, and duration. Decelerations may be benign depending on timing and frequency. Intermittent periodic decelerations occur in conjunction with fewer than half of contractions over a 20-minute period. Recurrent periodic decelerations occur in conjunction with half or more of contractions and are more concerning (Fig. 16.24).

Early Decelerations. Early decelerations are typically symmetric, which means that the FHR returns to baseline in approximately the same amount of time it took to reach its nadir (the point of lowest bpm of the deceleration). When differentiating between an early deceleration and a late deceleration, it is critical to consider the location of the nadir. The nadir of an early deceleration lines up with the peak, or apex, of the contraction. In other words, when the contraction is at its strongest, the FHR is at its slowest.

Early decelerations are benign and occur because of pressure on the top of the fetal head stimulating the vagus nerve. Pressure on the top of the head of an older human has a similar effect on the pulse rate. No interventions are required. As with any significant change appearing on a fetal monitoring strip, early decelerations should be documented (Fig. 16.25).

Variable Decelerations. Variable decelerations may be episodic, meaning that they happen at random times and not in conjunction with a contraction, or periodic, meaning that they happen in conjunction with a contraction. Acceleration "shoulders" are part of the classic variable deceleration and occur on either side of the variable deceleration. A shoulder acceleration is an increase of the

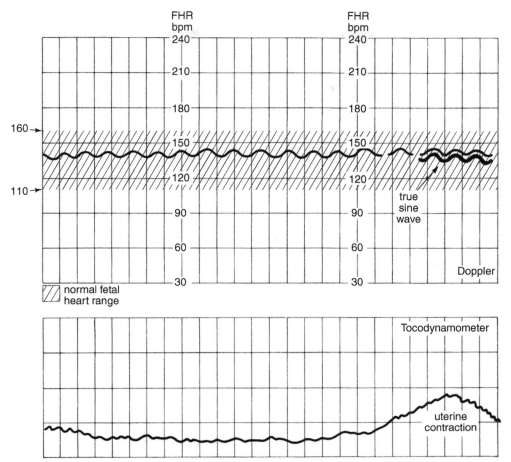

Figure 16.23. **FHR pattern characteristic: Sinusoidal, associated with fetal anemia.** FHR, fetal heart rate. (Reprinted with permission from Cabaniss, M. L., & Ross, M. G. [2009]. *Fetal monitoring interpretation* [2nd ed., Fig. 3.3]. Philadelphia, PA: Lippincott Williams & Wilkins.)

FHR by 20 bpm or more for less than 20 seconds. The mark of a variable contraction is a quick decrease in FHR of 15 bpm or less that lasts for 15 seconds to 2 minutes (Fig. 16.26). Variable decelerations often are alarming because of their precipitous drop and descent to lower FHRs than other types of decelerations. Occasional variable decelerations are not concerning clinically, and the depth of a variable deceleration has not been correlated with negative fetal outcomes. The shape of the tracing of a variable deceleration is often a U or V but may also be a W.

Variable decelerations are associated with abrupt disruption in blood flow, as with compression of the cord. Variable decelerations are thus most common during the transition phase of the first and second stages of labor, when there is a greater likelihood of cord compression and/or traction.

Late Decelerations. A deceleration is deemed late if the nadir of deceleration occurs after the peak of the contraction. The shape of the tracing of a late deceleration is similar to that of an early deceleration, with a gradual decrease from and return to baseline (Fig. 16.27). Late decelerations indicate a disruption in the transfer of oxygen to the fetus, which is exacerbated at the time of the contraction. A pregnancy with good oxygen reserves is not likely to experience a deceleration at the time of

a contraction, when oxygen from the mother's circulation to the placenta is temporarily decreased. Conditions that cause a decrease in this baseline oxygenation, however, can result in late decelerations. Examples of conditions associated with this lower baseline oxygen perfusion include placental insufficiency, uterine tachysystole, maternal cardiac disease, and postterm pregnancy, among others. Late decelerations may be transient and reversible with intervention (Table 16.2). Late decelerations are particularly concerning when seen with decreased or absent variability.

Prolonged Decelerations. A prolonged deceleration is a decrease in FHR of 15 bpm or more below the baseline for more than 2 minutes but less than 10 minutes (Fig. 16.28). A decrease of the FHR for more than 10 minutes would be classified as a change in baseline heart rate. Unlike with other types of decelerations, the shape of the tracing of a prolonged deceleration is not important. The identification of a prolonged deceleration is made by evaluation of the duration. Unlike with variable decelerations, the depth of a prolonged deceleration is thought to reflect the significance of the hypoxia, as is the duration of the prolonged deceleration. As with late decelerations and variable decelerations, the addition of diminished or lost variability to a prolonged deceleration increases concern.

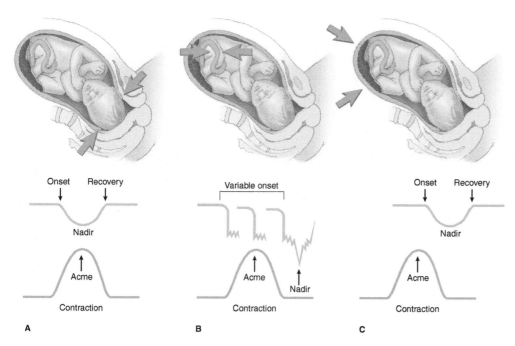

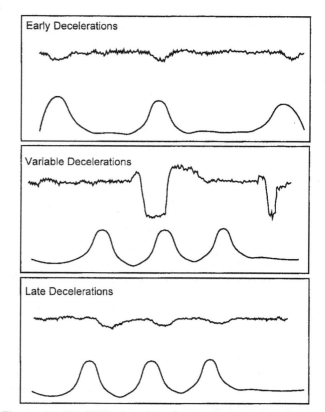

Figure 16.24. Fetal heart rate decelerations. (A) Early deceleration. **(B)** Variable deceleration. **(C)** Late deceleration. (Reprinted with permission from Evans, R. J., Brown, Y. M., & Evans, M. K. [2014]. *Canadian maternity, newborn, and women's health nursing* [2nd ed., Fig. 15.16]. Philadelphia, PA: Lippincott Williams & Wilkins.)

Care and Management

Types and Frequency of FHR Tracings

The aspects of a fetal tracing that must be evaluated are baseline FHR, variability of the FHR, accelerations, decelerations, and changes over time, such as changes in baseline, variability, or the nature or frequency of accelerations or decelerations. In low-risk pregnancies, review of these tracings occurs every half hour in the first stage of labor and every 15 minutes in the second stage of labor ("ACOG Practice Bulletin No. 106," 2009).

Categories of Abnormal FHR Patterns

FHR patterns are grouped into three broad categories (Box 16.2). Category I includes patterns not associated with fetal hypoxia, as measured by a postpartum evaluation of acid-base balance. Category III includes patterns that are associated with fetal hypoxia, and Category II includes indeterminate patterns that bear further observation and evaluation but may or may not require intervention, as determined by the obstetric provider.

It was explained to Rebecca and Russ in Chapter 6 that a category II pattern means, "We don't know for sure that the baby is in trouble, but we're also not sure it's not in trouble." They also learned that a category III tracing indicates there's a high chance of fetal distress.

Conditions Associated With Abnormal FHR Patterns

Fetal Hypoxia

Interventions aimed to correct fetal hypoxia, or low oxygenation, and thus concerning FHR patterns are often referred to as **intrauterine resuscitation**. Although the term implies

Figure 16.25. FHR decelerations relative to maternal contraction. The top section of each graph represents the FHR; the bottom section of each graph represents uterine contractions. The top graph indicates an early deceleration that is concurrent with the uterine contraction. The middle graph demonstrates variable fetal heart decelerations that are due to umbilical cord compression. The bottom graph indicates a late deceleration that occurs after the uterine contraction. FHR, fetal heart rate. (Reprinted with permission from Stephenson, S. R. [2015]. *Obstetrics and gynecology* [3rd ed., Fig. 25.7]. Philadelphia, PA: Lippincott Williams & Wilkins.)

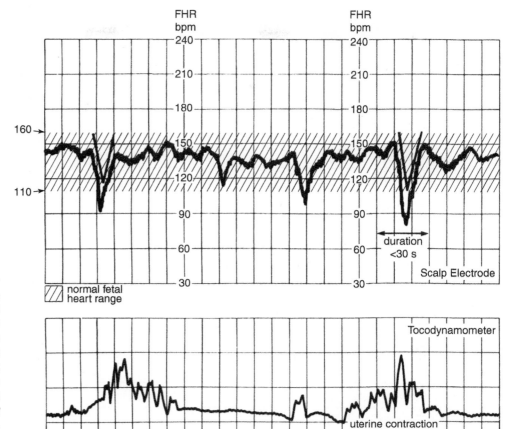

Figure 16.26. FHR pattern characteristic: Variable decelerations, V-shaped. Note that the fetal heart monitoring in this case is with a scalp electrode, which may be used when external monitoring is insufficient. bpm, beats per minute; FHR, fetal heart rate. (Reprinted with permission from Cabaniss, M. L., & Ross, M. G. [2009]. *Fetal monitoring interpretation* [2nd ed., Fig. 2.122]. Philadelphia, PA: Lippincott Williams & Wilkins.)

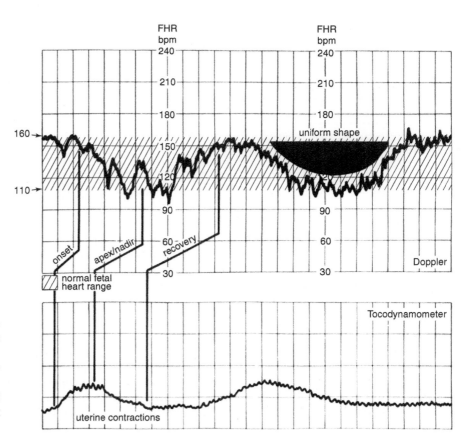

Figure 16.27. FHR pattern characteristic: Late decelerations with moderate variability. bpm, beats per minute; FHR, fetal heart rate. (Reprinted with permission from Cabaniss, M. L., & Ross, M. G. [2009]. *Fetal monitoring interpretation* [2nd ed., Fig. 2.82]. Philadelphia, PA: Lippincott Williams & Wilkins.)

Table 16.2   Causes of Fetal Heart Rate Pattern Changes

Cause	Heart Rate		Variability		Deceleration		
	Fast	Slow	Absent	Minimal	Variable	Late	Prolonged
Maternal Causes							
Maternal fever	X						
Infection	X						
Dehydration	X	X					
Anxiety	X						
Tachysystole			X	X		X	X
Hypotension		X				X	X
Anemia	X					X	
Medications or drugs	X		X	X		X	
Supine position		X	X	X		X	
Fetal Causes							
Infection	X						
Activity	X						
Placental insufficiency			X	X		X	
Chronic hypoxemia	X						
Prematurity			X	X			
Stimulation	X						
Vagal stimulation							X
Abnormal heart rhythm	X						
Placental problems						X	X
Anemia	X						
Cardiac abnormalities	X						
Cord compression			X	X	X		X
Sleep			X	X			

direct action in the fetus in the uterus, the interventions are actually directed at the laboring woman to the benefit of the fetus. Common interventions include a change in maternal position, typically to a lateral side-lying position, oxygen administration, and IV hydration (Table 16.3). Additionally, in the case of maternal hypotension, a medication such as epinephrine may be ordered by the obstetric provider and administered by the nurse.

Uterine tachysystole is defined as either five or more or six or more contractions every 10 minutes for a half hour. Uterine tachysystole may happen with oxytocin augmentation of labor or spontaneously (Ahmed et al., 2016). If it occurs with oxytocin and results in FHR abnormalities, the oxytocin may be reduced

or discontinued. Tocolytics that relax the uterus may also be prescribed by an obstetric provider and administered by a nurse.

In the second stage of labor, abnormal FHR tracings may require different nursing interventions. Open glottis pushing provides better oxygenation for the mother and the fetus and therefore should be encouraged. The nurse may advise the laboring woman to push for a shorter duration or to not push with every contraction. The nurse may also advise women to allow for passive descent, to push only when they feel the urge to do so, and to maintain a position other than lithotomy if supine hypotension is suspected.

Further evaluation beyond that of the FHR tracing may also be warranted. Stimulation of the fetal scalp through the cervix

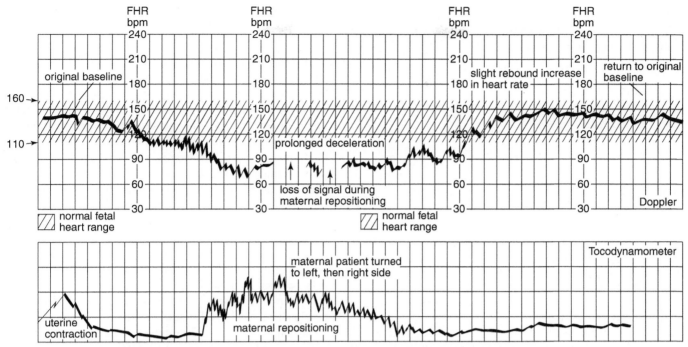

Figure 16.28. FHR pattern characteristic: Prolonged deceleration after epidural anesthesia. bpm, beats per minute; FHR, fetal heart rate. (Reprinted with permission from Cabaniss, M. L., & Ross, M. G. [2009]. *Fetal monitoring interpretation* [2nd ed., Fig. 2.162]. Philadelphia, PA: Lippincott Williams & Wilkins.)

with a gloved finger or vibroacoustic stimulation through the uterine wall at the level of the fetal head for 1 to 5 seconds may produce an acceleration of the FHR. An acceleration (a rise of at least 15 bpm for at least 15 seconds) is reassuring of fetal oxygen status, although a lack of an acceleration is not diagnostic of fetal compromise. Stimulation should be applied only when the heart rate is at baseline and should not be done in the case of bradycardia.

Acidemia

The fetal acid-base balance is often assessed after the birth as a supplementary evaluation to Apgar scoring to evaluate neonatal well-being. The assessment is performed on cord blood, as ordered by the obstetric provider. Blood obtained from the umbilical artery reflects fetal usage of oxygen, whereas blood from the umbilical vein reflects oxygen available to the fetus. Laboratory tests ordered for this evaluation include pH, P_{CO_2}, P_{O_2}, and base excess. Optimally, the arterial pH should be from 7.2 to 7.3 and the venous pH should be from 7.3 to 7.4. The base deficit for both should be below 12. If acidemia is diagnosed, the type (metabolic, respiratory, or mixed) is determined by further analysis of the blood gasses (P_{CO_2} and P_{O_2}); respiratory acidemia has a base deficit below 12, whereas metabolic and mixed acidemia have a base deficit at or above 12.

Low Volume of Amniotic Fluid

Although rupture of the amniotic sac is a normal part of labor, the absence of amniotic fluid can sometimes contribute to the compression of the cord between the fetus and the walls of the uterus. This compression occludes the flow of blood between the placenta and the fetus and may be identified by the presence of variable decelerations. In some cases, the obstetric provider may decide to artificially expand the volume of amniotic fluid by instilling Ringer's lactate or normal saline into the amniotic sac (Hofmeyr & Lawrie, 2012).

In this procedure, the fluid is instilled through a catheter by gravity flow or an infusion pump. The typical volume instilled is 100 to 1,000 mL. Common practice is to start the infusion at 10 to 16 mL/min, although practice varies by obstetric provider and birthing venue. Fluid may be instilled at room temperature or it may be warmed first. The nurse should continually monitor contractions throughout instillation, as well as uterine tone via a uterine pressure catheter. The resting tone during the procedure should not exceed 15 mm Hg, as measured with an internal pressure catheter. The volume of fluid instilled as well as that of fluid returned should be documented.

Pain and Discomfort of Labor and Delivery

Pain threshold is the point at which people interpret a sensation as pain, and pain tolerance is the degree of pain that a patient is able to bear. In labor and delivery, as at all other times, pain is what the patient says it is. Many different factors can play into pain tolerance. The presence of a supportive, knowledgeable, reassuring team can contribute positively to a woman's pain tolerance, whereas negative or sporadic support can do the opposite. Stress, anxiety, and fatigue can all increase the perception of pain, as can fear and uncertainty. Previous experience of pain, long term or short term, can also impact pain tolerance.

Box 16.2 Continuous Electronic FHR Monitoring Categories

Category I

Includes *all* of the following:

- Baseline fetal heart rate (FHR) of 110–160 bpm
- Moderate variability
- With or without accelerations
- With or without early decelerations
- No variable decelerations
- No late decelerations

Category II

Includes any tracing that is not a Category I or Category III and may include *any* of the following:

- Bradycardia with variability
- Tachycardia
- Minimal variability
- Absent variability without recurrent decelerations
- Marked variability
- Absence of accelerations with fetal scalp stimulation
- Recurrent variable decelerations with minimal or moderate variability
- Prolonged deceleration
- Recurrent late decelerations with moderate variability

Category III

Includes *any* of the following:

- Absent variability with recurrent late decelerations
- Absent variability with recurrent variable decelerations
- Absent variability and bradycardia
- Sinusoidal pattern

Adapted from American Congress of Obstetricians and Gynecologists. (2009). ACOG Practice Bulletin No. 106: Intrapartum fetal heart rate monitoring: Nomenclature, interpretation, and general management principles. *Obstetrics and Gynecology, 114*(1), 192–202.

How women manifest pain tolerance may vary. In some Asian and Native American cultures, women are expected to bear pain stoically without vocalization. The nurse should not interpret this silence as a lack of pain. Other cultures may encourage women to vocalize during labor. Conversely, the nurse should not interpret this vocalization as a sign of lower pain tolerance. Women who are prepared for childbirth through methods such as Lamaze, Hypnobirthing, and Birthing from Within may report a significantly higher pain tolerance than those who are not (Chaillet et al., 2014).

The pain of labor is both visceral and somatic. Visceral pain comes from actual or threatened injury to internal organs, whereas somatic pain arises from actual or threatened insult to muscle, ligaments, tendons, skin, and bone. Visceral pain in labor comes not only from mechanical pressure but also from ischemia (reduced oxygen perfusion) of the uterus during contractions. Visceral pain tends to be generalized, whereas the location of somatic pain can be pinpointed. Pain may also be referred to other parts of the body, such as the hips, back, and thighs.

Manifestation of Pain

First Stage

In the first stage of labor, the sensations of pain and discomfort are typically experienced as wrapping around the lower maternal torso like a broad belt and are most acute in the lower middle abdomen and the lower back. These sensations result from ischemia to the uterine muscle during a contraction and from the dilation and effacement of the cervix. This pain is visceral because it originates in an internal organ. The woman may also experience referred pain, meaning that the pain originates in the uterus but may be felt in the thighs, buttocks, back, or iliac crests. In general, pain subsides completely between contractions. An exception is when a fetus is in the "sunny side" up or occiput-posterior position, in which the fetus faces the mother's front. In this case, lower back pain may persist between contractions as the fetal head pushes against the maternal sacrum. Continuous abdominal pain between contractions would be concerning for placental abruption. The sensations of contraction pain and discomfort build and then ebb, and simple visualization exercises, such as visualizing walking up and running down a mountain or waves coming in and going out, may be helpful metaphors that aid in coping for some women.

Second Stage and Beyond

In the second stage of labor, the discomfort resulting from ischemia is still present, but much of the focus and location of sensation is on the perineum as the fetus progresses down through the now open cervix, to the introitus, and out of the vagina. There is a sensation of acute stretching, pulling, and even tearing as maternal tissue yields. Some women may find that bearing down lessens the intensity of the pain. The third stage of labor and the afterpains of the fourth stage and beyond include visceral pain of a quality similar to that of the first stage of labor, although the degree of pain felt in these final two stages is rarely as acute as that of the first or second stages.

Management

Pharmacologic Management

Most women elect to receive medication to manage the discomfort and pain of labor and delivery. Optimally, a woman will make this decision in consultation with an obstetric provider prior to labor, although she may make it at any time. Women may receive an analgesic, which provides pain relief, or anesthesia, which blocks all sensation, or both. Medications to manage pain and discomfort are generally not provided until labor is established. As with the administration of any pain medication, the nurse should use a pain scale to assess the woman's pain level prior to and after administration.

Parenteral Medications

Opioids are a type of analgesia used during labor and may be administered intramuscularly or IV alone or in combination with other medications. Parenteral opioids in childbirth

Table 16.3 Nursing Actions for Fetal Heart Pattern Changes

Nursing Action	Heart Rate		Variability		Deceleration		
	Fast	Slow	Absent	Minimal	Variable	Late	Prolonged
Inform the obstetric provider	X	X	X	X	X	X	X
Prepare for delivery	X	X	X	X	X	X	X
Perform or assist with amnioinfusion*					X	X	X
Assist with artificial rupture of membranes*			X	X			
Verify monitor placement		X					
Simulate the fetal scalp*		X	X	X	X		X
Perform or assist with vaginal or speculum examination		X			X	X	X
Medicate as ordered	X				X	X	X
Maintain maternal hydration	X	X	X	X		X	X
Assess maternal vital signs	X	X					
Turn the woman to a side-lying position	X	X	X	X	X	X	X
Stop oxytocin infusion	X	X	X	X	X	X	X
Administer oxygen	X	X	X	X	X	X	X
Increase intravenous fluids	X	X	X	X		X	X

*Interventions
- Amnioinfusion: Infusion of lactated Ringer's solution or normal saline into the uterus after rupture of membranes via a catheter inserted through the cervix to relieve cord compression. Infusion may be by pump or gravity. Fluid is commonly warmed prior to instillation.
- Artificial rupture of membranes: Rupture of fetal membranes through the cervix using a tool
- Fetal scalp stimulation: A gentle digital pressure or pinch on the fetal scalp. A fetal heart rate acceleration of 15 beats per minute for 15 seconds is reassuring. Alternatively, in some cases, noninvasive vibroacoustic stimulation may be done.

do not eliminate sensation but rather dull pain. They also induce a somnolence that may cause a woman to appear to sleep between contractions. Medications introduced into the maternal bloodstream do pass the placenta to the fetus; consequently, the neonate may have depressed respirations at and immediately after the birth. The Pharmacy 16.1 summarizes some commonly used analgesics and adjunct medications.

In Chapter 7, Hannah had nalbuphine IV for pain management. She was somnolent between contractions, waking up at their apex confused.

Neuraxial Analgesia and Anesthesia

In 2008, the most recent year the Centers for Disease Control has reported data, 61% of women in the United States who had vaginal births did so with the assistance of neuraxial analgesia (Osterman & Martin, 2011). Neuraxial drug administration is the delivery of medication to an area in close proximity to the spinal cord and nerve roots and includes the epidural and intrathecal routes of drug administration. Epidural administration is the delivery of medication to the epidural space, which is the space between the inside of the vertebral column and the dura mater, which is the outer membrane that surrounds the brain and spinal cord. Intrathecal or spinal administration is the delivery of medication to the subarachnoid space, which is the space filled with cerebrospinal fluid that immediately surrounds the spinal cord.

Because of their ability to deliver medication so close to the spinal cord and nerve roots, which transmit pain, and thus to rapidly and effectively relieve or block pain, the epidural and spinal routes of administration are commonly used during labor (see Box 4.16). The use of both of these routes together to administer pain medication is known as combined spinal-epidural (CSE) administration. Epidurals, spinals, and CSEs may be used to deliver analgesic (pain-relieving) medications, anesthetic (pain-blocking) medications, or a combination of the two. Medications used include opioid analgesics such as fentanyl and anesthetics such as bupivacaine.

Epidurals, spinals, and CSEs relieve or block pain in a specific region of the body, such as the pelvis, and so are known as a

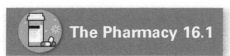

The Pharmacy 16.1   Opioids, Mixed Opioid Agonist/Antagonists, and Adjunct Medications for Nausea

Medication	Route and Dosing	Onset	Notes
Opioids			
Meperidine (Demerol)	50–100 mg IM 25–50 mg IV	40 min IM 5 min IV	• Single dose lasts 3–4 h • Neonate respiratory depression is most common if the birth is within 4 h after dosing. • Monitor for maternal respiratory and CNS depression
Sublimaze (Fentanyl)	100 µg IM 25–50 µg IV	7–10 min IM 1–3 min IV	• Short acting • IV dose lasts 30–60 min, IM dose lasts 1–2 h • Crosses the placenta • Monitor for maternal and fetal CNS depression, FHR changes • May cause maternal and neonatal respiratory depression • Maternal nausea, vomiting, and pruritus are common.
Mixed Opioid Agonist/Antagonists			
Nalbuphine (Nubain)	10–20 mg IM 10–20 mg IV	10–15 min IM 2–3 min IV	• Single dose lasts 3–6 h • Less risk for respiratory depression than with opioids • Should not be used in women dependent on opioids or may cause withdrawal • Less nausea and vomiting than with opioids
Butorphanol (Stadol)	1–2 mg IV or IM	10–15 min IM 5–10 min IV	• Single dose lasts 3–4 h • Less risk for respiratory depression than with opioids • CNS sedation similar to that for opioids • Should not be used in women dependent on opioids or may cause withdrawal • Dysphoria is common.
Pentazocine (Talwin)	20–40 mg IV or IM	5–20 min IM 2–3 min IV	• Single dose lasts 2–3 h • Less risk for respiratory depression than with opioids • Should not be used in women dependent on opioids or may cause withdrawal • Dysphoria is common.
Adjunct Medications for Nausea			
Promethazine (Phenergan)	25–75 mg IV or IM	10–20 min	• Antiemetic often used with opioids • Single dose lasts 3–4 h • Monitor for hypotension
Hydroxyzine (Vistaril)	25–50 mg IM	30 min	• Antiemetic often used with opioids • Single dose lasts 3 h • IM only, no IV dosing

CNS, central nervous system; FHR, fetal heart rate; IM, intramuscular; IV, intravenous.

type of regional analgesia or anesthesia. Neuraxial analgesia is commonly used for both vaginal and cesarean deliveries, but on occasion, general anesthesia may be required in cesarean deliveries, particularly in cases when rapid sedation is required or anesthesia by neuraxial methods cannot be sufficiently induced in a timely fashion. Epidurals and CSEs are by far the most popular pharmacologic interventions for labor pain. The most significant difference between the two methods is that the onset of relief following administration occurs approximately 5 minutes sooner with CSEs than with epidurals (Simmons, Taghizadeh, Dennis, Hughes, & Cyna, 2012). Relief provided and birth outcomes are comparable, although

the rates of maternal pruritus and fetal bradycardia are higher with a CSE than with an epidural (see Patient Teaching 2.4) (Simmons et al., 2012). Both may be placed at any point in labor, although some women may prefer to have them placed closer to the time of birth to shorten the period of time during which they may have impaired mobility.

Although nurses do not manage neuraxial analgesia or anesthesia, they do monitor it and have responsibilities prior to initiation and after administration. An anesthesiologist or nurse anesthetist is responsible for placing and managing the analgesia or anesthesia. Prior to administration, the anesthesiology provider or nurse follows certain steps to prepare for the procedure (Table 16.4).

Table 16.4 Procedures Prior to Neuraxial Analgesia

Action	Notes
Assess the patient's pain level.	There is no "right" amount of pain at which to start anesthesia in pregnancy. A pain assessment allows for the establishment of a baseline.
Assess the knowledge level of the patient and support person and provide teaching as needed.	The anesthesia provider or nurse may educate the patient and support person about options, side effects, and risks. Optimally, this education will be done prior to labor so that informed decisions may be made before the duress of labor.
Assess baseline vital signs.	A common side effect of neuraxial analgesia is maternal hypotension, which can cause a reduction in the perfusion of the placenta. It is important to establish a baseline blood pressure so that a rapid reduction may be noted. It is also not uncommon for women to experience a rise in temperature with neuraxial analgesia.
Examine the FHR.	Women who are starting neuraxial analgesia should always have continuous fetal monitoring in place. Because of the potential for maternal hypotension, it is important to also know the fetus' baseline.
Have the patient void prior to administration.	Because of reduced motor function, urine retention is common and may impair fetal descent because of a distended bladder. Catheterization is common.
Administer an IV bolus of IV fluid.	It is common practice to preload a laboring woman with a bolus of IV fluid prior to the administration of neuraxial analgesia to counteract the hypotension common to this method (see Box 4.17).
Collect blood for laboratory tests.	Low platelet levels are a contraindication to receiving neuraxial analgesia, and a platelet count may be ordered prior to administration. Similarly, blood type and Rh status may be verified if there is a high risk for hemorrhage.
Perform preprocedure verifications.	This varies by institution and is a process of verifying safety parameters including the correct patient, medication, method, timing, and patient consent.

FHR, fetal heart rate; IV, intravenous.

Adapted from Association of Women's Health, Obstetric and Neonatal Nurses. (2011). *Nursing care of the woman receiving regional analgesia/ anesthesia in labor* (2nd ed.). Washington, DC: Author.

For placement of neuraxial analgesia or anesthesia, a woman should either be in a lateral side-lying position or sitting. With either position, the woman should arch her torso forward over her abdomen to allow for separation of the vertebrae (see Fig. 6.6A), where the anesthesia provider will be inserting a needle or catheter for administration of the medication or medications. Monitoring of the patient and fetus by the nurse after administration is critical and is described in Table 16.5.

When Sophie got an epidural in Chapter 4, the nurse, Fiona, was careful to move her to a side-lying position and to frequently check her blood pressure immediately afterward. Fiona also kept a close eye on the fetal monitoring strip.

Pudendal Block

A pudendal block is a form of local anesthesia that provides numbing to a small area. A pudendal block involves the injection of a local anesthetic into the pudendal nerve, thus numbing the perineum (Fig. 16.29). A pudendal block may be used during operative vaginal births, for episiotomies, and for repairs after the birth, such as repair of lacerations.

Nitrous Oxide

Nitrous oxide, a gas mixed with oxygen that is administered by the patient, is becoming more popular as an analgesic for labor pain in the United States..

Nitrous oxide is a self-administered analgesic gas that, in childbirth, is typically delivered in a 50/50 mix with oxygen (Fig. 16.30). It has been used as analgesia since the middle of the 19th century. Although the use of nitrous oxide has been out of regular use for laboring women in the United States for many years, it is once again becoming popular here and has always been commonly used in Europe and Canada.

Nitrous oxide is short acting, with an onset approximately 15 to 30 seconds after it is started, a peak at about a minute, and a resolution of effects about a minute after use has ceased. Although it does not eliminate pain, it does help increase the pain threshold. Because it is self-administered, women may use it as they feel necessary. For best effect, the nurse should instruct the patient to start inhaling the gas 15 to 30 seconds before a contraction is expected to start or, in the case of irregular contractions, as soon as the contraction starts. This prevents the woman from having to breathe the gas between contractions. The side effects are a temporary deepening of the voice, possible nausea and vomiting, a sensation of vertigo or lightheadedness, and giddiness. It is from the giddiness

Table 16.5 Monitoring with Neuraxial Analgesia

Aspect to Monitor or Monitor For	Notes
Maternal and fetal vital signs, every 5–15 min or per protocols	• Approximately 40% of women experience hypotension, defined as a systolic BP of 100 mm Hg or less, or 20% of preanesthesia BP.
Maternal position (maintain lateral or upright position)	• Prevent supine hypotension leading to poor uteroplacental perfusion.
Sedation	• If an opioid is used, approximately half of women experience drowsiness.
Motor function	• If a woman was provided neuraxial analgesia that allows for ambulation, motor blockade needs to be ascertained prior to ambulation to avoid falls.
Pruritus (itching)	• Itching is common with any neuraxial analgesia and is more common with CSEs than epidurals. Medicate per orders.
Nausea and vomiting	• About half of women experience nausea with or without vomiting after neuraxial analgesia, which may be treated per orders with an antiemetic.
Headache	• A small percentage of women will develop a headache because of leakage of spinal fluid, in which case the anesthesia provider should be informed.
Uterine contractions	• Contractions may become less active for up to an hour after placement of neuraxial analgesia. Oxytocin may be given per orders.
Pain	• If pain control is insufficient, adjustments may be necessary by the anesthesia provider.
Rare complication of intravascular injection, or accidental injection into the blood	Requires notification of obstetric and anesthesia provider, oxygen, fluids, medications as ordered. Clinical signs of intravascular injection are: • Tinnitus (ringing in the ears) • Dizziness • Hypertension • Maternal bradycardia or tachycardia • Loss of consciousness • Metallic taste in mouth

BP, blood pressure; CSE, combined spinal-epidural.

Adapted from Association of Women's Health, Obstetric and Neonatal Nurses. (2011). *Nursing care of the woman receiving regional analgesia/anesthesia in labor* (2nd ed.). Washington, DC: Author.

that nitrous oxide gets its familiar name "laughing gas" (Likis et al., 2014).

The United States Food and Drug Administration approved nitrous oxide for use in childbirth in 2011. Since then, the number of hospitals providing the gas has increased from a few across the country to several hundred. No ill effects on the mother are known other than those mentioned above, and nitrous oxide does not impact uterine contractions. Although the fetal concentration of nitrous oxide is 80% of that of the mother, no ill effects on the fetus are known, either, and the gas dissipates quickly, within a minute, after it is no longer breathed. The ability to rapidly discontinue administration also has the advantage of making it easy to switch from nitrous oxide to another method of analgesia if nitrous oxide proves insufficient to control pain and discomfort.

Nitrous oxide is also significantly less expensive than other methods. An epidural may cost thousands of dollars and requires an anesthesiologist, whereas nitrous oxide administration may cost less than $100 and is self-administered under the supervision of the obstetric provider (Likis et al., 2014).

Nonpharmacologic Management

Approximately 17% of women give birth without an epidural, parenteral opioid, nitrous oxide, or general anesthesia (Declercq et al., 2013). Nonpharmacologic strategies to cope with labor pain include focused breathing techniques, cutaneous stimulation, aromatherapy, music therapy, hydrotherapy, and counter pressure (Figs. 16.31 to 16.34; Table 16.6). Often a combination

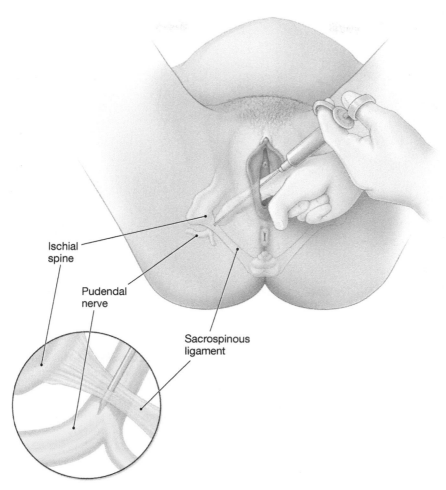

Ischial
spine

Pudendal
nerve

Sacrospinous
ligament

Figure 16.29. Pudendal block. Local anesthesia can be administered easily at the time of delivery to provide perineal anesthesia for a vaginal delivery. (Reprinted with permission from Beckmann, C. R., Herbert, W., Laube, D., Ling, F., & Smith, R. [2013]. *Obstetrics and gynecology* [7th ed., Fig. 8.7]. Philadelphia, PA: Lippincott Williams & Wilkins.)

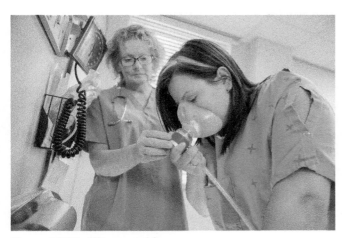

Figure 16.30. Nitrous oxide.

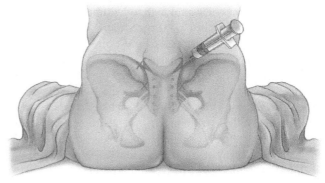

Figure 16.31. Location of intradermal water injections. The nurse administers four sterile water injections to relieve the pain of back labor. (Reprinted with permission from Hatfield, N. T., & Kincheloe, C. A. [2017]. *Introductory maternity and pediatric nursing* [4th ed., Fig. 9-4]. Philadelphia, PA: Lippincott Williams & Wilkins.)

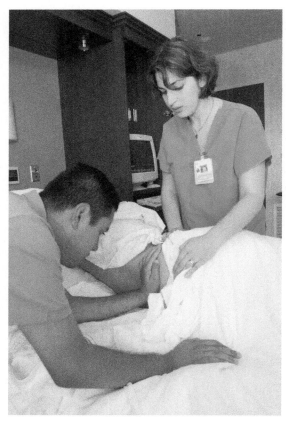

Figure 16.32. Counter pressure. With a posterior fetal position, the woman may feel extensive back pressure. Application of pressure on her lower back by her support person may help relieve this problem. (Reprinted with permission from Hatfield, N. T., & Kincheloe, C. A. [2017]. *Introductory maternity and pediatric nursing* [4th ed., Fig. 9-3]. Philadelphia, PA: Lippincott Williams & Wilkins.)

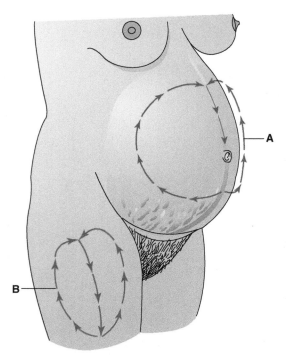

Figure 16.33. Effleurage. (A) During uterine contractions, a laboring woman or support person traces the pattern shown on her bare abdomen with her fingers. **(B)** If electronic fetal monitoring is being used, effleurage may be performed on the thigh. (Reprinted with permission from Nettina, S. M. [2014]. *Lippincott manual of nursing practice* [10th ed., Fig. 37-10]. Philadelphia, PA: Lippincott Williams & Wilkins.)

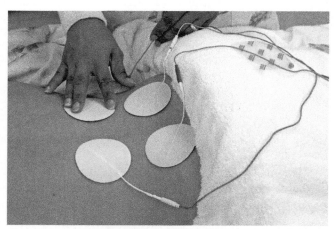

Figure 16.34. Transcutaneous electrical nerve stimulation electrode placement when used for labor analgesia. (Reprinted with permission from Craven, R. F., Hirnle, C. J., & Jensen, S. [2013]. *Fundamentals of nursing* [7th ed., Fig. 34.10A]. Philadelphia, PA: Lippincott Williams & Wilkins.)

of strategies is needed, and nurses should be prepared to change out one strategy for another.

The gate control theory of pain states that a limited number of sensations, or messages, can be transmitted and processed by the brain at one time. Distractions from pain, such as music, guided imagery, massage, stroking, and aromatherapy, "crowd out" pain signals, diminishing the perception of pain. Imagine a livestock pen filled with black sheep and white sheep. The black sheep represent pain. The white sheep represent other sensations. All of them are trying to leave the pen by the same gate at the same time. Some black sheep will get out, but some white sheep will leave at the same time. Without the white sheep, only black sheep escape. Similarly, without the aforementioned distractions or others, only the pain remains to be perceived, undiluted by other sensations. Many of the strategies for mitigating the pain and discomfort of childbirth are based on this idea (Mendell, 2014).

Table 16.6 Nonpharmacologic Strategies for Managing Pain During Labor

Strategy	Notes
Cognitive Strategies	

Childbirth education	• Participation in a childbirth class is associated with a higher rate of vaginal rather than cesarean births (Afshar et al., 2016)
	• Methods provide a focus on confidence and coping strategies
	• Distraction techniques and methods of moving the mental focus away from the contraction and onto an object, sound, or other stimulus are covered
	• Different breathing patterns may be taught, with each beginning with a deep, cleansing breath Different breathing techniques may offer distraction and a sense of control while also optimizing oxygenation and relaxation
	• Related websites:
	  ○ www.birthingfromwithin.com
	  ○ www.cappa.net
	  ○ https://www.lamaze.org

Hypnosis	• Hypnosis is often taught as a form of guided imagery that allows for distraction and dissociation from or reframing of the sensations of labor to make it more tolerable • Goal is to be relaxed, awake, and fully in control • Related website: https://us.hypnobirthing.com/
Biofeedback	• Taught as part of some childbirth classes, biofeedback is a method of relaxation that informs a woman of physiologic processes and helps her optimize her reaction to them. For example, a woman might be taught to recognize an elevated heartbeat or area of muscle tension and to control her response to it • Breathing techniques may be considered a form of biofeedback
Cutaneous Stimulation Strategies	
Intradermal water block	• The injection of 0.5–0.1 mL of sterile water subcutaneously in four locations in the lower back • Intense stinging similar to a bee sting for 20–30 s • May provide relief from back pain for up to 2 h
Counter pressure	• Often used in the case of back labor • Firm pressure at the location of the pain, to both hips or knees • Pressure may be applied with the fist, heel of hand, tennis ball, etc.
Effleurage	• A form of light, patterned touch over the abdomen, thigh, or chest • May be irritating later in labor as a greater sensitivity to touch is experienced
Transcutaneous electrical nerve stimulation	• Used for lower back pain, most effective in early labor • Electrodes placed on the lower back provide a buzzing vibration that appears to improve pain tolerance
Acupressure and acupuncture	• Acupuncture involves the placement of special needles into particular areas of the skin • Acupressure involves placement of pressure, cold, or heat to the same areas • Used for labor pain and contraction stimulation
Touch and massage	• Touch may be used to communicate comfort or presence • Touch may also be used to indicate tense muscles that the laboring woman can consciously relax • Massage may be most acceptable in the hands and feet, as the hyperesthesia (sensitivity to touch) of later labor makes touch less welcome

(continued)

Table 16.6 Nonpharmacologic Strategies for Managing Pain During Labor (continued)

Strategy	Notes
Water therapy	• Shower, bath, whirlpool, or birthing pool • May contribute to relaxation • May aid in faster labor, less medication, and the rotation of the fetus into a more optimal position • Women may elect to give birth in water in accordance with the policies of the birthing venue and the judgment of the obstetric provider
Other Sensory Stimulation	
Aromatherapy	• Scents may be used alone or in conjunction with massage • May be added to lotions or creams before cutaneous use • Scented oils may be used in baths according to policy • May promote relaxation and improved pain tolerance • Peppermint and fresh lemon scents may help mitigate nausea
Music	• May distract from sensations of labor and reduce stress

Think Critically

1. You are discussing home birth with a friend. Using what you learned in this chapter, how do you discuss the pros and cons of this birthing venue?

2. List from memory the five Ps of labor and provide a brief description of each.

3. A patient comes to labor and delivery with suspected labor. What questions are important to ask to determine whether this is likely? What exam elements would be helpful?

4. You suspect your patient may be in transition. What would make you suspect this and how would your suspicion be verified?

5. Your patient is holding her breath when pushing. You recommend open glottis pushing and your patient asks why. What should you tell her?

6. Your patient elects not to have continuous electronic fetal monitoring during labor, opting instead for intermittent monitoring. How often should you monitor her and for how long?

7. On a piece of graph or lined paper, draw the following variations of fetal heart rates: late deceleration, early deceleration, and variable deceleration.

8. Your patient is experiencing late decelerations with 50% or more of her contractions. What are your responsibilities as a nurse?

9. Your patient asks you to describe the difference between an epidural and a combined spinal/epidural. How would you explain this to her?

10. Your patient has elected to use nitrous oxide during labor. How would you coach her in its use?

11. Your patient is determined not to use any pharmaceutical pain relief while laboring. What methods of nonpharmacologic relief could you direct her and her support person to try?

References

Afshar, Y., Wang, E. T., Mei, J., Esakoff, T. F., Pisarska, M. D., & Gregory, K. D. (2016, November 15). Childbirth education class and birth plans are associated with a vaginal delivery. *Birth, 44*(1), 29–34. doi:10.1111/birt.12263

Ahmed, A. I., Zhu, L., Aldhaheri, S., Sakr, S., Minkoff, H., & Haberman, S. (2016). Uterine tachysystole in spontaneous labor at term. *The Journal of Maternal-Fetal and Neonatal Medicine, 29*(20), 3335–3339.

Alfirevic, Z., Devane, D., & Gyte, G. (2013). Comparing continuous electronic fetal monitoring in labour (cardiotocography, CTG) with intermittent listening (intermittent auscultation, IA). *The Cochrane Database of Systematic Reviews.*

Alfirevic, Z., Devane, D., Gyte, G., & Cuthbert, A. (2017). Continuous cardiotocography (CTG) as a form of electronic fetal monitoring (EFM) for fetal assessment during labour. *The Cochrane Database of Systematic Reviews*, (2), CD006066.

American Academy of Nursing. (2015). *Electronic fetal heart rate monitoring*. Retrieved from https://aannet.connectedcommunity.org/initiatives/choosing-wisely/electronic-fetal-heart-rate-monitoring

Begley, C., Gyte, G., Devane, D., McGuire, W., & Weeks, A. (2015). Active versus expectant management for women in the third stage of labour. *The Cochrane Database of Systematic Reviews*, (11), CD007412. doi:10.1002/14651858.CD007412.pub4

Chaillet, N., Belaid, L., Crochetière, C., Roy, L., Gagné, G.-P., Moutquin, J. M., . . . Bonapace, J. (2014). Nonpharmacologic approaches for pain management during labor compared with usual care: A meta-analysis. *Birth, 41*(2), 122–137.

Cox, K. J., & King, T. L. (2015). Preventing primary cesarean births: Midwifery care. *Clinical Obstetrics and Gynecology, 58*(2), 282–293.

Declercq, E., Sakala, C., Corry, M., Applebaum, S., & Herrlich, A. (2013). *Listening to Mothers(SM) III: New mothers speak out.* New York, NY: Childbirth Connection.

Gao, L., Rabbitt, E. H., Condon, J. C., Renthal, N. E., Johnston, J. M., Mitsche, M. A., . . . Mendelson, C. R. (2015). Steroid receptor coactivators 1 and 2 mediate fetal-to-maternal signaling that initiates parturition. *Journal of Clinical Investigation, 125*(1), 2808–2824.

Gizzo, S., Gangi, S. D., Noventa, M., Bacile, V., Zambon, A., & Nardelli, G. B. (2014). Women's choice of positions during labour: Return to the past or a modern way to give birth? A cohort study in Italy. *BioMed Research International, 2014,* 7.

Hodnett, E., Gates, S., Hofmeyr, G., & Sakala, C. (2013). Continuous support for women during childbirth (Review). *The Cochrane Database of Systematic Reviews,* (7), CD003766.

Hofmeyr, G., & Lawrie, T. (2012). Amnioinfusion for potential or suspected umbilical cord compression in labour. *The Cochrane Database of Systematic Reviews,* (1), CD000013.

Korhonen, U., & Heinonen, P. T. (2014). The diagnostic accuracy of pelvic measurements: Threshold values and fetal size. *Archives of Gynecology and Obstetrics, 290*(4), 643–648.

Korhonen, U., Taipale, P., & Heinonen, S. (2013). Assessment of bony pelvis and vaginally assisted deliveries. *ISRN Obstetrics and Gynecology, 2013,* 763782.

Lawrence, A., Lewis, L., Hofmeyr, G. J., & Styles, C. (2013). Maternal positions and mobility during first stage labour. *The Cochrane Database of Systematic Reviews,* (8), CD003934.

Lemos, A., Amorim, M. D., de Souza, A., Cabral Filho, J., & Correia, J. (2015). Pushing/bearing down methods for the second stage of labour (Review). *The Cochrane Database of Systematic Reviews,* (10), CD009124.

Likis, F. E., Andrews, J. C., Collins, M., Lewis, R. M., Starr, S. A., Walden, R. R., & McPheeters, M. (2014). Nitrous oxide for the management of labor pain: A systematic review. *Anesthesia and Analgesia, 118*(1), 153–167.

MacDorman, M. F., Mathews, T., & Declercq, E. (2014). Trends in out-of-hospital births in the United States, 1990–2012. *NCHS Data Brief, 144,* 1–8.

Martin, J., Hamilton, B., Osterman, M., Curtin, S., & Mathews, T. (2015). Births: Final data for 2014. *National Vital Statistics Reports, 64*(12), 1–64.

Mendell, L. M. (2014). Constructing and deconstructing the gate theory of pain. *Pain, 155*(2), 210–216.

Menon, R., Bonney, E. A., Condon, J., Mesiano, S., & Taylor, R. N. (2016). Novel concepts on pregnancy clocks and alarms: Redundancy and synergy in human parturition. *Human Reproduction Update, 22*(5), 535–560.

Osterman, M. J., & Martin, J. A. (2011). Epidural and spinal anesthesia use during labor: 27-State reporting area, 2008. *National Vital Statistics Reports, 50*(9).

Pattinson, R., Cuthbert, A., & Vannevel, V. (2017). Pelvimetry for fetal cephalic presentations at or near term for deciding on mode of delivery. *The Cochrane Database of Systematic Reviews,* (3), CD000161.

Simmons, S., Taghizadeh, N., Dennis, A., Hughes, D., & Cyna, A. (2012). Combined spinal-epidural versus epidural analgesia in labour. *The Cochrane Database of Systematic Reviews,* (10), CD003401.

Stapleton, S., Osborne, C., & Illuzzi, J. (2013). Outcomes of care in birth centers: Demonstration of a durable model. *Journal of Midwifery and Women's Health, 58*(1), 3–14.

Stark, M. A., Remynse, M., & Zwelling, E. (2016). Importance of the birth environment to support physiologic birth. *Journal of Obstetric, Gynecologic, & Neonatal Nursing, 45*(2), 285–294.

Wax, J. R., & Barth, W. H., Jr. (2016). Planned home birth. *Obstetrics and Gynecology, 128,* e26–e31.

Wojcieszek, A., Stock, O., & Flenady, V. (2014). Antibiotics for prelabour rupture of membranes at or near term. *The Cochrane Database of Systematic Reviews,* (10), CD001807.

Zielinski, R., Ackerson, K., & Low, L. K. (2015). Planned home birth: Benefits, risks, and opportunities. *International Journal of Women's Health, 7,* 361–377.

Suggested Readings

Adams, E. D., Stark, M. A., & Low, L. K. (2016). A nurse's guide to supporting physiologic birth. *Nursing for Women's Health, 20*(1), 76–86.

Wisner, K. (2015). Intermittent auscultation in low-risk labor. *American Journal of Maternal Child Nursing, 40*(1), 58.

17 After Delivery

Objectives

1. Describe the anticipated physiologic and psychosocial changes in the mother in the immediate postpartum period.
2. Identify pertinent postpartum nursing assessments and care considerations.
3. Identify variations in postpartum care required by patients with vaginal births when compared with those with cesarean births.
4. Discuss the important aspects of discharge instructions.

Key Terms

Afterpains
Approximation
Boggy uterus
Ecchymosis
Ileus
Involution

Lochia
Prolactin
Rugae
Subinvolution
Thrombus

Although the fourth stage of labor typically consists of only the first 4 hours after a birth, the entire postpartum period encompasses the first 6 weeks after delivery. It is a time of physical, mental, and emotional change for the new mother, with a relatively low risk of complications. Complications, when they do occur, however, can be far-reaching. Meaningful nursing presence and support can be critical to a positive outcome in the life of a new family during this time (Fig. 17.1). Assessments generally occur according to a regular schedule: every 15 minutes for the first hour, every 30 minutes for the second hour, every 4 hours for the remaining 22 of the 24 hours of the first day, and then once every 8-hour shift. New learners may find the BUBBLE-EE mnemonic helpful for organizing care (Box 17.1).

Postpartum Physiologic Changes and Care

Most of the profound physical changes that occurred during pregnancy reverse almost completely in just 6 weeks after the birth. Some women may begin the postpartum period with the expectation that their bodies will return to their prepregnancy state more quickly than can reasonably be expected. Other short-term changes, such as diaphoresis, increased diuresis, and lochia, may be unanticipated by the patient. Educational interventions about her changing body are often just as important as physical interventions and routine assessments.

Simple things, such as the wardrobe of the immediate postpartum period, may seem unfamiliar to a first-time mother. Hospital gowns with shoulder snaps are useful for the evaluation of breasts and for breastfeeding access but can be difficult to reassemble. Hospital-provided undergarments, stretchy nets that hold absorbent pads in place, are rarely seen outside of the postpartum unit. The pads themselves are designed to hold a higher volume of discharge than the typical menstrual bleed and may seem oversized and even comedic. A walk-through of these unfamiliar items and their use can be reassuring and empowering for a new mother.

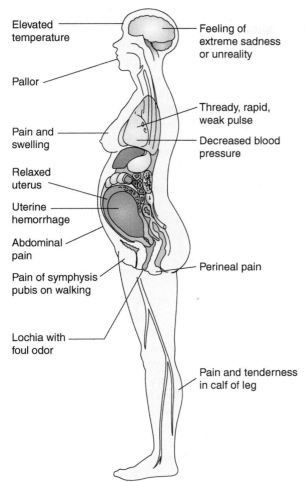

Elevated temperature

Feeling of extreme sadness or unreality

Pallor

Thready, rapid, weak pulse

Pain and swelling

Decreased blood pressure

Relaxed uterus

Uterine hemorrhage

Abdominal pain

Pain of symphysis pubis on walking

Perineal pain

Lochia with foul odor

Pain and tenderness in calf of leg

Figure 17.1. Assessment of the postpartum woman for complications. (Reprinted with permission from Pillitteri, A. [2002]. *Maternal and child health nursing: Care of the childbearing and childrearing family* [4th ed., Fig. 25-1]. Philadelphia, PA: Lippincott Williams & Wilkins.)

Reproductive System

Within the reproductive system, major changes occur in the uterus, perineum, cervix, vagina, pelvic muscles, and breasts during the postpartum period.

Uterus

Physiologic Changes

The shrinkage of the uterus, called **involution**, begins immediately after the birth. The uterus grows during pregnancy because of a combination of hypertrophy and hyperplasia. Postpartum, the hypertrophied cells shrink and the muscles of the uterus atrophy. The hyperplasia, or new cell growth, remains. Because of this, the woman's uterus will not completely regress to the size it was previous to the pregnancy. Additionally, the contraction of the uterus aids the involution process. If the uterus does not contract sufficiently, uterine atony occurs, which can cause hemorrhage from the site of the placenta. This compression of the contracted uterus, is primarily responsible for the prevention of postpartum hemorrhage.

Box 17.1 BUBBLE-EE Mnemonic for Postpartum Nursing Care

Breasts: Breasts should be symmetrically soft and nontender for the first 24 h postpartum, becoming slowly and progressively more full until milk comes in sometime between postpartum days 2 and 5. Engorgement manifests as breast fullness and tenderness.

Uterus: The uterus should be firm and midline, descending from the umbilicus toward the pelvis at a predictable rate.

Bladder: Encourage frequent emptying of the bladder, because a full bladder can displace the uterus and cause atony. Infrequent emptying of the bladder may also predispose a woman to cystitis.

Bowels: Bowel motility may be slow to recover from the birth and the hormones of pregnancy. Women who delivered by cesarean section are more likely to experience an ileus (lack of movement of intestines). Women may not have a bowel movement before discharge. Passing flatus and positive bowel sounds are sufficient proof of bowel function.

Lochia: Assess and record the amount of lochia per the protocols of the institution.

Episiotomy/perineum: Assess any episiotomy wound or other laceration, as well as the general condition of the perineum. Assess for hemorrhoids.

Extremities: Assess the patient's legs for unilateral edema, warmth, induration, or tenderness, any of which may suggest a thromboembolism.

Emotional status: Extreme mood swings, anxiety, and depression are causes for concern.

In Chapter 4, the nurse taking care of Sophie postpartum, Mary, was careful to explain uterine involution to her. At that time, the fundus of Sophie's uterus was located at the umbilicus, an anticipated location in the first few hours after birth.

The failure of the uterus to shrink at the expected rate is called **subinvolution**. Immediately after the birth, the top, or fundus, of the uterus is usually about 2 cm, or two fingerbreadths, below the level of the umbilicus. In the first several hours it may rise to a fingerbreadth above the umbilicus, after which it begins the steady process of involution. By 24 hours after the birth, the uterus is at the umbilicus—the same position as it was at 20 weeks of gestation. After the first 24 hours, the appropriately involuting uterus has descended from the level of the umbilicus by 1 to 2 cm (see Fig. 16.18). By 2 weeks postpartum, the uterus should again be a pelvic organ, and by 6 weeks, it should have involuted completely. In the immediate postpartum period, the uterus weighs about 1,000 g, or as much as a 1-L bottle of soda. By week 6 postpartum, it should weigh about 70 g, or less than a bar of soap.

Because the contraction of the uterus is so important, oxytocin may be administered postpartum to promote it. Women who have an intravenous (IV) line or saline lock usually receive oxytocin IV, whereas others receive oxytocin intramuscularly (IM). Breast stimulation by breastfeeding promotes endogenous release of oxytocin, leading to uterine contractions. In the case of field births (usually unanticipated births outside the hospital), immediate and frequent breastfeeding is often endorsed to promote this process. Women may not perceive these contractions or may feel them only minimally, particularly after the first pregnancy. When these contractions are painful, they are referred to as **afterpains**. Women who have given birth previously or had a multifetal pregnancy, a large baby, or uterine distention related to polyhydramnios are more likely to experience afterpains and to have them for up to a week. These pains are typically most pronounced while breastfeeding.

A distended bladder may at times contribute to the discomfort of afterpains and will increase the risk for uterine atony. Women experiencing afterpains may benefit from warmth applied to the abdomen and analgesics, most often ibuprofen and acetaminophen. The timing of medication should take into the account the role of breastfeeding in afterpains. Many women may prefer to take medication prior to breastfeeding to help prevent or lessen afterpains, whereas others may be concerned about the medication passing from the breast milk to the infant and may take medication after nursing or not at all (see Chapter 18).

In addition to these afterpains, which aid in uterine contraction and vascular constriction at the placental site, thus promoting hemostasis and preventing hemorrhage, other changes are also occurring that directly impact the placental site (which was previously referred to as the decidua basalis during pregnancy). Scar tissue does not stretch, move, or function as well as the tissue it replaces. For the sake of future placental implantation and the maintenance of future pregnancies, therefore, it is important that

the placental site not scar. To prevent healing by scarring, the endometrium instead sloughs the necrotic decidua. This process of regeneration and replacement of the decidua with the endometrium is completed by the end of the 6-week postpartum period.

The sloughing of the decidua as well as other debris is responsible for the uterine discharge that persists for 1 to 2 months after the birth. The nature and composition of this discharge, called **lochia**, change throughout this period of time (Table 17.1).

In Chapter 8, the nurse taking care of Gracie, Bethany, was careful to explain the different kinds of lochia to her and what kind she should anticipate at what time. When Gracie learned how long lochia can last, she was glad that she received an employee discount on feminine hygiene products.

Women who have given birth by cesarean section typically have more scant lochia than do those who deliver vaginally. Perfuse or persistent lochia rubra, on the other hand, is concerning for hemorrhage and/or retained placenta or fetal membranes. Afterpains from breastfeeding can cause an increase in lochia, as can ambulation. It is also common for lochia rubra to reappear a week or two after the birth for a few hours as part of the healing process of the placenta site. Lochia rubra that returns and persists for more than a few hours, however, is concerning for secondary postpartum hemorrhage.

Nurses must be alert for postpartum bleeding that may not be lochia. Lochia is typically a slow trickle but may become a brief gush with afterpains, uterine massage, or assuming an upright position after a prolonged period of lying down. It is typically dark in color. Blood that appears to spurt or pump or is persistently bright red in a woman with a contracted uterus is not likely to be lochia. This type of bleeding is suspicious for a laceration of the cervix or vagina, is typically identified shortly after the birth, and warrants assessment by the obstetric provider (Fig. 17.2).

Table 17.1 Types of Lochia

Lochia Type	Appearance	Composition	Duration	Abnormalities
Lochia rubra (Rubra means "red" in Latin.)	Dark red	Blood, decidua, and other pregnancy debris	3–4 d	• Foul odor (suggests infection) • Saturation of pad in 15 min or less • Tissue • Clots larger than plums • Duration more than 4 d
Lochia serosa (Serosa means "serum" in Latin.)	Lighter red, pink, or brown	Debris, old blood, white blood cells, and serum	10–14 d	• Saturation of pad in 15 min or less • Foul odor (suggests infection) • Bright red blood for more than 1–2 h
Lochia alba (Alba means "white" in Latin.)	Yellow or white	White blood cells, serum, mucus, and bacteria	2–4 wk	• Foul odor (suggests infection) • Bright red blood for more than 1–2 h

must be checked during scheduled assessments. The frequency of the assessments, which is greater in the first few hours and then is reduced to once per shift later, reflects the peak risk for postpartum hemorrhage in the first hour after the birth. Postpartum hemorrhage in the first 24 hours after birth is primary postpartum hemorrhage, whereas hemorrhage between 24 hours and 12 weeks after birth is referred to as secondary (see Chapter 23).

In Chapter 1, Bess's postpartum hemorrhage was early, and she required a hysterectomy to control bleeding. (In Chapter 2, Tatiana experienced late postpartum hemorrhage, which resolved with conservative measures.)

As for any patient, the nurse must inform the postpartum patient of the rationale for the exam and the exam procedure before it is started. The nurse should ask her about her last void of urine, whether she has changed a pad, and, if so, how saturated it was (Fig. 17.4). The nurse should ask her whether she has breastfed, experienced afterpains, or recently ambulated. If the patient has not voided recently or cannot remember when she last voided, the nurse should instruct her to use the bathroom before assessment and to set her used pad aside for evaluation of lochia. A full bladder may displace the uterus, which could cause uterine atony and hemorrhage. A uterus that is not midline when palpated is often displaced to one side or the other by a full bladder.

If a woman has not recently ambulated and has been lying down, she may have accumulated pooled lochia that will then leak profusely when she is upright. The nurse should warn the recumbent patient that this may happen, and place chux pads on the floor near the bedside in case of leakage. It is important to assist the patient to ensure she does not slip on the chux pad or any lochia on the pad or the floor.

To assess the progress of uterine involution, the nurse should stabilize the lower uterus with one hand while feeling for the fundus of the uterus with the other (Fig. 17.5). Uterine inversion, a condition in which the fundus of the uterus prolapses toward or even through the cervix, is an extremely rare condition but a theoretical risk of applying force to the fundus without also providing support to the lower uterine segment. When feeling for the fundus, the nurse should start at the umbilicus and move down, palpating deeply but gently until locating it.

The expected finding for a fundal exam is a uterus that is midline, firm, and involuted to the degree anticipated by the time of birth (Fig. 17.6). A uterus that is not firm, a **boggy uterus**, indicates uterine atony and a risk for hemorrhage. The nurse should massage the uterus with the palm of one hand while stabilizing the lower uterine segment with the other hand. Fundal massage stimulates the uterus to contract. The obstetric provider may order oxytocin or another medication to enhance contractions. The nurse should report ongoing atony to the obstetric provider (see Chapter 23). If the uterus is firm but the lochia is heavy, the nurse should replace the pad and assess it again after 15 minutes. If after 15 minutes the uterus is still firm and the lochia still heavy, the bleeding is likely not lochia and may indicate a laceration or ruptured vulvar or vaginal hematoma. In this case, urgent consultation with the obstetric provider is warranted.

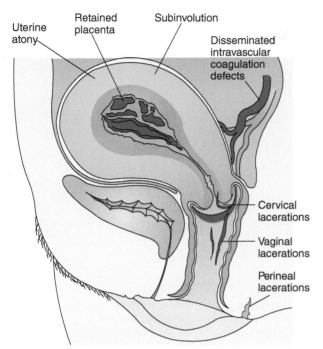

Figure 17.2. Postpartum hemorrhage from various causes. (Reprinted with permission from Evans, R. J., Brown, Y. M., & Evans, M. K. [2014]. *Canadian maternity, newborn, and women's health nursing* [2nd ed., Fig. 19.1]. Philadelphia, PA: Lippincott Williams & Wilkins.)

Nursing Care

Because assessment of the reproductive organs may involve contact with bodily fluids, nurses on the postpartum unit must wear gloves throughout the exam (Fig. 17.3).

A critical physical aspect of postpartum care is a thorough assessment of the uterus, including assessment of involution, uterine tone and position, and lochia. Each of these elements

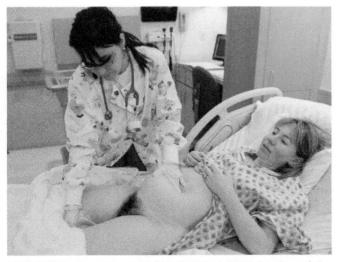

Figure 17.3. Assessment of the lochia with palpation of the fundus. Ideally, when performing this assessment, one hand supports the lower uterine segment, whereas the other palpates the fundus. (Reprinted with permission from Ricci, S. S. [2009]. *Essentials of maternity, newborn, & women's health nursing* [2nd ed., Fig. 16.3]. Philadelphia, PA: Lippincott Williams & Wilkins.)

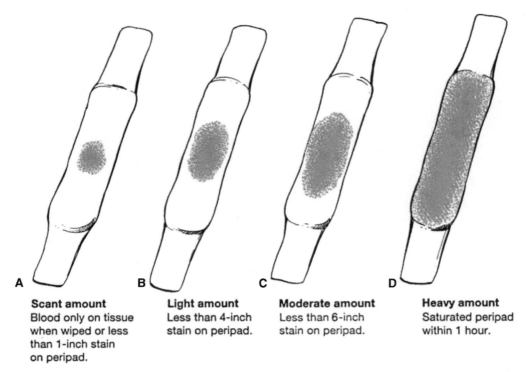

Scant amount
Blood only on tissue when wiped or less than 1-inch stain on peripad.

Light amount
Less than 4-inch stain on peripad.

Moderate amount
Less than 6-inch stain on peripad.

Heavy amount
Saturated peripad within 1 hour.

Figure 17.4. **Lochia of varying degrees. (A)** Scant: slight coloring or darkening appears on the top of the pad, with no soaking through the absorbent material. **(B)** Light: approximately one third of the pad is covered centrally. **(C)** Moderate: approximately two thirds of the pad is covered centrally. **(D)** Heavy: the whole pad is covered. (Reprinted with permission from Evans, R. J., Brown, Y. M., & Evans, M. K. [2014]. *Canadian maternity, newborn, and women's health nursing* [2nd ed., Fig. 18.7]. Philadelphia, PA: Lippincott Williams & Wilkins.)

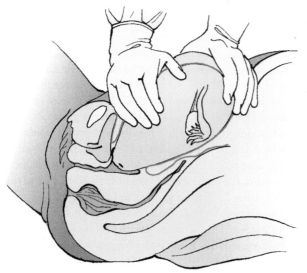

Figure 17.5. **Hand placement for fundal palpation and massage.** (Reprinted with permission from Lippincott's Nursing Procedures and Skills, 2007.)

The nurse determines the degree of uterine involution by assessing the level of the uterine fundus in relation to the midline of the abdomen and the umbilicus. A woman with a uterus that deviates from midline who did not urinate prior to the exam should do so, and the nurse should reassess afterward. The position

of the uterine fundus in relation to the umbilicus is recorded in centimeters, with a centimeter equivalent to a fingerbreadth. "U-2," for example, would indicate a fundal height 2 cm below the umbilicus, which is appropriate for a few days after a birth.

While assessing the patient's uterine fundus, the nurse should ask the patient's permission to slide down her pad, so that the discharge of lochia may be observed at the same time. An increase of lochia during the exam is not uncommon, and it is useful for the nurse to observe if heavy discharge has occurred normally over time or is due to the exam process.

The nurse should determine the amount of lochia flow over the course of an hour. A pad being saturated over the course of an hour, for example, should be considered heavy flow. If the saturation occurs over 4 hours, however, it would not indicate heavy flow. Four different descriptions of lochia amount are generally used. Lochia should be reported with each exam as one of the following:

- Scant: an inch or less on the pad in an hour
- Light: 4 in or less on the pad in an hour
- Moderate: 6 in or less on the pad in an hour
- Heavy: the pad is completely saturated in an hour

Clots are a normal part of lochia rubra if small, particularly if the postpartum patient has been lying down for a period of time, allowing the blood to pool and congeal. Clots larger than a plum, however, particularly in conjunction with heavy lochia, are more concerning, because larger clots may prevent the uterus from

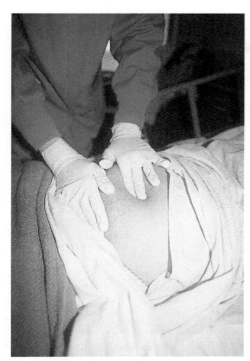

Figure 17.6. Evaluation of uterine firmness. (Reprinted with permission from Lippincott's Nursing Procedures and Skills, 2007.)

contracting down adequately, thus causing uterine atony. Clots should be examined carefully to ensure they do not contain tissue, because retained placenta can cause subinvolution and hemorrhage. A blood clot will dissolve in water, whereas placental tissue and membranes will not. Therefore, to determine whether a clot is actually placental tissue, the nurse should carefully run the clot under warm water.

Perineum

Physiologic Changes

The perineum refers to the anatomic area between the pubic symphysis and the coccyx and includes skin, muscle, and connective tissue. Trauma to the perineum may occur as a result of stretching, tearing (laceration), and sometimes cutting (episiotomy). Varicosities of the vulva and rectum may have their onset during pregnancy. Vulvar varicosities typically resolve quickly after the birth, whereas rectal varicosities (hemorrhoids), which may result from bearing down during delivery, take longer to resolve. Edema (swelling), **ecchymosis** (bruising), and discomfort of the perineum are common and can typically be managed with ibuprofen, acetaminophen, and ice packs. Worsening pain and discomfort is suspicious for a perineal hematoma (see Chapter 23).

In Chapter 11, Edie developed a vulvar hematoma after sustaining a significant laceration with the birth. Her nurse, Marnie, first suspected it when Edie developed severe perineal pain 6 hours after the birth.

Nursing Care

The nurse should check the perineum every time he or she assesses the uterus and lochia. Points of assessment include erythema (redness), edema, ecchymosis, discharge, and approximation of repaired wound edges, if present. **Approximation** pertains to the proximity of the wound edges to each other. With a well-approximated wound, the two edges line up with no space between them. With a poorly approximated wound, the two edges of the wound do not meet and healing is compromised.

The nurse should perform the perineal exam with the patient in the side-lying position (Fig. 17.7). The patient may require assistance from the nurse in moving into this position. The nurse should wear gloves for this exam and ensure the patient's privacy and the availability of good lighting. While explaining the exam, the nurse should lower the patient's panties and pad and separate her buttocks and labia for better visualization of the area. Findings such as mild-to-moderate edema and some ecchymosis are expected.

The nurse should evaluate repaired lacerations and episiotomies for approximation and infection. Although some redness and swelling are not unexpected at the site of the healing wound, persistent redness, purulent discharge, and worsening pain are unexpected and suspicious for infection (Fig. 17.8). Initial healing of lacerations and episiotomies takes approximately 2 to 3 weeks.

If the patient reports perineal pain, the nurse should have the patient rate the pain and then record the score. If the nurse plans to perform an intervention to address the patient's pain, the former should record a pain score prior to and after the intervention.

Tylenol and ibuprofen are common standing orders for women postpartum and are typically given according to a regular schedule unless declined. Ice packs are common first-line interventions for perineal pain, and topical anesthetics may be used if ordered. The side-lying position may provide some positional relief from discomfort. Perineal pads should fit closely to avoid rubbing with movement.

Wiping after urination or defecation is often uncomfortable, and spraying warm water from a perineal irrigation, or peri bottle, over the perineum can provide a more comfortable method of

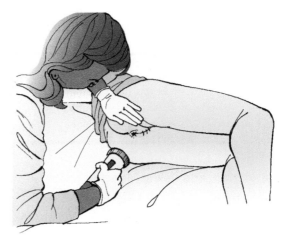

Figure 17.7. Assessment of the perineum. (Reprinted with permission from Lippincott's Nursing Procedures and Skills, 2007.)

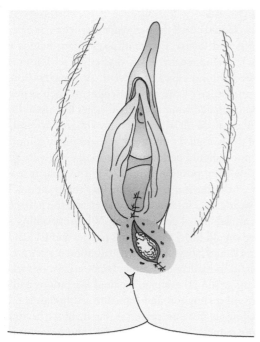

Figure 17.8. An infected suture line. Infected suture lines typically appear reddened and edematous and often contain purulent secretions. Note the poor approximation of the wound edges. (Reprinted with permission from Pillitteri, A. [2002]. *Maternal and child health nursing: Care of the childbearing and childrearing family* [4th ed., Fig. 25-3]. Philadelphia, PA: Lippincott Williams & Wilkins.)

maintaining cleanliness and mitigate the risk for infection. Warm sitz baths (Fig. 17.9), witch hazel pads, and topical anesthetics may provide temporary relief from pain and pruritus, which may occur with hemorrhoids (Eshkevari, Trout, & Damore, 2013). Hemorrhoids typically regress within 6 weeks of the birth.

Women may express anxiety about voiding and defecating after a birth for fear of creating or worsening perineal pain. Docusate sodium is a medication commonly given to patients to ensure that stool is soft and less likely to cause pain or require uncomfortable pushing (see The Pharmacy 9.2). The peri bottle may be used over the perineum during voiding to dilute urine. Women may also void into a sitz bath (see Box 9.9).

In Chapter 8, Gracie's postpartum nurse, Raven, was concerned that Gracie was not voiding. With Raven's help, Gracie used the peri bottle to help promote urination, as well as hygiene.

Cervix, Vagina, and Pelvic Muscles

Physiologic Changes

By 2 to 3 days postpartum, the opening of the cervix (the os) has contracted from 10 cm to 2 or 3 cm, and within a week it has contracted to 1 cm. It appears bruised in the immediate postpartum period and may be lacerated. Small lacerations usually

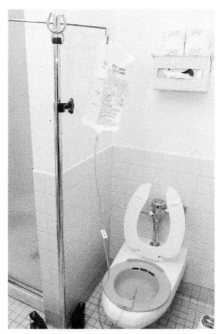

Figure 17.9. Sitz bath setup. (Reprinted with permission from Ricci, S. S. [2013]. *Essentials of maternity, newborn, & women's health nursing* [3rd ed., Fig. 16.6]. Philadelphia, PA: Lippincott Williams & Wilkins.)

heal without intervention, although larger lacerations may bleed bright red blood profusely and require intervention. After a vaginal birth, the external cervical os changes from a round or ovoid shape to an elongated slit (Fig. 17.10).

The vagina involutes and regains tone after the birth but never returns completely to its postpartum state. The **rugae**, or internal folds and ridges of the vagina, return, but are less abundant than prior to pregnancy. The rugae of breastfeeding women do not return until after lactation has ceased because estrogen is required to stimulate their return and lactation suppresses estrogen. Low estrogen levels during lactation are also responsible for atrophy (thinning) of the vaginal mucosa and reduced vaginal secretions and lubrication, making dryness and discomfort with sex common

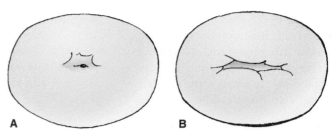

Figure 17.10. Appearance of the cervix in nulliparous and multiparous women. (A) The cervix of a nulliparous woman, showing the dimple-like structure of the external os. **(B)** The cervix of a multiparous woman, showing the slit-like external os. (Reprinted with permission from Klossner, N. J. [2005]. *Introductory maternity nursing* [1st ed., Fig. 12.2]. Philadelphia, PA: Lippincott Williams & Wilkins.)

among lactating women. Silicone- or water-based lubricants can make sex more comfortable and pleasurable, and natural lubrication returns with ovulation and menses.

The pelvic floor muscles that support the pelvic structures regain tone within 6 months of birth. This progression and the degree of tone regained may be aided by Kegel exercises (see Patient Teaching 15.1). A late postpartum complication that occurs years after the birth is further relaxation of the pelvic floor muscles. Although this can happen in any woman, it is more common in women who have experienced one or more vaginal births. This laxity can cause the uterus to prolapse into or even out of the vagina. Prolapse of the urinary bladder into the vagina is called a cystocele. Prolapse of the bowel into the vaginal space is called a rectocele. Herniation of the bowel into the rectovaginal space, which is between the posterior vagina and the anterior rectum, is an enterocele (see Chapter 27). Pain, urinary incontinence, retention of stool, and other complications may happen as a result of these changes. Different strategies to mitigate these changes may be tried, including pelvic physical therapy, surgery, and space-occupying devices called pessaries (Fig. 17.11).

Nursing Care

Assessment of the vagina, cervix, and pelvic floor muscles is not routine during the postpartum period in the absence of a suspected complication, such as hemorrhage from a laceration of the cervix or vagina or a vaginal hematoma. A role of the postpartum nurse, however, is that of an educator.

The nurse should discuss with the patient the differences she may note as she heals, especially vaginal dryness and a need for lubrication with sex. The nurse should teach her how to perform Kegel exercises, emphasizing that the benefits of the exercises may take many weeks to become evident.

Breasts

Physiologic Changes

Women's breasts begin producing small amounts of colostrum, which is rich in nutrients and antibodies, in the second trimester of pregnancy. Colostrum production continues into the early postpartum period and then evolves into milk production, which occurs in higher volume, at approximately 2 to 5 days after the birth. Milk production starts earlier if labor is spontaneous and later if the birth is induced or by scheduled cesarean section prior to the onset of labor.

Primary engorgement is due to swelling of the breast tissue and filling of the ducts with milk, which contains more carbohydrates, less protein, and more water than colostrum. Over the course of several hours, breasts that were previously soft become firm, larger, warm, and tender. Women may experience a pulsing sensation in their breasts and report tender axillary lymph nodes. Some women develop a low-grade fever, with a temperature up to 38°C (100.4°F). Depending on the degree of engorgement, the nipple may flatten, making it difficult or impossible for the infant to achieve an adequate latch (Fig. 17.12).

In Chapter 2, a lactation consultant, Donna, was careful to explain engorgement to Tatiana. She described it as a sensation of the breasts being overly full when the milk first comes in.

Nursing Care

The nurse can encourage a patient whose breasts are engorged to express the milk with a pump to provide relief and allow for

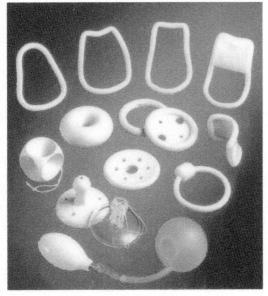

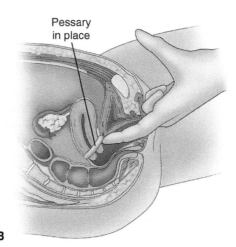

Pessary in place

A   **B**

Figure 17.11. Pessaries. (A) Various shapes and sizes of pessaries available. **(B)** Insertion of one type of pessary. (Reprinted with permission from Hinkle, J. L., & Cheever, K. H. [2017]. *Brunner & Suddarth's textbook of medical-surgical nursing* [14th ed., Fig. 57-4]. Philadelphia, PA: Lippincott Williams & Wilkins.)

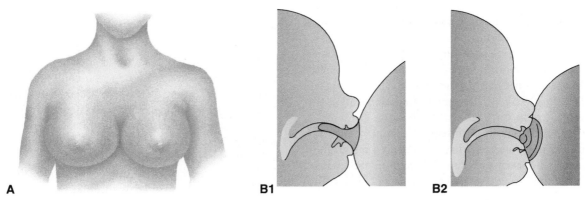

Figure 17.12. Engorged breasts. (A) Note the swelling and inflammation of both breasts. **(B)** Breast engorgement can disrupt breastfeeding: **(1)** When sucking at a normal breast, the infant's lips compress the areola and fit neatly against the sides of the nipple. The infant also has adequate room to breathe. **(2)** When a breast is engorged, however, the infant has difficulty grasping the nipple and its breathing ability is compromised. (Reprinted with permission from Pillitteri, A. [2010]. *Maternal and child health nursing: Care of the childbearing and childrearing family* [6th ed., Fig. 19-6]. Philadelphia, PA: Lippincott Williams & Wilkins.)

latch attainment. The nurse should also check the patient's nipples regularly for bruising, blood blisters, and chapping, which can occur as the mother and baby grow accustomed to breastfeeding and the latch is not yet perfected.

Women who are not planning to breastfeed should avoid nipple stimulation, as it encourages ongoing lactation. The nurse should instruct these mothers to avoid stimuli such as facing toward the water while showering. The nurse should instruct women choosing not to breastfeed to wear a supportive bra all day as well as at night until their breasts no longer feel engorged. Ice packs may be helpful for relief of the discomfort of engorgement but should not be left on for more than 15 minutes at a time in any given hour to avoid a rebound effect. Heat may further stimulate milk production, so its use should be discouraged.

Cardiovascular System

Blood Volume and Cardiac Function

Physiologic Changes

The most overt cardiovascular change in the postpartum period is a dramatic drop in the circulating blood volume. Blood volume increases by up to 45% during pregnancy. The typical blood loss for a vaginal birth is between 200 and 500 mL and for a cesarean section is 500 to 1,000 mL, accounting for a total reduction in blood volume of 10% to 30%. The remaining excess blood volume resolves over the first few postpartum days by a combination of increased diuresis and diaphoresis.

The stroke volume, cardiac output, and pulse all increased during pregnancy. In the immediate postpartum period, the woman's cardiac output and stroke volume increase again. Within an hour after the birth, the heart rate is expected to decrease, whereas the cardiac output and stroke volume remain high, although slightly lower than immediately after the birth, and blood pressure remains unchanged. The cardiac output gradually decreases

over time, returning to prepregnancy output by approximately 3 months postpartum.

Nursing Care

The nurse should review the patient's vital signs with each assessment. Heart rate is typically elevated for the first hour postpartum but then decreases, with bradycardia (usually 40 to 50 beats per minute) being common in the first few days postpartum. A rapid pulse rate is concerning for hemorrhage but may also indicate pain or anxiety.

Blood pressure initially remains unchanged from levels during pregnancy and returns to prepregnancy levels over a period of weeks and months following the pregnancy. A low blood pressure reading is a late sign of hemorrhage. Postpartum blood pressure readings of 140/90 or greater on two occasions at least 6 hours apart is concerning for continuing preeclampsia or the postpartum onset of preeclampsia.

Many women experience orthostatic hypotension in the first few postpartum days. The nurse should encourage the patient to sit up slowly before standing from lying down and to rise slowly from the sitting position.

Blood Composition

Physiologic Changes

Because the extra volume of plasma of the blood that is gained during pregnancy dilutes the red blood cell concentration and thus the hematocrit, interpretation of these results postpartum can be challenging. Hemoglobin and hematocrit tests are rarely done in the absence of known or suspected excessive bleeding. Leukocytosis, a condition of elevated white blood cell count, is a common finding postpartum and can make the diagnosis of infection more challenging. The leukocyte count may be as high as 30,000/mm³ during labor and the immediate postpartum period even in the absence of infection.

The increased clotting risk of pregnancy continues into the postpartum period. Exacerbated by immobility and the tissue damage that occurs in labor and delivery, **thrombus** formation (blood clots) continues to be a danger for as long as 6 weeks postpartum, particularly in the presence of varicosities that allow blood to pool (Fig. 17.13).

In Chapter 3, Susan developed a deep vein thrombosis and a pulmonary embolism directly related to the increased risk of clotting for women who are pregnant or in the immediate postpartum period. Susan's obesity also contributed to her risk for thrombus formation.

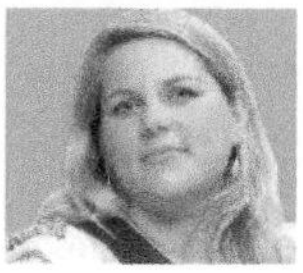

Nursing Care

The nurse should encourage patients to ambulate early and frequently in the postpartum period to encourage blood flow and reduce the risk of clot formation. Women who cannot ambulate

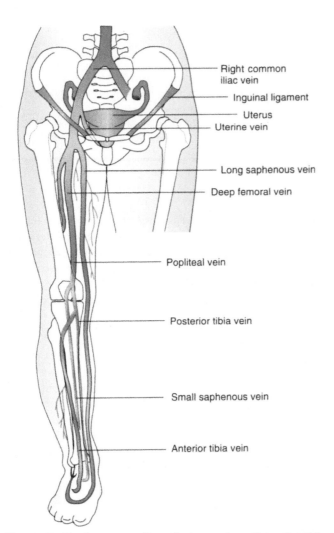

Figure 17.13. Common sites of postpartum thrombophlebitis. (Reprinted with permission from Evans, R. J., Brown, Y. M., & Evans, M. K. [2014]. *Canadian maternity, newborn, and women's health nursing* [2nd ed., Fig. 19.8]. Philadelphia, PA: Lippincott Williams & Wilkins.)

Labels in figure:
- Right common iliac vein
- Inguinal ligament
- Uterus
- Uterine vein
- Long saphenous vein
- Deep femoral vein
- Popliteal vein
- Posterior tibia vein
- Small saphenous vein
- Anterior tibia vein

often have compression devices on their legs and may be encouraged to perform gentle exercises in bed.

The nurse should evaluate the patient's legs at every assessment for signs of clotting, which include tenderness, focal warmth, unilateral swelling, discoloration or redness, and distension of superficial veins of the affected leg. However, about half of people with thrombi experience no symptoms. Homan's sign is a test for deep vein thrombosis that requires the examiner to sharply dorsiflex the foot. Resistance to dorsiflexion, calf pain, pain behind the knee, and involuntary knee flexion are all considered positive tests. Homan's sign has a sensitivity of less than 50% and a specificity of 20%, making it a poor test; a positive test is not diagnostic and a negative test does not rule out deep vein thrombosis. However, many examiners still routinely use the test during postpartum exams (Ambesh, 2017; McGee, 2012).

Immune System

Physiologic Changes

A slightly elevated temperature—up to 38°C (100.4°F)—is common in the first 24 hours after birth and is likely due to dehydration. Women may also have a similarly elevated temperature with primary engorgement of the breasts as the milk supply increases between 2 and 5 days postpartum.

A woman who is Rh negative requires specific follow-up postpartum. If her baby tests Rh negative, no further action is necessary, because the fetal Rh is compatible with the maternal Rh. If the infant is Rh positive, however, an injection of Rh_o (D) immune globulin must be administered to the mother within 72 hours. In the event that Rh-positive fetal blood mixed with the mother's blood during delivery this intervention will prevent the mother from being sensitized to Rh-positive blood, which would endanger any future pregnancies with an Rh-positive fetus. Some providers routinely perform a Kleihauer-Betke test on maternal blood to determine the correct dose of Rh_o (D) immune globulin needed, whereas others may only order the test in the case of known or suspected fetal-maternal hemorrhage. The Kleihauer-Betke test determines the amount of fetal hemoglobin in the maternal circulation. A circulating fetal hemoglobin level above 15 mL requires a larger dose of Rh_o (D) immune globulin, but in most cases a dose of 300 μg IM is sufficient.

In Chapter 5, Letitia was found to be Rh negative. She was given a dose of Rh_o (D) immune globulin when she had a spontaneous abortion in early pregnancy. With her next pregnancy, she received a dose of Rh_o (D) immune globulin at 28 weeks of gestation. She was given her final dose of Rh_o (D) immune globulin prior to 72 hours postpartum because her baby, Laci, was Rh positive.

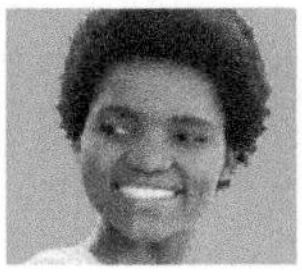

The rubella immunization is contraindicated during pregnancy because it contains a live virus and thus poses a theoretical risk to the fetus, particularly in early pregnancy. Women who are screened for rubella immunity during pregnancy and found to be not immune will be vaccinated in the immediate postpartum period unless they opt out. Women who are vaccinated should avoid pregnancy for 4 weeks after the injection is given.

Nursing Care

Temperature elevation above 38°C after the first 24 hours postpartum is suspicious for infection and warrants further investigation and notification of the obstetric provider. Temperature should be evaluated at the same time as other routine assessments: every 15 minutes for the first hour, every 30 minutes for the second hour, every 4 hours after the second hour for the first day, and then once every shift or per institution protocols.

Endocrine System

Physiologic Changes

Circulating levels of estrogen, progesterone, beta-human chorionic gonadotropin (β-hCG), human placental lactogen (hPL), and relaxin all drop quickly after the detachment and birth of the placenta. For women who are not breastfeeding, estrogen levels begin to rebound to prepregnancy levels within approximately 2 weeks postpartum. Breastfeeding women do not experience a similar rebound in estrogen levels until breastfeeding frequency decreases. Beta-hCG level is generally undetectable within a month after the birth, and circulating hPL is absent within 24 hours of the birth. Normalization of progesterone levels occurs with the first menses.

Prolactin, in addition to stimulating breast milk production, inhibits menses and ovulation. Prolactin release from the anterior pituitary is cued by the drop in estrogen. Women who do not breastfeed have a drop in prolactin level as they experience a rise in estrogen level. Breastfeeding and other types of nipple stimulation enhance prolactin release. In women who are not lactating and do not have sustained increased levels of prolactin, the first menses after the birth usually occurs within 4 weeks, although it may not be associated with ovulation for a few cycles. For women who are lactating, the return of menses and ovulation is unpredictable. Women who are with their infants all of the time and breastfeed whenever the infant cues hunger return to their regular cycle later than women who are not breastfeeding on demand and who supplement infant feeds. Although lactating women may not be ovulating, lactational amenorrhea (lack of menses due to lactation) is not a reliably effective method of birth control (Van der Wijden & Manion, 2015). This is an important consideration, because women who have births that are less than 18 months apart face a higher risk of adverse outcomes (Appareddy, Pryor, & Bailey, 2016).

Nursing Care

The nurse should discuss contraception options with the patient prior to discharge, regardless of whether the patient intends to breastfeed, to avoid an untimely or unintended pregnancy (see Chapter 29). The nurse should also encourage women who are

breastfeeding to feed the infant frequently, particularly early on, to ensure sustained increased levels of prolactin and establishment of a robust milk supply.

Respiratory System

Physiologic Changes

The birth of the neonate and placenta and the involution of the uterus make room for the abdominal organs, and the diaphragm returns to its prepregnancy position. The dimensions of the rib cage regress, as well, although some women may note a permanent increase in chest girth. Tidal volume and other variables return to prepregnancy values within 3 weeks. Pulmonary embolism resulting from the breaking off of a clot from the lower extremities is a very rare complication of the postpartum period and the sixth-leading cause of pregnancy-related deaths, accounting for just over 9% of pregnancy-related deaths (Centers for Disease Control and Prevention, 2017). There are many different ways in which a pulmonary embolism may manifest, but dyspnea and chest pain are common.

Although the pulmonary embolism Susan experienced postpartum is rare, her clinical manifestations were not. Dyspnea, chest pain, and anxiety are classic manifestations of a pulmonary embolism.

Nursing Care

The nurse should evaluate respiratory rate and breath sounds at the same time as other regular assessments. The respiratory rate should be within the normal adult range of 16 to 24 breaths per minute, and lung sounds should be clear. The nurse should encourage the patient to inform the nurse or another healthcare provider if she experiences sudden shortness of breath or chest pain.

Urinary System

Physiologic Changes

The drop in estrogen level that occurs after the birth contributes to increased diaphoresis and prolactin levels and, together with the drop in oxytocin level, causes increased diuresis within about 12 hours after the birth. Like diaphoresis, diuresis helps offload the extra fluid accumulated in pregnancy. Complicating the increased filling of the bladder, however, is a change in voiding urge sensation that frequently occurs as a result of the removal of the pressure of the gravid uterus from the bladder. Bladder trauma during the birth and anesthesia may also impair the voiding urge sensation. Some women may also have edema of the urethra after the birth that causes urinary retention. Many women experience anxiety about urinating for fear that urine splashing against the vulva may be painful, particularly in the presence of a laceration or episiotomy.

In Chapter 9, Nancy was unable to void spontaneously for 12 hours because of swelling of the perineum as well as anxiety that urination might be painful. Because an empty bladder is important postpartum in preventing postpartum hemorrhage, she was catheterized on two different occasions to empty her bladder.

It is important that women void within the first 6 or so hours after the birth for a few reasons. Distention of the bladder can lead to displacement of the uterus, which may cause uterine atony and bleeding. Retention of urine may lead to an infection that causes inflammation of the urinary bladder, called cystitis. Symptoms of cystitis include pain with voiding, urinary frequency, and a sense of urgency with urination without voiding a large amount. Urinary frequency is common during the postpartum period, however, and should not be considered concerning if a substantial amount is voided.

Nursing Care

Early in the postpartum period, the nurse should instruct the patient to void into a urine collection device known as a hat, which is placed in the toilet, so that the volume of each void may be assessed to verify that urine is not being retained (Fig. 17.14). An adequate void is 150 mL or more. The patient initially may find it easier to void if she is given extra privacy, runs water from the faucet, and sprays warm water over her perineum from the peri bottle. Placing peppermint oil drops in the hat may help the urinary sphincter to relax, promoting urination (see Box 9.6). Women who have not voided spontaneously within 12 hours after the birth may need to be catheterized with a Foley or a straight (in and out) catheter. Voiding issues related to edema should resolve within 24 hours after the birth.

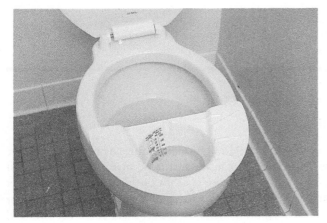

Figure 17.14. A calibrated urine collection container, sometimes referred to as a "hat." (Photo by B. Proud.)

Gastrointestinal System

Physiologic Changes

Postpartum patients may not have a bowel movement for a few days after the birth because of having had diarrhea in early labor or passing stool during the second stage of labor. Although progesterone levels drop quickly after the birth of the placenta, the action of progesterone to reduce peristalsis of the bowel can still slow stool transit. The dehydration that often raises the maternal temperature in the first 24 hours of the birth can also contribute to constipation, as can the modified bed rest common to many women in the immediate postpartum period. As with urinary retention, women may fear the pain of a bowel movement after experiencing perineal trauma during the birth. Reduced intraabdominal pressure resulting from the birth of the fetus relieves pressure on the bowels, which can also slow stool transit. Analgesics, particularly opioids, also contribute to constipation. Stool softeners are given routinely to make bowel movements less dense and painful (see The Pharmacy 9.2). Adequate hydration and a diet higher in fiber can help increase the bulk of the stool and counteract or even prevent constipation.

In Chapter 9, Nancy was just as daunted by the idea of a bowel movement as she was by urination. She was concerned that she would tear through her stitches. She tried drinking warm liquids, including prune juice and peppermint tea, and eating fiber. She ambulated regularly to stimulate her bowels. She wanted to avoid taking a laxative if possible.

Approximately 10 to 13 lb are lost during childbirth, which includes the weight of the neonate, uterus, blood, and fetal membranes. An additional 5 to 8 lb is lost because of uterine involution and the resolution of extra interstitial and intravascular fluids. The fat gained during pregnancy is lost more slowly, over a period of months, and women who breastfeed for 6 months or more tend to lose more weight than those who do not (Martin, MacDonald-Wicks, Hure, Smith, & Collins, 2015).

Nursing Care

To prevent constipation, the nurse should administer any ordered stool softener, such as docusate, and explain to the patient its purpose. During routine assessments, the nurse should ask whether the patient is passing gas or stool and listen to the patient's bowel sounds. A lack of bowel sounds indicates an **ileus** (lack of peristalsis), which is more common after a cesarean section. The nurse should be prepared to address a postpartum woman's hunger by making sure the patient receives sufficient nutrition. Women may be hungry immediately after the birth and for several days afterward and may eat and drink a regular diet unless otherwise indicated.

Musculoskeletal System

Physiologic Changes

Joints that became more lax during pregnancy because of the effects of estrogen, progestin, and relaxin begin to return to their prepregnancy state postpartum, although some women may report permanently requiring a larger shoe size. Within 6 to 8 weeks, the joints should be entirely stabilized and any residual pain associated with joint laxity should resolve. Muscles that were stretched out by the growing uterus during pregnancy remain soft and flabby in the postpartum period until muscle tone is regained through muscle atrophy and exercise of the abdominal muscles.

Nursing Care

Some women may anticipate a quick return to a flat abdomen postpartum and may require reassurance that their muscles will become more toned over time, although work may be required. Often, women find they may not be able to exercise as they wish for several weeks postpartum either because of surgical recovery, muscle laxity, or both. Some women who experienced pain related to joint laxity may continue to have discomfort in the immediate postpartum period and may require reassurance and support.

Neurologic System

Physiologic Changes

Women who have an epidural, spinal-epidural, or spinal, (collectively known as intrathecal anesthesia or local anesthesia) should have a full return of sensation within a few hours after the last administration of the medication. Rarely, epidural and spinal anesthesia can result in an acute and very painful headache because of leakage of the cerebrospinal fluid. Such headaches are usually worse when the patient is upright and improve somewhat when lying down. The anesthesia provider should be informed if a cerebrospinal leak is suspected.

Headaches postpartum are not uncommon and, like headaches at other times, may have different causes. A headache in conjunction with a blood pressure reading of over 140/90 mm Hg is concerning for preeclampsia that has continued from the pregnancy or is of new onset, and the nurse should notify the obstetric provider of such findings.

Nursing Care

Pain assessment and management are a critical part of nursing. Nurses should be alert for maternal discomfort and the need for postpartum analgesia, particularly for women who had traumatic or surgical births. Women who have received intrathecal anesthesia should initially ambulate with assistance until full sensation has returned and they can do so without presenting a fall risk.

As previously mentioned, most patients have scheduled ibuprofen and acetaminophen available. Prior to dispensing pain medication, the nurse should assess the patient's pain using a pain scale. A half hour after the administration, the nurse should assess the patient's pain again to determine whether the intervention had its intended effect. In addition, patients may be prescribed opioid medications. Nurses should inform patients receiving opioids that the medication may make them drowsy and that constipation is a common side effect. Nurses should also inform patients that small amounts of the analgesics they take may pass to the baby via breast milk, although this is unlikely to be harmful.

Postpartum Psychosocial Changes and Care

The postpartum period is a time of tremendous adjustment for the new mother, the partner of the pregnancy, and other family members. Often, postpartum nurses see only a brief portion of this transition in the first few days postpartum. The process of attachment, which in most cases starts prior to the birth, is enhanced by sustained contact between the newborn and his or her family. The mother's active involvement in the care of the newborn and skin-to-skin contact can facilitate this process. Equally, situations that restrict contact with the newborn may impede the process (see Chapter 24).

Although usually a joyful event, the birth and the integration of a new demanding, helpless person can be tremendously stressful and draining. The nurse should encourage the woman and her family to process the birth by talking and discussing their fears, frustrations, and challenges in caring for a newborn. She may observe the new mother's emotional status by watching how she interacts with the new infant, visitors, and any support people and observing her level of independence and energy. Crying, mood swings, irritability, or a flattened affect may indicate a continuation or exacerbation of an existing psychosocial issue or the emergence of a new problem. The nurse should communicate any concerns to the obstetric provider or an institutional social worker (see Chapter 23).

In Chapter 11, Marnie was concerned that Edie might be depressed. She encouraged her to talk about her birth experience and her concerns about her baby and her own body. Marnie encouraged her to talk with a social worker to develop a plan for her mental health. Edie was concerned that her husband, Frank, wouldn't approve.

Psychosocial Changes

Bonding

Bonding is the unidirectional attraction a new parent has to the newborn beginning in the first hour after the birth. For most newborns, this first hour after the birth is a time of being quiet and alert, often looking directly at the person holding him or her. Of note, the distance between the face of the newborn and the face of the person holding him or her is the distance of the newborn's optimal visual acuity.

Attachment

Although bonding is attraction, attachment is affection. This is a reciprocal process that occurs over time and is a much longer process than bonding. Providing routine care and activities that seek to stimulate a reaction, such as soothing and singing, can facilitate attachment. As infants mature and grow, they respond to stimulation with smiles, coos, and other actions. Bonding is the beginning part of this process.

The backgrounds, culture, and upbringing of the parents may impact the process of attachment, because the expectations and experiences of interaction may encourage or discourage behaviors that facilitate attachment. The health, appearance, and temperament of the newborn may also affect attachment. If the newborn does not meet the expectations held prior to and throughout the pregnancy, attachment may be slowed or prevented. Care practices, too, may have a direct impact on attachment. Institutional practice or the health of the newborn or mother may call for separation of the infant from the parents, negatively impacting attachment. A restrictive visitor policy that does not allow the parents to share their newborn with friends and family may impact attachment. A lack of support from staff and others may also preclude attachment.

Maternal Adaptation Phases

As described by Reva Rubin, the phases of maternal adaptation are taking in, taking hold, and letting go (Sluetal, 2002). The taking-in phase is marked by dependent behavior on the part of the mother, in which she, recovering from pregnancy and birth, takes a passive role in her own care and that of the newborn. In this phase, the mother often processes the birth experience by talking it through with one or more people. The taking-hold phase is a period of transition from dependent to independent behavior and may last several weeks. In this phase, the mother is growing used to her new reality and is focused on taking charge of the care of herself and her newborn. She may require reassurance that her actions are correct and her care of herself and the newborn is sufficient. The last phase, the letting-go phase, is more inclusive of other people. She acknowledges the new normal, the baby as a person instead of a much-speculated upon idea, and her altered position in her new life.

Partner Adaptation Phases

The partner of the pregnancy is also likely to progress through the predictable stages of adjustment (Goodman, 2005). Just as with the maternal phases, however, not all partners have the same experience of adjustment, any more than all mothers have the same experience. Timing of the phases and how a phase is perceived and managed may differ among individuals, couples, and particular situations.

The first phase starts prior to the birth and even prior to the pregnancy. It is a time when a partner considers how he or she was parented and what kind of parent he or she wants to be. The partner's lived experience of being parented may be quite different from his or her own expectations of a desirable parenting strategy. This may be perceived as a time of an idealized imagining of parenting.

The second phase incorporates the reality of infant care and the changes in the relationship with his or her partner. The incorporation of new responsibilities with old ones can be overwhelming and isolating. The expectations of the first phase may be swiftly dwarfed in the second stage. Partners may want to have an active role but have limited ability to do so. A mother's preoccupation with the newborn and her own healing may provoke a sense of aloneness in the partner.

In the third phase, the partner of the pregnancy learns to take hold of the new role. Positive reinforcement from the mother can help build confidence and allay anxiety about infant care. In the final phase, signs of reciprocity at 6 to 8 weeks of age begin to enhance the parent–child relationship as the infant responds to overtures from other people with eye contact, cooing, calming, smiling, and laughing.

Nursing Care

Parents often expect that they will fall instantly in love and become immediately attached to the newborn at birth. In truth, for most people attachment is more of a process, and the nurse should reassure parents if they don't immediately feel it. Some new parents report that they feel immediately protective and nurturing of the newborn but that the process of falling in love and becoming attached takes much longer.

As parents adapt to parenthood, encouragement from healthcare providers can help parents gain the skills and confidence necessary for their success. The nurse can teach parents simple essential skills, such as swaddling and soothing of the infant, that are helpful from a practical perspective but also aid in the attachment and role attainment process. A new infant can be overwhelming, and the nurse should reassure parents that this is a normal feeling and that rest and accepting help from friends and family can be important coping strategies.

Through all stages of pregnancy, infancy, and childhood, partners may feel marginalized and excluded by healthcare providers and professional support people. Such exclusion can be discouraging for partners and make them question the importance of their role in the life of the infant and family. It is a nursing responsibility to encourage partners to participate in care as much as possible. Partners should be educated along with partners about infant and self-care measures. The concept of teamwork should be integrated into all teaching.

Variations in Postpartum Care After a Cesarean Section

Women recovering from a cesarean section are coping with the changes that come with the birth in addition to recovering from major abdominal surgery. Initial hospitalization following a cesarean section is usually 3 to 5 days, as opposed to 48 hours after an uncomplicated vaginal birth. Full recovery from the surgery can take 6 weeks. Complications are more likely with a cesarean section than with a vaginal birth, particularly if the procedure was emergent rather than planned (Creanga et al., 2015) (Table 17.2; see Chapter 23).

Table 17.2 Common Complications of Cesarean Delivery

Complication	Description	Occurrence Rate in Birth (%) Cesarean	Vaginal	Signs and Symptoms
Endometritis	Inflammation of the inner lining of the uterus, usually from infection	6–11*	<3[†]	• Fever after first 24 h • Midline pelvic pain • Tachycardia • Uterine tenderness
Wound	Dehiscence, infection, hematoma, or seroma	1–2*	NA	• Usually manifests 4–10 d after surgery but may occur in first 48 h • Cellulitis • Fever • Poor wound approximation • Purulent discharge • Swelling
Hemorrhage	>500 mL of blood loss with a vaginal birth; >1,000 mL with a cesarean birth	0.43[‡]	0.23[‡]	• Vaginal bleeding greater than expected • Pallor • Tachycardia • Air hunger • Weakness • Confusion • Syncope • Palpitations • Hypotension
Surgical injury	Injury to the maternal bowel or urinary tract	0.2–0.5*	NA	• Fever • Anuria or oliguria • Hematuria • Flank pain • Nausea and/or vomiting • Ileus • Abdominal distension or pain
Blood clot	A mass of coagulated blood that can occlude a blood vessel, leading to deep vein thrombosis, pulmonary embolism, stroke, or myocardial infarction	0.246**	0.165**	Of deep vein thrombosis: • Leg pain • Leg swelling • Area of warmth and induration on the leg Of pulmonary embolism and myocardial infarction: • Shortness of breath • Chest pain Of stroke: • Sudden unilateral numbness or weakness • Sudden confusion or difficulty with communication or comprehension • Sudden vision change • Sudden problem with balance, coordination, or ambulation • Sudden severe headache
Ileus	Diminished peristalsis that leads to a buildup of waste, liquid, and gas	10–20*	NA	• No passage of stool or flatus • Nausea or vomiting • Abdominal distention

NA, not available.
*Data adapted from Hammad, I., Chauhan, S., Magann, E., & Abuhamad, A. (2014). Peripartum complications with cesarean delivery: A review of maternal-fetal medicine units network publications. *Journal of Maternal, Fetal, and Neonatal Medicine, 27*(5), 463–474.
[†]Data adapted from Burrows, L., Meyn, L., & Weber, A. (2004). Maternal morbidity associated with vaginal versus cesarean delivery. *Obstetrics and Gynecolocy, 103*(5), 907.
[‡]Data adapted from Kramer, M. S., Berg, C., Abenhaim, H., Dahhou, M., Rouleaud, J., Mehrabadi, A., & Joseph, K. (2013). Incidence, risk factors, and temporal trends in severe postpartum hemorrhage. *American Journal of Obstetrics and Gynecology, 209*(5), 449.e1–449.e7.
**Data adapted from Kamel, H., Navi, B., Sriram, N., Hovsepian, D., Devereux, R., & Elkind, M. (2014). Risk of a thrombotic event after the 6-week postpartum period. *New England Journal of Medicine, 370*(14), 1307.

Immediate Postoperative, Postpartum Care

Care after a cesarean section is in some ways more akin to the care in a postanesthesia care unit than care after a vaginal delivery. Care includes one-on-one nursing for the mother, with another nurse assigned to her newborn. As per the protocols of the institution, postoperative vaginal bleeding onto chux and eventually pads is often weighed. A gram of blood loss equals 1 mL, and there are 1,000 mL/L. The nurse should carefully monitor the patient's oral and IV intake and urinary output.

Most cesarean births are performed with anesthesia in place rather than general anesthesia. Hypothermia is common after the spinal anesthesia, and that it's also not uncommon for women not to recognize that their temperature has dropped (Shawa, Steelmana, DeBergb, & Schweizer, 2017). The nurse may dress a woman who experiences hypothermia in a thermal gown and infuse her with warmed IV fluids.

The First 24 Hours

After a cesarean section, the nurse should check vital signs every hour for the first 4 hours, then every 4 hours until stable, and then once every 8-hour shift. The nurse should assess the patient regularly for pain and a return of sensation after discontinuation of spinal anesthesia. After a cesarean section, most patients have a standing order for an oral opioid, as well as ibuprofen and acetaminophen. A bandage should remain in place over the cesarean section incision for 24 hours, and the nurse should check it regularly for seepage. Because these women are at a higher risk for blood clots after surgery, they often require compression boots on their legs to stimulate blood flow until they can ambulate regularly.

Morphine is a common component of spinal anesthesia and may be provided IV for some patients after discontinuation of spinal anesthesia. Like all opioids, morphine can cause respiratory depression, making the evaluation of respirations and level of consciousness particularly important. Morphine can also cause pruritus, nausea and vomiting, and urinary retention after removal of the catheter. All of these side effects may be treated with naloxone, which reverses the effect of opioids. Pruritus may also be treated with diphenhydramine. Urinary retention may be treated with periodic catheterization, and the nausea and vomiting may be treated with an antiemetic. A woman with respiratory depression may be given oxygen in addition to or instead of naloxone (The Pharmacy 17.1).

As with a vaginal birth, routine lochia and fundal checks are indicated for cesarean births. Oxytocin is regularly administered IV after a cesarean section because anesthesia increases the risk for uterine atony and hemorrhage. After an abdominal surgery, a portion of the bowel may stop moving, a condition referred to as an ileus. An ileus can cause acute abdominal pain and nausea. Flatus is generally considered evidence of a functioning bowel, as are normal bowel sounds by auscultation with a stethoscope.

A Foley catheter is placed prior to a cesarean section and is generally left in place until the patient can safely ambulate to the

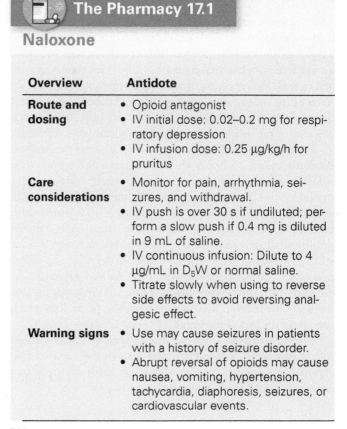

The Pharmacy 17.1

Naloxone

Overview	Antidote
Route and dosing	• Opioid antagonist • IV initial dose: 0.02–0.2 mg for respiratory depression • IV infusion dose: 0.25 µg/kg/h for pruritus
Care considerations	• Monitor for pain, arrhythmia, seizures, and withdrawal. • IV push is over 30 s if undiluted; perform a slow push if 0.4 mg is diluted in 9 mL of saline. • IV continuous infusion: Dilute to 4 µg/mL in D_5W or normal saline. • Titrate slowly when using to reverse side effects to avoid reversing analgesic effect.
Warning signs	• Use may cause seizures in patients with a history of seizure disorder. • Abrupt reversal of opioids may cause nausea, vomiting, hypertension, tachycardia, diaphoresis, seizures, or cardiovascular events.

IV, intravenous.

bathroom independently. For early trips to the bathroom, the nurse should assist the patient to ensure safety.

In Chapter 3, Susan gave birth by planned cesarean section. She didn't like having the compression devices on her legs and was eager to ambulate to the bathroom with Betty, a nurse, so she could stop using them.

Patients who are breastfeeding should take extra care when positioning the infant to avoid putting uncomfortable pressure on the abdomen and incision.

Women who deliver by cesarean section, particularly if the surgery was unplanned, may feel a sense of letdown. They may be disappointed that their birth did not go as planned or feel that their body failed in an essential task. The nurse should encourage women who are struggling with such feelings after a cesarean birth to talk about their experience. Although few women would disagree that the birth of a healthy infant is the ultimate goal of any birth, it does not mean there isn't room for a woman to have negative feelings about the birth itself. Facilitating the expression of such feelings by the nurse can be therapeutic.

Until Discharge

After approximately 24 hours, the care of a woman who has given birth by cesarean section is similar to the care of a woman who has had an uncomplicated vaginal delivery. Her fundus and lochia are assessed with her vital signs every shift. Her pain is assessed and treated. She's encouraged to ambulate and stay hydrated. She starts eating shortly after her surgery, after her bowel sounds and flatus return. The patient may require more help with self-care and care of the infant while in the hospital and after discharge.

The nurse generally removes the dressing over the cesarean section incision 24 hours after the surgery and inspects the wound; it should show minimal signs of seepage. After removing this bulky dressing, the nurse places a lighter dressing that can be easily removed for incision checks. The incision is closed either with stitches or staples. Staples and stitches are usually removed prior to discharge on day 4 or 5 postpartum, although internal stitches, as well as some stitches that close the skin, will absorb over time. Timing of the removal of sutures and staples is a decision of the obstetric provider, however, who may opt for later removal. The incision itself is approximately 12 cm long and is just above the line of the pubic hair (Fig. 17.15).

Women are advised to avoid lifting anything heavier than the infant for 4 to 6 weeks and to slowly increase their activity level according to comfort. Women should not drive as long as they are taking opioid medications such as oxytocin.

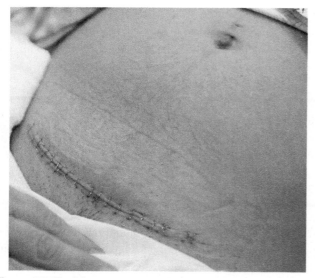

Figure 17.15. A low-transverse incision for a cesarean birth (also called a Pfannenstiel incision). In this type of incision, both the skin and the uterus are cut horizontally, which minimizes the risk for uterine rupture with future pregnancies and labors. A vertical incision of the uterus, conversely, makes uterine rupture more likely with future pregnancies and labors. This wound is closed with staples. Many wounds are closed with stitches, which minimize scarring. (Reprinted with permission from Evans, R. J., Brown, Y. M., & Evans, M. K. [2014]. *Canadian maternity, newborn, and women's health nursing* [2nd ed., Fig. 16.26]. Philadelphia, PA: Lippincott Williams & Wilkins.)

Postpartum Discharge Planning

Discharge planning starts from the moment a family is admitted. A woman may be discharged within 48 hours of an uncomplicated vaginal birth and within 72 hours of an uncomplicated cesarean birth. Although an early discharge may be advantageous for families wishing to go home and settle into their new roles, they may also feel they are ill-prepared to deal with all of the physical, emotional, and lifestyle changes the birth has brought with it. The need to assimilate information about infant care and feeding, maternal discomfort, maternal nutrition and activity, contraception, immunizations, and any variations that may complicate any of these considerations may seem overwhelming. Discharge teaching regarding the infant is discussed in Chapter 18.

As shown in Patient Teaching 17.1, the nurse should be aware of and communicate to the patient clinical signs of common postpartum complications that indicate the need for further assessment. The nurse should instruct the patient to contact her obstetric provider should she note these signs after discharge.

The nurse should also provide discharge instructions concerning anticipated postpartum physical changes (Patient Teaching 17.2) and self-care measures (Patient Teaching 17.3), such as good nutrition and the appropriate use of contraception.

✚ Patient Teaching 17.1

Signs of Postpartum Complications That Should Be Reported

Sign	Possible Complication
New onset pain, burning, urgency, or frequency of urination	Urinary tract infection
New onset focal leg pain and warmth	Deep vein thrombosis
Chest pain and shortness of breath	Pulmonary embolism
Localized, firm area of redness on the breast, especially with flu-like symptoms	Mastitis
Pelvic pain	Infection of pelvic organs or urinary tract
Elevated temperature	Infection
Foul-smelling lochia	Infection
Return of heavy, bright red lochia lasting for more than a few hours	Secondary postpartum hemorrhage
Sustained depressed mood or sadness; thoughts of hurting self or infant	Postpartum depression or postpartum psychosis

Note: See Chapter 23 for a detailed discussion of postpartum complications.

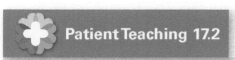

Change	Significance
Breast engorgement	• Primary breast engorgement occurs as lactation transitions from colostrum to milk and the volume increases. • If breast fullness prevents latch, express milk before feeding. • If not breastfeeding, avoid breast stimulation and wear a supportive bra around the clock for several days.
Diaphoresis and diuresis	• Expect increased sweating and urinary frequency for several days postpartum as your body eliminates fluid accumulated in pregnancy. Drink plenty of fluids. • If clothes become wet because of sweating, change them frequently to avoid chills. • Urinate frequently to avoid uterine atony.
Weight loss	• Approximately 12 lb of the weight gained in pregnancy is lost at the time of birth. • An additional 5–8 lb is lost because of elimination of fluid and uterine involution.
Uterine involution and lochia	• Education about expected involution • Education about expected progression of lochia

Patient Teaching 17.3   Postpartum Self-Care

Aspect of Care	Instructions and Education
Perineal care	• Continue to use the peri bottle, as desired. • Change your pad frequently.
Breast care	• If not breastfeeding, avoid nipple stimulation and wear a supportive bra night and day. Engorgement should resolve within a week. • If breastfeeding, monitor for nipple breakdown and symptoms suggesting mastitis. • Consult with an outpatient lactation specialist, as needed.
Pain control	To alleviate pain, take acetaminophen or ibuprofen and apply ice or heat.
Discharge medications	Review all medications prescribed for use after discharge, including the purpose of the medication, correct use, dosing, and common potential side effects.
Nutrition needs	If lactating, stay well hydrated and eat approximately 500 calories more than when not lactating.
Activity and exercise	• Start exercise gradually, as tolerated. • An increase in lochia may result from exercising too much, too early. • Abdominal exercises may not be possible in the early postpartum period due to muscle weakness or recent abdominal surgery (in the case of cesarean delivery). • Walk regularly to reduce the risk of a thrombus or constipation.
Rest	Learn to rest when the baby does and to accept help from others to care for the baby and take care of other activities of daily living.
Contraception	• Remember that it's possible for you to get pregnant even before your first scheduled postpartum visit with the obstetric provider. • Make a plan for contraception use prior to discharge.
Sexual activity	• Resume sexual activity when you feel ready both physically and emotionally. • You may need to use additional lubrication because of hormonal changes to increase comfort.
Smoking	• Avoid smoking near your newborn and exposing your newborn to the secondhand smoke of others. • If you stopped smoking during the pregnancy, continue smoking cessation. • If you currently smoke, strongly consider stopping. • Consider using counseling services, medications, and peer support programs to help you stop smoking.

Think Critically

1. You are checking your patient's lochia. Before drawing any conclusions about her saturated pad, what factors must be considered?
2. Why is it important for a woman to empty her bladder frequently postpartum?
3. You patient is having difficulty urinating spontaneously. What measures do you try prior to catheterization?
4. What factors do you think would inhibit bonding and attachment between parents and their newborn?
5. Your patient sits up to ambulate to the bathroom and tells you she feels light-headed. What do you do?
6. Your patient complains of calf pain. What questions do you ask? What physical assessments are important for her?
7. Your patient's partner takes you aside because he's concerned the patient is acting very passively, which is unusual for her. He's wondering if something's wrong. What do you say or do?
8. You are changing the diaper of a newborn and making it a point to include the partner of the pregnancy in the process. Why is this a good idea?
9. Your patient gave birth an hour ago by cesarean section. How do you expect you'll time her future assessments?
10. You are discussing discharge with a patient. What would you tell her are reasons to call her obstetric provider?

References

Ambesh, P. (2017). Homan's sign for deep vein thrombosis: A grain of salt? *Indian Heart Journal, 69*(3), 418–419.

Appareddy, S., Pryor, J., & Bailey, B. (2016). Inter-pregnancy interval and adverse outcomes: Evidence for an additional risk in health disparate populations. *The Journal of Maternal-Fetal and Neonatal Medicine*, 1–5.

Centers for Disease Control and Prevention. (2017, November 9). *Pregnancy mortality surveillance system.* Retrieved from https://www.cdc.gov/reproductivehealth/maternalinfanthealth/pmss.html

Creanga, A., Bateman, B., Butwick, A., Raleigh, L., Maeda, A., Kuklina, E., & Callaghan, W. (2015). Morbidity associated with cesarean delivery in the United States: Is placenta accreta an increasingly important contributor? *American Journal of Obstetrics and Gynecology, 231*(3), 384.e1–384.e11.

Eshkevari, L., Trout, K. K., & Damore, J. (2013). Management of postpartum pain. *Journal of Women's Health and Midwifery, 58*(6), 622–631.

Goodman, J. (2005). Becoming an involved father of an infant. *Journal of Obstetric and Gynecologic Nursing, 34*(2), 190–200.

Martin, J., MacDonald-Wicks, L., Hure, A., Smith, R., & Collins, C. E. (2015). Reducing postpartum weight retention and improving breastfeeding outcomes in overweight women: A pilot randomised controlled trial. *Nutrients, 7*(3), 1464–1479.

McGee, S. (2012). *Evidence-based physical diagnosis.* Philadelphia, PA: Saunders.

Shawa, C. A., Steelmana, V. M., DeBergb, J., & Schweizer, M. L. (2017). Effectiveness of active and passive warming for the prevention of inadvertent hypothermia in patients receiving neuraxial anesthesia: A systematic review and meta-analysis of randomized controlled trials. *Journal of Clinical Anesthesia, 38*, 93–104.

Sluetal, M. R. (2002). Intrapartum nursing: Integrating Rubin's framework with social support theory. *Journal of Obstetric, Gynecologic, and Neonatal Nursing, 32*(1), 76–82.

Van der Wijden, C., & Manion, C. (2015). Lactational amenorrhoea method for family planning. *Cochrane Database of Systematic Reviews,* (10), CD001329.

Suggested Readings

Chan, Z. C., Wong, K. S., Lam, W. M., Wong, K. Y., & Kwok, Y. C. (2013). An exploration of postpartum women's perspective on desired obstetric nursing qualities. *Journal of Clinical Nursing, 23*(1–2), 103–112.

Harrington, D. (2013). Preventing and recognizing venous thromboembolism after obstetric and gynecologic surgery. *Nursing for Women's Health, 17*(4), 325–329.

Lai, Y.-L., Hung, C.-H., Stocker, J., Chan, T.-F., & Liu, Y. (2015). Postpartum fatigue, baby-care activities, and maternal–infant attachment of vaginal and cesarean births following rooming-in. *Applied Nursing Research, 28*(2), 116–120.

Martins, H. E., Souza, M. D., Khanum, S., Naz, N., & Souza, A. C. (2016). The practice of nursing in the prevention and control of postpartum hemorrhage: An integrative review. *American Journal of Nursing Science, 5*, 8–15.

18 The Newborn

For infants born at term, the transition to life outside the uterus is typically low risk and straightforward. Essential early physiologic changes include establishing and maintaining respiratory function, temperature regulation, initiation of nutrition and passage of waste via the bowel, weight maintenance, circulatory changes, and extrauterine adaptations to stimuli outside of the womb. The important aspects of the newborn's care to support an uneventful transition in the first 28 days outside the womb (known as the **neonatal period**) include assisting parents and caregivers in providing infant nutrition and other care of the newborn, maintaining neonatal body heat, monitoring respiratory function, and minimizing the risk of neonatal infection through action and education.

Anatomic and Physiologic Changes in the Newborn

The clamping of the umbilical cord and the first breath of the neonate begin the transition to extrauterine life. The placenta, which had functioned as the lungs, nutrition source, and temporary endocrine gland of pregnancy, is no longer available, and the neonate must adapt quickly to a new environment away from the warmth and protection of the womb. This transition period typically lasts 6 to 8 hours after the birth.

At birth, the healthy term infant is active and alert. The heart rate is 120 to 160 beats per minute (bpm), and respirations are rapid and irregular (40 to 60 breaths per minute). Neonates in this period may appear particularly likely to startle, and crying and tremors are not unexpected. Bowel sounds are active and it is common for the first meconium to pass at this time. This period typically lasts up to 30 minutes, although the alertness of the neonate may persist for as long as 1 to 2 hours. This phase is referred to as the first period of reactivity (Cavaliere, 2016; Desmond, Rudolph, & Phitaksphraiwan, 1966). This is an optimal time for early bonding and initiation of breastfeeding.

The second phase is a time of sleep and may last several hours. The respiratory and heart rates slow to within normal parameters. The neonate's breathing should be unlabored, with no grunting, retractions, or crackles. The neonate should be allowed to sleep and is unlikely to show interest in feeding if awoken.

The final phase of transition is the second period of reactivity, which occurs any time between 2 hours after the birth to 8 hours. It may last minutes or several hours. During this phase, the newborn is alert and has increased heart rate, respiratory rate, and muscle tone. Mucus production increases, and neonates can gag more easily and require suction of their mouths and nares as respiratory secretions break up. Meconium is often passed at this time.

Respiratory System

Changes

The cues to start breathing are mechanical, chemical, and thermal. The fetus starts "practice breathing" as early as the first trimester, although the lungs are not completely functional until the end of a term pregnancy.

The chemicals that cue breathing in the neonate are CO_2 and O_2. When the cord is clamped and the placenta can no longer provide the exchange of CO_2 and O_2, this creates a mild state of hypoxia, similar to that produced when holding one's breath. This increase in CO_2 causes acidosis, which stimulates the respiratory center of the medulla oblongata of the brain, which in turn stimulates breathing. Repeated mild hypoxia throughout labor as the uterus contracts and temporarily restricts the exchange of CO_2 and O_2 may also contribute to this process.

The lungs of the neonate have fluid in them, despite the fluid having decreased as the pregnancy neared term and during labor (because some is expelled from the lungs as the fetus squeezes through the birth canal) and after delivery and despite an increase in catecholamines, which promote clearance of fluid from the lungs. The lymphatic system also absorbs some of the fluid.

The squeeze through the birth canal is the mechanical mechanism that helps initiate breathing. In addition to helping to clear fluid from the lungs, this event causes a rebound of thoracic expansion as the chest leaves the birth canal. This rebound of the chest to its previous dimensions pulls in air, much like a set of bellows. The surfactant that lines the alveoli of mature neonatal lungs keeps the alveoli from collapsing completely while reducing the surface tension of the alveoli, thus minimizing the amount of pressure necessary to keep the lungs open. Crying encourages expansion of the alveoli, as well.

When leaving the mother's body, the neonate goes from a liquid environment to one that is dry. The temperature drops, and the newborn, who, as a fetus, was typically 0.5°C warmer than the mother, is now losing heat by convection, conduction, evaporation, and radiation. This change in temperature is also believed to stimulate the respiratory center of the medulla oblongata; thus the change of temperature is the thermal mechanism that helps initiate breathing. Lights, smells, sounds, handling of the newborn, suctioning, and other stimuli may excite the respiratory center of the medulla.

The breathing of the neonate is fast and shallow, typically ranging from 40 to 60 breaths per minute. Pauses in breathing that last up to 20 seconds are considered normal, but longer periods of apnea are concerning. In healthy newborns, the chest and abdomen rise and fall synchronously during breathing. Seesaw breathing, a type of breathing in which the abdomen rises as the chest falls, is abnormal and should be reported (Table 18.1). Patent nares must be maintained, as newborns are preferential nose breathers.

Care Considerations

Monitoring of neonatal breathing and oxygenation is a critical task of the nurse postpartum. The nurse should evaluate respirations at the time of each assessment and address any signs of respiratory distress promptly (see Table 18.1). It is best to assess the respiratory rate when the newborn is not crying. The nurse should observe both the chest and abdomen for retractions and seesaw breathing. Some nurses, particularly new learners, may find it helpful to lightly lay a hand on an infant's torso when counting respirations to have tactile confirmation of individual breaths, which can be challenging to visualize and count accurately.

In Chapter 8, the pediatrician caring for Gracie's baby recognized that he was in respiratory distress because he was tachypneic, with flaring of the nares and intercostal and subcostal retractions. He made a grunting noises with expiration.

Cardiovascular System

Changes

Just as significant physiologic changes must occur to initiate and sustain breathing, major anatomic changes must occur at birth for the successful establishment of a mature circulatory system. The two are not mutually exclusive, because respiratory changes influence changes in the circulatory system. The newborn's first breaths expand the lungs, but they also dilate the pulmonary vasculature, reducing pulmonary vascular resistance. This results in an increase in blood return from the lungs to the left atrium. The left atrium is now higher in pressure than the right atrium, causing the foramen ovale, a small hole in the wall between the two atria, to close. At the same time, systemic vascular resistance increases because of the clamping of the umbilical cord. The clamping of the cord also eliminates

Table 18.1 Signs of Respiratory Distress

Sign	Clinical Considerations
Cyanosis	Acrocyanosis, a blue color of the neonate's hands and feet, is normal in the first 24 h postpartum. Central cyanosis, which is indicated by bluing of the lips and chest, is abnormal. Transient cyanosis when crying is not uncommon immediately after birth.
Apnea	Cessation of breathing for 20 s or more is concerning. Shorter periods of apnea in the absence of other signs of distress are considered normal. Apnea over 20 s may indicate sepsis, hypothermia, hypoglycemia, or another problem.
Tachypnea	Neonates typically take 30–60 breaths per minute. Sustained tachypnea is abnormal and may indicate respiratory distress syndrome (see Chapter 24) or fluid in the lungs. It may also indicate infection or cardiac or metabolic illness.
Intercostal or substernal retractions (see Fig. 5.11)	Retractions are the pulling in of tissue with each breath and indicate reduced pressure inside the lungs, likely because of occlusion of the upper airways.
Grunting	Grunting with expiration occurs with a partially closed glottis. This partial occlusion increases the pressure within the lungs so more oxygen can diffuse into the bloodstream. Grunting may be auscultated with a stethoscope or, in more severe cases, heard without assistance.
Nasal flaring	Nasal flaring expands the airway and reduces airway resistance.
Seesaw breathing	The chest and abdomen rise simultaneously in the absence of respiratory distress. Seesaw breathing, like retractions, suggests partial blockage of the airways.
Stridor	Stridor, which is an abnormal, high-pitched breath sound, is a sign of upper airway obstruction.
Gasping	Gasping is a sign of upper airway obstruction.

the blood flow through the ductus venosus, which begins to atrophy. Closure of the ductus arteriosus, which shunts blood from the pulmonary artery to the aorta, happens more slowly, over days or weeks, likely influenced by hormonal, chemical, and pressure processes.

Ultimately, when all of the adaptations are complete, deoxygenated blood enters the heart through the superior and inferior vena cava into the right atrium. The blood then travels into the right ventricle, then the pulmonary artery, and then into the vascular bed of the lungs, where oxygen and carbon dioxide are exchanged. The oxygenated blood then travels through the pulmonary veins into the left atrium, then into the left ventricle, and then through the aorta to the systemic circulation.

Term neonates have a higher hemoglobin concentration (14 to 24 g/dL) than do adults (12.1 to 17.2 g/dL) or even older infants (9.5 to 13 g/dL). Their hematocrit levels are typically between 51% and 56%. Fetal hemoglobin differs from adult hemoglobin and has a shorter life span, thus the hemoglobin and hematocrit levels drop quickly after birth. The fetal red blood cell of a term infant has a life span of 60 to 90 days, compared with 120 days in an adult. By 20 weeks, only 5% of hemoglobin is fetal and the remainder is mature (Christensen & Yaish, 2016).

Leukocytosis, or a condition of elevated white blood cell count, is normal at birth, with the typical term neonate having a white blood cell count between 9,000 and 30,000/mm³. This count usually increases in the day after the birth before decreasing to 12,000/mm³. For context, a count above 11,000/mm³ is typically considered high in an adult. Therefore, white blood cell count is not considered a reliable indicator of infection in the neonate. Some infants may have a rise in neutrophils with infection, whereas others may not. Further complicating the situation, the infant's white blood cell count may go up for reasons unrelated to infection, such as exposure to oxytocin during labor, birth at high altitude, prolonged crying, and other causes. In contrast with red blood cell and white blood cell counts, the platelet count for the neonate is similar to that of an adult: 150,000 to 300,000. However, clotting factors are low during the first days of extrauterine life due to a low level of vitamin K. Vitamin K is usually obtained as a by-product of gut bacteria and through diet. The gut of the neonate is sterile and does not yet have bacteria present to create vitamin K. In addition, vitamin K does not cross the placenta, and there is little of it in breast milk. The bacteria in the gut of the newborn are not sufficient for the infant's needs for several weeks postpartum.

Care Considerations

At birth, newborns are given a shot of vitamin K so that the liver will create the clotting factors necessary to prevent a pathologic bleed that may be life-threatening (Fig. 18.1). The injection is usually done with a 5/8-in 25-gauge needle in the vastus lateralis muscle of the anterior thigh. Since 1961, a vitamin K injection

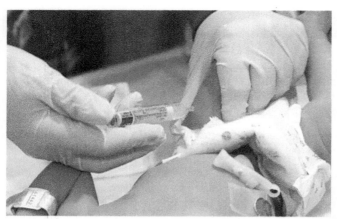

Figure 18.1. Vitamin K injection to the neonate's thigh. (Reprinted with permission from Ricci, S. S. [2009]. *Essentials of maternity, newborn, & women's health nursing* [2nd ed., Fig. 18.5]. Philadelphia, PA: Lippincott Williams & Wilkins.)

between 0.5 and 1 mg has been recommended for every infant within 6 hours following birth. The parental rejection of vitamin K for neonates is becoming increasingly common, however, and is associated with a rise in major hemorrhagic complications of the newborn (Schulte et al., 2014).

The newborn heart rate is typically assessed by auscultation of the apical pulse (in the fourth intercostal space, left midclavicular line). The neonatal heart rate is normally rapid, ranging from 120 to 160 bpm at rest, with brief extremes, such as with sleep when the apical rate may dip as low as 85 bpm or with crying or distress when it may reach as high as 180 bpm, which makes an accurate count challenging. The apical pulse must be assessed for one full minute, preferably while the infant is asleep or quiet. Dysrhythmia is common in neonates in the first hours of life and is not generally considered concerning in the absence of other symptoms such as cyanosis or pallor. Heart rates below 120 bpm or above 160 bpm should be reevaluated in 30 to 60 minutes or with changes in activity (e.g., the waking of a sleeping infant or breastfeeding of an infant who had been previously crying). It is not unusual to auscultate heart murmurs in the neonate. Most of these murmurs are physiologic and resolve within 6 months. Murmurs associated with feeding difficulties, cyanosis, pallor, and

neonatal apnea for more than 15 to 20 seconds may indicate a cardiac defect.

Blood pressure in most institutions is not routinely evaluated in the newborn in the absence of a known or suspected problem. Reasons that a blood pressure measurement may be ordered for a neonate include prematurity, tachycardia, a symptomatic murmur, pallor, or cyanosis indicating poor perfusion. If a cardiac defect is suspected, blood pressure is measured in both the upper and lower extremities. When measuring the neonatal blood pressure, the cuff is wrapped around the upper arm or leg and should cover two thirds of that appendage. At birth, the normal neonatal blood pressure is 50 to 70/30 to 45 mm Hg, rising to 90/50 mm Hg at approximately 10 days of life. Blood pressure should be measured with the infant at rest. Crying and movement can cause artificially high values in systolic blood pressure.

Temperature Regulation

Changes

Neonates have a higher ratio of body surface to body mass than adults and blood vessels that are closer to the surface of the skin, putting them at particular risk for hypothermia. Infants rarely shiver and do not have fully functional sweat glands, which also contributes to the problem of optimal thermoregulation. Infants may lose heat by evaporation, conduction, convection, and radiation (Table 18.2; Fig. 18.2). Neonates work to retain heat by maintaining a flexed position to reduce body surface and by increased body movement. A hypothermic infant may be cool to the touch and display acrocyanosis.

Although infants do not typically shiver, they do produce heat by a process called nonshivering thermogenesis. Nonshivering thermogenesis is the mobilization of stores of brown fat that can double heat production. Brown fat reserves are most abundant in term infants, and stores of the fat are depleted within several weeks after birth, more quickly in the case of acute cold stress (see Chapter 24).

Because neonates do not have fully developed sweat glands, they do not sweat to a degree sufficient to aid in cooling. An infant

Table 18.2	Neonatal Heat Loss	
Means of Heat Loss	**Explanation**	**Care Considerations**
Evaporation	Heat loss due to evaporation of liquid from the body	Dry neonates thoroughly after the birth. Stabilize their temperature prior to the bath, and bathe them in a warm environment.
Conduction	Transfer of heat by direct contact with a cooler object	Place infants on prewarmed surfaces or keep them skin to skin with the mother.
Convection	Heat transfer from the newborn to the surrounding air	Keep the ambient room temperature at least 72°F. Avoid having air currents from open windows and fans.
Radiation	Transfer of heat from or to the newborn from or to nearby surfaces	Keep the infant away from cool windows and exterior walls.

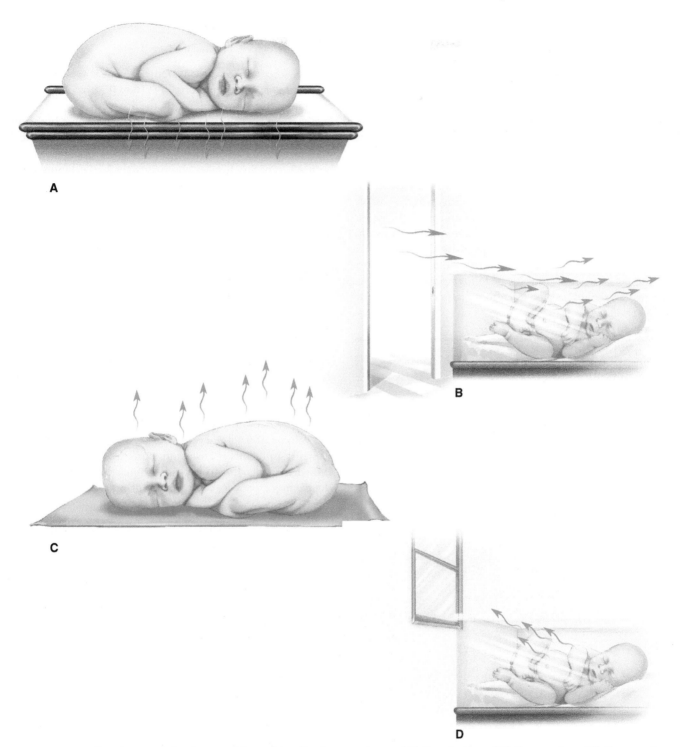

Figure 18.2. The four mechanisms of heat loss in the newborn. (A) Conduction. **(B)** Convection. **(C)** Evaporation. **(D)** Radiation. (Reprinted with permission from Chow, J., Ateah, C. A., Scott, S. D., Ricci, S. S., & Kyle, T. [2013]. *Canadian maternity and pediatric nursing* [Fig. 17.2]. Philadelphia, PA: Lippincott Williams & Wilkins.)

who is hyperthermic for reasons other than sepsis appears flushed and assumes an extended posture to increase surface area and facilitate the radiation of heat away from the body. The infant's hands and feet are warm to touch. In contrast, an infant who is hyperthermic due to sepsis may instead appear pale with cool hands and feet. A septic neonate may present with hypothermia instead of hyperthermia, however. Hyperthermia may result in seizures, brain damage, and death.

Care Considerations

A primary care goal for neonates is to provide a thermoneutral environment wherein the infant is less subject to hypothermia or hyperthermia. Skin-to-skin contact with the parent under a warmed blanket with or without a hat minimizes heat loss by all methods. The neonate should be dried quickly and thoroughly after birth and after bathing. If the neonate must be unwrapped for an assessment or intervention for longer than the time needed to change a diaper, the nurse should use a warmer. However, the nurse should unwrap the newborn as little as is necessary. For example, if the nurse is auscultating the apical pulse, only the newborn's left torso should be exposed. An infant may become overheated, however, from inappropriate use of external heat sources or overdressing. A common pointer for new parents is to dress the neonate in the same number of layers as the parents themselves intend to wear for the temperature, plus one. So, for instance, if the father is planning to wear a t-shirt and a sweatshirt, he should dress his newborn in a onesie, t-shirt, and sweatshirt to promote a neutral thermal environment. The newborn's first bath should be delayed until his or her temperature is stable. The newborn should be kept away from drafts and cold outside walls and windows.

In Chapter 10, baby Kylie was premature, which made her particularly susceptible to temperature instability. Because of this, she was kept in an isolette to help better regulate the ambient temperature and, in turn, Kylie's temperature. Eric, the nurse practitioner in the neonatal intensive care unit, also strongly encouraged skin-to-skin care, which can help regulate body temperature as well as blood glucose levels.

Gastrointestinal System

Changes

At birth, the stomach capacity of the neonate is approximately 5 to 10 mL, or 1 to 2 teaspoons, or 0.16 to 0.32 oz. The stomach volume increases to 60 mL within the first week. On average, the infant receives a half ounce of colostrum per feeding in the first 24 hours, two thirds of an ounce per feeding on days 2 and 3, and about an ounce per feeding after 3 days, roughly mirroring stomach capacity. It takes approximately 2 to 4 hours for the neonate's stomach to empty, and this is about as often as he or she should be fed, per infant demand.

Meconium—the first infant stool, which appears thick, green, and tarry—is typically passed in the first 24 hours, often during one of the two early periods of reactivity described earlier (Fig. 18.3). Meconium may also be passed in utero, particularly in the case of infants born postterm or who experienced distress in utero. The stool changes from greenish-black to a greenish-brown or greenish-yellow by the third day, at which time it is called transitional stool. By the end of the first week, the stool of breastfed infants appears yellow and seedy and has a sour odor and a pasty consistency. The stool of formula-fed infants by the end of the first week, on the other hand, is browner, has an unpleasant rather than a sour odor, and is more formed.

Breastfed infants pass stool four to eight times daily, more frequently than do formula-fed infants. Reassure parents that the volume of stool does not indicate gastrointestinal distress. Diarrhea in infants is green and loose. Constipation is rare in breastfed infants. Infants fed with formula that is not sufficiently diluted may experience constipation. Infants typically pass a single

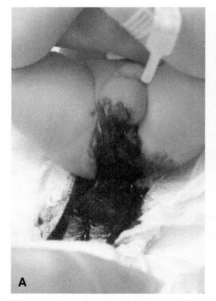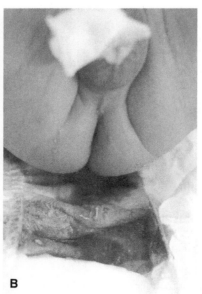

Figure 18.3. Newborn stool. (A) Meconium stool, typically passed in the first 24 hours postpartum. **(B)** Stool of a breastfed infant, 3 or 4 days postpartum. Note the seedy appearance. (Reprinted with permission from Kyle, T., & Carman, S. [2013]. *Essentials of pediatric nursing* [2nd ed., Fig. 3.2]. Philadelphia, PA: Lippincott Williams & Wilkins.)

meconium stool in the first 24 hours and three stools daily for the remainder of the neonatal period.

Care Considerations

Particularly to new parents, meconium can look alarming. Assure caregivers of the normalcy of meconium stool and inform them of the anticipated timetable for the transition of stool color, consistency, and odor. Encourage parents to check diapers frequently and change them immediately after the production of stool to protect skin integrity. Advise them to cleanse the infant's perineal area thoroughly with a warm, moist cloth and to liberally apply a barrier cream such as petroleum jelly or zinc oxide to the perineum with each diaper change.

In Chapter 4, Sophie's nurse, Kylie, told her not to be alarmed by the appearance of meconium. She taught her to put barrier cream on baby Gabi's bottom with every change and watched as Sophie changed the diaper, ready to offer assistance as needed.

Urinary System

Changes

Neonates typically lose 5% to 10% of their birth weight within 3 to 5 days after birth because of diuresis, defecation, respiration, and limited fluid intake. This weight is regained within 2 weeks after birth, more quickly in formula-fed infants than in breastfed infants. Neonates are often born with a small amount of urine in their bladders, and they may urinate at the time of birth. In the first 48 hours postpartum, newborns usually urinate two to six times, but by the middle of the first week, they urinate six to eight times daily.

The urine of a newborn is less concentrated and has a lower specific gravity than that of an adult for approximately the first 3 months of life. The urine is thus a very pale straw color, which may be difficult to visualize, even against a white diaper. Unlike more concentrated urine, it is nearly odorless. Uric acid crystals that look like red brick dust are often found in the diaper in the first week and are not concerning. After the first week, however, they may be a sign of dehydration.

Care Considerations

Change wet diapers promptly, clean the skin with a warm, damp cloth, and replace barrier cream as needed. Educate parents about the anticipated volume of urine. Record the number of wet diapers a newborn has, including those reported by caregivers and not changed by the nurse. Educate parents about uric acid crystals and about how their red color can be alarming and can make it easy to mistake them for blood. Report fewer than five wet diapers in 24 hours to the pediatric provider.

Hepatic System

Changes

The liver of the neonate is disproportionately large in comparison with the liver of an adult, taking up 40% of the abdominal cavity. The liver of the term newborn contains enough iron to contribute to the production of red blood cells for 4 to 6 months. These stores are replenished with each feeding, as both breast milk and formula contain iron, although the iron in breast milk has superior bioavailability. This means that although breast milk has less total iron, the form of iron it has is used more efficiently than the form in formula. Despite this increased bioavailability, however, the American Academy of Pediatrics recommends that infants receive an iron supplement beginning at the age of 4 months until the regular feeding of iron-containing solids begins (Wang, 2016).

Gluconeogenesis, the production of new glucose from noncarbohydrate sources, happens primarily in the liver. In utero, maternal glucose passes the placenta into the fetus's circulation, but insulin does not. After birth, the newborn continues to produce insulin from the pancreas as prior to birth, but without the regular incoming supply of the mother's glucose. This causes an immediate drop in the newborn's blood glucose level, which bottoms out between 30 and 90 minutes after birth before beginning to rise again because of gluconeogenesis in the liver. Glucose levels typically stabilize between 50 and 60 mg/dL after the initial drop, and measure between 60 and 80 mg/dL within the first week postpartum. Infants born to diabetic mothers are at particular risk for hypoglycemia because of continued overproduction of insulin from the neonate's pancreas after birth.

Physiologic jaundice is common to some degree in most term newborns (see Chapter 25 for information about pathologic jaundice) and is even more common in preterm infants. It resolves without treatment. Jaundice is the visible yellowing of the skin and the sclera of the eyes. It is caused by a rise in unconjugated bilirubin. Bilirubin is a normal product of the breakdown of red blood cells. This bilirubin is normally conjugated, or joined, with glucuronic acid in the liver. This conjugated form can then be excreted. When not enough bilirubin is excreted, jaundice occurs, first in the sclera and face and then descending down to the chest, abdomen, and extremities. Neonates are particularly at risk for high levels of unconjugated bilirubin because of a high volume of red blood cells at birth, the short life span of fetal red blood cells, and a limited ability of the liver to conjugate sufficient bilirubin in the first days postpartum. In addition, conjugated bilirubin in the neonate's intestines may become unconjugated, with the bilirubin being reabsorbed by the intestinal mucosa and returned to the neonate's circulation.

Breastfeeding-associated jaundice occurs in the first week and is caused not by breastfeeding in general or by breast milk itself but by ineffective feeding. Colostrum works as a laxative, and less colostrum consumed means less peristalsis and fewer stools. Fewer stools means that unconjugated bilirubin is more likely to be reabsorbed by the intestinal mucosa and returned to the neonatal circulation.

A slightly later-onset form of jaundice, **breast milk jaundice**, may appear on days 4 through 7 and last for up to 4 months. In this case bilirubin levels peak in the second week after birth and then gradually diminish. The etiology of this form of jaundice is unclear, and it is rarely dangerous. Approximately 20% to 30% of breastfed newborns have breast milk jaundice at the age of 1 month (Maisels et al., 2014).

Care Considerations

Glucose screening protocols and treatment thresholds may vary among organizations. Newborns at risk for hypoglycemia (Box 18.1) are typically screened a half hour to an hour after birth and after the first feeding. Then, blood glucose is rechecked every 3 to 6 hours for the first 24 to 48 hours (Harris, Weston, & Harding, 2012). Monitoring is continued until the neonate consistently maintains blood glucose in the normal range. Many institution protocols call for treatment of infants with a blood glucose level of less than 40 mg/dL or when symptomatic (see Box 3.10 and 5.7). Treatment generally starts with breast or formula feeding and kangaroo care, which is the practice of the caregiver holding the infant with skin-to-skin contact. Breastfed infants with resistant hypoglycemia may be fed formula, and infants with hypoglycemia resistant to formula may be treated with intravenous glucose or medications per orders (see Chapter 24 for more information about neonatal hypoglycemia).

In Chapter 9, baby Jonathan was considered at risk for neonatal hypoglycemia because he was large for gestational age and because Nancy had gestational diabetes during his pregnancy.

With physiologic jaundice in infants of European and African ancestry, bilirubin peaks between 5 and 6 mg/dL by 72 to 96 hours after the birth and then decreases to 2 to 3 mg/dL by day 5. Infants of Asian ancestry may take as long as 120 hours to reach the same peak, and the bilirubin levels for these infants may not fall to 2 to 3 mg/dL until between days 7 and 10. Frequent infant

---

Box 18.1   Risk Factors for Hypoglycemia

- Maternal diabetes
- Maternal obesity
- Gestational age < 37 wk
- Gestational age > 42 wk
- Newborn is large for gestational age
- Intrauterine growth restriction
- Admission to the neonatal intensive care unit
- Perinatal stress

---

feedings help stimulate peristalsis and the passage of meconium, thus reducing the opportunity for unconjugated bilirubin to become reabsorbed.

Initial evaluation of jaundice may be by visual inspection with reflex testing by transcutaneous monitoring and/or blood test. Jaundice after 24 hours postpartum that is limited to the face is generally considered an expected finding, whereas jaundice that extends below the umbilicus is concerning for significant hyperbilirubinemia. Institutions may also require a single transcutaneous screening prior to discharge for all infants (see Chapter 25). Levels of bilirubin as assessed transcutaneously or by blood draw are compared with those on a nomogram to help guide care (see Fig. 5.9).

Immune System

Changes

The human immune system does not fully develop until well into childhood. Term infants are born with some protections in place, less so preterm infants.

- Immunoglobulin (Ig) G provides protection against viruses and bacteria to which the host, in this case the mother, has been exposed. The infant is born with IgG that passes the placenta into the fetal bloodstream. This is a form of passive immunity, which means the protection offered is temporary, lasting about 3 months. The immunity generated by the administration of the hepatitis B vaccine in infancy, however, is an example of active immunity.
- IgM is the first antibody type produced in response to an infection and also the first produced by the fetus. It helps destroy foreign substances in the body.
- IgA is found in tears, blood, and saliva and on mucus membranes in places such as the nose, vagina, and gastrointestinal tract. Neonates are not born with a complement of IgA, but can acquire IgA to protect the gastrointestinal tract from bacterial and viral pathogens via breast milk.
- Leukocyte (white blood cell) function is immature in neonates, leaving them more vulnerable to infection.
- Lymphocytes are a type of leukocyte responsible for antibody production. If lymphocytes are repeatedly exposed to a pathogen, they destroy the pathogen. Because newborns do not have prior exposure to pathogens, lymphocyte response is delayed.

Care Considerations

Because neonates are less able to fight infection than they will be when they are more mature, good infection protection measures are crucial. Excellent handwashing and aseptic techniques must be used. Infection is one of the leading causes of neonatal illness and death, and infants remain at higher risk for several months. Educate caregivers about the importance of limiting the newborn's exposure to large crowds and individuals known to have a readily infectious illness, such as an upper respiratory infection.

Neonates may have a fever with an infection but may alternately have hypothermia or an unstable temperature. Some symptoms of infection are typical of what you may see late in life, such as lethargy, vomiting, diarrhea, irritability, and poor feeding. Other symptoms of infection, such as reduced reflexes, pallor, and mottled skin, are more specific to the ill newborn. Symptoms of respiratory distress, such as retractions, grunting, apnea for 20 seconds or more, and tachypnea, may be seen with pneumonia. Unusual discharge from any orifice and rashes should be investigated.

Integumentary System

Changes

In the third trimester, vernix, a thick, white, creamy substance, is secreted by the fetal sebaceous gland. This substance is fused with the epithelium and forms a waterproof barrier in utero and a barrier against bacteria and dehydration after birth (Míková et al., 2014). At birth, the vernix is often limited to skin folds but may be distributed more diffusely and can be rubbed into the skin or washed off in the bath (Fig. 18.4).

In Chapter 4, baby Gabi had vernix in her creases, which Kylie washed away during her first bath. Kylie wore gloves when caring for baby Gabi until after her bath was complete.

Lanugo is a fine, downy hair that covers the body and face of the fetus from week 16 of gestation on. It is most abundant in week 20 and then begins to shed into the amniotic fluid. The fetus, swallowing the amniotic fluid, also swallows the lanugo,

which makes up a large part of the meconium. Lanugo in utero helps anchor the vernix and has mostly been replaced by a different fine hair, vellus hair, by term. Some term infants, however, may still have some lanugo, which is often noted over the shoulders, forehead, and temples. Lanugo is typically shed within the first few weeks after birth. Lanugo is seen more often and in greater abundance in preterm infants (Fig. 18.5).

Several skin variations that may be present at birth or seen in the early postpartum period can be alarming to parents. Education about the nature of the variations and anticipated resolution is an important part of effective infant care (Table 18.3).

Care Considerations

Some parents may opt not to have their infant bathed in the hospital to prolong the vernix. Note that infants must not be handled without gloves if they have not been bathed. Skin variations are common and are important points for education. Central cyanosis and pallor are reasons for further assessment, documentation, and reporting, as is diffuse petechiae. Skin variations, including Mongolian spots and erythema toxicum, should be documented.

Reproductive System

Breasts

Many infants have swelling of the breast tissue as a response to the high estrogen environment of the uterus. Because of the withdrawal of this estrogen at the time of birth, a small number of infants may produce some nipple discharge (witch's milk). No intervention is required, and both the breast enlargement and nipple discharge resolve spontaneously.

Female Genitalia

In term female neonates, the labia cover the vestibule, although in preterm infants, the clitoris appears more prominent and the

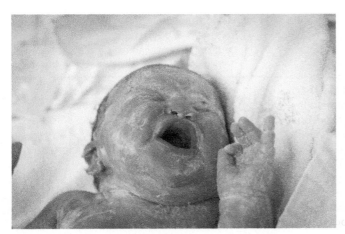

Figure 18.4. A newborn with vernix coating the skin. (Reprinted with permission from Hatfield, N. T. [2014]. *Introductory maternity and pediatric nursing* [3rd ed., Fig. 13-4]. Philadelphia, PA: Lippincott Williams & Wilkins.)

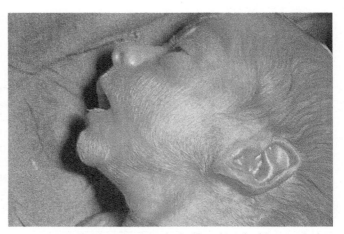

Figure 18.5. Profuse lanugo hair. (Reprinted with permission from Stedman, T. L. [2006]. *Stedman's medical dictionary* [28th ed.]. Philadelphia, PA: Lippincott Williams & Wilkins.)

Table 18.3 Neonatal Skin Variations

Variation	Appearance	Care Considerations
Milia 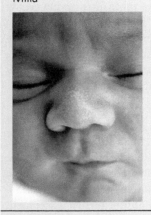	Small white sebaceous glands	• Typically resolve in 2–4 wk without treatment. • Discourage attempts to remove.
Desquamation (peeling)	Peeling primarily of the palms, ankles, and soles within a few days after birth	• May be a sign of postmaturity. • Advise caregivers to avoid removing the skin.
Acrocyanosis 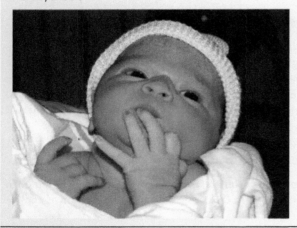 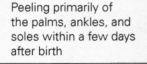	Bluish tint to the hands and feet, particularly when cold, due to immature circulation	A common normal finding during the first 7–10 d postpartum.
Circumoral cyanosis	Bluish tint around the mouth	• Normal during the transition period (first 6–8 h postpartum). • If persistent, can indicate a cardiac problem.
Mongolian spots 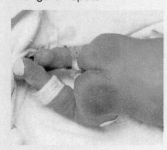	Area of bluish-black pigmentation that can appear like a bruise; more common in infants with darker skin and on the back and buttocks, but may also appear in infants with lighter skin and on other parts of the body	• Not associated with trauma. • Document carefully to avoid suspicion of physical abuse with future exams. • May expand for first year before it begins to resolve.
Mottling	Pattern of pale and dark splotchiness that occurs with cold	• Keep the infant swaddled or under a warmer when in a cold environment to prevent

Table 18.3 Neonatal Skin Variations (continued)

Variation	Appearance	Care Considerations
Harlequin sign	A transient condition in which one side of the body is blanched, whereas the other is erythematous	• Associated with low birth weight. • Benign • Often occurs on day 3 or 4 postpartum and resolves by 3 wk of age.
Erythema toxicum 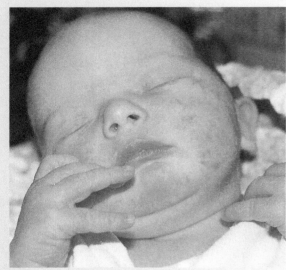	A red rash with white papules and red macules that may occur over any part of the body but most commonly occurs on the trunk	• Appears between 24 h and 2 wk postpartum. • Benign • May last up to 3 wk. • Does not appear to be uncomfortable for the infant. • No treatment is indicated.
Nevi simplex (salmon patches, stork bites, angel kisses, telangiectatic nevi) 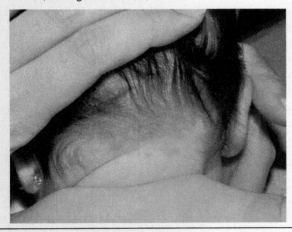	Flat, pink, blanchable areas of skin that most commonly occur on the nape of the neck, nose, eyelids, and upper lip and are usually symmetric (e.g., on both eyelids or on both sides of the midline)	• Facial lesions resolve in the first few years. • Neck lesions may persist into adulthood. • Benign
Nevus flammeus (port-wine stain) 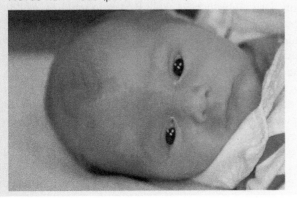	A nonblanchable discoloration of the skin mostly found on the neck and face that is typically flat and pink at birth but darkens and becomes textured with time	• Often removed by surgery or laser treatment.

(continued)

Table 18.3   Neonatal Skin Variations (continued)

Variation	Appearance	Care Considerations
Nevus vascularis (strawberry hemangioma) 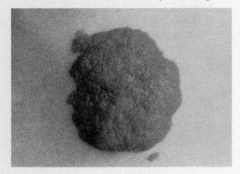	An area of the skin that is raised and sharply demarcated and may be present at birth or appear in the first several weeks postpartum	• May grow for up to 2 y and then shrink and fade. • Typically resolve in the first decade of life.

Images reprinted with permission from: Milia: Jensen, S. (2011). *Nursing health assessment: A best practice approach* (1st ed., Fig. 17.25). Philadelphia, PA: Lippincott Williams & Wilkins; Acrocyanosis: Kyle, T., & Carman, S. (2012). *Essentials of pediatric nursing* (2nd ed., Fig. 3.3A). Philadelphia, PA: Lippincott Williams & Wilkins; Mongolian spots: Weber, J. R. (2014). *Nurses' handbook of health assessment* (8th ed., Fig. 25.7). Philadelphia, PA: Lippincott Williams & Wilkins; Erythema toxicum: Bowden, V. R., & Greenberg, C. S. (2013). *Children and their families: The continuum of nursing care* (3rd ed., Fig. 25.7). Philadelphia, PA: Lippincott Williams & Wilkins; Nevi simplex: Goodheart, H. P., & Gonzalez, M. E. (2016). *Goodheart's photoguide to common pediatric and adult skin disorders: Diagnosis and management* (4th ed., Fig. 1.9). Philadelphia, PA: Lippincott Williams & Wilkins; Nevus flammeus: Johnson, J. T., & Rosen, C. A. (Eds.). (2014). *Bailey's head and neck surgery—Otolaryngology* (5th ed., Vol. 1, Fig. 104.88). Philadelphia, PA: Lippincott Williams & Wilkins; Nevus vascularis: Weber, J. R., & Kelley, J. H. (2014). *Health assessment in nursing* (5th ed., Fig. 30.15F). Philadelphia, PA: Lippincott Williams & Wilkins.

labia smaller. The labia are typically edematous and are more so with a breech birth, when they appear bruised, as well. Note when assessing the female genitalia that the urethra is located posterior to the clitoris, closer to the vestibule. A different location of the urethra is suspicious for ambiguous genitalia, with the apparent clitoris actually a small penis.

Some female infants have pseudomenstruation shortly after birth as a result of the withdrawal of estrogen, similar to what can happen with nipple discharge. This is a normal finding and resolves spontaneously.

Male Genitalia

The foreskin of the male neonate completely covers the glans of the penis and is not retractable. The urethral opening normally is at the tip of the penis. If it occurs in the ventral aspect of the penis or scrotum, it is known as **hypospadias**, and, more rarely, if it is located on the dorsum of the penis, it is known as **epispadias**. A form of epithelial cyst is found rarely on the tip of the prepuce and is a benign finding. These cysts, also called **Epstein's pearls**, may also be found on the gums and palate of the mouth. Regardless of location, they typically disappear within a few weeks after birth without intervention.

The neonate's scrotum is more darkly pigmented than the rest of the neonate's skin. The scrotum of a near-term infant is smoother than that of a term or postterm neonate, who will have more rugae on the scrotal sack. By the time of birth, most male term infants have testes that have descended into the scrotum. A neonate who is delivered breech will have an edematous and possibly bruised scrotum.

Care Considerations

Like the "brick dust" that can appear in the urine, pseudomenses can be alarming to new parents worried that their infant is bleeding. In uncircumcised infants, do not retract the foreskin, because it is not fully retractable until the age of 3 or 4 years, and attempting to do so prematurely may cause injury. The decision to circumcise the foreskin of the male infant is the parents', although certain medical conditions, such as hypospadias and epispadias, may be a contradiction to the procedure.

Head

The neonate's head accounts for approximately a quarter of its length, and the face appears small in relation to the head. The neck is proportionately smaller and weaker, and neonates can lift and turn their heads for brief periods only when lying prone. Infants born vaginally have skulls subject to molding. Molding is a process by which the shape of the head changes temporarily because of mobility of the skull sutures and overlapping of the bones of the skull during passage through the vagina. The shape of the head is restored within a few days (see Fig. 16.7).

In addition to mobile sutures, the infant skull also has fontanels or soft spots. They are the frontal or anterior fontanel and occipital or posterior fontanel. The posterior fontanel is covered by tough connective tissue and occurs as a triangular opening where the occipital bone meets the parietal bones. It usually closes within a few months after the birth. The anterior fontanel is diamond-shaped and located at the top of the head where the parietal bones meet the frontal bones. It closes within 18 months to 2 years after birth. Two pairs of smaller fontanels are located on each side of the head and close between 6 and 18 months. Like the mobile sutures, fontanels aid with passage through the birth canal. They also allow for more rapid brain growth than would the closed skull.

Caput Succedaneum

Caput succedaneum is a generalized edema of the occiput common in infants born vaginally in the vertex position. It is not painful and resolves spontaneously in the first week postpartum. Caput crosses the suture line, and the swelling is superficial. Caput is more common in infants who have been born with the assistance of a vacuum device (Fig. 18.6).

Cephalhematoma

A cephalhematoma is deeper than the edema of caput succedaneum and occurs between the skull and the periosteum, the layer of tissue that surrounds the bone. It does not consist of interstitial fluid but rather blood. Unlike caput, which is generalized, a cephalhematoma is more defined and, because it is specific to a particular bone of the skull, does not cross suture lines. It is not uncommon for a cephalhematoma to occur at the same time as caput succedaneum. Cephalhematoma takes 2 to 8 weeks to resolve, however, rather than 3 to 4 days for caput. Because resolution includes the hemolysis of accumulated red blood cells, hyperbilirubinemia is a potential complication of this condition.

In Chapter 9, the nurse caring for Nancy and Jonathan, Rae, told Nancy and her partner Missy that baby Jonathan had a cephalhematoma. She explained that the fact that the swelling didn't cross the suture line was reassuring, and that the condition was unlikely to become dangerous.

Subgaleal Hemorrhage

A subgaleal hemorrhage is more superficial yet more dangerous than a cephalhematoma. It occurs under the galea aponeurosis, a tendinous sheath that forms the inner layer of the scalp. It is not associated with a single bone of the scalp, so the bleeding does cross the suture line. Blood loss can be severe and may lead to dangerous complications, including shock and death. It is most common after a challenging operative vaginal birth.

The first step in distinguishing a subgaleal hemorrhage from a cephalhematoma is assessment of the suture lines. Swelling that does not cross the suture line is unlikely to be a subgaleal hemorrhage. In addition, a cephalhematoma tends to be firm, whereas a subgaleal hemorrhage is more boggy on palpation. Blood from a cephalhematoma pools at the back of the neck and head, pushing the ears forward. Serial head measurements that increase are highly suspicious for subgaleal hemorrhage, and tachycardia and pallor also contribute to a suspicion of hemorrhage. Serial hematocrits may be ordered, as well as

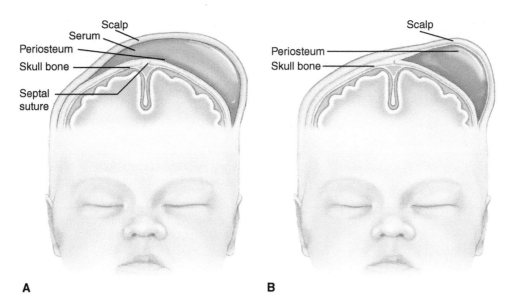

A   **B**

Figure 18.6. Comparison of caput succedaneum with cephalhematoma. (A) Caput is a collection of serous fluid (edema) between the periosteum and the scalp caused by the pressure of the fetal head against a partially dilated cervix. Caput often crosses suture lines. **(B)** Cephalhematoma is a collection of blood between the periosteum and the skull. It does not cross suture lines. (Reprinted with permission from Hatfield, N. T. [2014]. *Introductory maternity and pediatric nursing* [3rd ed., Fig. 13-6]. Philadelphia, PA: Lippincott Williams & Wilkins.)

repeat assessments for the level of consciousness. As with cephalhematoma, hemolysis can lead to hyperbilirubinemia as the blood degrades.

Care Considerations

New parents may find normal molding alarming and should be reassured of its speedy resolution. Swelling of the soft tissues should be examined thoroughly to differentiate between caput succedaneum, cephalhematoma, and subgaleal hemorrhage. A suspicion of subgaleal hemorrhage should be brought to the immediate attention of the pediatric provider.

Neurologic System

Changes

Tremors are common to almost all newborns, particularly in the hands and chin. Tremors occur at times of agitation and are usually accompanied by crying and end within a month. Tremors that occur when the infant is at rest are not normal and may be due to hypoglycemia (especially if they occur in the first 48 hours after birth), hypocalcemia, or an underlying neurologic condition. Moreover, tremors of any type that last

beyond a month are not normal and may indicate one of the conditions just listed.

Newborns have various reflexes. Some of these reflexes persist throughout the lifetime, whereas others are limited to months or even weeks (Table 18.4).

Care Considerations

Assessment of reflexes is part of a full exam of the neonate. Educating parents about reflexes such as the grasp-and-suck reflex can help parents interact with their newborn and feel more bonded. The rooting reflex is very helpful for establishing breastfeeding. Educate parents about the extrusion reflex, which they may later in the infant's life interpret as a rejection of food.

Newborn Behavior

The Brazelton Neonatal Behavioral Scale is a method of explaining, describing, and categorizing infant behavior as the infant progresses through the four different levels of developmental challenges. The first level is autonomic regulation, which includes the capacity for controlling breathing, heart rate, and temperature.

Table 18.4 Neonatal Reflexes

Reflex	Assessment and Normal Response	Other Considerations
Rooting	When the mouth or cheek is touched, the infant turns toward the stimulus and opens the mouth.	• Is weak or absent if the infant is sated. • Disappears in 3–12 mo.
Swallowing	When fed, the neonate successfully coordinates sucking, swallowing, and breathing.	May be uncoordinated in prematurity.
Extrusion	The neonate sticks out the tongue if the tip of the tongue is touched or pushed.	• Lasts for the first 4–5 mo of life. • May be interpreted by parents as a rejection of nourishment.

Table 18.4 Neonatal Reflexes (continued)

Reflex	Assessment and Normal Response	Other Considerations
Grasp: palmar (shown in figure) and plantar 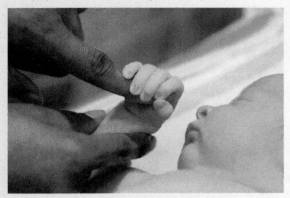	• *Palmar:* The infant curls the fingers around an object placed in the hand. • *Plantar:* The infant curls the toes against an object placed at the base of the toes.	• *Palmar:* lasts 3–4 mo • *Plantar:* lasts about 8 mo
Tonic neck (fencing) 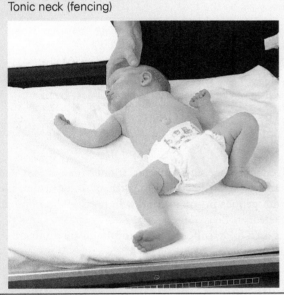	Turning the infant's head quickly to one side causes the infant to extend the arm and leg on that side and to flex the arm and leg on the other side.	Lasts for 3–4 mo; if longer, is concerning for cerebral palsy.
Moro (often called the startle reflex when there is a response to sound)	• When startled by a loud noise or a small, controlled drop of the head and neck (supported), the infant abducts and extends the arms with the hands forming the shape of a C. • The legs may also respond. • After the initial startle, the limbs adduct and relax.	• Complete response until 8 wk. • Partial response for as long as 6 mo. • Any response beyond 6 mo is suspicious for neurodevelopmental problem. • Asymmetric response is concerning for injury to the upper extremity. • A preterm infant may have an incomplete response because of muscle weakness. • An exaggerated response with central nervous system excitability, as with neonatal abstinence syndrome.

(continued)

Table 18.4	Neonatal Reflexes (continued)	
Reflex	**Assessment and Normal Response**	**Other Considerations**
Babinski	When a finger or hard instrument strokes along the plantar lateral aspect of the sole and then across the ball of the foot in a continuous motion, the newborn extends the toes and dorsiflexes the large toe.	A lack of response warrants neurologic assessment. This reflex normally goes away by 1 y of age. In adults, anticipate curling of the toes. Extension of the toes in adults is concerning for neurologic injury or disease.
Stepping	• When held upright by the torso, such that the feet touch the surface, the infant simulates the walking movement. • Term infants walk on the soles; preterm infants walk on the toes.	This reflex disappears within a month postpartum.
Crawling	When placed in the prone position, the infant moves the arms and legs in a crawling motion.	This reflex resolves within about 6 wk.

Images reprinted with permission from: Rooting and palmar grasp: Chow, J., Ateah, C. A., Scott, S. D., Ricci, S. S., & Kyle, T. (2013). *Canadian maternity and pediatric nursing* (Figs. 25.9 [rooting] and 18.14G [palmar grasp]). Philadelphia, PA: Lippincott Williams & Wilkins; Extrusion and tonic neck: Pillitteri, A. (2014). *Maternal and child health nursing: Care of the childbearing and childrearing family* (7th ed., Figs. 29-18 [extrusion] and 18-7 [tonic neck]). Philadelphia, PA: Lippincott Williams & Wilkins.

The second level is motor control. The third is state regulation, or the development of a regular sleep/wake cycle and communication through crying and consolation by a caregiver. The last level is that in which the infant has the capacity to interact socially, staying alert, engaged, and responsive to a stimulus. The scale evaluates 28 different items clustered into five different categories (Box 18.2). Assessment using the scale provides a means for clinicians and caregivers to evaluate and discuss infant behavior through the third month and plan care (The Brazelton Institute,

2013). Gestational age, environmental stimuli, time elapsed, and the maternal use of medication in the prenatal, intrapartum, and postpartum periods in conjunction with breastfeeding may all influence neonate behavior.

Terms used to describe responses to stimuli are summarized in Box 18.3.

Newborn Senses

Newborns see best when the object they are viewing is about 17 to 20 cm away from the eyes, the approximate distance between the face of the infant and the face of the caregiver when cuddling or nursing. Infants prefer faces and high contrast patterns to other images. Neonates are routinely assessed for hearing deficits prior to

---

Box 18.2 Brazelton Neonatal Behavioral Assessment Scale Assessment Categories

• *Habituation (sleep protection):* the ability to adjust to audio and light stimulation in relation to sleep
• *Motor:* the maturity of muscle tone and control
• *Self-regulation:* the ability to self-console and to be consoled when crying
• *Stress response:* the newborn's threshold of stimulation in response to stress
• *Social interactive capacity:* alertness and responsiveness to human and other stimuli

Adapted from The Brazelton Institute. (2013). *The newborn behavioral observations system: What is it?* Retrieved from http://www.brazelton-institute.com/clnbas.html.

Box 18.3 Response to Stimuli

• *Temperament:* an infant's habitual response to stimuli; often described in terms such as "calm" or "active"
• *Crying:* the amount of crying and stimuli that trigger crying
• *Consolability:* the ease with which the crying infant may be self-soothed or soothed by a caregiver
• *Irritability:* the threshold at which the infant begins to cry
• *Cuddliness:* the degree to which an infant relaxes into an embrace

discharge. Newborns prefer higher-pitched noises and often find rhythmic noises soothing, likely as a result of habituation to the maternal heartbeat in utero. Neonates have a keen sense of smell and can recognize their mother's odor at 2 days of age (Marin, Rapisardi, & Tani, 2015). Infants who can smell breast milk after a painful procedure have a lower level of stress hormones and calm more readily (Badiee, Asghari, & Mohammadizadeh, 2013). Newborns prefer sweet tastes, and, as with the smell of breast milk, sweet tastes appear to reduce pain from procedures (Stevens, Yamada, Ohlsson, Haliburton, & Shorke, 2016). The neonate's sense of touch is well developed. Human touch is a critical component of normal infant and child development. Like sweet tastes and the smell of breast milk, gentle human touch can mitigate the pain experience of the neonate (Herrington & Chiodo, 2014).

Sleep–Wake States

The different states of consciousness, from deep sleep to high irritability, are described as the six sleep–wake states. There are two identified sleep states (deep sleep and light sleep) and four identified wake states (drowsy, quiet alert, active alert, and crying; Box 18.4). The sleep–wake states identified by The Brazleton Institute (2013) are part of the third level of identified behavior, state regulation.

Assessment and Care of the Newborn

The first 4 hours of life outside the womb are a critical time of assessment and intervention for the neonate. Assessment and prevention of cold stress, assessment and support of respirations, assessment of Apgar score and appropriate interventions, as well as other important tasks, are priorities, as are early implementation of skin-to-skin contact and breastfeeding. Subsequent assessment and care until discharge is informed by the findings of assessment during the first 4 hours postpartum.

The First 4 Hours After Birth

Care starts with review of the prenatal records and birth whenever possible. Evidence of pregnancy complications such as preeclampsia, gestational diabetes, premature rupture of membranes, intrapartum medications, and prematurity may alter how care is prioritized. The nurse must use universal precautions during care of a neonate until after bathing to avoid exposure to pathogens that may have been in the amniotic fluid or maternal blood.

Immediately after the birth, the nurse dries the infant places him or her under a warmer or in direct contact with the mother's skin under a warmed blanket to prevent heat loss by conduction or radiation. Drying prevents heat loss by evaporation. Placement of a cap on the neonate's head reduces heat loss by convection. If necessary, the nurse should clear the neonate's airways of mucus and fluid using a bulb syringe. In some cases, wall suction may be indicated and implemented per institution protocol.

Apgar Score

The nurse assesses and records the Apgar score at 1 minute and at 5 minutes after delivery and performs interventions as indicated. The Apgar score is a useful assessment tool to inform care providers about infant status and the efficacy of interventions in the early postpartum period but does not predict long-term outcomes (see Table 1.4). Apgar refers to the physician who invented the assessment, Virginia Apgar, but also serves as a helpful mnemonic (Box 18.5; Fig. 18.7). The Apgar score scale is between 0 and 10. A score between 7 and 10 suggests excellent condition of the neonate, whereas lower scores may indicate a need for warming, clearance of the airways, vigorous stimulation of the skin, and other interventions.

In Chapter 8, the pediatrician reported that Gracie's baby, Eddie, had a 1-minute and 5-minute Apgar score of 5, indicating moderate depression. He lost points for color and grimace. He was diagnosed with neonatal respiratory distress syndrome.

> ### Box 18.4   Sleep–Wake States
>
> - *Deep sleep:* possible startle reflex but no other movement; regular breathing; no eye movement or change in state due to external stimuli.
> - *Light sleep:* some body movement; irregular breathing; rapid eye movement; possible change in state due to external stimuli.
> - *Drowsy:* muscle movement; irregular breathing; eyes open and close; external stimuli typically results in change of state.
> - *Quiet alert:* regular respirations; eyes open, may focus on stimuli; optimal time to attempt breastfeeding.
> - *Active alert:* body movements and possible fussiness; increased startle reflex and motor activity; eyes open; irregular respirations.
> - *Crying:* intense crying, difficult to calm, ample body movement. Breathing irregular.
>
> Adapted from The Brazelton Institute. (2013). *The newborn behavioral observations system: What is it?* Retrieved from http://www.brazelton-institute.com/clnbas.html.

> ### Box 18.5   APGAR Mnemonic
>
> - Activity and muscle tone
> - Pulse
> - Grimace with stimulation (such as suctioning the nares)
> - Appearance (skin color)
> - Respirations

	Score 0	Score 1	Score 2
Appearance			
Pulse	No pulse	<100/min	>100/min
Grimace			
Activity			
Respirations	No respirations	Weak, slow	Strong cry

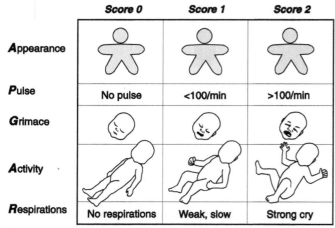

Figure 18.7. APGAR chart. (Reprinted with permission from LifeART image © 2018 Lippincott Williams & Wilkins. All rights reserved.)

Gestational Age Assessment

Gestational age is usually assessed early in the prenatal period and may be calculated using Naegele's rule (see Fig. 2.4), according to the first day of the last menstrual period, or determined via ultrasound, as indicated. At times, however, this early assessment must be compared with indicators of neonate maturity after the birth. Assessment of gestational age is also appropriate for situations in which prenatal care was not sought or is incomplete. According to institutional policy, a postnatal gestational age assessment should be done in cases of premature or postterm pregnancies, infants weighing under 2,500 g or over 4,000 g, infants admitted to the neonatal intensive care unit, and infants of mothers with diabetes.

A commonly used means of assessing gestational age is the New Ballard Score (www.ballardscore.com), which can be used from 20 weeks of gestation and later. This tool involves performing the following assessments:

- *Posture:* Observe the flexion of the infant's arms and legs when the infant is quiet and supine.
- *Square window:* Apply gentle pressure using the index and third fingers to the back of the infant's hand while supporting the wrist.
- *Arm recoil:* Flex and then extend the infant's arms and observe the rate and strength of recoil while the infant is in the supine position.
- *Popliteal angle:* Flex the infant's thigh onto the abdomen. Extend the infant's knee and measure the popliteal angle (behind the knee).
- *Scarf sign:* Move the infant's arm across the body. Observe the point to which the elbow moves readily in relation to the midline.
- *Heel to ear:* With the infant supine, grasp the infant's foot and pull it toward the ear on the same side using minimal force. Observe the popliteal angle.

Infants up to 26 weeks of gestation should be assessed within 12 hours after delivery, and older infants should be screened within 48 hours after delivery. An accurate exam requires an alert, rested infant, which may delay the exam. It should be noted, however, that prenatal dating remains more accurate (Lee et al., 2017).

Additional Assessments

The nurse should take vital signs within the first 30 minutes after delivery, again at the first hour, and then hourly until the end of the **fourth stage of labor** (the first 4 hours after the birth). Infants in distress may have vital signs taken more frequently, as often as once every 5 minutes.

The cord is inspected to determine the number of vessels present (having two arteries and one vein is normal, although having only one artery occurs in a small number of pregnancies). The number of cord arteries is typically identified prior to birth by ultrasound, however.

The nurse should perform an initial newborn assessment within the first few hours postpartum that covers the respiratory, cardiovascular, neurologic (including reflexes), gastrointestinal, and genitourinary systems, as well as the skin, ears, nose, eyes, and general appearance. The nurse completes an additional assessment prior to discharge (Table 18.5).

Infants at risk for hypoglycemia undergo blood glucose screening in the first half hour to an hour after birth. Infants displaying signs of hypoglycemia, such as jitteriness, temperature instability, and apnea, also have blood glucose assessed (see Box 3.10).

In Chapter 3, baby Winston was large for gestational age due to Susan's gestational diabetes. Susan talked with her nurse, Betty, about her disappointment that her gestational diabetes affected her baby, despite her hard work to control her blood glucose level through diet and exercise during pregnancy.

The nurse typically takes baseline measurements of size in this earliest period, as well, documenting weight, head circumference, and body length and comparing these findings with average measurements in a growth chart. Infants appropriate for gestational age have a weight between the 10th and 90th percentiles (see Fig. 1.16). Prior to weighing the infant, the nurse should take care to zero the scale and place the infant on a warm blanket and not directly in contact with the cool surface of the scale. The head circumference is measured at the widest point, the occipitofrontal diameter (Fig. 18.8; see Fig. 1.16). The length of the newborn is measured with the infant's leg extended. The measurement is from the top of the head to the heel (Fig. 18.9).

Early Routine Interventions

According to institution policy, mothers, infants, and often support people must wear bracelets with matching identification codes. An ophthalmic ointment, usually erythromycin 0.5%, is

Table 18.5 Newborn Assessment

Assessment	Technique	Expected Findings	Clinical Considerations
Posture	Inspect prior to disruption. Consider the context of fetal position and presentation as well as the type of birth.	Arms and legs should be flexed and hands fisted. The newborn should resist extension.	• Hypertonia may indicate CNS disorder or chronic intrauterine exposure to opioids, nicotine, or some medications, including opioid replacements. • Hypotonia may indicate exposure to some maternal medications, prematurity, hypoxia in utero, or some congenital defects. • Birth injuries may cause paralysis or postural asymmetry. • A frank breech presentation results in temporary extension of the legs at the knee.
Pulse	Auscultate for the apical pulse rather than palpate for a peripheral pulse. Auscultate pulse for a full minute, preferably with a neonate stethoscope. Although challenging to assess rhythm, strive to count an accurate heart rate.	At rest: 120–160 bpm When crying: tachycardia to 180 bpm In deep sleep: 100 bpm or less Murmurs are typically physiologic and resolve in early infancy. Further assessment of murmurs is rarely indicated in the absence of other cardiac or respiratory difficulties.	• Prolonged tachycardia that does not resolve over multiple auscultations over a designated period of time is concerning for respiratory distress, sepsis, and cardiac defects. • Bradycardia that is similarly assessed is concerning for sepsis, hypoxemia, and increased intracranial pressure.
Respirations	As for the apical pulse, assess respirations over a full minute by visualizing the chest and abdomen. Lightly resting a hand on the neonate's abdomen may aid in this assessment.	30–60 bpm, irregular The chest and abdomen should rise simultaneously. Occasional apnea, up to 15–20 s with compensatory tachypnea, is normal.	• Apnea over 20 s is concerning for respiratory or cardiac problems. • Tachypnea may indicate hypothermia, hypoglycemia, respiratory distress syndrome, or sepsis.
Blood pressure	Not part of routine assessment. Assess upper and lower extremities simultaneously when the infant is at rest. Special equipment is required.	50–70/30–45 mm Hg is normal for the first 10 d.	Artificially high systolic values are obtained if the infant is moving or crying.
Temperature	Temperature may be taken with an axillary or temporal thermometer, depending on institution protocol.	36.5°C–37.2°C	Sepsis, a hot or cold environment, and neurologic disorders may cause abnormally high or low temperatures.
Weight	Place a warmed blanket or other protective cover on the scale to protect the neonate from heat loss from conduction. Set the scale to zero after placing the protective cover and before placing the naked neonate on the scale. Never leave a neonate unattended on the scale.	Refer to a weight chart for AGA weight. Weight loss up to 10% is anticipated in the first week because of normal fluid loss, limited fluid intake, and metabolic changes. The weight is typically regained within 2 wk.	• SGA (weight below the 10th percentile) may reflect prematurity, intrauterine growth restriction, maternal calorie restriction in pregnancy, maternal infections, or congenital defects. • LGA (weight above the 90th percentile) is common in infants of diabetic mothers. • Failure to regain weight within 2 wk indicates the need for breastfeeding assessment.

(continued)

Table 18.5 Newborn Assessment (continued)

Assessment	Technique	Expected Findings	Clinical Considerations
Head circumference	Measure around the head, with the tape measure above the ears and eyebrows. A repeat measurement may be required after the third day in case of excessive molding.	Consult a growth chart for expected head circumference for gestational age. A finding between the 10th and 90th percentiles is considered normal.	• Microcephaly (head circumference below the 10th percentile) occurs with maternal infections such as Zika, drug and alcohol use, and congenital conditions. • Macrocephaly (head circumference above the 90th percentile) is concerning for hydrocephaly, particularly if the sutures are widely spaced and the head circumference is 4 cm or more larger than the chest.
Length	Measure from the top of the head to the heel of the extended leg. To facilitate measuring, extend the neonate's leg and mark the surface on which the neonate is lying, and then measure on the surface from the top of the head to the mark.	Assess according to a growth chart.	• Molding may cause the infant to measure longer than is accurate. • Longer measures may also result from congenital defects or genetic inheritance (e.g., tall parents). • Assess infants who measure as shorter for prematurity and intrauterine growth restriction. • Longer measures may also occur from congenital defects or genetic inheritance.
Chest circumference	Measure by placing the tape around the torso at the nipple line.	Anticipate the chest measuring 2–3 cm smaller than the head circumference.	• Smaller in prematurity
Chest general assessment	Assess for shape and symmetry. Assess breasts for swelling and discharge. Assess lung sounds. Assess the clavicle.	The chest should be symmetrical and barrel-shaped. Common findings include breasts swollen due to maternal hormones and milky fluid leaking from the nipples. Lung sounds should be equal and may be clear or have scattered crackles for the first few hours after birth. The clavicle should be intact.	• Variations besides barrel chest, such as funnel or pigeon chest, are abnormal. • Persistent crackles, reduced breath sounds, stridor, wheezing, and grunting are concerning for respiratory distress. • Preterm infants may lack breast swelling. • A broken clavicle may result from birth trauma.
Integumentary	Inspect for color, bruising, birth marks, lanugo, vernix, temperature, and rashes. Inspect the nails for length. Inspect the infant in a warm area, only exposing as much skin as necessary at one time. Use a good lighting source.	Pink, possibly with blue hands and feet. Mottling, harlequin sign, erythema toxicum, telangiectases, milia, and physiologic jaundice are normal findings. Petechiae may be seen over the presenting part, and ecchymoses of the presenting part is common in breech births and with forceps use in vertex births. Postterm infants may have nails that extend beyond the fingertips. They may scratch their skin in utero or postpartum.	• Deeper pink or red coloration may indicate polycythemia or prematurity. • Central cyanosis may indicate hypoglycemia, hypothermia, cardiopulmonary disease, infection, or congenital disease. • Pallor may indicate blood loss, infection, or a cardiovascular problem. • Gray coloration may indicate poor perfusion. • Generalized petechiae (not just in the presenting part) may indicate infection or a clotting disorder. • Generalized ecchymoses may indicate hemorrhagic disease. • Jaundice prior to 24 h postpartum is pathologic and results from increased hemolysis. • Excessive lanugo suggests prematurity.

Table 18.5 Newborn Assessment (continued)

Assessment	Technique	Expected Findings	Clinical Considerations
Head	Inspect for molding, caput succedaneum, cephalohematoma, and subgaleal hemorrhage. Inspect the fontanels and suture lines.	Molding is common and resolves in the first week. Fontanels may be slightly depressed at rest but may bulge with crying. Lacerations caused by a scalp electrode may be visualized. Bruising and localized scalp edema are common with vacuum extraction. Caput succedaneum and cephalohematoma are common benign findings that resolve spontaneously.	• Depressed fontanels may indicate dehydration. • Bulging fontanels that are not associated with crying may indicate hydrocephaly, particularly when the sutures are separated. • Subgaleal hemorrhage requires prompt assessment and intervention.
Eyes	Assess eye symmetry and placement in the face. Assess for eye discharge. Evaluate eyeballs for presence, lens opacity, movement, and sclera color.	Eyes should be symmetrical and equal. The distance between the eyes should be roughly equivalent to the distance between the inner and outer canthus of each eye. Some tears or discharge from ocular medications may be present. Subconjunctival hemorrhage is common. Eye movement is typically random and jerky.	• Epicanthal folds in patients not of an ethnicity that typically has epicanthal folds are concerning for a congenital disorder. • Purulent discharge is abnormal and suggests infection. • Opaque lenses may indicate congenital cataracts. • Yellow sclera occur with jaundice, and blue sclera occur with osteogenesis imperfecta.
Nose	Observe the patency and placement of the nares and the shape of the nose.	The nose should be located midline and have minimal mucosal discharge. Sneezing is common. Both nares should be patent.	• A malformed nose and copious drainage are concerning for syphilis. • Malformation may also indicate a chromosomal disorder or birth trauma. • Nasal flaring is a sign of respiratory distress.
Ears	Assess for placement and cartilage. Assess hearing prior to discharge.	The corners of the eyes should align with the tops of the ears where they attach to the scalp. The cartilage should be firm. The infant should startle to loud sounds and respond to high-pitched noises.	• Low placement of the ears is associated with congenital abnormalities. • Incomplete cartilage formation is associated with prematurity. • Failure of a hearing test in the early newborn period necessitates further assessment after discharge.
Mouth	Inspect the palate, assess the suck reflex by inserting a gloved finger into the mouth. Inspect the lips, gums, and tongue.	All structures should be symmetric, intact, moist, and pink. Epstein's pearls are a common benign finding.	• Natal teeth may be benign or associated with a congenital aberration. • Cleft lip and palate are neural tube defects.
Neck	Assess for flexibility, movement, and bruising.	The neck should be short, thick, and mobile, with no webbing.	• Webbing is suspicious for Turner syndrome. • Torticollis is a condition in which the neck is twisted to the side. It typically resolves over a period of months.

(continued)

Table 18.5 Newborn Assessment (continued)

Assessment	Technique	Expected Findings	Clinical Considerations
Abdomen	Inspect the umbilical stump. Inspect, auscultate, and palpate the abdomen. Observe movement with respiration.	The umbilical stump should be white or gray and odorless. Remove the clamp after 24 h. The cord stump falls off within 2 wk. The abdomen should be soft, round, and nondistended. Bowel sounds should be present. The abdomen should rise with the chest when breathing.	• Drainage and redness around the cord are concerning for infection. • Bleeding from the cord is suspicious for a bleeding disorder. • Herniation of the abdominal contents into the stump is abnormal. • A firm, distended abdomen should be reported to pediatric provider. • An absence of the rise of the abdomen or a rise of the abdomen that occurs with the fall of the chest is concerning.
Rectum	Inspect for placement and patency.	Passage of meconium should occur within 24 h. An anal wink is present.	• The absence of an anus or the presence of an imperforate anus requires urgent evaluation and intervention.
Male genitals	Assess the placement of the urinary meatus. Palpate the scrotum to assess for the descent of the testicles while occluding the inguinal canal with fingers of the opposite hand.	The urinary meatus should be located at the tip of the penis. The scrotum should be large and rugated in term neonates. Both testes should be palpable within the scrotum.	• Hypospadias and epispadias may occur independently or with other congenital defects. • Undescended testes are not palpable and typically "drop" into the scrotum in the first year of life. • An inguinal hernia may present as a groin or scrotal mass.
Female genitals	Gently separate the labia to assess for the presence of the clitoris, labia minora, and vaginal opening.	In term infants, the labia majora covers the labia minora, clitoris, and introitus. Pseudomenses (mucosal or bloody discharge) is normal.	• A prominent clitoris and small labia that do not cover the introitus can indicate prematurity. • In term babies, ambiguous genitalia may require genetic testing to determine sex. • Urethral placement above or on top of the clitoris instead of beneath also suggests ambiguous genitalia.
Musculoskeletal	Inspect the spine, extremities, and gluteal folds at the hips.	Arms and legs should be of symmetrical length and strength, with full range of motion and no clicks with movement. The spine should curl into the shape of a C with no dimple, cyst, or tuft of hair at the base of the spine above the buttocks. The infant should have 10 fingers and 10 toes.	• Nonsymmetrical gluteal folds or clicks with joint movement are associated with hip dislocation. • The pediatric provider and not the nurse should perform the Barlow-Ortolani maneuver because of the risk of injury. • Polydactyly (too many digits) or syndactyly (fewer than 10 of each type of digit) may happen independently or with other congenital disorders. • Reduced muscle tone or range of motion may occur in prematurity, birth injury, and neurologic disorder.

CNS, central nervous system; bpm, beats per minute; AGA, appropriate for gestational age; SGA, small for gestational age; LGA, large for gestational age.

placed in the infant's eyes shortly after birth. Parents may opt for placement after the first period of reactivity to facilitate eye contact and bonding. Vitamin K is injected into the thigh. The nurse should cluster assessment and intervention activities to minimize the disruption of bonding.

Four Hours After Birth to Discharge

Subsequent care of the newborn after the first 4 hours continues to focus on the transition to life outside of the uterus, assessment of overall health, and educating parents to care for the neonate

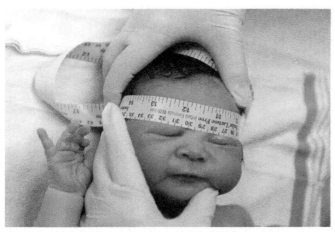

Figure 18.8. Measuring the head circumference of a newborn. (Reprinted with permission from Evans, R. J., Brown, Y. M., & Evans, M. K. [2014]. *Canadian maternity, newborn, and women's health nursing* [2nd ed., Fig. 20.9]. Philadelphia, PA: Lippincott Williams & Wilkins.)

In Chapter 9, Missy brought Teddy to meet his new baby brother in the hospital. Missy gave Teddy a book she said was from the baby, but Teddy was unimpressed and thought his new brother looked like a snap pea and smelled weird.

Periodic Assessments and Care

The nurse should complete a basic newborn assessment according to the schedule set by the institution, typically once per shift. Infant apical pulse, respiratory rate, and temperature are evaluated at this time, but not blood pressure, unless ordered, because it is challenging for infants to maintain a stable body temperature, and the nurse should instruct parents to keep the infant swaddled and capped or to provide skin-to-skin contact. Infants who are swaddled (Fig. 18.10; Step-by-Step Skills 18.1) and capped with a temperature below 36.5°C should be placed skin to skin and covered with a warm blanket. In the absence of other problems, abnormal vital signs may be reassessed after a short interval of time. If the temperature remains low, warming under a radiant warmer set at 1.5°C warmer than the neonate's temperature is warranted. Persistent hypothermia may result in hypoglycemia, and glucose levels should be checked per protocol. Persistent abnormal vital signs should be reported to the pediatric provider.

Although some parents are knowledgeable about infant care, others need more support. The infant's diaper should be changed with each feeding and each assessment and if urine or stool is present. The presence of urine and meconium should be noted with each diaper change and charted. The nurse should communicate the normal number of wet diapers and stools to the parent. Before the stump of the cord falls off, which typically occurs spontaneously at or before 2 weeks postpartum, the infant's diaper should be affixed so it is not snug at the top or overlying the stump. The stump should otherwise be left alone in the absence of signs of infection, such as redness or seepage.

through teaching, example, guidance, and supervision of tasks such as diapering and infant feeding.

Upon admittance to the postpartum unit, or after the birth in the case of an institution in which labor and postpartum care are provided in the same room, the infant is often fitted with a tracking device. This device triggers an alarm if removed from the infant prior to deactivation, or if the infant moves out of a predetermined zone. This measure is designed to prevent infant abduction. Maternity wards are typically locked, secure units.

The nurse orients the parents to the unit upon admission, including explaining to them the visiting policies. Some institutions have different policies for different units, and it's important to be familiar with each. A unit may temporarily alter its policies, as well, as may be the case during a particularly virulent flu season as infants' immature immune system can make such infections particularly dangerous. Unless prohibited by policy, the nurse should encourage sibling visits to promote family bonding.

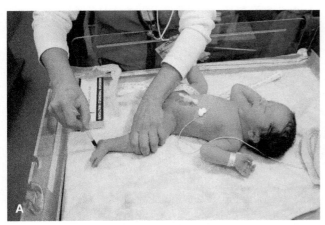
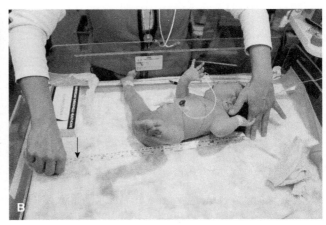

Figure 18.9. Measuring a newborn's length. (A) The nurse extends the newborn's leg and marks the pad at the heel. **(B)** The nurse measures from the newborn's head to the heel mark. (Reprinted with permission from Ricci, S. S. [2009]. *Essentials of maternity, newborn, & women's health nursing* [2nd ed., Fig. 18.1]. Philadelphia, PA: Lippincott Williams & Wilkins.)

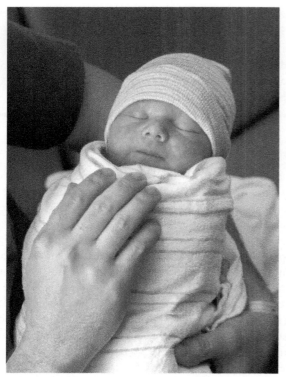

Figure 18.10. A swaddled newborn. Note that the nostrils and mouth are well clear of the blanket. The newborn is wearing a hospital-issued cap to help maintain thermostasis.

Although the perineal area of the newborn should be wiped thoroughly with a clean, moist cloth with each cleaning and a protective barrier cream applied, daily bathing with soap is not necessary. Bathing of the face and hands with soap is also not recommended, and any soap used on other body parts should be gentle with a neutral pH. Newborns are typically bathed prior to discharge, although it is not a condition of discharge. New parents often benefit from witnessing the first bath after newborn temperature stability is achieved (Fig. 18.11; Step-by-Step Skills 18.2).

Step-by-Step Skills 18.1

Swaddling

1. Place a blanket on a flat surface.
2. Fold down the corner furthest from you.
3. Place the newborn on the blanket with the top of the fold in line with the neck.
4. Fold the left corner across the infant and pull snugly, tucking the extra length under the infant's back.
5. Bring the bottom corner up and fold loosely over the chest of the infant.
6. Fold the right corner over the infant and tuck it under the opposite side, making sure both arms are snug against the body and that none of the blanket covers the mouth or nose.

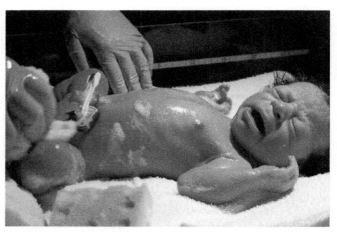

Figure 18.11. A newborn receiving his first bath in the hospital. Note that the nurse is wearing gloves and the cord clamp is in place.

Step-by-Step Skills 18.2

Newborn Bath

1. Bathe the newborn in a warm room free of drafts. In an institutional setting, baths are often done under a warmer.
2. You must wear gloves when handling an infant until the bath is complete.
3. Start with bathing the eyes using a cloth moistened with warm water. Do not use soap. Clean from the inner canthus to the outer canthus using a different part of the cloth for each eye. Put the cloth aside.
4. Using a fresh cloth, wash the rest of the face. Moisten the cloth with warm water only, no soap.
5. Wash the hands using a warm, moist cloth with no soap.
6. Cleanse the neck, focusing on the folds, and the upper body using a moist cloth and soap. Rinse off the clean areas using warm water in a peri bottle.
7. Using a fresh cloth, similarly wash and rinse the lower extremities.
8. Using a different cloth, bathe and rinse the perineal area. Wash female genitals front to back, and lift the male scrotum when bathing, paying special attention to the creases.
9. Shift the newborn into the prone position, and similarly wash and rinse the back with a clean cloth.
10. Dry the newborn, dress in a fresh diaper and clothing, and swaddle.
11. With the infant in a secure football hold under your arm with the head supported, gently scrub the scalp with a soapy cloth. Rinse over the sink with warm water from a peri bottle.
12. Completely dry the head under a warmer and replace the swaddling blanket, which may have become wet.
13. Place a cap on the head.

Note: This process varies among institutions and care providers.

Soothing Newborns

Crying is the means by which newborns communicate. They may cry to indicate hunger, physical discomfort, illness, or boredom. Often the reason for the crying is unknown—a fact that can be distressing to caregivers. Infants who are less consolable can be a source of frustration for parents and may make them feel less successful in their parenting role. The nurse should explain to the parent that having an infant who is difficult to console is not a reflection of parenting. The amount of infant crying generally increases until approximately 6 weeks postpartum and then gradually decreases. Infants who cry for at least 3 hours a day, 3 days a week, for 3 weeks are considered colicky (Wolke, Bilgin, & Samara, 2017).

A common cause of infant distress is hunger. Ideally, signs of hunger will be identified prior to crying because, particularly for young infants, establishing a productive latch is far more difficult with a distressed infant. Hunger cues include rooting, moving the hand to the mouth, and opening the mouth.

Most infants find swaddling comforting, likely because the snug fit is similar to the physical sensation of being in the womb. Infants may find the sound of a heartbeat soothing, as well as the warmth of a caregiver. Thus, cuddling against the chest is often effective for calming a crying newborn. Many infants are at their most calm when being worn in a sling or other infant carrier (Fig. 18.12). This is often referred to as "baby wearing."

Infants often find movement soothing. Infant swings and vibrating chairs are designed with this in mind. Cradles should be used with caution, because a vigorously rocked cradle may result in injury. Going for walks often soothes newborns. In the hospital setting, parents can be encouraged to walk with their infants in the hallways, either holding them or pushing them in their cribs, according to institution protocol. Walking outside with a stroller or carriage may also be an effective strategy after discharge, and many infants find rides in cars while in a secured car seat soothing.

Newborn Screening

Newborn screening is done to detect disorders that may be debilitating or deadly before the infant is symptomatic. The disorders screened for may be metabolic, endocrine, cardiac, immunologic, hematologic, or other. Newborn screening is routine in all states and territories in the United States, and about four million newborns are screened annually. Approximately one in 4,000 infants screens positive (Centers for Disease Control and Prevention, 2012). Currently, the Advisory Committee on Heritable Disorders in Newborns and Children recommends screening for 34 different conditions (Advisory Committee on Heritable Disorders in Newborns and Children, 2016). Different states, however, may choose to include or exclude different disorders in the screening panel.

For most newborns, the screening blood specimen is obtained close to the time of discharge and must be collected at 24 hours to 7 days after the birth. Because many of the disorders are metabolic in nature, the nurse must be allowed time for the initiation of metabolic processes prior to screening. The nurse should collect blood via a heel stick (see Step-by-Step Skills 3.1; Fig.18.13; see Fig. 5.12) and deposit it into the circles printed on special paper designated for this purpose. The nurse should explain to the parents the process of the blood collection and its purpose. In some states, a signature of consent may be required. A positive screening test needs to be confirmed with diagnostic testing.

Hearing Screening

Significant hearing impairment is detected in as many as one or two out of every 1,000 newborns (Tran et al., 2016). Newborns are routinely screened for hearing loss prior to discharge either by nursing staff or by an audiologist. The two hearing tests that are done routinely are automated auditory brainstem responses (Fig. 18.14) and otoacoustic emissions (Fig. 18.15). Both are nonpainful and are performed when the infant is asleep or quiet alert. Both rely on a physiologic measure rather than a behavioral response. Neither provides information about the type (conductive or sensorineural) or degree of hearing loss. A positive screening requires follow-up diagnostic testing.

Circumcision

Male circumcision is an elective procedure performed primarily on neonates that involves removal of the foreskin of the penis. It may be done for cultural, religious, or medical reasons. The

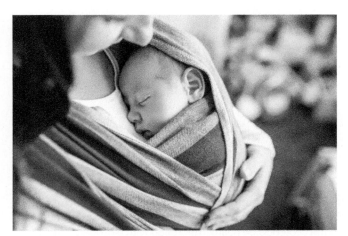

Figure 18.12. Infant in a sling or carrier. Many infants find it comforting to be carried in a sling or other carrier by a caregiver.

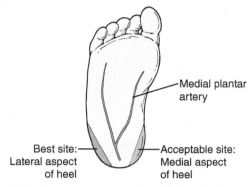

Medial plantar artery

Best site:
Lateral aspect
of heel

Acceptable site:
Medial aspect
of heel

Figure 18.13. Approximate sites for the heel-stick procedure. (Reprinted with permission from Rosdahl, C. B., & Kowalski, M. T. [2016]. *Textbook of basic nursing* [10th ed., unnumbered figure in Chapter 67]. Philadelphia, PA: Lippincott Williams & Wilkins.)

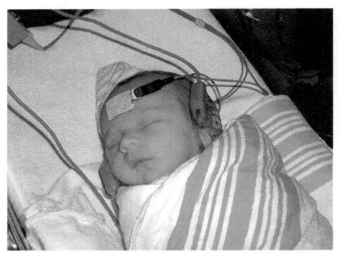

Figure 18.14. An infant undergoing automated auditory brainstem responses hearing screening. With electrodes placed on the neonate's forehead and mastoid, the test assesses electrical activity of the brainstem, auditory nerve, and cochlea. (Reprinted with permission from MacDonald, M. G., Ramasethu, J., & Rais-Bahrami, K. [2012]. *Atlas of procedures in neonatology* [5th ed., Fig. 54-2]. Philadelphia, PA: Lippincott Williams & Wilkins.)

American Academy of Pediatrics has issued a statement that the health protection circumcision offers outweighs any risk of the procedure (Freedman, 2016). The procedure is typically performed between 1 and 8 days after the birth. Major contraindications to the procedure include penile anomalies, bleeding abnormalities, or medical instability of the neonate.

Neonates should be at least 12 hours old and have voided at least once before undergoing circumcision. Voiding provides reassurance that no penile abnormality is present. To avoid vomiting and aspiration, feeding of the infant should be avoided for at least

an hour prior to the procedure. Verification of infant identity is critical prior to starting the procedure. The American Academy of Pediatrics recommends confirmation of vitamin K administration prior to the procedure to avoid excessive bleeding (American Academy of Pediatrics Task Force on Circumcision, 2012).

Parental consent is necessary for the procedure. Parents should be aware that not all insurance plans cover circumcision. Parents should also be aware that circumcision is associated with a reduced incidence of penile cancer and a reduction in cervical cancer in partners. Circumcision is associated with a reduced rate of HIV and other sexually transmitted diseases as well as a reduction in inflammatory penile disorders and disorders of foreskin retraction. Penile hygiene is also easier to maintain with circumcision. Potential complications include bleeding, infection, adhesions, injury, and amputation. Studies do not support changes in sexual satisfaction (Morris & Krieger, 2013). Circumcision is a painful procedure, and anesthesia is necessary.

In Chapter 5, Letitia included in her birth plan that she did not want her baby to be circumcised if the baby was a boy.

Obstetric providers typically perform this procedure, but pediatric providers may perform it, as well. The nurse is responsible for preparing the procedure venue and supplies, as well as the infant. The infant is positioned on a specially designed circumcision board. Velcro affixes legs in an extended position, and the upper body remains swaddled (Fig. 18.16).

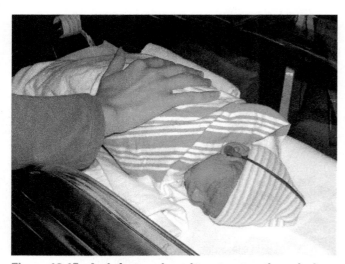

Figure 18.15. An infant undergoing otoacoustic emissions hearing screening. An ear probe detects responses of the hair cells of the cochlea. (Reprinted with permission from MacDonald, M. G., Ramasethu, J., & Rais-Bahrami, K. [2012]. *Atlas of procedures in neonatology* [5th ed., Fig. 54-1]. Philadelphia, PA: Lippincott Williams & Wilkins.)

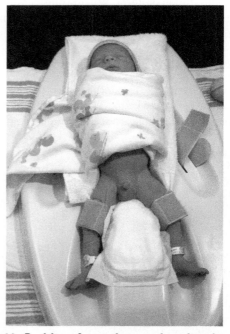

Figure 18.16. Position of a newborn undergoing circumcision. The newborn's upper body is swaddled, and his legs are strapped to the circumcision board. (Reprinted with permission from Hatfield, N. T. [2008]. *Broadribb's introductory pediatric nursing* [7th ed., Fig. 12-6A]. Philadelphia, PA: Lippincott Williams & Wilkins.)

Pain control may be by topical local anesthesia or anesthesia injected into the base of the penis. Infants often find an oral solution of 24% sucrose and nonnutritive sucking on a pacifier or gloved finger soothing. The person performing the procedure is responsible for applying the anesthesia and for draping. The three most common procedures use a Gomco clamp, a Plastibell, or a Mogen clamp (Fig. 18.17). Bleeding after the procedure is typically managed by applying pressure on the area or superficial stitches, as necessary.

Immediately after the procedure, the penis is wrapped in gauze thickly covered with petroleum jelly to avoid friction with and adhesion to the diaper and to minimize the contact the wound has with urine and meconium. This gauze should be replaced with each diaper change for 3 to 5 days. Some swelling should be expected. A yellowish crust develops over the penile glans and should not be wiped or washed off. Blood in the diaper larger than a quarter or a lack of urination within 12 hours should be reported to the person who performed the procedure.

Immunization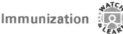

Hepatitis B is passed through blood and sexual contact. Immunity is conferred through a series of three vaccinations. The infant should receive the first dose before discharge, the second dose at 2 months of age, and the final dose at 6 months of age. Additionally, neonates who were exposed to hepatitis B by an infected mother should be given a dose of hepatitis B immune globulin within 12 hours after the birth. Like vitamin K, the hepatitis B immunization is intramuscular and injected into the muscle of the thigh. Parents may opt out of the hepatitis B vaccination or defer it until the infant is older.

Newborn Feeding

Infants may be fed human breast milk or formula. Breast milk may be delivered either directly from the breast, by bottle, or by gavage. Formula may be delivered by bottle or gavage. Human

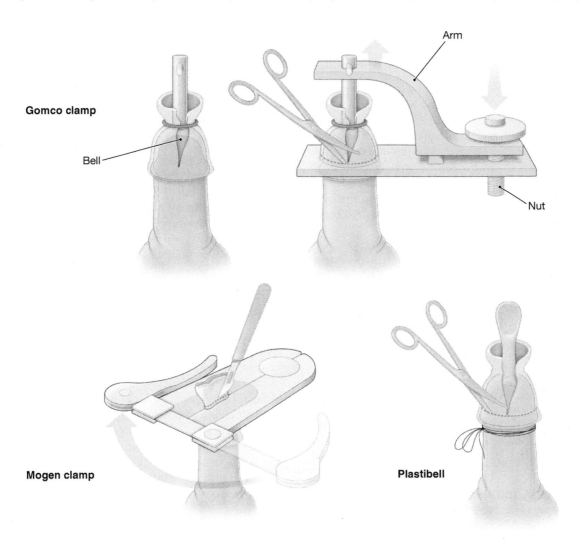

Figure 18.17. Surgical instruments for circumcision. Instruments used for circumcision include the Gomco clamp, Plastibell device, and Mogen clamp. (Reprinted with permission from Beckmann, C. R., Herbert, W., Laube, D., Ling, F., & Smith, R. [2013]. *Obstetrics and gynecology* [7th ed., Fig. 10.4]. Philadelphia, PA: Lippincott Williams & Wilkins.)

breast milk is considered the optimal exclusive form of nutrition for infants up to 6 months old (Hauk, 2015; Section on Breastfeeding, 2012). Optimally, breastfeeding should continue after 6 months with the introduction of solid foods.

The decision to breast or formula feed is a deeply personal one. The nurse should explain the benefits of breastfeeding to families but should respect a woman's choice to formula feed, if that is what she's decided to do. Women may choose to formula feed for many reasons, including fear of pain from breastfeeding or a perception that it will be difficult, the need to return to work soon after the birth, lack of education, lack of support, and the perceived convenience of formula feeding. Of these concerns, the lack of support of the partner, friends, and family is likely the most crucial (Fischer & Olson, 2014). Healthy People 2020 goals include targets of increasing any breastfeeding from 74% to 81.9% of infants, exclusive breastfeeding for 3 months from 33.6% to 46.2%, some breastfeeding for 6 months from 45.5% to 60.6%, exclusive breastfeeding through 6 months from 14.1% to 25.5%, and some breastfeeding for a full year from 22.7% to 34.1% (Healthy People 2020, 2017).

Breastfeeding

There are many advantages to breastfeeding for both the mother and the baby, some of which are itemized in Box 12.3. Contraindications to breastfeeding are few and rare; these are itemized in Box 18.6. The composition of breast milk is outlined in Box 2.8.

Preparation for lactation begins in puberty with the formation of lobules and alveolar glands, which eventually produce the milk that travels through the lactiferous ducts and to the nipple (Fig. 18.18). After puberty, breasts do not mature further until pregnancy, during which time the maturation and proliferation

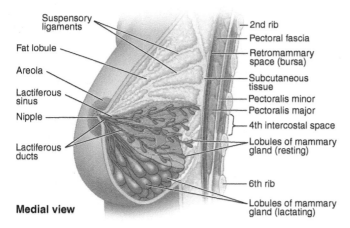

Medial view

Figure 18.18. Sagittal section of a female breast and anterior thoracic wall. The superior two thirds of the figure demonstrate the suspensory ligaments and alveoli of the breast with resting lobules of the mammary gland; the inferior part shows lactating lobules of the mammary gland. (Reprinted with permission from Moore, K. L., Dalley, A. F., & Agur, A. M. R. [2014]. *Clinically oriented anatomy* [7th ed., Fig. 1.22]. Philadelphia, PA: Lippincott Williams & Wilkins.)

Box 18.6 Contraindications to Breastfeeding

- Infant diagnosed with galactosemia (a metabolic disorder)
- Infant diagnosed with phenylketonuria (cannot be exclusively breastfed; feeding with a mix of breast milk and specialized formula is optimal)
- Mother with human immunodeficiency virus in a high-resource setting (formula and clean water are accessible)
- Mother with active tuberculosis infection prior to treatment for 2 full weeks
- Mother with active herpes outbreak on the breast, varicella, or H1N1 (may use pumped milk)
- Mother with untreated brucellosis bacterial infection
- Mother infected with human T-lymphotropic virus
- Maternal use of PCP, cannabis, or cocaine
- Mother who consumed alcohol less than 2 h ago
- Maternal use of amphetamines
- Maternal use of chemotherapeutic agents
- Maternal use of ergotamines
- Maternal use of statins
- Maternal treatment with radiation

Adapted from Section on Breastfeeding. (2012). Breastfeeding and the use of human milk. *Pediatrics, 129*(3), e827.

---

of secretory breast tissue continues. Some milk production starts in pregnancy at approximately 16 weeks of gestation (stage I lactogenesis). The birth of the placenta, the decrease of progesterone postpartum, and a rise in prolactin cue the onset of copious milk production postpartum (stage II lactogenesis). This copious milk production comes with breast swelling and often engorgement of the breasts and normally occurs 2 to 3 days postpartum but may happen as late as 7 days postpartum. Cesarean birth is associated with later stage II lactogenesis, and women who have just had their first birth tend to experience it later than women with subsequent births (Kendall-Tackett, 2015).

The ejection of milk (letdown reflex) from the alveolar lumen into the lactiferous ducts is stimulated by oxytocin, which is in turn released by stimulation of the nipple by suckling or pumping. Failure to cue milk ejection and distention of the alveolar lumen lead to a series of chemical events that results in a reduction and eventual cessation of milk production. Regular stimulation of the nipples and production of oxytocin, as well as emptying of the breasts by direct nursing or pumping, maintains an adequate milk supply. The letdown reflex may also be stimulated by infant crying, visualizing the infant, and sexual arousal. The reflex may be inhibited by fatigue, stress, or anxiety.

Initiating Breastfeeding

Lack of skin-to-skin contact in the first hour after the birth and supplementation with formula are major reasons cited for lack of success with breastfeeding and early breastfeeding cessation (Box

18.7; Chantry, Dewey, Peerson, Wagner, & Nommsen-Rivers, 2014). As of 2017, only 20.26% of hospitals had implemented all of the 10 steps recognized to contribute to breastfeeding success, up from 9% in 2015 (Baby-Friendly USA, 2017).

In keeping with the Ten Steps, nurses should ensure that skin-to-skin contact and the first feeding happen in the delivery room, whenever possible, and should delay nonessential tasks such as weighing and measuring, if possible (Section on Breastfeeding, 2012). Whenever possible, the mother and baby should be roomed together, with the infant being placed on a different sleep surface than the mother when not being held by an alert caregiver. The nurse should monitor and explain to the patient the progression of lactogenesis as evidenced by breast swelling. The nurse should also thoroughly communicate to the mother infant feeding positions, latch, letdown, and reasonable expectations.

Positioning

The mother should be in a comfortable position for breastfeeding, either upright or side-lying. The infant should be positioned facing toward the mother with the neck, hip, and spine aligned in a neutral position. The infant's neck should be slightly extended, giving the appearance of the nose in a "sniffing position." The four classic positions for breastfeeding are cradle, cross-cradle, football, and side-lying holds (Box 18.8). The infant and the mother's arms are generally supported by pillows to allow for greater comfort.

Box 18.7 Ten Steps to Successful Breastfeeding, Developed by the World Health Organization and the United Nations Children's Fund

1. Have a written policy on breastfeeding that is communicated routinely to all staff.
2. Train all healthcare staff in the skills needed to implement the policy.
3. Inform all pregnant women of the benefits and management of breastfeeding.
4. Help mothers start breastfeeding within 1 h after birth.
5. Show mothers how to breastfeed and maintain lactation, even if they are separated from their infants.
6. Give newborns no food or drink other than breast milk, unless other feedings are medically indicated. Hospitals must pay a fair market price for formula and feeding supplies.
7. Allow mothers and infants to remain together at all times (continuous rooming-in).
8. Encourage breastfeeding on demand.
9. Provide no pacifiers or artificial teats to nursing infants.
10. Foster the establishment of breastfeeding support groups and refer mothers to them.

Adapted from Section on Breastfeeding. (2012). Breastfeeding and the use of human milk. *Pediatrics, 129*(3), e827.

Box 18.8 Breastfeeding Positions

Cradle position:

In this classic position, the newborn's head is placed in the crook of the mother's elbow. The newborn's back is supported by the mother's arm and the buttocks are supported by her hand. The mother and newborn are positioned with abdomens touching. Although this position often becomes the default for older infants, it can be challenging to achieve a good latch with couplets who are first learning to nurse.

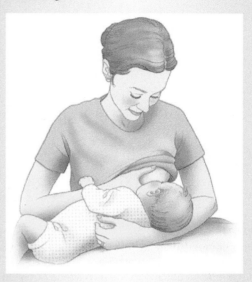

Cross-cradle position:

This position is a variation of the cradle position. The infant's head, instead of being positioned in the crook of the mother's elbow, is supported by her hand. As with the cradle position, the infant's back is supported by the mother's forearm and the abdomens of the mother and newborn touch. It is an easier position for obtaining a good latch than the cradle position.

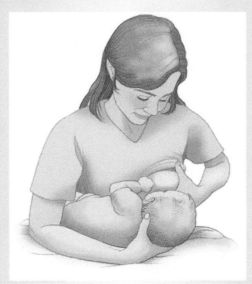

Box 18.8 Breastfeeding Positions (continued)

Football hold position:

The newborn is positioned to the side of the mother under her arm. The head is supported by mother's hand. Many mothers feel this position gives them the best support and control.

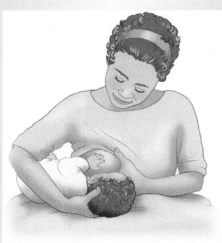

Side-lying position:

The mother and infant lie side by side facing each other. The mother can help support the infant's head and align the infant's body with the arm she is not lying on. Caution is warranted, as the mother may fall asleep during the feed, which risks infant suffocation.

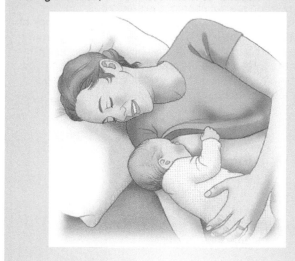

Images from the Office on Women's Health, U.S. Department of Health and Human Services, 2014. Available at: http://www.womenshealth.gov/breastfeeding/learning-to-breastfeed.html.

Latch

The latch, or latch-on, is the process of the newborn attaching to the breast. The mother should bring the infant to the breast rather than bring the breast to the infant. The mother can facilitate the latch by gathering the breast tissue gently with the fingers of the hand under the breast and the thumb on top, well back from the nipple. Grasping the breast too close to the nipple may inadvertently break the seal of the latch. This hold allows the mother to guide the nipple into the infant's mouth as the infant's mouth comes level with her breast (Fig. 18.19). A frequent challenge to achieving a good latch is ensuring the infant's mouth is open wide enough. Touching the infant's chin to the breast causes the infant to reflexively open the mouth because of the rooting reflex.

A good latch has the following qualities:

- Upper and lower lips flanged out rather than curled under
- Chin and the tip of the nose pushed into breast
- Wide-open mouth, approximately 120°
- Full cheeks
- Asymmetry of the exposed areola: more areola should be observable at the top of the breast above the upper lip than under the flanged lower lip
- Tongue pushed out over the lower gums and touching the breast (cannot visualize without pulling away the lower lip and risking losing the latch)

A good latch comes with practice. Factors that can impede a good latch are breast engorgement, inverted nipples, nipples that are slippery with emollient used to help avoid or heal chapping, and a breast hold too close to the nipple. An infant with neurologic difficulties or a short frenulum (ankyloglossia; the tissue attaching the tongue to the floor of the mouth; Fig. 18.20) may also have difficulty achieving a good latch. Infants who are overly agitated and crying may also have difficulty latching. Infants, particularly hungry ones, often bring their hands to their mouths, which can also make achieving and keeping a good latch challenging.

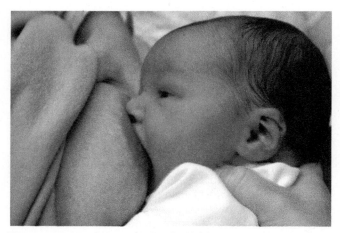

Figure 18.19. A proper latch. With correct latching, the newborn's lips flange out over the mother's areola, and the newborn's nose and chin touch the mother's breast. (Reprinted with permission from Evans, R. J., Brown, Y. M., & Evans, M. K. [2014]. *Canadian maternity, newborn, and women's health nursing* [2nd ed., Fig. 21.6]. Philadelphia, PA: Lippincott Williams & Wilkins.)

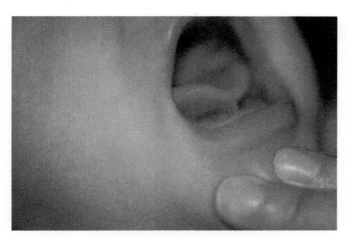

Figure 18.20. Ankyloglossia in an infant. (Reprinted with permission from Salimpour, R. R., Salimpour, P., & Salimpour, P. [2014]. *Photographic atlas of pediatric disorders and diagnosis* [1st ed., unnumbered figure in Section A]. Philadelphia, PA: Lippincott Williams & Wilkins.)

Signs of a poor latch include the following:

- Sunken cheeks instead of full
- Upper and lower lips touching at the corners of the mouth, indicating that the mouth is not open wide enough
- Creased nipple after the latch is broken
- Tongue not visible if the lower lip is moved aside

In Chapter 2, Tatiana was helped by a lactation consultant, Donna. She was surprised by how challenging breastfeeding was; she expected it to be a natural and intuitive task.

Nonnutritive Sucking

Infants often find sucking pleasurable, even when it's not associated with feeding. Some may suck on their fingers, fists, or thumbs, and others may enjoy pacifiers. Some neonates may be comforted by sucking on the finger of a caregiver. Sucking not associated with feeding is referred to as nonnutritive sucking.

Parents often feel strongly about the use of a pacifier, and the nurse should respect their wishes. In 2009, the American Academy of Pediatrics advised the use of pacifiers to help prevent sudden infant death syndrome (Zimmerman & Thompson, 2015). Parents may be concerned, however, that pacifiers may interfere with the newborn's interaction with other stimuli or that they may become "addicted" to the pacifier and use it longer than may be socially acceptable. Parents may also be concerned about nipple confusion.

Nipple confusion is the inability of an infant to change sucking patterns between different kinds of nipples. The sucking pattern used for breastfeeding differs from that used for bottle-feeding and with a pacifier (Fig. 18.21). With nipple confusion, infants may reject the breast in favor of the easier sucking pattern required for the bottle or pacifier. Evidence is mixed as to whether

concern about nipple confusion is warranted, but the World Health Organization recommends never giving breastfeeding infants artificial nipples (Zimmerman & Thompson, 2015).

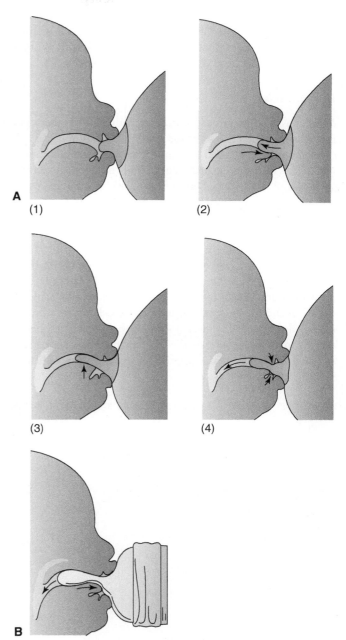

Figure 18.21. Differences in the sucking mechanism. (A) Breastfeeding. **(1)** Lips of the infant clamp in a C shape. The cheek muscles contract. **(2)** The tongue thrusts forward to grasp the nipple and areola. **(3)** The nipple is brought against the hard palate as the tongue pulls backward, bringing the areola into the mouth. **(4)** The gums compress the areola, squeezing milk into the back of the throat. **(B)** Formula feeding. The large rubber nipple of a bottle strikes the soft palate and interferes with the action of the tongue. The tongue moves forward against the gums to control the overflow of milk into the esophagus. (Reprinted with permission from Pillitteri, A. [2014]. *Maternal and child health nursing: Care of the childbearing and childrearing family* [7th ed., Fig. 19-2]. Philadelphia, PA: Lippincott Williams & Wilkins.)

Parents are often advised not to give artificial nipples to breastfed infants prior to 1 month of age.

Whenever possible, pacifiers should not be used to delay feedings or as a replacement for interaction with caregivers. Pacifiers should not be hung around the infant's neck, as the cord presents a risk for strangulation. Silicone pacifiers that are made in a single piece are considered safer than pacifiers made with multiple pieces, which may break and pose a choking risk (Fig. 18.22).

Milk Transfer

Milk transfer is the process of the milk moving from the breast into the infant. For this to be successful, the infant must be able to maintain an organized suck and swallow. Premature infants and infants with neurologic deficits may not be able to coordinate sucking and swallowing. Signs of disorganized sucking are premature break of the latch by the infant, gagging, and coughing. Often infant swallowing can be heard as a regular clicking noise. Parents can be assured that wet diapers and weight gain are both good signs of adequate intake.

Infants who are sated often break the latch spontaneously, no longer respond with the rooting reflex when the cheek or chin is touched, and appear calm, if not asleep. Infants who come off the breast and still indicate hunger by rooting should be switched to the other breast. The mother should empty one breast before moving to the second breast. The next feeding should start on the second breast to ensure it is emptied completely before returning

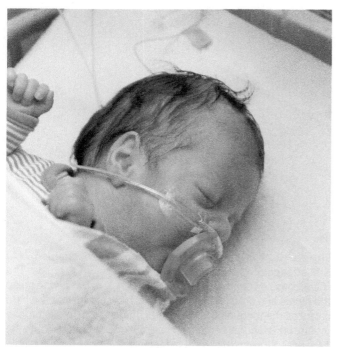

Figure 18.22. A preterm newborn receiving nonnutritive sucking with a pacifier. This type of pacifier is made from a single piece of silicone to minimize the risk of breakage and choking. (Reprinted with permission from Ricci, S. S. [2013]. *Essentials of maternity, newborn, & women's health nursing* [3rd ed., Fig. 23.6]. Philadelphia, PA: Lippincott Williams & Wilkins.)

the infant to the first breast. Some mothers use a bracelet or pin they move from one side to another to help them remember which breast the newborn nursed from last.

At times, particularly if the latch is uncomfortable, the mother or the nurse will need to break it. Simply pulling the infant from the nipple can be painful and may damage the nipple. To break a latch safely, place a gloved finger into the corner of the infant's mouth, breaking the suction.

Feeding Frequency

Optimally, the mother feeds the infant on demand, offering both breasts each feeding. The frequency with which infants demand feeding depends on the efficiency of milk transfer and milk supply. Infants often have discrete days when they feed more frequently before going back to their more typical schedule. Neonates feed as often as hourly, with frequency of feedings diminishing to 8 to 12 times daily by the time the infant is a week old. Milk transfer takes approximately 5 to 20 minutes per breast, depending on the mother–baby couplet and such factors as milk supply and infant age.

Infants tell parents when they are hungry, and it is a role of the nurse to help parents recognize these cues. Infants who are hungry often move their fists and fingers to their mouths and suck on them. They may smack their lips, become fussy and agitated, and flail their limbs. A loud persistent cry is generally a late sign of hunger. It is more difficult to achieve a latch with an agitated crying baby, and, optimally, hunger cues will be identified before this stage. Newborns who are ill or premature may not show later signs of hunger because of lack of reserves. Infants who do not wake naturally at least every 4 hours should be woken and fed until the milk supply is well established.

Breastfeeding Assessment

Successful breastfeeding can require some time, help, and ample reassurance. Many women cite their perception of inadequate milk intake as a reason for stopping breastfeeding (Odom, Li, Scanlon, Perrine, & Grummer-Strawn, 2013). Inadequate milk intake by an infant may be caused by issues with milk supply or milk extraction. Reasons for inadequate milk supply include previous breast surgery, insufficient development of breast tissue in pregnancy, and use of medications, such as decongestants, that reduce milk supply. Lactogenesis stage II (mature breast milk production) may be delayed as a result of retained placental fragments, preeclampsia, gestational hypertension, maternal obesity, prolactin insufficiency, or polycystic ovarian syndrome. Poor milk extraction may be caused by a poor latch, separation of the mother and baby, neurologic immaturity or abnormalities of the newborn, or excessive newborn sleepiness (American Academy of Pediatrics Committee on Nutrition, 2014).

Newborns lose an average of 7% of their birth weight within the first 5 days of life and usually regain this weight within 2 weeks. After lactogenesis stage II, no further infant weight loss is anticipated. Continuing weight loss and failure to gain weight are concerning, particularly if weight loss exceeds 10% of the birth weight. Newborns who are feeding well should have 6 to 8 wet diapers and three stools daily.

Several different scoring systems are used frequently to assess breastfeeding adequacy. None, however, have been thoroughly tested for validity and reliability, and thus they must be used with caution (Pados, Park, Estrem, & Awotwi, 2016). Scores may vary widely among users, so these assessments should not replace regular infant weighing, which provides the most accurate means of assessing intake.

The nurse should instruct the mother to observe the infant for evidence of feeding. Swallowing can often be heard as a click and viewed as a movement at the base of the throat. A well-fed infant spontaneously breaks the latch when sated and falls asleep or appears drowsy. Early on, mothers often find that the release of oxytocin during successful suckling causes them to become sleepy, as well. The nurse should instruct mothers to return infants to a firm surface absent of blankets, soft toys, and other suffocation risks prior to sleeping herself.

Nipple Discomfort

Nipple discomfort is a normal part of early breastfeeding. Normal nipple discomfort occurs for the first few sucks, may last for up to a minute, and is likely due to negative pressure acting on ducts that have yet to fill with milk. It typically resolves within a few weeks of the delivery (Lawrence & Lawrence, 2011). Nipple pain that lasts throughout the feeding and even worsens and pain that persists beyond a week or two is more likely associated with nipple injury due to poor positioning and/or latch. Common injuries include cracking, bruising, blistering, and abrasions.

Preventing Nipple Trauma

Strategies to prevent such injuries include optimized latch and the referral of women with flat or inverted nipples for prompt consultation with a lactation consultant. Abnormalities of the infant's mouth, such as a short frenulum, also require prompt evaluation. Women should defer the use of soap on the nipples and allow them to air dry. There is likely no benefit for preventing or healing nipple injuries from the use of lanolin, although it remains a popular routine intervention. No intervention or applying expressed breast milk to nipples after nursing may be equally or more effective (Dennis, Jackson, & Watson, 2014). Other breast problems associated with lactation are described in Table 18.6.

Care of Nipple Trauma

Primary actions for a patient with nipple trauma include evaluation of the latch and feeding the infant on the undamaged side first with each feeding. Infants suck more vigorously at the beginning of a feeding and may retraumatize a healing nipple more easily if the injured nipple is offered first. Traumatized nipples should be treated similarly to any other moist wound, with antibacterial ointments and nonstick pads to avoid the nipple sticking to the bra cup. Women may elect to pump their milk and feed their infant with a bottle in the short or long term if a traumatic latch continues to be challenging.

Milk Expression and Storage

Women often choose to pump milk. Pumped milk is typically stored but may be provided to the infant by bottle or gavage

Table 18.6 Breast Issues Associated With Lactation

Diagnosis	Symptoms	Interventions
Mastitis	• Area of localized pain and redness • Fever • Myalgia	• Anti-inflammatories • Cold compresses • Continuation of breastfeeding with complete emptying of the breast • Antibiotics
Abscess	• Tender breast mass • Typically proceeded by mastitis • Other symptoms, as with mastitis	• Drainage • Antibiotics • Continued emptying of the breasts by nursing or pumping
Candidal infection	• Deep, sharp, shooting pain • May be associated with infant candida infection • May have flaky or shiny nipple skin	• Topical antifungal • Gentian violet • Systemic antifungal
Bloody nipple discharge	• Pink-to-red milk in first days or weeks • Most common with first lactation	• Provide reassurance
Plugged duct	• Area of localized redness and tenderness • No systemic symptoms	• Optimize feeding technique • Breast massage • Warm compresses and showers • Analgesics
Galactoceles	• Milk-filled cysts • Nontender • Diagnosed by ultrasound and/or aspiration	• May be removed by surgery or aspiration if bothersome

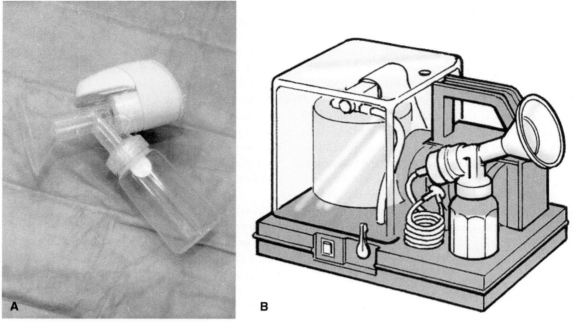

Figure 18.23. **Breast pumps. (A)** A handheld breast pump. **(B)** An electric breast pump. (Reprinted with permission from Ricci, S. S. [2013]. *Essentials of maternity, newborn, & women's health nursing* [3rd ed., Fig. 18.25]. Philadelphia, PA: Lippincott Williams & Wilkins.)

immediately. Rarely, pumped milk may be pumped to be discarded, as may be the case for a woman who needs to take a medication that is incompatible with breastfeeding. In these cases normal breastfeeding can resume per the instructions of the provider directing the patient's care. Most women who pump their milk do so to store it for later use when they will not be present to feed, as is the case for a mother returning to work before the infant is weaned. Women often pump when they are away from their infant for a period of time. When building the supply of milk for later use, many women pump immediately after feeding an infant.

Pumps may be electric or manual and may empty one breast at a time or both breasts (Figs. 18.23 and 18.24). Hospital pumps that closely simulate the suckling of infants are often available for rent. Some health insurance plans cover the cost of breast pumps for purchase or rent. Some women are able to manually empty their breasts without the use of a pump (Fig. 18.25).

Expressed milk may be stored at room temperature, in the refrigerator, in the freezer attached to a refrigerator, or in a deep freezer (Box 18.9). Milk may be stored in special bags or glass or BPA-free bottles. Stored milk should be labeled with the date the milk was expressed. When freezing milk, at least an inch of space should be left at the top of the storage container to allow for expansion during freezing. Frozen milk should be stored at the back of the freezer or refrigerator rather than the front to avoid temperature variation. Milk may be thawed overnight in the refrigerator and may be warmed or thawed under warm running water or in a bowl of warm water. Milk should not be warmed in the microwave or on the stovetop, because these processes may destroy maternal antibodies. Milk that has been thawed should be used within a few hours if left at room temperature and within

24 hours if refrigerated. It should not be refrozen (Office on Women's Health, 2016).

Formula Feeding

Infants not fed breast milk are fed formula, most often by bottle. Reasons for formula feeding may be health related, personal, or circumstantial. Women who need to go back to a job where they are unlikely to have the opportunity or space to pump, for example, may elect to bottle-feed with formula. In some cultures, formula feeding may be seen as a sign of affluence. Some women

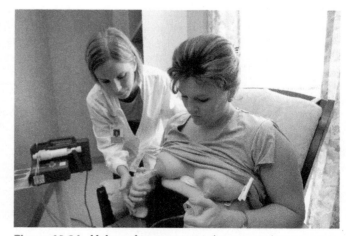

Figure 18.24. **Using a breast pump.** A nurse assists a woman in using a hospital pump to pump milk from both breasts at the same time. (Reprinted with permission from Hatfield, N. T. [2008]. *Broadribb's introductory pediatric nursing* [7th ed., Fig. 11-4]. Philadelphia, PA: Lippincott Williams & Wilkins.)

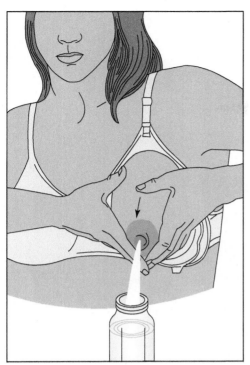

Figure 18.25. Manual breast milk expression. Instruct the mother to massage her breasts in a circular motion prior to starting expression (similar to a breast self-exam). Then, place her hand on her breast in a C shape, about an inch back from the areola. Have the mother press backward toward the chest wall, compress her breast between her fingers, and relax. It may take multiple cycles of pressing, compressing, and relaxing to see milk begin to flow. (Reprinted with permission from MacDonald, M. G., & Seshia, M. M. K. [2016]. *Avery's neonatology* [7th ed., Fig. 21.6B]. Philadelphia, PA: Lippincott Williams & Wilkins.)

may perceive formula feeding as more convenient or as a way to share the care of and bonding with the infant with partners and other caregivers. Women may be embarrassed by the idea of breastfeeding in public or in front of others in private spaces and thus believe breastfeeding is isolating. Women may be averse to the idea of breastfeeding or may not have good support from family, friends, or healthcare providers to breastfeed. They may perceive breastfeeding as difficult and lack the confidence to attempt it (Anstey, Chen, Elam-Evans, & Perrine, 2017; Bonia et al., 2014).

Box 18.9 Breast Milk Storage

- Room temperature: up to 6 h
- Insulated cooler: up to 1 d
- Refrigerator: up to 5 d
- Freezer: 3–6 mo
- Deep freezer: 6–12 mo

Adapted from Office on Women's Health. (2016, November). *Your guide to breastfeeding.* Retrieved from womenshealth.gov: https://www.womenshealth.gov/publications/our-publications/breastfeeding-guide/.

In Chapter 3, a nurse, Betty, asked whether Susan could pump breast milk for baby Winston. Susan explained she could stay home only for a few weeks with the baby before returning to work and that there was no place at work for her to pump. Susan became frustrated because she felt like formula was the best she could do and Betty was pushing her to do something that was not possible with her current work and life situation.

Infants digest formula more slowly than breast milk, and caregivers can anticipate less frequent feeding. Unlike breastfeeding, which is the task of the woman who was pregnant, formula feeding by bottle may be done by multiple caregivers. Women may feel that traveling with prepared formula and having others provide formula when she is absent are more convenient than pumping and planning activities around breastfeeding.

Formula does not have the same antibodies as those of breast milk, and formula-fed infants are more prone to infections. Parents of formula-fed infants miss more work because of childhood illnesses than do parents of breastfed infants. Formula-fed infants are more prone to childhood obesity and diabetes later in life. Although breastfeeding women require 500 additional calories a day when breastfeeding, formula feeding remains a more expensive option and, unlike breastfeeding, creates environmental waste (Office of Women's Health, 2014).

Infants should always be held during bottle-feeding, keeping the head elevated above the body (Fig. 18.26). Infants should

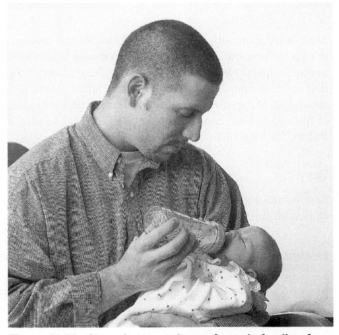

Figure 18.26. A newborn receives a formula feeding from her father. Notice the correct positioning. (Reprinted with permission from Hatfield, N. T. [2014]. *Introductory maternity and pediatric nursing* [3rd ed., Fig. 15-6]. Philadelphia, PA: Lippincott Williams & Wilkins.)

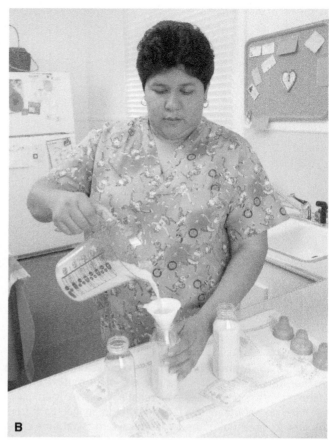

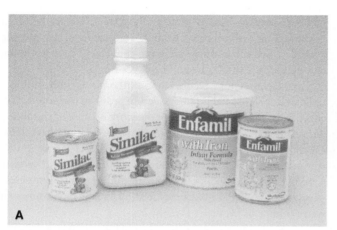

Figure 18.27. Bottle-feeding with formula. (A) Many types of prepared formulas are available for bottle-feeding. **(B)** When preparing bottles, always be sure to mix the formula according to the label instructions if the formula is not "ready-to-feed." (Reprinted with permission from Carter, P. J. [2016]. *Lippincott textbook for nursing assistants: A humanistic approach to caregiving* [4th ed., Fig. 44-12]. Philadelphia, PA: Lippincott Williams & Wilkins.)

never be fed alone with the bottle braced, because this presents a risk for choking and aspiration. Caregivers should be instructed to stop feeding the infant when the infant indicates satiety rather than trying to complete the remainder of the bottle. Information about types of formula, formula preparation, anticipated volume of formula needed, and feeding considerations are detailed in Patient Teaching 12.1 (Fig. 18.27).

Burping

Both bottle- and breastfeeding infants often swallow air along with nourishment. Burping infants is often believed to prevent colic from trapped gas and to minimize regurgitation. This practice is not well studied and was not found effective by a small study done recently but is frequently recommended for all infants regardless of feeding method. Burping at least twice, halfway through feeding (between breasts or halfway through the bottle) as well as after feeding (Kaur, Bharti, & Saini, 2015), is a typical recommendation.

To burp an infant, have a cloth ready to catch any fluid that may be regurgitated during the process. Infants can be burped with their body face down over the caregiver's lap, over the caregiver's shoulder, or in the sitting position. The infant's back should be lightly patted and/or rubbed until the infant burps (see Fig. 12.3).

Think Critically

1. What factors cause a neonate to initiate respirations?
2. Describe how an infant in respiratory distress might present.
3. From memory draw two pictures: one of fetal circulation and one of newborn circulation. What are the critical components?

4. An infant appears jaundiced. What factors would make the jaundice more concerning?
5. An infant has a red patch on his or her skin. How would you identify this mark, differentiating it from other types of markings? How would you discuss anticipated clinical outcomes with his or her parents?

6. Describe how infant senses differ from mature senses.
7. Identify and explain the different aspects of Apgar screening.
8. How would you explain the purpose of newborn screening and the method of sample collection to a new parent?
9. You are teaching a mother about infant feeding cues. How do you describe a hungry infant?
10. You are caring for a mother–baby couplet who are learning to breastfeed. The mother complains of nipple pain. What would cause you to suspect that the nipple pain is due to a poor latch or nipple damage?

References

Advisory Committee on Heritable Disorders in Newborns and Children. (2016, November). *Recommended uniform screening panel*. Retrieved from U.S. Department of Health and Human Services: https://www.hrsa.gov/advisory-committees/mchbadvisory/heritabledisorders/recommendedpanel/index.html

American Academy of Pediatrics Committee on Nutrition. (2014). Breastfeeding. In R. Kleinman, & F. Greer (Eds.), *Pediatric nutrition* (7th ed., p. 41). Elk Grove Village, IL: Author.

American Academy of Pediatrics Task Force on Circumcision. (2012). Male circumcision. *Pediatrics, 130*(3), e756.

Anstey, E., Chen, J., Elam-Evans, L., & Perrine, C. (2017). Racial and geographic differences in breastfeeding—United States, 2011–2015. *Morbidity and Mortality Weekly Report, 66*(27), 723.

Baby-Friendly USA. (2017, March 2). *Find facilities*. Retrieved from http://www.babyfriendlyusa.org/find-facilities

Badiee, Z., Asghari, M., & Mohammadizadeh, M. (2013). The calming effect of maternal breast milk odor on premature infants. *Pediatrics and Neonatology, 54*(5), 322–325.

Bonia, K., Twells, L., Halfyard, B., Ludlow, V., Newhook, L. A., & Murphy-Goodridge, J. (2014). A qualitative study exploring factors associated with mothers' decisions to formula-feed their infants in Newfoundland and Labrador, Canada. *BMC Public Health, 13*, 645.

Cavaliere, T. (2016). From fetus to neonate: A sensational journey. *Newborn and Infant Nursing Reviews, 16*(2), 43–47.

Centers for Disease Control and Prevention. (2012). CDC grand rounds: Newborn screening and improved outcomes. *Morbidity and Mortality Weekly Report, 61*(21), 390.

Chantry, C., Dewey, K., Peerson, J., Wagner, E., & Nommsen-Rivers, L. (2014). In-hospital formula use increases early breastfeeding cessation among first-time mothers intending to exclusively breastfeed. *The Journal of Pediatrics, 164*(6), 1339.e5–1345.e5.

Christensen, R. D., & Yaish, H. M. (2016). Hemolysis in preterm neonates. *Clinics in Perinatology, 43*(2), 233–240.

Dennis, C., Jackson, K., & Watson, J. (2014). Interventions for treating painful nipples among breastfeeding women. *Cochrane Database of Systematic Reviews,* (12), CD007366.

Desmond, M. M., Rudolph, A. J., & Phitaksphraiwan, P. (1966). The transitional care nursery: A mechanism for preventive medicine in the newborn. *Pediatric Clinics of North America, 13*(3), 651–668.

Fischer, T. P., & Olson, B. H. (2014). A qualitative study to understand cultural factors affecting a mother's decision to breast or formula feed. *Journal of Human Lactation, 30*(2), 209–216.

Freedman, A. L. (2016). The circumcision debate: Beyond benefits and risks. *Pediatrics, 137*(5). doi:10.1542/peds.2016-0594

Harris, D., Weston, P., & Harding, J. (2012). Incidence of neonatal hypoglycemia in babies identified as at risk. *The Journal of Pediatrics, 161*(5), 787–791.

Hauk, L. (2015). AAFP releases position paper on breastfeeding. *American Family Physician, 91*(1), 56–57.

Healthy People 2020. (2017, March 7). *Maternal, infant, and child health*. Retrieved from HealthyPeople.gov: https://www.healthypeople.gov/2020/topics-objectives/topic/maternal-infant-and-child-health/objectives

Herrington, C. J., & Chiodo, L. M. (2014). Human touch effectively and safely reduces pain in the newborn intensive care unit. *Pain Management Nursing, 15*(1), 107–115.

Kaur, R., Bharti, B., & Saini, S. K. (2015). A randomized controlled trial of burping for the prevention of colic and regurgitation in healthy infants. *Child: Care Health and Development, 41*(1), 52–56.

Kendall-Tackett, K. (2015). Birth interventions, postpartum depression, and breastfeeding. *Clinical Lactation, 6*(3), 85–86.

Lawrence, R., & Lawrence, R. (2011). *Breastfeeding: A guide for the medical professions* (7th ed.). Maryland Heights, MO: Mosby Elsevier.

Lee, A. C., Panchal, P., Folger, L., Whelan, H., Whelan, R., Rosner, B., … Lawn, J. E. (2017). Diagnostic accuracy of neonatal assessment for gestational age determination: A systematic review. *Pediatrics, 140*(6), e20171423.

Maisels, M. J., Clune, S., Coleman, K., Gendelman, B., Kendall, A., McManus, S., & Smyth, M. (2014). The natural history of jaundice in predominantly breastfed infants. *Pediatrics, 134*(2), e340–e345.

Marin, M. M., Rapisardi, G., & Tani, F. (2015). Two-day-old newborn infants recognise their mother by her axillary odour. *Acta Paediatrica, 104*(3), 237–240.

Míková, R., Vrkoslav, V., Hanus, R., Háková, E., Hábová, Z., Doležal, A., … Cvačka, J. (2014, June 9). Newborn boys and girls differ in the lipid composition of vernix caseosa. *PLoS One, 9*(6), e99173.

Morris, B., & Krieger, J. (2013). Does male circumcision affect sexual function, sensitivity, or satisfaction?—A systematic review. *Journal of Sexual Medicine, 10*(11), 2644–2657.

Odom, E., Li, R., Scanlon, K., Perrine, C., & Grummer-Strawn, L. (2013). Reasons for earlier than desired cessation of breastfeeding. *Pediatrics, 131*(3), e726–e732.

Office of Women's Health. (2014, July 21). *Why breastfeeding is important*. Retrieved from womenshealth.gov: https://www.womenshealth.gov/breastfeeding/breastfeeding-benefits.html

Office on Women's Health. (2016, November). *Your guide to breastfeeding*. Retrieved from womenshealth.gov: https://www.womenshealth.gov/publications/our-publications/breastfeeding-guide/

Pados, B. F., Park, J., Estrem, H., & Awotwi, A. (2016). Assessment tools for evaluation of oral feeding in infants younger than 6 months. *Advances in Neonatal Care, 16*(2), 143–150.

Schulte, R., Jordan, L. C., Morad, A., Nafte, R. P., Wellons, O. C., & Sidonio, R. (2014). Rise in late onset vitamin K deficiency bleeding in young infants because of omission or refusal of prophylaxis at birth. *Pediatric Neurology, 50*(6), 564–568.

Section on Breastfeeding. (2012). Breastfeeding and the use of human milk. *Pediatrics, 129*(3), e827.

Stevens, B., Yamada, J., Ohlsson, A., Haliburton, S., & Shorke, A. (2016, July 15). Sucrose for analgesia in newborn infants undergoing painful procedures. *Cochrane Database of Systematic Reviews, 7*, CD001069.

The Brazelton Institute. (2013). *The newborn behavioral observations system: What is it?*

Tran, T., Ng, I., Choojitarom, T., Webb, J., Jumonville, W., Smith, M., … Berry, S. (2016). Late newborn hearing screening, late follow-up, and multiple follow-ups increase the risk of incomplete audiologic diagnosis evaluation. *Journal of Early Hearing Detection and Intervention, 1*(2), 49–55.

Wang, M. (2016). Iron deficiency and other types of anemia in infants and children. *American Family Medicine, 93*(4), 270–278.

Wolke, D., Bilgin, A., & Samara, M. (2017). Systematic review and meta-analysis: Fussing and crying durations and prevalence of colic in infants. *The Journal of Pediatrics, 185*, 55–61.

Zimmerman, E., & Thompson, K. (2015). Clarifying nipple confusion. *Journal of Perinatology, 35*, 895–899.

Suggested Readings

Baby-Friendly USA. Retrieved from https://www.babyfriendlyusa.org/

Hillman, N., Kallapur, S. G., & Jobe, A. (2012). Physiology of transition from intrauterine to extrauterine life. *Clinics in Perinatology, 39*(4), 769–783.

National Association of Neonatal Nurses. Retrieved from http://nann.org/

Office on Women's Health, U.S. Department of Health and Human Services. (2017). *Breastfeeding*. Retrieved from https://www.womenshealth.gov/breastfeeding/

Unit 3
High-Risk Conditions and Complications

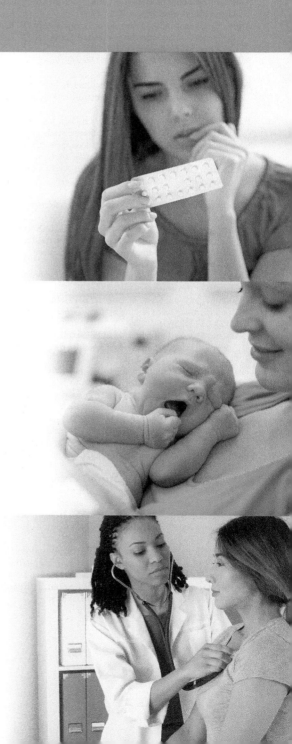

19 Conditions Existing Before Conception

Objectives

1. Identify preexisting conditions associated with increased pregnancy risk and explain why they increase risk.
2. Describe assessments related to preexisting conditions that nurses should be prepared to perform during pregnancy.
3. Discuss the major treatment options available for women with preexisting conditions during pregnancy and the effect of those treatments on the pregnancy.
4. Identify the key aspects of nursing care for common conditions that predate pregnancy.

Key Terms

Anorectal atresia
Contraction stress test
Diabetic ketoacidosis
Graves disease
Hashimoto thyroiditis
Hydrops fetalis

Multiple sclerosis (MS)
Ophthalmopathy
Phenylketonuria (PKU)
Systemic lupus erythematosus (SLE)
Vasculopathy

Conditions that complicate a pregnancy may start during the pregnancy, such as preeclampsia or gestational diabetes, or they may preexist the pregnancy. This chapter reviews some of the more common preexisting conditions that can complicate a pregnancy and the care considerations associated with them.

Asthma

Asthma is a chronic inflammatory disease of the airways.

Prevalence

Asthma complicates approximately 3% to 8% of pregnancies and is by far the most common pulmonary complication in pregnancy (Namazy & Schatz, 2016).

Signs and Symptoms

Symptoms are recurrent and highly variable. Some people with asthma rarely have symptoms, whereas others are frequently symptomatic and require medication throughout the day to suppress exacerbations. The signs and symptoms of an asthma attack include shortness of breath, a reported sensation of tightness in the chest, a cough that may be productive or nonproductive, wheezing, and a respiratory rate above 20 breaths per minute. Airways may become so restricted that hypoxia occurs. The signs of hypoxia include a respiratory rate over 30 breaths per minute, lethargy or agitation, confusion, intercostal retractions, and cyanosis.

Course in Pregnancy

Asthma overall tends to improve in the last 4 weeks of pregnancy, and asthma exacerbations in labor and delivery are rare. Some women experience an overall worsening of their asthma in pregnancy, whereas others note an improvement. Women who experience a worsening of their asthma in pregnancy tend to do so between weeks 29 and 36 of the pregnancy, and women who experience an improvement in their asthma tend to do so gradually throughout the course of the pregnancy. Up to one third of women experience an acute exacerbation of their asthma in pregnancy, and this may be attributed at least partly to women stopping or reducing their medications in a misguided effort to protect their pregnancies. Women with asthma are more likely to experience the following complications in pregnancy: antepartum and postpartum hemorrhage, preeclampsia, miscarriage, pulmonary embolism, preterm birth, low birth weight, and cesarean delivery. Such complications are increasingly likely with more severe asthma (Mendola et al., 2013).

Treatment

The goals of asthma management in pregnancy are the same as those outside of pregnancy: to optimize control of asthma and to limit or even eliminate exacerbations. Many of the medications used to treat asthma in pregnancy, including systemic corticosteroids, have minimal or no effects on a pregnancy (Bain et al., 2014; Namazy, Chambers, & Schatz, 2014). The great risks to the life of the mother and the health of the pregnancy that an acute asthma exacerbation poses typically outweigh the small risks of treatment (American College of Obstetricians and Gynecologists [ACOG], 2008, reaffirmed 2016a).

Care Considerations

Women may be concerned that medications taken in pregnancy may harm the fetus. The nurse should reassure these women that the benefits of limiting asthma exacerbations outweigh any potential harm and that taking the medications as directed will limit the potential for pregnancy complications (Namazy & Schatz, 2016).

Smoking cessation is important for everyone, especially for pregnant women, because smoking is associated with pregnancy loss, placenta previa, preterm labor, low birth weight, ectopic pregnancy, and preterm premature rupture of membranes. Smoking cessation is even more critical for pregnant women with asthma, as smoking increases the risk for asthma exacerbations and the need for medication.

Asthma is, in part, a response to the environment, and people with asthma can be hyperresponsive to allergens, exercise, cold air exposure, cigarette smoke, and other individual factors. The nurse should instruct all people with asthma to identify their triggers and avoid them as much as possible.

Women with asthma may require more frequent follow-up, generally determined by the severity of the disease and how well controlled it is. Visits at least every 4 weeks throughout pregnancy may help improve compliance with medication and overall asthma control (Baarnes, Hansen, & Ulrik, 2016).

Dyspnea is common with many pregnant women, but dyspnea with wheezing or a cough suggests an exacerbation of disease in women with asthma. Such women take control medications, as ordered, on a regular schedule to prevent exacerbations and rescue medications to stop them once they occur. Exacerbations in pregnancy that do not respond fully to rescue medications are medical emergencies. Although asthma itself is a risk to a pregnancy,

exacerbations further increase the risk for placental abruption, gestational diabetes, preeclampsia, and placenta previa (Ali, Hansen, & Ulrik, 2016).

A woman who is admitted with an exacerbation of asthma in pregnancy should have continuous pulse oximetry, with a goal of maintaining an oxygen saturation level (Spo_2) of 95% or higher. The nurse should deliver oxygen per orders to maintain this Spo_2. Spirometry, peak flow, or both are used to objectively assess the severity of the exacerbation. When evaluating the blood gasses during an asthma exacerbation in pregnancy, it is important to remember that some respiratory alkalosis is normal in pregnancy. A $Paco_2$ over 35 mm Hg or a Pao_2 below 70 mm Hg is more significant in a pregnant woman than in someone who is not pregnant and suggests more severe compromise. Women experiencing an acute attack are often more comfortable in a seated position than lying down.

The nurse should assess the fetal heart rate to verify fetal well-being. A heart rate between 110 and 160 beats per minute is reassuring of good fetal oxygenation. A nonstress test may be used to confirm fetal well-being, but not prior to 24 weeks of gestation. After 24 weeks, 50% of fetuses show accelerations using a nonstress test, and at 30 weeks, over 95% show accelerations (Pillai & James, 1990; see Box 3.6).

Epilepsy

Epilepsy is a disorder of the brain that causes recurrent seizures and is the most common neurologic disorder of women in pregnancy.

Prevalence

Approximately 1.2% of the total population of the United States has epilepsy (also called seizure disorder; Zack & Kobau, 2017). Offspring of mothers with epilepsy are at increased risk for developing a seizure disorder (Peljto et al., 2014).

Course in Pregnancy

Although 90% of women with epilepsy have an uneventful pregnancy, the condition presents a small increased risk for preterm labor, placental abruption, fetal growth restriction, prematurity, fetal death, and preeclampsia (MacDonald, Bateman, McElrath, & Hernandez-Diaz, 2015). Women who have not had a seizure for 9 months prior to the pregnancy are at a low risk for a seizure during pregnancy. However, a woman with epilepsy who smokes is at a considerably higher risk for preterm delivery (Harden, Pennell et al., 2009). The risk of maternal death during delivery is more than 10 times greater in women with epilepsy than those without it, with 80 deaths per 100,000 pregnant women with epilepsy compared with 6 deaths per 100,000 women in the general pregnant population (MacDonald et al., 2015). Women with epilepsy do not have more seizures during pregnancy than they would when not pregnant, and most do not have any seizures during pregnancy.

Treatment

Many medications are available to treat epilepsy and, in particular, to prevent seizures. Unfortunately, women who take these medications during pregnancy are at an increased risk for having children with minor or major congenital disorders. Untreated individuals do not have an increased risk for similar defects (Veiby, Daltveit, Engelsen, & Gilhus, 2014). The antiseizure drug valproate is particularly implicated in congenital anomalies, although the drugs phenytoin, carbamazepine, topiramate, and phenobarbital have also been associated with birth defects. Malformations of the neural tube, ear, urinary tract, palate, and skeleton are the common malformations among infants born to women taking these medications, and the use of multiple agents and high doses is associated with increased risk. Cognitive and verbal impairments in these children may be noted later in life. An increased risk of autism has been noted with the use of valproate in pregnancy (Christensen et al., 2013).

Care Considerations

Despite the potential risks to the fetus of taking medications, the nurse should encourage women to take the recommended doses to avoid seizure activity. The nurse should also instruct patients to get adequate sleep and to avoid individual triggers associated with seizure activity.

Many antiseizure drugs used to treat epilepsy—including phenytoin, lamotrigine, primidone, topiramate, carbamazepine, and oxcarbazepine—are cytochrome P-450 inducers, which means that they change the metabolism of some medications, including hormonal contraceptive methods, in such a way that either the contraceptive or the anti-seizure medication is less effective. Experts recommend against contraceptive pills, patches, and rings for women taking these medications (Curtis et al., 2016). Methods such as intrauterine contraception and contraceptive implants, which are considered more reliable in general, are especially recommended for women taking the above medications to treat epilepsy.

Because the use of antiseizure medications, especially valproate and carbamazepine, is associated with neural tube defects, as well as other congenital defects, a high intake of folic acid is recommended for women who take these medications. Preconception folic acid intake of 0.4 to 0.8 mg daily is recommended for all women, but women taking high-risk antiseizure medications should take 4 mg of supplemental folic acid daily, from 3 months before conception through at least 1 month after conception (ACOG Practice Bulletin, 2017).

A maternal serum alpha-fetoprotein (AFP) test based on blood drawn between 14 and 16 weeks of gestation is 80% to 90% sensitive for open neural tube defects (spina bifida and anencephaly). The addition of an ultrasound increases the accuracy of assessment to 94% to 100%. An amniocentesis may be performed to detect AFP from the amniotic fluid and acetylcholinesterase, as high levels of both are highly predictive of an open neural tube defect. Ultrasonography at 18 to 20 weeks of gestation, known as the fetal survey, can assess more broadly for anatomic defects (see Box 1.8).

Prescribing providers should carefully evaluate women taking an antiseizure medication for their continuing need for the medication, the type of medication, and the dose. Optimally, this evaluation should be done months before a woman attempts pregnancy. Because of changes in metabolism, renal clearance, gastrointestinal absorption, plasma protein, and maternal size and body composition,

medication monitoring and adjustment is warranted for several antiseizure medications, including topiramate, phenytoin, oxcarbazepine, levetiracetam, and lamotrigine. Ideally, plasma samples for the assessment of drug levels, if indicated, should be drawn consistently at the same interval since the last dose, preferably during the trough, which is usually first thing in the morning.

The neonates of mothers who have been taking antiseizure medications, particularly phenytoin, phenobarbital, and carbamazepine, are at an increased risk for bleeding (Cornelissen et al., 1993). To mitigate this effect, many providers recommend a maternal supplementation of 10 to 20 mg/d of vitamin K in the last month of pregnancy. However, evidence of the efficacy of this intervention is lacking in the literature (Harden, Hopp et al., 2009). In any case, all newborns receive a 1-mg intramuscular injection of vitamin K at birth and are monitored for bleeding. Fresh frozen plasma may be ordered in the event of a bleed.

Although a vaginal birth is generally preferred, even among women with epilepsy, a cesarean section may be done for a woman who experienced frequent seizures in her third trimester or who experiences high stress as a seizure trigger. It is important to maintain the therapeutic plasma levels of antiseizure medications during labor and delivery and the postpartum period. Women who do experience a seizure are treated with an intravenous (IV) benzodiazepine or phenytoin. Note that benzodiazepines may cause sedation and withdrawal symptoms in the neonate.

As the maternal physiology reverts to the prepregnant state, medication doses need to be titrated again. As during pregnancy, women with epilepsy should rest and avoid seizure triggers postpartum. To lessen the chance of injury to the neonate in the case of a maternal seizure, the mother should change the infant's diaper on the floor or in another low-risk position. Someone other than the mother should bathe the infant or be present when the mother is bathing the infant. It may be prudent for the mother to limit her carrying of the infant. Breastfeeding is not contraindicated with the maternal use of antiseizure medications.

Thyroid Conditions

The thyroid is a gland located in the neck that plays an important role in the maintenance of metabolism. A person with a hypoactive thyroid may feel cold and tired and experience hair loss and dry skin, among other symptoms. A person with hyperthyroidism may have difficulty keeping on weight and sleeping, emotional lability, and heat intolerance, as well as other complaints.

A hormone called thyrotropin-releasing hormone (TRH) is released from the hypothalamus in the brain, which stimulates the release of thyroid-stimulating hormone (TSH) from the pituitary gland (Fig. 19.1). TSH, in turn, stimulates the thyroid to release the hormones thyroxine (T4) and triiodothyronine (T3), which then stimulate tissue metabolism. Some conditions, such as the autoimmune condition Graves disease, cause the thyroid to overproduce T4 and T3. The hypothalamus, sensing the overabundance of these hormones, releases less TRH, and the pituitary, likewise, releases less TSH. A low plasma level of TSH, therefore, suggests hyperthyroidism. A sluggish thyroid that produces little T4 and T3, however, causes abundant secretion of TRH and TSH in an effort to stimulate greater production

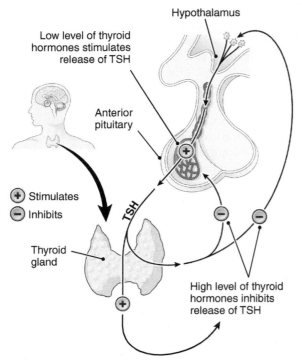

Figure 19.1. Negative feedback control of thyroid hormones. The anterior pituitary releases thyroid-stimulating hormone (TSH) when the blood levels of thyroid hormones are low. High levels of thyroid hormones inhibit the release of TSH, causing thyroid hormone levels to fall. (Reprinted with permission from Taylor, J. J., & Cohen, B. J. [2013]. *Memmler's structure and function of the human body* [10th ed., Fig. 11.1]. Philadelphia, PA: Lippincott Williams & Wilkins.)

of T4 and T3 from the thyroid. A high TSH level, therefore, suggests hypothyroidism.

Universal screening for thyroid disease in pregnancy is controversial. Often TSH is checked only in women with a personal or family history of thyroid disease, a personal history of pregnancy loss or preterm delivery, type 1 diabetes, obesity, infertility, or a history of radiation to the head or neck. Because a lack of screening may result in hyper- or hypothyroidism going undetected in over half the women who have it, however, others advocate for broader screening in the absence of signs, symptoms, and risk factors (Alexander et al., 2017).

Hypothyroidism

Etiology

The most common cause of hypothyroidism in countries with adequate dietary iodine is the autoimmune condition **Hashimoto thyroiditis**, also referred to as chronic autoimmune thyroiditis. Expected lab findings for hypothyroidism include a high TSH level and a low T4 level. A subclinical form of hypothyroidism would include a high TSH level and a normal T4 level. Rarely, a woman will have a form of central hypothyroidism that affects the hypothalamus or pituitary gland and is characterized by a normal TSH level and a low T4 level.

Signs and Symptoms

Many women with hypothyroidism have no symptoms or symptoms that are very similar to those seen in a normal pregnancy. Fatigue is a common finding for both, as are constipation, weight gain, and sensitivity to cold.

Course in Pregnancy

Hypothyroidism complicates only 0.3% to 0.5% of pregnancies despite being present in approximately 5% of women in the population (Garber et al., 2012). When complications do arise, however, they can pose considerable risks to the pregnancy. These include preeclampsia and gestational hypertension, postpartum hemorrhage, increased incidence of cesarean section, low birth weight, preterm delivery, placental abruption, infertility, and early pregnancy loss (Mannisto et al., 2013).

Cognitive impairment and neuropsychological damage of the neonate are thought to be particularly risks when the mother has hypothyroidism in the first trimester, as normal T4 levels are critical to fetal brain development and the fetus does not start to produce its own thyroid hormones until midway through the pregnancy. Not all studies agree with this conclusion, however, and hypothyroidism may, in fact, not pose a significant risk for cognitive or neuropsychological compromise (Fan & Wu, 2016).

Treatment

Treatment of hypothyroidism involves replacement of the thyroid hormones, usually only T4, as the liver converts T4 to T3, although some providers and patients also prefer to supplement T3. The adequacy of thyroid replacement treatment is measured by TSH serum levels according to trimester. The serum-level goals for TSH are as follows: 0.1 to 2.5 mU/L for the first trimester, 0.2 to 2 mU/L for the second trimester, and 0.3 to 3 mU/L for the third trimester (Stagnaro-Green et al., 2011). To meet these goals, the dose of T4 may need to be increased as early as the fifth week of pregnancy and by as much as 50%.

Women diagnosed with hypothyroidism typically receive a starting dose of 1 to 1.6 μg/kg/d of levothyroxine (a T4 replacement). The dose is evaluated by a TSH draw every 4 to 6 weeks and adjusted, typically by 25 to 50 μg, as indicated. Monitoring may be spaced out to every 2 or 3 months after the first trimester, as more dose adjustments are typically required in early pregnancy than in later pregnancy. Women with preexisting hypothyroidism should have their dose optimized prior to pregnancy, and as many as 85% require a dose adjustment in pregnancy (Vadiveloo, Mires, Donnan, & Leese, 2013).

Care Considerations

Levothyroxine should be taken on waking in the morning on an empty stomach, with no further oral intake for an hour. The nurse should emphasize to the patient the importance of taking the medication correctly. Some women just starting levothyroxine at a higher dose may initially feel anxious as a result of the medication and should be reassured that this is not an uncommon side effect and is transient.

Hyperthyroidism

Hyperthyroidism is a condition of overactivity of the thyroid.

Prevalence

Approximately 0.1% to 0.4% of pregnant women are diagnosed with hyperthyroidism (Lo et al., 2015).

Etiology

This condition is most often caused by **Graves disease** or by human chorionic gonadotropin (hCG)–mediated hyperthyroidism, which is generally more mild than the hyperthyroidism seen with Graves disease and is transient in pregnancy. Thyroid-stimulating immunoglobulins in the blood may be tested to determine the etiology of the hyperthyroidism, and are typically specific to Graves disease. In a pregnancy complicated by hyperthyroidism, maternal TSH level is either lower than anticipated or undetectable. Although it is normal for the total serum levels of T4 and T3 to be high in pregnancy, free levels of T4 and T3 should not rise.

If the hyperthyroidism is mediated by hCG, it is typically transient and does not require treatment. If the condition is caused by Graves disease, treatment is indicated.

Signs and Symptoms

Common discomforts of pregnancy, including poor heat tolerance, diaphoresis, and tachycardia, may also be signs and symptoms of hyperthyroidism. Weight loss with normal eating, a tremor, and anxiety are more suspicious for hyperthyroidism. Signs of Graves disease include a goiter and **ophthalmopathy**, an inflammatory condition of the eye that can cause retraction of the eyelid, conjunctivitis, swelling, and bulging eyes.

Course in Pregnancy

Pregnancy complications of hyperthyroidism, if not controlled, may include pregnancy loss, low birth weight, preterm labor, preeclampsia, and maternal heart failure (Alexander et al., 2017).

Rarely, infants of mothers with Graves disease are born with hyperthyroidism because of the transport of maternal thyroid-stimulating antibodies across the placenta. Tachycardia of the infant, goiter, poor growth, advanced bone development, premature fusion of the cranial sutures, heart failure, and an abnormal accumulation of fluid, called **hydrops fetalis**, are all potential signs and complications of the condition.

Treatment

Although there are multiple options to treat hyperthyroidism outside of pregnancy, the most common method is suppression of thyroid hormone synthesis with a class of medications called thioamides, which includes methimazole and propylthiouracil (PTU). Both methimazole and PTU cross the placenta and suppress fetal thyroid hormone synthesis, and both have been associated with fetal anomalies, including scalp defects, gastrointestinal abnormalities, and urinary tract abnormalities (Andersen, Olsen, Wu, & Laurberg, 2013). PTU is generally preferred in the first trimester and methimazole for the remainder of the pregnancy (Alexander et al., 2017; Ross et al., 2016).

The treatment goal for hyperthyroidism is to maintain mild hyperthyroidism to avoid hypothyroidism in the fetus (Alexander et al., 2017). Free T4 levels should be maintained at or slightly above the normal range for pregnancy, and total T4 levels should stay at 1.5 times the nonpregnant standard (Ross et al., 2016). A common starting dose for PTU is 50 mg two or three times daily and for methimazole 5 to 10 mg daily. Higher starting doses may be indicated for women with severe hyperthyroidism (Alexander et al., 2017; Ross et al., 2016). Thyroid tests should be done monthly, with the frequency increased to every 2 weeks when switching medications. Medication can often be discontinued in the third trimester for patients with Graves disease. Women often relapse postpartum and need continued monitoring, approximately every 6 weeks.

Providers may elect not to treat subclinical or mild hyperthyroidism, hCG-mediated hyperthyroidism, or a form of hyperthyroidism associated with hyperemesis gravidarum. Such women may instead be monitored by an assessment for serial T4 and TSH values every 4 to 6 weeks. Women with hyperthyroidism who are unable to take or tolerate medications may instead opt for a thyroidectomy during pregnancy. Women who are symptomatic may be offered a short course of beta blockers to mitigate symptoms until the thioamide prescribed is effective.

Care Considerations

PTU is associated with sudden and progressive liver damage. Women should be advised to report new-onset light-colored stools, dark urine, jaundice, weakness, malaise, nausea, and vomiting. Thioamides do pass into the breast milk, but mothers can be reassured that there is no evidence of a significant impact on the neonate. As with women diagnosed with and treated for hypothyroidism, the importance of consistent medication use must be emphasized.

Pregestational Diabetes

Many women start pregnancy with a diagnosis of type 1 or 2 diabetes. In other cases, particularly with type 2 diabetes, women are diagnosed early in the pregnancy. Women diagnosed with diabetes either before or early in pregnancy have pregestational diabetes, not gestational diabetes. Ideally, women with diabetes prior to pregnancy should receive preconception care and achieve excellent glycemic control prior to attempting pregnancy. Many pregnancies are unplanned, however, and prenatal visits are often the first chance for providers to assess patients for diabetes and provide education and interventions. Pregnancies complicated by preexisting diabetes are at a higher risk for preeclampsia, perinatal death, macrosomia of the infant, congenital anomalies, polyhydramnios, fetal loss, and spontaneous and indicated preterm birth, among other risks.

The more severe the diabetes, the more high risk is the pregnancy. The White classification (Table 19.1) is a commonly used tool to guide diabetes assessment and counseling, although other

Table 19.1 Modified White Classification of Diabetes in Pregnancy

Class	Description
Pregestational Diabetes	
A	Abnormal glucose tolerance test before pregnancy at any age or of any duration treated only by diet therapy
B	Onset at age 20 y or older and duration of less than 10 y
C	Onset at age 10–19 y or duration of 10–19 y
D	Onset before 10 y of age, duration over 20 y, benign retinopathy, or hypertension (not preeclampsia)
R	Proliferative retinopathy or vitreous hemorrhage
F	Nephropathy with over 500 mg/d proteinuria
RF	Criteria for both classes R and F
G	Many pregnancy failures
H	Evidence of arteriosclerotic heart disease
T	Prior renal transplantation
Gestational Diabetes	
A1	Diet controlled
A2	Insulin required for control

Adapted from White, P. (1978). Classification of obstetric diabetes. *American Journal of Obstetrics and Gynecology, 130*(2), 228–230; Bennett, S. N., Tita, A., Owen, J., Biggio, J. R., & Harper, L. M. (2015). Assessing White's classification of pregestational diabetes in a contemporary diabetic population. *Obstetrics and Gynecology, 125*(5), 1217–1223. doi:10.1097/AOG.0000000000000820

Box 19.1 Alternate Diabetes Risk Classification in Pregnancy

Type 1 Diabetes

Cause: Beta cell destruction and lack of insulin production
Subtypes:
a. Without vascular complications
b. With vascular complications (specify nephropathy, retinopathy, hypertension, arteriosclerotic heart disease, transplant, etc.)

Type 2 Diabetes

Cause: Inadequate insulin secretion and increased insulin resistance of cells
Subtypes:
a. Without vascular complications
b. With vascular complications (specify nephropathy, retinopathy, hypertension, arteriosclerotic heart disease, transplant, etc.)

Gestational Diabetes

Cause: Similar to that for type 2 diabetes, except that it develops only during pregnancy and typically resolves after pregnancy

Other Types of Diabetes

Causes:
• Genetic trait
• Drug or chemical induced

Adapted from Sacks, D. A., & Metzger, B. E. (2013). Classification of diabetes in pregnancy: Time to reassess the alphabet. *Obstetrics and Gynecology, 121*(2 Pt. 1), 345–348. doi: 10.1097/AOG.0b013e31827f09b5

criteria are sometimes used to conceptualize the severity of the diabetes and the risk it poses in pregnancy (Box 19.1; Sacks & Metzger, 2013). Women with an R or F designation by the White classification, for example, are at a significantly higher risk for preeclampsia than are women with a designation of B, C, or D (Sibai et al., 2000).

Assessment and Treatment Throughout the Pregnancy

First Trimester

Unlike women classified as low risk in pregnancy, who are generally screened only once for asymptomatic bacteriuria in pregnancy, women with diabetes, who are considered high risk,

may be screened frequently for bacteriuria throughout pregnancy, beginning in the first trimester.

Women with diabetes, particularly those who did not have preconception counseling or who do not have an established record of tight glycemic control, also undergo hemoglobin A_{1c} testing in the first trimester. The hemoglobin A_{1c} test provides information about the patient's average blood glucose level for the past 2 to 3 months.

If not done prior to conception, the mother undergoes an evaluation in the first trimester to determine any end-organ damage to the kidneys, thyroid, heart, and eyes resulting from the diabetes as well as comorbidities. An assessment of urine protein content, either by a 24-hour urine collection or by a single urine sample evaluated for the protein:creatinine ratio, is performed to provide information about baseline kidney function. Women with type 1 diabetes are often screened for thyroid dysfunction during pregnancy with tests of blood levels of TSH and T4. Ischemic heart disease is common in women who have pregestational diabetes with hypertension and/or evidence of vascular damage from diabetes (diabetic vasculopathy). An electrocardiogram can screen for this damage (Blumer et al., 2013). Diabetic retinopathy is a common complication of diabetes, and the American Diabetes Association recommends a comprehensive dilated eye exam by an ophthalmologist starting in the first trimester and then regularly throughout the pregnancy and the first-year postpartum at intervals determined by exam findings (American Diabetes Association, 2017).

An early ultrasound is often ordered because women with poor glycemic control miscarry more frequently and because careful dating of the pregnancy is important in the event that an early delivery is indicated.

Second and Third Trimesters

In the second trimester, visits for women with diabetes are often 2 to 4 weeks apart. In the third trimester, visits may be scheduled every 1 or 2 weeks to monitor maternal glycemic control and fetal well-being. Also in the third trimester, more frequent dosing adjustments are commonly required for women who are insulin-dependent. In the event of good glycemic control, fetal demise is rare. With poor glycemic control, fetal hypoxia may result from maternal hyperglycemia that leads to fetal hyperglycemia and increased insulin production and oxygen consumption, or from a reduction in uteroplacental perfusion resulting from diabetic **vasculopathy**. Vasculopathy may first be evidenced by fetal growth restriction. Prepregnancy obesity and poor glycemic control, in addition to gaining more weight than recommended, are associated with macrosomia (see Box 1.5; Siegel, Tita, Biggio, & Harper, 2015).

Antepartum testing for fetal well-being usually begins between 32 and 34 weeks of gestation (ACOG, 2005, reaffirmed 2016). Evaluations may include nonstress tests, biophysical profiles, fetal movement counts, and contraction stress tests (see Box 3.6; Table 1.2; Box 5.4).

A **contraction stress test** is similar to a nonstress test in that both monitor uterine activity and fetal heart rate. By definition, however, a nonstress test is done in the absence of contractions, and a contraction stress test can be done only in the presence of contractions (Figs. 19.2 and 19.3; Table 19.2). The choice of a nonstress test or a contraction stress test is at the discretion of the obstetric provider. One is not clearly more predictive than the other. A contraction stress test requires uterine contractions induced either with oxytocin or with stimulation of the maternal nipples and is thus risker, typically making the nonstress test the evaluation of choice. The contraction stress test is contraindicated with any condition in which labor is a contraindication, including placenta previa and a high risk for preterm delivery. Nonreassuring results may occur with maternal ketoacidosis or maternal hyperglycemia and may be reversible. If the cause of the nonreassuring test is not reversible, the pregnancy may be delivered promptly or after a course of glucocorticoids if the pregnancy is less than 34 weeks of gestation (see The Pharmacy 8.2).

Delivery

Diabetes also affects considerations regarding the timing and type of delivery. In births occurring prior to 39 weeks of gestation,

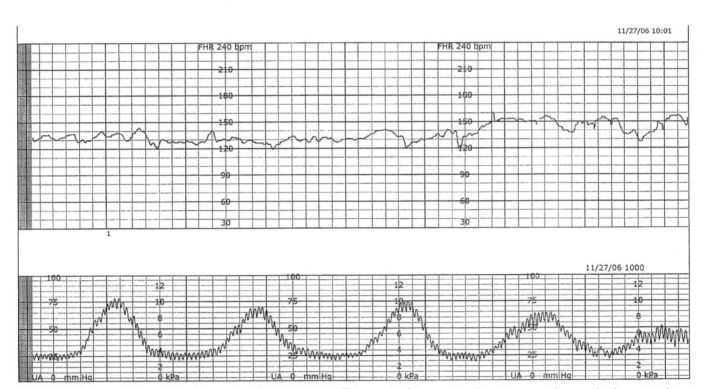

Figure 19.2. A negative result of a contraction stress test. This result of the contraction stress test is negative because there are no early decelerations, indicating good fetal reserve. FHR, fetal heart rate; bpm, beats per minute. (Reprinted with permission from Gabrielli, A., Layon, A. J., & Yu, M. [2008]. *Civetta, Taylor, and Kirby's critical care* [4th ed., Fig. 101.5]. Philadelphia, PA: Lippincott Williams & Wilkins.)

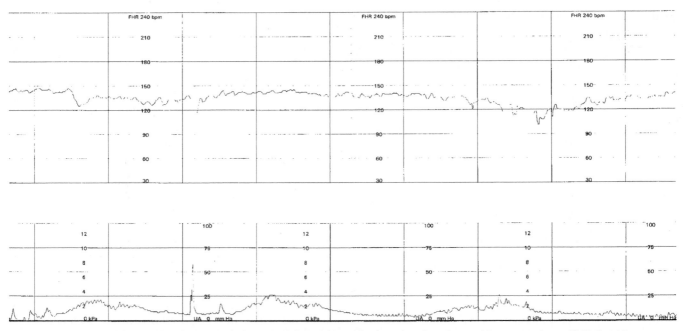

Figure 19.3. A positive result of a contraction stress test. Note the late decelerations with contractions. FHR, fetal heart rate; bpm, beats per minute. (Reprinted with permission from Menihan, C. A., & Kopel, E. [2014]. *Point-of-care assessment in pregnancy and women's health: Electronic fetal monitoring and sonography* [1st ed., Fig. 4.7]. Philadelphia, PA: Lippincott Williams & Wilkins.)

Table 19.2   Comparison of Nonstress Tests With Contraction Stress Tests: Procedure and Interpretation of Findings

	Nonstress Test	Contraction Stress Test
Procedure	1. Place a fetal heart monitor on the woman's abdomen at the level of the fetal heart. 2. Place a tocotransducer at the fundus of the uterus to detect any spontaneous uterine activity.	1. Place a fetal heart monitor on the woman's abdomen at the level of the fetal heart. 2. Place a tocotransducer at the fundus of the uterus to detect any spontaneous uterine activity. 3. Induce contractions by administering dilute oxytocin or having the woman directly stimulate her nipples until three uterine contractions occur in 10 min.
Reassuring findings	• *Reactive, fetus 32 wk or older:* Two or more fetal heart rate accelerations of 15 bpm or more for 15 s or more in 20 min • *Reactive, fetus younger than 32 wk:* Two accelerations or more of at least 10 bpm lasting 10 s or more in 20 min	*Negative:* No late decelerations or frequent variable decelerations
Indeterminate findings	N/A	• *Equivocal:* Some late decelerations or several variable decelerations • *Unsatisfactory:* Three contractions in 10 min could not be achieved.
Nonreassuring findings	*Nonreactive:* Does not meet standards of reactivity. The test should continue for at least 40 min and as long as 120 min before the findings are determined to be nonreactive.	*Positive:* Decelerations with at least 50% of contractions, even if three contractions in 10 min have not been achieved
Possible causes of nonreassuring findings	• Fetal hypoxemia • Fetal sleep • Maternal smoking just prior to the test • Fetal immaturity • Sepsis • Fetal abnormalities • Drugs with cardiac effects	Fetal hypoxemia (up to 40% correlation)

Table 19.2 Comparison of Nonstress Tests With Contraction Stress Tests: Procedure and Interpretation of Findings (continued)

	Nonstress Test	Contraction Stress Test
Further evaluation	• Biophysical profile • Vibroacoustic stimulation • Repeat test after half hour • Contraction stress test	Biophysical profile

bpm, beats per minute; NA, not applicable.

infants of mothers with pregestational diabetes are more likely to experience respiratory distress because of the maternal endocrine changes associated with diabetes impacting fetal lung development. Although it was once common to test amniotic fluid collected by amniocentesis to assess fetal lung maturity, this practice is now far less prevalent and rarely done for pregnancies that have reached 39 weeks by reliable dates. Although births before 39 weeks are avoided in the case of good glycemic control and no apparent complications, induction between 39 and 40 weeks is common practice (ACOG, 2005, reaffirmed 2016). Indications for an earlier delivery include nonreassuring antepartum fetal testing (nonstress test, biophysical profile, and/or contraction stress test), poor maternal glycemic control, abnormal fetal growth, vascular disease, preeclampsia, and/or history of stillbirth in a prior pregnancy (ACOG, 2005, reaffirmed 2016).

Pregestational diabetes is not a contraindication to vaginal birth, although some providers may opt to recommend a cesarean birth for a fetal macrosomia assessed by ultrasound, despite the limited correlation between ultrasound size estimates and actual birth weight. Although a strong suspicion of fetal macrosomia is always a potential indication for cesarean section, the increased chest and shoulder proportions of the macrosomic infants of diabetic mothers make these deliveries particularly high risk for shoulder dystocia (ACOG, 2016).

After Delivery

The mother's insulin needs drop sharply after the birth and are recalculated according to serial assessments of blood glucose level (see Fig. 9.5). For women with type 1 diabetes, glucose level should be checked every 4 to 6 hours, with insulin doses titrated accordingly. Within 48 hours after delivery, the required dose of insulin is approximately half of what it was prior to delivery and the patient can typically resume a calculated dose of 0.6 U/kg of her current weight.

Women with type 2 diabetes who still make endogenous insulin require different care. Like women with type 1 diabetes, women with type 2 diabetes who require insulin have insulin prescribed according to glucose results, but serial checks are done fasting, before meals, and after meals. Their blood glucose level should also normalize within 48 hours, and the standard care they required prior to pregnancy (management by diet, exercise, or medications) can resume.

Neither diabetes nor the medications used to treat it are contraindications for breastfeeding. Breastfeeding should be encouraged. Breastfeeding requires about 500 kcal/d and can be counted as 100 g of carbohydrates and 20 g of protein for the purposes of dietary tracking and glycemic control.

Care Considerations

It is important that women with diabetes adhere closely to prescribed diet, exercise, and medications during pregnancy. Regular blood glucose readings are often part of prescribed self-care and may be new for patients without a prior diagnosis or who are early in the disease process. Patients often need more frequent prenatal visits to regularly and routinely evaluate self-care.

When a birth prior to 34 weeks of gestation is anticipated, the administration of glucocorticoids is indicated to improve fetal outcomes. Glucocorticoids, however, cause a kind of transient hyperglycemia that can be particularly concerning in women with diabetes, regardless of the adequacy of their glucose control. The hyperglycemic effect begins approximately 12 hours after the administration of the first injection and lasts for approximately 5 days. Frequent glucose monitoring and the titration of insulin doses are required during this time. Women whose diabetes cannot be managed adequately with subcutaneous (SQ) insulin may require IV insulin. A common plan of care includes hourly glucose monitoring starting 12 hours after the first steroid injection and lasting through 24 hours after the final dose. After this, glucose monitoring continues at gradually widening intervals until the glucose level is stable.

Because the pregnancies of women with diabetes are at a higher risk for nonreassuring fetal statuses, continuous rather than intermittent fetal monitoring is indicated. Monitoring and maintenance of maternal blood glucose level is important. Maternal blood glucose level is typically monitored at the time of admission and then every 2 to 6 hours, depending on her degree of glycemic control in pregnancy. Many women can be maintained with SQ insulin during labor and delivery, although both glucose and insulin are available for IV administration as indicated by blood glucose results. The goal for maternal blood glucose level during labor and delivery is generally between 70 and 126 mg/dL (ACOG, 2005, reaffirmed 2016; Blumer et al., 2013). Maternal hyperglycemia as low as 140 to 180 mg/dL can result in maternal ketoacidosis or fetal hyperglycemia. Fetal hyperglycemia results in a higher fetal need for oxygen and an increased risk for fetal hypoxia.

Complications and Comorbidities of Diabetes During Pregnancy

Besides the usual concerns associated with diabetes outside of pregnancy, diabetes is also associated with significant complications and comorbidities during pregnancy, which are discussed below.

Hypertension and Preeclampsia

Women with diabetes often also have hypertension. Some medications used to treat hypertension, such as angiotensin-converting enzyme inhibitors and angiotensin receptor blockers, are known teratogens and must be discontinued during pregnancy and replaced with other medications. The blood pressure of women who do not have end-organ damage is maintained below 160/105 mm Hg, and that of women with evidence of organ damage is maintained below 140/90 mm Hg (ACOG, 2005, reaffirmed 2016; American Diabetes Association, 2017). Pregestational diabetes is a risk factor for preeclampsia, and taking an 81-mg aspirin daily after 12 weeks of gestation can significantly reduce that risk by as much as 24% in this population (Henderson et al., 2014).

Congenital Anomalies

Poor preconception glycemic control as measured by hemoglobin A_{1c} is associated with a higher rate of miscarriage and more congenital anomalies. The most common anomalies associated with poor preconception glycemic control are neural tube and cardiac defects, and the risk of perinatal death is higher in this population (Tennant, Glinianaia, Bilous, Rankin, & Bell, 2014). A maternal AFP test and ultrasound in the late first trimester screen for neural tube defects, and a second trimester fetal survey can detect cardiac and other anatomic defects. Because of the higher risk of neural tube defects, supplementation with 4 to 5 mg of folic acid is indicated (Blumer et al., 2013).

Accelerated Fetal Growth

Pregnancies complicated by diabetes may also be complicated by accelerated fetal growth. Less common is impaired growth associated with preeclampsia and/or diabetic vasculopathy. Fundal height measurements are done regularly (see Fig. 4.4). Generally, a measurement that is more than 2 cm greater or smaller than anticipated requires further evaluation. Fundal height measurement is often supplemented by ultrasound evaluations of fetal size in the third trimester.

Although maternal glucose passes the placenta to the fetus, maternal insulin does not. Fetuses exposed to excess maternal glucose produce extra insulin. Insulin is a growth hormone, which acts to accelerate fetal growth and can lead to infants being large for gestational age (greater than 90th percentile for gestational age) or macrosomic (over 4,000 g; Hewapathirana & Murphy, 2014). These infants, in addition to being large, have disproportionately accelerated growth of the shoulders and chest. Thus, maternal diabetes increases the risk for shoulder dystocia significantly, in addition to increasing the risk for surgical delivery, birth trauma for the mother and baby, perinatal death, and a prolonged second stage (pushing stage) of labor.

Diabetes is not the only risk factor for shoulder dystocia. Edie, in Chapter 11, was not diabetic. Her risk factor for shoulder dystocia was the rapid speed of her labor and delivery.

Diabetic Ketoacidosis

Diabetic ketoacidosis is a life-threatening complication of diabetes in which acidic ketones accumulate in the blood as a result of the metabolizing of stored fats, causing a state of acidosis. Common symptoms include polyuria, polydipsia (thirst), abdominal pain, nausea and vomiting, and mental status changes. In the nonpregnant population, diabetic ketoacidosis usually manifests with a blood glucose level of 250 mg/dL or more. In the pregnant population, however, it may appear with a blood glucose level as low as 200 mg/dL. Because of the abnormal diuresis that occurs with this condition, maternal plasma volume decreases, resulting in hypoperfusion of the uterus and placenta, which can, in turn, lead to fetal hypoxemia and hypoxia. The rate of fetal mortality with diabetic ketoacidosis is as high as 36% (Sibai & Viteri, 2014). Management priorities include glycemic control, volume replacement, electrolyte replacement, and close fetal monitoring. Ketoacidosis is not an indication for emergent delivery, and the fetal heart tracing taken during this complication (which often shows no or minimal variability, no accelerations, and decelerations) typically returns to normal as the condition of the mother improves (Sibai & Viteri, 2014). See Chapter 25 for care of the neonate of a diabetic mother.

Systemic Lupus Erythematosus

Systemic lupus erythematosus (SLE) is an autoimmune disease in which the immune system attacks various parts of the body. It has multiple presentations (Fig. 19.4). The disease is treatable but has no cure and is most common in women. Most people diagnosed with SLE live a normal life span and will have times when their disease is active, referred to as "flares," and quiescent times referred to as "remission."

Course in Pregnancy

SLE poses a risk for both the mother and fetus in pregnancy, and it is safest to attempt pregnancy when the disease has been in remission for at least 6 months. Women who have had active disease in the 6 months prior to pregnancy or have renal involvement are most likely to experience disease exacerbation in pregnancy, and overall, between 25% and 60% of women living with SLE in pregnancy experience these flares (Lateef & Petri, 2013). More severe maternal disease that includes cardiac, lung, or renal involvement or stroke indicates a higher-risk pregnancy, as does the presence of antiphospholipid antibodies (Lateef & Petri, 2013).

Women with SLE have two to seven times the risk of pregnancy complications, including hypertensive disorders of pregnancy (gestational hypertension, preeclampsia, and eclampsia), preterm labor and birth, cesarean section, blood clots, infection, thrombocytopenia (low platelets), and the need for a blood transfusion. The risk for maternal death is also approximately 20 times that of the general pregnant population (Clowse, Jamison, Myers, & James, 2008). Up to 30% of pregnant women with SLE develop preeclampsia (Abalos, Cuesta, Grosso, Chou, & Say, 2013). Up to 50% of women with SLE deliver prematurely, and up to 30%

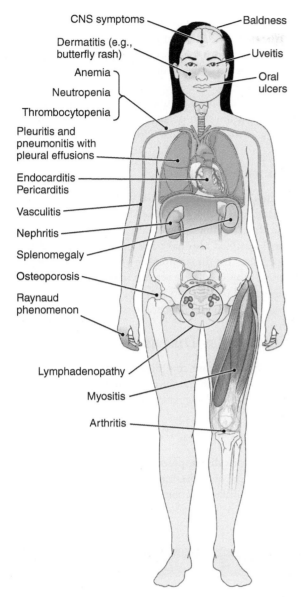

Figure 19.4. Clinical findings in systemic lupus erythematosus. (Reprinted with permission from McConnell, T. H. [2014]. *The nature of disease: Pathology for the health professions* [2nd ed., Fig. 3.12]. Philadelphia, PA: Lippincott Williams & Wilkins.)

of fetuses of mothers with SLE are growth restricted and born small for gestational age (Saavedra et al., 2012). Some infants of mothers carrying the anti-Rh/SSA or anti-LA/SAA antibodies associated with lupus and another autoimmune disease, Sjogren syndrome, develop neonatal lupus. The manifestations of neonatal lupus are usually cutaneous and/or cardiac but may also present as abnormalities of the blood or liver.

Additionally, fetuses of women who test positive for anti-Ro/SSA and anti-La-SSB antibodies are at a high risk for developing a heart block, usually between 16 and 24 weeks of gestation. Some degrees of heart block may be reversible by the use of glucocorticoids during pregnancy, but the overall combined fetal and infant mortality rate resulting from SLE-related heart block is over 17% (Izmirly et al., 2011). Overall, however, the risk is quite low, with only approximately 1% to 2% of infants born to women with anti-Ro/SSA and anti-La-SSB antibodies developing neonatal lupus with heart block (Brito-Zeron, Izmirly, Ramos-Casals, Buyon, & Khamashta, 2015).

Assessment

Ideally, assessment should be done prior to pregnancy to evaluate disease status and the functioning of target organs. Laboratory tests will be performed to examine renal and liver function, complete blood count, antibodies, and complement levels (low or decreasing levels of complement are associated with SLE flares).

Because of the frequency of intrauterine growth restriction, serial ultrasounds for fetal growth start in the first trimester and are repeated approximately monthly or more frequently depending on findings. Fetal testing by nonstress test, biophysical profile, and/or contraction stress test is routine in the final 4 to 6 weeks of pregnancy. Fetuses of women who test positive for anti-Ro/SSA and anti-La-SSB antibodies should undergo antepartum heart monitoring by weekly echocardiograms between 16 and 38 weeks of gestation (Donofrio et al., 2014).

Treatment

Some medications used to treat SLE are contraindicated in pregnancy, and others may be considered safer with reduced dosing.

Care Considerations

Mothers with a diagnosis of SLE typically require additional laboratory tests to monitor kidney function, complete blood count, and disease activity as indicated by the clinical presentation. Postpartum flares of the disease are not uncommon, particularly in women with significant SLE-related organ damage who were not in remission at the time that pregnancy was achieved. Postpartum laboratory tests are performed at 1 month after the birth and are generally the same as those used to monitor the disease process and kidney function during pregnancy. Because of the high risk for preeclampsia, low-dose aspirin therapy (81 mg daily) is recommended starting between 12 and 20 weeks postpartum (Henderson et al., 2014). Fetal growth monitoring and antepartum screening of neonatal well-being are critical components of care. Women with SLE may still breastfeed, although some of the medications used to treat the disease are contraindicated while they are breastfeeding, including cyclophosphamide and high doses of methotrexate.

It is essential for nurses to educate patients with SLE prior to conception about the importance of waiting to attempt pregnancy until the patient has had six consecutive symptom-free months and about the risks associated with not doing so, particularly in the presence of renal involvement. The nurse should take care to provide contraception education to the patient during riskier periods to help prevent pregnancies. Women with SLE require frequent prenatal visits and close monitoring during pregnancy, and the nurse should provide clear instructions to the patient and emphasize the importance of receiving this care and complying with instructions to help optimize pregnancy outcomes.

Multiple Sclerosis

Multiple sclerosis (MS) is a chronic immune-modulated demyelinating disease of the central nervous system. Most people with MS are women and, at least initially, have a form of the disease that includes both relapses and remissions (Compston & Coles, 2008).

Signs and Symptoms

Common symptoms of relapse include changes in sensation, loss of vision, weakness, motor changes, gate disturbances, sphincter and bowel dysfunction, pain, and others. In general, pregnancy is a time of disease remission, whereas the postpartum period is significant for relapse (Bove et al., 2014). Pregnancy does not appear to increase the risk for long-term disability from MS (Ramagopalan et al., 2012). Artificial reproductive technology, however, appears to dramatically heighten the risk for increased MS disease activity (Hellwig & Correale, 2013).

Course in Pregnancy

The risks that MS poses to pregnancy include a modest increase in rate of cesarean section and a decrease in birth weight. There is likely no increased risk for stillbirth, birth defects, preterm birth, pregnancy loss, or pregnancy complications (Bove et al., 2014).

Treatment

Some drugs used to treat MS are teratogenic and contraindicated in pregnancy. Other medications have limited safety information available. Prescribing clinicians may opt to continue the use of disease-modifying medications during pregnancy, whereas others, based on the clinical situation, may opt to discontinue medications. When the medications are discontinued prior to pregnancy, a washout period is often advised during which a woman should not attempt pregnancy. Depending on the medication, the washout period may last for 1 to 6 months (Coyle, 2014). Although the rate of relapse is lower in pregnancy, relapses do occur during pregnancy and are often treated with IV glucocorticoids.

Care Considerations

Breastfeeding is not contraindicated with MS. Although studies suggest that disease activity is reduced for women who breastfeed, it may be that the numbers actually reflect that women who choose to breastfeed also have less disease activity, although. Others speculate that the suppression of menses by breastfeeding may, in turn, suppress disease activity (Hellwig et al., 2015). The medications used to treat MS may not be safe for the breastfed infant, and most women choose not to take them during this time.

Cardiovascular Disease

Although cardiac disease complicates only a small number of pregnancies, it is a significant cause of nonobstetric maternal morbidity and mortality in pregnancy (Gaddipati & Troiano, 2013).

Course in Pregnancy

The risk that cardiac disease poses to the pregnant woman depends on the specific type of cardiac anomaly (Table 19.3), the effect the disease has on cardiac function (Tables 19.4 and 19.5), and the

Table 19.3   Heart Conditions That Complicate Pregnancy

Condition	Description	Care
Congenital Cardiac Disorders: Left-to-Right Shunts*		

Ventricular septal defect	• Congenital opening between the right and left ventricles
	• Rarely, part of the sequelae after an MI
	• Small and repaired defects: no impact on pregnancy
		Potential complications with large defects:
		• Heart failure
		• Pulmonary hypertension
		• Arrhythmias
		• Shunting (deoxygenated blood reenters the systemic circulation)
		• Increased risk for:
		  ○ Congenital heart defects in offspring
		  ○ Emboli
		Nursing considerations:
		• Be alert for blood clots
		• Use venous compression devices during labor and delivery and postpartum
		• Administer heparin per orders

Patent ductus arteriosus	• Persistence of ductus arteriosus after birth, causing shunting between the aorta and the pulmonary artery • Routinely repaired in childhood • Small defects: no related complications in pregnancy	Potential complications with large, unrepaired defects: • Congestive heart failure • Pulmonary hypertension

Table 19.3 Heart Conditions That Complicate Pregnancy (continued)

Condition	Description	Care
Atrial septal defect	• The most common congenital cardiac lesion in pregnancy • An opening between the right and left atria	Increased risk for emboli Nursing considerations: • Pulmonary hypertension rare • Be alert for blood clots • Use venous compression devices during labor and delivery and postpartum • Administer heparin per orders
Other Congenital Cardiac Lesions		

Tetralogy of Fallot	• The most common congenital heart defect causing cyanosis
	• Features include:
	  ○ Pulmonary stenosis
	  ○ Ventricular septal defect
	  ○ An overriding aorta
	  ○ Hypertrophy of the right ventricle
	• Major outcome: Shunting of the blood into the systemic circulation without it first passing through the lungs to be oxygenated
	• Pregnancy outcomes usually good if defect corrected prior to pregnancy
		Cardiologist consultation advised prior to pregnancy, even with correction
		If unrepaired, higher risk for:
		• Tachycardia
		• Right-sided heart failure
		• Congenital cardiac anomalies of offspring (thus echocardiogram of fetus recommended in second trimester)

Coarctation of the aorta	• Narrowing of the aorta, usually distal to the left subclavian artery • Often repaired in childhood	Monitor for development of hypertension and aortic dissection
Acquired Cardiac Disorders		
Mitral valve stenosis	• Narrowing of the mitral valve • Reduced function of the valve, causing slowed filling of the left ventricle • Most commonly caused by rheumatic heart disease caused by a group A strep infection • May be congenital	Treatment: • Beta blockers (increase diastolic filling time) • Anticoagulants (in case of atrial fibrillation from distention of the atrium or pooling of blood in a left atrium that is not emptying completely) • Diuretics (in case of heart failure) • Valve replacement (rare)
Aortic stenosis	• Narrowing of the aortic valve • Most often rheumatic in origin • Patients may have difficulty keeping up with increased cardiac output demands of pregnancy • Risk minimal until valve is one third or less normal size • May be repaired prior to or even during pregnancy	Increased risk for: • Heart failure • Pulmonary edema • Arrhythmias Nursing considerations: • Hypovolemia presents more risk than hypervolemia • Maintain blood volume
Peripartum cardiomyopathy	• A form of heart failure that appears late in pregnancy or in the first 5 mo postpartum • Partial or complete recovery possible	Increased risk for: • Maternal mortality in the 2 y following diagnosis • Recurrence with future pregnancies Treatment: • Oxygen and symptom relief • Anticoagulants (if elevated clotting risk) • Beta blockers (if arrhythmia) • Diuretics (to reduce preload) • Vasodilators (to reduce afterload) • Sodium, fluid, and activity restriction

(continued)

Table 19.3 Heart Conditions That Complicate Pregnancy (continued)

Condition	Description	Care
Marfan syndrome	An autosomal dominant disorder that affects: • Heart • Musculoskeletal system • Eyes • Central nervous system • Skin • Lungs Aortic root diameter <40 mm associated with less risk	Increased risk for: • Aortic dissection and rupture • Preterm delivery • Offspring inheriting syndrome (50% chance) Treatment: • Beta blockers (to minimize aortic dilation and keep BP <130 mm Hg systolic) • Corrective surgery or termination of the pregnancy (large aortic root diameter) • Regional anesthesia and avoidance of Valsalva in labor • Cesarean section Nursing considerations: • Observe for chest pain (classic symptom of aortic dissection, typically in the third trimester or postpartum) • Frequent echocardiograms • Close monitoring for 4–6 wk postpartum
Chronic hypertension	BP > 140/90 mm Hg that meets any of the following criteria: • Predates pregnancy • Presents in first 20 wk of gestation • Persists past 12 wk postpartum	Increased risk for (Bramham et al., 2014): • Preeclampsia • Placental abruption • Fetal growth restriction • Preterm birth • Cesarean delivery • Perinatal death • NICU admission Treatment: Antihypertensives (for BP > 160/110 mm Hg, with goal of 140/90 mm Hg or less; lower BP treated depending on clinical picture) Nursing considerations: • Some medications contraindicated in pregnancy • Diet without significant salt restriction (Regitz-Zagrosek et al., 2011) • Bed rest not recommended • Moderate exercise (ACOG, 2013b) • Baseline evaluations for renal disease and diabetes

MI	Rare during pregnancy
	Risk factors:
	• Age > 35 y
	• High BP
	• Diabetes
	• Obesity
	• Smoking
	• High cholesterol (Elkayam et al., 2014)
		Highest risk for maternal death in third trimester
		When MI experienced prior to pregnancy, high risk for:
		• Angina
		• Repeat MI
		• Heart failure
		• Arrhythmia
		• Adverse obstetric and neonatal outcomes (Burchill et al., 2015)
		
		Nursing considerations:
		• Care similar to that outside of pregnancy
		• Minimize cardiac workload during delivery:
		  ○ Side-lying position
		  ○ Oxygen supplementation
		  ○ Cesarean or operative vaginal birth

*Left-to-right shunts are lesions that allow blood from the left side of the heart (systemic circulation) to reenter the right side of the heart (pulmonary circulation). This causes abnormally high pressure on the pulmonary vasculature and can lead to pulmonary hypertension. If the pulmonary pressure exceeds the systemic pressure, it can lead to Eisenmenger syndrome, in which the left-to-right shunt becomes a right-to-left shunt, resulting in a dangerously reduced oxygen saturation of the blood.

MI, myocardial infarction; BP, blood pressure; NICU, neonatal intensive care unit.

Table 19.4 Cardiac Risk Classifications in Pregnancy

Class	Description	Examples	Actions
I	• No association with increased risk for maternal mortality • No or mildly increased risk for morbidity	• Small patent ductus arteriosus • Mild pulmonic stenosis • Mitral valve prolapse • Successfully repaired cardiac lesions • Isolated ectopic beats	One to two visits with a cardiologist during pregnancy
II	• Small increased risk for maternal mortality • Moderately increased risk for maternal morbidity	• Unrepaired atrial or ventricular septal defect • Repaired tetralogy of Fallot • Most arrhythmias	Visits with a cardiologist each trimester
II or III	Classification depends on individual circumstances	• Mild left ventricular impairment • Hypertrophic cardiomyopathy • Repaired coarctation • Marfan syndrome with aortic dimension <40 mm, no aortic dissection • Bicuspid aortic valve with ascending aorta <45 mm	Depending on the individual, visits with a cardiologist monthly or each trimester
III	• Significantly increased risk for maternal mortality • Severely increased risk for maternal morbidity	• Mechanical valve • Unrepaired cyanotic heart disease • Bicuspid aortic valve with ascending aortic • Marfan syndrome with an aortic root diameter of 45–50 mm	• Monthly or twice monthly visits with a cardiologist • Consideration of therapeutic abortion
IV	Pregnancy contraindicated because of extreme risk for maternal morbidity and mortality	• Mitral stenosis • Marfan syndrome with aortic root diameter >45 mm • Ejection fraction < 30% • Bicuspid aortic valve with ascending aorta diameter >50 mm • Significant pulmonary hypertension • Severe coarctation	• Therapeutic abortion should be considered. • If not, cardiologist involvement as in Class III

Adapted from Regitz-Zagrosek, V., Blomstrom Lundqvist, C., Borghi, C., Cifkova, R., Ferreira, R., Foidart, J. M., ... Torracca, L.; European Society of Gynecology; Association for European Paediatric Cardiology; German Society for Gender Medicine; E. S. C. Committee for Practice Guidelines. (2011). ESC Guidelines on the management of cardiovascular diseases during pregnancy: The Task Force on the Management of Cardiovascular Diseases during Pregnancy of the European Society of Cardiology (ESC). *European Heart Journal, 32*(24), 3147–3197. doi:10.1093/eurheartj/ehr218; Thorne, S., MacGregor, A., & Nelson-Piercy, C. (2006). Risks of contraception and pregnancy in heart disease. *Heart, 92*(10), 1520–1525. doi:10.1136/hrt.2006.095240

Table 19.5 Classification of Cardiac Disability

Class	Explanation of Scale
I	• Diagnosis of cardiac disease but no limitations of physical activity • No unusual fatigue, dyspnea, palpitations, or anginal pain with normal activity • Activity examples: running or walking for 5 miles, snow shoveling, walking up eight steps carrying 24 lb of weight
II	• Slight activity limitation • Activity examples: gardening or walking 4 mph over level ground
III	• Marked activity limitations • Activity examples: showering independently, making a bed, walking 2.5 mph over level ground
IV	All activities uncomfortable Cannot carry out any of the example activities listed for Class I, II, or III

Adapted from Goldman, L., Hashimoto, B., Cook, E. F., & Loscalzo, A. (1981). Comparative reproducibility and validity of systems for assessing cardiovascular functional class: Advantages of a new specific activity scale. *Circulation, 64*(6), 1227–1234; The Criteria Committee of the New York Heart Association, 1994 #21874.

development of complications, such as hypertension or infection, that may further tax cardiac functioning. Normal changes of pregnancy (Box 19.2) that are well tolerated in women without previous cardiac compromise can have a devastating impact on women with preexisting cardiac conditions. Risks include congestive heart failure, arrhythmias, pulmonary hypertension and edema, stroke, and maternal or fetal death. Conditions causing maternal cyanosis are a major risk factor for compromised fetal growth, prematurity, and fetal loss, with fewer than half of such pregnancies resulting in a live birth.

The demand for cardiac output increases throughout pregnancy. As the pregnancy progresses, the demands on the heart may increase by as much as 50%, exacerbating any underlying condition that may compromise the heart.

By the eighth week of pregnancy, approximately half of the anticipated increase in cardiac output has occurred, and therefore, the risk for cardiac decompensation increases. The patient and care team should be aware of the signs and symptoms of cardiac decompensation that indicate a worsening of cardiac disease (Box 19.3). Cardiac decompensation means that the heart can no longer compensate for the congenital or acquired compromise and cannot maintain adequate circulation.

Cardiac output levels off at 20 to 24 weeks of gestation and continues at this level until labor and delivery. Comorbidities

that put further demands on the heart, such as hypothyroidism, obesity, anemia, infection, and hypertension, should be minimized.

During labor and delivery, cardiac output increases even more: 15% in the latent phase and 30% in the active phase of the first stage, 45% in the second stage, 65% in the immediate postpartum period, and then back down to a 40% increase above baseline 60 minutes postpartum. In addition, each contraction increases cardiac output by 15% for its duration (Gaddipati & Troiano, 2013).

Assessment

Antepartum fetal monitoring by nonstress test, biophysical profile, or, more rarely, contraction stress test typically begins between 26 and 32 weeks of gestation for all patients with cardiovascular disease because of the high risk for poor uteroplacental perfusion and fetal hypoxia. During labor, invasive hemodynamic assessment, often within the pulmonary artery, may be ordered, which measures blood pressure, blood flow, and blood oxygen content. Serial arterial blood gas tests may be ordered to assess for oxygenation of the maternal blood. Continuous blood pressure and oxygen saturation monitoring are routine, as is electrocardiographic monitoring. Continuous monitoring of the fetal heart rate and uterine contractions is indicated.

Treatment

Medical management of cardiac disease in pregnancy depends on the disease type, severity, and complications and often involves collaboration between several disciplines, including obstetrics, cardiology, and neonatology. Inotropic drugs that modify the muscular activity of the heart to increase or decrease contractions of the heart may be ordered. For conditions that include incomplete emptying of a chamber of the heart or atrial fibrillation, the anticoagulant heparin is often administered. The anticoagulant warfarin is rarely given in pregnancy because it freely passes the placenta and is a known teratogen. Antiarrhythmics may be prescribed in the event of a dangerously irregular heartbeat. Diuretics may be used to treat pulmonary edema or to reduce preload. Antibiotic prophylaxis may be administered to protect select high-risk patients from infective endocarditis.

A spontaneous vaginal birth is preferred. Oxytocin and cervical ripening agents are generally well tolerated but should be used at the lowest effective dose to minimize maternal hemodynamic effects. Preterm delivery may be indicated in the case of deterioration of the status of the mother or fetus.

Because a pain-free labor is associated with superior cardiac outcomes, epidural analgesia is routine. Epidural anesthesia, however, often causes vasodilation, which can reduce preload, which, in turn, reduces cardiac output. Administration of an IV fluid bolus before and after the epidural as needed can help mitigate this effect.

Passive descent in the lateral position in the second stage rather than pushing is preferred to limit maternal effort, optimize placental perfusion, and reduce oxygen needs (Arafeh, 2014). Open-glottis pushing may be attempted according to the clinical circumstances, but Valsalva pushing should be discouraged. Operative birth by forceps or vacuum is common.

Care Considerations

The nurse should continue monitoring for the signs and symptoms of decompensation for 48 to 72 hours after the birth, and be particularly attentive for the signs of pulmonary edema and hemorrhage. As the normal mobilizing of interstitial fluid occurs over the first 3 to 5 days postpartum, women with cardiac disease are at particular risk for pulmonary edema. Women on anticoagulants are most at risk for postpartum hemorrhage. Hypovolemia is particularly dangerous for these patients, and replacement of blood volume is a priority.

Cardiac decompensation continues to be a risk for up to 6 months postpartum, and the patient and care providers must continue monitoring for its signs and symptoms (Arafeh, 2014). Women who are decompensated may require additional support with hygiene, ambulation, and other activities of daily living.

Breastfeeding is not contraindicated by disease but may be compromised by the status of the mother. The nurse may have to be creative in facilitating the bonding process between the mother and baby, as the mother may be unable to hold or interact with her infant for long periods of time. As with all women, the nurse should discuss contraception and family planning and, when possible, implement a plan prior to discharge, as further pregnancies, particularly closely spaced, would also be high risk.

Chronic Hypertension

Course in Pregnancy

Maternal chronic hypertension is associated with a higher rate of poor pregnancy outcomes, including preterm birth, intrauterine growth restriction, and stillbirth. Women with chronic hypertension are more likely to develop pulmonary edema, preeclampsia, and stroke during their pregnancy than the general pregnant population and are more likely to be delivered by cesarean section (Bramham et al., 2014; Orbach et al., 2013).

Pregnancy-associated strokes are rare but primarily happen in the first 2 days postpartum and are associated with hypertension (Kuklina, Tong, Bansil, George, & Callaghan, 2011).

Assessment

Ideally, chronic hypertension is diagnosed prior to pregnancy. Although most hypertension is primary hypertension, secondary hypertension may occur in pregnant women. If suspected in patients who do not have clear risk factors, it should be ruled out. If a woman is suspected of having secondary hypertension, her provider typically orders laboratory tests to evaluate her kidneys and thyroid gland and to assess for diabetes, a common comorbidity.

Chronic (preexisting) hypertension is defined diagnostically as having a systolic blood pressure of 140 mm Hg or greater and/or a diastolic blood pressure equal to or greater than 90 mm Hg that predates the pregnancy, appears before the 20th week of pregnancy, or persists past 12 weeks postpartum. Mild-to-moderate chronic hypertension in pregnancy is defined as having a systolic blood pressure of 140 to 159 mm Hg and/or a diastolic blood pressure of 90 to 109 mm Hg. Severe chronic hypertension in pregnancy is defined as having a systolic blood pressure equal to or greater than 160 mm Hg and/or a diastolic blood pressure equal to or greater than 110 mm Hg,

Frequent prenatal visits are indicated to assess maternal blood pressure and to screen for proteinuria, which can indicate the onset of preeclampsia, as these patients are at a higher risk for this complication. Fetal size should be regularly evaluated, first clinically by fundal height measurements and then by ultrasound evaluation as needed in the third trimester. Antepartum fetal assessment by nonstress test, biophysical profile, and/or contraction stress test may not be indicated in the absence of clinical features suggesting preeclampsia or intrauterine growth restriction.

Careful monitoring for pregnancy-associated disorders, including preeclampsia and **H** (hemolysis, which is the breaking down of red blood cells) **EL** (elevated liver enzymes) **LP** (low platelet count), should continue postpartum.

Treatment

There is no clear benefit to the mother or fetus of treating women with blood pressures under 150 mm Hg systolic or under 100 mm Hg diastolic. Similarly, the benefit of treating women with moderate chronic hypertension in pregnancy, which is defined as having a systolic blood pressure from 150 to 160 mm Hg or a diastolic blood pressure from 100 to 109 mm Hg, is not certain. Available evidence does not indicate that treating these blood pressures reduces preeclampsia, placental abruption, or severe hypertension (Abalos, Duley, & Steyn, 2014).

Women with severe chronic hypertension, however, should be treated with the goal of maintaining a blood pressure of 140 to 150 mm Hg systolic and 90 to 100 mm Hg diastolic to avoid hypertension complications such as stroke, renal failure, and heart failure. It may be desirable for women with evidence of target-organ damage from chronic hypertension to maintain a lower blood pressure (ACOG, 2013b; Magee, Singer, von Dadelszen, & Group, 2015).

Preferred antihypertensives in pregnancy include labetalol, methyldopa, and nifedipine. Blood pressure in a pregnancy uncomplicated by pregnancy-induced hypertensive disorders may go down to a value below that seen prior to pregnancy, and women who started pregnancy taking an antihypertensive medication may have it discontinued or have the dose reduced. Aspirin therapy starting between 12 and 20 weeks of gestation is indicated to reduce preeclampsia risk (Henderson et al., 2014).

The American College of Obstetricians and Gynecologists recommends delivery at the following gestational ages for women with varying degrees of hypertension:

- 38 to 39 6/7 weeks for women with hypertension who do not require medication
- 37 to 39 6/7 weeks for women with hypertension who do require medication
- 36 to 37 6/7 for women with difficult-to-control, severe hypertension (ACOG, 2013a)

If medications were started in pregnancy, they may be continued into the postpartum period.

Care Considerations

Nonsteroidal antiinflammatory drugs (NSAIDs) such as ibuprofen should be used cautiously for these patients postpartum as they are associated with increased blood pressure readings. Breastfeeding is not contraindicated with chronic hypertension and is safe with the medications used to treat this condition, although they do pass into the breast milk. The use of methyldopa may increase the risk for postpartum depression (Castro, Billick, Kleiman, Chiechi, & Al-Rashdan, 2014).

Obesity

Prevalence

From 2011 to 2014, 35.4% of women between the ages of 20 and 39 years in the United States were classified as obese (Ogden, Carroll, Fryar, & Flegal, 2015).

Course in Pregnancy

Obesity is associated with increased complications. Because fat has an endocrine function, when in excess it can have a detrimental effect on inflammatory pathways, vasculature, and the metabolism, which have been linked to poor obstetric outcomes (Lisonkova et al., 2017).

Many women with obesity ovulate less frequently, but even those who ovulate regularly are at a higher risk for subfertility. The rate of repeat early pregnancy loss is higher in obese women: 1.7 to 3.5 times the rate of women with a normal body mass index (BMI) (18.5 to 24.9 kg/m^2; Sugiura-Ogasawara, 2015). This increased rate of loss may be associated with hormonal changes that lessen the ability of the endometrium to sustain a pregnancy. In the case of women with polycystic ovarian syndrome, which often co-occurs with obesity, low-grade chronic inflammation common to the disease may contribute (Palomba et al., 2014). In addition, women who are obese are at a higher risk for dizygotic (fraternal) twinning.

In Chapter 2, Tatiana worked diligently through diet and exercise to lose and maintain her weight after her diagnosis of polycystic ovarian syndrome. She was able to become pregnant without medical intervention.

Women with obesity are more likely to begin the pregnancy prediabetic or diabetic. Those who are not diabetic are more likely to develop gestational diabetes than women with a normal BMI. A progressively higher BMI is associated with an increased risk for gestational diabetes. For every 1 kg/m^2 increase in BMI, there is an almost 1% increase in the occurrence of gestational diabetes. Overall, women with a BMI between 35.0–39.9 kg/m^2 (class II obesity) are three times as likely to develop gestational diabetes as women of normal weight, and women with class III obesity (a BMI ≥ 40.0) are more than five and a half times as likely to develop gestational diabetes (Torloni et al., 2009).

Regardless of other risk factors, women who are obese experience double the risk for developing preeclampsia and other hypertensive disorders of pregnancy with every 5 to 7 kg/m^2 increase in BMI above normal (O'Brien, Ray, & Chan, 2003). Because of the complications associated with diabetes and hypertensive disorders, in particular, women who are obese in pregnancy also have an increased risk for a medically induced preterm birth (induction or cesarean section; Cnattingius et al., 2013). Although obese women who also have a diagnosis of polycystic ovarian syndrome are at a higher risk for a spontaneous preterm birth, it is less clear whether obese women without this diagnosis also carry this risk, although it is speculated that inflammatory changes related to polycystic ovarian syndrome are the root cause (Palomba et al., 2014).

Although women who are obese are more likely to have labor induced, they are also twice as likely to experience induction failure, with the risk increasing with higher BMIs (Wolfe, Rossi, & Warshak, 2011). Women who are overweight or obese experience a slower first stage of labor, with full cervical dilation taking an average of 1 to 2 hours longer than for women of normal weight. The duration of the second stage is similar among women of all BMI categories (Robinson et al., 2011). Women who are obese are also more likely to undergo planned or emergency cesarean section. Although women who are obese are more likely to have macrosomic infants, which is an indication for cesarean section, the obesity itself appears to be an independent risk factor for the procedure.

Postpartum, women with obesity are more likely to develop a thromboembolism. Although the higher rate of cesarean section contributes to the increased rate, obesity appears to be an independent risk factor for this complication, as well. Higher BMI is associated with higher risk, and women with class III obesity have a four-times higher risk for a postpartum thromboembolism than women with normal BMIs (Blondon et al., 2016). Women who are obese are also more subject to infection during the postpartum period. In addition, these women are at a higher risk for postpartum depression, anxiety, and eating disorders than peers with normal BMIs (Molyneaux, Poston, Ashurst-Williams, & Howard, 2014).

In Chapter 3, Susan developed a deep vein thrombosis as well as a pulmonary embolism. One of her risk factors for developing blood clots was obesity.

The offspring of women who are obese are at a higher risk for neural tube defects, cleft palate, cardiac defects, limb reductions, and **anorectal atresia** (a condition in which the anus is absent or abnormally positioned). As the severity of the obesity increases, the risk for fetal anomalies increases. Obesity also presents an increased risk for stillbirth, perinatal death, and death of the infant postpartum, with risks increasing with the increasing class of obesity (women with class III obesity are at a higher risk for fetal and infant loss than women with class II obesity; ACOG 2015a).

Fetal exposure to the endocrine variations of excessive adiposity, including elevated glucose, insulin, and inflammatory factors, may contribute to changes in the fetal metabolism that result in lifelong health implications. This research is ongoing, however, and it is challenging to differentiate between the effects of genetics, lifestyle, upbringing, and obesity exposure in utero (Catalano & Shankar, 2017). Obesity in pregnancy is also associated with a higher risk for asthma in offspring (Forno, Young, Kumar, Simhan, & Celedon, 2014). In addition, offspring may be at a higher risk for neurodevelopmental and psychological issues, including cerebral palsy, depression, schizophrenia, cognitive impairment, and autism (Edlow, 2017).

Assessment

Obesity is defined as having a BMI of 30 kg/m² or greater (see Box 1.4). Obesity is classified according to severity by BMI range:

- Class I: 30 to 34.9 kg/m²
- Class II: 35 to 39.9 kg/m²
- Class III: 40 kg/m² or greater

Prior to conception, patients with obesity are ideally screened for obesity-associated comorbidities, particularly hypertension and diabetes. The nurse should note that people who are obese often require a larger cuff for an accurate blood pressure reading.

Early in pregnancy, an ultrasound may be ordered for accurate dating in the event that an induced birth is warranted and to confirm the number of fetuses, as multiple pregnancies are more common in obese women. Women who had bariatric surgery for weight loss may be assessed prior to pregnancy or in early pregnancy for nutritional deficits common after such surgery. Obstetric providers may choose to order baseline laboratory tests evaluating kidney and liver function.

A routine fetal survey is recommended in the second trimester with special emphasis on the fetal heart because of the higher risk of fetal cardiac defects. Maternal obesity, however, can make ultrasound less sensitive, and repeat ultrasounds and/or a fetal echocardiogram may be ordered. Maternal obesity also makes fundal height measurements less accurate, and obstetric providers may instead rely on serial monthly ultrasounds to track fetal growth.

During labor and delivery, isolation of the fetal heart may be difficult with an obese mother. Internal monitoring may instead be indicated.

Treatment

Prior to conception, medical treatment options for obesity include weight-loss medications, contraindicated in pregnancy but safe prior to conception, and bariatric surgery for weight loss. Lifestyle counseling for weight loss including a healthy diet and regular exercise as first-line interventions. Prepregnancy weight loss is associated with a reduced risk for macrosomia, cesarean section, gestational diabetes, and stillbirth (Cnattingius & Villamor, 2016).

Care Considerations

As with all preexisting conditions, it is optimal for the patient to seek care prior to pregnancy. During such visits, the nurse should inform the patient of the effect of obesity on fertility and the complications of pregnancy associated with obesity. As part of an interprofessional team that includes a nutritionist, the nurse should encourage the patient to make changes in diet, behavior, and exercise before conception, changes that are recommended for ensuring a successful weight loss.

Weight loss during pregnancy rather than prior to pregnancy is associated with an increased risk for infants who are small for gestational age and is, therefore, not generally recommended (Kapadia et al., 2015). Limiting weight gain, however, is associated with some reduction of the risks of obesity in pregnancy (see Box 1.5). Exercise in pregnancy can help control pregnancy weight gain and reduces the risk for preterm birth and gestational diabetes (Magro-Malosso, Saccone, Di Mascio, Di Tommaso, & Berghella, 2017).

In Chapter 3, Dr. Cheema recommended that Susan exercise regularly and gain less than 20 lb in pregnancy. Susan was fatigued and found that a healthy diet and exercise were difficult to fit into her life and her budget. A nurse, Valerie, encouraged her to start walking just 10 minutes a day for starters.

Because women who are obese are at a higher risk for preeclampsia, low-dose aspirin is often started in the second trimester. Anesthesia consults are often ordered prior to labor as obesity can make the administration of anesthesia more challenging.

Eating Disorders

Eating disorders, including anorexia nervosa, bulimia nervosa, and binge eating disorder, are common in female adolescents and young women of reproductive age and are associated with poor health and psychosocial outcomes (Box 19.4). Women with eating disorders often try to hide their illness, making assessment and diagnosis challenging (Box 19.5). Although women with anorexia nervosa are below normal weight, those with bulimia nervosa or binge eating disorder are often of normal weight or even overweight. Women with all types of eating disorders typically find the normal changes of pregnancy more distressing than do their peers who do not have an eating disorder. Women with eating disorders are also more likely to report that their infant is fussy and has a difficult temperament (Zerwas et al., 2012).

Box 19.4 Types of Eating Disorders

Anorexia Nervosa

- Restricted energy intake leading to a significantly low body weight
- Intense fear of weight gain
- Disturbed self-perception of one's body, heavily influenced by weight
- Minimization of risk of low weight

Bulimia Nervosa

- Recurrent binge eating with a feeling of loss of control
- Compensatory actions (vomiting, laxatives, extreme exercise, etc.)
- Self-perception heavily influenced by weight

Binge Eating Disorder

- Binge eating with feeling of loss of control
- Unlike bulimia nervosa, no compensatory actions

Women with eating disorders are more likely to smoke during the pregnancy and to suffer from antepartum as well as postpartum depression (Easter et al., 2015; Solmi et al., 2016).

Anorexia Nervosa

Most women with anorexia nervosa do not ovulate, but a history of anorexia nervosa does not impact fertility. Both unplanned

Box 19.5 Evaluation for Eating Disorders

Warning Signs

- History of an eating disorder
- Abnormally low body mass index
- Lack of weight gain over two prenatal visits
- Electrolyte abnormalities
- Problems with tooth enamel from vomiting (bulimia nervosa only)
- Hyperemesis gravidarum
- Anxiety or mood disorder

Questions to Ask

- Are you trying to restrict what you eat?
- Do you sometimes feel out of control of your eating?
- Do you eat secretly?
- Are you concerned about gaining weight in pregnancy?
- How do you feel about your weight?
- Do you feel guilty about how you eat?
- Do you ever vomit after eating or take medications such as laxatives or water pills?
- When do you exercise, how often, for how long, and at what intensity?

pregnancy and abortion are more common in women who have been diagnosed with anorexia nervosa at some point in their life (Easter, Treasure, & Micali, 2011).

Women with anorexia nervosa are at a higher risk for miscarriage, antepartum hemorrhage, preeclampsia, preterm delivery, and cesarean delivery. Infants born to women with anorexia nervosa are more likely to be either small for gestational age or large for gestational age (Linna et al., 2014). A woman's anorexia nervosa may go into remission during pregnancy and the postpartum period, but it may also progress or cross over to a different eating disorder, such as bulimia nervosa.

Bulimia Nervosa

Women with bulimia nervosa do not have reduced fertility compared with peers who do not have eating disorders, although women with active disease are more likely to miscarry. Induced abortion is also more common in this population (Linna et al., 2013). Approximately 60% of women with this condition gain more weight in pregnancy than is recommended, whereas 20% gain less (Siega-Riz et al., 2011). Unlike women with anorexia nervosa, women with bulimia nervosa do not appear to be at increased risk for large or small neonates, preeclampsia, or cesarean or preterm delivery. Postpartum, women may experience remission of the bulimia, cross over to a different eating disorder (usually binge eating disorder), or continue to suffer from bulimia (Knoph et al., 2013).

Binge Eating Disorder

Approximately 5% of women have a binge eating disorder, many of whom first develop this condition during pregnancy (Watson et al., 2013). Women with binge eating disorder are about three times as likely to miscarry and are more likely to smoke during pregnancy (Linna et al., 2013). Most gain an excessive amount of weight in pregnancy (Siega-Riz et al., 2011). They are no more likely than peers without eating disorders to experience preeclampsia, preterm delivery, or cesarean section, and their infants are not more likely to be either large or small for gestational age at birth (Linna et al., 2014). As with anorexia nervosa and bulimia nervosa, binge eating disorder may continue, go into remission, or cross over to a different eating disorder (most commonly bulimia nervosa).

Care Considerations

Women with anorexia nervosa may not menstruate or may menstruate irregularly, as may women with bulimia nervosa or binge eating disorder who are overweight or obese. The nurse should inform patients with eating disorders who do not menstruate regularly that a lack of menses does not necessarily indicate a lack of ovulation and that they may still be fertile. If they do not wish to be pregnant, the nurse should offer education about the methods of contraception.

As with many chronic illnesses, pregnancy should optimally be planned for a time of disease remission. Because women with eating disorders are more likely to experience depression both during and after pregnancy and to be more distressed by normal changes of pregnancy, the nurse should help establish access to counseling services for such patients early in pregnancy. A team that includes a nutritionist and mental health provider, as well as an obstetric provider, often manages the care of women with an eating disorder.

Because of the frequency of crossover between eating disorders, the nurse should question all women diagnosed with an eating disorder about medications often used for bulimic compensation and appetite suppression and discourage their use in pregnancy. Such medications include diuretics and laxatives, as well as appetite suppressants, including cocaine, nicotine, amphetamines, and other medications available over the counter, by prescription, or illegally. The nurse should weigh women with anorexia nervosa in hospital gowns, as they may pad or add weight to their clothing. The nurse should not inform women who find weight gain distressing of weight changes unless weight gain is insufficient or by patient request.

Maternal Phenylketonuria

Phenylketonuria (PKU) is an autosomal recessive amino acid disorder in which phenylalanine is not converted to tyrosine. This leads to high serum levels of phenylalanine and its metabolites that can result in intellectual disability in individuals with the condition if not managed appropriately.

Course in Pregnancy

Women with PKU whose disease is not controlled by dietary interventions can have pregnancies complicated by phenylalanine embryopathy (PE). PE can result in cardiac malformations, microcephaly, intrauterine growth restriction, and intellectual disability. Phenylalanine levels should be monitored prior to conception and managed to a goal of 2 to 6 mg/dL during pregnancy. Levels should be rechecked once or twice weekly and diet adjusted accordingly.

Assessment

Neonates are screened for PKU within the first few days of life, and the disease rarely goes undetected (see Step-by-Step Skills 5.2; see Fig. 18.13).

Treatment

To prevent PE, women with PKU must carefully adhere to a phenylalanine-restricted diet prior to conception and during pregnancy. Low concentrations of 6 mg/dL of maternal phenylalanine for at least 3 months prior to conception and throughout pregnancy are associated with superior outcomes for offspring. Plasma phenylalanine levels are typically monitored at least once weekly.

For newborns diagnosed with PKU, dietary interventions typically begin in the first week of life and include a low-protein diet and supplementation with protein substitutes. Dietary management for life is recommended.

Care Considerations

A mother with PKU and a baby who does not have PKU can breastfeed without fear of harming the infant, although the mother should continue her phenylalanine-restricted diet. If both the mother and baby have PKU, close monitoring of phenylalanine serum levels is indicated for both the mother and infant if breastfeeding is initiated and a tight phenylalanine-restricted diet is required for the mother. Partial breastfeeding and supplementation with a phenylalanine-restricted formula may be initiated to mitigate risks to the newborn of developing the complications of PKU in this scenario (Banta-Wright, Press, Knafl, Steiner, & Houck, 2014).

Iron Deficiency Anemia

Prevalence

The onset of iron deficiency anemia may be prior to or during a pregnancy. Approximately 16% to 29% of women will become anemic in pregnancy, usually in the third trimester (Bailit, Doty, & Todia, 2007).

Course in Pregnancy

Although rare in developed countries, severe anemia (hemoglobin level less than 7 g/dL) is associated with nonreassuring fetal heart rate, depletion of amniotic fluid volume, low birth weight, prematurity, fetal loss, and maternal death (Cantor, Bougatsos, Dana, Blazina, & McDonagh, 2015). There is also evidence of cognitive deficits in children who were anemic as infants (Congdon et al., 2012). Such severe anemia can typically be attributed to poor nutrition and disease that causes lysis of red blood cells. Other risk factors for anemia include close spacing of pregnancies, a pregnancy with more than one fetus, disordered eating such as anorexia nervosa, heavy bleeding, and adolescence.

Assessment

Because of the increase in plasma volume during pregnancy, hemoglobin levels decrease slightly. This change is often referred to as physiologic anemia or dilutional anemia of pregnancy because it is a normal, expected finding caused by dilution of the red blood cells by plasma. The expected hemoglobin level in nonpregnant women who are not anemic is 12.1 to 15.1 g/dL. In pregnant women, however, the normal range is lower, from 11 to 14 g/dL, and the expected hematocrit level is 33%. According to the Centers for Disease Control and Prevention, in the second trimester, a hemoglobin level as low as 10.5 g/dL and a hematocrit level below 32% is still considered normal, whereas values below these are diagnostic for anemia (Centers for Disease Control and Prevention, 1989). Hemoglobin and hematocrit levels are lower in people of African descent, however, and in this population, the cutoff for anemia can be lowered by 0.8 g/dL: 10.2 g/dL in the first and third trimesters and 9.7 g/dL in the second trimester (Ioannou, Spector, Scott, & Rockey, 2002). The hemoglobin trough in pregnancy is typically reached from about 28 to 36 weeks of gestation, after which the plasma volume stabilizes and the hemoglobin volume increases modestly.

Women who are diagnosed with anemia often undergo further laboratory tests, typically including a ferritin level to evaluate iron stores.

Treatment

Although there is good evidence that supplementing with iron improves maternal hemoglobin and hematocrit levels, there is insufficient evidence to suggest that routine screening for anemia and supplementation with iron improves clinical outcomes (Cantor et al., 2015). Routine supplementation, typically as part of a prenatal vitamin, is common, however. Oral iron is associated with the side effects of pruritus and rash, as well as frequent gastrointestinal symptoms, including cramps, constipation, nausea, and vomiting. Some women may, therefore, prefer IV iron supplementation. A common dose for oral dosing with the diagnosis of anemia is 60 to 200 mg of elemental iron daily.

Care Considerations

The nurse should inform patients that iron is best absorbed orally if taken on an empty stomach but that this may lead to gastrointestinal distress. The nurse should advise patients to avoid consuming milk, antacids, high-fiber foods, and caffeine for 2 hours after taking iron for superior absorption. The nurse should also warn patients that iron is often constipating and black stools are common with iron supplementation.

Beta Thalassemia

Beta thalassemia has two forms: major and minor. Beta thalassemia minor is the heterozygous form, and beta thalassemia major, also called Cooley's anemia, is the homozygous form. Women with beta thalassemia should undergo genetic counseling, preferably prior to pregnancy, as the homozygous form of beta thalassemia, beta thalassemia major, can have profound health implications for any offspring. If both parents are heterozygous, there is a 25% chance that the offspring will have beta thalassemia major and a 50% chance that any offspring will have beta thalassemia minor.

People with beta thalassemia minor have microcytic, hypochromic red blood cells (blood cells that are small and pale). Their bodies compensate, however, by producing a large number of the cells, thus their blood may not have a reduced oxygen carrying capacity. When anemia occurs in such people, it tends to be minor, and the disease has little or no health impact. Women with beta thalassemia minor should not be treated with supplemental iron unless further testing of ferritin levels indicates that they are iron deficient. These patients are more likely to develop a more pronounced form of diffusion anemia of pregnancy, however, and in rare cases, may require a blood transfusion.

Beta thalassemia major, in contrast, is a serious disease condition, and until the advent of routine repeat blood transfusions, it was not considered compatible with life past infancy. Even with modern therapy, beta thalassemia major has profound implications for health that are beyond the scope of this chapter. Patients with this condition routinely undergo periodic blood transfusions and chelation therapy. Cardiac abnormalities are common in this population, and a woman should not attempt pregnancy if her cardiac function is abnormal (ACOG, 2007, reaffirmed 2015). A woman with beta thalassemia major will pass the gene for the disease on to all offspring. If the partner of the pregnancy does not carry the gene for beta thalassemia, all offspring will have beta thalassemia minor. If the partner is a heterozygous carrier, offspring have a 50% chance of developing beta thalassemia major.

Sickle Cell Anemia

Sickle cell anemia is a genetic disorder in which the red blood cells have an abnormal "sickle" shape, which, depending on the type of disease, can be either a minor concern with few if any symptoms or a major concern with serious implications for the mother and baby.

Prevalence

Certain populations, particularly those of African, Indian, Middle Eastern, and Caribbean descent, have a sickle cell trait prevalence as high as 10% to 30%, making genetic counseling an important aspect of preconception screening for this condition (Ojodu, Hulihan, Pope, & Grant, 2014). If two people with sickle cell trait reproduce, the chance of an offspring developing sickle cell disease is 25%.

Etiology

Sickle cell anemia is categorized as either sickle cell trait or sickle cell disease. People with the sickle cell trait have a single copy of a gene responsible for sickle cell, whereas people with sickle cell disease have two copies of the gene. With sickle cell trait, some red blood cells are sickle-shaped but have a typical life span. Sickle cell trait is considered a carrier state rather than a disease but may still have some subtle heath implications. In the case of sickle cell disease, the cells have a sickle configuration, as with sickle cell trait, but the life span of the cells is as short as 5 to 10 days, compared with the typical 120 days, leading to far greater consequences.

Course in Pregnancy

As with beta thalassemia minor, most of the people with sickle cell trait in the United States are asymptomatic. Women with sickle cell trait may be at a higher risk for blood clots in pregnancy and the postpartum period and are at a higher risk for urinary tract infections in pregnancy as well as other times. The trait appears to be protective against fetal demise and preterm birth, but there is a small increased risk for anemia in pregnancy (Jans, de Jonge, & Lagro-Janssen, 2010). Blood clots associated with the use of estrogen methods of birth control do not increase for women with sickle cell trait (Haddad, Curtis, Legardy-Williams, Cwiak, & Jamieson, 2012).

Sickle cell disease, however, affects almost all organ systems of the body. People with sickle cell disease are more likely to have hypertension due to nephropathy, which results from the disease, and retinitis, which may worsen in pregnancy. Moreover, they often have excess stores of iron and thus require chelation therapy, which in the case of women who are planning to attempt pregnancy, should be done prior to conception. Women with sickle cell disease are at a higher risk for pulmonary hypertension, cardiac dysfunction, and embolism. They are prone to recurrent crises of fever and pain, which can occur in any part of the body but most commonly occur in joints and the abdomen. These crises are caused by the occlusion of blood vessels by sickle-shaped red blood cells and are typically triggered by dehydration, low blood oxygen level, or acidosis. Approximately half of women with sickle cell disease experience a crisis related to pregnancy, usually in the last months of pregnancy or postpartum.

The maternal mortality rate for women with sickle cell disease is 72 per 100,000 births. These women are at a higher risk for thrombosis, infection, sepsis, transfusion, and systemic inflammatory response syndrome. Obstetric risks for this population include hypertensive disorders of pregnancy, placental abruption, antepartal bleeding, fetal growth restriction, preterm labor, and infection postpartum. They do, however, have a lower rate of postpartum hemorrhage (Oteng-Ntim, 2017).

Assessment

In the case of a woman with sickle cell disease, preconception counseling is particularly important because all of her offspring will at least have the sickle cell trait, and if the partner of the pregnancy is also a carrier of the trait, there is a 50% risk for sickle cell disease.

Treatment

For women with the sickle cell trait, no special treatment is required. Those with sickle cell disease, however, require the following treatment considerations. They may need a higher dose of folic acid, up to 5 mg daily, prior to and during pregnancy, as recommended. Their providers may need to change their medications or adjust their doses, preferably prior to conception. Chelation therapy is usually discontinued with, but not prior to, conception, and angiotensin-converting enzymes and angiotensin II receptor blockers used to treat hypertension, which are teratogenic, are contraindicated in pregnancy. NSAIDs for pain management should be avoided after week 30 of pregnancy because of the risk for premature closure of the fetal ductus arteriosus.

Care Considerations

Dehydration is a common event in pregnancy, labor and delivery, and postpartum. Although for most women this has few, if any, implications, for women with sickle cell disease, dehydration can lead to extremely painful, debilitating attacks. It is critical that the nurse monitor for dehydration and maternal hypoxia when caring for these patients. Because of the higher clot risk for women with sickle cell trait and sickle cell disease, the nurse should promote early ambulation and implement other clot prevention measures as indicated. Breastfeeding is not contraindicated with this condition.

Intimate Partner Violence

It is not unusual for intimate partner violence to begin or progress in pregnancy or immediately following a pregnancy (see Chapter 30).

Prevalence and Risk Factors

An estimated 7% to 20% of pregnancies are complicated by physical abuse, but women also experience psychological and sexual abuse during pregnancy, which are often underreported. Approximately 5% of women report that their partners tried to get them pregnant when they did not want to be (Breiding et al., 2014). Women who have pregnancies that are unplanned are approximately three times as likely to be abused by their intimate partners than are women with planned pregnancies. Women who are either pregnant or recently gave birth are almost twice as likely as other women to be victims of homicide (Wallace, Hoyert, Williams, & Mendola, 2016).

Various risk factors have been identified that make women more likely to be victims of intimate partner violence (see Box 12.1), including youth, community norms, poverty, and diminished opportunities due to poverty, and lack of education. People are more likely to act abusively toward partners if they were exposed to similar behavior in childhood, are economically unstable, or abuse substances (Gracia, Lopez-Quilez, Marco, Lladosa, & Lila, 2015; Renner & Whitney, 2012).

In Chapter 12, Loretta was a victim of intimate partner violence. She witnessed violence in her home as a child and thought of it as a normal part of life. She was also young, poor, and poorly educated. Intimate partner violence was a risk factor for the depression she experienced.

Course in Pregnancy

In addition to a higher risk of homicide, abuse by an intimate partner in the year prior to pregnancy is associated with a greater likelihood for severe nausea and vomiting during pregnancy, urinary tract infection, hypertension, preterm delivery, low birth weight, placental abruption, perinatal death, and fractures to the bones of the fetus in utero. Women who experience abuse, particularly psychological abuse, during the pregnancy are at least twice as likely to suffer from depression postpartum (Han & Stewart, 2014).

Care Considerations

Women who experience abuse by a partner often do not disclose the fact because of shame, guilt, a poor sense of self-worth, and many other reasons and may require a long period of trust-building before they will tell a nurse or another healthcare provider about the abuse. For this reason and because the abuse may start before, during, or after the pregnancy, the nurse should screen patients for intimate partner violence during the first prenatal visit and then every trimester and postpartum. Many labor and delivery units now make this part of the required patient intake, as well. Screening is associated with improved pregnancy outcomes and lower rates of recurrent abuse in the pregnant population (Taft et al., 2013).

Asking patients questions about intimate partner violence can be difficult and intimidating, and some nurses may find it useful to use a standard screening questionnaire. Institution protocols may require the nurse to screen patients via such a written questionnaire, verbally during the intake process, or both. The nurse should question patients about abuse only when alone, with no one else present, whenever possible. Nurses should be prepared with information about appropriate referrals in the event of a positive screen, including social workers and intimate partner violence nonprofit organizations, including the National Domestic Violence Hotline (Box 19.6).

Substance Abuse

Substances commonly abused in pregnancy include nicotine, alcohol, opioids, marijuana, cocaine, hallucinogens, methamphetamine, and inhalants. Pregnancy is a prime time to implement healthful changes, but many women, particularly those using illegal substances, may feel shame and guilt about their substance use and fail to seek prenatal care. They may also fear that seeking help may risk social service involvement and offspring being removed from their care. In some states, the abuse of substances in pregnancy is classified as child abuse (ACOG, 2011). Nurses must be aware of locally mandated reporting requirements.

Prevalence

According to one survey, 15.4% of pregnant women smoke, 9.4% drink alcohol, and 5.4% use illegal drugs in pregnancy. Teens are at a higher risk for substance abuse, with 14.6% of teens between 15 and 17 years old using illegal drugs in pregnancy when compared with 3.2% of pregnant women aged 26 to 44 years (SAMHSA/CSAT Treatment Improvement Protocols, 2005).

Course in Pregnancy

Infants exposed to opioids and opioid replacement drugs such as buprenorphine in pregnancy are at a high risk for neonatal abstinence syndrome (withdrawal from opioids by the neonate

after birth; see Chapter 25), a growing problem. Between 2004 and 2013, the rate of admission to the neonatal intensive care unit for neonatal abstinence syndrome went from 7 per 1,000 admissions to 27 per 1,000 admissions (Tolia et al., 2015).

There is no known safe amount of alcohol that may be consumed in pregnancy. Alcohol is a known teratogen, and consuming it during pregnancy can lead to fetal alcohol spectrum disorder, which includes effects that are physical, mental, behavioral, and cognitive. Alcohol can impact fetal growth and development at any point in pregnancy, and there is no "safe" time during the pregnancy for women to consume it (Williams & Smith, 2015).

Smoking in pregnancy is associated with preterm birth, intrauterine growth restriction, subfertility, miscarriage, stillbirth, preeclampsia, placental abruption, and sudden infant death syndrome (the unexpected death of a healthy-seeming infant), as well as other adverse outcomes (Centers for Disease Control and Prevention, 2016).

Assessment

The nurse should screen all pregnant women verbally for substance abuse, including alcohol use and smoking, during the first prenatal visit and then periodically. Substance use in pregnancy is not limited to any one population group, hence the recommendation for universal screening. Universal laboratory screening is not commonly done because of cost and limitations of the tests (e.g., eating poppy seeds can cause a positive opioid screen), although such screening may be indicated in some circumstances (Box 19.7). Obtaining informed consent prior to laboratory screening is essential, and failure to do so is unethical (ACOG, 2015b). The nurse should inform women of all potential ramifications of a positive laboratory test for drug use before initiating one.

A positive screening and intervention is associated with improved outcomes for the couplet (ACOG Committee on Health Care for Underserved Women & American Society of Addiction Medicine, 2012). Several screening tools exist, and institutions often adopt one or more of them for use. Examples include the 4P's Plus screen, the CRAFFT Screening Tool for substance abuse in adolescents and young adults, the National Institute on

---

Box 19.6 National Domestic Violence Hotline

http://www.thehotline.org
1-800-799-7233
1-800-787-3224 (TTY)

Box 19.7 Indications for Laboratory Drug Screening

- Previous positive screen
- Monitoring for compliance with opioid replacement therapy
- Lack of adherence with prenatal care
- Prescription requests for opioids
- Placental abruption
- Fetal growth restriction with no known cause
- Preterm labor with no known cause
- Fetal demise with no known cause

Drug Abuse Quick Screen, and others. Screening often begins with an assessment of abuse of legal substances, such as tobacco and alcohol, and then progresses to a misuse of over-the-counter medications, then to a misuse of prescription drugs, and last of all to the use of illegal substances.

The nurse should use neutral and nonjudgmental language and tone during verbal screening. In addition to the substance used, the nurse should determine and record the patient's frequency and duration of use, route of administration, quantity of use, substance source, and time of last use.

Treatment

Counseling about the negative impact of substance abuse in pregnancy in a factual, nonjudgmental manner is the first-line intervention, followed by referral for treatment for patients who are willing to explore cessation or reduction of use (Table 19.6). Women using opioids are often treated with opioid replacement (methadone or buprenorphine) throughout pregnancy, as abrupt cessation of opioids is associated with pregnancy loss.

Stopping the consumption of alcohol at any point in pregnancy is associated with improved outcomes. Even brief educational interventions during pregnancy may reduce maternal alcohol consumption and improve pregnancy outcomes. Some women may benefit from the use of naltrexone to minimize alcohol use. Naltrexone may modestly decrease the volume of alcohol consumed as well as the number of days during which alcohol is consumed.

The nurse may successfully support smoking cessation by counseling, incentives, and health education, with monetary incentives being particularly effective (Chamberlain et al., 2017). The use of nicotine replacement products such as patches or gum may also facilitate smoking cessation or reduction (ACOG, 2017). The use of bupropion is another strategy to facilitate the reduction and cessation of tobacco use. Because of concerns about teratogenicity, use may be delayed until the second trimester of pregnancy (Berard, Zhao, & Sheehy, 2016).

Care Considerations

Women with a substance use disorder often also have comorbid conditions and psychosocial challenges, such as homelessness, poor nutrition, depression, sexually transmitted infections, and intimate partner violence, which should ideally be screened for

Table 19.6 Risks Associated with Substance Use

Substance	Obstetric Risks	Risks to Offspring
Opioids	Note: risks may be due to the opioid or withdrawal from it. • Subfertility • Pregnancy loss • Chorioamnionitis • Placental abruption • Preeclampsia • Premature rupture of membranes • Preterm birth • Fetal growth restriction • Postpartum hemorrhage • Meconium-stained amniotic fluid	• Neonatal abstinence syndrome (see Chapter 25) • Reduced cognitive functioning (however, may be due to disruptions in childhood and not intrauterine exposure to opioids)
Alcohol	• Low birth weight • Small for gestational age • Preterm birth • Stillbirth	Fetal alcohol spectrum disorders (cognitive, behavioral, physical, and mental problems; see Chapter 25)
Smoking	• Subfertility • Ectopic pregnancy • Pregnancy loss • Premature rupture of membranes • Placental abruption • Preterm birth • Preeclampsia • Decreased milk volume	• Small for gestational age • Cleft lip and pallet • Gastrointestinal defects • Cardiac defects • Limb reductions • Kidney agenesis • Digital anomalies • Sudden infant death syndrome • Type 2 diabetes • Behavioral problems • Asthma • Schizophrenia

(continued)

Table 19.6	Risks Associated with Substance Use (continued)	
Substance	**Obstetric Risks**	**Risks to Offspring**
Cocaine	• Preterm birth • Low birth weight • Short for gestational age • Small for gestational age • Miscarriage • Placental abruption	• Behavioral issues • Problems with sustained attention
Methamphetamines	• Fetal growth restriction • Gestational hypertension • Preeclampsia • Neonatal death • Fetal demise • Preterm birth	None known

Adapted from Maeda, A., Bateman, B. T., Clancy, C. R., Creanga, A. A., & Leffert, L. R. (2014). Opioid abuse and dependence during pregnancy: Temporal trends and obstetrical outcomes. *Anesthesiology, 121*(6), 1158–1165. doi:10.1097/ALN.0000000000000472; Ross, E. J., Graham, D. L., Money, K. M., & Stanwood, G. D. (2015). Developmental consequences of fetal exposure to drugs: What we know and what we still must learn. *Neuropsychopharmacology, 40*(1), 61–87. doi:10.1038/npp.2014.147; Nygaard, E., Slinning, K., Moe, V., & Walhovd, K. B. (2017). Cognitive function of youths born to mothers with opioid and poly-substance abuse problems during pregnancy. *Child Neuropsychology, 23*(2), 159–187. doi:10.1080/09297049.2015.1092509; Kesmodel, U., Wisborg, K., Olsen, S. F., Henriksen, T. B., & Secher, N. J. (2002). Moderate alcohol intake during pregnancy and the risk of stillbirth and death in the first year of life. *American Journal of Epidemiology, 155*(4), 305–312; Patra, J., Bakker, R., Irving, H., Jaddoe, V. W., Malini, S., & Rehm, J. (2011). Dose-response relationship between alcohol consumption before and during pregnancy and the risks of low birthweight, preterm birth and small for gestational age (SGA)—A systematic review and meta-analyses. *British Journal of Obstetrics and Gynaecology, 118*(12), 1411–1421. doi:10.1111/j.1471-0528.2011.03050.x; Practice Committee of the American Society for Reproductive Medicine. (2012). Smoking and infertility: A committee opinion. *Fertility and Sterility, 98*(6), 1400–1406. doi:10.1016/j.fertnstert.2012.07.1146; Sullivan, P. M., Dervan, L. A., Reiger, S., Buddhe, S., & Schwartz, S. M. (2015). Risk of congenital heart defects in the offspring of smoking mothers: A population-based study. *Journal of Pediatrics, 166*(4), 978.e2–984.e2. doi:10.1016/j.jpeds.2014.11.042; Cain, M. A., Bornick, P., & Whiteman, V. (2013). The maternal, fetal, and neonatal effects of cocaine exposure in pregnancy. *Clinical Obstetrics and Gynecology, 56*(1), 124–132. doi:10.1097/GRF.0b013e31827ae167; Cornelius, M. D. (2014). People with schizophrenia are more likely to have a mother who smoked during pregnancy than people without the condition. *Evidence-Based Nursing, 17*(3), 80. doi:10.1136/eb-2013-101549; Ackerman, J. P., Riggins, T., & Black, M. M. (2010). A review of the effects of prenatal cocaine exposure among school-aged children. *Pediatrics, 125*(3), 554–565. doi:10.1542/peds.2009-0637; Eze, N., Smith, L. M., LaGasse, L. L., Derauf, C., Newman, E., Arria, A., ... Lester, B. M. (2016). School-aged outcomes following prenatal methamphetamine exposure: 7.5-year follow-up from the infant development, environment, and lifestyle study. *Journal of Pediatrics, 170*, 34.e1–38.e1. doi:10.1016/j.jpeds.2015.11.070

and treated concurrently with substance abuse treatment. Wrap-around, interprofessional management with physicians, nurses, social workers, and other care providers is an important strategy for maximizing the chance of positive outcomes for these families. Women using opioids or opioid replacements postpartum often have an abundant milk supply, and providing education about pumping and safe milk storage may be particularly helpful for these mothers.

Depression

Depression may begin before, during, or after pregnancy. The focus in this section is on depression that begins before conception. Postpartum depression is covered in Chapter 23.

Course in Pregnancy

Preexisting depression and antepartum depression (depression that begins during the pregnancy) are associated with a small increased risk for pregnancy loss, preterm birth, bleeding in pregnancy and postpartum hemorrhage, and cesarean section (Chaudron, 2013). There may also be a modest increase in the

incidence of birth defects among the offspring of women with depression (Raisanen et al., 2014). Women with depression are less likely to start or continue breastfeeding (Figueiredo, Canario, & Field, 2014).

Maternal depression is associated with a mild-to-moderate increase in developmental disturbances in the woman's offspring, including a challenging temperament, excessive crying, childhood sleep problems, and behavioral problems. There may be a modest decrease in cognition for offspring. Children of women with antepartum and preexisting depression are more likely to exhibit depression, anxiety, and antisocial behavior (Stein et al., 2014). Offspring may have a small language delay (Skurtveit, Selmer, Roth, Hernandez-Diaz, & Handal, 2014). Maternal depression is also associated with an increased risk for sudden infant death syndrome (National Institute for Health and Care Excellence, 2017).

Assessment

The Patient Health Questionnaire nine-item scale (PHQ-9) is often used clinically to screen for and diagnose depression before and during pregnancy (Fig. 19.5).

PATIENT HEALTH QUESTIONNAIRE-9 (PHQ-9)

Over the <u>last 2 weeks</u>, how often have you been bothered by any of the following problems? *(Use "☒" to indicate your answer)*	Not at all	Several days	More than half the days	Nearly every day
1. Little interest or pleasure in doing things	0	1	2	3
2. Feeling down, depressed, or hopeless	0	1	2	3
3. Trouble falling or staying asleep, or sleeping too much	0	1	2	3
4. Feeling tired or having little energy	0	1	2	3
5. Poor appetite or overeating	0	1	2	3
6. Feeling bad about yourself—or that you are a failure or have let yourself or your family down	0	1	2	3
7. Trouble concentrating on things, such as reading the newspaper or watching television	0	1	2	3
8. Moving or speaking so slowly that other people could have noticed? Or the opposite—being so fidgety or restless that you have been moving around a lot more than usual	0	1	2	3
9. Thoughts that you would be better off dead or of hurting yourself in some way	0	1	2	3

FOR OFFICE CODING _0_ + _____ + _____ + _____

=Total Score: _____

If you checked off <u>any</u> problems, how <u>difficult</u> have these problems made it for you to do your work, take care of things at home, or get along with other people?

Not difficult at all	Somewhat difficult	Very difficult	Extremely difficult
☐	☐	☐	☐

Figure 19.5. Patient Health Questionnaire nine-item scale. (Developed by Drs. Robert L. Spitzer, Janet B.W. Williams, Kurt Kroenke and colleagues, with an educational grant from Pfizer Inc. No permission required to reproduce, translate, display, or distribute.)

Treatment

Major depression is not treated in pregnancy in up to half of women diagnosed because of cost, stigma, fear of harming the fetus, and a lack of clinical expertise in providers. Many women overestimate the risk of taking antidepressants in pregnancy (Osborne et al., 2015). Left untreated, depression can lead to substance abuse, poor adherence to care, less access to prenatal care, poor nutrition, impaired relationships, and suicide risk. Antidepressants and psychotherapy are the cornerstones of treatment for depression. Generally, if a woman was successful on an antidepressant previous to the pregnancy, she continues taking that medication (or restarts it, if she has stopped taking it), with the exception of monoamine oxidase inhibitors (MAOIs), because of a risk for fetal growth restriction associated with these medications (Vigod, Wilson, & Howard, 2016).

Antidepressants, usually selective serotonin reuptake inhibitors (SSRIs), are used in approximately 1 in 12 pregnancies in the United States (Huybrechts et al., 2013). Although SSRIs do pass the placenta and into the fetal circulation, they may have no significant teratogenic effect (Malm et al., 2015). The use of SSRIs in the second and third trimesters of pregnancy is associated with lower Apgar scores (see Table 1.4), although the clinical significance of this is unclear (Malm et al., 2015). Women taking SSRIs also have a higher risk for postpartum hemorrhage (Grzeskowiak, McBain, Dekker, & Clifton, 2016).

Fewer pregnant women use other types of antidepressants, such as serotonin-norepinephrine reuptake inhibitors (SNRIs), bupropion, and serotonin modulators such as trazodone, tricyclic antidepressants, or MAOIs. SNRIs may increase the risk for hypertensive disorders of pregnancy, preterm birth, and, like SSRIs, postpartum hemorrhage (Palmsten et al., 2013). Although there are fewer studies on antidepressants other than SSRIs, existing evidence suggests that the risk for fetal harm is low. Antidepressants are not a contraindication in breastfeeding (Kim, Epperson, Weiss, & Wisner, 2014).

Care Considerations

Depression is an illness and should be treated as such. The nurse should educate a patient with depression about the potential harms to herself and her fetus of foregoing treatment and inform her that depression is very common, even in pregnancy, and does not reflect her love for her offspring. Stigma is common to all mental illness, and a woman may feel significant shame and may be reticent to discuss the problem. If a patient shows signs of progressing or poorly managed depression, such as a report of poor nutrition, poor adherence to prenatal care, or a stagnant or worsening PHQ-9 score, the nurse should evaluate the patient further, including her compliance with treatment, and consider making changes to her plan of care, as needed. Nurses may help form a care team for the patient that includes identification of a counselor who works well for this particular patient.

Anxiety

Anxiety disorders include generalized anxiety disorder (GAD), phobias, obsessive compulsive disorder, posttraumatic stress disorder (PTSD), panic disorder, and agoraphobia. Often a person will have multiple anxiety disorders, and a codiagnosis with depression is common.

Prevalence

GAD affects as many as 12% of people in the United States, and women are twice as likely to be diagnosed as men (Kessler et al., 2008). Approximately 4% to 8% of people are diagnosed with a panic disorder, and as many as a third of individuals report having had an isolated panic attack at some point in their lives (Kessler et al., 2006).

Signs and Symptoms

The characteristics of GAD include excessive, difficult-to-control worry that causes significant impairment and/or distress on more days than not for at least 6 months. People with GAD may also report fatigue, tension, irritability, and a pervasive sense of apprehension.

Panic attacks are intense periods of severe anxiety lasting for several minutes to an hour. Patients often report cardiac, respiratory, and gastrointestinal features during attacks. Panic attacks may occur independently or with other anxiety disorders. In the case of a panic disorder, the attacks may be triggered by circumstances or occur spontaneously, and patients with this disorder often worry about experiencing new attacks and avoid situations they think may have precipitated them.

Agoraphobia includes anxiety and/or avoidance of entering into situations that may be difficult to leave or in which help may be unavailable. This used to be considered a form of a panic disorder but is currently understood to be an independent anxiety disorder (American Psychiatric Association, 2013).

Assessment

The GAD seven-item scale (GAD-7) is a frequently used tool to assess for GAD. The tool is also frequently used to assess for panic disorder, social anxiety disorder, and PTSD.

Treatment

Anxiety in pregnancy, like depression, is often treated with antidepressants, particularly SSRIs, and counseling. Occasionally, benzodiazepines, such as clonazepam or lorazepam, may be used for severe anxiety, although they carry with them risks for dependence and complications for the neonate, including withdrawal symptoms (ACOG, 2008, reaffirmed 2016b). In addition, benzodiazepine use in pregnancy is associated with fetal loss and preterm birth. Studies are mixed about the teratogenicity of benzodiazepines, with some studies finding a weak association between the medications and birth defects, such as cleft palates, and others finding no association (National Institute for Health and Clinical Excellence, 2014).

Care Considerations

Nurses can do much to facilitate a sense of patient empowerment that may help mitigate the symptoms of anxiety. The nurse can help the patient with anxiety make wise decisions by providing meticulous and realistic education about the risks of different therapies. Also, the nurse can facilitate a sense of well-being and minimize anxiety symptoms in the patient by teaching self-care measures, such as mindfulness, exercise, and good nutrition. As with depression, cognitive behavioral therapy can be tremendously beneficial for the treatment of anxiety, and nurses may facilitate a therapeutic relationship with an appropriate care provider.

Think Critically

1. Recalling what you know about diabetes and without referring to your text, make a list of common complications associated with this disease. Make a second list of indicated assessments and a third of interventions. Refer back to your text to see whether you missed anything.

2. Draw three pictures from memory: tetralogy of Fallot, atrial septal defect, and ventricular septal defect. Refer back to your text to check your work.

3. List the signs of cardiac decompensation as well as you can from memory.

4. Draw a diagram illustrating how one sibling might inherit the sickle cell trait while another inherits sickle cell disease when they have the same parents.

5. Write a brief dialogue you imagine having with a client you think may be in an abusive relationship. How will you help?

6. On the basis of your reading, what do you consider the most dangerous substance of abuse in pregnancy? How would you discuss the risk with a patient who is using this substance during pregnancy?

Unfolding Patient Stories: Fatime Sanago • Part 2

Fatime Sanogo, the primiparous 23-year-old you met in Unit 2. Fatime is now at 41 4/7 weeks gestation and admitted to the hospital for induction of labor. What physical findings should be present before labor is induced? What nursing assessments are performed and what nursing interventions are implemented to safely manage induction of labor with an oxytocin infusion? What assessment data should be documented when artificial rupture of membranes is performed?

Care for Fatime and other patients in a realistic virtual environment: *vSim for Nursing* (thepoint.lww.com/vSimMaternity). Practice documenting these patients' care in DocuCare (thepoint.lww.com/DocuCareEHR).

Unfolding Patient Stories: Amelia Sung • Part 2

Think back to Amelia Sung, who, as you learned in Unit 1, is 36 years old and Gravida 2 Para 1. She is diagnosed with gestational diabetes mellitus at 26 weeks. Explain the areas of education the nurse should provide on diabetes management. How does the nurse evaluate Amelia's understanding of the information provided and her ability to manage diabetes and maintain normal glucose levels?

Care for Amelia and other patients in a realistic virtual environment: *vSim for Nursing* (thepoint.lww.com/vSimMaternity). Practice documenting these patients' care in DocuCare (thepoint.lww.com/DocuCareEHR).

References

Abalos, E., Cuesta, C., Grosso, A. L., Chou, D., & Say, L. (2013). Global and regional estimates of preeclampsia and eclampsia: A systematic review. *European Journal of Obstetrics and Gynecology and Reproductive Biology, 170*(1), 1–7. doi:10.1016/j.ejogrb.2013.05.005

Abalos, E., Duley, L., & Steyn, D. W. (2014). Antihypertensive drug therapy for mild to moderate hypertension during pregnancy. *Cochrane Database of Systematic Reviews,* (2), CD002252. doi:10.1002/14651858.CD002252.pub3

Alexander, E. K., Pearce, E. N., Brent, G. A., Brown, R. S., Chen, H., Dosiou, C., ... Sullivan, S. (2017). 2017 Guidelines of the American Thyroid Association for the diagnosis and management of thyroid disease during pregnancy and the postpartum. *Thyroid, 27*(3), 315–389. doi:10.1089/thy.2016.0457

Ali, Z., Hansen, A. V., & Ulrik, C. S. (2016). Exacerbations of asthma during pregnancy: Impact on pregnancy complications and outcome. *Journal of Obstetrics and Gynaecology, 36*(4), 455–461. doi:10.3109/01443615.2015.1065800

American College of Obstetricians and Gynecologists. (2005, reaffirmed 2016). Practice bulletin no. 60: Pregestational diabetes mellitus. *Obstetrics and Gynecology, 105*(3), 675–685.

American College of Obstetricians and Gynecologists. (2007, reaffirmed 2015). ACOG practice bulletin no. 78: Hemoglobinopathies in pregnancy. *Obstetrics and Gynecology, 109*(1), 229–237.

American College of Obstetricians and Gynecologists. (2008, reaffirmed 2016a). ACOG practice bulletin: Clinical management guidelines for obstetrician-gynecologists number 90, February 2008: Asthma in pregnancy. *Obstetrics and Gynecology, 111*(2 Pt. 1), 457–464. doi:10.1097/AOG.0b013e3181665ff4

American College of Obstetricians and Gynecologists. (2008, reaffirmed 2016b). ACOG practice bulletin: Clinical management guidelines for obstetrician-gynecologists number 92, April 2008 (replaces practice bulletin number 87, November

2007). Use of psychiatric medications during pregnancy and lactation. *Obstetrics and Gynecology, 111*(4), 1001–1020. doi:10.1097/AOG.0b013e31816fd910

American College of Obstetricians and Gynecologists. (2011). AGOG committee opinion no. 473: Substance abuse reporting and pregnancy: The role of the obstetrician-gynecologist. *Obstetrics and Gynecology, 117*(1), 200–201. doi:10.1097/AOG.0b013e31820a6216

American College of Obstetricians and Gynecologists. (2013a). ACOG committee opinion no. 560: Medically indicated late-preterm and early-term deliveries. *Obstetrics and Gynecology, 121*(4), 908–910. doi:10.1097/01.AOG.0000428648.75548.00

American College of Obstetricians and Gynecologists. (2013b). Hypertension in pregnancy. Report of the American College of Obstetricians and Gynecologists' Task Force on Hypertension in Pregnancy. *Obstetrics and Gynecology, 122*(5), 1122–1131. doi:10.1097/01.AOG.0000437382.03963.88

American College of Obstetricians and Gynecologists. (2015a). ACOG practice bulletin no. 156: Obesity in pregnancy. *Obstetrics and Gynecology, 126*(6), e112–e126. doi:10.1097/AOG.0000000000001211

American College of Obstetricians and Gynecologists. (2015b). Committee opinion no. 633: Alcohol abuse and other substance use disorders: Ethical issues in obstetric and gynecologic practice. *Obstetrics and Gynecology, 125*(6), 1529–1537. doi:10.1097/01.AOG.0000466371.86393.9b

American College of Obstetricians and Gynecologists. (2016). Practice bulletin no. 173: Fetal macrosomia. *Obstetrics and Gynecology, 128*(5), e195–e209. doi:10.1097/AOG.0000000000001767

American College of Obstetricians and Gynecologists Committee on Health Care for Underserved Women & American Society of Addiction Medicine. (2012). ACOG committee opinion no. 524: Opioid abuse, dependence, and addiction in pregnancy. *Obstetrics and Gynecology, 119*(5), 1070–1076. doi:10.1097/AOG.0b013e318256496e

ACOG practice bulletin. (2017). Neural tube defects. *Obstet Gynecol, 130*, e279.

American Diabetes Association. (2017). 13. Management of diabetes in pregnancy. *Diabetes Care, 40*(Suppl. 1), S114–S119. doi:10.2337/dc17-S016

American Psychiatric Association. (2013). *Diagnostic and statistical manual of mental disorders, fifth edition (DSM-5)*. Arlington, VA: Author.

Andersen, S. L., Olsen, J., Wu, C. S., & Laurberg, P. (2013). Birth defects after early pregnancy use of antithyroid drugs: A Danish nationwide study. *Journal of Clinical Endocrinology and Metabolism, 98*(11), 4373–4381. doi:10.1210/jc.2013-2831

Arafeh, J. (2014). Cardiac disease in pregnancy. In K. R. Simpson & P. A. Creehan (Eds.), *Perinatal nursing* (4th ed.). Philadelphia, PA: Wolters Kluwer.

Baarnes, C. B., Hansen, A. V., & Ulrik, C. S. (2016). Enrolment in an asthma management program during pregnancy and adherence with inhaled corticosteroids: The 'Management of Asthma during Pregnancy' program. *Respiration, 92*(1), 9–15. doi:10.1159/000447244

Bailit, J. L., Doty, E., & Todia, W. (2007). Repeated hematocrit measurements in low-risk pregnant women. *Journal of Reproductive Medicine, 52*(7), 619–622.

Bain, E., Pierides, K. L., Clifton, V. L., Hodyl, N. A., Stark, M. J., Crowther, C. A., & Middleton, P. (2014). Interventions for managing asthma in pregnancy. *Cochrane Database of Systematic Reviews,* (10), CD010660. doi:10.1002/14651858.CD010660.pub2

Banta-Wright, S. A., Press, N., Knafl, K. A., Steiner, R. D., & Houck, G. M. (2014). Breastfeeding infants with phenylketonuria in the United States and Canada. *Breastfeeding Medicine, 9*(3), 142–148. doi:10.1089/bfm.2013.0092

Berard, A., Zhao, J. P., & Sheehy, O. (2016). Success of smoking cessation interventions during pregnancy. *American Journal of Obstetrics and Gynecology, 215*(5), 611.e1–611.e8. doi:10.1016/j.ajog.2016.06.059

Blondon, M., Harrington, L. B., Boehlen, F., Robert-Ebadi, H., Righini, M., & Smith, N. L. (2016). Pre-pregnancy BMI, delivery BMI, gestational weight gain and the risk of postpartum venous thrombosis. *Thrombosis Research, 145*, 151–156. doi:10.1016/j.thromres.2016.06.026

Blumer, I., Hadar, E., Hadden, D. R., Jovanovic, L., Mestman, J. H., Murad, M. H., & Yogev, Y. (2013). Diabetes and pregnancy: An endocrine society clinical practice guideline. *Journal of Clinical Endocrinology and Metabolism, 98*(11), 4227–4249. doi:10.1210/jc.2013-2465

Bove, R., Alwan, S., Friedman, J. M., Hellwig, K., Houtchens, M., Koren, G., ... Sadovnick, A. D. (2014). Management of multiple sclerosis during pregnancy and the reproductive years: A systematic review. *Obstetrics and Gynecology, 124*(6), 1157–1168. doi:10.1097/AOG.0000000000000541

Bramham, K., Parnell, B., Nelson-Piercy, C., Seed, P. T., Poston, L., & Chappell, L. C. (2014). Chronic hypertension and pregnancy outcomes: Systematic review and meta-analysis. *BMJ, 348*, g2301. doi:10.1136/bmj.g2301

Breiding, M. J., Smith, S. G., Basile, K. C., Walters, M. L., Chen, J., & Merrick, M. T. (2014). Prevalence and characteristics of sexual violence, stalking, and intimate partner violence victimization—National intimate partner and sexual violence survey, United States, 2011. *MMWR Surveillance Summaries, 63*(8), 1–18.

Brito-Zeron, P., Izmirly, P. M., Ramos-Casals, M., Buyon, J. P., & Khamashta, M. A. (2015). The clinical spectrum of autoimmune congenital heart block. *Nature Reviews, 11*(5), 301–312. doi:10.1038/nrrheum.2015.29

Burchill, L. J., Lameijer, H., Roos-Hesselink, J. W., Grewal, J., Ruys, T. P., Kulikowski, J. D., ... Silversides, C. K. (2015). Pregnancy risks in women with pre-existing coronary artery disease, or following acute coronary syndrome. *Heart, 101*(7), 525–529. doi:10.1136/heartjnl-2014-306676

Cantor, A. G., Bougatsos, C., Dana, T., Blazina, I., & McDonagh, M. (2015). Routine iron supplementation and screening for iron deficiency anemia in pregnancy: A systematic review for the U.S. Preventive Services Task Force. *Annals of Internal Medicine, 162*(8), 566–576. doi:10.7326/M14-2932

Castro, J., Billick, S., Kleiman, A., Chiechi, M., & Al-Rashdan, M. (2014). Confounding psychosis in the postpartum period. *Psychiatric Quarterly, 85*(1), 91–96. doi:10.1007/s11126-013-9271-5

Catalano, P. M., & Shankar, K. (2017). Obesity and pregnancy: Mechanisms of short term and long term adverse consequences for mother and child. *BMJ, 356*, j1. doi:10.1136/bmj.j1

Centers for Disease Control and Prevention. (1989). CDC criteria for anemia in children and childbearing-aged women. *Morbidity and Mortality Weekly Report, 38*(22), 400–404.

Centers for Disease Control and Prevention. (2016). *Smoking in pregnancy.* Retrieved from https://www.cdc.gov/tobacco/basic_information/health_effects/pregnancy/index.htm

Chamberlain, C., O'Mara-Eves, A., Porter, J., Coleman, T., Perlen, S. M., Thomas, J., & McKenzie, J. E. (2017). Psychosocial interventions for supporting women to stop smoking in pregnancy. *Cochrane Database of Systematic Reviews, 2*, CD001055. doi:10.1002/14651858.CD001055.pub5

Chaudron, L. H. (2013). Complex challenges in treating depression during pregnancy. *American Journal of Psychiatry, 170*(1), 12–20. doi:10.1176/appi.ajp.2012.12040440

Christensen, J., Gronborg, T. K., Sorensen, M. J., Schendel, D., Parner, E. T., Pedersen, L. H., & Vestergaard, M. (2013). Prenatal valproate exposure and risk of autism spectrum disorders and childhood autism. *JAMA, 309*(16), 1696–1703. doi:10.1001/jama.2013.2270

Clowse, M. E., Jamison, M., Myers, E., & James, A. H. (2008). A national study of the complications of lupus in pregnancy. *American Journal of Obstetrics and Gynecology, 199*(2), 127.e1–127.e6. doi:10.1016/j.ajog.2008.03.012

Cnattingius, S., & Villamor, E. (2016). Weight change between successive pregnancies and risks of stillbirth and infant mortality: A nationwide cohort study. *The Lancet, 387*(10018), 558–565. doi:10.1016/S0140-6736(15)00990-3

Cnattingius, S., Villamor, E., Johansson, S., Edstedt Bonamy, A. K., Persson, M., Wikstrom, A. K., & Granath, F. (2013). Maternal obesity and risk of preterm delivery. *JAMA, 309*(22), 2362–2370. doi:10.1001/jama.2013.6295

Compston, A., & Coles, A. (2008). Multiple sclerosis. *The Lancet, 372*(9648), 1502–1517. doi:10.1016/S0140-6736(08)61620-7

Congdon, E. L., Westerlund, A., Algarin, C. R., Peirano, P. D., Gregas, M., Lozoff, B., & Nelson, C. A. (2012). Iron deficiency in infancy is associated with altered neural correlates of recognition memory at 10 years. *Journal of Pediatrics, 160*(6), 1027–1033. doi:10.1016/j.jpeds.2011.12.011

Cornelissen, M., Steegers-Theunissen, R., Kollee, L., Eskes, T., Motohara, K., & Monnens, L. (1993). Supplementation of vitamin K in pregnant women receiving anticonvulsant therapy prevents neonatal vitamin K deficiency. *American Journal of Obstetrics and Gynecology, 168*(3 Pt. 1), 884–888.

Coyle, P. K. (2014). Multiple sclerosis and pregnancy prescriptions. *Expert Opinion on Drug Safety, 13*(12), 1565–1568. doi:10.1517/14740338.2014.973848

Curtis, K. M., Tepper, N. K., Jatlaoui, T. C., Berry-Bibee, E., Horton, L. G., Zapata, L. B., ... Whiteman, M. K. (2016). U.S. medical eligibility criteria for contraceptive use, 2016. *MMWR Recommendations and Reports, 65*(3), 1–103. doi:10.15585/mmwr.rr6503a1

Dolgin M, Association NYH, Fox AC, Gorlin R, Levin RI, New York Heart Association. Criteria Committee. Nomenclature and criteria for diagnosis of diseases of the heart and great vessels. 9th ed. Boston, MA: Lippincott Williams and Wilkins; March 1, 1994.

Donofrio, M. T., Moon-Grady, A. J., Hornberger, L. K., Copel, J. A., Sklansky, M. S., Abuhamad, A., ... Stroke, N. (2014). Diagnosis and treatment of fetal cardiac disease: A scientific statement from the American Heart Association. *Circulation, 129*(21), 2183–2242. doi:10.1161/01.cir.0000437597.44550.5d

Easter, A., Solmi, F., Bye, A., Taborelli, E., Corfield, F., Schmidt, U., ... Micali, N. (2015). Antenatal and postnatal psychopathology among women with current and past eating disorders: Longitudinal patterns. *European Eating Disorders Review, 23*(1), 19–27. doi:10.1002/erv.2328

Easter, A., Treasure, J., & Micali, N. (2011). Fertility and prenatal attitudes towards pregnancy in women with eating disorders: Results from the Avon Longitudinal Study of Parents and Children. *British Journal of Obstetrics and Gynaecology, 118*(12), 1491–1498. doi:10.1111/j.1471-0528.2011.03077.x

Edlow, A. G. (2017). Maternal obesity and neurodevelopmental and psychiatric disorders in offspring. *Prenatal Diagnosis, 37*(1), 95–110. doi:10.1002/pd.4932

Elkayam, U., Jalnapurkar, S., Barakkat, M. N., Khatri, N., Kealey, A. J., Mehra, A., & Roth, A. (2014). Pregnancy-associated acute myocardial infarction: A review of contemporary experience in 150 cases between 2006 and 2011. *Circulation, 129*(16), 1695–1702. doi:10.1161/CIRCULATIONAHA.113.002054

Fan, X., & Wu, L. (2016). The impact of thyroid abnormalities during pregnancy on subsequent neuropsychological development of the offspring: A meta-analysis. *Journal of Maternal-Fetal and Neonatal Medicine, 29*(24), 3971–3976. doi:10.3109/14767058.2016.1152248

Figueiredo, B., Canario, C., & Field, T. (2014). Breastfeeding is negatively affected by prenatal depression and reduces postpartum depression. *Psychological Medicine, 44*(5), 927–936. doi:10.1017/S0033291713001530

Forno, E., Young, O. M., Kumar, R., Simhan, H., & Celedon, J. C. (2014). Maternal obesity in pregnancy, gestational weight gain, and risk of childhood asthma. *Pediatrics, 134*(2), e535–e546. doi:10.1542/peds.2014-0439

Gaddipati, S. T., Troiano, N. H. (2013). Cardiac disorders in pregnancy. In N. H. Troiano, C. J. Harvey, & B. F. Chez (Eds.), *High-risk & critical care obstetrics* (3rd ed.). Philadelphia, PA: Wolters Kluwer.

Garber, J. R., Cobin, R. H., Gharib, H., Hennessey, J. V., Klein, I., Mechanick, J. I., ... Woeber, K. A.; American Thyroid Association Taskforce On Hypothyroidism In Adults. (2012). Clinical practice guidelines for hypothyroidism in adults: Cosponsored by the American Association of Clinical Endocrinologists and the American Thyroid Association. *Thyroid, 22*(12), 1200–1235. doi:10.1089/thy.2012.0205

Gracia, E., Lopez-Quilez, A., Marco, M., Lladosa, S., & Lila, M. (2015). The spatial epidemiology of intimate partner violence: Do neighborhoods matter? *American Journal of Epidemiology, 182*(1), 58–66. doi:10.1093/aje/kwv016

Grzeskowiak, L. E., McBain, R., Dekker, G. A., & Clifton, V. L. (2016). Antidepressant use in late gestation and risk of postpartum haemorrhage: A retrospective cohort study. *British Journal of Obstetrics and Gynaecology, 123*(12), 1929–1936. doi:10.1111/1471-0528.13612

Haddad, L. B., Curtis, K. M., Legardy-Williams, J. K., Cwiak, C., & Jamieson, D. J. (2012). Contraception for individuals with sickle cell disease: A systematic review of the literature. *Contraception, 85*(6), 527–537. doi:10.1016/j.contraception.2011.10.008

Han, A., & Stewart, D. E. (2014). Maternal and fetal outcomes of intimate partner violence associated with pregnancy in the Latin American and Caribbean region. *International Journal of Gynaecology and Obstetrics, 124*(1), 6–11. doi:10.1016/j.ijgo.2013.06.037

Harden, C. L., Hopp, J., Ting, T. Y., Pennell, P. B., French, J. A., Hauser, W. A., ... American Epilepsy Society. (2009). Practice parameter update: Management issues for women with epilepsy—Focus on pregnancy (an evidence-based review): Obstetrical complications and change in seizure frequency: Report of the Quality Standards Subcommittee and Therapeutics and Technology Assessment Subcommittee of the American Academy of Neurology and American Epilepsy Society. *Neurology, 73*(2), 126–132. doi:10.1212/WNL.0b013e3181a6b2f8

Harden, C. L., Pennell, P. B., Koppel, B. S., Hovinga, C. A., Gidal, B., Meador, K. J., ... American Epilepsy Society. (2009). Practice parameter update: Management issues for women with epilepsy—Focus on pregnancy (an evidence-based review): Vitamin K, folic acid, blood levels, and breastfeeding: Report of the Quality Standards Subcommittee and Therapeutics and Technology Assessment Subcommittee of the American Academy of Neurology and American Epilepsy Society. *Neurology, 73*(2), 142–149. doi:10.1212/WNL.0b013e3181a6b325

Hellwig, K., & Correale, J. (2013). Artificial reproductive techniques in multiple sclerosis. *Clinical Immunology, 149*(2), 219–224. doi:10.1016/j.clim.2013.02.001

Hellwig, K., Rockhoff, M., Herbstritt, S., Borisow, N., Haghikia, A., Elias-Hamp, B., ... Langer-Gould, A. (2015). Exclusive breastfeeding and the effect on postpartum multiple sclerosis relapses. *JAMA Neurology, 72*(10), 1132–1138. doi:10.1001/jamaneurol.2015.1806

Henderson, J. T., Whitlock, E. P., O'Conner, E., Senger, C. A., Thompson, J. H., Rowland, M. G. (2014). *Low-dose aspirin for the prevention of morbidity and mortality from preeclampsia: A systematic evidence review for the U.S. Preventive Services Task Force.* Retrieved from https://www.ncbi.nlm.nih.gov/books/NBK196392/

Hewapathirana, N., & Murphy, H. (2014). Perinatal outcomes in type 2 diabetes. *Curr Diab Rep, 14*(2), 461.

Huybrechts, K. F., Palmsten, K., Mogun, H., Kowal, M., Avorn, J., Setoguchi-Iwata, S., & Hernandez-Diaz, S. (2013). National trends in antidepressant medication treatment among publicly insured pregnant women. *General Hospital Psychiatry, 35*(3), 265–271. doi:10.1016/j.genhosppsych.2012.12.010

Ioannou, G. N., Spector, J., Scott, K., & Rockey, D. C. (2002). Prospective evaluation of a clinical guideline for the diagnosis and management of iron deficiency anemia. *American Journal of Medicine, 113*(4), 281–287.

Izmirly, P. M., Saxena, A., Kim, M. Y., Wang, D., Sahl, S. K., Llanos, C., ... Buyon, J. P. (2011). Maternal and fetal factors associated with mortality and morbidity in a multi-racial/ethnic registry of anti-SSA/Ro-associated cardiac neonatal lupus. *Circulation, 124*(18), 1927–1935. doi:10.1161/CIRCULATIONAHA.111.033894

Jans, S. M., de Jonge, A., & Lagro-Janssen, A. L. (2010). Maternal and perinatal outcomes amongst haemoglobinopathy carriers: A systematic review. *International Journal of Clinical Practice, 64*(12), 1688–1698. doi:10.1111/j.1742-1241.2010.02451.x

Kapadia, M. Z., Park, C. K., Beyene, J., Giglia, L., Maxwell, C., & McDonald, S. D. (2015). Weight loss instead of weight gain within the guidelines in obese women during pregnancy: A systematic review and meta-analyses of maternal and infant outcomes. *PLoS One, 10*(7), e0132650. doi:10.1371/journal.pone.0132650

Kessler, R. C., Chiu, W. T., Jin, R., Ruscio, A. M., Shear, K., & Walters, E. E. (2006). The epidemiology of panic attacks, panic disorder, and agoraphobia in the National Comorbidity Survey Replication. *Archives of General Psychiatry, 63*(4), 415–424. doi:10.1001/archpsyc.63.4.415

Kessler, R. C., Gruber, M., Hettema, J. M., Hwang, I., Sampson, N., & Yonkers, K. A. (2008). Co-morbid major depression and generalized anxiety disorders in the National Comorbidity Survey follow-up. *Psychological Medicine, 38*(3), 365–374. doi:10.1017/S0033291707002012

Kim, D. R., Epperson, C. N., Weiss, A. R., & Wisner, K. L. (2014). Pharmacotherapy of postpartum depression: An update. *Expert Opinion on Pharmacotherapy, 15*(9), 1223–1234. doi:10.1517/14656566.2014.911842

Knoph, C., Von Holle, A., Zerwas, S., Torgersen, L., Tambs, K., Stoltenberg, C., ... Reichborn-Kjennerud, T. (2013). Course and predictors of maternal eating disorders in the postpartum period. *International Journal of Eating Disorders, 46*(4), 355–368. doi:10.1002/eat.22088

Kuklina, E. V., Tong, X., Bansil, P., George, M. G., & Callaghan, W. M. (2011). Trends in pregnancy hospitalizations that included a stroke in the United States from 1994 to 2007: Reasons for concern? *Stroke, 42*(9), 2564–2570. doi:10.1161/STROKEAHA.110.610592

Lateef, A., & Petri, M. (2013). Managing lupus patients during pregnancy. *Best Practice and Research. Clinical Rheumatology, 27*(3), 435–447. doi:10.1016/j.berh.2013.07.005

Linna, M. S., Raevuori, A., Haukka, J., Suvisaari, J. M., Suokas, J. T., & Gissler, M. (2013). Reproductive health outcomes in eating disorders. *International Journal of Eating Disorders, 46*(8), 826–833. doi:10.1002/eat.22179

Linna, M. S., Raevuori, A., Haukka, J., Suvisaari, J. M., Suokas, J. T., & Gissler, M. (2014). Pregnancy, obstetric, and perinatal health outcomes in eating disorders. *American Journal of Obstetrics and Gynecology, 211*(4), 392.e1–392.e8. doi:10.1016/j.ajog.2014.03.067

Lisonkova, S., Muraca, G. M., Potts, J., Liauw, J., Chan, W. S., Skoll, A., & Lim, K. I. (2017). Association between prepregnancy body mass index and severe maternal morbidity. *JAMA, 318*(18), 1777–1786. doi:10.1001/jama.2017.16191

Lo, J. C., Rivkees, S. A., Chandra, M., Gonzalez, J. R., Korelitz, J. J., & Kuzniewicz, M. W. (2015). Gestational thyrotoxicosis, antithyroid drug use and neonatal outcomes within an integrated healthcare delivery system. *Thyroid, 25*(6), 698–705. doi:10.1089/thy.2014.0434

MacDonald, S. C., Bateman, B. T., McElrath, T. F., & Hernandez-Diaz, S. (2015). Mortality and morbidity during delivery hospitalization among pregnant women with epilepsy in the United States. *JAMA Neurology, 72*(9), 981–988. doi:10.1001/jamaneurol.2015.1017

Magee, L. A., Singer, J., von Dadelszen, P., & Group, C. S. (2015). Less-tight versus tight control of hypertension in pregnancy. *New England Journal of Medicine, 372*(24), 2367–2368. doi:10.1056/NEJMc1503870

Magro-Malosso, E. R., Saccone, G., Di Mascio, D., Di Tommaso, M., & Berghella, V. (2017). Exercise during pregnancy and risk of preterm birth in overweight and obese women: A systematic review and meta-analysis of randomized controlled trials. *Acta Obstetricia et Gynecologica Scandinavica, 96*(3), 263–273. doi:10.1111/aogs.13087

Malm, H., Sourander, A., Gissler, M., Gyllenberg, D., Hinkka-Yli-Salomaki, S., McKeague, I. W., ... Brown, A. S. (2015). Pregnancy complications following prenatal exposure to SSRIs or maternal psychiatric disorders: Results from population-based national register data. *American Journal of Psychiatry, 172*(12), 1224–1232. doi:10.1176/appi.ajp.2015.14121575

Mannisto, T., Mendola, P., Grewal, J., Xie, Y., Chen, Z., & Laughon, S. K. (2013). Thyroid diseases and adverse pregnancy outcomes in a contemporary US cohort. *Journal of Clinical Endocrinology and Metabolism, 98*(7), 2725–2733. doi:10.1210/jc.2012-4233

Mendola, P., Laughon, S. K., Mannisto, T. I., Leishear, K., Reddy, U. M., Chen, Z., & Zhang, J. (2013). Obstetric complications among US women with asthma. *American Journal of Obstetrics and Gynecology, 208*(2), 127.e1–127.e8. doi:10.1016/j.ajog.2012.11.007

Molyneaux, E., Poston, L., Ashurst-Williams, S., & Howard, L. M. (2014). Obesity and mental disorders during pregnancy and postpartum: A systematic review and meta-analysis. *Obstetrics and Gynecology, 123*(4), 857–867. doi:10.1097/AOG.0000000000000170

Namazy, J. A., Chambers, C., & Schatz, M. (2014). Safety of therapeutic options for treating asthma in pregnancy. *Expert Opinion on Drug Safety, 13*(12), 1613–1621. doi:10.1517/14740338.2014.975203

Namazy, J., & Schatz, M. (2016). The treatment of allergic respiratory disease during pregnancy. *Journal of Investigational Allergology and Clinical Immunology, 26*(1), 1–7; quiz 2p following 7.

National Institute for Health and Care Excellence. (2017). *Antenatal and postnatal mental health: Clinical management and service guidance.* Retrieved from https://www.nice.org.uk/guidance/cg192

National Institute for Health and Clinical Excellence. (2014). In *Antenatal and postnatal mental health: Clinical management and service guidance: Updated edition.* Leicester, England: British Psychological Society.

O'Brien, T. E., Ray, J. G., & Chan, W. S. (2003). Maternal body mass index and the risk of preeclampsia: A systematic overview. *Epidemiology, 14*(3), 368–374.

Ogden, C. L., Carroll, M. D., Fryar, C. D., & Flegal, K. M. (2015). *Prevalence of obesity among adults and youth: United States, 2011–2014.* https://www.cdc.gov/nchs/data/databriefs/db219.pdf.

Ojodu, J., Hulihan, M. M., Pope, S. N., Grant, A. M.; Centers for Disease Control and Prevention. (2014). Incidence of sickle cell trait—United States, 2010. *Morbidity and Mortality Weekly Report, 63*(49), 1155–1158.

Orbach, H., Matok, I., Gorodischer, R., Sheiner, E., Daniel, S., Wiznitzer, A., ... Levy, A. (2013). Hypertension and antihypertensive drugs in pregnancy and perinatal outcomes. *American Journal of Obstetrics and Gynecology, 208*(4), 301.e1–301.e6. doi:10.1016/j.ajog.2012.11.011

Osborne, L. M., Hermann, A., Burt, V., Driscoll, K., Fitelson, E., Meltzer-Brody, S., ... Miller, L.; National Task Force on Women's Reproductive Mental Health. (2015). Reproductive psychiatry: The gap between clinical need and education. *Am J Psychiatry, 172*(10), 946–948. doi:10.1176/appi.ajp.2015.15060837

Oteng-Ntim, E. (2017). Pregnancy in women with sickle cell disease is associated with risk of maternal and perinatal mortality and severe morbidity. *Evidence-Based Nursing, 20*(2), 43. doi:10.1136/eb-2016-102450

Palmsten, K., Hernandez-Diaz, S., Huybrechts, K. F., Williams, P. L., Michels, K. B., Achtyes, E. D., ... Setoguchi, S. (2013). Use of antidepressants near delivery and risk of postpartum hemorrhage: Cohort study of low income women in the United States. *BMJ, 347*, f4877. doi:10.1136/bmj.f4877

Palomba, S., Falbo, A., Chiossi, G., Orio, F., Tolino, A., Colao, A., ... Zullo, F. (2014). Low-grade chronic inflammation in pregnant women with polycystic ovary syndrome: A prospective controlled clinical study. *Journal of Clinical Endocrinology and Metabolism, 99*(8), 2942–2951. doi:10.1210/jc.2014-1214

Peljto, A. L., Barker-Cummings, C., Vasoli, V. M., Leibson, C. L., Hauser, W. A., Buchhalter, J. R., & Ottman, R. (2014). Familial risk of epilepsy: A population-based study. *Brain, 137*(Pt. 3), 795–805. doi:10.1093/brain/awt368

Pillai, M., & James, D. (1990). The development of fetal heart rate patterns during normal pregnancy. *Obstetrics and Gynecology, 76*(5 Pt. 1), 812–816.

Raisanen, S., Lehto, S. M., Nielsen, H. S., Gissler, M., Kramer, M. R., & Heinonen, S. (2014). Risk factors for and perinatal outcomes of major depression during pregnancy: A population-based analysis during 2002–2010 in Finland. *BMJ Open, 4*(11), e004883. doi:10.1136/bmjopen-2014-004883

Ramagopalan, S., Yee, I., Byrnes, J., Guimond, C., Ebers, G., & Sadovnick, D. (2012). Term pregnancies and the clinical characteristics of multiple sclerosis: A population based study. *Journal of Neurology, Neurosurgery, and Psychiatry, 83*(8), 793–795. doi:10.1136/jnnp-2012-302848

Regitz-Zagrosek, V., Blomstrom Lundqvist, C., Borghi, C., Cifkova, R., Ferreira, R., Foidart, J.M., ... Torracca, L.; European Society of Gynecology; Association for European Paediatric Cardiology; German Society for Gender Medicine; E. S. C. Committee for Practice Guidelines. (2011). ESC Guidelines on the management of cardiovascular diseases during pregnancy: The Task Force on the Management of Cardiovascular Diseases during Pregnancy of the European Society of Cardiology (ESC). *European Heart Journal, 32*(24), 3147–3197. doi:10.1093/eurheartj/ehr218

Renner, L. M., & Whitney, S. D. (2012). Risk factors for unidirectional and bidirectional intimate partner violence among young adults. *Child Abuse and Neglect, 36*(1), 40–52. doi:10.1016/j.chiabu.2011.07.007

Robinson, B. K., Mapp, D. C., Bloom, S. L., Rouse, D. J., Spong, C. Y., Varner, M. W., ... Ehrenberg, H.; Human Development of the Maternal-Fetal Medicine Units Network. (2011). Increasing maternal body mass index and characteristics of the second stage of labor. *Obstetrics and Gynecology, 118*(6), 1309–1313. doi:10.1097/AOG.0b013e318236fbd1

Ross, D. S., Burch, H. B., Cooper, D. S., Greenlee, M. C., Laurberg, P., Maia, A. L., ... Walter, M. A. (2016). 2016 American Thyroid Association Guidelines for diagnosis and management of hyperthyroidism and other causes of thyrotoxicosis. *Thyroid, 26*(10), 1343–1421. doi:10.1089/thy.2016.0229

Saavedra, M. A., Cruz-Reyes, C., Vera-Lastra, O., Romero, G. T., Cruz-Cruz, P., Arias-Flores, R., & Jara, L. J. (2012). Impact of previous lupus nephritis on maternal and fetal outcomes during pregnancy. *Clinical Rheumatology, 31*(5), 813–819. doi:10.1007/s10067-012-1941-4

Sacks, D. A., & Metzger, B. E. (2013). Classification of diabetes in pregnancy: Time to reassess the alphabet. *Obstetrics and Gynecology, 121*(2 Pt. 1), 345–348. doi:10.1097/AOG.0b013e31827f09b5

SAMHSA/CSAT Treatment Improvement Protocols. (2005). In *Medication-assisted treatment for opioid addiction in opioid treatment programs*. Rockville, MD: Substance Abuse and Mental Health Services Administration.

Sibai, B. M., Caritis, S., Hauth, J., Lindheimer, M., VanDorsten, J. P., MacPherson, C., ... McNellis, D. (2000). Risks of preeclampsia and adverse neonatal outcomes among women with pregestational diabetes mellitus. National Institute of Child Health and Human Development Network of Maternal-Fetal Medicine Units. *American Journal of Obstetrics and Gynecology, 182*(2), 364–369.

Sibai, B. M., & Viteri, O. A. (2014). Diabetic ketoacidosis in pregnancy. *Obstetrics and Gynecology, 123*(1), 167–178. doi:10.1097/AOG.0000000000000060

Siega-Riz, A. M., Von Holle, A., Haugen, M., Meltzer, H. M., Hamer, R., Torgersen, L., ... Bulik, C. M. (2011). Gestational weight gain of women with eating disorders in the Norwegian pregnancy cohort. *International Journal of Eating Disorders, 44*(5), 428–434. doi:10.1002/eat.20835

Siegel, A. M., Tita, A., Biggio, J. R., & Harper, L. M. (2015). Evaluating gestational weight gain recommendations in pregestational diabetes. *American Journal of Obstetrics and Gynecology, 213*(4), 563.e1–563.e5. doi:10.1016/j.ajog.2015.07.030

Skurtveit, S., Selmer, R., Roth, C., Hernandez-Diaz, S., & Handal, M. (2014). Prenatal exposure to antidepressants and language competence at age three: Results from a large population-based pregnancy cohort in Norway. *British Journal of Obstetrics and Gynaecology, 121*(13), 1621–1631. doi:10.1111/1471-0528.12821

Solmi, M., Veronese, N., Sergi, G., Luchini, C., Favaro, A., Santonastaso, P., ... Stubbs, B. (2016). The association between smoking prevalence and eating disorders: A systematic review and meta-analysis. *Addiction, 111*(11), 1914–1922. doi:10.1111/add.13457

Stagnaro-Green, A., Abalovich, M., Alexander, E., Azizi, F., Mestman, J., Negro, R., ... Wiersinga, W. (2011). Guidelines of the American Thyroid Association for the diagnosis and management of thyroid disease during pregnancy and postpartum. *Thyroid, 21*(10), 1081–1125. doi:10.1089/thy.2011.0087

Stein, A., Pearson, R. M., Goodman, S. H., Rapa, E., Rahman, A., McCallum, M., ... Pariante, C. M. (2014). Effects of perinatal mental disorders on the fetus and child. *The Lancet, 384*(9956), 1800–1819. doi:10.1016/S0140-6736(14)61277-0

Sugiura-Ogasawara, M. (2015). Recurrent pregnancy loss and obesity. *Best Practice and Research. Clinical Obstetrics and Gynaecology, 29*(4), 489–497. doi:10.1016/j.bpobgyn.2014.12.001

Taft, A., O'Doherty, L., Hegarty, K., Ramsay, J., Davidson, L., & Feder, G. (2013). Screening women for intimate partner violence in healthcare settings. *Cochrane Database of Systematic Reviews, (4)*, CD007007. doi:10.1002/14651858.CD007007.pub2

Tennant, P. W., Glinianaia, S. V., Bilous, R. W., Rankin, J., & Bell, R. (2014). Pre-existing diabetes, maternal glycated haemoglobin, and the risks of fetal and infant death: A population-based study. *Diabetologia, 57*(2), 285–294. doi:10.1007/s00125-013-3108-5

Tolia, V. N., Patrick, S. W., Bennett, M. M., Murthy, K., Sousa, J., Smith, P. B., ... Spitzer, A. R. (2015). Increasing incidence of the neonatal abstinence syndrome in U.S. neonatal ICUs. *New England Journal of Medicine, 372*(22), 2118–2126. doi:10.1056/NEJMsa1500439

Torloni, M. R., Betran, A. P., Horta, B. L., Nakamura, M. U., Atallah, A. N., Moron, A. F., & Valente, O. (2009). Prepregnancy BMI and the risk of gestational diabetes: A systematic review of the literature with meta-analysis. *Obesity Reviews, 10*(2), 194–203. doi:10.1111/j.1467-789X.2008.00541.x

Vadiveloo, T., Mires, G. J., Donnan, P. T., & Leese, G. P. (2013). Thyroid testing in pregnant women with thyroid dysfunction in Tayside, Scotland: The thyroid epidemiology, audit and research study (TEARS). *Clinical Endocrinology (Oxford), 78*(3), 466–471. doi:10.1111/j.1365-2265.2012.04426.x

Veiby, G., Daltveit, A. K., Engelsen, B. A., & Gilhus, N. E. (2014). Fetal growth restriction and birth defects with newer and older antiepileptic drugs during pregnancy. *Journal of Neurology, 261*(3), 579–588. doi:10.1007/s00415-013-7239-x

Vigod, S. N., Wilson, C. A., & Howard, L. M. (2016). Depression in pregnancy. *BMJ, 352*, i1547. doi:10.1136/bmj.i1547

Wallace, M. E., Hoyert, D., Williams, C., & Mendola, P. (2016). Pregnancy-associated homicide and suicide in 37 US states with enhanced pregnancy surveillance. *American Journal of Obstetrics and Gynecology, 215*(3), 364.e1–364.e10. doi:10.1016/j.ajog.2016.03.040

Watson, H. J., Von Holle, A., Hamer, R. M., Knoph Berg, C., Torgersen, L., Magnus, P., ... Bulik, C. M. (2013). Remission, continuation and incidence of eating disorders during early pregnancy: A validation study in a population-based birth cohort. *Psychological Medicine, 43*(8), 1723–1734. doi:10.1017/S0033291712002516

Williams, J. F., & Smith, V. C.; Committee on Substance Abuse. (2015). Fetal alcohol spectrum disorders. *Pediatrics, 136*(5), e1395–e1406. doi:10.1542/peds.2015-3113

Wolfe, K. B., Rossi, R. A., & Warshak, C. R. (2011). The effect of maternal obesity on the rate of failed induction of labor. *American Journal of Obstetrics and Gynecology, 205*(2), 128.e1–128.e7. doi:10.1016/j.ajog.2011.03.051

Zack, M. M., & Kobau, R. (2017). National and state estimates of the numbers of adults and children with active epilepsy—United States, 2015. *Morbidity and Mortality Weekly Report, 66*(31), 821–825. doi:10.15585/mmwr.mm6631a1

Zerwas, S., Von Holle, A., Torgersen, L., Reichborn-Kjennerud, T., Stoltenberg, C., & Bulik, C. M. (2012). Maternal eating disorders and infant temperament: Findings from the Norwegian mother and child cohort study. *International Journal of Eating Disorders, 45*(4), 546–555. doi:10.1002/eat.20983

Suggested Readings

Bianchi, A. L., Cesario, S. K., & McFarlane, J. (2016). Interrupting intimate partner violence during pregnancy with an effective screening and assessment program. *Journal of Obstetric, Gynecologic, and Neonatal Nursing, 45*(4), 579–591. doi:10.1016/j.jogn.2016.02.012

Diabetes and Pregnancy. Retrieved from https://www.cdc.gov/pregnancy/diabetes.html

LactMed Drugs and Lactation Database. Retrieved from https://toxnet.nlm.nih.gov/newtoxnet/lactmed.htm

Smeltzer, S. C., Mitra, M., Iezzoni, L. I., Long-Bellil, L., & Smith, L. D. (2016). Perinatal experiences of women with physical disabilities and their recommendations for clinicians. *Journal of Obstetric, Gynecologic, and Neonatal Nursing, 45*(6), 781–789. doi:10.1016/j.jogn.2016.07.007

20 Conditions Occurring During Pregnancy

Perinatal
Pessary
Placenta previa
Placental abruption
Placentation
Polycystic ovarian syndrome
Polycythemia
Polyzygotic
Pruritic urticarial papules and plaques of pregnancy
   (PUPPP)
Pustular psoriasis of pregnancy (PPP)

Retinopathy of prematurity
Scotomata
Spiral arteries
Teratogenic
Tocolytic
Tonic-clonic seizure
Total parenteral nutrition
Twin-to-twin transfusion syndrome
   (TTTS)
Vertical transmission
Wernicke's encephalopathy

Pregnancy complications can happen at any time. Some complications, such as multiple gestation, occur at, or shortly after, conception. Others, such as preeclampsia, almost exclusively occur in the second half of pregnancy. By considering pregnancy complications in the context of time of onset, we are more likely to accurately identify problems as they occur. Although some complications do span the whole pregnancy and may be identified at various times, this chapter presents complications by the trimester in which they are most likely to be diagnosed.

Conditions That Typically Occur in the First Trimester

Conditions that commonly occur in the first trimester, which is from conception to 13 weeks of gestation, include multiple pregnancy, hyperemesis gravidarum (HG), bleeding, miscarriage, ectopic pregnancy, and gestational trophoblastic disease (GTD).

Multiple Pregnancy

A multiple pregnancy is one in which more than one fetus is present. It may also be referred to as a multiple gestation pregnancy, twin pregnancy, triplet pregnancy, etc.

Prevalence

The rate of multiple pregnancies has been rising steadily for a number of years (Hamilton, Martin, Osterman, Curtin, & Mathews, 2015). Overall, there has been a 76% increase in twinning over the past three decades (Kulkarni et al., 2013). At this time approximately 3% of births are of twins (Hehir et al., 2015).

Etiology

There are three kinds of multiple pregnancies. The first, a multizygotic pregnancy, happens when two or more eggs are fertilized at the same time. When two eggs are fertilized, this is referred to as dizygotic or fraternal twins. These twins are never identical and may be of different genders or even, very rarely, from different fathers. A multiple pregnancy with different fathers is referred to as heteropaternal superfecundation.

Approximately 70% of multiple pregnancies are multizygotic. Risk factors include the use of artificial reproductive technology (ART; including the use of some fertility drugs and in vitro fertilization), ethnicity (particularly African descent), and a family history of prior fraternal twinning. In the case of ART, a multizygotic pregnancy may result from the introduction and implantation of multiple embryos or the simultaneous fertilization of multiple eggs in situ. Another major contributor to the rising rate of multizygotic pregnancies is advanced maternal age. As a woman approaches menopause, she is more likely to release more than one egg at ovulation because of a rise in follicle-stimulating hormone. Each fetus in a multizygotic pregnancy has a separate amnion and chorion. However, the fetus' placentas may grow together.

Another kind of multiple pregnancy is monozygotic, meaning all of the fetuses came from the same ovum. These siblings, almost always twins rather than triplets or a higher-order multiple, are identical. The sharing of structures, such as the amnion, chorion, and placenta, is determined by when after fertilization the ovum divides (Fig. 20.1).

- If the cleavage of the pregnancy happens from days 1 to 3 after fertilization during the morula phase, the twins are unlikely to share any structures.
- If the split happens from days 4 to 8, the blastocyst phase, they are likely to have two amnions, one chorion, and one placenta.
- Twins that split after implantation but before the formation of the embryonic disk are sometimes referred to as monoamniotic-monochorionic (MoMo) twins. They share a chorion, amnion, and placenta.
- Conjoined twins occur when the split happens from days 13 to 15 after fertilization, after formation of the embryonic disk (see Chapter 15 to review embryology and fetal development).

Monozygotic twinning is considered a random, spontaneous event. It is not associated with a genetically inherited trait and is not seen with any greater frequency in any ethnic group. Monozygotic twins occur with a slightly higher frequency with the use of ART. Of every 1,000 twin pregnancies born in 2014,

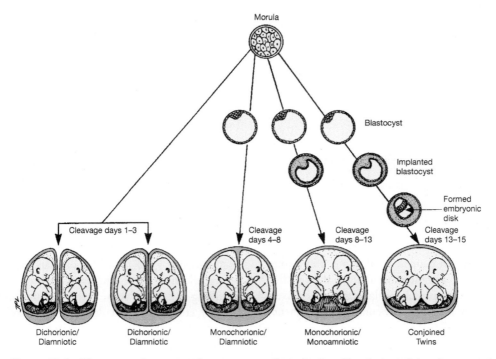

Figure 20.1. Cleavage of an ovum in monozygotic twinning. The timing of the cleavage of the ovum in monozygotic twinning significantly determines the amnionicity and chorionicity of the resulting embryos. (Reprinted with permission from LifeART image copyright © 2018 Lippincott Williams & Wilkins. All rights reserved.)

about 3 were monozygotic (Kanter, Boulet, Kawwass, Jamieson, & Kissin, 2015).

Triplets and higher-order multiple pregnancies (quadruplets, sextuplets, and so on) typically result from multiple ova but may occasionally occur from a single ovum. Rarely, higher-order multiples result from a combination of a monozygotic split and multiple fertilized ova. These pregnancies account for the third category of multiple pregnancy and are often referred to as **polyzygotic**.

Course in Pregnancy

Multiple pregnancies are always considered high-risk pregnancies for both the mother and fetuses. The discomforts of pregnancy are often amplified for women pregnant with more than one fetus and include greater urinary frequency, increased nausea, backache, and swelling (edema). More serious risks for the mother include a higher occurrence of gestational diabetes, hypertensive disorders of pregnancy including preeclampsia, and a higher rate of pulmonary embolism during pregnancy and in the postpartum period (Jordan, Engstrom, Marfell, & Farley, 2014).

Perinatal mortality rate (death immediately before or after a birth) is about three times greater for twins and four times greater for triplets and higher-order multiples than for a pregnancy with a single fetus (Blackburn, 2014). The most frequent contributor to the death of the neonate is complications of prematurity, and approximately 50% of twins are born prematurely (Hehir et al., 2015; King et al., 2015). Other risks include fetal growth restriction, fetal anomalies, early pregnancy loss, stillbirth, and **placenta previa**.

MoMo twins account for about 1% of twinning. These twins are at a particular risk for entanglement in the umbilical cords, umbilical cord compression, and a phenomenon called **twin-to-twin transfusion syndrome (TTTS)**, wherein one twin receives a majority of the nutrition from the shared placenta, whereas the other is undernourished. Twins with TTTS have a mortality rate of 50% or higher, even with treatment (Simpson, 2013).

Assessment

Once a multiple pregnancy is identified, typically by ultrasound, it is usually closely followed by ultrasound every 2 to 4 weeks, and more frequent prenatal visits are recommended. Women may discover they require more rest as the pregnancy progresses (King et al., 2015).

Treatment

Although bed rest was at one time prescribed routinely for many problems of pregnancy, it has not been found to be effective for preventing preterm births for twin pregnancies or for any other problems that occur in pregnancy. In addition, it has real physical, psychological, social, and economic consequences that should not be discounted (Lorenz, 2014; McCall, Grimes, & Lyerly, 2013).

Care Considerations

Women who are pregnant with multiple fetuses need more calories, protein, vitamins, and minerals than do those pregnant with one fetus. In general, a woman who is pregnant with twins with a normal body mass index (BMI) should gain 37 to 54 lb, a woman with a BMI from 25 to 29.9 should gain 31 to 50 lb, and a woman with a BMI of 30 or higher should gain 25 to 42 lb. Recommended gestational weight gain for higher-order multiples is generally individualized (American College of Obstetricians and Gynecologists [ACOG], 2013, reaffirmed 2016). Anticipation of welcoming more than one baby may be a cause of joy in the family but may also be a reason for increased anxiety with the anticipation of overstretched personal and economic resources. The nurse should pay attention to these concerns. Twins may be born by vaginal or cesarean delivery depending on the position of the fetuses, the expertise of the care provider, and other clinical considerations. The cesarean rate for twins is approximately 75% and for triplets is 95% (Monson & Silver, 2015).

Hyperemesis Gravidarum

Hyperemesis gravidarum (HG) is a condition specific to pregnancy characterized by unusually acute nausea and vomiting. Although approximately 50% of women experience some nausea and even vomiting, particularly in weeks 12 through 14 of pregnancy (Jordan et al., 2014), women with HG have symptoms so severe that they lead to weight loss, malnutrition, dehydration, **ketonuria**, and electrolyte imbalances.

Prevalence

Approximately 0.5% to 2% of women are diagnosed with this condition, which typically starts around week 10 and ends by week 20. For an unfortunate 20% to 45% of these women, however, symptoms last throughout the pregnancy (Fletcher et al., 2015). HG has a high rate of recurrence in subsequent pregnancies.

Etiology

The root cause of HG is not completely clear, but it may be related to hormonal changes; physical variations of the inner

---

> ### Box 20.1 Risk Factors for Hyperemesis Gravidarum
>
> - History of hyperemesis gravidarum
> - Gestational trophoblastic disease
> - Multiple pregnancy
> - Hyperthyroidism (overactive thyroid)
> - Gastrointestinal disease prior to pregnancy
> - Depression and anxiety
> - Female fetus
>
> Adapted from King, T., Brucker, M., Kriebs, J., Fahey, J., Gregor, C., & Varney, H. (2015). *Varney's midwifery.* Burlington, MA: Jones & Bartlett; Fletcher, S., Watermanb, H., Nelsona, L., Carterc, L., Dwyerd, L., Robertsc, C., . . . Kitchener, H. (2015). Holistic assessment of women with hyperemesis gravidarum: A randomised controlled trial. *International Journal of Nursing Studies, 52*(11), 1669–1677.

---

ear, gastrointestinal tract, or **corpus luteum**; or psychological factors (King et al., 2015). It should be particularly noted, however, that a more modern interpretation of correlation between psychological factors and HG is that the depression, anxiety, and even posttraumatic stress disorder is a product of the HG and not a cause (Box 20.1). Preexisting anxiety or depression may also amplify the severity of symptoms or a patient's perception of symptoms (Mitchell-Jones et al., 2017).

Course in Pregnancy

HG is the second-most common cause for hospitalization in pregnancy after preterm labor (King et al., 2015) and the single most common cause of hospital admission in early pregnancy (Grooten et al., 2016).

In Chapter 6, Rebecca had nausea and even daily vomiting in early pregnancy. However, she was able to eat well and gain weight and thus did not meet the criteria for HG.

Assessment

Nurses must carefully evaluate patients for signs of dehydration, such as tenting of the skin and dry mucous membranes. Signs of malnutrition may include ketones in the urine and weight loss. Other laboratory tests may be ordered to evaluate for conditions such as hyperthyroidism, gastrointestinal disease, liver disease, and infection, which may be contributing to or causing the HG. Ultrasound studies may be done to evaluate for a multiple pregnancy and to rule out gestational trophoblastic disease (GTD) (see Chapter 13).

In Chapter 13 Tanya had GTD. She had nausea, which was unusual for her, compared with her previous pregnancies. Although HG is a later symptom of GTD, her nausea occurred earlier in the disease process and was not as severe.

Treatment

Providers must always use caution when prescribing medication in pregnancy. Some medications have a known **teratogenic** effect, whereas the long- and short-term effects of most medications on a fetus remain unknown. Some medications, such as higher doses of corticosteroids, have a known teratogenic effect and limited proven efficacy for treatment of HG but may still be used as a last resort (Grooten, Vinke, Roseboom, & Painter, 2015).

A class of drugs commonly used to treat HG is **antiemetics** (The Pharmacy 20.1). Ondansetron (Zofran) is a medication in this class that has relatively few side effects, but its safety in pregnancy and efficacy for HG have not been proven (Abas, Tan,

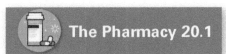

The Pharmacy 20.1 — Medications Commonly Used to Treat Hyperemesis Gravidarum

Medications (Class and Drugs)	Overview
Antihistamines	
H$_1$-receptor antagonists	
• Doxylamine (Unisom)	
• Diphenhydramine (Benadryl)	
• Hydroxyzine (Vistaril)	
H$_2$-receptor antagonists	May work by minimizing reflux
• Famotidine (Pepcid)	• May be used in combination with vitamin B$_6$
• Ranitidine (Zantac)	• Sedating
	• Nonsedating
Dopamine Antagonists	
Metoclopramide (Reglan)	May work by enhancing peristalsis of the gut that was slowed by the progesterone of pregnancy
Promethazine (Phenergan)	Likely works centrally on the part of the brain that stimulates vomiting
Serotonin Antagonists	
Ondansetron (Zofran)	• Limited information about safety and efficacy
	• May not be any more effective than promethazine
Corticosteroids	
	• Mixed evidence about efficacy
	• Evidence of oral cleft malformations when used in early pregnancy
	• Medication of last resort

Adapted from Boelig, R. C., Berghella, V., Kelly, A. J., Barton, S. J., & Edwards, S. J. (2013). Interventions for treating hyperemesis gravidarum. *Cochrane Database of Systematic Reviews*, (6).

Azmi, & Omar, 2014). Metoclopramide (Reglan), a dopamine antagonist used for its antiemetic properties, has a long record of use for HG and is considered generally safe, particularly with short-term use (less than 12 weeks). Many women report that it is not effective for the treatment of HG, however (Taylor, 2014). Promethazine (Phenergan) is another dopamine antagonist that may be used for HG and is believed safe for the fetus if not taken later in pregnancy. None of these medications is universally effective, however, and many women have little to no relief from pharmaceutical interventions. Some women may also try complementary therapies for relief (Box 20.2).

Care Considerations

As there is no one factor that is understood to cause HG, there is also no one care intervention to treat it. Priorities for caring for a woman with HG are maximizing patient comfort and minimizing potential complications resulting from dehydration and malnutrition.

Box 20.2 Complementary Medicine Treatments for Hyperemesis Gravidarum

• *Acupuncture:* Trials for both nausea and vomiting of pregnancy and hyperemesis gravidarum (HG) have yielded mixed results.
• *Ginger:* Trials of ginger have demonstrated improvement of the symptoms of HG with no ill effects.
• *Vitamin B$_6$:* It is also a standard medically prescribed treatment, often in conjunction with an H$_1$-receptor antagonist. It has some effect on nausea, but not vomiting, in pregnancy. Trials have not shown efficacy for the treatment of HG.

Adapted from Boelig, R. C., Berghella, V., Kelly, A. J., Barton, S. J., & Edwards, S. J. (2013). Interventions for treating hyperemesis gravidarum. *Cochrane Database of Systematic Reviews*, (6).

The dietary and lifestyle changes that may work for less acute nausea and vomiting typical of early pregnancy (see Box 13.2) are unlikely to be helpful for HG. Patients often require intravenous (IV) rehydration, usually with normal saline, on either an inpatient or outpatient basis. Patients may also require the administration of parenteral electrolytes and even carbohydrates, amino acids, and vitamins, most crucially thiamine. A rare but potentially fatal effect of prolonged (three or more weeks) vomiting and the resulting thiamine deficiency is **Wernicke's encephalopathy**. Food, when reintroduced following parenteral nutrition, is typically bland and low fat. In some cases, **total parenteral nutrition** may be started. In the most severe cases, the pregnancy may be terminated.

Bleeding in the Early Pregnancy

Bleeding in early pregnancy is exceedingly common, with up to 10% to 20% of women reporting at least one episode. Many women experience implantation bleeding, typically about 6 to 11 days after fertilization, which is bright red or dark brown bleeding lasting a day on average. Other women experience spotting throughout early pregnancy because of infection, sex, or increased blood flow to the cervix. Bleeding for all of these reasons is typically brief and painless.

A subset of women, however, experience bleeding in pregnancy that heralds the end of the pregnancy, danger for the mother, or both. Specifically bleeding may occur as a significant symptom of miscarriage, ectopic pregnancy, or GTD, each of which is discussed as a separate condition below. Thus, the nurse should carefully evaluate all bleeding in pregnancy.

Miscarriage

A miscarriage, also referred to as spontaneous abortion or spontaneous pregnancy loss, is any loss of pregnancy before 20 weeks of gestation without deliberate surgical or medical induction. Although "spontaneous abortion" is the technically correct term, "miscarriage" is generally preferred when discussing an unplanned loss with a patient.

In Chapter 5, Letitia had a miscarriage at 8 weeks of gestation. Her provider, Dr. Janachek, initially referred to the event as a "spontaneous abortion," which Letitia found upsetting.

Prevalence

Spontaneous pregnancy loss is exceedingly common, with an estimated 15% to 20% of pregnancies ending spontaneously prior to 20 weeks of gestation. When preimplantation losses are considered, approximately half of pregnancies end spontaneously prior to 20 weeks of gestation (Kutteh, 2014).

Etiology

The peak time in pregnancy for loss is from 5 to 8 weeks of gestation, and a majority of these losses are believed to be due to chromosomal abnormalities of the fetus (Bardos, Hercz, Friedenthal, Missmer, & Williams, 2015). Approximately 70% of pregnancy losses, which accounts for 22% of all pregnancies, occur before the pregnancy can be detected by ultrasound (Wilcox et al., 1988). Once a heartbeat is seen by ultrasound, typically about 6 weeks after a woman's last menstrual period, and the embryo measures about 2 mm, the risk of a spontaneous abortion is approximately 3% to 6% (Bardos et al., 2015). Risk factors for early loss of a pregnancy are advanced age of parents, drug and alcohol use, poor maternal nutrition, the use of teratogenic medications, and certain maternal health conditions, such as diabetes, lupus, and uterine abnormalities. The cause or causes of recurrent spontaneous abortions, defined variably as the spontaneous loss of two or three consecutive pregnancies, remain poorly understood (Practice Committee of American Society for Reproductive Medicine, 2013).

Course in Pregnancy

Women may have mixed feelings about their pregnancy and may have equally mixed feelings about the end of the pregnancy. Even a wanted pregnancy can be met with various feelings as a woman copes with changes in her body and role identity, as well as stressors related to psychosocial and economic considerations. All of these feelings are normal and reasonable.

Although most spontaneous abortions are caused by genetic abnormalities, many patients may think that stress, arguing, falls, lifting heavy objects, and previous use of oral contraception and intrauterine contraceptive devices can cause spontaneous abortions (Bardos et al., 2015). Because of this, women may feel guilty about the loss of the pregnancy. This guilt may make any grief they feel more acute.

Assessment

When assessing a woman for a suspected spontaneous abortion, the nurse should take a careful history of the symptoms of cramping, bleeding, and passage of tissue, as well as the common symptoms of early pregnancy, such as nausea, fatigue, and breast tenderness. An ultrasound may be ordered to evaluate for the continuing presence of a pregnancy and fetal heartbeat, as well as confirm the location of the pregnancy inside the uterus. In the case of a threatened abortion, the patient undergoes serial serum draws for laboratory testing of beta human chorionic gonadotropin (hCG) levels. Beta hCG is a hormone produced by trophoblast cells of the placenta, and its levels double every 29 to 53 hours during the first 30 days post implantation with a healthy, progressing pregnancy. Numbers that do not double as expected or drop are associated with a failing or ectopic pregnancy. A laboratory test to evaluate hemoglobin level or complete blood count (CBC) may be performed to assess for anemia from blood loss associated with the miscarriage.

Treatment

The management of a spontaneous abortion depends on what kind it is (Table 20.1). It is essential that women who are Rh negative receive Rh_o (D) immune globulin within 72 hours of a pregnancy loss (see The Pharmacy 5.1). Women who are less than 12 weeks pregnant require a lower dose of the medication than that used later in pregnancy and postpartum. Patients may need to be treated with an iron supplement to help the body correct any anemia discovered. On rare occasions, a blood transfusion may be indicated.

Care Considerations

Nursing care considerations for women with various types of spontaneous abortion are shown in Table 20.1. The nurse should encourage women to process the pregnancy loss as they see fit and should offer them support as needed and desired.

Ectopic Pregnancy

An ectopic pregnancy is one that occurs outside of the uterus.

Etiology

The most common location for an ectopic pregnancy is in the middle third of the fallopian tubes, called the ampulla. These pregnancies can implant in various locations, however, including the ovaries, intestines, and cervix (Fig. 20.2).

Course in Pregnancy

Ectopic pregnancies cannot be safely continued. Although there are rare cases of ectopic pregnancies that come to term and are successfully delivered by cesarean section, an ectopic pregnancy is considered a life-threatening situation for the pregnant woman and must be ended urgently.

Assessment

Classic clinical signs of ectopic pregnancy are severe pelvic pain that may refer to one shoulder and bleeding. Signs may be subtle, however. Some mild pelvic midline cramping in early pregnancy as the uterus starts to grow is normal, but worsening pain, particularly if it is off to one side or the other, is concerning. Ectopic pregnancies may also be asymptomatic. Some mild spotting is normal in pregnancy, but bleeding that is recurrent or persistent should always be evaluated (Box 20.3). As with miscarriage, bleeding in women with ectopic pregnancies who are Rh negative requires the administration of Rh_o (D) immune globulin.

Table 20.1 Types of Spontaneous Abortion

Type of Spontaneous Abortion	Clinical Findings	Care Considerations
Complete	• Patient report of passing clots and tissue accompanied by heavy cramping and bleeding that quickly decrease • On exam, cervix closed and possible residual blood is present in the vagina	• Supportive measures • Medical intervention is rarely required if all tissue passes and no infection or signs of hemorrhage are present.
Missed	• Patient report of amenorrhea • On exam, cervix closed • Pregnancy not developing but has not passed out of the cervix	• Option of watchful waiting for as long as 6 wk in early pregnancy to allow the products of conception to pass spontaneously • Alternate treatment with misoprostol, which dilates the cervix, or dilation and curettage to mechanically empty the uterus • A second trimester loss may require dilation and evacuation.
Inevitable	• Heavy cramping and bleeding • Some passage of clots and tissue • Unlike a complete abortion, cramping and bleeding may persist and the cervix is open.	• Supportive measures • Dilation and curettage or dilation and evacuation
Threatened	• On exam, cervix closed but bleeding evident • Patient report of cramping possible	• Careful monitoring by laboratory testing of beta human chorionic gonadotropin and/or ultrasound • Supportive measures
Recurrent	• Defined as two losses of clinically documented or three pregnancies in a row	

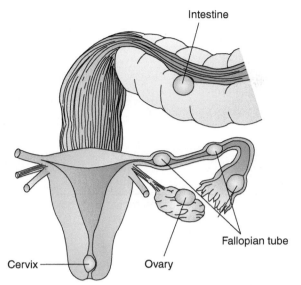

Figure 20.2. Locations where an ectopic pregnancy can occur. Show your patient the locations other than the uterine wall where the fertilized egg can implant. (Reprinted with permission issue from *Lippincott Advisor*. [2016, May]. Philadelphia, PA: Wolters Kluwer.)

Ectopic pregnancies are typically identified in two ways. The first is the serial laboratory tests of beta hCG mentioned previously. Blood is drawn on the first visit and then 48 to 72 hours later. Beta hCG values that rise by at least 35% every 48 hours within the first 40 days of pregnancy are consistent with a normally implanted pregnancy at least 90% of the time (Kirk, Bottomley, & Bourne, 2014; Morse et al., 2012). Beta hCG levels should at least double within 72 hours. The second means of evaluation is by transvaginal ultrasound. A gestational sac is evident by transvaginal ultrasound by the fifth week of pregnancy (3 weeks after ovulation and fertilization). A pregnancy should almost always be visible in the uterus on ultrasound by the time the beta hCG level reaches 3,500 mIU/mL.

Box 20.3   Risk Factors for Ectopic Pregnancy

- History of ectopic pregnancy
- History of pelvic infection
- History of pelvic surgery
- Advanced maternal age
- Cigarette smoking
- Current use of intrauterine contraception
- History of sexually transmitted infection, particularly gonorrhea and/or chlamydia

Adapted from Moini, A., Hosseini, R., Jahangiri, N., Shiva, M., & Akhoond, M. R. (2014). Risk factors for ectopic pregnancy: A case–control study. *Journal of Research in Medical Sciences, 19*(9), 844–849.

Treatment

Depending on the gestation of the pregnancy at the time of its discovery, an ectopic pregnancy may be managed medically or surgically. Medical treatment typically involves the administration of methotrexate, which ends the pregnancy (The Pharmacy 20.2). The embryo and other tissues of pregnancy then over time reabsorb into the woman's body. Eligibility for the treatment of ectopic pregnancy by methotrexate typically requires low levels of beta hCG, no cardiac activity of the embryo, and an ectopic pregnancy size less than 3 to 4 cm (Menon, Colins, & Barnhart, 2007).

An ectopic pregnancy may, however, require surgical intervention, particularly if the pregnancy is more progressed, is higher risk, or shows evidence of hemorrhage or a high risk of hemorrhage (Capmas, Bouyer, & Fernandez, 2014). In some cases, just the pregnancy may be removed safely. In other cases, the structure in which the pregnancy is implanted, such as the ovary or fallopian tube, may need to be removed, as well. This can have permanent implications for future fertility.

Care Considerations

Because an ectopic pregnancy can be life-threatening, frightening, and emotionally and physically traumatizing to the woman, the nurse should be prepared to provide her with emotional as well as physical care.

Gestational Trophoblastic Disease

Another rare but concerning cause of bleeding in early pregnancy is **gestational trophoblastic disease**, in which a fertilized egg fails to develop properly, leading to a nonviable mass of trophoblastic tissue.

Etiology

GTD begins at the moment of conception in one of two ways (see Table 13.1). A complete molar pregnancy occurs when an egg that contains no genetic material is fertilized. The products of conception include no fetal parts but instead consist of grape-like fluid-filled vesicles (see Fig. 13.1).

A partial molar pregnancy occurs when two sperm, rather than the usual one, simultaneously fertilize one egg with normal genetic material. This kind of molar pregnancy can consist of fetal parts as well as fluid-filled vesicles.

In Chapter 13, Tanya had a complete molar pregnancy. Dr. Wickham explained that sperm fertilized an ovum that contained no genetic material, and no fetal parts were present.

Course in Pregnancy

GTD pregnancies are never viable, meaning that in no case can they result in a successful birth. Moreover, unlike a miscarriage

The Pharmacy 20.2 Methotrexate

Overview	A folic acid antagonist that inhibits cell reproduction and DNA synthesis. Besides being used as a treatment for ectopic pregnancy, it is also used to treat psoriasis, rheumatoid arthritis, and certain neoplasms.
Route and dosing	Commonly given IM but may be IV or PO for ectopic pregnancy management Common ectopic pregnancy protocol: • 50 mg/m^2 IM single dose • Patients may require a second dose or even a third. • A 4-d dose of 1 mg/m^2 IV or IM is an alternative.
Care considerations	• Common side effects are conjunctivitis and stomatitis (inflammation of the mouth and lips). • Dermatitis related to methotrexate may occur with sun exposure. • Patients should avoid foods containing folic acid. • Patients should avoid new conception until hCG levels are undetectable. • Patients should avoid sexual intercourse and pelvic examinations until therapy is complete because of the risk of tubal rupture. • Gloves must be worn when handling this medication. • When preparing medication for injection, double gloves, a gown, and a ventilation cabinet should be used. • NSAIDs should be avoided during use to minimize the risk of gastrointestinal toxicity.
Warning signs	• Monitor for hypersensitivity (anaphylaxis), including shortness of breath, swelling of tongue or throat, vomiting, itchy rash, low blood pressure, and lightheadedness.

IM, intramuscular; IV, intravenous; PO, by mouth; hCG, human chorionic gonadotropin; NSAIDs, nonsteroidal anti-inflammatory drugs.

or ectopic pregnancy, GTD can become malignant and change into a highly treatable form of cancer, gestational trophoblastic neoplasia (GTN). Approximately 1% to 5% of partial molar pregnancies and 20% of complete molar pregnancies evolve into GTN (Berkowitz & Goldstein, 2013). However, GTD accounts for only 50% of GTN. One in 150,000 term pregnancies and one in 15,000 miscarriages result in GTN (Ngan & Seckl, 2007). If GTN stays limited to the myometrium (the muscular layer of the uterus), it is called a **gestational trophoblastic invasive mole**. If it spreads beyond the myometrium, it is called **gestational choriocarcinoma**. The most common sites of metastases for gestational choriocarcinoma are the lungs, vagina, and central nervous system, and the most common presentation is bleeding at the site of metastasis.

Assessment

A molar pregnancy grows at an abnormally rapid rate and produces an abnormally high level of beta hCG. With a complete molar pregnancy, this rapid growth rate causes a woman's uterus to measure larger than expected for gestational age in a minority of patients. A partial molar pregnancy may result in a smaller-than-expected uterus. A small minority of women with a molar pregnancy experience HG.

On ultrasound, a complete molar pregnancy resembles a "snowstorm," lacking the expected structures of the gestation sac, fetus, and yolk sac or placenta. On occasion, some of the vesicles may spontaneously pass through the cervix and out of the vagina. Most women with GTD experience vaginal bleeding.

Ovarian cysts, early-onset preeclampsia, and hyperthyroidism are later complications of GTD. For some time now, however, molar pregnancies in the United States have been commonly detected in the first trimester prior to the development of late symptoms. The presenting symptoms of most women may include vaginal bleeding or only the common symptoms of early pregnancy, such as pelvic pressure, uterine growth, and nausea.

GTNs produce an abnormally high level of beta hCG in the absence of a viable pregnancy. Thus, laboratory testing of beta hCG level is the primary method of evaluating for an invasive mole or choriocarcinoma. Typically, beta hCG levels are monitored until they normalize to nonpregnant levels and stay there for 3 to 4 weeks. After this they are monitored monthly for 6 months to a year, because most invasive moles and choriocarcinomas appear within the first 6 months postpartum, if at all (see Box 13.5).

Treatment

The uterus of a woman with a molar pregnancy must be evacuated by **dilation and curettage** if the products of conception do not pass spontaneously.

Care Considerations

Because a new pregnancy following GTD could make it difficult to determine whether a rise in beta hCG is the normal rise to be expected from the new pregnancy or an indicator of GTN, the nurse should advise the woman to avoid getting pregnant again for at least 6 months to 1 year after the end of the molar pregnancy.

Atopic Eruption of Pregnancy

Atopic eruption of pregnancy (AEP) usually starts in early pregnancy and recurs in any future pregnancies. It is the most common kind of dermatoses in pregnancy and is associated with a personal or familial predisposition to other forms of atopy, such as asthma, environmental allergies, and atopic dermatitis. It may present as a new or recurrent atopic dermatitis or a worsening of an existing atopic dermatitis. It typically appears as eczematous patches but may also present as nodules, papules, or folliculitis. Diagnosis is clinical and the treatment is topical corticosteroids or an antihistamine such as loratadine or cetirizine. AEP is not associated with poor pregnancy outcomes, and symptoms usually resolve within weeks after the birth.

Conditions That Typically Occur in the Second Trimester

Conditions that commonly occur in the second trimester, which is from 13 through 26 weeks of gestation, include hypertensive disorders of pregnancy, gestational diabetes, infections, and cervical insufficiency.

Hypertensive Disorders of Pregnancy

Hypertensive disorders of pregnancy include chronic hypertension, which predates the pregnancy or occurs in the first 20 weeks of pregnancy (covered in Chapter 19), as well as gestational hypertension, preeclampsia, eclampsia, and HELLP syndrome which by definition occur only in pregnancy. Approximately 5% to 10% of women are diagnosed with a hypertensive disorder in pregnancy (Lo, Mission, & Caughey, 2013).

Gestational Hypertension

Gestational hypertension is hypertension (a systolic blood pressure of 140 mm Hg or higher and/or a diastolic blood pressure of 90 mm Hg or higher) without protein in the urine or signs of end-organ dysfunction diagnosed at 20 weeks of gestation or later (ACOG, Task Force on Hypertension in Pregnancy, 2013). For care considerations pertinent to this condition, see the section on preeclampsia and eclampsia.

Prevalence

Women are more likely to be diagnosed with gestational hypertension with first pregnancies, if they were diagnosed with preeclampsia with a previous pregnancy, if they are overweight or obese, or if they are pregnant with more than one fetus. Women are less likely to develop gestational hypertension if they are multiparous and no previous pregnancy was complicated by preeclampsia.

Course in Pregnancy

As many as half of women with gestational hypertension go on to develop preeclampsia (Melamed, Ray, Hladunewich, Cox, & Kingdom, 2014). Offspring are more likely to be delivered preterm, and small for gestational age (SGA). Placental abruption is more common with gestational hypertension.

Assessment

Critically, women who develop gestational hypertension must have preeclampsia ruled out (Box 20.4). A diagnosis of gestational hypertension requires that the blood pressure be elevated and documented for at least two different readings taken at least 4 hours apart (Step-by-Step Skills 20.1). A very high blood pressure, meaning a systolic measurement of 160 mm Hg or higher or a diastolic of 110 mm Hg, may be confirmed within minutes instead of waiting for 4 hours (ACOG, Task Force on Hypertension in Pregnancy, 2013). Later, if there is new evidence of end-organ dysfunction or protein in the urine, the diagnosis is changed to preeclampsia. If the high blood pressure persists past 12 weeks postpartum, the diagnosis is changed to chronic hypertension. If the woman's blood pressure returns to normal before 12 weeks postpartum, the end diagnosis is transient hypertension of pregnancy.

Women with gestational hypertension undergo frequent evaluations of fetal well-being by ultrasound, nonstress test (see Box 3.6), and/or biophysical profile (BPP; see Table 1.2). During delivery, and postpartum they are continued to be monitored closely for the development of preeclampsia.

Treatment

Women with a blood pressure below 160/110 mm Hg can generally maintain their regular activities with monitoring by obstetric providers once or twice weekly and education about the signs and symptoms of preeclampsia, such as persistent headaches, visual

---

Box 20.4 Diagnostic Criteria for Preeclampsia

Systolic blood pressure (BP) of 140 mm Hg or higher and/or diastolic BP of 90 mm Hg or higher on two occasions at least 4 h apart at, or after, 20 wk of gestation in a patient with previously normal BP (Note: A systolic BP of 160 mm Hg or higher and/or a diastolic BP of 110 mm Hg does not require a 4-h wait between readings.)
AND
Proteinuria of 300 mg or higher in a 24-h sample OR a protein:creatinine ratio of 0.3 or higher OR a dipstick reading of 1+ or higher if previous tests unavailable.
OR
New-onset hypertension, as described above, with or without proteinuria
AND
- Platelet count: <100,000
- Serum creatinine level: >1.1 mg/dL
- Liver transaminases level: two times the normal limits
- Pulmonary edema
- New-onset visual or cerebral symptoms (i.e., blurred vision, flashing lights, new blind spot, headache refractory to analgesics)

Adapted from American College of Obstetricians and Gynecologists, Task Force on Hypertension in Pregnancy. (2013). Hypertension in pregnancy. Report of the American College of Obstetricians and Gynecologists' Task Force on Hypertension in Pregnancy. *Obstetrics and Gynecology, 122*(5), 1122.

Step-by-Step Skills 20.1

Blood Pressure Assessment

1. Have the patient sit or lie down, with the upper arm on one side level with heart and free of clothing.
2. If the patient is sitting, the legs should be uncrossed and the feet flat on the floor.
3. Position the blood pressure cuff snugly about an inch above the brachial pulsation.
4. Close the valve on the sphygmomanometer by turning it clockwise.
5. Palpate the radial or brachial pulse, inflate the cuff, note when the pulse can no longer be palpated, and inflate it 20 to 30 mm Hg higher.
6. Place the diaphragm of stethoscope over the brachial artery, and slowly deflate the cuff (2 to 3 mm Hg per second).
7. Listen for the appearance of sound (systolic) and the disappearance of sound (diastolic).
8. Deflate the cuff completely, and remove it from the arm.

changes, and right upper quadrant or epigastric pain (ACOG, Task Force on Hypertension in Pregnancy, 2013). The fetus may be delivered early.

Women with a blood pressure of 160/110 mm Hg or higher are usually treated with antihypertensive medications and delivered early. They may be given magnesium sulfate as a prophylaxis against eclampsia (Boxes 20.6 and 20.7).

Preeclampsia and Eclampsia

Preeclampsia typically develops subsequent to gestational hypertension and, like this condition, involves hypertension that develops in pregnancy in or after the 20th week of gestation, though it may be superimposed on chronic hypertension. What distinguishes preeclampsia from gestational hypertension diagnostically is the presence of protein in the urine, known as proteinuria, or other evidence of end-organ dysfunction (Box 20.4).

Eclampsia is preeclampsia with tonic-clonic seizure activity that has no other known cause.

Prevalence

Preeclampsia occurs in approximately 3% to 5% of pregnancies (Abalos, Cuesta, Grosso, Chou, & Say, 2013; Lo et al., 2013). Approximately 2% to 3% of women with severe preeclampsia who are not treated with seizure prophylaxis develop eclampsia, as will about 1 out of every 200 women who do (Fong, Chau, Pan, & Ogunyemi, 2013). Approximately 60% of eclamptic seizures occur antepartum, 21% postpartum, and 20% during labor (Berhan & Berhan, 2015).

Etiology

Although the etiology of preeclampsia and eclampsia is still not perfectly understood, it is believed to be associated with abnormal

placentation, (attachment of the placenta). In a normal pregnancy, not complicated by preeclampsia, arteries in the uterus called spiral arteries change to allow for increased blood flow to the placenta. In a pregnancy complicated by preeclampsia, this change does not occur or occurs imperfectly, and, as a result, the placenta is not as well perfused by maternal blood. Thus, preeclampsia and eclampsia may be the effect of the placenta attempting to overcome the consequences of this poor placentation (Kobayashi, 2015). Other models propose abnormal pregestational maternal inflammation and/or epithelial cell functioning as an alternate disease pathway.

This underperfusion of the tissue by oxygen-carrying red blood cells, known as ischemia, causes the placenta to chemically cue the epithelial cells that line the maternal blood vessels to constrict in such a way as to cause increased peripheral resistance and permeability of the blood vessels. This increased permeability causes the blood vessels to leak plasma, making the blood, which is diluted by the normal processes of pregnancy, more concentrated with oxygen-carrying red blood cells, a phenomenon known as hemoconcentration. The increased peripheral resistance increases the blood pressure, which makes the blood move more forcefully through the insufficiently altered arteries of the uterus, thus increasing placental perfusion.

Course in Pregnancy

This poor placentation alone may contribute to problems with the fetus as the pregnancy progresses, such as oligohydramnios (a low volume of amniotic fluid), placental abruption (premature detachment of the placenta from the wall of the uterus), and intrauterine growth restriction (IUGR), although later changes in maternal vascularization have traditionally been thought to cause these complications.

Moreover, all of the compensatory changes described above that help improve perfusion for the placenta and fetus can lead maternal organs to be less perfused and can cause the following problems for the pregnant woman:

- Renal damage leading to renal failure
- Pulmonary and peripheral edema (as plasma leaks from the blood vessels into the surrounding tissue)
- Liver damage and impaired liver function
- Blurry vision and scotomata (blind spots), typically completely reversible
- Cerebral edema and hemorrhage, leading to headaches, hyperreflexia (reflexes above 2+), clonus, and, with eclampsia, seizures
- Thrombocytopenia (a platelet count $<100,000/mm^3$)

Assessment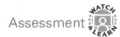

As noted above, a diagnosis of preeclampsia requires assessment of the woman's blood pressure and laboratory testing for proteinuria and evidence of end-organ dysfunction. The characteristic proteinuria of this condition results from the placenta chemically cueing the epithelial cells of glomeruli of the kidneys to constrict, increasing permeability, which causes the kidney to spill protein, particularly albumin, into the urine. And increased levels of liver enzymes may indicate damage to the liver caused by the lack of maternal perfusion associated with preeclampsia.

Peripheral edema was once considered an important component of preeclampsia but is no longer part of the diagnostic criteria. A rapid onset or worsening of edema and associated weight gain may be significant, however, and should not be ignored, particularly if the edema is facial. Risk factors for preeclampsia can be found in Box 4.11.

Oliguria, or decreased urine production, is another potential sign of preeclampsia, as it indicates renal damage caused by a lack of perfusion to the kidneys. Similarly, right upper quadrant or epigastric pain may indicate edema of the liver, which is one of the complications of preeclampsia.

Beyond the initial diagnosis, ongoing assessment of a woman with preeclampsia includes symptom evaluation, accurate blood pressure readings, 24-hour urine and other laboratory tests, and accurate assessment of weight. An ultrasound of the pregnancy may be ordered at the time of diagnosis and then every 3 weeks to evaluate fetal growth, and fundal height is assessed with each visit. Evaluation typically includes fetal evaluation by a nonstress test (see Box 3.6) and BPP (see Table 1.2) once or twice weekly. Laboratory testing of CBC with platelets, liver enzyme level, and serum creatinine level is done weekly to monitor for thrombocytopenia, liver dysfunction, and renal dysfunction, respectively. The nurse should monitor the woman's blood pressure and assess her urine for proteinuria twice weekly. The nurse should also encourage the woman to measure her blood pressure at home, in addition to the in-clinic measurements (ACOG, Task Force on Hypertension in Pregnancy, 2013).

The nurse must be able to recognize signs of severe preeclampsia (Box 20.5). In addition to the parameters outlined in Box 20.5, preeclampsia may also be considered severe with a blood pressure elevated to a systolic reading of 140 to 160 mm Hg and/or a diastolic blood pressure of 90 to 100 mm Hg plus evidence of liver impairment, renal insufficiency, vision loss, pulmonary edema, thrombocytopenia, or cerebral dysfunction. A higher quantity of protein in the urine, however, does not necessarily indicate

severe preeclampsia (ACOG, Task Force on Hypertension in Pregnancy, 2013).

Ongoing assessment for a woman with severe preeclampsia is similar to that for a woman with mild preeclampsia. The nurse must assess the woman's blood pressure and urine output per orders and collect blood for laboratory testing (most frequently CBC with platelets, liver enzyme level, and serum creatinine level). The nurse should regularly interview the patient to assess for epigastric and right upper quadrant pain, signs of labor, vaginal bleeding or unusual vaginal discharge, vision changes, and mental status changes. Per orders, the nurse may also perform intermittent or continuous fetal heart rate monitoring. Initial and serial ultrasounds, and fundal height measurements to assess fetal size, as well as nonstress tests and BPPs are performed to assess fetal well-being.

Throughout labor and delivery, women with a hypertensive disorder typically have an IV in place as well as continuous fetal monitoring. Because of a continuing risk for placental abruption, the nurse should regularly assess for vaginal bleeding, persistent uterine tone, and abdominal pain between contractions.

Postpartum, as for all patients, the nurse should regularly evaluate the vital signs, fluid intake, and urine output of women with preeclampsia and gestational hypertension. In the initial postpartum period, the nurse should also continue to assess for evidence of worsening preeclampsia, such as headache, vision changes, and epigastric pain.

For patients taking magnesium sulfate, the nurse should continue to assess their deep tendon reflexes and level of consciousness postpartum and, because of the increased risk for uterine atony and postpartum hemorrhage with the use of magnesium sulfate, assess their uterine tone and lochia.

Treatment

Patients at a high risk for preeclampsia may be advised to start taking aspirin in the first trimester of pregnancy, which has been associated with a 24% reduction in the development of preeclampsia (Henderson et al., 2014). Calcium supplementation in pregnancy may also be helpful for preventing preeclampsia, but likely only for those who are calcium deficient (Patrelli et al., 2012).

Women with mild preeclampsia and gestational hypertension typically receive care on an outpatient basis. Women with mild preeclampsia may be initially evaluated on an inpatient basis, and carry their pregnancies to term. They also do not usually require medications.

Women suspected of having progressed to severe preeclampsia are monitored at least initially as inpatients and may need to be induced and delivered early to protect their health and that of their offspring. Immediate delivery is recommended for women with severe preeclampsia who are at 34 or more weeks of gestation or who are prior to 34 weeks of gestation and have unstable maternal-fetal conditions (ACOG, Task Force on Hypertension in Pregnancy, 2013). Women with severe preeclampsia who are not delivered immediately are often given IV magnesium sulfate to prevent eclampsia (tonic-clonic seizures resulting from preeclampsia). This medication reduces central nervous system irritability caused by cerebral edema and brings down

---

Box 20.5 Features of Severe Preeclampsia

- *Blood pressure (BP):* A systolic BP of 160 mm Hg or higher and/or a diastolic BP of 110 mm Hg or higher on two occasions at least 4 h apart in the absence of antihypertensive treatment
- *Thrombocytopenia:* platelet count < 100,000
- *Impaired liver function:* liver enzymes twice the normal concentration and/or severe right upper quadrant or epigastric pain that does not improve with analgesics
- *Progressive renal insufficiency:* doubling of serum creatinine and/or serum creatinine level (>1.1 mg/dL)
- *Pulmonary edema*
- *New-onset cerebral or visual changes:* headaches, blurred vision, blind spots, etc.

seizure activity by an estimated 50% (Berzan, Doyle, & Brown, 2014). It may also help protect the fetal brain (Crowther, Brown, McKinlay, & Middleton, 2014). It is administered throughout labor and the immediate postpartum period (ACOG, Task Force on Hypertension in Pregnancy, 2013).

However, at higher doses, magnesium sulfate can be toxic, so it is critical for the nurse to regularly screen patients who are on this medication for signs of magnesium toxicity. These signs include bradypnea (slow breathing rate), bradycardia, slurred speech, muscle weakness, lethargy, and hyporeflexia (deep tendon reflexes that are absent or under 2+; see The Pharmacy 4.1; Boxes 20.6 and 20.7).

Also, although no longer believed to be a **tocolytic**, which is a medication used to delay preterm labor (McNamara, Crowther, & Brown, 2015), magnesium sulfate may cause the uterus to contract less forcefully and thus prolong labor. In such cases, oxytocin may be given simultaneously to induce and strengthen uterine contractions.

Women with severe preeclampsia also typically receive IV antihypertensive medications to protect them from complications of hypertension, such as stroke, renal damage, and heart failure. These medications include nifedipine, labetalol, methyldopa, and hydralazine. Additionally, women under 34 weeks pregnant may be given a series of corticosteroid injections to promote fetal maturity and reduce the risk of perinatal death (see The Pharmacy 8.2). A woman may remain hypertensive for up to 12 weeks postpartum with all forms of gestation-specific hypertension and thus may remain on hypertensive medications in the short term.

Box 20.6 Roles and Responsibilities in the Administration of Magnesium Sulfate

- It is the responsibility of the *physician* to provide the orders for the magnesium sulfate administration.
- It is the responsibility of the *nurse* to verify the dose of the medication.
- If the *nurse* has questions about a medication or dosage, she may consult with the *physician* and/or the *pharmacist*.
- The hanging of the magnesium sulfate as a "piggyback" is a *nursing* responsibility, as is setting the pump to the rate ordered.
- Regular patient assessments specific to magnesium sulfate administration, including deep tendon reflexes, are a *nursing* responsibility.
- Immediate stoppage of magnesium sulfate administration due to suspected toxicity is a *nursing* responsibility.
- Calcium gluconate administration as an antidote to magnesium toxicity is usually a *physician* responsibility.

Box 20.7 Magnesium Sulfate Administration: Dosing, Assessments, and Interventions for Toxicity

Dosing
- Administered as a secondary infusion by pump
- Loading dose: 4–6 g over 15–30 min
- Maintenance dose: 1–3 g/h to maintain a serum magnesium level of 4–7 mEq/L

Assessments
- Urine output
- Respirations
- Deep tendon reflexes
- Heart rate

Signs of Toxicity
- Respiratory depression
- Oliguria
- Absent reflexes
- Lethargy
- Slurred speech
- Muscle weakness
- Loss of consciousness

Risks of Toxicity
- Acute respiratory arrest
- Acute cardiac arrest

Interventions to Address Toxicity
- Stop infusion immediately
- Administer calcium gluconate (the antidote to magnesium sulfate toxicity) as ordered (typically, 1 g is given by slow push over 3 min)

Should preeclampsia develop into eclampsia, the woman experiences tonic-clonic seizures or coma. As with any seizure disorder, the primary concern is the safety of the patient (Box 20.8). The nurse should strive to rapidly control seizure activity, typically by administering a bolus of 4 to 6 g of magnesium sulfate, followed by a maintenance dose that continues until 48 hours postpartum, with relevant adjustments to maintain the therapeutic range and avoid toxicity. If the diastolic blood pressure is not between 90 and 100 mm Hg, adjustments are made to correct it with hypertensive medications. Also, the nurse should administer supplemental oxygen at 8 to 10 L/h by nonrebreather mask to avoid hypoxia due to hypoventilation.

Box 20.8 Warning Signs of a Pending Eclamptic Seizure

- Headache
- Blurred vision
- Restlessness

Care Considerations

The goals of therapy for all hypertensive disorders of pregnancy are to provide supportive care but also to mitigate clinical manifestations to protect the lives and the health of the pregnant woman and the fetus in the long and short terms.

Perhaps the most critical aspect of care for a woman diagnosed with mild preeclampsia and gestational hypertension is education. The nurse should counsel women to monitor fetal movement at home and rest frequently. The nurse should also encourage women when lying down to lie on the left side to encourage blood flow to the uterus and avoid pressure of the pregnancy on the vena cava. Although complete bed rest was at one time considered a critical part of the care of preeclampsia, this practice has not been associated with improved outcomes and presents increased risks of blood clots, maternal deconditioning, and psychological distress, among other harms (Biggio, 2013; McCall et al., 2013). A woman may elect to stop working if this is financially an option for her. As with all pregnancies, the nurse should recommend a balanced diet. However, salt restriction has not been found to be an effective intervention (ACOG, Task Force on Hypertension in Pregnancy, 2013).

In Chapter 4, Sophie was diagnosed with preeclampsia. Although Dr. Riley initially recommended bed rest, she conceded that there's not good evidence to support the practice. Sophie was anxious to work because she was worried about losing her job and needed the money.

The nurse must instruct patients with mild preeclampsia to immediately report symptoms associated with a progression to severe preeclampsia and HELLP (see the next section). These include epigastric pain, a severe persistent headache, visual changes, malaise, and shortness of breath. Patients should also report immediately any signs of fetal distress, further complications of pregnancy, and impending birth, including reduced fetal movement, contractions, vaginal bleeding, leakage of fluid from the vagina, and abdominal pain (ACOG, Task Force on Hypertension in Pregnancy, 2013).

HELLP Syndrome

HELLP syndrome is a hypertensive disorder of pregnancy that occurs most often as a complication of preeclampsia. HELLP is an acronym for *H*emolysis, *E*levated *L*iver enzymes, and *L*ow *P*latelet count, which are the key findings associated with this condition. The diagnosis of HELLP is based on the results of a CBC with platelet count, a peripheral smear, and aspartate aminotransferase and bilirubin levels. For care considerations pertinent to this condition, see the section on preeclampsia and eclampsia.

Prevalence

HELLP syndrome occurs in 10% to 20% of women with preeclampsia, although as many as 20% of women with HELLP syndrome are not first diagnosed with preeclampsia (Sibai, 1990).

Thus, although it is generally considered a more severe form of preeclampsia, it may be an independent disorder.

Course in Pregnancy

HELLP syndrome poses considerable risks to both the pregnancy and the pregnant woman. Women diagnosed with HELLP are at risk for serious complications, including disseminated intravascular coagulation, placental abruption, acute renal failure, pulmonary edema, hematoma of the liver, and retinal detachment. Most require transfusion with blood or blood products. Prematurity and IUGR and associated complications, as well as perinatal death, are common in the infant of a pregnancy complicated by HELLP.

Assessment

In the absence of proteinuria and hypertension, the first indication of HELLP may be symptomatic. Associated symptoms reflect cerebral edema and include a severe (typically frontal) headache, blurred vision, and scotomata. Patients may also first present with the epigastric or right upper quadrant pain that results from edema and the subsequent distension of the liver capsule. Symptoms can also be less specific and include malaise, flu-like symptoms, and nausea and vomiting.

Treatment

As with other hypertensive disorders specific to pregnancy, the only true cure for HELLP syndrome is delivery. If this condition develops after 34 weeks of gestation, the woman is delivered immediately. If it develops prior to this gestational age, delivery may be delayed for 48 hours to complete a course of intramuscular (IM) corticosteroids to facilitate fetal lung development (see The Pharmacy 8.2).

In Chapter 10, Dr. Stone diagnosed Lexi with HELLP syndrome after she was found to have a blood pressure of 148/98 mm Hg, protein in her urine, and symptoms of headache, abdominal pain, and vomiting and lab results consistent with the condition. Because of developing this condition, she had to have a preterm cesarean delivery. Being 37 years old, her advanced maternal age was a risk factor for developing HELLP syndrome.

Gestational Diabetes

Gestational diabetes is a form of diabetes mellitus that has its onset in pregnancy (see Chapter 9). It is associated with insulin resistance and results in high blood glucose levels.

Prevalence

More than 90% of pregnancies complicated by diabetes are complicated by a form of diabetes that is specific to pregnancy. Gestational diabetes occurs in about 6% to 7% of pregnancies and is on the rise, likely due to the increased prevalence of obesity as well as higher birth rates for members of ethnic groups more prone to gestational diabetes, including African Americans, Native Americans, Latinas, and Asians (Moyer, 2014).

Etiology

Insulin is like a fist knocking on the front door of a cell. It is the job of insulin to tell the cells when they should open and let glucose in. Insulin resistance happens when cells become more resistant to answering the door to the insulin knock. Type 1 diabetes is a disease in which the pancreas produces no insulin: the cells don't answer the door because there isn't any insulin knocking. The person with type 1 diabetes is dependent on insulin injections. Type 2 diabetes is a condition in which cells become resistant to answering insulin's knock. The pancreas of a person with type 2 diabetes releases more and more insulin to knock harder and harder to try to overcome the resistance of the cells to taking in glucose. Over time, many people with type 2 diabetes also become dependent on insulin, because their pancreas is no longer able to keep up with the increased demand for insulin.

Gestational diabetes is most similar to type 2 diabetes. It is normal for the hormones of pregnancy to create a form of insulin resistance in the second and third trimesters of pregnancy. For most women, this is not problematic as the pancreatic beta cells increase their production of insulin. A woman who has gestational diabetes, however, is not able to produce enough insulin to overcome the insulin resistance of the cells caused by the pregnancy. This leaves a high circulating volume of glucose in the blood, resulting in the hyperglycemia that is characteristic of diabetes.

Course in Pregnancy

Many of the most common problems and complications of gestational diabetes are directly related to large fetal size, although women with gestational diabetes are also at a higher risk for preeclampsia (Box 20.9). Unlike diabetes that preexists the

---

Box 20.9 Risks Associated with Gestational Diabetes

- Preeclampsia
- Fetal macrosomia
- Polyhydramnios
- Fetal organomegaly
- Operative delivery (cesarean section or surgical vaginal delivery)
- Birth trauma to the mother and/or fetus (shoulder dystocia, perineal trauma, etc.)
- Neonatal respiratory problems
- Neonatal metabolic problems (particularly hypoglycemia, hypocalcemia, and jaundice)
- Perinatal mortality

Adapted from Ovesen, P. G., Jensen, D. M., Damm, P., Rasmussen, S., & Kesmodel, U. S. (2015). Maternal and neonatal outcomes in pregnancies complicated by gestational diabetes. A nation-wide study. *The Journal of Maternal-Fetal and Neonatal Medicine, 28*(14), 1720–1724.

---

pregnancy, however, gestational diabetes is not associated with birth defects.

The large fetal size associated with gestational diabetes occurs as a result of the excess glucose in the maternal circulation passing the placenta and entering the fetal circulation. Maternal insulin does not pass the placenta, however. The fetus now needs to produce a large amount of insulin to address this high circulating volume of glucose. Insulin is an anabolic hormone, meaning that it works to build up body mass. The extra insulin production results in a fetus that is **large for gestational age** (weight in the top 90th percentile for gestational age) or has **macrosomia** (a condition in which the fetus is large regardless of gestational age). Some sources define macrosomia as having a birth weight of 4,000 g (8 lb 13 oz) or more, whereas others define it as having a birth weight of 4,500 g (10 lb) or more.

Most of this extra growth in the fetus is not skeletal but rather excessive adipose tissue (fat), particularly in the shoulders and trunk. This sort of extra mass in this location increases the risk for the infant becoming lodged in the birth canal, with the anterior shoulder getting caught behind the mother's pelvic bone. This condition is called shoulder dystocia and can result in a surgical birth and birth trauma.

In Chapter 11, the birth of Edie's baby was complicated by shoulder dystocia. Her infant had a brachial plexus injury, and she incurred significant injury to her perineum.

Assessment

Assessment related to gestational diabetes includes initial screening and ongoing evaluation with fetal surveillance.

Screening

Gestational diabetes is typically recognized during routine screening. In the United States, it is routine to screen all patients in pregnancy. High-risk patients may be screened at their first prenatal visit for preexisting diabetes, and all patients are screened at 24 to 28 weeks of gestation for gestational diabetes (Boxes 20.10 and 20.11). The initial screening of high-risk women in the first trimester is to diagnose nongestational diabetes rather than to find gestational diabetes. As discussed in Chapter 19, screening in the initial visit may be by one of the three following methods:

- *Fasting glucose:* A glucose level of 126 mg/dL or more indicates nongestational diabetes, whereas a glucose level from 92 to 125 mg/dL indicates gestational diabetes.
- *Hemoglobin A$_{1c}$ (HbA$_{1c}$):* A HbA$_{1c}$ level equal to or greater than 6.5% indicates nongestational diabetes.
- *Random glucose:* A glucose level equal to or greater than 200 mg/dL is suspicious for nongestational diabetes but must be confirmed by fasting glucose or HbA$_{1c}$ testing.

Screening for gestational diabetes from 24 to 28 weeks of gestation is nearly universal. Two different protocols may be used to screen for gestational diabetes in the second trimester, between

Box 20.10 Risk Factors for Gestational Diabetes

- Body mass index > 25 (overweight or obese)
- Prior history of gestational diabetes
- Family history of type 2 diabetes
- Previous unexplained fetal demise
- Previous birth with macrosomia
- Infant with congenital anomalies
- Maternal age >40 y
- Hispanic, African American, Native American, Asian, or Pacific Islander ethnicity
- Polycystic ovarian syndrome
- Hypertension

Box 20.11 Protective Factors for Gestational Diabetes

- Maternal age < 25 y
- Not of Hispanic, African American, Native American, Asian, or Pacific Islander ethnicity
- Body mass index < 25
- No known history of diabetes among immediate family members
- No history of adverse obstetric outcomes, such as macrosomia or stillbirth
- No history of abnormal glucose tolerance

24 and 28 weeks of gestation (see Lab Values 3.2): the two-step 1-hour and 3-hour oral glucose tolerance test (OGTT) and the one-step 2-hour OGTT.

For the 1-hour phase of the two-step OGTT, a woman does not need to fast before the test. However, the nurse should advise her that a high-carbohydrate meal or snack prior to the test may make her blood glucose level appear higher than it is, resulting in a false positive. For this test, a woman consumes a 50-g oral glucose load, usually as a flat orange liquid. Some women do not tolerate the glucose drink well and may experience nausea or even vomiting. An hour after drinking the solution, the woman has her blood glucose level tested. A blood glucose level of 130 to 140 mg/dL or greater indicates a need for further evaluation with the 3-hour phase of the two-step OGTT.

Unlike with the 1-hour phase of the two-step OGTT, the 3-hour phase requires the woman to fast overnight prior to the test, have blood drawn just before the test for fasting glucose level testing, and drink 100 g of glucose rather than just 50 g. After drinking the 100 g of glucose, the woman's blood glucose level is checked again at 1 hour, 2 hours, and 3 hours. Two different criteria are currently used clinically to determine the diagnostic ceiling for this test. Values above those presented in the table are considered diagnostic for gestational diabetes. The pregnant woman must have at least two of the four values (fasting, 1-hour, 2-hour, or 3-hour blood glucose level) elevated to be diagnosed with gestational diabetes.

Although the two-step 1-hour and 3-hour OGTT is most common in the United States, in other countries, the one-step 2-hour OGTT is used instead. For this test, a 75-g bolus of glucose is consumed. The patient's blood glucose level is evaluated before the glucose drink (fasting), 1 hour after the drink, and 2 hours after the drink. Although the 3-hour phase of the two-step OGTT requires at least two elevated levels, the single-step 2-hour OGTT requires only one elevated level.

Fetal Surveillance

Women who have good blood glucose control with diet and exercise alone generally do not require fetal monitoring beyond what is standard for a woman with a pregnancy uncomplicated by gestational diabetes, although practice may vary as there is no current consensus regarding fetal monitoring with well-controlled gestational diabetes. Women who do require metformin, glyburide, or insulin and those with additional risks, such as obesity, hypertension, or a history of fetal demise, may be monitored more closely (Committee on Practice Bulletins-Obstetrics, 2013).

Management of a woman with comorbidities or poor glycemic control is similar to monitoring for a woman with diabetes that preexists the pregnancy. Additional testing is usually started no earlier than the third trimester of pregnancy. Nonstress tests may begin at 32 weeks of gestation and are performed as often as twice weekly until the birth. BPPs may also be ordered. The size of the fetus is of particular interest and concern, although there is currently no reliable way of accurately gauging fetal size. A fetus estimated by ultrasound to weigh 4,800 g (10.5 lb) has only about a 50% chance at birth of weighing 4,500 g (9.9 lb) or more (Little, Edlow, Thomas, & Smith, 2012).

Treatment

The primary intervention for gestational diabetes is usually management of diet, regular exercise, and home glucose monitoring. For patients who continue to demonstrate poor control of blood glucose level, however, medication and induced or cesarean delivery may be necessary.

Diet

Although patients with gestational diabetes are often referred to nutritionists and dieticians, these appointments can be difficult to get or may not occur for weeks or months after the diagnosis of gestational diabetes is made. Therefore, it is the nurse's responsibility to provide the patient with accurate dietary advice. Closely following a diet normalizes blood glucose levels in about 75% to 80% of women with gestational diabetes, in which case no additional intervention is required (Patient Teaching 20.1; see Box 3.5).

Exercise

Exercise has many benefits, one of which is that it increases the sensitivity of cells to insulin; in other words, cells are more likely to answer the knock of insulin at the door if the person has been exercising. As a result, less insulin is required overall and less glucose circulates in the blood because it is entering the cells.

Patient Teaching 20.1

Nutrition and Gestational Diabetes

Instruct patients to do the following:

- Follow the weight gain recommendations relevant to your body mass index previous to pregnancy.
- Carefully monitor your intake of carbohydrates, which cause the greatest rise in blood sugar. About 35%–40% of your calories should come from complex carbohydrates, and you should eliminate simple sugars.
- Protein should make up an additional 20%–30% of your diet. The remaining 40%–45% of your diet should consist of fats.
- Avoid spikes and dips in your blood glucose level. Eat three meals and two to three snacks per day, all of which except for breakfast should contain carbohydrates (eating carbohydrates with breakfast can create a higher spike in blood sugar than can eating carbohydrates with other meals).
- One of the snacks should be just before bedtime and should contain carbohydrates.
- Don't go for longer than 10 h without eating.
- Keep a food log that includes your finger stick glucose test results in either a written journal or a smart phone app.
- Check out the American Diabetes Association website to learn more about nutrition and diabetes, including resources for easy methods of counting carbohydrates.

Adapted from Phillips, C., & Boyd, M. (2015). Intrahepatic cholestasis of pregnancy. *Nursing for Women's Health, 19*(1), 46–57. doi:10.1111/1751-486X.12175

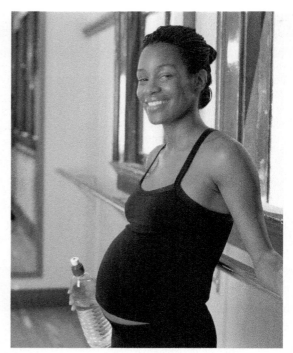

Figure 20.3. Exercise during pregnancy. Pregnant women are urged to get at least 30 minutes of moderate, safe exercise three times a week throughout their pregnancies. Exercise is particularly important for women diagnosed with gestational diabetes. Women should consult their obstetric providers prior to beginning any exercise program during pregnancy. (Reprinted with permission from Dudek, S. G. [2014]. *Nutrition essentials for nursing practice* [7th ed., Fig. 11.2]. Philadelphia, PA: Lippincott Williams & Wilkins.)

Low-intensity, moderate-intensity, and even short periods of high-intensity activity are all effective in producing these results (Fig. 20.3). However, chest pain, bleeding, dizziness, preterm labor, vaginal leakage of fluid, headache, muscle weakness, and reduced fetal movement are all reasons to stop activity (Coombes, 2015).

Exercise guidelines include the following:

- Exercise should occur at least 3 days per week with no more than 48 hours between exercise sessions.
- Patients are encouraged to exercise at 60% to 90% of maximum heart rate for at least 30 minutes 3 days a week.

Blood Glucose Monitoring

An important aspect of gestational diabetes care is the patient's self-monitoring of blood glucose level at home. A typical initial frequency for monitoring is at least four times daily. This frequency may be reduced with good evidence of control. Typical monitoring times are before and after breakfast, before and after lunch, after dinner, and before bed (see Step-by-Step Skills 9.1). Schedules should be customized to the individual woman. Some experts advise that the postprandial (after eating) blood glucose level test be taken an hour after the first bite of a meal, whereas others advocate for 2 hours. Patients should be aware that the insulin

needs of pregnancy, after an early drop, climb steadily until the birth. Because of this, they may find their blood glucose more challenging to control as the pregnancy progresses (see Fig. 9.5).

Guidelines for blood glucose monitoring include the following:

- Fasting glucose levels should remain <95 mg/dL.
- One-hour postprandial glucose levels should remain under 140 mg/dL with 2-hour testing.
- Two-hour postprandial glucose levels should remain <120 mg/dL.

Although there is no standard threshold for starting medication to enhance glucose control, levels that exceed the guidelines may prompt pharmacologic intervention (Brown, Martis, Hughes, Rowan, & Crowther, 2017).

Medications

Continued poor control of blood glucose level is an indication for starting medications. One of two oral medications are frequently used in pregnancy to manage blood glucose level: glyburide and metformin (see The Pharmacy 3.2).

Glyburide, a sulfonylurea, stimulates the pancreas to release more insulin. Typical dosing in pregnancy is 20 to 60 minutes before breakfast and a possible second dose 20 to 60 minutes before dinner (Caritis & Hebert, 2013). This medication is contraindicated in patients with an allergy to sulfa or with kidney failure.

Very little of the medication is believed to cross the placenta to the fetus. Glyburide can cause **hypoglycemia** (low blood sugar). The nurse should teach patients about the signs and symptoms of hypoglycemia and encourage them to always carry a source of fast sugar, such as candy or juice, in the event that this condition occurs.

Metformin is often used as first-line treatment in patients with type 2 diabetes. It increases the sensitivity of cells to insulin. It also decreases the release of glucose from the liver. It is known to cross the placenta but is still believed to be safe in pregnancy. Patients using metformin are more likely to require supplemental insulin, but metformin is associated with lower birth weight (Balsells, García-Patterson, Solà Roqué, Gich, & Corcoy, 2015; Brown et al., 2017).

Injectable insulin is often the medication of last resort for correcting blood glucose level, although some healthcare providers may choose to use it over the oral medications as there are no lingering concerns about it having a teratogenic effect on the fetus. Insulin can be challenging to manage from the perspective of the patient and the provider. The delivery method of injection can be a particularly unattractive option for patients.

In Chapter 9, Nancy, whose risk factors for gestational diabetes included obesity and Asian ethnicity, was advised to start insulin by her provider, Ron. Ron preferred to manage his patients who have gestational diabetes with insulin. (In contrast, in Chapter 3, Susan's gestational diabetes was successfully managed with metformin by Dr. Cheema.)

Induced or Cesarean Birth

Spontaneous vaginal birth is the preferred method of delivery rather than an induced vaginal birth or cesarean birth for reasons of safety and superior birth outcomes. In women who have good glycemic control and no comorbidities or indications of fetal or maternal stress, there is little reason for an induced or surgical birth to be pursued prior to 40 weeks of gestation.

Suboptimal maternal glucose control, maternal comorbidities, and evidence of fetal distress or macrosomia, however, can be indications for an induced vaginal birth or cesarean section at 39 weeks of gestation due to the high risk for stillbirth. A woman with a fetus estimated by ultrasound or physical examination to be macrosomic may be offered a cesarean section without first having a trial of labor. This practice is controversial, however, due to the noted lack of reliability of fetal size estimates by ultrasound (American Congress of Obstetricians and Gynecologists' Committee on Practice Bulletins—Obstetrics, 2016).

Care Considerations

The nurse should monitor the blood glucose level of women with gestational diabetes regularly during labor according to orders and institution protocol with a goal of maintaining euglycemia. This is primarily done to reduce the occurrence of hypoglycemia in the infant after birth. The nurse may need to administer IV insulin, as ordered (Ryan & Al-Agha, 2014).

Women with gestational diabetes typically have resolution of the condition shortly after the placenta is delivered. These women should be aware, however, that they are at a greater risk for developing gestational diabetes again with any future pregnancies. They are also at a high risk for developing type 2 diabetes later in life, particularly if they are obese. Breastfeeding and regular exercise may delay or even prevent the onset of disease. Women should be screened for type 2 diabetes by OGTT 6 to 12 weeks after the end of pregnancy (Blumer et al., 2013).

Infections

Many different infections commonly occur during pregnancy, including sexually transmitted infections (STIs), vaginitis, TORCH infections, and urinary tract infections, all of which are covered in detail below. The presentation of an infection may be different in a woman who is pregnant, and the implications can be severe. For example, it's not uncommon for a pregnant woman with bacteria in her bladder to not experience symptoms of a urinary tract infection during pregnancy. Genital herpes, a common and relatively benign condition in a woman who is not pregnant, may be devastating for a neonate who comes in contact with a herpetic lesion at the time of birth.

Sexually Transmitted Infections

The impact of an STI in pregnancy varies depending on the STI and when it is diagnosed (see Chapter 28). An STI diagnosis may complicate an intimate relationship or impair fertility. The STI may cause minor short-term or severe long-term complications for the fetus. Risk factors for contracting an STI include multiple sexual partners, unprotected sex, and, for STIs that are also bloodborne, IV drug use.

Chlamydia

Chlamydia is a bacterial infection and one of the most common STIs. It is screened for during the first prenatal visit routinely. Women who test positive are generally treated with an antibiotic and retested at 1 and at 3 to 4 months after the initial diagnosis. The infection is typically asymptomatic in both men and women. Regardless of the initial diagnosis, women who are high risk or under the age of 25 should be rescreened for chlamydia in the third trimester. Chlamydia in pregnancy poses a risk for premature rupture of membranes (PROM), postpartum endometritis (inflammation of the lining of the uterus), preterm labor, and low birth weight.

Gonorrhea

Gonorrhea is also a common bacterial infection and carries the same risks for preterm labor, PROM, and postpartum endometritis. In addition, gonorrhea may contribute to IUGR, postpartum sepsis, and direct infection of the membranes surrounding the pregnancy (chorioamnionitis). Infants may also be born with conjunctivitis, arthritis, and pharyngitis (Liu et al., 2013). Screening is performed routinely during the first prenatal visit. Women who screen positive are treated and then retested 3 months later.

Herpes Simplex Virus

Herpes is an exceedingly common infection. An estimated 70% of pregnant women are carriers of the herpes simplex virus 1, and 16% are carriers of the herpes simplex virus 2 (Delaney, Gardella, Saracino, Magaret, & Wald, 2014). People with herpes are infectious sporadically and unpredictably, and many have few or no outbreaks and are often unaware of the infection (Workowski & Bolan, 2015). The primary concern of herpes in pregnancy is transmission to the fetus. Neonates exposed to herpetic lesions during the delivery are at risk for severe infection that could lead to death. Neonates are most at risk for damage from herpes if the woman is first exposed to the virus late in pregnancy. A less likely means of harm to the neonate is from a recurrent lesion from an infection acquired prior to pregnancy. Herpes is not a contraindication to a vaginal birth in the absence of an active genital lesion, however. Women known to have genital herpes are typically prescribed an antiviral medication, usually acyclovir, to take during the month prior to the pregnancy's due date to minimize the chance of an intrapartum herpes outbreak. The presence of lesions at the time of birth is an indication for a cesarean section. The virus is not screened for routinely in pregnancy.

Human Papillomavirus

Human papillomavirus (HPV) is not one virus but a group of over 100 viruses. High-risk strains of HPV can cause the cell changes that may lead to cancer of the cervix, rectum, or head and neck. Other, low-risk strains can cause genital warts. The high-risk forms are not known to contribute to changes in pregnancy outcomes. The low-risk kind can thrive in pregnancy, creating genital warts that may bleed excessively during and after the birth or even block the birth passage. Treatment to remove the warts is indicated to prevent these complications. Rarely, the virus may be transmitted to the neonate during delivery, manifesting later in life as lesions on the conjunctiva, mucosa, or throat. However, the presence of warts is not considered an indication for cesarean section (Workowski & Bolan, 2015).

Syphilis

Although syphilis, a bacterial infection, is not as common or as widespread as it once was, it is still screened for routinely in the first trimester, and, if present, prompt treatment is critical. The Centers for Disease Control and Prevention also recommends rescreening in the third trimester and at the time of delivery for women who are at a high risk for acquiring the disease in pregnancy (Workowski & Bolan, 2015). Syphilis has many of the same potential complications associated with chlamydia and gonorrhea, and it may also lead to stillbirth, premature delivery, low birth weight, and considerable congenital anomalies.

Trichomoniasis

Trichomoniasis is a flagellated, microscopic parasite that is sexually transmitted and may be found in the genital tracts of males and females. It is often asymptomatic but may present as vaginal irritation and discharge. It is associated with poor pregnancy outcomes, including PROM, premature labor, and low birth weight. It can be resolved in pregnancy with a single dose of the antibiotic metronidazole. Screening for trichomoniasis at the time of the first prenatal visit is recommended for women who are positive for human immunodeficiency virus (HIV), because coinfection with trichomoniasis increases the risk of HIV transmission to the fetus (Workowski & Bolan, 2015).

Human Immunodeficiency Virus

Pregnancy is not contraindicated in women with HIV. With modern treatments, people diagnosed with HIV may lead long, productive, and relatively healthy lives. A pregnant women who takes antiretroviral medications to suppress her viral load during pregnancy reduces her chance of transmitting the virus to the fetus to less than 2% (Forbes et al., 2012). Although most women with HIV may give birth vaginally, cesarean section may reduce the chance for HIV transmission to the fetus for women with a high viral load. Infants born to women who are HIV positive are typically treated with antiretroviral medications for 4 to 6 weeks following the birth starting at between 6 and 12 hours of life to prevent infection (Mandelbrot et al., 2015). Infants who are not infected with HIV may continue to test positive for HIV for as long as 18 months after the birth because of the persistence of maternal antibodies. Thus, serial testing for the virus itself is preferred to testing of antibodies to HIV. Breastfeeding increases the risk of transmission. All women should be screened for HIV at the time of their first visit. Women considered high risk should be rescreened during the third trimester of pregnancy.

Hepatitis B Virus

Approximately 5% of adults who contract the hepatitis B virus develop a chronic disease that creates a risk for cancer and other liver disease. Of the neonates who contract hepatitis B from their mothers, however, 90% develop chronic liver disease (Tassopoulos et al., 1987). It is essential that infants born to mothers who test positive for hepatitis B receive both the hepatitis B vaccination and hepatitis B immune globulin within 12 hours of birth. All pregnant women should be screened in the first trimester and again later in pregnancy if there are risk factors. The hepatitis B vaccination is considered safe in pregnancy. Breastfeeding does not increase the risk of transmission.

Hepatitis C Virus

The hepatitis C virus does not transmit easily by sexual intercourse and today is typically passed by the use of shared needles (Denniston et al., 2014). Risk factors for infection with hepatitis C before 1992 included receiving blood transfusions and organ transplants. Approximately 80% of people with hepatitis C were born from 1945 to 1965 (Denniston et al., 2014). The incidence of **vertical transmission** (transmission from the mother to the fetus) is about 6%, in general, and 11% if the mother is also HIV positive (Benova, Mohamoud, Calvert, & Abu-Raddad, 2014). As with HIV, children should be screened for viral RNA rather than antibodies to hepatitis C in the first 18 months to avoid false positives from maternal antibodies. Currently, no vaccination or method to reduce transmission is available for hepatitis C. Breastfeeding does not increase the risk of transmission. Women should be screened in pregnancy if they were born between 1945 and 1965 or if they are considered high risk.

Vaginal Infections

In addition to the STIs discussed above, the vagina may also be affected by microorganisms that are normally present in a healthy woman, known as normal vaginal flora. Bacterial vaginosis refers to an overgrowth of normal vaginal bacteria. Candidiasis is a fungal infection with yeasts from the genus *Candida*. Women are often colonized with yeast, meaning that the organisms are present but are not creating uncomfortable symptoms. Uncomfortable vaginal symptoms caused by yeast are often referred to as a yeast infection. Neither bacterial vaginosis nor candidiasis is considered an STI, and both often present as a change in vaginal discharge. The nurse should advise women that changes in vaginal discharge in pregnancy should always be evaluated to rule out leakage of amniotic fluid, bacterial vaginosis, or an infectious process.

Bacterial Vaginosis

Bacterial vaginosis often presents as a thin, watery vaginal discharge with a fishy smell. Women with this condition may also experience some mild vulvar irritation because of this increased discharge. Although this condition is benign and often self-limiting in women who are not pregnant, it may present an additional risk of preterm birth, postpartum pelvic infection, and late miscarriage in women who are pregnant. Women with bacterial vaginosis are most often treated with oral or vaginal clindamycin or metronidazole (see Chapter 28). There is little evidence, however, that treatment is effective for improving pregnancy outcomes, and screening and treatment of asymptomatic infections is not currently recommended (Workowski & Bolan, 2015).

Candidiasis Vaginitis

Pregnant women are prone to vaginal yeast infections because of the increased glucose in the vaginal secretions, hormonal changes, and slightly higher overall body temperature that typically occur in pregnancy. Yeast infections usually present as vaginal itching and irritation, and women often report a clumpy white discharge, which may be seen on exam, as well. Although irritating, vaginal yeast is not believed to cause poor pregnancy outcomes (Workowski & Bolan, 2015). Women can usually be successfully treated with topical vaginal preparations (see Chapter 28).

TORCH Infections

TORCH infections are a group of infections commonly implicated in congenital anomalies. They typically cause few or flu-like symptoms for the mother but may pass the placenta and cause congenital infection of the fetus that can have devastating effects. The acronym TORCH stands for Toxoplasmosis, Other, Rubella, Cytomegalovirus (CMV), and genital herpes (HSV-1 and HSV-2), which are the primary pathogenic microorganisms that form this group. "Other" may refer to various infections, most commonly syphilis, but also varicella, parvovirus, mumps, and HIV. Below, only toxoplasmosis, rubella, and CMV are covered. For information on herpes, see the STI section.

Toxoplasmosis

Toxoplasmosis is a disease caused by infection with a protozoan, a type of parasite, that is transmitted in oocyte form to a pregnant woman by exposure to the litter of an infected cat, gardening without gloves, or eating raw or rare meat, most commonly (see Box 15.3). Antibodies to the protozoan persist for years, and their presence in a single test without a previous negative test is not diagnostic of a new infection. Instead, diagnosis of a new infection is based on results from two blood tests taken at least 2 weeks apart. A negative antibody test followed by a positive antibody test is diagnostic of a new infection. Routine screening is not recommended in pregnancy (ACOG, 2015). Risk to the fetus is greatest when the mother's exposure to the parasite occurs during the first trimester of pregnancy. A woman who was exposed to toxoplasmosis three or more months prior to the pregnancy is not believed to be at risk for passing the infection to the fetus. Damage to the fetus is most common in, but not limited to, the central nervous system, skin, and ears. Treatment of a new infection with antibiotics in pregnancy likely does not stop transmission from the mother to the fetus but may reduce damage to the central nervous system.

Rubella Virus

Most people are vaccinated for the rubella virus in childhood. Some parents, however, may choose not to vaccinate their children, or vaccination may be contraindicated for health reasons. In addition, vaccines are not always completely effective. Usually people who are not vaccinated or for whom the vaccination has not worked are protected regardless because most of the people around them are vaccinated, a phenomenon known as herd immunity. When too small a proportion of people in a given community are vaccinated, however, this herd immunity is lost and those who are not effectively vaccinated are more vulnerable to the illness. Vaccination for rubella is contraindicated in pregnancy. Women who are not immune should be offered the rubella vaccination in the immediate postpartum period.

Maternal symptoms of rubella include a rash, fever, and flu-like symptoms. If a woman contracts the virus in the first 12 weeks of pregnancy, there is up to an 81% chance that the fetus is congenitally infected. Fetuses exposed to the virus in the second trimester have a 25% chance of congenital infection, and there is a 35% chance of congenital infection with exposure from 27 to 30 weeks of gestation and an almost 100% infection rate with exposure after 36 weeks. A majority of congenital defects, however, result from maternal infections in the first 16 weeks of pregnancy. Fetal anomalies that commonly occur as a result of rubella infection include central nervous system, cardiac, ocular, endocrine, and other damage (Miller, Cradock-Watson, & Pollock, 1982).

Cytomegalovirus

CMV is the most common cause of congenital infections in developed countries and the leading cause of nonhereditary hearing loss. It can also result in other neurodevelopmental disabilities, including vision impairment and **cerebral palsy**. Most women who contract the virus experience no or flu-like symptoms.

The implications of congenital infection are broad and include damage to the liver and the central nervous system. Hearing loss is the most common effect. Almost 60% of women are infected with CMV by age 44 years (Staras et al., 2006), and approximately 2.3% of these women are infected during pregnancy (Hyde, Schmid, & Cannon, 2010). Maternal exposure in the 2 months prior to pregnancy poses a 5% to 15% chance of transmission to the fetus, whereas exposure in pregnancy poses a 35.5% to 65% chance of fetal infection, with the chances of transmission highest in the third trimester (Picone et al., 2013). Fetal infection may be detected by amniocentesis or cord blood sampling, and some fetal anomalies resulting from CMV may be detected by ultrasound or magnetic resonance imaging.

Urinary Tract Infections

Urinary tract infections include cystitis, asymptomatic bacteriuria, and pyelonephritis. As in the nonpregnant population, these infections often result from bacteria originating in the gut. All types of urinary tract infections should always be treated with an antibiotic during pregnancy.

Cystitis

Cystitis is an infection of the urinary bladder. Acute cystitis occurs in about 1% to 2% of pregnancies (Wing, Fassett, & Getahun, 2014). Common symptoms are frequent urination, a sensation of incomplete emptying, pain with urination, and lower abdominal or pelvic pain.

Asymptomatic Bacteriuria

Asymptomatic bacteriuria is a condition of bacteria in the urine that occurs in about 2% to 7% of pregnancies. Although patients with this condition by definition have no symptoms, the chance of the bacteriuria progressing to a symptomatic urinary tract infection in pregnancy is 30% to 40% (Smaill & Vazquez, 2015). Some studies have also found a correlation between asymptomatic bacteriuria and preeclampsia, preterm birth, and low birth weight, although these same results were not found in other studies (Minassian, Thomas, Williams, Campbell, & Smeeth, 2013; Smaill & Vazquez, 2015). For this reason, routine screening for this condition by urine culture is recommended from 12 to 16 weeks of gestation or at the time of the first prenatal visit, with no repeat screening indicated in low-risk women (Lin & Fajardo, 2008).

Pyelonephritis

Pyelonephritis is a condition of infection and inflammation of the kidneys. It complicates about 0.5% to 2% of pregnancies (Wing et al., 2014). Women are more likely to get pyelonephritis in pregnancy because of the smooth muscle relaxation that occurs during this time. Symptoms may include those associated with cystitis as well as systemic symptoms such as fever, chills, nausea, vomiting, and lower back pain. Women may look acutely ill. Pyelonephritis is associated with preterm birth (Wing et al., 2014). Pyelonephritis can also progress to sepsis, kidney failure, respiratory failure, and even maternal and/or fetal death.

Cervical Insufficiency

Cervical insufficiency, previously referred to as incompetent cervix, refers to the painless, premature dilation of the cervix in the second trimester of pregnancy.

Etiology

Cervical insufficiency may be caused by congenital or acquired cervical or uterine defects. Acquired causes include a history of rapid mechanical dilation of the cervix prior to this pregnancy, repeat second- or third-trimester pregnancy terminations, and a treatment for cervical cancer called a cone biopsy, which can involve removal of a large portion of the cervix. Other factors, such as infection, inflammation, multiple pregnancy, and placental abruption, may cause premature dilation of the cervix, but dilation for these reasons is not considered cervical insufficiency, and thus these are not considered risk factors for future pregnancies.

Course in Pregnancy

A cervix measuring less than 25 mm prior to 24 weeks of gestation is considered short and indicates a pregnancy that is at a high risk for ending in miscarriage or premature birth (Iams, Cebrik, Lynch, Behrendt, & Das, 2011). In pregnancies with a maternal cervix measuring less than 25 mm at 24 weeks of gestation, approximately 18% end prior to 35 weeks. For pregnancies with a cervix half this length, 13 mm, at 24 weeks of gestation, 50% end before 35 weeks (Iams et al., 2011).

Assessment

Diagnosis of this condition requires a preexisting congenital or acquired structural defect of the cervix and may be made in one of two ways:

- *History-based diagnosis:* two or more pregnancy losses in a row in the second trimester of pregnancy OR three or more previous births occurring before 34 weeks of gestation
- *History- and exam-based diagnosis:* one or more prior pregnancy losses in the second trimester AND cervical length by ultrasound shorter than 25 mm prior to 24 weeks of pregnancy in the current pregnancy

Although painless dilation of the cervix is the classic presentation of cervical insufficiency, the pregnant woman may report other symptoms that should be further investigated. These symptoms include unusual vaginal discharge and/or spotting, pelvic cramping, and pelvic pressure. Women with risk factors for cervical insufficiency or a diagnosis of cervical insufficiency in a prior pregnancy are generally evaluated by transvaginal ultrasound from 12 to 24 weeks of gestation. Depending on risk factors, history, and ultrasound findings, this exam may be repeated every 1 to 2 weeks. The purpose of this ultrasound exam is to measure the length of the cervix.

Treatment

Two common strategies are used to address cervical insufficiency and may be used individually or in combination: maternal progesterone supplementation and cervical cerclage.

Supplemental progesterone may be administered to the mother by the IM or vaginal route starting at 16 to 20 weeks of gestation and continuing through 36 weeks.

Cervical cerclage is a procedure whereby the cervix is stitched closed. This reinforces the cervix and keeps it from dilating prematurely. It may also help protect the fetal membranes from exposure and keep the **mucus plug** intact. Cerclage placement may significantly extend the duration of a pregnancy and reduce the occurrence of preterm birth (Alfirevic, Stampalija, Roberts, & Jorgensen, 2012). The cerclage may be placed through the vagina (transvaginally) or by the transabdominal route. The transabdominal route may be preferred if a transvaginal cerclage failed previously. Often, a cerclage placed transvaginally will be removed in the 37th week of pregnancy. A transabdominal cerclage is an indication for a cesarean birth (Fig. 20.4).

Patients may have cramping, spotting, or mild pain with urination immediately after placement of a cerclage. Increased uterine activity (contractions) is an expected finding for the remainder of their pregnancy. The nurse should encourage women to report any signs of infection or change in vaginal fluid. Amniotic fluid volume may be verified by ultrasound prior to discharge after placement of the cerclage.

Other interventions may be tried despite not being well supported by the evidence. These interventions include the use of a **pessary** (a space-filling device that is inserted into the vagina and left in place and that supports and changes the angle of the cervix) (see Fig. 17.1), indomethacin (a nonsteroidal anti-inflammatory drug [NSAID]), antibiotics, and lifestyle modifications such as bed rest and activity restrictions.

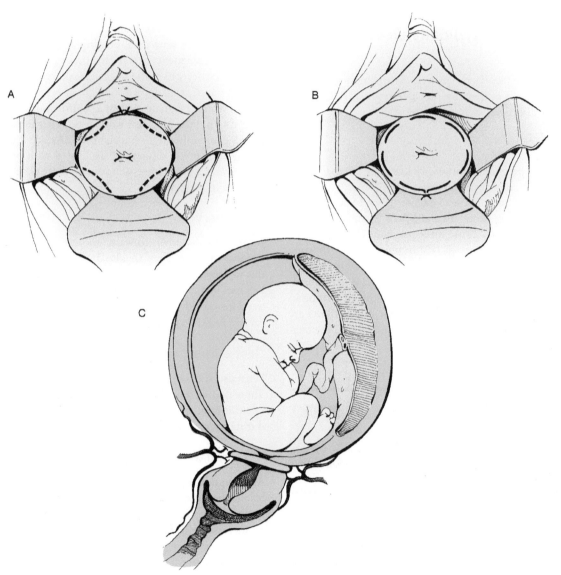

Figure 20.4. Types of cervical cerclage. (A) McDonald cerclage. **(B)** Shirodkar cerclage. **(C)** Transabdominal cerclage. (Reprinted with permission from Ling, F. W., Carson, S. A., Fowler, W. C., Jr., & Snyder, R. R. [2015]. *Step-up to obstetrics and gynecology* [1st ed., Fig. 26.6]. Philadelphia, PA: Lippincott Williams & Wilkins.)

Care Considerations

The diagnosis of cervical insufficiency can be frightening for families. Women with this diagnosis, particularly those with a history of a prior pregnancy loss, may feel responsible. The nurse must inform women of their care options, as well as the risks and benefits of each. For instance, bed rest and activity restriction are still commonly prescribed for women with cervical insufficiency despite a lack of evidence to support this practice. If these interventions are prescribed, the nurse should inform the patient of the limitations of the evidence supporting their use, particularly as bed rest is not a benign intervention and can cause significant physical, emotional, social, and financial hardships (Sosa, Althabe, Belizán, & Bergel, 2015). The nurse should also discuss with families the implications of a preterm birth and the care options and realistic outcomes for premature infants (see chapter 25), which allows them to make informed decisions in advance of preterm birth regarding the care of the neonate.

Conditions That Typically Occur in the Third Trimester

Conditions that commonly occur in the first trimester, which is from 27 to 40 weeks of gestation, include trauma, IUGR, and amniotic fluid disorders.

Trauma

Women who are pregnant continue to live their lives. They are still subject to falls, motor vehicle accidents (MVAs), gun shots, stab wounds, and intimate partner violence (IPV). In fact, women are more likely to suffer from falls and MVAs (Redelmeier, May, Thiruchelvam, & Barrett, 2014) while pregnant. There is mixed evidence about the prevalence of IPV in pregnancy, with some studies finding a rise and others finding little correlation between pregnancy and increased risk of IPV (Box 20.12). When considering the evaluation, treatment, and implications of trauma in pregnancy, the nurse should remember that two patients are potentially at risk (the mother and the fetus), and that the anatomic and physiologic changes of pregnancy may dramatically change the clinical picture.

Although Loretta's IPV was primarily psychological rather than physical, it still impacted her pregnancy and her life. Although it is a form of trauma, Loretta did not perceive herself as being in immediate danger.

Cardiovascular

Nurses providing trauma care for women must be aware of the cardiovascular changes that occur throughout pregnancy. Cardiac output increases by as much as 50% in pregnancy and peaks from 25 to 30 weeks of gestation, and maternal blood volume increases by 40% to 45%. The pulse rate in pregnancy is approximately

---

Box 20.12 Intimate Partner Violence

- Although intimate partner violence occurs across all groups, it is most common in poor women from ethnic minority groups. These women also typically experience worse outcomes.
- African American women may show greater resilience, even in the face of extreme intimate partner violence, than women from other ethnic groups.
- African American and Latina women may be more likely to use aggression to fight back against their abusers.

Adapted from Mechanic, M. B., & Pole, N. (2013). Methodological considerations in conducting ethnoculturally sensitive research on intimate partner abuse and its multidimensional consequences. *Sex Roles, 69,* 205–225.

15 to 20 beats per minute faster than before pregnancy. From mid pregnancy on, the woman lying supine can put excessive pressure on her vena cava, causing symptoms such as nausea and lightheadedness. This means that the proportion of blood lost may be deceptive, and vital signs, particularly the pulse rate, may be out of range for a nonpregnant person but normal for a person who is pregnant. When a supine position is required for care, rotating the pregnant woman onto her left side or placing a wedge under her right hip can help displace the weight of the uterus and correct discomfort associated with occlusion of the vena cava. Chest compressions can be more challenging and ineffective in pregnancy.

Pulmonary

In pregnancy, women consume more oxygen and have reduced residual capacity. They are also at an increased risk for acidosis due to decreased blood-buffering capacity. Oxygen consumption increases by approximately 20%. Nurses must be aware that hypoxia develops quickly in pregnant women and should be monitored for carefully. Oxygen should be used liberally.

Gastrointestinal

Peristalsis slows in pregnancy and abdominal pressure increases. These two factors may cause the lower esophageal sphincter to open, increasing the risk for the aspiration of gastric contents during trauma and interventions.

Abdominal

As a pregnancy progresses past the first trimester, the uterus and bladder become abdominal organs instead of pelvic organs. When no longer protected by the bony pelvis, these organs may be at an increased risk for trauma. Blunt force trauma, even minor, presents a risk for placental abruption, and women should be thoroughly evaluated for abdominal pain, contractions, and vaginal bleeding. Rupture of the uterus from trauma is rare. Any abdominal trauma may also be an indication for providing Rh_o (D) immune globulin to an Rh-unsensitized woman who is Rh negative in the event of a bleed that introduces fetal blood into the maternal circulation.

Joint

Nurses should be aware that relaxin, as well as other hormones that peak in pregnancy, causes a laxity of ligaments that may create a greater potential for injury of unstable joints (Dehghan et al., 2014).

Assessment

In the event that a pregnant woman sustains major trauma, the nurse or other first responder should evaluate the woman's airway, breathing, and circulation (ABC). Next, the nurse should immediately assess the pregnancy and fetus, determining the gestational age, fetal status, and uterine size. Continuous fetal monitoring is routine for women who have sustained major trauma and whose fetuses have reached viability and could be reasonably expected to live outside of the womb. Contraction monitoring is also indicated. An ultrasound is typically performed to assess the fetus and the attachment of the placenta. If a preterm birth may be imminent or indicated, the nurse, per orders, may administer IM glucocorticoids to the mother to hasten fetal lung development.

Whenever appropriate, if imaging is required of the pregnant woman, ultrasound should be used to avoid ionizing radiation from radiography and computed tomography, although the risk to the fetus is believed to be minimal. Imaging by a method that risks fetal exposure to ionizing radiation should not be deferred if delay would endanger the pregnant woman.

Treatment

Delivery by cesarean is optimally done within 5 minutes in the event of the start of unsuccessful cardiopulmonary resuscitation of the pregnant woman, with the incision for delivery made at minute four. This rapid intervention has been found to benefit mothers in about a third of cases and to have caused no harm in the remaining two thirds. Approximately 98% of neonates born within this window do not suffer ill effects from hypoxia (Lipman et al., 2014). Additional possible reasons for emergent cesarean are nonreassuring fetal heart rate and imminent maternal death.

Intrauterine Growth Restriction

IUGR is not a disease itself but rather a condition that indicates a complication of pregnancy.

Prevalence

Approximately 20% of stillborn infants are diagnosed with IUGR. IUGR complicates 10% to 15% of all pregnancies (Suhag & Berghella, 2013).

Etiology

The root cause of IUGR may be maternal, placental, or fetal in origin and may be associated with a combination of factors (Box 20.13). Although a fetus measuring under the 10th percentile for weight is referred to as SGA, the designation of IUGR is made when there is a pathologic process in place that is causing the fetus not to meet its growth potential (Lausman et al., 2014). It is important to note that SGA and IUGR should not be used interchangeably. Although 30% of SGA fetuses have IUGR, 70% do not (Suhag & Berghella, 2013).

There are two kinds of IUGR. The most common is asymmetric IUGR, with approximately 70% of cases falling into this category. With asymmetric IUGR, the growth restriction happens mostly or entirely in the third trimester of pregnancy. The fetal head continues to grow normally while the body grows at a slower rate, hence the asymmetry. With symmetric IUGR, both the head and the body grow at the same slower rate and thus remain symmetric. Symmetric IUGR is also referred to as global growth restriction and is almost always associated with significant neurologic problems for the neonate. Symmetric IUGR, because of the nature of the insults causing the problem, may be seen on ultrasound in the second trimester of pregnancy.

Course in Pregnancy

After prematurity, IUGR is the second-most common cause of perinatal death (Jordan et al., 2014). Infants with IUGR may have various health problems early on in the days immediately after the birth, but also in the long term.

Short Term

Infants with IUGR are at a high risk for hypoglycemia in the days immediately following the birth. These infants may also have problems with thermoregulation, and the nurse must pay careful attention to maintaining their body temperature. Infants with IUGR are more at risk for **neonatal respiratory distress syndrome** (see Box 8.4). They are also at an increased risk for **necrotizing enterocolitis**, **retinopathy of prematurity**, and death. They are at risk for

---

Box 20.13 Select Causes of Intrauterine Growth Restriction

Asymmetric Intrauterine Growth Restriction

- Uteroplacental insufficiency
- Maternal hypertensive disorders
- Severe maternal malnutrition
- Select maternal genetic disorders
- Select maternal acquired disease
- Abnormal placentation
- Multiple gestation

Symmetric Intrauterine Growth Restriction

- TORCH infection
- Maternal substance abuse
- Maternal anemia
- Chromosomal abnormality of the fetus
- Smoking
- Teratogenic medications

polycythemia (a high red blood cell count), which, in turn, increases their risk for elevated circulating **bilirubin**, resulting in neonatal **jaundice** (Longo et al., 2013).

Long Term

Infants with IUGR are at an increased risk later in life for chronic conditions such as hypertension, type 2 diabetes, metabolic syndrome, high cholesterol, and cardiovascular disease. Females are at a higher risk for developing **polycystic ovarian syndrome**. Long- and short-term motor and cognitive delays may also be evident (Longo et al., 2013). See Chapter 24 for more about the complications and care considerations for an infant with IUGR.

Assessment

Initial screening for IUGR is made by measurement of the uterus. Starting at 20 weeks of gestation, the distance from the maternal pubic symphysis to the uterine fundus in centimeters should be equivalent to the gestational age of the pregnancy: a 24-week pregnancy, for example, should measure 24 cm. A pregnancy that is measuring 3 cm or less than expected has screened positive for IUGR. The diagnosis is confirmed by multiple ultrasounds for fetal size, typically done at least 2 weeks apart. A fetal survey (see Box 1.8) is also done by ultrasound to assess for any fetal anomalies that may speak to the cause of the restricted growth.

Once IUGR has been diagnosed, fetal well-being is carefully monitored with several different tests. Regular ultrasounds for fetal size may be ordered, as well as ultrasound evaluation of the umbilical cord. In the third trimester, routine nonstress tests (see Box 3.6) and BPPs (see Table 1.2) are ordered to assess for fetal well-being.

Treatment

If the fetus is compromised and there is imminent concern for fetal demise, the decision may be made to end the pregnancy prematurely. If imminent birth seems advisable prior to 34 weeks, maternal glucocorticoids are administered to encourage more rapid fetal lung development (Lausman et al., 2014).

Care Considerations

The diagnosis of IUGR is frightening for families, who worry about the fetus and are uncertain about pregnancy outcomes as well as the long- and short-term implications for the offspring once born. It is a nursing responsibility to ensure that families have the information they need to aid them to make the required care decisions both during and after pregnancy.

Amniotic Fluid Volume Disorders

Amniotic fluid starts forming approximately 12 days after conception. It serves as a protective buffer for the pregnancy and allows for relative freedom of fetal growth and movement. Initially, the source of the fluid is not the fetus but rather the mother via the placenta. At about mid pregnancy, a primary

contributor of amniotic fluid is the fetal kidneys. Fetal lungs also excrete fluid that contributes to the volume of the amniotic fluid. As the pregnancy progresses, the amniotic fluid is cycled out by the fetus swallowing it, as well as through the intramembranous pathway between the amniotic fluid and the maternal circulation. Amniotic fluid volume increases until week 34 to 36 of gestation, after which it either stabilizes or gradually declines. It is completely replaced on a daily basis.

Under certain circumstances, however, amniotic fluid volume can exceed or fall below expected values. Two concerning disorders related to amniotic fluid volume are polyhydramnios and oligohydramnios.

Polyhydramnios

Polyhydramnios, also sometimes referred to as **hydramnios**, is a condition of excessive amniotic fluid.

Prevalence

It may be diagnosed in the second or the third trimester and complicates 1% to 2% of pregnancies (Pri-Paz, Khalek, Fuchs, & Simpson, 2012).

Etiology

Polyhydramnios results from a mismatch between the production and the absorption of amniotic fluid, generally between fetal swallowing and fetal urinary elimination. Approximately 40% of cases of polyhydramnios are **idiopathic**, which means the cause of the problem is unknown (Abele et al., 2012). Most known causes of polyhydramnios are fetal in origin, the most common of these being congenital anomalies of the fetal gut, heart, and neural tube. Macrosomia is also associated with polyhydramnios and is likely a complication of diabetes. When polyhydramnios is diagnosed with a twin pregnancy, the suspected cause is twin-to-twin transfusion.

Course in Pregnancy

Polyhydramnios is associated with poor outcomes for the fetus and for the mother. Overall, the rate of perinatal death increases 5-fold with polyhydramnios (Pilliod et al., 2015). Other problems resulting from polyhydramnios include preterm labor, birth defects, postpartum hemorrhage due to uterine overdistension, and placental abruption. Poor fetal outcomes include meconium-stained fluid, poor tolerance of labor, low Apgar scores, and increased neonatal intensive care unit admissions related to fetal hypoxia in utero. Other complications may include maternal respiratory problems from overdistension of the uterus, poor fetal positioning for labor, and cord prolapse.

Assessment

Amniotic fluid volume can be assessed in two ways. The first is by measuring the vertical depth of the four largest pockets of amniotic fluid during ultrasound and then totaling the results to produce the amniotic fluid index (AFI). Values greater than 20 to 25 cm are considered abnormal. A second method requires measuring only the largest vertical pocket (LVP). A value of equal to or greater than 8 cm is considered polyhydramnios.

Polyhydramnios that is asymptomatic is categorized as mild or moderate and is followed by serial BPPs and nonstress tests weekly or biweekly.

Treatment

If the polyhydramnios is severe and causes symptoms such as maternal discomfort or uterine contractions, two interventions may be offered through 34 weeks of pregnancy. The first intervention, **amnioreduction**, removes some of the excess amniotic fluid. The procedure may need to be repeated every 24 to 72 hours as the fluid regenerates. The second intervention, administration of the NSAID indomethacin, may help reduce and stabilize amniotic fluid, although it should not be used past 34 weeks of gestation because of concerns about constriction of the fetal ductus arteriosus (this is a class effect, meaning that it is a side effect of all NSAIDs). After 34 weeks of gestation, fetal lungs are assessed for maturity and maternal corticosteroids given as necessary. Typically, labor is induced or a cesarean section performed.

Oligohydramnios

In contrast to polyhydramnios, oligohydramnios is a condition of less amniotic fluid than anticipated for gestational age.

Etiology

The cause of the oligohydramnios often goes unidentified with moderately low or borderline AFI and LVP measurements. Common reasons for moderate or severe oligohydramnios in the second trimester of pregnancy are fetal anomalies and PROM. In the third trimester, PROM and fetal anomalies continue to contribute to oligohydramnios, as does uteroplacental insufficiency, in which there is insufficient blood flow to the placenta to keep up with the needs of the pregnancy. Not surprisingly, given the association with uteroplacental insufficiency, IUGR commonly co-occurs.

Course in Pregnancy

Pregnancies with oligohydramnios generally have a poor prognosis. Oligohydramnios in the third trimester is associated with preterm birth and early induction or cesarean section because of concerns about fetal well-being.

Assessment

Assessment for oligohydramnios is similar to that for polyhydramnios. In terms of a quantitative measurement, the diagnostic AFI for oligohydramnios is equal to or less than 5 cm, and the LVP is equal to or less than 2 cm. Often, the first indication of oligohydramnios is a pregnancy that measures smaller than expected on a routine examination.

Treatment

Amnioinfusion is the process of adding fluid, often Ringer's lactate, into the amniotic sac to correct oligohydramnios. This may be done to optimize an ultrasound investigation or to aid in cephalic version (rotation of the fetus into a more optimal position for birth). It is not uncommon for a pregnancy complicated by oligohydramnios to involve a fetus that has failed to rotate into the vertex position for birth. Amnioinfusion may also be used during labor after the rupture of membranes to help "float" a compressed umbilical cord.

Care Considerations

Simple maternal hydration by drinking 2 L of water over 2 hours may help correct some cases of oligohydramnios, indicating maternal hydration is a factor in some cases (Gizzo et al., 2015).

Dermatoses of Late Pregnancy

Certain dermatologic conditions are specific to late pregnancy and the postpartum period. These include intrahepatic cholestasis of pregnancy, **pruritic urticarial papules and plaques of pregnancy** (PUPPP), pemphigoid gestationis, and **pustular psoriasis of pregnancy** (PPP).

Intrahepatic Cholestasis

Impaired bile flow from the liver, a condition known as **intrahepatic cholestasis**, occurs in 0.5% to 2.4% of pregnancies in the third trimester. Maternal bile acids pass the placenta, creating risks for preterm delivery, intrauterine demise, respiratory distress syndrome, and meconium-stained amniotic fluid (Phillips & Boyd, 2015).

Clinical manifestations of cholestasis in the pregnant woman include uncomfortable pruritus (particularly of the hands and feet), clay-colored stools, dark urine, fatigue, and, rarely, jaundice or right upper quadrant pain. Serum bile acid concentrations are almost always elevated with the condition, as are liver function tests.

Women may be treated with topical preparations to control pruritus and the oral medication ursodeoxycholic acid to reduce the concentration of bile acids. Women with cholestasis may find cold baths and compresses comforting. Women typically undergo antepartum fetal assessment by BPP or nonstress test twice weekly until delivery. The pregnancy is generally delivered by 36 or 37 weeks of gestation. Cholestasis and its symptoms resolve with the end of the pregnancy.

Pruritic Urticarial Papules and Plaques of Pregnancy

PUPPP is also referred to as polymorphic eruption of pregnancy. It affects women in the last few weeks of pregnancy or in the early postpartum period, most often in those who are experiencing their first pregnancy. PUPPP presents as highly pruritic papules within striae and may be associated with an inflammatory process caused by the stretching of the skin. It generally resolves within a few weeks after delivery. Treatment is typically a topical corticosteroid and an antihistamine such as loratadine or cetirizine. PUPPP is not harmful to the fetus.

Pemphigoid Gestationis

Pemphigoid gestationis is also referred to as herpes gestationis and is a rare autoimmune condition that typically occurs in the second or third trimester of pregnancy. It presents as acute pruritus followed by plaques or papules that typically appear on the abdomen but may appear over the entire body. Most cases resolve within a month or so after delivery but may recur with menstruation, the use of hormonal contraception, or in future pregnancies. It is diagnosed by biopsy. It is generally treated with topical or systemic corticosteroids. There is an increased risk for preterm birth and small-for-gestational-age neonates.

Pustular Psoriasis of Pregnancy

PPP generally presents in the third trimester, although it may manifest earlier in the pregnancy or postpartum. It is a form of psoriasis specific to pregnancy. Plaques typically start on the flexor surfaces but spread to the trunk and extremities. In some cases, erosions of the oral mucosa and esophagus may develop, and finger and toe nails may be affected. The condition is typically not pruritic as are other skin conditions of pregnancy, but systemic symptoms may include gastrointestinal distress, anorexia, malaise, fever, and tetany. Diagnosis is clinical or by biopsy. Often, leukocytosis, elevated erythrocyte sedimentation, and hypocalcemia are present. The fetus is monitored by BPP and/or nonstress test, and early delivery may be indicated as the condition is associated with placental insufficiency that may lead to stillbirth, respiratory distress, meconium aspiration syndrome, and fetal growth restriction. Maternal hypocalcemia must be corrected. Patients are generally treated with systemic corticosteroids, cyclosporine, or infliximab.

Think Critically

1. Draw a diagram that shows the anatomy of a twin pregnancy when the ovum divides, following fertilization.
2. Describe a nursing intervention that may be helpful for a patient with hyperemesis gravidarum.
3. How would you counsel a woman who is expressing guilt about a spontaneous abortion?
4. What aspects of a patient's history would make you concerned that she may have an ectopic pregnancy?
5. How would you explain to a patient with a recent history of molar pregnancy the importance of using a highly reliable form of birth control for the next 6 months to a year?
6. Your patient is being released from the hospital after evaluation for preeclampsia. How would you explain to her the warning signs that her preeclampsia has progressed and may cause serious complications?
7. You are working as a nurse in an outpatient clinic. You are caring for a patient with a new diagnosis of gestational diabetes. She is very concerned but states that she just doesn't know how she should change her diet. How do you help educate her?
8. You have a 30-year-old patient who is pregnant for the first time. She was diagnosed with genital herpes 10 years ago and has heard that she will not be able to give birth vaginally as a result. What do you tell her?
9. Your patient had a pregnancy loss at 18 weeks with her last pregnancy after an acute infection. She's wondering if her cervix "will need to be stitched up" with this pregnancy. What do you tell her?
10. Name three anatomic or physiologic changes in pregnancy that should be considered in a trauma situation involving a pregnant woman.
11. What's the difference between symmetric and asymmetric intrauterine growth restriction?
12. Why are pregnant women who are at risk for preterm birth given glucocorticoid injections?
13. On the basis of the reading about oligohydramnios, what might be a particularly important consideration for a woman who lives in a hot climate?

References

Abalos, E., Cuesta, C., Grosso, A., Chou, D., & Say, L. (2013). Global and regional estimates of preeclampsia and eclampsia: A systematic review. *European Journal of Obstetrics and Gynecology and Reproductive Biology, 170*(1), 1–7.

Abas, M. N., Tan, P. C., Azmi, N., & Omar, S. Z. (2014). Ondansetron compared with metoclopramide for hyperemesis gravidarum: A randomized controlled trial. *Obstetrics and Gynecology, 123*(6), 1272–1279.

Abele, H., Starz, S., Hoopmann, M., Yazdi, B., Rall, K., & Kagan, K. (2012). Idiopathic polyhydramnios and postnatal abnormalities. *Fetal Diagnosis and Therapy, 32*(4), 251.

Alfirevic, Z., Stampalija, T., Roberts, D., & Jorgensen, A. (2012). Cervical stitch (cerclage) for preventing preterm birth in singleton pregnancy. *Cochrane Database of Systematic Reviews,* (4), CD008991.

American College of Obstetricians and Gynecologists. (2013, reaffirmed 2016). Weight gain during pregnancy, committee opinion 548. *Obstetrics and Gynecology, 121,* 210–212.

American College of Obstetricians and Gynecologists. (2015). Practice bulletin no. 151: Cytomegalovirus, parvovirus B19, varicella zoster, and toxoplasmosis in pregnancy. *Obstetrics and Gynecology, 125*(6), 1510.

American Congress of Obstetricians and Gynecologists' Committee on Practice Bulletins—Obstetrics. (2016). Practice bulletin no. 173: Fetal macrosomia. *Obstetrics and Gynecology, 128*(5), e195.

American College of Obstetricians and Gynecologists, Task Force on Hypertension in Pregnancy. (2013). Hypertension in pregnancy. Report of the American College of Obstetricians and Gynecologists' Task Force on Hypertension in Pregnancy. *Obstetrics and Gynecology, 122*(5), 1122.

Balsells, M., García-Patterson, A., Solà I Roqué, M., Gich, I., & Corcoy, R. (2015). Glibenclamide, metformin, and insulin for the treatment of gestational diabetes: A systematic review and meta-analysis. *BMJ, 350,* h102.

Bardos, J., Hercz, D., Friedenthal, J., Missmer, S. A., & Williams, Z. (2015). A national survey on public perceptions of miscarriage. *Obstetrics and Gynecology, 125*(6), 1313–1320.

Benova, L., Mohamoud, Y., Calvert, C., & Abu-Raddad, L. (2014). Vertical transmission of hepatitis C virus: Systematic review and meta-analysis. *Clinical Infectious Diseases, 59*(6), 765.

Berhan, Y., & Berhan, A. (2015). Should magnesium sulfate be administered to women with mild pre-eclampsia? A systematic review of published reports on eclampsia. *Journal of Obstetrics and Gynaecology Research, 41*(6), 831.

Berkowitz, R., & Goldstein, D. (2013). Current advances in the management of gestational trophoblastic disease. *Gynecologic Oncology, 128*(1), 3–5.

Berzan, E., Doyle, R., & Brown, C. M. (2014). Treatment of preeclampsia: Current approach and future perspectives. *Current Hypertension Reports, 16,* 473.

Biggio, J. (2013). Bed rest in pregnancy: Time to put the issue to rest. *Obstetrics and Gynecology, 121*(6), 1158–1160.

Blackburn, S. (2014). *Maternal, fetal, and neonatal physiology: A clinical perspective* (4th ed.). Philadelphia, PA: Saunders.

Blumer, I., Hadar, E., Hadden, D., Jovanović, L., Mestman, J., Murad, M., & Yogev, Y. (2013). Diabetes and pregnancy: An endocrine society clinical practice guideline. *Journal of Clinical Endocrinology and Metabolism, 98*(11), 4227–4249.

Brown, J., Martis, R., Hughes, B., Rowan, J., & Crowther, C. (2017). Oral anti-diabetic pharmacological therapies for the treatment of women with gestational diabetes. *Cochrane Database of Systematic Reviews,* (1), CD011967.

Capmas, P., Bouyer, J., & Fernandez, H. (2014). Treatment of ectopic pregnancies in 2014: New answers to some old questions. *Fertility and Sterilization, 101*(3), 615–620.

Caritis, S., & Hebert, M. (2013). A pharmacologic approach to the use of glyburide in pregnancy. *Obstetrics and Gynecology, 121*(6), 1309.

Committee on Practice Bulletins-Obstetrics. (2013). Practice Bulletin No. 137: Gestational diabetes mellitus. *Obstetrics and Gynecology, 122*(2), 406.

Coombes, C. P. (2015). Exercise guidelines for gestational diabetes mellitus. *World Journal of Diabetes, 6*(8), 1033–1044.

Crowther, C., Brown, J., McKinlay, C., & Middleton, P. (2014). Magnesium sulphate for preventing preterm birth in threatened preterm labour. *Cochrane Database of Systematic Reviews,* (8), CD001060.

Dehghan, F., Haerian, B. S., Muniandy, S., Yusof, A., Dragoo, J. L., & Salleh, N. (2014). The effect of relaxin on the musculoskeletal system. *Scandinavian Journal of Medicine and Science in Sports, 24*(4), e220–e229.

Delaney, S., Gardella, C., Saracino, M., Magaret, A., & Wald, A. (2014). Seroprevalence of herpes simplex virus type 1 and 2 among pregnant women, 1989–2010. *JAMA, 312*(7), 746–748.

Denniston, M., Jiles, R., Drobeniuc, J., Klevens, R., Ward, J., McQuillan, G., & Holmberg, S. (2014). Chronic hepatitis C virus infection in the United States, National Health and Nutrition Examination Survey 2003 to 2010. *Annals of Internal Medicine, 160*(5), 293.

Fletcher, S., Watermanb, H., Nelsona, L., Carterc, L., Dwyerd, L., Robertsc, C., . . . Kitchener, H. (2015). Holistic assessment of women with hyperemesis gravidarum: A randomised controlled trial. *International Journal of Nursing Studies, 52*(11), 1669–1677.

Fong, A., Chau, C., Pan, D., & Ogunyemi, D. (2013). Clinical morbidities, trends, and demographics of eclampsia: A population-based study. *American Journal of Obstetrics and Gynecology, 209*(3), 229.e1.

Forbes, J., Alimenti, A., Singer, J., Brophy, J., Bitnun, A., Samson, L., . . . Read, S. (2012). A national review of vertical HIV transmission. *AIDS, 26*(6), 757–763.

Gizzo, S., Noventa, M., Vitagliano, A., Dall'Asta, A., D'Antona, D., Aldrich, C., . . . Patrelli, T. (2015). An update on maternal hydration strategies for amniotic fluid improvement in isolated oligohydramnios and normohydramnios: Evidence from a systematic review of literature and meta-analysis. *PLoS One, 10*(12), e0144334.

Grooten, I. J., Mol, B. W., van der Post, J. A., Ris-Stalpers, C., Kok, M., Bais, J. M., . . . Painter, R. C. (2016). Early nasogastric tube feeding in optimising treatment for hyperemesis gravidarum: the MOTHER randomised controlled trial (Maternal and Offspring outcomes after Treatment of HyperEmesis by Refeeding). *BMC Pregnancy and Childbirth, 16*(22).

Grooten, I. J., Vinke, M. E., Roseboom, T. J., & Painter, R. C. (2015). A systematic review and meta-analysis of the utility of corticosteroids in the treatment of hyperemesis gravidarum. *Nutrition and Metabolic Insights, 8*(Suppl. 1), 23–32.

Hamilton, B. E., Martin, J. A., Osterman, M. J., Curtin, S. C., & Mathews, T. (2015). Births: Final data for 2014. *National Vital Statistics Reports, 64*(12), 1–64.

Hehir, M. P., Mctiernan, A., Martin, A., Carroll, S., Gleeson, R., & Malone, F. D. (2015). Improved perinatal mortality in twins—Changing practice and technologies. *American Journal of Perinatology, 33*(1), 84–89.

Henderson, J. T., Whitlock, E. P., O'Connor, E., Senger, C. A., Thompson, J. H., & Rowland, M. G. (2014). Low-dose aspirin for prevention of morbidity

and mortality from preeclampsia: A systematic evidence review for the U.S. Preventive Services Task Force. *Annals of Internal Medicine, 160*(10), 695–703.

Hyde, T., Schmid, D., & Cannon, M. (2010). Cytomegalovirus seroconversion rates and risk factors: Implications for congenital CMV. *Reviews in Medical Virology, 20*(5), 311.

Iams, J., Cebrik, D., Lynch, C., Behrendt, N., & Das, A. (2011). The rate of cervical change and the phenotype of spontaneous preterm birth. *American Journal of Obstetrics and Gynecology, 205*(2), 130.e1.

Jordan, R., Engstrom, J., Marfell, J., & Farley, C. (2014). *Prenatal and postnatal care: A woman-centered approach.* Chichester, England: Wiley.

Kanter, J. R., Boulet, S. L., Kawwass, J. F., Jamieson, D. J., & Kissin, D. M. (2015). Trends and correlates of monozygotic twinning after single embryo transfer. *Obstetrics and Gynecology, 125*(1), 111–117.

King, T., Brucker, M., Kriebs, J., Fahey, J., Gregor, C., & Varney, H. (2015). *Varney's midwifery.* Burlington, MA: Jones & Bartlett.

Kirk, E., Bottomley, C., & Bourne, T. (2014). Diagnosing ectopic pregnancy and current concepts in the management of pregnancy of unknown location. *Human Reproduction Update, 20*(2), 250–261.

Kobayashi, H. (2015, October). The impact of maternal-fetal genetic conflict situations on the pathogenesis of preeclampsia. *Biochemical Genetics, 53*(9), 223–234.

Kulkarni, A., Jamieson, D. J., Kissi, N. D., Gallo, M., Macaluso, M., & Adashi, E. (2013). Fertility treatments and multiple births in the United States. *New England Journal of Medicine, 369*(23), 2218–2225.

Kutteh, W. H. (2014). Recurrent pregnancy loss. *Obstetrics and Gynecology Clinic, 41*(1), xi–xiii.

Lausman, A., Kingdom, J., Gagnon, R., Basso, M. H., Crane, J. G., Delisle, M.-F., . . . Sanderson, F. (2014). Intrauterine growth restriction: Screening, diagnosis, and management. *Journal of Obstetrics and Gynaecology Canada, 35*(8), 741–748.

Lin, K., & Fajardo, K. (2008). Screening for asymptomatic bacteriuria in adults: Evidence for the U.S. Preventive Services Task Force reaffirmation recommendation statement. *Annals of Internal Medicine, 149*(1), W20.

Lipman, S., Cohen, S., Einav, S., Jeejeebhoy, F., Mhyre, J. M., Morrison, L. J., . . . Carvalho, B. (2014). The Society for Obstetric Anesthesia and Perinatology consensus statement on the management of cardiac arrest in pregnancy. *Anesthesia and Analgesia, 118*(5), 1003–1016.

Little, S., Edlow, A., Thomas, A., & Smith, N. (2012). Estimated fetal weight by ultrasound: A modifiable risk factor for cesarean delivery? *American Journal of Obstetrics and Gynecology, 207*(4), 309.

Liu, B., Roberts, C., Clarke, M., Jorm, L., Hunt, J., & Ward, J. (2013). Chlamydia and gonorrhoea infections and the risk of adverse obstetric outcomes: A retrospective cohort study. *Sexually Transmitted Infections, 89*(8), 672–678.

Lo, J. O., Mission, J. F., & Caughey, A. B. (2013). Hypertensive disease of pregnancy and maternal mortality. *Current Opinion in Obstetrics and Gynecology, 25*(2), 124–132.

Longo, S., Bollani, L., Decembrino, L., Comite, A. D., Angelini, M., & Stronati, M. (2013). Short-term and long-term sequelae in intrauterine growth retardation (IUGR). *The Journal of Maternal-Fetal and Neonatal Medicine, 26*(3), 222–225.

Lorenz, R. P. (2014). What is new in bed rest in pregnancy? Best articles from the past year. *Obstetrics and Gynecology, 124*(2), 377–378.

Mandelbrot, L., Tubiana, R., Le Chenadec, J., Dollfus, C., Faye, A., Pannier, E., . . . S. (2015). No perinatal HIV-1 transmission from women with effective antiretroviral therapy starting before conception. *Clinical Infectious Diseases, 61*(11), 1715.

McCall, C. A., Grimes, D. A., & Lyerly, A. D. (2013, June). "Therapeutic" bed rest in pregnancy: Unethical and unsupported by data. *Obstetrics and Gynecology, 121*(6), 1305–1308.

McNamara, H., Crowther, C., & Brown, J. (2015). Different treatment regimens of magnesium sulphate for tocolysis in women in preterm labour. *Cochrane Database of Systematic Reviews,* (12), CD011200.

Melamed, N., Ray, J., Hladunewich, M., Cox, B., & Kingdom, J. (2014). Gestational hypertension and preeclampsia: Are they the same disease? *Journal of Obstetrics and Gynaecology Canada, 36*(7), 642–747.

Menon, S., Colins, J., & Barnhart, K. (2007). Establishing a human chorionic gonadotropin cutoff to guide methotrexate treatment of ectopic pregnancy: A systematic review. *Fertility and Sterility, 87*(3), 481.

Miller, E., Cradock-Watson, J., & Pollock, T. (1982). Consequences of confirmed maternal rubella at successive stages of pregnancy. *The Lancet, 1*(8302), 781.

Minassian, C., Thomas, S., Williams, D., Campbell, O., & Smeeth, L. (2013). Acute maternal infection and risk of pre-eclampsia: A population-based case-control study. *PLoS One, 8*(9), e73047.

Mitchell-Jones, N., Gallos, I., Farren, J., Tobias, A., Bottomley, C., & Bourne, T. (2017). Psychological morbidity associated with hyperemesis gravidarum: A systematic review and meta-analysis. *British Journal of Obstetrics and Gynaecology, 124*(1), 20–30.

Monson, M. S., & Silver, R. (2015). Multifetal gestation: Mode of delivery. *Clinical Obstetrics and Gynecology, 58*(3), 690–702.

Morse, C., Sammel, M., Shaunik, A., Allen-Taylor, L., Oberfoell, N., Takacs, P., . . . Barnhart, K. (2012). Performance of human chorionic gonadotropin curves in women at risk for ectopic pregnancy: exceptions to the rules. *Fertility and Sterility, 97*(1), 101.e2–106.e2.

Moyer, V. (2014). Screening for gestational diabetes mellitus: U.S. Preventive Services Task Force recommendation statement. *Annals of Internal Medicine, 160*(6), 414.

Ngan, S., & Seckl, M. (2007). Gestational trophoblastic neoplasia management: An update. *Current Opinion in Oncology, 19*(5), 486–491.

Patrelli, T. S., Dall'asta, A., Gizzoa, S., Pedrazzic, G., Piantellia, G., Jasonnibi, V. M., & Modenaa, A. B. (2012). Calcium supplementation and prevention of preeclampsia: A meta-analysis. *The Journal of Maternal-Fetal and Neonatal Medicine, 25*(12), 2570–2574.

Phillips, C., & Boyd, M. (2015). Intrahepatic cholestasis of pregnancy. *Nursing for Women's Health, 19*(1), 46–57. doi:10.1111/1751-486X.12175

Picone, O., Vauloup-Fellous, C., Cordier, A., Guitton, S., Senat, M., Fuchs, F., . . . Benachi, A. (2013). A series of 238 cytomegalovirus primary infections during pregnancy: Description and outcome. *Prenatal Diagnosis, 33*(8), 751–758.

Pilliod, R., Page, J., Burwick, R., Kaimal, A., Cheng, Y., & Caughey, A. (2015). The risk of fetal death in nonanomalous pregnancies affected by polyhydramnios. *American Journal of Obstetrics and Gynecology, 212*(1), S17–S18.

Practice Committee of American Society for Reproductive Medicine. (2013). Definitions of infertility and recurrent pregnancy loss: A committee opinion. *Fertility and Sterility, 99*(1), 63.

Pri-Paz, S., Khalek, N., Fuchs, K., & Simpson, L. (2012). Maximal amniotic fluid index as a prognostic factor in pregnancies complicated by polyhydramnios. *Ultrasound in Obstetrics and Gynecology, 39*(6), 648–653.

Redelmeier, D., May, S., Thiruchelvam, D., & Barrett, J. (2014). Pregnancy and the risk of a traffic crash. *Canadian Medical Association Journal, 186*(10), 742–750.

Ryan, E., & Al-Agha, R. (2014). Glucose control during labor and delivery. *Current Diabetes Reports, 14*(1), 450.

Sibai, B. (1990). The HELLP syndrome (hemolysis, elevated liver enzymes, and low platelets): Much ado about nothing? *American Journal of Obstetrics and Gynecology, 162*(2), 311.

Simpson, L. (2013). Twin-twin transfusion syndrome. *American Journal of Obstetrics and Gynecology, 208*(1), 3–18.

Smaill, F., & Vazquez, J. (2015). Antibiotics for asymptomatic bacteriuria in pregnancy. *Cochrane Database of Systematic Reviews,* (8), CD000490.

Sosa, C., Althabe, F., Belizán, J., & Bergel, E. (2015). Bed rest in singleton pregnancies for preventing preterm birth. *Cochrane Database of Systematic Reviews,* (3), CD003581.

Staras, S., Dollard, S., Radford, K., Flanders, W., Pass, R., & Cannon, M. (2006). Seroprevalence of cytomegalovirus infection in the United States, 1988–1994. *Clinical Infectious Diseases, 43*(9), 1143.

Suhag, A., & Berghella, V. (2013). Intrauterine Growth Restriction (IUGR): Etiology and diagnosis. *Current Obstetrics and Gynecology Reports, 2*(2), 102–111.

Tassopoulos, N., Papaevangelou, G., Sjogren, M., Roumeliotou-Karayannis, A., Gerin, J., & Purcell, R. (1987). Natural history of acute hepatitis B surface antigen-positive hepatitis in Greek adults. *Gastroenterology, 96*(2), 1844.

Taylor, T. (2014). Treatment of nausea and vomiting in pregnancy. *Australian Prescriber, 37*(2), 42–45.

Wilcox, A., Weinberg, C., O'Connor, J., Baird, D., Schlatterer, J., Canfield, R., . . . Nisula, B. (1988). Incidence of early loss of pregnancy. *New England Journal of Medicine, 319*(4), 189.

Wing, D., Fassett, M., & Getahun, D. (2014). Acute pyelonephritis in pregnancy: An 18-year retrospective analysis. *American Journal of Obstetrics and Gynecology, 310*(3), 219.e1–219.e6.

Workowski, K., & Bolan, G. (2015). Sexually transmitted diseases treatment guidelines, 2015. *MMWR Recommendations and Reports, 64*(RR-03), 1.

Suggested Readings

Pearce, C., & Martin, S. R. (2016). Trauma and considerations unique to pregnancy. *Obstetrics and Gynecology Clinics, 43*(4), 791–808.

Preeclampsia Foundation. Retrieved from https://www.preeclampsia.org

21 Complications Occurring Before Labor and Delivery

Approximately 90% of births happen after 37 weeks of gestation, and 76% of births result from spontaneous labor (Martin, Hamilton, Osterman, Driscoll, & Mathews, 2017). Birth is not always so straightforward, however. This chapter covers some variations of both preterm and term pregnancies as they approach birth.

Premature Rupture of Membranes

Premature rupture of membranes (PROM) is the rupture and leakage of the amniotic sac prior to the start of contractions at or after 37 weeks of gestation. When the rupture occurs prior to 37 weeks of gestation, it is called preterm premature rupture of membranes (PPROM).

Prognosis

An accurate diagnosis is important because PROM presents an increased risk for prolapse of the cord, abruption of the placenta, cord compression, neonatal intensive care unit (NICU) admissions, and chorioamnionitis (Middleton, Shepherd, Flenady, McBain, & Crowther, 2017).

Assessment

The classic presentation of PROM is a gush of fluid from the vagina, although the leak may be more gradual and experienced instead as a sensation of increased vaginal wetness.

Speculum Vaginal Examination

The nurse should not perform an internal digital examination of the cervix when PROM is suspected because of the risk of infection. The nurse or obstetric provider may, however, perform a sterile speculum examination to assess for pooling of fluid in the vaginal vault and/or leakage of fluid from the cervical os (see Step-by-Step Skills 7.1). If no fluid is visualized, asking the pregnant woman to cough or bear down may elicit the leakage of fluid from the cervical os.

Nitrazine pH Test

The nurse may also use Nitrazine paper or a Nitrazine swab to assess the pH level of the leaked fluid. The pH of the vagina is typically 3.8 to 4.2, or acidic, whereas the pH of amniotic fluid is typically 7.0 to 7.3, or alkaline. Normal vaginal fluid produces shades of yellow and light green on Nitrazine paper, whereas amniotic fluid and cervical mucus produce shades of darker green and blue (see Fig. 1.12). False positives occur rarely. A false negative may occur if the leakage is intermittent, and a false positive may occur in the presence of blood, soap, semen, and some infections.

Assessment for Meconium Staining

Once it is confirmed that the fluid is amniotic, the nurse should assess it for staining with meconium. Meconium-stained fluid is associated with an increased risk of chorioamnionitis, nonreassuring fetal heart rate patterns, fetal hypoxia, and meconium aspiration by the fetus. However, it is also produced as a normal function of fetal maturity and is present in 3% to 14% of births (Chettri, Adhisivam, & Bhat, 2015).

Arborization Testing

An additional test that is used to confirm the presence of amniotic fluid is for arborization (ferning; see Fig. 1.13). In arborization testing, the nurse takes a sample of fluid from the vaginal vault, places on a slide, and allows it to dry for 10 minutes. When examined microscopically, amniotic fluid has a delicate pattern (Fig. 1.13). A false negative may occur if the sample is heavily diluted.

Laboratory Tests

Laboratory tests are also available and may be used in cases in which the diagnosis is unclear, such as with negative clinical tests, a positive patient history, or an ultrasound evaluation revealing low fluid volume. Commercial tests for PROM include AmniSure, ACTIM PROM, and ROM Plus. Fetal fibronectin (fFN) in the vaginal fluid suggests PROM but may be present with any disruption of the connection between the decidua and chorion, not just membrane rupture. Alpha-fetoprotein in the vaginal fluids is also suggestive of rupture of membranes, but the presence of blood may cause a false-positive result. Other reasons a patient may report vaginal discharge are normal leukorrhea of pregnancy, vaginal infection, and involuntary loss of urine.

Other Considerations and Evaluations

If PROM is confirmed, the nurse confirms the gestational age of the pregnancy. Term PROM requires different care considerations and management than PPROM (see the next section). The nurse should assess fetal well-being by asking the mother to describe fetal movement and by evaluating the fetal heart rate. A nonstress test (NST) and/or biophysical profile (BPP) may be ordered. As occurs with the initial presentation of a laboring mother, fetal position is confirmed by Leopold's maneuvers (see Fig. 1.7). Ultrasound may be used in the case of an inconclusive examination. The nurse should also assess the mother for contractions as well as signs of chorioamnionitis, including uterine tenderness and fever.

Treatment

Approximately 90% of women with PROM at term go into labor within 24 hours of PROM, as do 50% of women with PPROM (Lyons, 2015). Active management involves induction of labor within 24 hours of PROM, whereas expectant management involves an intended delay of induction of over 24 hours. Active management is associated with a reduction in chorioamnionitis and NICU admissions. There is no difference in the rates of cesarean and operative vaginal delivery, neonatal sepsis, cord prolapse, and neonatal death or in Apgar scores at 5 minutes between active and expectant management for PROM (Middleton et al., 2017). Induction with oxytocin without further cervical ripening is common after PROM, although a ripening agent, such as misoprostol or dinoprostone, or a balloon cervical catheter may also be used for women with a Bishop score under 8 (see Analyze the Evidence 1.1).

In Chapter 7, Hannah's membranes ruptured at term. Because she was group B streptococcus (GBS)–positive, she was immediately started on intravenous (IV) antibiotics, and labor was induced because of the high risk for infection. Because of how ripe Hannah's cervix was, she received only oxytocin to induce labor and did not receive any cervical ripening agents. (Bess Gaskell, in Chapter 1, and Sophie Bloom, in Chapter 4, also experienced PROM and were given oxytocin to induce labor.)

Women without evidence of infection or other complications may instead choose, with their obstetric provider's support, not to induce within 24 hours. Women who choose expectant management over active management develop labor contractions spontaneously within 72 hours after PROM 95% of the time. The nurse should inform women, however, that the risk for chorioamnionitis and NICU admission does increase when labor is delayed for more than 24 hours (Middleton et al., 2017). Women who are being managed expectantly may choose, in consultation with their obstetric provider, to be hospitalized or to be managed at home. Women who are managed at home may be asked to monitor their temperature twice daily and report any changes in their discharge or fetal movement. Regardless of the choice of venue for management, additional fetal monitoring by NST and/or BPP may be ordered.

The use of antibiotic prophylaxis for PROM at term is not associated with improved outcomes (Saccone & Berghella, 2015a). Women who are GBS positive, however, should be treated (American College of Obstetricians and Gynecologists [ACOG], 2017).

Preterm Premature Rupture of Membranes

PPROM is spontaneous rupture of membranes prior to 37 weeks of gestation.

In Chapter 8, Gracie's waters broke at 33 weeks of gestation. Because her membranes ruptured prior to the start of contractions before the pregnancy was full term, this was considered PPROM.

Prevalence

PPROM complicates approximately 3% of pregnancies and is a factor in one third of preterm births (van der Heyden et al., 2013).

Etiology

Risk factors for PPROM include cigarette smoking, infections of the genital tract, previous PPROM, and any vaginal bleeding during the pregnancy. Most patients, however, do not have risk factors that are readily identifiable.

Prognosis

Infection related to PPROM, including chorioamnionitis, endometritis, and septicemia, is common. Infection with PPROM poses a greater overall risk for complications for the preterm newborn. A small number of PPROM pregnancies will be further complicated by placental abruption. It is not uncommon for a fetus to not assume a vertex position until after 34 weeks; thus, fetal malpresentation is common, particularly when complicated by oligohydramnios. This malpresentation also increases the risk for cord prolapse (see Chapter 22). Sustained PPROM earlier in pregnancy with oligohydramnios is associated with malformation of the lungs, bones, and face.

Assessment

The presentation of PPROM is similar to that of PROM. Monitoring is typically done in the hospital for women with PPROM, although it may occasionally be undertaken at home under close supervision. Major concerns are infection, cord prolapse, and precipitous labor. Regardless of the venue, the nurse must monitor women regularly for infection by assessing temperature

and uterine tenderness. The nurse should also regularly assess the woman's vital signs and contractions and the fetal heart rate.

If there is a question about fetal lung maturity (an uncertain gestational age, for example), amniotic fluid may be tested to assess for fetal lung maturity. Lung immaturity would be a reason to delay induction. Such testing is generally not performed prior to 32 weeks of gestation or after 39 weeks of gestation when the gestational age is reliable. All tests for fetal lung maturity are indirect measures of lung surfactant.

Treatment

Corticosteroids

Women with pregnancies under 34 weeks of gestation are given a course of steroid injections to promote lung maturity, prevent intraventricular hemorrhage brain bleeding, prevent necrotizing enterocolitis, and reduce the risk of neonatal death by 30% to 60% (Roberts, Brown, Medley, & Dalziel, 2017; see The Pharmacy 8.2). Routine administration of corticosteroids after 34 weeks of gestation is not well studied and is controversial (Saccone & Berghella, 2016).

Antibiotics

Because PPROM can be *caused* by infection but can also *result* in infection, a 1-week course of antibiotics is typically given for gestations of 37 weeks and under. The use of antibiotics results in a reduction of infection rates for both the mother and the offspring, a lesser need for surfactant and oxygen for the neonate after birth, and a reduction in abnormal ultrasounds of the fetal brain. The use of antibiotics may also help prolong the pregnancy (Kenyon, Boulvain, & Neilson, 2013). Multiple antibiotics are typically used, including azithromycin, ampicillin, and amoxicillin. Patients with a penicillin allergy should not use ampicillin or amoxicillin but may instead use a combination of other medications, including cephalexin and cefazolin or clindamycin and gentamicin. Azithromycin, however, is safe for patients with a penicillin allergy (Pierson, Gordon, & Haas, 2014). Women diagnosed with an infection, though, require therapeutic rather than prophylactic antibiotics.

Tocolytics

Tocolytics are medications used off label to prevent, suspend, or slow labor. They are often given for 48 hours to allow time for a full course of corticosteroid administration to the mother. Tocolytics are not associated with improved neonatal outcomes but are associated with an increased risk for chorioamnionitis. The use of tocolytics for PPROM is, thus, not universal and is somewhat controversial (Mackeen, Seibel-Seamon, Muhammad, Baxter, & Berghella, 2014). For further discussion of tocolytics, see the preterm labor and birth section.

Magnesium Sulfate

If delivery is anticipated within 24 hours, magnesium sulfate (the same medication used to prevent seizures with severe preeclampsia) is often administered to the mother if the gestation of the pregnancy is between 24 and 32 or 34 weeks. This brief period of administration is neuroprotective and is closely associated with a reduction in cerebral palsy for the neonate (Zeng, Xue, Tian, Sun, & An, 2016). Women receiving magnesium sulfate must be closely monitored for magnesium toxicity (see The Pharmacy 4.1 and Boxes 20.6 and 20.7).

Bed Rest

Although bed rest for PPROM has not been found efficacious for improving outcomes and is not believed by most physicians to be a useful intervention, a vast majority of women with PPROM will be put on bed rest (Bigelow, Factor, Miller, Weintraub, & Stone, 2016).

Preterm Delivery

Most women with a diagnosis of PPROM deliver within a week. It is relatively rare for the leakage to heal spontaneously, and artificial means of resealing the membranes are insufficiently supported by the evidence (Crowley, Grivell, & Dodd, 2016). A pregnancy complicated by PPROM may be delivered or managed expectantly. The patient and her obstetric care provider must consider many factors when deciding on their course of action, including especially gestational age, the presence of infection, fetal well-being, the degree of cervical ripening, the presence or absence of contractions, the availability of an NICU, and the presentation of the fetus. An induced delivery with PPROM is more likely in the presence of fetal compromise, maternal or fetal infection, or evidence of placental abruption. An earlier delivery may also be recommended if the fetal presentation creates a high risk for cord prolapse. In general, in the absence of these complications, delivery is not induced until 34 weeks of gestation, although labor and delivery may still occur spontaneously.

In the absence of other complications or contraindications, a vaginal birth is preferred. Induction may occur with oxytocin alone. In the case of an unripe cervix, misoprostol or dinoprostone may be used. Because of heightened concerns about infection with PPROM, clinicians may avoid using any means of mechanical ripening, such as a balloon catheter.

Midtrimester PPROM

Midtrimester PPROM is rupture of membranes before 23 weeks of gestation.

Prevalence

Midtrimester PPROM occurs in approximately 0.1% of pregnancies (Linehan et al., 2016).

Etiology

It may occur spontaneously or after an invasive procedure, such as amniocentesis.

Prognosis

Midtrimester PPROM is often followed by loss of the pregnancy, either induced or spontaneous (Linehan et al., 2016). Spontaneous "resealing" of the breech and accumulation of normal levels of amniotic fluid are rare, except in the case of a breech created during amniocentesis. Fewer than half of pregnancies with midtrimester PPROM are sustained for more than a week past the rupture.

The risks to the mother are the same as for later PPROM, and risks to the fetus are also similar. However, the risk of fetal demise is higher, with only half of fetuses born from 20 to 24 weeks of gestation with a pregnancy complicated by PPROM surviving. Of these, approximately a quarter have lifelong neurologic issues such as cerebral palsy, vision loss, deafness, and cognitive impairment (Kibel et al., 2016). Earlier gestational age of PPROM is also associated with a higher risk for placental abruption as well as placental retention after the birth of the fetus.

Care Considerations

This is a critical time of decision-making for families, who are called on to make decisions about the care of the neonate that may have lifelong implications for the offspring as well as the family. The nurse should provide compassionate counseling to the family about potential pregnancy outcomes. Information provided by the neonatology team both prior to and after the birth may be upsetting and confusing. Families may feel guilty and think that something they did caused the rupture. It is critical for the nurse to provide clear information and to practice active listening.

Preterm Labor and Birth

Preterm labor is defined as contractions that cervical change prior to 37 weeks. As many as 50% of women who experience labor preterm, however, go on to deliver at term. Preterm labor and birth may be induced or spontaneous. Indicated preterm births are intended to mitigate the problem that was endangering the mother and/or fetus. Common reasons for premature induction of labor are listed in Box 21.1.

Prevalence

In 2012, 7.7% of deliveries were prior to 37 weeks gestation. Of these births, 41.5% were indicated for the health of the mother

---

Box 21.1   Common Reasons for Premature Induction of Labor

- Placental problems
- History of uterine scarring
- Fetal grown restriction
- Chronic hypertension
- Preeclampsia
- Poorly controlled gestational diabetes
- Pregestational diabetes, poorly controlled or with vascular complications
- Preterm premature rupture of membranes

Adapted from American College of Obstetricians and Gynecologists. (2013b). ACOG committee opinion no. 560: Medically indicated late-preterm and early-term deliveries. *Obstet Gynecol, 121*(4), 908–910. doi:10.1097/01.AOG.0000428648.75548.00

and/or fetus and the remaining 58.5% occurred spontaneously (Gyamfi-Bannerman & Ananth, 2014). The preterm birth rate increased slightly from 9.57% of total births in 2014 to 9.63% in 2015. Prior to this, the rate of preterm births in the United States had been dropping steadily since 2007 (Martin et al., 2017). The Centers for Disease Control and Prevention categorizes preterm births as early (before 34 weeks of gestation) and late (from 34 to 36 weeks of gestation). The rate of early preterm births dropped slightly from 2.93% in 2007 to 2.76% in 2015. The rate of late-preterm births rose slightly from 6.82% to 6.87% during this same time (Martin et al., 2017). Pregnancies with twins, triplets, or higher-order multiples are far more likely to be delivered prematurely than singleton pregnancies, with half of twins and 9 out of 10 triplets being born prematurely (Martin et al., 2017).

Etiology

Common risk factors for spontaneous preterm birth are provided in Box 21.2. Whenever possible, the nurse should discuss risk factors with the woman prior to pregnancy and work to help mitigate them before the onset of preterm labor. Educating women about the increased risk of preterm birth associated with poor weight gain and smoking, for example, may encourage them to stop smoking and adopt a healthy diet. Approximately 40% pregnancies that end in preterm birth have no risk factors, however (Miller, Tita, & Grobman, 2015).

There are likely many different causes of preterm labor. Four that have been identified include an abnormally premature activation of a hormone cascade of the hypothalamic–pituitary–adrenal (HPA) axis of the mother or fetus, an exaggerated inflammatory response, placental bleeding (decidual hemorrhage or placental abruption), and uterine overdistension. These processes may be in place long before preterm labor is evident (Moroz & Simhan, 2014).

The HPA Axis

Women with abnormally high levels of physical or emotional stress may have twice the rate of preterm birth as those without, possibly because of stress hormones causing the premature activation of the HPA axis of the mother (Ding et al., 2014). A similar process may occur on the fetal side. A fetus subject to a stressor that leads to decreased perfusion of the placenta, such as abnormal placentation, may have premature activation of the HPA axis. Activation of the axis, either on the maternal or the fetal side, is thought to trigger a "placental clock" that limits the duration of the pregnancy and stimulates hormones that prompt uterine activity and initiate labor (Ding et al., 2014).

Inflammation

Inflammation caused by genitourinary infections and systemic inflammation from conditions such as periodontal disease are associated with preterm labor and birth. Up to half of the cases of preterm birth may be due to chorioamnionitis, either overt or occult (Donders et al., 2009). Features of the bacteria itself even in the absence of inflammation may promote preterm labor and birth. As mentioned previously, uteroplacental insufficiency and maternal stress may activate the HPA axis and prompt labor

---

Box 21.2 Risk Factors for Spontaneous Preterm Birth

- Low maternal education level
- Low maternal income level
- Infection
- Family history of preterm birth
- Pregnancy with more than one fetus
- Hypertension in pregnancy
- Substance abuse
- Tobacco and alcohol use
- Short maternal stature
- Poor weight gain in pregnancy
- Low or high body mass index
- Short duration between pregnancies
- High maternal stress
- Preexisting medical condition
- Fertility treatments
- First pregnancy
- Inadequate prenatal care
- Previous preterm birth
- Previous ectopic pregnancy or spontaneous or induced abortion
- Non-Hispanic black
- Adolescent pregnancy or pregnancy over the age of 35 y
- Uterine malformation
- Prior surgery on cervix

Adapted from Heaman, M., Kingston, D., Chalmers, B., Sauve, R., Lee, L., & Young, D. (2013). Risk factors for preterm birth and small-for-gestational-age births among Canadian women. *Paediatric and Perinatal Epidemiology, 27*(1), 54–61. doi:10.1111/ppe.12016; Prunet, C., Delnord, M., Saurel-Cubizolles, M. J., Goffinet, F., & Blondel, B. (2016). Risk factors of preterm birth in France in 2010 and changes since 1995: Results from the French National Perinatal Surveys. *Journal of Gynecology Obstetrics and Human Reproduction.* doi:10.1016/j.jgyn.2016.02.010; National Center for Chronic Disease Prevention and Health Promotion. (2016). *Premature birth.* Retrieved from https://www.cdc.gov/features/prematurebirth/index.html

---

prematurely, but they may also promote the production of proinflammatory mediators and an exaggerated inflammatory response that contributes to the initiation of labor (Christian, 2014).

Bleeding

Bleeding from the placenta and/or decidua may present as vaginal bleeding, may occur behind the placenta (retroplacental bleeding), or may be occult. Preterm birth associated with PPROM is particularly closely tied to placental bleeding and may result from hormonal cascades caused by the bleed, associated inflammation, or other causes (Buhimschi, Schatz, Krikun, Buhimschi, & Lockwood, 2010).

Uterine Overdistension

Uterine overdistension due to polyhydramnios, a multiple gestation, or other reasons is also associated with the initiation of preterm labor and birth. Distention of the uterus promotes activity of the uterine muscle, and it is likely the hormonal effects triggered by the distension cause an increase in oxytocin receptors and inflammation, which then increase contractions and cervical dilation (Adams Waldorf et al., 2015).

Prognosis

Preterm birth is the leading cause of death for children under the age of 5 years and resulted in nearly one million deaths in 2015 (World Health Organization, 2016). Death or lifelong health and developmental problems may be related to brain injury, infection, retinopathy of prematurity, and/or bronchopulmonary dysplasia (see Chapters 24 and 25). For reasons that are not clear, women who give birth spontaneously prematurely are at a higher risk for ischemic heart disease, stroke, and other cardiovascular disease for 12 to 35 years after the birth (Heida et al., 2016).

Assessment

Despite the many known risks for preterm labor and preterm birth, half of women who give birth prematurely have no risk factors, making it essential that the nurse educate all women about the signs and symptoms of preterm labor (Box 21.3). The symptoms of preterm labor, however, can be subtler than those for term labor and may feel similar to the discomforts of pregnancy. Although intense, regular, and progressive contractions are the subjective hallmark of labor, mild irregular contractions, known as Braxton Hicks contractions, are common throughout pregnancy and can be difficult to differentiate from the subtler presentation typical of preterm labor. Unlike Braxton Hicks contractions, however, contractions of preterm labor cause cervical changes. It is challenging for patients and providers to differentiate between contraction types, and of the women assessed for labor prior to 34 weeks of gestation due to contraction activity, only 13% deliver within the following week (Sotiriadis, Papatheodorou, Kavvadias, & Makrydimas, 2010).

When preterm labor is suspected, the nurse should assess for it promptly so that if it is occurring, there is time for interventions that may mitigate the harm of an early birth, such as the administration of glucocorticoids to reduce neonatal morbidity and mortality, magnesium sulfate to reduce the incidence of cerebral palsy, and antibiotics to prevent neonatal GBS infection and transfer to a hospital with adequate facilities to care for a preterm infant, as needed. Symptoms often abate with simple monitoring and self-care in the community, however (Patient Teaching 21.1).

Assessment for preterm labor can include taking a patient's history, conducting a physical examination, evaluating cervical length using ultrasound, and performing fFN testing, as well as follow-up evaluation for signs and symptoms.

Box 21.3 Symptoms of Preterm Labor

- Irregular contractions, often mild
- Report of "menstrual-like" cramping
- Low back pain
- Report of sensation of vaginal or pelvic pressure
- Light bleeding or spotting
- Bloody show

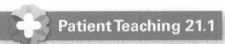

Patient Teaching 21.1

Self-Care for Symptoms of Preterm Labor

1. Call your obstetric provider or go to the birthing center right away if any of the following occur:
   a. Fluid leaking from your vagina
   b. Fishy or foul-smelling vaginal discharge
   c. Vaginal bleeding
   d. Contractions every 10 min or less for an hour
2. In the absence of the above symptoms, do the following:
   a. Drink two or three glasses of water: dehydration can cause Braxton Hicks contractions.
   b. Empty your bladder: a full bladder can cause the sensation of pelvic fullness and cramping.
   c. Lie on your side for an hour: Braxton Hicks contractions often resolve with rest.
3. If symptoms do not resolve, call your obstetric provider or go to the birthing center.
4. If symptoms DO resolve, resume light activity.
5. If symptoms return, call your obstetric provider or go to the birthing center.

Patient History and Physical Examination

The nurse should begin the assessment of the woman by taking a thorough history, as itemized in the PPROM section, and performing a physical examination. If PPROM is suspected, the examiner should take appropriate sterile cautions and not perform a digital examination to reduce the risk for infection. As with the assessment for PPROM, the examiner may perform a sterile speculum examination to examine the cervix. Cervical dilation of 3 cm or more supports a diagnosis of preterm labor. Blood from the cervical os supports the diagnosis of bleeding from the placenta, which is a trigger for preterm labor. An ultrasound is often done to assess for placental abruption and placenta previa and to assess cervical length.

Ultrasound Assessment of Cervical Length

The shorter the cervix as measured by ultrasound, usually transvaginal ultrasound, the greater the likelihood for labor. Similarly, the earlier the shortening is detected, the more likely preterm labor is to occur (Berghella, Baxter, & Hendrix, 2013). A longer cervix is associated with a reduced likelihood of an imminent birth. However, there is no threshold of length after which a birth is known to occur imminently, and even women with no measurable cervical length from 14 to 28 weeks of gestation may go on to deliver after 32 weeks 25% of the time (Vaisbuch et al., 2010).

Fetal Fibronectin Testing

fFN is a protein substance primarily concentrated in the area between the placenta and the decidua of the uterus that helps bond the amniotic sac to the uterus. From 22 to 35 weeks of gestation, a small amount, about 50 mg/mL, can normally be found in the cervical and vaginal secretions of the mother. Levels above 50 mg/mL, however, are 76.7% sensitive and 82.7% specific for birth within 10 days (Deshpande et al., 2013). Thus, fFN level is often tested to assess for imminent preterm labor and birth. The sources of false positives for an fFN test are similar to those for amniotic fluid testing: semen, blood, or a recent cervical examination (McLaren, Hezelgrave, Ayubi, Seed, & Shennan, 2015).

A common, qualitative protocol for fFN testing is to take an fFN swab for women under 34 weeks of gestation who are 3 or more cm dilated with a cervical length of 20 to 30 mm by transvaginal ultrasound. A negative result, meaning a lack of fFN in the maternal and cervical secretions, is reassuring and indicates a high likelihood that birth will not occur within the next 2 weeks. A positive result, however, is not diagnostic of preterm birth and only indicates a higher likelihood.

A second approach is to combine information about cervical length with a quantitative measurement of fFN. Although the qualitative test, discussed above, provides a simple positive or negative result, the quantitative test provides an fFN level for the sample, with higher levels being more predictive of impending birth (Bruijn et al., 2016).

Treatment

Interventions for actual or suspected preterm labor include suppression of labor, physical activity restriction, progesterone supplementation, and management of medications.

Should labor cease with or without intervention, little evidence is available as to optimal management. Women who had preterm labor but did not give birth and do not have significant cervical dilation are managed expectantly either in the hospital or in the community. Women with advanced cervical dilation or bleeding or who live some distance from adequate facilities are more likely to be hospitalized. A nonreassuring fetal status and other complications may also indicate hospitalization.

Suppression of Labor

Although preterm labor is true labor, featuring contractions with cervical changes, it does not always result in preterm birth. Preterm birth is challenging to predict and prevent, and 50% of women diagnosed with preterm labor continue their pregnancies to term without any intervention (Hackney, Olson-Chen, & Thornburg, 2013).

Tocolytics, discussed earlier, are medications that can delay delivery for up to 2 to 7 days, depending on the medication, but not until term. Their use, however, is not associated with significant improvements in clinical outcomes. In general, tocolysis is reserved for pregnancies that would benefit from a 48-hour delay in delivery, as when transport is needed to a different care facility or for the administration of corticosteroids as indicated to promote fetal lung maturity and reduce ventricular bleeding and necrotizing fasciitis (ACOG, 2016b). Tocolysis is not generally used before 24 weeks of gestation or beyond 34 weeks of gestation (ACOG, 2016a).

Contraindications to tocolysis are similar to indications for induced labor: nonreassuring fetal status, severe preeclampsia, and maternal hemorrhage with hemodynamic instability. Situations in which there would be no benefit to extending the pregnancy, such as intrauterine fetal demise and a lethal fetal anomaly, are also contraindications to tocolysis. Tocolysis is further contraindicated with an intraamniotic infection and in the case of a contraindication to the proposed tocolytic agent (The Pharmacy 21.1; ACOG, 2016b).

The Pharmacy 21.1 Tocolytics for the Temporary Suspension of Preterm Labor

Agent (Class)	Route and Dosing	Side Effects	Care Considerations
More Effective Agents			
Indomethacin (COX-2 inhibitor)	• Loading dose: 50–100 mg by mouth or rectally • Maintenance dose: 25 mg every 4–6 h for a total of 48 h	Maternal • Nausea • Vomiting • Reflux • Gastritis • Platelet dysfunction (rare) Fetal • Premature constriction or closure of the ductus arteriosus • Oligohydramnios	Courses limited to 48 h are associated with a reduced risk to the fetus. Maternal contraindications • Bleeding disorder • Gastric ulcer • Renal dysfunction • Asthma • Aspirin allergy
Nifedipine (calcium channel blocker)	• Loading dose: 30 mg by mouth • Maintenance dose: 10–20 mg by mouth every 4–5 h for a total of 48 h	Maternal • Headache • Palpitations • Dizziness • Nausea • Flushing • Hypotension	Maternal contraindications • Hypotension • Drug allergy • Certain cardiac conditions

(continued)

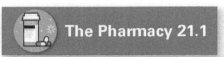

The Pharmacy 21.1 Tocolytics for the Temporary Suspension of Preterm Labor (continued)

Agent (Class)	Route and Dosing	Side Effects	Care Considerations
Terbutaline (beta-2 agonist)	• Initial dose: 2.5–5 µg/min every 20–30 min until contractions cease • Maintenance dose: minimum effective, ceasing at 48 h	Maternal • Tachycardia • Palpitations • Hypotension • Shortness of breath • Rarely, chest discomfort or pulmonary edema	Contraindications • Some cardiac disease • Poorly controlled diabetes • Placenta previa • Placental abruption Monitor for: • Shortness of breath • Chest pain • Tachycardia Monitor: • Intake and output • Glucose and potassium levels every 4–6 h Use for tocolysis recommended against because of lack of efficacy and safety concerns
Less Effective Agents			
Magnesium sulfate	Loading dose: 6 g IV over 20 min Maintenance dose: 2 g/h titrated to contractions and signs of maternal toxicity. See The Pharmacy 4.1.	Maternal Sweating and flushing most common. Drowsiness, lethargy, dry mouth, headache, blurred vision, shortness of breath, and hypotension possible.	Monitoring for magnesium toxicity is crucial. Effective for neuroprotection of fetus. Contraindicated with myasthenia gravis and some cardiac conditions. Dose adjustment indicated with renal dysfunction. When used with calcium channel blocker may cause respiratory depression. Calcium gluconate (1 g IV over 5–10 min) must be readily available to reverse toxicity. See Box 20.7
Nitrous oxide	10 mg patch on abdomen for 1 h; if ineffective add second patch. Patches left in place for 24 h, then removed and patient reassessed. OR 20 µg/min IV until tocolysis is achieved	Maternal Headache, hypotension	Contraindicated with hypotension and some cardiac problems.

COX-2, cyclooxygenase-2; IV, intravenous.

Adapted from Reinebrant, H. E., Pileggi-Castro, C., Romero, C. L., Dos Santos, R. A., Kumar, S., Souza, J. P., & Flenady, V. (2015). Cyclo-oxygenase (COX) inhibitors for treating preterm labour. *Cochrane Database of Systematic Reviews,* (6), CD001992. doi:10.1002/14651858.CD001992. pub3; Flenady, V., Wojcieszek, A. M., Papatsonis, D. N., Stock, O. M., Murray, L., Jardine, L. A., & Carbonne, B. (2014). Calcium channel blockers for inhibiting preterm labour and birth. *Cochrane Database of Systematic Reviews,* (6), CD002255. doi:10.1002/14651858.CD002255.pub2; Neilson, J. P., West, H. M., & Dowswell, T. (2014). Betamimetics for inhibiting preterm labour. *Cochrane Database of Systematic Reviews,* (2), CD004352. doi:10.1002/14651858.CD004352.pub3; Flenady, V., Reinebrant, H. E., Liley, H. G., Tambimuttu, E. G., & Papatsonis, D. N. (2014). Oxytocin receptor antagonists for inhibiting preterm labour. *Cochrane Database of Systematic Reviews,* (6), CD004452. doi:10.1002/14651858. CD004452.pub3; Crowther, C. A., Brown, J., McKinlay, C. J., & Middleton, P. (2014). Magnesium sulphate for preventing preterm birth in threatened preterm labour. *Cochrane Database of Systematic Reviews,* (8), CD001060. doi:10.1002/14651858.CD001060.pub2; Duckitt, K., Thornton, S., O'Donovan, O. P., & Dowswell, T. (2014). Nitric oxide donors for treating preterm labour. *Cochrane Database of Systematic Reviews,* (5), CD002860. doi:10.1002/14651858.CD002860.pub2; American College of Obstetricians and Gynecologists. (2016b). Practice bulletin no. 159: Management of preterm labor. *Obstetrics and Gynecology, 127*(1), e29–e38. doi:10.1097/AOG.0000000000001265

Although antibiotics are effective for treating GBS and for prolonging a pregnancy with PPROM and without labor, they are not effective for stopping contractions once they have started (Flenady, Hawley, Stock, Kenyon, & Badawi, 2013). Although hydration is sometimes helpful for quieting uterine activity not associated with cervical dilation, it cannot suppress labor contractions or stop preterm labor (Stan, Boulvain, Pfister, & Hirsbrunner-Almagbaly, 2013). Similarly, no evidence supports the use of bed rest to prevent preterm birth (Sosa, Althabe, Belizan, & Bergel, 2015).

Physical Activity Restriction

Although, as mentioned before, there is a lack of evidence supporting the practice, women who experience preterm labor pregnancy are often placed on bed rest either at home or in the hospital. Another common recommendation is that women who have had one or more episodes of preterm labor refrain from working more than 40 hours a week, working night shifts, and heavy lifting. Providers may also instruct them to avoid standing for longer than 8 hours in a 24-hour period or for more than 4 hours at a stretch (Bonzini, Coggon, & Palmer, 2007). Nurses should be aware that, although bed rest, activity restriction, and avoidance of exercise are common recommendations to prevent preterm birth, these recommendations are not evidence based (McCarty-Singleton & Sciscione, 2014; Satterfield, Newton, & May, 2016).

For some women with arrested preterm labor, sexual activity may trigger a resumption of contractions because of orgasm and prostaglandins in the semen. Women who report contractions after sexual activity should avoid intercourse (Hernandez-Diaz et al., 2014). Travel is not prohibited, but women should consider their access to care in the event of a status change while traveling.

Progesterone Supplementation

Women with a history of preterm birth with a prior pregnancy and a diagnosis of a short cervix by ultrasound in this pregnancy may receive progesterone to help extend the pregnancy. Supplementation with vaginal progesterone for women with a cervical length of 25 mm or less is associated with a reduction in preterm birth, neonate morbidity and mortality, increased birth rate, and fewer NICU admissions (Romero et al., 2016). Pregnancies with a positive fFN test result, however (see above), do not benefit from vaginal progesterone (Norman et al., 2016). For women in whom labor is threatened or established, progesterone supplementation does not extend the pregnancy (Martinez de Tejada et al., 2015). Dosing may be vaginal or intramuscular (IM). IM dosing is routinely 250 mg weekly, and vaginal dosing is 100 mg daily (Saccone et al., 2017).

Women on progesterone therapy due to a shortened cervix and previous preterm birth should continue this intervention, but a diagnosis of preterm labor alone is not a reason for progesterone supplementation.

Medication Management

As mentioned previously, for gestations from 23 to 34 weeks with imminent or actual preterm labor, a course of corticosteroids should be given to the mother to promote fetal lung maturity and reduce the occurrence of ventricular bleeding in the brain and necrotizing enterocolitis. The patient should complete the course of steroids even if labor resolves. If preterm labor stops and the threat of imminent delivery passes, a woman taking antibiotics for GBS will have them discontinued. If delivery is anticipated within 24 hours of a pregnancy of less than 32 to 34 weeks, magnesium sulfate administration is indicated for neuroprotection of the fetus.

In Chapter 10, Lexi developed HELLP syndrome and had to be delivered preterm. Prior to the delivery she was given magnesium sulfate to protect the fetal brain and corticosteroid injections to reduce the chances of her infant developing respiratory distress syndrome, necrotizing enterocolitis, and intraventricular hemorrhage. (Letitia Richford, in Chapter 5, had a late-preterm labor and delivery and had to undergo a cesarean section because of cord prolapse.)

Chorioamnionitis

Chorioamnionitis is infection of the amnion, chorion, or both. The term "intraamniotic infection" is now often preferred for this condition as it encompasses infections of the placenta, amniotic fluid, fetus, and umbilical cord and not just the fetal membranes. The term "triple I" has also been proposed, as it encompasses "intrauterine inflammation or infection or both" (Higgins et al., 2016).

In Chapter 7, Hannah was diagnosed with chorioamnionitis and was given antibiotics both during and after the birth. Despite treatment, she became feverish during labor, and her care team was concerned that her baby, Gaius, might develop sepsis.

Prevalence

However it is referred to, this condition complicates 1% to 2% of term births and as many as 50% of preterm births (Chapman, Reveiz, Illanes, & Bonfill Cosp, 2014).

Etiology

Most commonly, chorioamnionitis results from the ascent of bacterial flora through the cervix. Rarely, as in the cases of *Listeria monocytogenes*, *Staphylococcus aureus*, and *Streptococcus agalactiae*, a maternal infection may pass the placenta. Generally, however, the mucus plug, placenta, and membranes themselves prevent chorioamnionitis. PPROM is, thus, a significant risk factor for chorioamnionitis. Other risk factors include multiple digital vaginal examinations, PROM, prolonged labor, preterm labor, human immunodeficiency virus infection, first pregnancy, low socioeconomic status, meconium-stained fluid, genital tract infections, and internal fetal and contraction monitoring (see Box 7.5; Hofmeyr & Kiiza, 2016).

Prognosis

Chorioamnionitis can have serious implications for both the mother and the neonate.

Maternal Complications

Maternal complications include prolonged labor and, likely related to a similar mechanism, increased risk for postpartum hemorrhage. Women who undergo cesarean section or episiotomy or have a laceration are more likely to develop a wound infection if they also have chorioamnionitis. Postpartum infection of the endometrium, known as endometritis, is far more common with chorioamnionitis, as is venous thrombus. Nearly 20% of cases of maternal sepsis are associated with chorioamnionitis (Al-Ostad, Kezouh, Spence, & Abenhaim, 2015).

Neonatal Complications

Up to 40% of cases of neonatal sepsis are related to chorioamnionitis (Tita & Andrews, 2010). Besides sepsis and septic shock, intraamniotic infection can result in perinatal death, asphyxia, cerebral palsy, pneumonia, meningitis, intraventricular hemorrhage, neurodevelopmental delay, and problems related to prematurity if the pregnancy is delivered early.

Assessment

The diagnostic criteria for intraamniotic infection include a maternal fever of 38°C plus at least two of the following: fetal tachycardia (heart rate over 160 beats per minute [bpm]), maternal tachycardia (heart rate over 100 bpm), uterine tenderness, foul-smelling discharge, and maternal white blood cells over 15,000 cells/mm^3 (see Box 7.7; Hofmeyr & Kiiza, 2016). Subclinical chorioamnionitis may be present and not produce any of these signs or symptoms. It may instead manifest as preterm labor with or without PPROM.

Treatment

Prompt treatment with broad-spectrum IV antibiotics is necessary with the suspicion of chorioamnionitis. Ampicillin and gentamicin are common choices of medication. Clindamycin or metronidazole is often added in the case of cesarean delivery to mitigate the risk of postsurgical infection.

Postterm Pregnancy

A postterm pregnancy is one that has reached or exceeded 42 weeks of gestation, or 294 days since the first day of the mother's LMP (ACOG, 2013a).

Prevalence

In the United States in 2015, 0.4% of infants born were delivered post term and 6.51% were born late term at 41 weeks of gestation (Martin et al., 2017).

Etiology

There are likely multiple causes for postterm pregnancies, and the etiology for most is unknown. Up to a half of postterm births can likely be attributed to genetic factors influencing the duration of the pregnancy (Oberg, Frisell, Svensson, & Iliadou, 2013). A history of a previous postterm pregnancy is the most significant risk factor for future postterm pregnancies (Kortekaas et al., 2015). Other risk factors include first pregnancy, pregnancy with a male fetus, maternal obesity, advanced maternal age, and non-Hispanic white ethnicity (Oberg et al., 2013).

Prognosis

A key risk of a postterm pregnancy is fetal macrosomia due to the extra duration of intrauterine growth. The risk for macrosomia with a postterm pregnancy is almost 10 times what it is for a term pregnancy. Macrosomia creates a risk for protracted or arrested labor, dystocia, and birth injury, as well as maternal injury, including lacerations, infection, necessity for operative delivery, and postpartum hemorrhage (Boulvain, Irion, Dowswell, & Thornton, 2016). Postterm neonates often have peeling skin, starting on the palms and soles, along with decreased vernix caseosa, sparse lanugo, increased scalp hair, and longer nails.

Approximately 20% of postterm fetuses and infants have **dysmaturity**. Dysmaturity is a syndrome of intrauterine malnutrition due to the aging of the placenta. This diminishment of placental capacity means that the perinatal mortality rate at 42 weeks of gestation is twice what it is at term. Neonates with dysmaturity tend to have long, thin bodies and, instead of being macrosomic, are small for gestational age. Their skin may appear loose with prominent creases.

In addition to dysmaturity, cord compression is more common for postterm infants due to oliguria from the dysmaturity creating oligohydramnios. These factors combined can lead to nonreassuring fetal heart patterns. The passage of meconium in utero is more common for postterm pregnancies and may be due to fetal maturity or to hypoxia related to dysmaturity.

Assessment

Gestational age is typically estimated in the first trimester on the basis of the woman's LMP or ultrasound imaging. Early ultrasound is a more reliable tool for measuring gestation than LMP, and it's likely that the rates of postterm gestation are overstated when LMP is the standard measure rather than ultrasound.

Treatment

The two possible approaches to a postterm pregnancy are expectant management and induction, which may be preceded by a ripening of the cervix. Induction at 41 weeks of gestation is not associated with an increased rate of perinatal complications or cesarean section and is preferred by a majority of obstetric providers in the United States. An alternate approach is to induce from 42 to 42 6/7 weeks of gestation (ACOG, 2014).

Expectant Management

Expectant management of a postterm pregnancy involves close monitoring of the pregnancy for fetal and maternal well-being. Twice weekly assessment of the fetus, usually by NST with an assessment of amniotic fluid volume or by BPP, begins at 41 weeks of gestation. After 41 weeks, there is no significant difference between the induction and expectant management in terms of fetal asphyxia and admission of the newborn to the NICU (Gulmezoglu, Crowther, Middleton, & Heatley, 2012). Fetal distress and oligohydramnios are reasons to cease expectant management and induce labor.

Ripening the Unfavorable Cervix

For an induction of labor to be successful, the cervix must be physically distensible, soft, and, therefore, partly dilated. Contractions induced against an "unripe" cervix are less likely to result in a successful labor. Because of this, the cervix is generally assessed prior to induction for readiness, and, if necessary, mechanical or pharmaceutical means may be implemented to further ripen the cervix before beginning an oxytocin infusion.

Bishop Score

The Bishop score is a quantitative summary of information associated with cervical ripeness. The parameters evaluated include dilation, effacement, station, cervical consistency, and position of the cervix. The first three factors have been described earlier in the text, so only cervical consistency and the position of the cervix are described here. Cervical consistency may be firm, medium, or soft. A firm cervix has the consistency of a chin and a soft cervix feels mushy. Prior to delivery, the position of the cervix becomes more anterior and in line with the vaginal introitus. A Bishop score of 8 or higher is considered favorable, indicating a greater chance for a successful vaginal delivery. A score of 6 or less is unfavorable, indicating a lesser chance for a successful vaginal delivery (see Table 9.1).

Pharmaceutical Ripening

Prostaglandins are often used to ripen unscarred cervixes prior to the administration of oxytocin for labor induction. Prostaglandins for cervical ripening are contraindicated in women with a previous cesarean birth or a history of significant uterine surgery because of an increased risk for uterine rupture. Clinicians may also opt to delay use in the presence of contractions, as the addition of prostaglandins may induce uterine hyperstimulation.

Prostaglandins may also initiate contractions without the need for oxytocin.

A commonly used prostaglandin is misoprostol, which may be administered vaginally or orally (Alfirevic, Aflaifel, & Weeks, 2014). Vaginal dosing of misoprostol is typically from 25 to 50 μg every 3 to 6 hours. The 50 μg-dose, although more effective, is also associated with a higher rate of **uterine tachysystole** (referred to simply as tachysystole in the remainder of this chapter), which is a condition of excessively frequent uterine contractions during labor and delivery (McMaster, Sanchez-Ramos, & Kaunitz, 2015; Tang, Kapp, Dragoman, & de Souza, 2013). After administration, the nurse should monitor the fetal heart rate and uterine activity for at least 30 minutes or as long as uterine contractions are present (ACOG, 2014). Dosing of misoprostol may also be buccal or sublingual.

Another prostaglandin available for cervical ripening is dinoprostone. When marketed as Prepidil, 0.5 mg of dinoprostone in 2.5 mL of gel is inserted into the vagina and deposited near or in the cervix. A second dose may be provided 6 to 12 hours after the first, and oxytocin may be administered no sooner than 6 to 12 hours after the final dose to avoid tachysystole from the concurrent use of dinoprostone and oxytocin. A second preparation, Cervidil, contains 10 mg of dinoprostone that time releases at a rate of 0.3 mg/h. Cervidil comes as an insert and is removed when labor starts or after 12 hours. Unlike with Prepidil, which requires a wait of 6 to 12 hours prior to starting oxytocin, oxytocin may be initiated just a half hour after the Cervidil insert is removed.

Mechanical Ripening

Mechanical ripening may be done in addition to or instead of prostaglandin treatment. Although some women may experience gastrointestinal (GI) distress with prostaglandins, particularly misoprostol, mechanical ripening does not have systemic side effects. Also, mechanical methods of ripening pose a much lesser risk of tachysystole. In addition, mechanical ripening is less expensive. Mechanical ripening is associated with an increased risk for infection, however, as well as discomfort of the mother due to manipulation of the cervix. Oxytocin supplementation is needed more often with mechanical ripening than with prostaglandin ripening.

Mechanical dilation may be done by the insertion and expansion of a balloon catheter in the cervix or by the introduction of **hygroscopic dilators** into the cervical canal. Hygroscopic dilators may be made from various materials and are hydrophilic. They soak up surrounding moisture from the cervix and vagina and expand. Balloon catheters are generally removed after 12 hours, and hygroscopic dilators are removed after 6 to 24 hours, depending on the material used.

Membrane Sweeping

Membrane sweeping is a process during which the obstetric provider inserts a finger into the cervix and runs it between the fetal membranes and the wall of the uterus. It is more often used to stimulate cervical ripening when labor is safe and desired at term, as opposed to indicated imminently for the health and safety of the mother or the fetus. It is typically done during a routine office visit and requires no special monitoring.

Membrane sweeping causes a release of hormones that are thought to ripen the cervix. Although a 2005 meta-analysis found membrane sweeping ineffective to induce labor after 38 weeks of gestation, a 2006 study found that its use led to a 40% reduction in pregnancies progressing from 41 to 42 weeks of gestation (Boulvain, Stan, & Irion, 2005; de Miranda, van der Bom, Bonsel, Bleker, & Rosendaal, 2006).

Other less formal methods of labor induction often tried by patients are itemized in Box 21.4.

Induction of Labor

As of 2012, 23.3% of labors were induced (Osterman & Martin, 2014). An induction is indicated when the risks of continuing the pregnancy are considered greater than the risks of delivery prior to spontaneous labor. Common indications for the induction of labor are listed in Box 21.5. Elective, marginally indicated, or "social" inductions are performed for nonmedical reasons, such as to avoid potential scheduling challenges. Such inductions are not recommended prior to 39 weeks of gestation, as earlier inductions are associated with longer labor and increased neonatal

---

Box 21.4 Traditional and Home Methods of Labor Induction

- *Sex:* semen contains prostaglandins, which may aid in ripening the cervix
- *Nipple stimulation:* results in less postpartum hemorrhage; induces labor in some
- *Hypnosis:* no randomized, controlled studies available
- *Acupuncture:* some evidence of cervical change and shortened labor
- *Evening primrose oil, orally or vaginally:* associated with labor complications
- *Red raspberry leaf tea:* may shorten the second stage of labor
- *Castor oil:* a traditional method used at least since the time of ancient Egypt
- *Blue and black cohosh:* associated with adverse neonatal outcomes
- *Exercise:* little evidence to support that exercise of any kind induces labor
- *Acupressure:* has not been found effective in controlled studies
- *Spicy foods:* unlikely to promote labor
- *Bumpy car rides:* unlikely to promote labor

Adapted from Dante, G., Bellei, G., Neri, I., & Facchinetti, F. (2014). Herbal therapies in pregnancy: What works? *Current Opinion in Obstetrics and Gynecology, 26*(2), 83–91. doi:10.1097/GCO.0000000000000052; Torkzahrani, S., Mahmoudikohani, F., Saatchi, K., Sefidkar, R., & Banaei, M. (2017). The effect of acupressure on the initiation of labor: A randomized controlled trial. *Women and Birth, 30*(1), 46–50. doi:10.1016/j.wombi.2016.07.002; Bovbjerg, M. L., Evenson, K. R., Bradley, C., & Thorp, J. M. (2014). What started your labor? Responses from mothers in the third pregnancy, infection, and nutrition study. *Journal of Perinatal Education, 23*(3), 155–164. doi:10.1891/1058-1243.23.3.155

Box 21.5 Common Indications for Labor Induction

- Maternal diabetes
- Preeclampsia, eclampsia, or HELLP syndrome
- Twin pregnancy
- Preterm premature rupture of membranes
- Chorioamnionitis
- Placental abruption
- Oligohydramnios
- Cholestasis of pregnancy
- Alloimmunization (Rh sensitization)
- Fetal demise

---

morbidity. Labor induction for elective reasons after 39 weeks of gestation, however, is not currently believed to increase the rate of cesarean delivery, even with an unripe cervix, or adverse outcomes for the neonate (Bernardes et al., 2016; Saccone & Berghella, 2015b). Contraindications for induction and cervical ripening are provided in Box 21.6.

Oxytocin

Endogenous oxytocin is produced in the hypothalamus and excreted by the posterior pituitary. The synthetic form, commonly referred to as Pitocin, is chemically identical and is commonly used for labor induction. Oxytocin is inactivated in the gut and is thus typically given intravenously. An infusion pump is used to ensure precise administration.

A common dilution of oxytocin is 30 U in 500 mL of saline solution or another crystalloid IV fluid (Ringer's lactate, 5% dextrose in 1/2 normal saline, etc.). At this dilution, 1 mU/min is 1 mL/h. Initial dosing of oxytocin is 0.5 to 6 mU/min, the time between dose increases of 1 to 2 mU/min is 10 to 60 minutes, and the maximum dose is 16 to 64 mU/min according to institution protocol and as ordered by the obstetric provider (Budden, Chen, & Henry, 2014). Dosing is typically increased on a preset schedule until contractions are strong, regular, occurring three to five times in a 10-minute period, and lasting 40 to 90 seconds each. Alternatively, the dose may be titrated to 200 to 250 Montevideo units by internal contraction monitoring. (Montevideo

---

Box 21.6 Contraindications to Induction

High Risk for Rupture of the Uterus
- Vertical incision with prior cesarean section
- Previous uterine rupture
- Prior uterine surgery

Cesarean Indicated for Other Reasons
- Active genital herpes outbreak
- Umbilical cord prolapse
- Transverse fetal lie
- Placenta previa
- Vasa previa

units are the contractions in mm Hg multiplied by the number of contractions recorded in 10 minutes.) Oxytocin administration may also be pulsatile, occurring every 6 to 10 minutes.

After adequate uterine activity has been achieved, the dose may be sustained or discontinued. The fetal heart rate and uterine activity must be monitored continuously throughout an induction with oxytocin to assess the adequacy of contractions. A nonreassuring fetal heart rate is reason to stop the infusion.

Nurses should be aware that oxytocin may cause nausea, vomiting, headache, and flushing in the mother. Cardiovascular instability, manifested by tachycardia, hypotension, arrhythmias, and, rarely, myocardial infarction, is also possible. Water retention related to oxytocin administration has, rarely, led to hyponatremia, particularly if large volumes of oxytocin are administered in a hypotonic solution for 7 or more hours. The symptoms of hyponatremia may be similar to the side effects of oxytocin, including headache and GI distress, but can also include abdominal pain, mental status changes, and grand mal seizure.

The American Congress of Obstetricians and Gynecologists defines tachysystole as an average of five or more contractions every 10 minutes averaged over a half hour (ACOG, 2009; Fig. 21.1). Tachysystole may result from the administration of prostaglandins or oxytocin, and the use of both poses a cumulative risk. Because uterine contractions cause intermittent interruption in the perfusion of the placenta and, in turn, the fetus, tachysystole can result in fetal hypoxemia that may register as a category II or III fetal heart tracing (see Box 16.2). Rarely, tachysystole may result in uterine rupture.

The management of tachysystole depends on its cause. Tachysystole in a woman receiving oxytocin without a category II or III fetal heart tracing may have the oxytocin titrated down or stopped briefly. If a vaginal insert of prostaglandin is the source of the tachysystole, it should be removed if possible (the removal of Cervidil, an insert, is more feasible than the removal of Prepidil, a gel, or misoprostol, a tablet).

Tachysystole with oxytocin and a nonreassuring fetal heart change requires stoppage of the oxytocin infusion and notification of the obstetric care provider. Intrauterine resuscitation measures should be started immediately (Step-by-Step Skills 21.1). If

Step-by-Step Skills 21.1

Intrauterine Resuscitation

1. Stop administration of oxytocin.
2. Place the woman in the left, side-lying position.
3. Administer oxygen at 10 L/min via a nonrebreather mask.
4. Increase intravenous hydration.
5. Administer a tocolytic.

Adapted from Bullens, L. M., van Runnard Heimel, P. J., van der Hout-van der Jagt, M. B., & Oei, S. G. (2015). Interventions for intrauterine resuscitation in suspected fetal distress during term labor: A systematic review. *Obstetrical and Gynecological Survey, 70*(8), 524–539. doi:10.1097/OGX.0000000000000215

the tachysystole persists, a tocolytic may be provided IV, often terbutaline 250 mg subcutaneous or IV or nitroglycerin 60 to 90 µg IV. After the resolution of tachysystole, oxytocin may be restarted to achieve optimal contractions as needed. A common approach is to restart the infusion according to the time that has passed since discontinuation. If it has been less than 30 minutes, the starting dose is half of that administered at the time of tachysystole. If more than a half hour has passed, oxytocin is restarted at the initial starting dose.

Amniotomy

Amniotomy, the process of artificially rupturing the fetal membranes, is another method of inducing labor. Amniotomy may also be used to augment the effect of exogenous oxytocin or prostaglandins. This procedure requires that the cervix be partly dilated to accommodate the amniohook, a tool that is used to rupture the membranes. Care must be taken prior to the intervention to ensure the fetus is in the vertex position with the head engaged in the pelvis. Membrane rupture without fetal engagement is a risk for cord prolapse. A prolonged period of time after the rupture of the membranes prior to birth presents an increased risk for infection. The nurse should

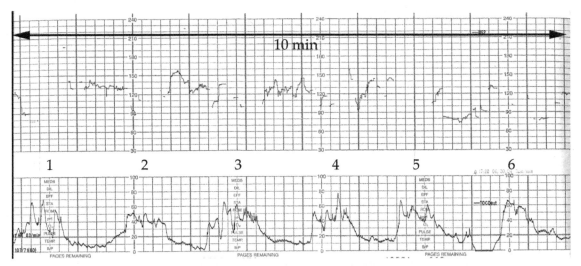

Figure 21.1. Fetal heart rate tracing demonstrating uterine tachysystole during induction of labor. (Reprinted with permission from Troiano, N. H., Harvey, C. J., & Chez, B. F. [2012]. *AWHONN's high risk and critical care obstetrics* [3rd ed., Fig. 12.2]. Philadelphia, PA: Lippincott Williams & Wilkins.)

monitor the fetal heart rate both prior to and after amniotomy to verify that the fetus has tolerated the procedure.

In Chapter 9, Ron ruptured Nancy's membranes with an amniohook. In Nancy's case, however, the procedure was done to hasten labor rather than to start it. The nurse caring for the family was relieved that the fluid released by the procedure did not contain meconium.

itself, however, with abnormalities in the spiral artery development (Avagliano, Bulfamante, Morabito, & Marconi, 2011).

In Chapter 6, Rebecca experienced placental abruption caused by blunt force trauma experienced during a traffic accident. She was 38 weeks pregnant and underwent a cesarean section after fetal distress was assessed. Despite this care, the fetus did not survive.

Placental Abruption

Placental abruption is the premature detachment of the placenta from the decidua of the uterus after 20 weeks of gestation.

Prevalence

Abruption complicates approximately 1% of pregnancies (Ananth et al., 2015). Approximately half of abruptions occur after 37 weeks and nearly one out of six occurs prior to 32 weeks. Occult placental abruption, in particular, is noted on a postpartum examination of the placenta in many pregnancies that deliver from 22 to 32 weeks of gestation with PPROM (Iams, 2014).

Etiology

Most placental abruptions have no known underlying cause. Blunt force trauma is the etiology for some. The placenta, unlike the wall of the uterus, is not flexible, so a sudden stretching or contraction of the uterine wall may cause the placenta to sheer from the decidua. Smoking and cocaine use are associated with placental abruption, as are structural uterine abnormalities. The process that leads to placental abruption may occur months in advance of the abruption

Whatever the underlying cause, bleeding is part of the sequelae of abruption. The bleeding typically starts on the maternal side of the placental interface, in the decidua basalis. Blood accumulates between the decidua and the villi of the placenta, causing the two to separate.

By far the greatest risk factor for placental abruption is a history of placental abruption with a previous pregnancy (Ruiter, Ravelli, de Graaf, Mol, & Pajkrt, 2015; see Box 6.2). Smoking, a modifiable risk factor, is particularly impactful in combination with hypertension. Hypertension alone is also a risk factor, though the administration of antihypertensives in pregnancy does not reduce the associated risk for placental abruption.

Prognosis

Placental abruption is often classified as mild or severe, although other grading systems exist, as well (Ananth et al., 2016; Table 21.1). Mild abruption is typically self-limiting, with limited impact on the mother or the fetus, whereas severe abruption may result in complete detachment of the placenta, thus endangering the life of both. Even when the placenta does not detach completely, gas and nutrient exchange between the mother and the placenta is disrupted at the area of separation. If sufficient attachment does

Table 21.1   Classification of Placental Abruption

	Class 0	Class 1	Class 2	Class 3
Severity	**Asymptomatic***	**Mild**	**Moderate**	**Severe**
% of abruptions	N/A	48%	27%	24%
Vaginal bleeding	N/A	None or little	None or little	None to heavy
Uterus	N/A	Slightly tender	Moderately to severely tender, contractions possible	Very painful, contracted
Cardiovascular and hemodynamic status	N/A	Stable	Tachycardia with orthostatic changes, low fibrinogen	Hypovolemic shock
DIC	N/A	None	None	Present
Fetal status	N/A	No fetal distress	Fetal distress	Fetal death

*Detected by examination of the placenta postpartum.
N/A, not applicable; DIC, disseminated intravascular coagulation.
Adapted from Deering, S. H. (2016). *Abruptio placentae.* Retrieved from http://emedicine.medscape.com/article/252810-overview

not remain, the pregnancy is compromised. When the abruption includes more than half the interface between the placenta and the decidua, fetal death is common, as is disseminated intravascular coagulation (DIC) in the mother.

In Chapter 1, Bess Gaskell experienced a mild placental abruption at 30 weeks of gestation and stayed a week in the hospital, where she was carefully monitored for any signs of hypovolemic shock. Fortunately, her placental abruption healed spontaneously and she was able to go home.

The impact of an abruption on the fetus is determined both by the severity of the abruption and by the gestational age at which it occurs. For the mother, the consequences are primarily based on only the severity of the bleeding. A mild abruption close to term may have little effect on mother or fetus, whereas a mild abruption earlier in pregnancy may pose little danger to the mother but have catastrophic consequences for the fetus.

A large loss of blood and DIC may lead to hypovolemic shock, multiorgan failure, and the need for transfusion. Surgical intervention may be required by emergency cesarean section and/or hysterectomy. For the fetus, an acute abruption can necessitate a preterm birth to prevent or mitigate hypoxemia and asphyxia. The rate of perinatal loss with abruption is 12%, with 50% due to death in utero as a result of asphyxia (Tikkanen et al., 2013).

Chronic abruption, discussed below, has been associated with preeclampsia and is a risk factor for preterm labor and birth with PPROM (Kobayashi et al., 2014). Oligohydramnios-associated abruption corresponds with a particularly high rate of preterm birth and fetal death when discovered in the second trimester of pregnancy (Kobayashi et al., 2014).

Presentation

Abruption may be acute or chronic. Presentation varies depending on the location and degree of abruption. Abruptions that happen centrally with the high-pressure arteries result in more life-threatening problems associated with severe bleeding. Abruption at the edges, however, is more likely to be venous and associated with more chronic issues of uterine hypoperfusion, such as oligohydramnios and fetal growth restriction (Fig. 21.2).

Acute Abruption

The classic presentation of an acute abruption is sudden onset of abdominal pain and vaginal bleeding and frequent, hypertonic uterine contractions (see Table 6.4). The uterus is rigid and may be tender. Up to 20% of women with an acute abruption experience only minor bleeding, however, as the blood remains trapped between the decidua and the placenta. Bleeding is considered a poor predictor of the severity of the abruption, and abdominal pain is considered more predictive (Kasai et al.,

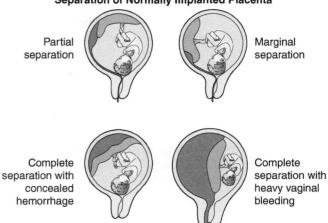

Placental Abruption: Various Degrees of Separation of Normally Implanted Placenta

Partial separation

Marginal separation

Complete separation with concealed hemorrhage

Complete separation with heavy vaginal bleeding

Figure 21.2. Classification of placental abruption. (Reprinted with permission from Suresh, M. [2012]. *Shnider and Levinson's anesthesia for obstetrics* [5th ed., Fig. 21.1]. Philadelphia, PA: Lippincott Williams & Wilkins.)

2015). Acute abruption related to trauma generally manifests within 24 hours.

Chronic Abruption

Unlike acute abruption, the presentation of chronic abruption tends to develop over time. Women may intermittently experience light bleeding as the only clinical sign. The fetus, however, may have intrauterine growth restriction and oligohydramnios. Maternal coagulation studies are usually unremarkable due to the slow rate of blood loss, and ultrasound may or may not reveal retroplacental hemorrhage. Findings on serial examinations of the fetus showing a pregnancy measuring small for gestational age may be the first clue. These findings during a fundal height measurement may be due to restricted fetal growth, oligohydramnios, or both. The diagnosis of abruption may be confirmed postpartum by a histologic examination of the placenta, although this may confirm only a third of cases (Elsasser, Ananth, Prasad, Vintzileos, & New Jersey-Placental Abruption Study, 2010).

Assessment

A blood clot visualized by ultrasound behind the placenta (a retroplacental hematoma) is a classic finding in placental abruption. Although outcomes are generally worse when the retroplacental hematoma is visualized, a severe abruption may still be present in its absence. Blood may escape via the cervix or bleeding may be chronic. Ultrasound may detect only 25% of cases of abruption, although when a retroplacental hematoma is visualized, the finding is highly predictive of an abruption (Shinde, Vaswani, Patange, Laddad, & Bhosale, 2016).

Once a diagnosis of placental abruption has been made, laboratory tests are typically ordered to evaluate coagulation for the manifestations of DIC, blood type, and crossmatch in case of a transfusion, and kidney function, as renal dysfunction is common with severe abruption. A complete blood count, including platelet count, is necessary to evaluate for anemia related to an acute bleed. Thrombocytopenia is also common with severe abruption. As preeclampsia and chronic abruption often happen together, women with preeclampsia are also likely to have their liver function evaluated.

The severity of the hemorrhage is generally reflected by the degree of abnormality seen in the maternal bloodwork. In particular, maternal fibrinogen levels at or below 200 mg/dL are highly predictive of severe hemorrhage, whereas values at or over 400 mg/dL strongly suggest a lack of severe hemorrhage (Wang et al., 2016). In the case of decreased fibrinogen and increased fibrinolysis (elevated D-dimer and fibrin degradation products), a diagnosis of DIC is highly probable (see the DIC section later in the chapter).

Treatment

Management largely depends on the gestational age and degree of abruption, as well as the complete clinical picture. A woman with a suspected minor abruption prior to 34 weeks with intact membranes, for example, may be monitored on an outpatient basis with regular antepartum assessments of the fetus.

Hospitalization and Monitoring

A woman with a suspected acute abruption, however, is likely to be admitted to labor and delivery for assessment, monitoring, and management (see Box 6.3). Critical points of care include the following:

- Continuous monitoring of fetal heart rate and uterine activity
- Wide-bore IV access in case a transfusion is needed, with the IV rate set to maintain a urine output above 30 mL/h
- Close monitoring of maternal hemodynamic status by urine output, heart rate, blood pressure, and blood loss

As mentioned previously, the amount of blood loss may be difficult to determine, as blood may be retained behind the placenta or within the uterus. When bleeding is frank, it should be collected and measured. Some institutions may also use visual aids to help staff assess what a particular amount of blood may look like when absorbed by a specific surface (Zuckerwise, Pettker, Illuzzi, Raab, & Lipkind, 2014).

Blood Transfusion

After an estimated blood loss of 500 to 1,000 mL, a transfusion may be ordered that includes platelets. Transfusion protocols may vary across institutions. The goals of transfusion are maintenance of a hematocrit level from 25% to 30%, a fibrinogen level at or above 100 mg/dL, and a platelet count at or above 75,000/μL.

Medications for Delivery

Medication considerations for delivery are similar to those for other births. Corticosteroids are administered for pregnancies less than 34 weeks of gestation. Tocolytics may be used to extend the pregnancy until the full course of corticosteroids is complete in the case of a subacute abruption with preterm labor. Magnesium

sulfate may be ordered in the 24-hour period prior to delivery for pregnancies less than 32 to 34 weeks of gestation for neuroprotection. Women who are GBS positive or for whom GBS status is unknown, prophylactic antibiotics are indicated during labor. Consultation with the anesthesiologist should occur early for planning and assessment purposes when possible.

Cesarean Section

Although a vaginal birth is typically preferred, a cesarean section may be indicated with maternal hemodynamic instability or coagulopathy. Because of the significant bleeding risk from the surgery, coagulopathy is corrected with blood products both prior to and during the cesarean section. In the case of a vaginal delivery, nurses should be aware that the situation can deteriorate quickly and dramatically with further abruption of the placenta. Close monitoring of the fetus and mother is essential.

Postpartum Care

After the birth of the neonate and placenta, the nurse administers oxytocin, as ordered, to firm the uterus and prevent further blood loss. In addition to the typical postpartum checks for hemodynamic stability, the nurse should expect to draw blood for hemoglobin, hematocrit, and coagulation studies (if previously abnormal) and monitor these levels regularly to guide the need for blood product replacement. If renal or other organ failure was evident during pregnancy due to hypovolemic shock or DIC, the nurse should provide support and monitoring until resolution.

In the case of severe abruption, the blood may penetrate the uterus, a condition referred to as a **Couvelaire uterus**. A Couvelaire uterus is particularly prone to postpartum hemorrhage and can result in DIC and hypovolemic shock. It is also less likely to respond to measures typically used to correct atony, such as oxytocin and uterine massage. Women with a Couvelaire uterus are at a high risk for hysterectomy postpartum.

DIC in Pregnancy

DIC is a disruption of hemostasis caused by a pathologic activation of the clotting cascade that results simultaneously in blood clots and platelet and clotting factor depletion and thus bleeding.

Etiology

DIC is always a complication of another condition. In pregnancy, common antecedent conditions include placental abruption, postpartum hemorrhage, preeclampsia/eclampsia/HELLP syndrome, acute fatty liver, amniotic fluid embolism, prolonged fetal demise, and maternal sepsis. Approximately a quarter of the fetuses of mother's with DIC will be stillborn (Cunningham & Nelson, 2015).

In Chapter 6, Rebecca was carefully monitored for DIC because of her placental abruption. Although she did not develop the condition, her team was acutely aware of the risk.

Prognosis

The combination of simultaneous clotting and depletion of circulating coagulants that occurs in DIC can lead to thrombosis, hemorrhage, and the failure of multiple organs. DIC is a challenging condition to manage at the best of times, but when it occurs in a pregnancy with a viable fetus, it presents additional challenges. Notably, a quarter of maternal deaths result from DIC (Callaghan, Creanga, & Kuklina, 2012). Approximately 20% of women with a diagnosis of DIC require a hysterectomy (Rattray, O'Connell, & Baskett, 2012).

Assessment

The presentation of DIC varies, but nurses should always be alert for the signs and symptoms in women with one of the antecedent conditions mentioned. Patients may display signs of shock (Box 21.7). Organ dysfunction may be evident in laboratory test results or clinical manifestations. Bleeding, whether overt and severe or slow, can be a sign of DIC. A more subtle bleed may be from an IV site, the gums, the nose, or the GI tract or in the form of hematuria, petechiae at the site of the blood pressure cuff, or bruising. Laboratory values for a person with DIC reveal thrombocytopenia and prolonged coagulation times. Other laboratory tests that may be ordered include a complete blood count and kidney and liver function tests to assess the underlying cause of the DIC and to evaluate for organ dysfunction. No one laboratory test is diagnostic for DIC, however, and a scoring system is often used to guide the diagnosis (Box 21.8).

Treatment

Interventions for a woman with DIC usually happen very rapidly, often with many aspects of care happening simultaneously to address both DIC and the underlying condition causing it. At least two large-bore IV lines should be started in anticipation of transfusion. The nurse should administer fluids and blood products per orders and institutional protocols. Oxygen administration by a nonrebreather mask may be necessary to keep the pulse oximetry above 95%.

Care Considerations

Nurses should be alert for signs of hypothermia and attentive to the amount of blood lost and evidence of sufficient urine production. The nurse should monitor fetal heart rate and uterine contractions continuously or per orders. In the case of fetal demise, the focus of care is only on the pregnant woman.

Box 21.7 Signs of Shock

- Tachycardia
- Hypotension
- Thready pulse
- Cool extremities
- Altered mental status
- Pulse pressure (the difference between the systolic and diastolic blood pressures) less than 25 mm Hg

Box 21.8 International Society on Thrombosis and Hemostasis DIC Scoring System

- Platelets
  - 1 Point: platelets < 100,000/μL
  - 2 Points: platelets < 50,000/μL
- Fibrin-related degradation marker (D-dimer and others)
  - 2 Points: greater than the upper limit of normal
  - 3 Points: over five times greater than the upper limit of normal
- Prothrombin time
  - 1 Point: prolonged by more than 3 and less than 6 s
  - 2 Points: prolonged by more than 6 s
- Fibrinogen
  - 1 Point: <100 mg/dL

A score of 5 or greater indicates overt DIC. A score of less than 5 may indicate developing DIC.
DIC, disseminated intravascular coagulation.
Adapted from Taylor, F. B., Jr., Toh, C. H., Hoots, W. K., Wada, H., & Levi, M.; Scientific Subcommittee on Disseminated Intravascular Coagulation of the International Society on Thrombosis and Haemostasis. (2001). Towards definition, clinical and laboratory criteria, and a scoring system for disseminated intravascular coagulation. *Thrombosis and Haemostasis, 86*(5), 1327–1330.

Placenta Previa

Placenta previa is a condition in which the placental tissue overlies the internal cervical os. The condition should be suspected for any woman of 20 weeks gestation or more with vaginal bleeding. In the case of a low lying placenta, the placenta is positioned in the lower uterine segment but does not overlie the os.

Prevalence

Placenta previa complicates approximately one out of every 200 pregnancies (Silver, 2015).

Etiology

Risk factors for placenta previa are listed in Box 21.9.

Prognosis

The major risk of placenta previa is maternal hemorrhage, and women with placenta previa experience bleeding 10 times as frequently as women without the condition (Silver, 2015). Of the women diagnosed with placenta previa, 22% develop postpartum hemorrhage. The lower portion of the uterus is less muscular than the fundus and cannot contract down at the site of a placenta previa or low-lying placenta as efficiently. This relative weakness of the myometrium at this location causes the increased susceptibility to hemorrhage in the postpartum period (Fan et al., 2017).

Box 21.9 Risk Factors for Placenta Previa

- Placenta previa in a prior pregnancy
- Multiple gestation
- Multiparity
- Prior cesarean section (risk increases with number)
- Advanced maternal age
- Treatment for infertility
- Previous intrauterine surgical procedure, including dilation and curettage for spontaneous or therapeutic abortion
- Maternal smoking
- Maternal cocaine use

Over 5% of women with placenta previa require a hysterectomy or ligation or embolization of the pelvic blood vessels to control bleeding postpartum (Rosenberg, Pariente, Sergienko, Wiznitzer, & Sheiner, 2011). Overall, however, the risk for maternal death in high-resource countries, such as the United States, is low.

The major complication for the fetus is prematurity, as over 44% of fetuses are delivered prior to 37 weeks, and the rate of perinatal mortality is 3- to 4-fold that of pregnancies not complicated by placenta previa (Silver, 2015). Fetuses are also at a higher risk for a nonvertex presentation, complicating delivery in the case of a low-lying placenta.

Assessment

Unlike with placental abruption, which classically presents as bleeding with pain, the bleeding from placenta previa is painless. Up to 20% of women presenting with bleeding and placenta previa in the second half of pregnancy, however, have pain and contractions similar to those in placental abruption, and 10% reach term having never bled (Ruiter et al., 2016). The condition is typically confirmed by routine ultrasound.

Placenta previa, in which the placenta overlies the os to any degree, must be distinguished from a low-lying placenta, which is very near the os but does not overlie it. The terms marginal and partial are no longer used to describe the relationship of the placenta to the internal cervical os (Silver, 2015).

Because the uterus is flexible whereas the placenta is not, the source of bleeding with placenta previa is likely from the sheering of the placenta from the cervix and the lower uterine segment as changes to these structures occur normally as the pregnancy progresses.

For most women, placenta previa is recognized by ultrasound during pregnancy and the condition does not persist until delivery. As the lower uterine segment lengthens and grows toward the fundus in pregnancy, the placenta attached to it moves away from the os. Thus, placenta previa only persists to delivery in 12% of cases identified at 19 weeks of gestation, 49% of those identified at 27 weeks of gestation, and 73% of those identified from 32 to 35 weeks of gestation (Dashe, McIntire, Ramus, Santos-Ramos, & Twickler, 2002).

Bess Gaskell, in Chapter 1, was found to have a low-lying placenta on ultrasound, which concerned Dr. Phillips. It never covered the cervical os, however, and so was not placenta previa.

Treatment

Palpation of the placenta through a partially dilated cervix is associated with acute bleeding. Thus, the nurse should not attempt a digital examination in patients with a known previa. Because of bleeding concerns, women are often instructed to avoid exercise and vaginal intercourse after 20 weeks of gestation because of the concern that uterine contractions caused by these activities may cause bleeding. The nurse should instruct women to seek care urgently if they experience bleeding or contractions.

Delivery is generally recommended from 36 to 37 weeks of gestation because of concerns for a greater likelihood for catastrophic bleeding if the pregnancy is prolonged (ACOG, 2013b). In the case of severe bleeding with evidence of maternal hemodynamic instability and/or a nonreassuring fetal heart pattern, expedited cesarean section is generally called for regardless of gestation. Less severe bleeding with apparent maternal and fetal stability may instead be managed expectantly prior to 34 weeks. As in other cases of anticipated preterm delivery, corticosteroids are given prior to 34 weeks of gestation to enhance the maturity of fetal organ systems, and magnesium sulfate may be administered for pregnancies prior to 32 to 34 weeks of gestation because of its neuroprotective effects for the fetus when given prior to delivery.

Because of the high rate of blood transfusions associated with the treatment of placenta previa, women generally have their blood typed and cross-matched at the time of admission, and blood is made available at the time of delivery. A cesarean section is almost always indicated for placenta previa, but women with a low-lying placenta may attempt a vaginal delivery. A placenta 20 mm from the cervix is associated with a better rate of successful vaginal birth than pregnancy with a placenta closer to the cervix.

Vasa Previa

Vasa previa occurs when fetal blood vessels overlie the internal cervical os. The occurrence of fetal blood vessels within 2 cm of the cervix is generally classified as vasa previa, as well.

Prevalence

Vasa previa occurs in approximately 1 out of every 2,500 births.

Etiology

Vasa previa generally occurs in two different ways. A type 1 vasa previa occurs with a velamentous cord insertion, in which blood

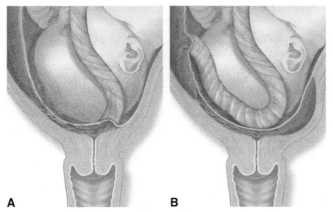

A   **B**

Figure 21.3. Vasa previa. (A) Type 1: Velamentous cord insertion. The umbilical cord inserts into the membranes at some distance from the placental mass, and the umbilical blood vessels course through the membranes to the placental disk. **(B)** Type 2: Succenturiate placentation. An accessory lobe of the placenta is present at a distance from the main placental disk, and umbilical blood vessels course through the membranes connecting the two placental masses. (Reprinted with permission from Stephenson, S. R. [2015]. *Obstetrics and gynecology* [3rd ed., Fig. 18.41]. Philadelphia, PA: Lippincott Williams & Wilkins.)

vessels between the umbilical cord and the placenta run along the fetal membranes overlying the cervix (Fig. 21.3). Pregnancies in which there is a resolved placenta previa are at a higher risk for a type 1 vasa previa. A type 2 vasa previa occurs with a succenturiate placenta, in which the placenta is made up of multiple lobes, usually two, with blood vessels connecting them.

Prognosis

Because the fetal blood vessels are attached to the chorion, membrane rupture in the presence of vasa previa creates a risk for vessel rupture resulting in fetal hemorrhage, exsanguination, asphyxia, and death. Asphyxia may also occur as a result of fetal pressure against the blood vessels even in the absence of a rupture. The survival rate for fetuses with a vasa previa diagnosed prenatally is 97.6%, whereas a vasa previa discovered during or after labor and delivery is associated with a neonatal mortality rate of over 55% (Sinkey, Odibo, Dashe, & Society of Maternal-Fetal Publications, 2015).

Assessment

Because of the higher risk of compression of the fetal vessels associated with vasa previa, antepartum testing with NST or BPP is often started at 32 weeks of gestation in such pregnancies.

Treatment

The treatment for vasa previa may include the administration of corticosteroids prior to 34 weeks of gestation to develop fetal lung maturity and admission of the pregnant woman in the hospital for surveillance. In these cases, NSTs may be performed multiple times a day. Immediate cesarean section is indicated with evidence of bleeding with a nonreassuring fetal heart pattern, labor contractions, rupture of membranes, or repeat variable decelerations of the fetal heart rate from cord compression. Even in the absence of any of these signs, a cesarean section is typically performed from 34 to 35 weeks of gestation (Hasegawa, Arakaki, Ichizuka, & Sekizawa, 2015).

Think Critically

1. Your patient has been diagnosed with a preterm premature rupture of membranes at 28 weeks of gestation. What medications do you anticipate seeing in the orders? How long do you expect they'll be administered for?
2. What are the three uses of magnesium sulfate in pregnancy?
3. Your patient is receiving oxytocin to augment labor and is experiencing six contractions every 10 minutes. The fetal heart tracing is now a category II. Draw a diagram to describe the interventions you anticipate using to address the tachysystole and the fetal heart tracing.
4. The patient described in question 2 no longer has tachysystole, and the fetal heart rate is now a category I. Unfortunately, she is no longer having regular uterine contractions. What next steps do you anticipate?
5. Why do you think placental abruption is more common with preeclampsia?

References

Adams Waldorf, K. M., Singh, N., Mohan, A. R., Young, R. C., Ngo, L., Das, A., . . . Johnson, M. R. (2015). Uterine overdistension induces preterm labor mediated by inflammation: Observations in pregnant women and nonhuman primates. *American Journal of Obstetrics and Gynecology, 213*(6), 830.e1–830.e19. doi:10.1016/j.ajog.2015.08.028

Alfirevic, Z., Aflaifel, N., & Weeks, A. (2014). Oral misoprostol for induction of labour. *Cochrane Database of Systematic Reviews,* (6), CD001338. doi:10.1002/14651858.CD001338.pub3

Al-Ostad, G., Kezouh, A., Spence, A. R., & Abenhaim, H. A. (2015). Incidence and risk factors of sepsis mortality in labor, delivery and after birth: Population-based study in the USA. *Journal of Obstetrics and Gynaecology Research, 41*(8), 1201–1206. doi:10.1111/jog.12710

American College of Obstetricians and Gynecologists. (2009). ACOG practice bulletin no. 106: Intrapartum fetal heart rate monitoring: Nomenclature, interpretation, and general management principles. *Obstetrics and Gynecology, 114*(1), 192–202. doi:10.1097/AOG.0b013e3181aef106

American College of Obstetricians and Gynecologists. (2013a). ACOG committee opinion no. 579: Definition of term pregnancy. *Obstetrics and Gynecology, 122*(5), 1139–1140. doi:10.1097/01.AOG.0000437385.88715.4a

American College of Obstetricians and Gynecologists. (2013b). ACOG committee opinion no. 560: Medically indicated late-preterm and early-term deliveries. *Obstetrics and Gynecology, 121*(4), 908–910. doi:10.1097/01.AOG.0000428648.75548.00

American College of Obstetricians and Gynecologists. (2014). Practice bulletin no. 146: Management of late-term and postterm pregnancies. *Obstetrics and Gynecology, 124*(2 Pt. 1), 390–396. doi:10.1097/01.AOG.0000452744.06088.48

American College of Obstetricians and Gynecologists. (2016a). Obstetric care consensus no. 3: Periviable birth. *Obstetrics and Gynecology, 127*(5), e82–e94. doi:10.1097/AOG.0000000000001105

ACOG. (2016b). Practice bulletin no. 159: Management of preterm labor. *Obstet Gynecol, 127*(1), e29-38. doi:10.1097/AOG.0000000000001265

American College of Obstetricians and Gynecologists. (2017). Committee opinion no. 687: Approaches to limit intervention during labor and birth. *Obstetrics and Gynecology, 129*(2), e20–e28. doi:10.1097/AOG.0000000000001905

Ananth, C. V., Keyes, K. M., Hamilton, A., Gissler, M., Wu, C., Liu, S., . . . Cnattingius, S. (2015). An international contrast of rates of placental abruption: An age-period-cohort analysis. *PLoS One, 10*(5), e0125246. doi:10.1371/journal.pone.0125246

Ananth, C. V., Lavery, J. A., Vintzileos, A. M., Skupski, D. W., Varner, M., Saade, G., . . . Wright, J. D. (2016). Severe placental abruption: Clinical definition and associations with maternal complications. *American Journal of Obstetrics and Gynecology, 214*(2), 272.e1–272.e9. doi:10.1016/j.ajog.2015.09.069

Avagliano, L., Bulfamante, G. P., Morabito, A., & Marconi, A. M. (2011). Abnormal spiral artery remodelling in the decidual segment during pregnancy: From histology to clinical correlation. *Journal of Clinical Pathology, 64*(12), 1064–1068. doi:10.1136/jclinpath-2011-200092

Berghella, V., Baxter, J. K., & Hendrix, N. W. (2013). Cervical assessment by ultrasound for preventing preterm delivery. *Cochrane Database of Systematic Reviews,* (1), CD007235. doi:10.1002/14651858.CD007235.pub3

Bernardes, T. P., Broekhuijsen, K., Koopmans, C. M., Boers, K. E., van Wyk, L., Tajik, P., . . . Groen, H. (2016). Caesarean section rates and adverse neonatal outcomes after induction of labour versus expectant management in women with an unripe cervix: A secondary analysis of the HYPITAT and DIGITAT trials. *British Journal of Obstetrics and Gynaecology, 123*(9), 1501–1508. doi:10.1111/1471-0528.14028

Bigelow, C. A., Factor, S. H., Miller, M., Weintraub, A., & Stone, J. (2016). Pilot randomized controlled trial to evaluate the impact of bed rest on maternal and fetal outcomes in women with preterm premature rupture of the membranes. *American Journal of Perinatology, 33*(4), 356–363. doi:10.1055/s-0035-1564427

Bonzini, M., Coggon, D., & Palmer, K. T. (2007). Risk of prematurity, low birthweight and pre-eclampsia in relation to working hours and physical activities: A systematic review. *Occupational and Environmental Medicine, 64*(4), 228–243. doi:10.1136/oem.2006.026872

Boulvain, M., Irion, O., Dowswell, T., & Thornton, J. G. (2016). Induction of labour at or near term for suspected fetal macrosomia. *Cochrane Database of Systematic Reviews,* (5), CD000938. doi:10.1002/14651858.CD000938.pub2

Boulvain, M., Stan, C., & Irion, O. (2005). Membrane sweeping for induction of labour. *Cochrane Database of Systematic Reviews,* (1), CD000451. doi:10.1002/14651858.CD000451.pub2

Bruijn, M. M., Kamphuis, E. I., Hoesli, I. M., Martinez de Tejada, B., Loccufier, A. R., Kuhnert, M., . . . van Baaren, G. J. (2016). The predictive value of quantitative fibronectin testing in combination with cervical length measurement in symptomatic women. *American Journal of Obstetrics and Gynecology, 215*(6), 793.e1–793.e8. doi:10.1016/j.ajog.2016.08.012

Budden, A., Chen, L. J., & Henry, A. (2014). High-dose versus low-dose oxytocin infusion regimens for induction of labour at term. *Cochrane Database of Systematic Reviews,* (10), CD009701. doi:10.1002/14651858.CD009701.pub2

Buhimschi, C. S., Schatz, F., Krikun, G., Buhimschi, I. A., & Lockwood, C. J. (2010). Novel insights into molecular mechanisms of abruption-induced preterm birth. *Expert Reviews in Molecular Medicine, 12*, e35. doi:10.1017/S1462399410001675

Callaghan, W. M., Creanga, A. A., & Kuklina, E. V. (2012). Severe maternal morbidity among delivery and postpartum hospitalizations in the United States. *Obstetrics and Gynecology, 120*(5), 1029–1036. doi:10.1097/AOG.0b013e31826d60c5

Chapman, E., Reveiz, L., Illanes, E., & Bonfill Cosp, X. (2014). Antibiotic regimens for management of intra-amniotic infection. *Cochrane Database of Systematic Reviews,* (12), CD010976. doi:10.1002/14651858.CD010976.pub2

Chettri, S., Adhisivam, B., & Bhat, B. V. (2015). Endotracheal suction for nonvigorous neonates born through meconium stained amniotic fluid: A randomized controlled trial. *Journal of Pediatrics, 166*(5), 1208.e1–1213.e1. doi:10.1016/j.jpeds.2014.12.076

Christian, L. M. (2014). Effects of stress and depression on inflammatory immune parameters in pregnancy. *American Journal of Obstetrics and Gynecology, 211*(3), 275–277. doi:10.1016/j.ajog.2014.06.042

Crowley, A. E., Grivell, R. M., & Dodd, J. M. (2016). Sealing procedures for preterm prelabour rupture of membranes. *Cochrane Database of Systematic Reviews, 7*, CD010218. doi:10.1002/14651858.CD010218.pub2

Cunningham, F. G., & Nelson, D. B. (2015). Disseminated intravascular coagulation syndromes in obstetrics. *Obstetrics and Gynecology, 126*(5), 999–1011. doi:10.1097/AOG.0000000000001110

Dashe, J. S., McIntire, D. D., Ramus, R. M., Santos-Ramos, R., & Twickler, D. M. (2002). Persistence of placenta previa according to gestational age at ultrasound detection. *Obstetrics and Gynecology, 99*(5 Pt. 1), 692–697.

de Miranda, E., van der Bom, J. G., Bonsel, G. J., Bleker, O. P., & Rosendaal, F. R. (2006). Membrane sweeping and prevention of post-term pregnancy in low-risk pregnancies: A randomised controlled trial. *British Journal of Obstetrics and Gynecology, 113*(4), 402–408. doi:10.1111/j.1471-0528.2006.00870.x

Deshpande, S. N., van Asselt, A. D., Tomini, F., Armstrong, N., Allen, A., Noake, C., . . . Westwood, M. E. (2013). Rapid fetal fibronectin testing to predict preterm birth in women with symptoms of premature labour: A systematic review and cost analysis. *Health Technology Assessment, 17*(40), 1–138. doi:10.3310/hta17400

Ding, X. X., Wu, Y. L., Xu, S. J., Zhu, R. P., Jia, X. M., Zhang, S. F., . . . Tao, F. B. (2014). Maternal anxiety during pregnancy and adverse birth outcomes: A systematic review and meta-analysis of prospective cohort studies. *Journal of Affective Disorders, 159*, 103–110. doi:10.1016/j.jad.2014.02.027

Donders, G. G., Van Calsteren, K., Bellen, G., Reybrouck, R., Van den Bosch, T., Riphagen, I., & Van Lierde, S. (2009). Predictive value for preterm birth of abnormal vaginal flora, bacterial vaginosis and aerobic vaginitis during the first trimester of pregnancy. *British Journal of Obstetrics and Gynecology, 116*(10), 1315–1324. doi:10.1111/j.1471-0528.2009.02237.x

Elsasser, D. A., Ananth, C. V., Prasad, V., Vintzileos, A. M., & New Jersey-Placental Abruption Study Investigators. (2010). Diagnosis of placental abruption: Relationship between clinical and histopathological findings. *European Journal of Obstetrics and Gynecology and Reproductive Biology, 148*(2), 125–130. doi:10.1016/j.ejogrb.2009.10.005

Fan, D., Xia, Q., Liu, L., Wu, S., Tian, G., Wang, W., . . . Liu, Z. (2017). The incidence of postpartum hemorrhage in pregnant women with placenta previa: A systematic review and meta-analysis. *PLoS One, 12*(1), e0170194. doi:10.1371/journal.pone.0170194

Flenady, V., Hawley, G., Stock, O. M., Kenyon, S., & Badawi, N. (2013). Prophylactic antibiotics for inhibiting preterm labour with intact membranes. *Cochrane Database of Systematic Reviews,* (12), CD000246. doi:10.1002/14651858.CD000246.pub2

Gulmezoglu, A. M., Crowther, C. A., Middleton, P., & Heatley, E. (2012). Induction of labour for improving birth outcomes for women at or beyond term. *Cochrane Database of Systematic Reviews,* (6), CD004945. doi:10.1002/14651858.CD004945.pub3

Gyamfi-Bannerman, C., & Ananth, C. V. (2014). Trends in spontaneous and indicated preterm delivery among singleton gestations in the United States, 2005–2012. *Obstetrics and Gynecology, 124*(6), 1069–1074. doi:10.1097/AOG.0000000000000546

Hackney, D. N., Olson-Chen, C., & Thornburg, L. L. (2013). What do we know about the natural outcomes of preterm labour? A systematic review and meta-analysis of women without tocolysis in preterm labour. *Paediatric and Perinatal Epidemiology, 27*(5), 452–460. doi:10.1111/ppe.12070

Hasegawa, J., Arakaki, T., Ichizuka, K., & Sekizawa, A. (2015). Management of vasa previa during pregnancy. *Journal of Perinatal Medicine, 43*(6), 783–784. doi:10.1515/jpm-2014-0047

Heida, K. Y., Velthuis, B. K., Oudijk, M. A., Reitsma, J. B., Bots, M. L., Franx, A., & van Dunné, F. M.; Dutch Guideline Development Group on Cardiovascular Risk Management after Reproductive Disorders. (2016). Cardiovascular disease risk in women with a history of spontaneous preterm delivery: A systematic review and meta-analysis. *European Journal of Preventive Cardiology, 23*(3), 253–263. doi:10.1177/2047487314566758

Hernandez-Diaz, S., Boeke, C. E., Romans, A. T., Young, B., Margulis, A. V., McElrath, T. F., . . . Bateman, B. T. (2014). Triggers of spontaneous preterm delivery—Why today? *Paediatric and Perinatal Epidemiology, 28*(2), 79–87. doi:10.1111/ppe.12105

Higgins, R. D., Saade, G., Polin, R. A., Grobman, W. A., Buhimschi, I. A., Watterberg, K., . . . Raju, T. N.; Chorioamnionitis Workshop Participants. (2016). Evaluation and management of women and newborns with a maternal diagnosis of chorioamnionitis: Summary of a workshop. *Obstetrics and Gynecology, 127*(3), 426-436. doi:10.1097/AOG.0000000000001246

Hofmeyr, G. J., & Kiiza, J. A. (2016). Amnioinfusion for chorioamnionitis. *Cochrane Database of Systematic Reviews,* (8), CD011622. doi:10.1002/14651858.CD011622.pub2

Iams, J. D. (2014). Prevention of preterm parturition. *New England Journal of Medicine, 370*(19), 1861. doi:10.1056/NEJMc1402822

Kasai, M., Aoki, S., Ogawa, M., Kurasawa, K., Takahashi, T., & Hirahara, F. (2015). Prediction of perinatal outcomes based on primary symptoms in women with placental abruption. *Journal of Obstetrics and Gynaecology Research, 41*(6), 850–856. doi:10.1111/jog.12637

Kenyon, S., Boulvain, M., & Neilson, J. P. (2013). Antibiotics for preterm rupture of membranes. *Cochrane Database of Systematic Reviews,* (12), CD001058. doi:10.1002/14651858.CD001058.pub3

Kibel, M., Asztalos, E., Barrett, J., Dunn, M. S., Tward, C., Pittini, A., & Melamed, N. (2016). Outcomes of pregnancies complicated by preterm premature rupture of membranes between 20 and 24 weeks of gestation. *Obstetrics and Gynecology, 128*(2), 313–320. doi:10.1097/AOG.0000000000001530

Kobayashi, A., Minami, S., Tanizaki, Y., Shiro, M., Yamamoto, M., Yagi, S., . . . Ino, K. (2014). Adverse perinatal and neonatal outcomes in patients with chronic abruption-oligohydramnios sequence. *Journal of Obstetrics and Gynaecology Research, 40*(6), 1618–1624. doi:10.1111/jog.12395

Kortekaas, J. C., Kazemier, B. M., Ravelli, A. C., de Boer, K., van Dillen, J., Mol, B., & de Miranda, E. (2015). Recurrence rate and outcome of postterm pregnancy, a national cohort study. *European Journal of Obstetrics and Gynecology and Reproductive Biology, 193*, 70–74. doi:10.1016/j.ejogrb.2015.05.021

Linehan, L. A., Walsh, J., Morris, A., Kenny, L., O'Donoghue, K., Dempsey, E., & Russell, N. (2016). Neonatal and maternal outcomes following midtrimester preterm premature rupture of the membranes: A retrospective cohort study. *BMC Pregnancy and Childbirth, 16*, 25. doi:10.1186/s12884-016-0813-3

Lyons, P. (2015). Premature rupture of membranes. In *Obstetrics in family medicine. Current clinical practice*. Cham, Switzerland: Humana Press.

Mackeen, A. D., Seibel-Seamon, J., Muhammad, J., Baxter, J. K., & Berghella, V. (2014). Tocolytics for preterm premature rupture of membranes. *Cochrane Database of Systematic Reviews*, (2), CD007062. doi:10.1002/14651858.CD007062.pub3

Martin, J. A., Hamilton, B. E., Osterman, M. J., Driscoll, A. K., & Mathews, T. J. (2017). Births: Final data for 2015. *National Vital Statistics Reports, 66*(1), 1.

Martinez de Tejada, B., Karolinski, A., Ocampo, M. C., Laterra, C., Hosli, I., Fernandez, D., . . . Irion, O.; 4P Trial Group. (2015). Prevention of preterm delivery with vaginal progesterone in women with preterm labour (4P): Randomised double-blind placebo-controlled trial. *British Journal of Obstetrics and Gynecology, 122*(1), 80–91. doi:10.1111/1471-0528.13061

McCarty-Singleton, S., & Sciscione, A. C. (2014). Maternal activity restriction in pregnancy and the prevention of preterm birth: An evidence-based review. *Clinical Obstetrics and Gynecology, 57*(3), 616–627. doi:10.1097/GRF.0000000000000048

McLaren, J. S., Hezelgrave, N. L., Ayubi, H., Seed, P. T., & Shennan, A. H. (2015). Prediction of spontaneous preterm birth using quantitative fetal fibronectin after recent sexual intercourse. *American Journal of Obstetrics and Gynecology, 212*(1), 89.e1–89.e5. doi:10.1016/j.ajog.2014.06.055

McMaster, K., Sanchez-Ramos, L., & Kaunitz, A. M. (2015). Balancing the efficacy and safety of misoprostol: A meta-analysis comparing 25 versus 50 micrograms of intravaginal misoprostol for the induction of labour. *British Journal of Obstetrics and Gynecology, 122*(4), 468–476. doi:10.1111/1471-0528.12935

Middleton, P., Shepherd, E., Flenady, V., McBain, R. D., & Crowther, C. A. (2017). Planned early birth versus expectant management (waiting) for prelabour rupture of membranes at term (37 weeks or more). *Cochrane Database of Systematic Reviews, 1*, CD005302. doi:10.1002/14651858.CD005302.pub3

Miller, E. S., Tita, A. T., & Grobman, W. A. (2015). Second-trimester cervical length screening among asymptomatic women: An evaluation of risk-based strategies. *Obstetrics and Gynecology, 126*(1), 61–66. doi:10.1097/AOG.0000000000000864

Moroz, L. A., & Simhan, H. N. (2014). Rate of sonographic cervical shortening and biologic pathways of spontaneous preterm birth. *American Journal of Obstetrics and Gynecology, 210*(6), 555.e1–555.e5. doi:10.1016/j.ajog.2013.12.037

Norman, J. E., Marlow, N., Messow, C. M., Shennan, A., Bennett, P. R., Thornton, S., . . . Norrie, J.; OPPTIMUM Study Group. (2016). Vaginal progesterone prophylaxis for preterm birth (the OPPTIMUM study): A multicentre, randomised, double-blind trial. *The Lancet, 387*(10033), 2106–2116. doi:10.1016/S0140-6736(16)00350-0

Oberg, A. S., Frisell, T., Svensson, A. C., & Iliadou, A. N. (2013). Maternal and fetal genetic contributions to postterm birth: Familial clustering in a population-based sample of 475,429 Swedish births. *American Journal of Epidemiology, 177*(6), 531–537. doi:10.1093/aje/kws244

Osterman, M. J., & Martin, J. A. (2014). Recent declines in induction of labor by gestational age. *NCHS Data Brief*, (155), 1–8.

Pierson, R. C., Gordon, S. S., & Haas, D. M. (2014). A retrospective comparison of antibiotic regimens for preterm premature rupture of membranes. *Obstetrics and Gynecology, 124*(3), 515–519. doi:10.1097/AOG.0000000000000426

Rattray, D. D., O'Connell, C. M., & Baskett, T. F. (2012). Acute disseminated intravascular coagulation in obstetrics: A tertiary centre population review (1980 to 2009). *Journal of Obstetrics and Gynaecology Canada, 34*(4), 341–347.

Roberts, D., Brown, J., Medley, N., & Dalziel, S. R. (2017). Antenatal corticosteroids for accelerating fetal lung maturation for women at risk of preterm birth. *Cochrane Database of Systematic Reviews, 3*, CD004454. doi:10.1002/14651858.CD004454.pub3

Romero, R., Nicolaides, K. H., Conde-Agudelo, A., O'Brien, J. M., Cetingoz, E., Da Fonseca, E., . . . Hassan, S. S. (2016). Vaginal progesterone decreases preterm birth ≤ 34 weeks of gestation in women with a singleton pregnancy and a short cervix: An updated meta-analysis including data from the OPPTIMUM study. *Ultrasound in Obstetrics and Gynecology, 48*(3), 308–317. doi:10.1002/uog.15953

Rosenberg, T., Pariente, G., Sergienko, R., Wiznitzer, A., & Sheiner, E. (2011). Critical analysis of risk factors and outcome of placenta previa. *Archives of Gynecology and Obstetrics, 284*(1), 47–51. doi:10.1007/s00404-010-1598-7

Ruiter, L., Eschbach, S. J., Burgers, M., Rengerink, K. O., Pampus, M. G., Goes, B. Y., . . . Pajkrt, E. (2016). Predictors for emergency cesarean delivery in women with placenta previa. *American Journal of Perinatology, 33*(14), 1407–1414. doi:10.1055/s-0036-1584148

Ruiter, L., Ravelli, A. C., de Graaf, I. M., Mol, B. W., & Pajkrt, E. (2015). Incidence and recurrence rate of placental abruption: A longitudinal linked national cohort study in the Netherlands. *American Journal of Obstetrics and Gynecology, 213*(4), 573.e1–573.e8. doi:10.1016/j.ajog.2015.06.019

Saccone, G., & Berghella, V. (2015a). Antibiotic prophylaxis for term or near-term premature rupture of membranes: Metaanalysis of randomized trials. *American Journal of Obstetrics and Gynecology, 212*(5), 627.e1–627.e9. doi:10.1016/j.ajog.2014.12.034

Saccone, G., & Berghella, V. (2015b). Induction of labor at full term in uncomplicated singleton gestations: A systematic review and metaanalysis of randomized controlled trials. *American Journal of Obstetrics and Gynecology, 213*(5), 629–636. doi:10.1016/j.ajog.2015.04.004

Saccone, G., & Berghella, V. (2016). Antenatal corticosteroids for maturity of term or near term fetuses: Systematic review and meta-analysis of randomized controlled trials. *BMJ, 355*, i5044. doi:10.1136/bmj.i5044

Saccone, G., Khalifeh, A., Elimian, A., Bahrami, E., Chaman-Ara, K., Bahrami, M. A., & Berghella, V. (2017). Vaginal progesterone vs intramuscular 17alpha-hydroxyprogesterone caproate for prevention of recurrent spontaneous preterm birth in singleton gestations: Systematic review and meta-analysis of randomized controlled trials. *Ultrasound in Obstetrics and Gynecology, 49*(3), 315–321. doi:10.1002/uog.17245

Satterfield, N., Newton, E. R., & May, L. E. (2016). Activity in pregnancy for patients with a history of preterm birth. *Clinical Medicine Insights. Women's Health, 9*(Suppl. 1), 17–21. doi:10.4137/CMWH.S34684

Shinde, G. R., Vaswani, B. P., Patange, R. P., Laddad, M. M., & Bhosale, R. B. (2016). Diagnostic performance of ultrasonography for detection of abruption and its clinical correlation and maternal and foetal outcome. *Journal of Clinical and Diagnostic Research, 10*(8), QC04–QC07. doi:10.7860/JCDR/2016/19247.8288

Silver, R. M. (2015). Abnormal placentation: Placenta previa, vasa previa, and placenta accreta. *Obstetrics and Gynecology, 126*(3), 654–668. doi:10.1097/AOG.0000000000001005

Sinkey, R. G., Odibo, A. O., Dashe, J. S., & Society of Maternal-Fetal Publications. (2015). #37: Diagnosis and management of vasa previa. *American Journal of Obstetrics and Gynecology, 213*(5), 615–619. doi:10.1016/j.ajog.2015.08.031

Sosa, C. G., Althabe, F., Belizan, J. M., & Bergel, E. (2015). Bed rest in singleton pregnancies for preventing preterm birth. *Cochrane Database of Systematic Reviews*, (3), CD003581. doi:10.1002/14651858.CD003581.pub3

Sotiriadis, A., Papatheodorou, S., Kavvadias, A., & Makrydimas, G. (2010). Transvaginal cervical length measurement for prediction of preterm birth in women with threatened preterm labor: A meta-analysis. *Ultrasound in Obstetrics and Gynecology, 35*(1), 54–64. doi:10.1002/uog.7457

Stan, C. M., Boulvain, M., Pfister, R., & Hirsbrunner-Almagbaly, P. (2013). Hydration for treatment of preterm labour. *Cochrane Database of Systematic Reviews*, (11), CD003096. doi:10.1002/14651858.CD003096.pub2

Tang, J., Kapp, N., Dragoman, M., & de Souza, J. P. (2013). WHO recommendations for misoprostol use for obstetric and gynecologic indications. *International Journal of Gynaecology and Obstetrics, 121*(2), 186–189. doi:10.1016/j.ijgo.2012.12.009

Tikkanen, M., Luukkaala, T., Gissler, M., Ritvanen, A., Ylikorkala, O., Paavonen, J., . . . Metsaranta, M. (2013). Decreasing perinatal mortality in placental abruption. *Acta Obstetricia et Gynecologica Scandinavica, 92*(3), 298–305. doi:10.1111/aogs.12030

Tita, A. T., & Andrews, W. W. (2010). Diagnosis and management of clinical chorioamnionitis. *Clinics in Perinatology, 37*(2), 339–354. doi:10.1016/j.clp.2010.02.003

Vaisbuch, E., Romero, R., Mazaki-Tovi, S., Erez, O., Kusanovic, J. P., Mittal, P., . . . Hassan, S. S. (2010). The risk of impending preterm delivery in asymptomatic patients with a nonmeasurable cervical length in the second trimester. *American Journal of Obstetrics and Gynecology, 203*(5), 446.e1–446.e9. doi:10.1016/j.ajog.2010.05.040

van der Heyden, J. L., van Kuijk, S. M., van der Ham, D. P., Notten, K. J., Janssen, T., Nijhuis, J. G., . . . Mol, B. W. (2013). Subsequent pregnancy after preterm prelabor rupture of membranes before 27 weeks' gestation. *AJP Reports, 3*(2), 113–118. doi:10.1055/s-0033-1353389

Wang, L., Matsunaga, S., Mikami, Y., Takai, Y., Terui, K., & Seki, H. (2016). Pre-delivery fibrinogen predicts adverse maternal or neonatal outcomes in patients with placental abruption. *Journal of Obstetrics and Gynaecology Research, 42*(7), 796–802. doi:10.1111/jog.12988

World Health Organization. (2016). *Preterm birth*. Retrieved from http://www.who.int/mediacentre/factsheets/fs363/en/

Zeng, X., Xue, Y., Tian, Q., Sun, R., & An, R. (2016). Effects and safety of magnesium sulfate on neuroprotection: A meta-analysis based on PRISMA guidelines. *Medicine (Baltimore), 95*(1), e2451. doi:10.1097/MD.0000000000002451

Zuckerwise, L. C., Pettker, C. M., Illuzzi, J., Raab, C. R., & Lipkind, H. S. (2014). Use of a novel visual aid to improve estimation of obstetric blood loss. *Obstetrics and Gynecology, 123*(5), 982–986. doi:10.1097/AOG.0000000000000233

Suggested Readings

Burke, C., & Chin, E. G. (2016). Chorioamnionitis at term: Definition, diagnosis, and implications for practice. *Journal of Perinatal and Neonatal Nursing, 30*(2), 106–114. doi:10.1097/JPN.0000000000000163

Doyle, J., & Silber, A. (2015). Preterm labor: Role of the nurse practitioner. *Nurse Practitioner, 40*(3), 49–54. doi:10.1097/01.NPR.0000445957.28669.51

Heavey, E., & Dahl Maher, M. (2015). Placental abruption: Are we going to lose them both? *Nursing, 45*(5), 54–59. doi:10.1097/01.NURSE.0000463662.37982.73

Main, E. K., Goffman, D., Scavone, B. M., Low, L. K., Bingham, D., Fontaine, P. L., . . . Levy, B. S. (2015). National partnership for maternal safety: Consensus bundle on obstetric hemorrhage. *Journal of Obstetric, Gynecologic, and Neonatal Nursing, 44*(4), 462–470. doi:10.1111/1552-6909.12723

22 Complications Occurring During Labor and Delivery

Labor and delivery is also known as the intrapartum period. Although most follow a predictable course and progress without incident, labor and delivery is not without risks. Care of the laboring woman includes care of the fetus. Labor and delivery care is acute care and requires careful preparation, specialized knowledge, and keen evaluation skills. Teamwork is an essential component of intrapartum care.

Group B Streptococcus

Prevalence

The urogenital tracts of approximately a quarter of pregnant women are colonized with group B streptococcus (GBS; Brigtsen et al., 2015). While this colonization is benign outside of pregnancy, it can be dangerous to the neonate exposed intrapartum.

Prognosis

Although GBS itself can be treated with antibiotics and is not a complication, GBS colonization of a woman, particularly if untreated or treated inadequately, can have a devastating effect on the neonate. GBS infection in the neonate typically manifests as sepsis, pneumonia, or meningitis. Neonates born to mothers who are colonized with GBS and are not treated with intravenous (IV) antibiotics intrapartum have an approximately 50% chance of being infected via intrapartum transmission. Of these infants, only a small number develop GBS disease.

The good news, however, is that intrapartum GBS treatment has resulted in a reduction of more than 80% in neonatal GBS disease before 6 days of age and a reduction in neonatal deaths. Prior to routine GBS prophylaxis during labor for pregnant women colonized with GBS, the incidence of early-onset neonatal GBS disease was as high as 1.8 per 1,000 births. In 2015, the rate of GBS disease in neonates was 0.15 per 1,000 births (Centers for Disease Control and Prevention, 2017).

Assessment

In the pregnant woman, GBS is usually asymptomatic. Women are routinely checked for GBS colonization of the urogenital tract in the 36th week of pregnancy. The Centers for Disease Control and Prevention (CDC) recommends that a maternal GBS culture be collected from 35 to 37 weeks of gestation (see Chapter 15). Colonization tends to come and go, and a woman who is not colonized in early pregnancy may still be positive later, and vice versa. Women who have GBS in their urine at any point during pregnancy and women who previously delivered infants who developed GBS in the first week after birth are typically treated with antibiotics in labor regardless of the results of the culture test (see Box 7.2). The culture is taken from the vaginal introitus and the rectum, using either one swab for each site or a single swab.

In Chapter 7, Hannah was diagnosed with GBS and treated with IV antibiotics when she was admitted to labor and delivery. Because she was GBS positive, when she experienced premature rupture of membranes, she was induced right away rather than managed expectantly to minimize the chance of GBS disease in Hannah's newborn.

Treatment

The administration of antibiotics during labor protects newborns from developing a GBS infection before 6 days of age. Because of the grave risk GBS infection poses to the neonate, this care has been routinely recommended by the CDC since 1996 for women who test positive for GBS.

Because the time of delivery is not predictable, antibiotics are begun at the time of admission for rupture of membranes or labor and administered every 4 hours until delivery (see Box 7.4). Women in preterm labor are treated with GBS prophylaxis without screening, and treatment is stopped if labor stops. GBS prophylaxis is provided for preterm premature rupture of membranes unless and until results from a GBS culture test are negative.

Antibiotics are given IV to create a high maternal serum level of the antibiotic that then crosses the placenta for fetal uptake. Antibiotics must be started 4 or more hours prior to delivery to be considered adequate. Treatment for a shorter amount of time is considered inadequate and puts the infant at risk for GBS disease. Moreover, only treatment with penicillin G, ampicillin, or cefazolin is considered adequate; these antibiotics, however, are contraindicated in people with severe allergies to penicillin. Treatment with other antibiotics is considered inadequate, and the neonate remains at an increased risk for GBS disease, although less so than it would be without any antibiotic prophylaxis.

Dystocia

Dystocia is any labor with an abnormally slow or fast progression. A 2006 study identified that as many as one in five labors are complicated by dystocia (Zhu et al., 2006), and dystocia is the most common reason for primary (first-time) cesarean sections. Causes of dystocia are diverse and include problems with any of the main components of labor, known as the five Ps—powers, passageway, passenger, psyche, and position of the mother (see Chapter 16)—or a combination of them. Factors associated with dystocia include the following (Tana, Rachel, & Kamalini, 2017):

- Asian, African, or Hispanic descent
- Diabetes
- Oxytocin augmentation
- History of operative delivery with previous pregnancy
- Increased fetal weight

Powers

As discussed in Chapter 16, the powers of labor refer to the forces that open the cervix and push the newborn through the birth canal. Contractions are considered primary powers, whereas voluntary pushing by the mother is a secondary power. A problem with either of these powers can result in dystocia.

Dysfunctional Uterine Contractions

Labor is defined as the presence of contractions that result in cervical effacement and dilation. In early labor, the latent phase of the first stage, irregular contractions and gradual cervical changes are expected. As labor progresses, however, contractions should become stronger and more productive, progressing from a rate of two to four every 10 minutes in the latent phase of the first stage of labor to four to five every 10 minutes in the active phase. During transition at the end of the first stage of labor, contractions are normally particularly strong and closely spaced as the cervix achieves its final dilation and effacement.

Dysfunctional uterine contractions, however, are irregular in timing, strength, or both and do not contribute to cervical changes or fetal descent. They may be either hypotonic or hypertonic.

Hypotonic Uterine Dysfunction

Hypotonic uterine dysfunction (also referred to as hypotonic labor patterns, secondary uterine inertia, or hypocontractile uterine activity) is a condition in which uterine contractions are either too uncoordinated or insufficiently strong to effectively dilate the cervix. This condition occurs in the active phase of the first stage of labor.

Factors contributing to hypotonic uterine dysfunction include overdistention of the uterus from polyhydramnios, macrosomia, a multiple pregnancy, or a history of multiple pregnancies. Women with hypotonic uterine dysfunction experience productive contractions initially, which then become weaker and less effective and may stop all together. The most common reasons for this reduction in uterine activity are malposition of the fetus and cephalopelvic disproportion.

Women with ruptured membranes whose duration of labor is prolonged due to hypotonic contractions or any other cause are at an increased risk for infection. Postpartum, women who experienced hypotonic uterine dysfunction are at a higher risk for postpartum hemorrhage.

The nurse may monitor contraction frequency and duration by external tocodynamometer or palpation of the uterus. Hypotonic contractions feel soft on palpation and occur at a rate of less than three or four every 10 minutes. A hypotonic contraction lasts for less than 50 seconds. In the case of internal monitoring of contractions, cumulative contraction pressure within 10 minutes of less than 200 to 250 Montevideo units (MVUs) is considered hypotonic (contraction pressure in MVUs is calculated by subtracting the baseline uterine pressure from the peak pressure of each contraction that occurs within a 10-minute period and then adding together the differences). Mothers may report that these contractions cause little discomfort.

The management of hypotonic contractions typically includes ruling out cephalopelvic disproportion and fetal malposition. The nurse should regularly monitor the well-being of both the fetus and the mother. In the absence of contraindications (vaginal birth being contraindicated, hypertonic uterus, etc.), oxytocin is typically administered to augment labor. Other measures used to augment labor include nipple stimulation to increase the endogenous production of oxytocin, ambulation, and rupture of intact membranes.

Hypertonic Uterine Dysfunction

Hypertonic uterine dysfunction describes a contraction pattern seen in the latent phase of the first stage of labor, primarily in women experiencing their first birth (nulliparas). In this condition, contractions are frequent, have irregular tone, and do not contribute to cervical effacement or dilation or fetal descent. Often, the uterus does not relax completely between contractions. The contractions, rather than occurring mostly in the fundus of the uterus, as they do in normal labor, occur in the midsection of the uterus. Fundal contractions apply downward pressure that contributes to cervical changes and fetal descent. Midsection contractions, in contrast, do not.

The intensity of the contractions in combination with their lack of efficacy can be overwhelming and exhausting for the laboring woman. Because of the frequency of contractions and the failure of the uterus to relax between contractions, the fetal heart rate may be category II (indeterminate) or category III (abnormal) (see Table 6.5).

Hypertonic uterine contractions of the latent phase of the first stage should not be confused with uterine tachysystole, also referred to as hyperstimulation or hypertonus. Tachysystole is more than five contractions over 10 minutes within a 30-minute window with or without fetal heart rate changes. Unlike hypertonic uterine contractions, the contractions of tachysystole are strong, organized, and fundal. Tachysystole is associated with labor augmentation medications such as oxytocin and prostaglandin preparations but may also happen spontaneously.

The nurse may facilitate a period of rest for the mother, which is desirable, by conservative measures, such as providing a warm bath, or by the administration of an opioid, as ordered, such as morphine or meperidine to reduce pain and lessen contractions. A sleep medication may also be ordered to encourage a period of rest. After a period of 4 to 6 hours of rest, a normal contraction pattern often ensues.

Prognosis

Whatever the type or cause of dysfunctional uterine contractions, the resulting abnormal labor patterns are associated with increased risks for both the mother and the infant. The risk for operative delivery increases, as do the risks for perineal lacerations, postpartum urinary retention and hemorrhage, and chorioamnionitis (Miller et al., 2017; Stephansson, Sandstrom, Petersson, Wikstrom, & Cnattingius, 2016). A protracted first stage is associated with an increased rate of neonatal intensive care unit (NICU) admissions and lower 5-minute Apgar scores. A prolonged second stage is associated with a small increase in the incidence of complications related to fetal asphyxia (Sandstrom et al., 2017).

Assessment

The standards for normal labor, still used today, were established by Emanuel Friedman in the 1950s on the basis of the observations of 500 women at a single institution. However, more modern studies, including one by Zhang and colleagues in 2010 that included 65,415 women at 19 different institutions, indicate that labor today is generally slower than the Friedman observations suggested. These changes may be attributed to births later in life, heavier mothers, changes in labor practices, and changes in anesthesia use. At this time, however, an updated standard has not been universally adopted (Cohen & Friedman, 2015; Friedman, 1954). According to a 2011 study, the average time it takes for a woman with a body mass index (BMI) of less than 25 kg/m^2 to dilate from 4 to 10 cm is 5.4 hours, whereas for a woman with a BMI of greater than 40 kg/m^2 it is 7.7 hours (Kominiarek et al., 2011).

Friedman recognized six different classifications of abnormal labor (Table 22.1):

1. Prolonged latent phase
2. Protracted active-phase dilation
3. Secondary arrest: no change
4. Protracted descent
5. Arrest of descent
6. Failure of descent

These classifications, along with their more modern interpretations, are discussed below.

The latent phase of labor has a wide range of normal. A **prolonged latent phase** is classically considered to be one that lasts more than 20 hours for a nulliparous woman or 14 hours for a woman who has given birth previously. Contemporary parameters, however, assign more similar prolonged durations: over 9.6 hours to dilate from 4 to 6 cm for a woman who has not given birth before and over 10.7 hours for a woman who has.

Protracted active-phase dilation, or **protracted active dilation** during the active phase, is, according to the classic model, dilation of less than 1.2 cm/h for first births and less than 1.5 cm/h for subsequent births. The newer model allows slightly more nuance, with different rates anticipated for different degrees of dilation. Thus, today, **protracted active labor** refers to women in the active phase who are dilating less than 1 to 2 cm/h after a

Table 22.1 Abnormal Labor Patterns

Classification of Abnormal Labor Pattern	Classic Criteria		Contemporary Criteria		
	Nulliparas	**Multiparas**	**All Women: Cervical Dilation/ Status of Contractions/ Epidural Use**	**Nulliparas**	**Multiparas**
Prolonged latent phase	>20 h	>14 h	4–5 cm	>6.4 h	>7.3 h
			5–6 cm	>3.2 h	>3.4 h
Total			4–6 cm	>9.6 h	>10.7 h
Protracted active-phase dilation	<1.2 cm/h	<1.5 cm/h	6–7 cm	>2.2 h	>1.9 h
			7–8 cm	>1.6 h	>1.3 h
			8–9 cm	>1.4 h	>1 h
			9–10 cm	>1.8 h	>0.9 h
Total			6–10 cm	<1.75 cm/h	<1.28 cm/h
Secondary arrest: no change	2+ h	2+ h	With adequate contractions	4+ h	
			Without adequate contractions	6+ h	
Protracted descent	<1 cm/h	<2 cm/h	With an epidural	>3.6 h second stage	>2 h second stage
			Without an epidural	>2.8 h second stage	>1.3 h second stage
Arrest of descent	1+ h	0.5+ h	N/A	N/A	N/A
Failure of descent	No fetal descent during deceleration phase of first stage or in second stage		N/A	N/A	N/A

N/A, not applicable.
Adapted from Zhang, J., Landy, H. J., Branch, D. W., Burkman, R., Haberman, S., Gregory, K. D., . . . Consortium on Safe Labor. (2010). Contemporary patterns of spontaneous labor with normal neonatal outcomes. *Obstetrics and Gynecology, 116*(6), 1281–1287. doi:10.1097/AOG.0b013e3181fdef6e; Friedman, E. (1989). Normal and dysfunctional labor. In W. Cohen, D. Ackers, & E. Friedman (Eds.), *Management of Labor* (6th. ed.). Rockville, MD: Aspen.

dilation of 6 cm or more (Spong, Berghella, Wenstrom, Mercer, & Saade, 2012; Zhang et al., 2010).

Friedman determined that no change in cervical dilation with adequate uterine contractions for more than 2 hours qualified as "secondary arrest: no change." Today, however, an **arrest of the active phase** is diagnosed in two circumstances: (1) when contractions are adequate and no cervical change has occurred for 4 or more hours or (2) contractions are inadequate and no cervical change has occurred for 6 or more hours.

Fetal descent in the second phase in the classic model should be faster than 1 cm/h with the first vaginal birth and faster than 2 cm/h for subsequent births, and rates less than these would indicate **protracted descent**. The newer model, however, assigns different values for women receiving epidural anesthesia and those who are not when determining cases of protracted descent. The classic model also provides parameters for arrest of descent and failure of descent.

Treatment

The management of dysfunctional uterine contractions depends on their timing. A prolonged latent period may be treated conservatively with rest or more actively with an amniotomy, if the fetal head in engaged, or with oxytocin or a prostaglandin to stimulate greater uterine activity. Therapeutic rest may be facilitated with medications such as morphine or a sedative (Mackeen, Fehnel, Berghella, & Klein, 2014).

A protracted active phase is often treated with the administration of oxytocin. If the fetal head is engaged, an amniotomy in conjunction with oxytocin is associated with superior outcomes to either method of augmentation alone (Wei et al., 2013). Amniotomy without the use of oxytocin does not appear to improve outcomes (Smyth, Markham, & Dowswell, 2013). Active-phase arrest is treated with cesarean section.

Although it's challenging to know from the information provided whether Nancy in Chapter 9 technically had protracted active labor, her obstetric provider elected to perform an amniotomy in the hopes of shortening the active phase of the first stage. Her nurse thought that this intervention worked. Nancy was also receiving oxytocin IV.

In the second stage of labor, allowing pushing for at least 3 hours for first births and for at least 2 hours with second births is recommended prior to surgical intervention (American College of Obstetricians and Gynecologists [ACOG] & Society for Maternal-Fetal Medicine, 2014). Extra time may be allowed for individual circumstances, including epidural anesthesia (Spong, Berghella, Wenstrom, Mercer, & Saade, 2013). Although a mechanical problem such as fetal malposition or macrosomia is a more likely cause for arrest than are inadequate contractions in the second stage, some providers may use oxytocin augmentation if they observe slow descent of the fetus.

In the case of slow or arrested fetal descent in a woman with an epidural, decreasing the dose of the epidural medication is not currently understood to reduce the need for surgical interventions.

Care Considerations

Changes in maternal position for women without an epidural and variations in pushing technique are also unlikely to facilitate a significantly more rapid birth, and thus the nurse should encourage women to find the positions most comfortable for them (Gupta, Sood, Hofmeyr, & Vogel, 2017). Although obstetric providers commonly apply additional manual pressure to the fundus to augment the action of contractions, little evidence suggests it improves outcomes (Hofmeyr, Vogel, Cuthbert, & Singata, 2017).

Ineffective Pushing

Ineffective pushing by the mother during labor can also lead to dystocia. **Laboring down** is a process of allowing the primary powers to slowly facilitate fetal descent in the second stage of labor without augmentation by maternal pushing. Delaying pushing in this way may decrease the amount of time a woman pushes but may also extend the duration of the second stage of labor. There is no clear evidence of a difference in outcomes between laboring down and voluntary bearing down (Lemos et al., 2017). Women with epidurals typically have the urge to bear down diminished along with pain, which can impact the timing of pushing as well as the efficacy. Fatigue from an extended labor with little nutrition and rest may also impede secondary powers.

Precipitous Labor

Problems with the powers of labor can result not only in a prolonged labor but in a **precipitous labor**. A labor that lasts 3 hours or less from the onset of regular contractions until fetal expulsion is classified as precipitous. In the United States, the reported occurrence rate is from 0.1% to 3%, whereas in Japan, the rate is closer to 14% (Suzuki, 2015a). In this condition, contractions are strong and frequent, typically in the absence of medications such as oxytocin. Precipitous labor is most common in women who have given birth previously, women who are under the age of 20 years, preterm births, women with hypertensive disorders in pregnancy, and births of neonates weighing less than 2,500 g.

The primary complication associated with precipitous delivery is placental abruption, which is attributed to the uterine tachysystole typical of a precipitous birth. Some research has associated precipitous delivery with perineal lacerations, postpartum hemorrhage, placental retention after the birth, prolonged hospitalization, and more frequent blood transfusions, although these findings are not universal (Suzuki, 2015a). Because of the intensity of the contractions and the briefer intervals of relaxation between contractions, there is an increased risk of fetal hypoxia and intracranial trauma for the fetus. Such births do not typically present a significant increase in infant or maternal morbidity or mortality, however.

Because of their rapid nature, precipitous births often happen someplace other than the labor and delivery unit, such as at home or during transit to the hospital. The nurse should encourage women with a history of precipitous birth to seek care early in labor to optimize the chance of access to trained care providers.

In Chapter 11, Edie had a precipitous birth, which may have contributed to her baby having shoulder dystocia and, most likely, to sustaining a brachial plexus injury. All of these things left Edie feeling overwhelmed.

Passageway

The second of the five Ps of labor is passageway. Passageway refers to the maternal bony pelvis and soft tissues. Although passageway complications most often occur in conjunction with those of the third P, passenger, discreet complications related to the maternal anatomy alone can also present challenges.

Bony Pelvis Dystocia

A maternal pelvis that is smaller than normal, or contracted, can lead to dystocia. Reduced pelvic dimensions may be due to genetic variations, nutritional deficiencies, trauma, neoplasms, or spinal problems. For a pelvis to be classified as contracted, it must have one or more dimensions that are at least 1 cm below normal. The contraction of the pelvis may be at the pelvic inlet, through which the fetal head first passes; the midpelvis, often at the level of the ischial spines; or the pelvic outlet. Pelvimetry, the assessment of the maternal bony pelvis to determine its sufficiency for vaginal birth, may be done clinically or by X-ray, computed tomography, or magnetic resonance imaging. There is currently little compelling research to support its use for decision-making. Pelvimetry is associated with a higher rate of cesarean section but not overall improved outcomes (Pattinson, Cuthbert, & Vannevel, 2017). Pelvic dystocia may be suspected with failure of descent of the fetal head.

Soft Tissue Dystocia

Soft tissue dystocia occurs when the soft tissues of or surrounding the birth canal impede delivery of the fetus. Some forms of soft tissue dystocia, such as an impediment caused by a full bladder or bowel, may be easily addressed, whereas others, such as placenta previa (see Chapter 21) or occasionally a large fibroid in the lower uterine segment, preclude a vaginal birth. Another form of soft tissue dystocia, cervical edema, can result from voluntarily bearing down against a cervix that is not fully dilated. Scarring of the cervix, however, as occurs with a loop electrosurgical excision procedure for the treatment of high-grade cervical dysplasia, does not appear to increase the risk for soft tissue dystocia or cesarean section (Frey et al., 2013).

Bandl's Ring

Bandl's ring, also called Bandl's constriction or a pathologic retraction ring, occurs at the junction of the upper and lower uterine segments (Fig. 22.1). It is a rare complication that occurs during the first or second stage of labor. It occurs in one in 5,000 births, and it's not clear whether it is a cause or a result of dystocia. There is not a clear correlation between Bandl's ring and premature rupture of membranes, oxytocin use, fetal position, prolonged labor, or a contracted pelvis. The ring may, in fact, be present prior to the onset of labor, although it is typically identified at the time of cesarean section. It may also be identified by ultrasonography during labor. The ring may compress the fetal thorax, neck, or head and can rarely cause injury due to compression. A further danger of Bandl's ring is that a stretched, thin lower uterine segment is at an increased risk for uterine rupture (Tinelli, Di Renzo, & Malvasi, 2015).

Passenger

Dystocia related to the fetus, the passenger, may be caused by fetal anomalies such as hydrocephalus, fetal size, or malposition of the fetus. Fetal dystocia is associated with an increased risk of soft tissue injuries to the mother and fetal injuries such as fractures and brachial plexus injuries. Vaginal surgical procedures such as forceps-assisted and vacuum-assisted interventions or a cesarean delivery may be required.

Cephalopelvic Disproportion

Cephalopelvic disproportion (CPD) is a mismatch between the size of the fetal head and the size of the maternal pelvis. True CPD may be related to issues with the maternal bony pelvis or soft tissue, but it is more commonly associated with macrosomia (a fetus weighing 4,000 g or more). Fetuses are more likely to be macrosomic with maternal diabetes and obesity, advanced maternal age, and excessive weight gain in pregnancy, among other factors. Although a risk for CPD may be suspected with fetal weight estimates by ultrasound in late pregnancy and risk factors, CPD cannot be accurately predicted. Many cases classified as CPD may, in fact, instead be fetal malposition or malpresentation.

In Chapter 9, the delivery of Nancy's baby was complicated by his weight: 4,400 g (9 lb 7 oz)! The infant's weight was likely related to Nancy's gestational diabetes. The baby's large size made CPD a concern for delivery.

Fetal Malposition

The fetal position is the position of the presenting fetal part in relation to the maternal pelvis (see Chapter 16). The most common fetal positions are left occiput anterior and right occiput anterior, meaning that the occiput (the back of the fetal head) is at the front left or right of the maternal pelvis. The most common **fetal malposition** is the occiput posterior (OP) position, sometimes referred to as "sunnyside up" because the fetus is facing toward the front of the mother and appears faceup if the birth occurs with the mother in the lithotomy position.

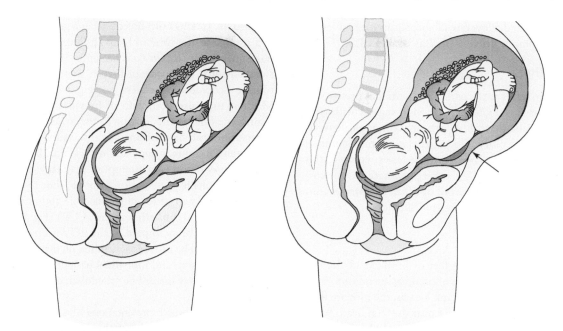

Figure 22.1. Bandl's ring. (A) A normal uterus in the second stage of labor. Notice how the upper uterine segment is becoming thicker and the lower uterine segment is thinning. Bandl's ring is normally formed at the division of the upper and lower uterine segments. **(B)** A uterus with a Bandl's ring. The wall below the ring is thin and the abdomen shows an indentation. (Reprinted with permission from Pillitteri, A. [2002]. *Maternal and child health nursing: Care of the childbearing and childrearing family* [4th ed., Fig. 21-4]. Philadelphia, PA: Lippincott Williams & Wilkins.)

Etiology

Maternal risk factors for having a fetus in the OP position include first birth, previous birth complicated by OP, advanced maternal age, obesity, small pelvic outlet, advanced gestation, macrosomic infant, anterior implantation of the placenta, and African American ethnicity. Although epidural anesthesia is often identified as a risk factor, births of fetuses with an OP presentation include severe maternal back pain and a greater use of anesthesia, and it is not clear whether the epidurals contribute to the risk for an OP position or women with OP fetuses are simply more likely to require epidurals (Ghi et al., 2016).

Prognosis

In 89% of pregnancies with an OP fetal position in the first stage of labor, the fetus rotates into an occiput anterior position before the head reaches the −2 station. Rotation after the −2 station is unlikely (Vitner et al., 2015).

An OP fetal position is associated with longer first and second stages of labor. Compared with those with occiput anterior fetal positions, patients with an OP fetal position are more likely to undergo interventions to hasten labor, such as amniotomy and oxytocin administration, are twice as likely to have a vaginal surgical birth, and are four times as likely to have a cesarean delivery (Simpson, Chambers, Sharshiner, & Caughey, 2015).

Assessment

An OP fetal position can generally be identified during a digital vaginal examination on the basis of the location of the fontanels of the fetal skull (Fig. 22.2).

Treatment

Antepartum and in the first stage of labor, changes in maternal position and attempts to manually rotate the fetus are ineffective for resolving the OP position (Le Ray et al., 2016). In the case of a persistent OP position and a prolonged second stage, the obstetric provider may attempt a manual rotation, which has a

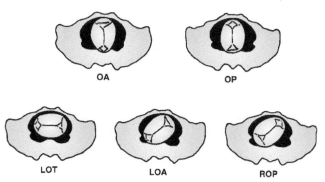

Figure 22.2. Position of the fetal head. The nurse should palpate the sutures of the fetal head and record the fetal head position to ensure that the normal cardinal movements of labor are being followed. The fetal occiput and the maternal pelvic inlet are the reference points. Hence, OA refers to the occiput anterior position; OP, occiput posterior; LOT, left occiput transverse; LOA, left occiput anterior; ROP, right occiput posterior. (Reprinted with permission from Gibbs, R. S., Karlan, B. Y., Haney, A. F., & Nygaard, I. E. [2008]. *Danforth's obstetrics and gynecology* [10th ed., Fig. 24-7]. Philadelphia, PA: Lippincott Williams & Wilkins.)

high rate of success and a low rate of complications and reduces the risk for an operative delivery (Le Ray et al., 2013).

Malpresentation

Fetal presentation refers to the part of the fetus that presents first to the maternal pelvis (see Chapter 16). Most vaginal births are of fetuses in the cephalic (head-first) presentation, typically vertex (crown of the head first). In addition to being the most common, vertex presentation is associated with the fewest complications and thus is considered normal. All other presentations are known as **malpresentations**, as they are not optimal. Malpresentations include breech, nonvertex cephalic, and shoulder.

Breech Presentation

With a breech presentation, the feet or buttocks of the fetus present first. There are three types of breech presentation: frank, footling, and complete. With a frank breech, the hips are flexed and knees extended with the feet up near the fetal head. With a footling breech, one or both feet present before the buttocks. With a complete breech, both hips and knees are flexed (see Fig. 16.8).
Prevalence. Breech is by far the most common malpresentation, occurring in 1 out of 33 births.
Etiology. Although most breech presentations occur spontaneously without known risk factors, they are more likely to occur with preterm gestation, uterine and placental abnormalities, some fetal abnormalities, a contracted maternal pelvis, multiple gestation, fetal growth restriction, a short umbilical cord, oligohydramnios, polyhydramnios, fetal neurologic impairment, and advanced maternal age, among other factors (Fruscalzo et al., 2014).

Prognosis. Infants born breech are at a greater risk for asphyxia and trauma at the time of birth. Infants born footling breech pose a particular risk for cord prolapse.
Assessment. Diagnosis of breech presentation is usually by routine Leopold's maneuvers (see Fig 1.7) in later pregnancy. Mothers may also complain of pressure from the fetal head against the fundus and kicking in the lower abdomen. Clinical observations can be confirmed by ultrasound.
Treatment. A common approach in the United States to addressing breech presentation is to attempt to manually rotate the breech fetus to a cephalic presentation prior to labor by externally manipulating fetal parts through the mother's abdomen, a procedure called an **external cephalic version (ECV)** (Fig. 22.3). A trial of labor may then be attempted. If the ECV is unsuccessful, a trial of labor may still be offered, depending on institutional protocol, provider judgment, and individual patient circumstances. A cesarean section may instead be scheduled, either with or without a trial of labor.

Women with breech presentations who undergo an ECV have approximately 50% lower risk of a breech presentation at the time of birth and of cesarean delivery than do those who do not undergo this procedure (Hofmeyr, Kulier, & West, 2015). The risk for cesarean section is still twice that of women with nonbreech presentations, however, due to both nonreassuring fetal heart rate patterns and dystocia (de Hundt, Velzel, de Groot, Mol, & Kok, 2014). The ECV is more likely to be successful with a fetus in a transverse rather than breech presentation, in people of African descent, in pregnancies with the placenta on the posterior wall of the uterus, with fetuses in a complete breech position (hips and knees flexed), and with an amniotic fluid index above 10 (Ebner et al., 2016).

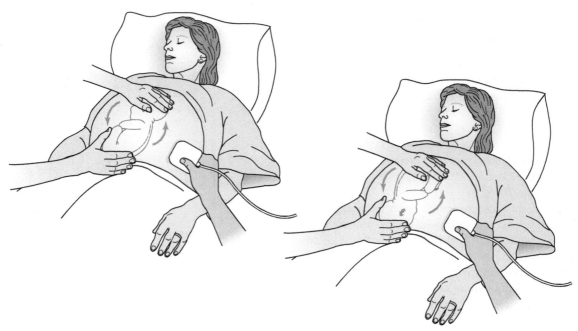

Figure 22.3. External cephalic version. The obstetric provider rotates the fetus by external pressure to a cephalic lie. An ultrasound helps guide a safe result. (Reprinted with permission from Pillitteri, A. [2014]. *Maternal and child health nursing: Care of the childbearing and childrearing family* [7th ed., Fig. 23-11]. Philadelphia, PA: Lippincott Williams & Wilkins.)

Contraindications to ECV include conditions such as placenta previa that would contraindicate a vaginal birth, hyperextension of the fetal neck, rupture of membranes or oligohydramnios, placental abruption, a nonreassuring nonstress test (NST) or biophysical profile (BPP), or a significant fetal or uterine anomaly. Overall, complications from ECV are rare and include fetal heart rate changes, transfer of fetal blood to the maternal circulation, emergency cesarean delivery, rupture of membranes, vaginal bleeding, placental abruption, cord prolapse, and fetal death (Grootscholten, Kok, Oei, Mol, & van der Post, 2008).

An internal version, also called an internal podalic version, is a more unusual procedure that involves the obstetric provider inserting a hand into the uterus to change the orientation of the fetus (Fig. 22.4). It is typically used in vaginal twin births to deliver a malpresenting second fetus. Contraindications include an estimated weight disparity between twins of 20% or more, a prolonged second stage or pronounced molding of the head of the firstborn twin, or a gestational age under 28 weeks (Society for Maternal-Fetal Medicine, 2016). Many obstetric providers, however, have little experience with the procedure and are more comfortable performing a cesarean delivery for both twins when one is breech.

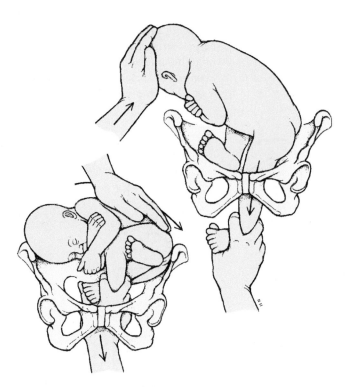

Figure 22.4. Internal podalic version: conversion from a dorsoposterior transverse lie to a breech presentation. (A) The obstetric provider's right hand grasps the fetal foot within the uterus while the left hand applies pressure externally to rotate the fetus into a breech presentation toward the pelvic inlet. **(B)** The obstetric provider maneuvers the fetus into a longitudinal orientation by applying traction to foot while externally directing the head into fundus, so that delivery can proceed as in breech presentation. (Credit: Neil O. Hardy, Westpoint, CT.)

Care Considerations. Because of a small risk for emergency cesarean delivery and precipitous vaginal delivery with ECV, the procedure is typically attempted in a location with ready access to the resources necessary for this type of care. It is usually attempted after 36 weeks of gestation. It may occasionally be attempted in early labor with intact membranes.

Prior to the procedure, the patient is assessed by ultrasound to confirm the position of the fetus and the placenta and to is assessed amniotic fluid volume. Fetal well-being by NST or BPP and patient education regarding the procedure is provided. In particular, the patient must understand why the procedure is being done, possible risks, the success rate, the chance that the fetus will revert to breech even after a successful ECV, benefits, and alternatives.

Tocolysis is often administered to relax the uterine muscle as well as the muscles of the anterior abdominal wall. Typically, the nurse administers as ordered a single dose of terbutaline, 0.25 mg subcutaneously, 15 to 30 minutes prior to the procedure. Fetal vibroacoustic stimulation, such as that used with an NST may be used, to improve the likelihood of a successful ECV (Cluver, Gyte, Sinclair, Dowswell, & Hofmeyr, 2015). ECV is generally only mildly uncomfortable for women, but the nurse may provide as ordered an analgesic for women reporting unusual distress.

The nurse should monitor the fetus throughout the procedure and until the fetal heart rate is reactive and stable after the procedure. It is not unusual for the fetal heart rate to be nonreactive for up to 40 minutes after the procedure. Bradycardia and variable decelerations are unexpected, and the nurse should report them to the obstetric provider should they arise. The nurse should also obtain the maternal vital signs during and after the procedure and assess for vaginal bleeding and discharge suggestive of amniotic fluid. The nurse should administer Rh_o (D) immune globulin to women who are Rh negative after the procedure because of the small risk of fetomaternal transfusion.

Nonvertex Cephalic Presentations

Cephalic presentations other than vertex include sinciput (forehead), brow (eyebrows), face, and chin (Fig. 22.5).

Prevalence. Nonvertex cephalic presentations occur in 1 out of 500 to 1 out of 1,000 births.

Etiology. Nonvertex presentations occur when the fetal neck is extended rather than flexed. This alternate orientation means that a wider cephalic diameter needs to pass through the pelvis (Fig. 22.6). This increased diameter can be enough to inhibit both engagement and fetal descent through the birth canal. Risk factors associated with an increased occurrence of fetal neck extension in the cephalic presentation include both low birth weight and macrosomia, along with fetal head and neck abnormalities, twin pregnancy, and polyhydramnios. Women with a contracted pelvis, a platypelloid pelvis, or a history of cesarean delivery or who are of African descent are also at greater risk. Poor maternal abdominal tone may also contribute (Tapisiz et al., 2014).

Prognosis. Neonates born face first generally have significant facial bruising and edema and skull molding that resolves within 48 hours. Tracheal trauma due to hyperextension of the neck can cause problems with resuscitation if needed. Occasional facial

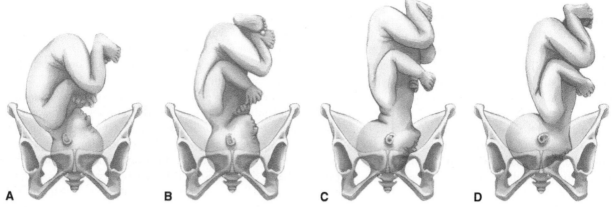

Figure 22.5. Cephalic presentations. Fetal attitude affects the type of presentation in cephalic (head-first) presentations. The degree of fetal flexion affects whether the presentation is classified as **(A)** vertex, **(B)** sinciput, **(C)** brow, or **(D)** face. (Reprinted with permission from Hatfield, N. T. [2014]. *Introductory maternity and pediatric nursing* [3rd ed., Fig. 8-7]. Philadelphia, PA: Lippincott Williams & Wilkins.)

trauma and injury to the spinal cord is possible, although serious problems for either mother or baby are rare.

Assessment. As with an OP position, an alternate cephalic presentation is usually diagnosed by a digital examination during labor. The diagnosis may be confirmed by ultrasound.

Treatment. Fetuses with a face (mentum) presentation with the chin anterior are more likely to be successfully born vaginally than are fetuses with the presenting part posterior, because of the dimensions of the pelvis. Fetuses with mentum posterior presentation are almost always delivered by cesarean section if spontaneous rotation of the fetus does not occur. Approximately

half of fetuses with a brow presentation convert to a facial or vertex presentation in the second stage of labor. Protracted or arrested descent with an alternate cephalic presentation is an indication for cesarean section.

Shoulder Presentation

With shoulder presentation with a fetal transverse lie, the shoulder, arm, or trunk is the presenting part (Fig. 22.7). Shoulder presentations are present at the time of delivery with 1 in every 300 births (Gardberg, Leonova, & Laakkonen, 2011). Risk factors are similar to those of a breech presentation. Fetuses with

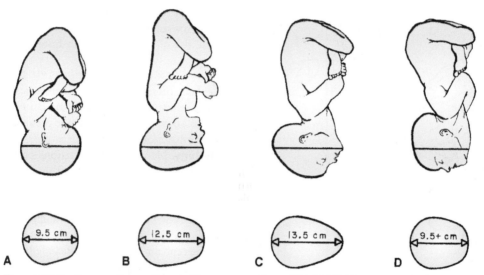

Figure 22.6. Comparison of cephalic presentations. (A) Full-flexion, vertex presentation presents the smallest circumference of the fetal head to the narrower planes of the pelvis. **(B)** Military attitude, sinciput presentation usually changes to full flexion with descent into the pelvis. **(C)** Brow presentation usually converts to full flexion or a face presentation, as the occipitomental diameter is too large for all except the largest pelves to accommodate. **(D)** Face presentation shows dimensions that allow descent through the pelvis, unless the chin is posterior. A fetus in persistent mentum posterior presentation must be delivered by cesarean section. (Reprinted with permission from Gibbs, R. S., Karlan, B. Y., Haney, A. F., & Nygaard, I. E. [2008]. *Danforth's obstetrics and gynecology* [10th ed., Fig. 2-11]. Philadelphia, PA: Lippincott Williams & Wilkins.)

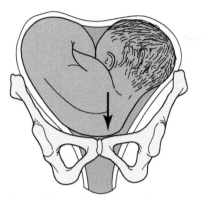

Figure 22.7. Shoulder presentation. (Reprinted with permission from Kennedy, B. B., & Baird, S. M. [2017]. *Intrapartum management modules* [5th ed., Fig. 2-14]. Philadelphia, PA: Lippincott Williams & Wilkins.)

a shoulder presentation must have their presentation converted by in order for a vaginal birth to be attempted. In the event that ECV is not attempted or is contraindicated, a cesarean section must be performed. ECV considerations and procedures are the same as for a breech presentation.

Shoulder Dystocia

Shoulder dystocia is obstruction of fetal descent by the shoulders after the birth of the fetal head. The shoulders, and thus the remainder of the fetus, fail to deliver spontaneously.

Etiology

In half of the cases, no risk factors exist, although macrosomia and maternal diabetes are often associated with shoulder dystocia (see Box 11.6).

Prognosis

Approximately 5% of neonates with shoulder dystocia experience complications as a result of the prolonged descent and obstetric interventions associated with this condition, including hypoxia and injury to the brachial plexus, which may be either temporary or permanent. Risks to the mother include lacerations and postpartum hemorrhage due to uterine atony (see Box 11.7).

In Chapter 11, the birth of Edie's baby was complicated by shoulder dystocia, which likely contributed to the brachial plexus injury that her newborn sustained as well as Edie's perineal injury.

Assessment

Turtle sign is often the first indication of shoulder dystocia. With turtle sign, the fetal head is born, but the cheeks of the newborn rest on the maternal introitus as the anterior shoulder is unable to pass beneath the maternal symphysis pubis.

Treatment

Common first interventions to attempt to relieve the shoulder dystocia are McRoberts' maneuver (see Fig. 11.5) and the application of suprapubic pressure (see Fig. 11.6). To perform McRoberts' maneuver, the nurse sharply flexes the mother's hips with her knees pulled back toward her chest. To perform suprapubic pressure, the nurse pushes downward on the maternal abdomen just above the level of the pubic bone in an attempt to dislodge the fetal anterior shoulder. At the same time, the obstetric provider guides the fetal head downward toward the maternal anus. Other obstetric interventions to relieve shoulder dystocia are itemized in Table 11.1.

Psyche

The patient's psyche or psychological state can also contribute to dystocia. Anxiety increases catecholamine levels, which may have a negative impact on normal labor progress and fetal outcomes. Support from others, particularly continuous one-on-one support, can help allay anxiety and is generally desired by most women. One-on-one support can reduce the rate of cesarean delivery, need for pain medication, use of epidural and spinal anesthesia, reports of negative childbirth experiences, and length of labor (Hodnett, Gates, Hofmeyr, & Sakala, 2013). The partner of the pregnancy, a friend or family member designated as a birthing partner, a labor doula, or a nurse may play this support role. A labor doula is trained to provide emotional and physical support as well as information to women before, during, and after birth (Fig. 22.8). Doulas may be paid or may act on a volunteer basis.

Position

Maternal position can also affect the progress of labor. Common positions in labor are typically either upright or supine. Upright positions include sitting, kneeling, squatting, and standing. Supine positions include lateral side-lying (Sims'), semirecumbent (upper body tilted up 30°), lithotomy, and Trendelenburg

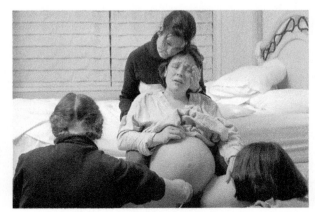

Figure 22.8. A woman having a home birth, assisted by a doula and a midwife. (Reprinted with permission from Evans, R. J., Brown, Y. M., & Evans, M. K. [2014]. *Canadian maternity, newborn, and women's health nursing* [2nd ed., Fig. 14.2]. Philadelphia, PA: Lippincott Williams & Wilkins.)

positions (head lower than the pelvis; see Fig. 16.12). A neutral position suggests that the angle of the maternal torso is more recumbent than upright.

An upright instead of horizontal position may shorten the first stage of labor by as much as 90 minutes, particularly for women who have given birth before. An upright position also shortens the second stage of labor by approximately 4 minutes and reduces the rate of surgical vaginal deliveries. The upright positions may also play a small role in improving uteroplacental profusion. An upright position likely increases the rate of second-degree or higher lacerations and postpartum hemorrhage, but decreases the episiotomy rate. An upright position may also help reduce labor pain. As mentioned previously, variations of maternal position likely do not affect fetal position (Desseauve, Fradet, Lacouture, & Pierre, 2017).

The use of a peanut-shaped exercise ball in labor has been shown to reduce the duration of the first stage of labor for primiparous women but not for multiparous women. It does not impact the duration of the second stage. It may reduce the rate of cesarean section (Roth, Dent, Parfitt, Hering, & Bay, 2016; Tussey et al., 2015). The peanut ball has been best studied and is most often used in women who have received epidural anesthesia with ambulation restrictions. The laboring woman assumes a side-lying position with the peanut placed between her thighs as close to her hips as is comfortable. Sitting and/or gently bouncing on a round exercise ball or curling forward around one during labor may help reduce labor pain (Fig. 22.9; Makvandi, Latifnejad Roudsari, Sadeghi, & Karimi, 2015).

Second-Stage Intrapartum Procedures

Some procedures that are used to facilitate birth, such as episiotomy and assistance with forceps and vacuum suction, pose their own risk for complications to the mother and fetus.

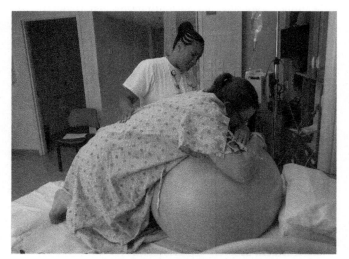

Figure 22.9. A woman kneeling in bed using a birthing ball. (Reprinted with permission from Simpson, K. R., & Creehan, P. A. [2014]. *AWHONN's perinatal nursing* [4th ed., Fig. 14.10F]. Philadelphia, PA: Lippincott Williams & Wilkins.)

Episiotomy

An **episiotomy** is a surgical incision of the posterior aspect of the vulva made during the second stage of labor (see Fig. 16.16).

Prevalence

Although it was once a routine procedure, this practice has gone out of routine use because of a risk for complications. In the United States, the rate of episiotomy dropped from 17.3% in 2006 to 11.6% in 2012, and the World Health Organization recommends an episiotomy rate of 10%. Women are less likely to receive an episiotomy when attended by a midwife or a physician associated with an academic training facility (Friedman, Ananth, Prendergast, D'Alton, & Wright, 2015b).

Indications

Episiotomy is now typically done if the patient is judged to be at a high risk for a third- or fourth-degree perineal tear or if an expedited delivery is necessary because of evidence of fetal compromise. An episiotomy may also be performed to allow more room for a forceps-assisted delivery, a vacuum-assisted delivery, or manipulation by an obstetric provider in the case of shoulder dystocia.

Risks

A midline incision is more closely associated with extension of the cut into a third- or fourth-degree laceration, whereas the more common mediolateral incision is associated with a lower risk of extending lacerations. There is no evidence that episiotomy reduces trauma to the fetal head, improves wound healing when compared with a naturally occurring laceration, protects the musculature of the pelvic floor or sphincter, or prevents shoulder dystocia (Pergialiotis, Vlachos, Protopapas, Pappa, & Vlachos, 2014; Sagi-Dain & Sagi, 2015). Besides possible wound extension, episiotomy creates a risk for unanticipated injury to the maternal perineum, increased blood loss, infection, wound dehiscence, and perineal injury with future births (Muhleman et al., 2017).

Procedure

Women with neuraxial anesthesia (a spinal or epidural) do not require any further anesthesia for an episiotomy. Women who do not have neuraxial anesthesia in place may instead be given a pudendal block (see Fig. 16.29) or local anesthesia such as lidocaine at the planned incision site. An episiotomy done prior to the fetal head crowning is associated with greater vulva trauma and blood loss, and thus the episiotomy is typically done after crowning, when delivery is anticipated within the next several contractions. The obstetric provider typically makes an incision of about 3 to 5 cm with a scalpel or scissors. After delivery, the obstetric provider thoroughly evaluates the perineum and sutures the incision. The sutures are generally absorbable, so later removal is not required. Although infection and dehiscence (wound separation) are uncommon following an episiotomy, nurses should assess the repaired incision regularly postpartum. The administration of prophylactic antibiotics is rarely indicated.

Operative Vaginal Birth

An operative vaginal birth may be attempted in the case of a prolonged second stage of labor, fetal compromise, or a maternal disorder that limits the mother's ability to push. Contraindications to an operative vaginal birth include a brow or face presentation, an unknown fetal position, a gestation of less than 34 weeks, fetal bleeding disorders, CPD, an unengaged fetal head, and a fetal osteogenesis imperfecta. Generally, fetuses estimated to weigh either less than 2,000 g or more than 4,000 g are not eligible for a surgical vaginal birth (ACOG, 2015). In 2015, 3.1% of deliveries were operative vaginal births. Approximately 18% of these were forceps assisted and the remaining 82% were vacuum assisted (Martin, Hamilton, Osterman, Driscoll, & Mathews, 2017).

For an operative vaginal delivery to be attempted, the membranes must be ruptured and the cervix must be fully dilated. The head should be engaged and the fetal presentation known. In most cases the fetus must be in a cephalic position, although rarely a specific kind of forceps delivery may be attempted to assist the delivery of the head of a breech infant. Patient consent must be obtained, and the maternal bladder must be emptied to reduce the chance of bladder injury and to increase the room for the fetus (ACOG, 2015).

Forceps-Assisted Birth

Forceps are a form of tongs. They are made of stainless steel and come in different sizes and shapes designed to fit around the fetal head (Fig. 22.10). The blades of the forceps may be solid or have cutouts in the center. The choice of forceps type is up to the obstetric provider. Forceps delivery may be outlet, low, or midforceps depending on the station of the fetus (see Fig. 16.5) and position (see Fig. 16.11; Box 22.1). In general, outlet forceps delivery is associated with the lowest risk for maternal and fetal injury, and midforceps delivery is the highest risk. Neuraxial anesthesia is preferred, although a pudendal block may be sufficient. Episiotomy is not performed routinely. In general, operative vaginal delivery attempts are abandoned in preference for a cesarean section if the descent is not aided by the forceps, if it becomes difficult to apply the forceps safely, or if delivery

---

Box 22.1 Forceps Classifications

Outlet Forceps

Indicated when

- the top of the fetal scalp can be visualized at the introitus without separating the labia.
- the fetal position is right occiput anterior, left occiput anterior, right OP, or left OP.
- fetal rotation is not more than 45°.

Low Forceps

Indicated when the fetal station is +2 or lower

Midforceps

Indicated when the leading point of the fetal skull is between 0 and +2 station

---

does not occur in a timely fashion (usually 15 to 20 minutes). Approximately 91% of forceps deliveries are successful, with the remainder converting to cesarean section or vaginal births without forceps assistance (O'Mahony, Hofmeyr, & Menon, 2010).

Neonatal complications of a forceps delivery include scalp and facial lacerations, eye trauma, intracranial or subgaleal hemorrhage, nerve damage, skull fracture, facial palsies, skull fractures, and death (O'Mahony et al., 2010). Maternal complications include damage to the vulva, vagina, urinary tract, and anal sphincter, with the OP position of the fetus creating the greatest risk (Friedman, Ananth, Prendergast, D'Alton, & Wright, 2015a). Because of these risks for injury, the labor and delivery nurse must report the use of instrumentation to the postpartum nurse to whom she transfers the patient.

Vacuum-Assisted Birth

Vacuum-assisted birth involves the use of a device that creates suction against the fetal head and aids in extraction. Obstetric providers are more likely to use vacuum assistance rather than forceps because of their greater level of comfort and expertise with the method and greater instrument availability. Providers trained

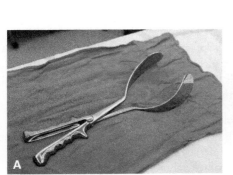
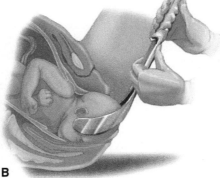
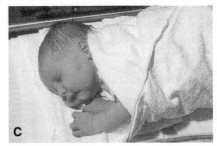

Figure 22.10. Use of forceps during birth. (A) A pair of forceps. **(B)** Forceps being applied to the fetal head. **(C)** Forceps marks on a newborn's head. (Reprinted with permission from Ricci, S. S. [2013]. *Essentials of maternity, newborn, & women's health nursing* [3rd ed., Fig. 21.6]. Philadelphia, PA: Lippincott Williams & Wilkins.)

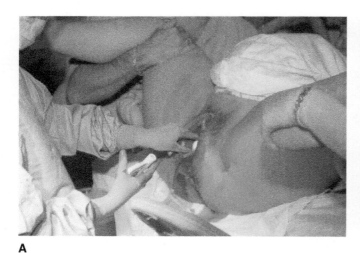

A

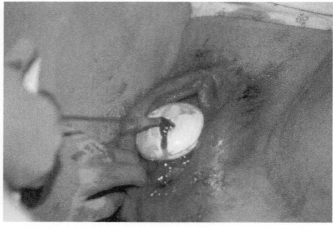

B

Figure 22.11. A delivery assisted by vacuum extraction. (A) The birth attendant has just placed the suction cup on the fetal head and is using the hand pump to increase the pressure. **(B)** Gentle traction is placed on the fetal head to assist it through the last maneuvers of delivery. (Reprinted with permission from Hatfield, N. T. [2014]. *Introductory maternity and pediatric nursing* [3rd ed., Fig. 11-2]. Philadelphia, PA: Lippincott Williams & Wilkins.)

in both methods may be more likely to select vacuum extraction for births that are anticipated to be easier and forceps for more challenging deliveries. Vacuum extraction is associated with a lower rate of maternal injury than forceps delivery (O'Mahony et al., 2010). Potential complications for the fetus include hemorrhage that is intraventricular, subgaleal, or intracranial, as well as cephalohematoma, brachial plexus injury from traction, retinal hemorrhage, and abrasions and lacerations of the fetal scalp.

Vacuum cups attach to the fetal head by suction provided by an attached pump. The cups may be soft or rigid (Fig. 22.11). Soft cups are frequently chosen for occiput anterior presentations, whereas the rigid cups, which are less likely to detach when traction is applied, are preferred for OP and occiput transverse positions. The suction may be produced either manually or electronically. Suction pressure is set to a point that minimizes the likelihood of the cup coming off the fetal head when traction is applied, which occurs when the pressure is too low, or the risk for fetal scalp or cerebral trauma, which occurs when the suction is too high.

The obstetric provider applies traction on the cup and co-ordinates the traction with contractions and maternal pushing. Fetal descent is expected each time traction is applied to the cup. Different guidelines suggest different thresholds for stopping vacuum extraction attempts, including one or two pop-offs of the cup from the fetal head, three sets of pulls (traction), and a total vacuum application time of 15 to 30 minutes (Ghidini, Stewart, Pezzullo, & Locatelli, 2017).

Cesarean Birth

Cesarean birth is the delivery of the fetus through an incision in the abdominal wall and the anterior wall of the uterus. A primary cesarean section refers to the first delivery of this kind for the woman and accounts for approximately 70% of the procedures. The remaining 30% are secondary cesarean sections, meaning the patient has previously delivered by this method (Boyle et al., 2013).

Prevalence

The rate of cesarean delivery in the United States was 32% in 2015, down from its peak of 32.9% in 2009 (Martin et al., 2017). It is the most common operating room procedure performed in this country. In 1965, the rate of cesarean delivery was 4.5% (National Partnership for Women and Families, 2016). A suggested optimal cesarean delivery rate of 10% to 15% has been proposed (Makvandi et al., 2015).

Indications

Approximately 35% of cesarean sections are done because of failure to progress in labor, 24% because of a nonreassuring fetal heart tracing, and 19% because of malpresentation of the fetus. More rare reasons for cesarean section include abnormal placentation, cord prolapse, and suspected macrosomia, among others (Boyle et al., 2013). Approximately 1% of primary cesarean deliveries are performed at the request of the pregnant woman in the absence of a medical necessity. Although it is often assumed that changes in pregnant women have led to the change in practice (such as increased maternal obesity and older birthing mothers), the rate of cesarean delivery has gone up for all groups, not just those associated with higher-risk pregnancies and births. In addition, the fear of medical malpractice by obstetric providers likely has little or no role in the increased rate of cesarean deliveries. Instead, the increased rate is likely the result of a combination of several factors, including the following:

- Low provider tolerance for prolonged labor
- The increased risk for cesarean section as a consequence of certain obstetric interventions, such as labor induction and continuous electronic fetal monitoring
- An unwillingness of many institutions and obstetric providers to offer a vaginal birth after cesarean section
- A high societal tolerance for surgery

- Limited awareness of the risks for cesarean section
- Lack of financial incentive for obstetric providers to attend a prolonged birth
- Patients' trust in the advice and recommendations of their obstetric providers (National Partnership for Women and Families, 2016).

Risks and Complications

A cesarean delivery is major abdominal surgery and carries with it the risks of such a procedure. Women are at risk for complications related to anesthesia, bowel and bladder injury during the surgery, hemorrhage, and air or amniotic fluid embolism. Postpartum, women are at a higher risk for infection at the wound site, urinary tract infection, and endometritis. They are at a higher risk for atelectasis and bowel dysfunction related to the surgery. Complications such as wound hematoma, wound dehiscence, necrotizing fasciitis, and thromboembolism, although rare, are far more likely with a cesarean section than a vaginal birth. Women are typically hospitalized for at least twice as many days after a cesarean section and experience a slowed recovery. Maternal-infant bonding may be disrupted or delayed.

In 2013, the average total charges for a pregnancy ending in vaginal birth were $30,000 and the charges for a cesarean delivery were $50,000. Out-of-pocket charges to patients with commercial insurance averaged 12% of the total cost (Truven Health Analytics, 2013). In any subsequent pregnancies, abnormal placentation such as placenta previa or placental accreta is more common after cesarean section. If a trial of labor is attempted with a future pregnancy, uterine rupture is more likely than for women without a previous cesarean delivery.

Birth trauma such as lacerations of the fetus by surgical tools is rare. Respiratory complications leading to NICU admission are more common after cesarean section (Dodd, Crowther, Huertas, Guise, & Horey, 2013). Emerging evidence suggests that infants born by cesarean section may be at a higher risk for obesity later in life (Mueller et al., 2015), immune system compromise in the short term, and diabetes, allergies, and asthma in the long term (Azad et al., 2015; Cho & Norman, 2013).

Types

A cesarean delivery may be scheduled prior to labor because of known risk factors or complications or it may be performed emergently because of complications of labor and delivery. More rarely a cesarean section may be performed at the request of the mother. Very rarely a cesarean section may be legally ordered at the behest of the obstetric provider if a cesarean section is deemed necessary for the well-being of the fetus but is declined by the mother. Such dilemmas are a form of maternal–fetal conflict, as what is best for the fetus may not be best for the mother. Actively listening to the mother's concerns and seeking alternatives when possible may best diffuse such cases. An institution's ethics board would then be consulted if no solution is found. Legal action is rare in such cases and sought only in unusual circumstances.

Unplanned

Most cesarean deliveries are unplanned and are done because of a failure to progress, a nonreassuring fetal tracing, or a malpresentation of the fetus (Boyle et al., 2013; Fig. 22.12). Although malpresentation may be detected prior to birth, it may also present during labor, and thus lead to an unplanned cesarean delivery. Rupture of the uterus is also a cause for an unplanned cesarean section, as is cord prolapse. A cesarean section that occurs after the onset of labor is referred to as an emergency cesarean section and, as dictated by national standards, must begin within 30 minutes of the decision to operate. However, many such procedures are performed after the 30-minute mark, and the clinical significance of this delay is unknown (Tolcher, Johnson, El-Nashar, & West, 2014).

An unplanned cesarean section may occur after a long labor and considerable effort. Women and families are often deeply invested in their birth process and may express frustration and disappointment or even a sense of failure about the need for a cesarean section. Because of the emergent nature of an unplanned cesarean section, obtaining consent and providing education are often rushed, and the nurse may have to repeatedly review instructions and other details, as needed.

Lexi, in Chapter 10, had wanted to attempt a vaginal delivery even though the delivery of her previous pregnancy was by cesarean. Dr. Stone was initially willing to attempt this, but once Lexi was diagnosed with HELLP syndrome, he strongly urged her to deliver by cesarean again. (Letitia, in Chapter 5, also had to undergo an cesarean delivery, this time because of cord prolapse.)

Scheduled

A cesarean birth may be scheduled because of a known obstetric complication that precludes a vaginal birth, such as placenta previa, an active genital herpes outbreak, or a strong suspicion of fetal macrosomia. A cesarean delivery may also be scheduled in the case of a cesarean section with a previous pregnancy, although, depending on the obstetric provider, institutional policy, and patient preference, a trial of labor may be preferred.

Because Susan, in Chapter 3, had undergone a cesarean section with the birth of her first child, Dr. Cheema explained that she would have to deliver her current pregnancy via cesarean section, as it was the hospital's policy.

Elective

A cesarean birth may be performed without an obstetric or medical indication for the procedure at the request of the mother. Because the procedure is associated with more risks for the couplet, it is

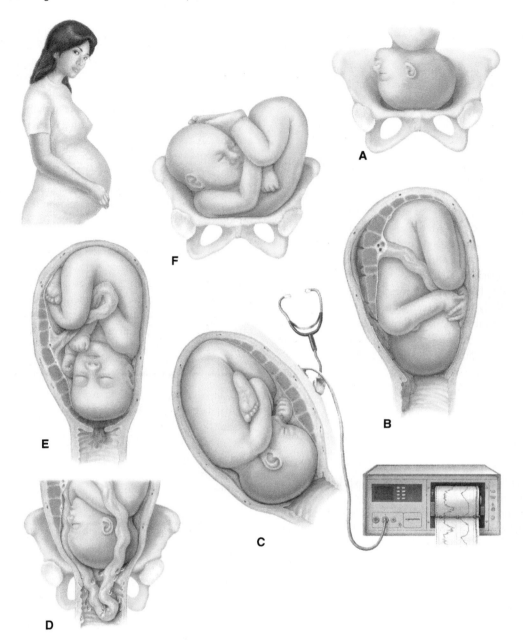

Figure 22.12. Conditions indicating the need for cesarean section. Starting in the upper right and moving clockwise: **(A)** cephalopelvic disproportion, **(B)** placental abruption with severe hemorrhage and maternal or fetal compromise, **(C)** nonreassuring fetal status, **(D)** cord prolapse, **(E)** placenta previa, and **(F)** fetal malpresentation. (Reprinted with permission from Anatomical Chart Company.)

imperative that the nurse inform the mother of potential complications. However, the care team must also respect the woman's bodily autonomy and delivery preferences. As with all births, it is desirable that the pregnancy progress to at least 39 weeks of gestation to minimize the risks of prematurity for the neonate. A woman may request a cesarean birth for many reasons, including fear of labor and the associated pain, planning purposes, helping retain a sense of control, and concerns about future problems with sexual functioning and pelvic floor dysfunction, including incontinence and pelvic organ prolapse.

Preoperative Care

Prior to a cesarean section, the patient must be educated about the risks, benefits, and alternatives to the cesarean section and sign a consent form. Although it is the responsibility of the obstetric provider to obtain consent, it is often the role of the nurse to provide the education. A cesarean delivery is a technical procedure, and team members must be proficient in a number of skills. Particularly in the case of an unplanned cesarean delivery, events may move very quickly. The nurse must focus on the patient's care and inform the patient and her support person or team of what's happening. When possible, the nurse should minimize extraneous noise, play music of the patient's choosing, and dim the lights. In many cases the birthing partner stays with the woman. If not, the nurse should provide the partner with information updates when possible. Like other team members, partners should be dressed appropriately for the operating room.

In the case of planned cesarean delivery, the procedure is typically scheduled for week 39 of gestation to avoid complications of prematurity. When possible, the patient consults with the anesthesiologist prior to admission to plan care. Standard fasting guidelines are recommended, including no clear liquids for 2 hours, no solids for 6 hours, and no fatty meals for 8 hours prior to the procedure. A medication, or a combination of medications, is often provided orally or IV to further minimize the risk of aspiration of gastric contents.

At least one 16- to 18-gauge IV line is placed prior to a cesarean delivery. A second IV line may be placed if the patient is at a particularly high risk for hemorrhage or requires magnesium sulfate. When possible, the mother's nondominant hand or arm is used so her dominant hand may be free to hold and nurse the infant after the birth. A hemoglobin, blood type, and antibody screen is performed if no current record exists. If the patient is deemed low risk for transfusion, the surgeon may instead opt for a "hold clot" in which the patient's blood is drawn but no tests are performed unless her risk for transfusion rises (Box 22.2). A woman is considered at a higher risk for transfusion during the delivery under the following conditions:

- General anesthesia is used
- History of multiple cesarean sections
- Anemic prior to the birth
- Severe preeclampsia, eclampsia, or HELLP syndrome
- Placental complications, such as placenta previa, placental abruption, or placenta accreta

Because a woman undergoing a cesarean delivery has up to 20 times the risk of infection as a woman who gives birth vaginally, antibiotic prophylaxis is indicated (Smaill & Grivell, 2014). A common strategy is a single dose of a narrow-spectrum antibiotic IV within 1 hour before the primary incision is made. Women who are already receiving antibiotics for GBS prophylaxis or chorioamnionitis may or may not require an additional antibiotic.

It is the standard of care in the United States for women undergoing a cesarean delivery to have mechanical thromboembolism prophylaxis with pneumatic compression boots during and after the surgery, until regular ambulation is established. Women who are obese, have a history of a thromboembolism, or are otherwise deemed to be at a higher risk for a blood clot may in addition receive pharmacologic prophylaxis, usually with heparin. The nurse should start administering heparin, if indicated, 6 to 12 hours after the delivery to minimize the chance of hemorrhage and continue it until the patient is ambulating regularly.

If the cesarean delivery is planned, the nurse should assess and document the fetal heart rate at the time of admission, along with maternal vital signs. In the case of a high-risk pregnancy with

Box 22.2 Cesarean Section Preoperative Care Considerations

- Laboratory testing
  - Hemoglobin (must be within the last month)
  - Blood type and antibody screen on file or a "hold clot" (blood has been drawn but no tests are performed unless indicated)
- Antibiotics administration
  - Single-dose antibiotic given within 60 min before incision
- Thromboembolism prophylaxis
  - Pneumatic compression devices for women at low risk
  - Pneumatic compression device and pharmacologic prophylaxis (heparin) for women at high risk
- Fetal heart rate monitoring
  - Heart rate recording on admission for a planned cesarean section
  - Continuous monitoring for women in labor
    - Discontinue external monitoring when preparation of the incision site begins.
    - Discontinue internal monitoring prior to incision.
- Placental location and fetal position assessment
  - Ultrasound
  - Leopold's maneuvers
- Bladder catheterization
- Skin preparation
  - Scrub with chlorhexidine or iodine.
  - If hair removal is indicated, clip (don't shave) the patient's hair just prior to the procedure.
- Vaginal preparation
  - Scrub with chlorhexidine or iodine for women with ruptured membranes (Haas, Morgan, & Contreras, 2014).
- Draping around the surgical site
- Displacement of the uterus to avoid supine hypotension
  - Use a wedge, rolled blanket, or pillow or tilt the table.

previous antepartum testing, the single fetal heart rate recording may be replaced by NST. If the patient is already in labor when the decision is made to deliver by cesarean section, monitoring continues into the operating room. In the case of external monitoring, assessment of the fetal heart rate ceases when preparation of the abdomen begins. Internal monitoring is discontinued just prior to the incision. In addition, an ultrasound may be performed by the operating physician to confirm fetal position and the location of the placenta.

Catheterization of the urinary bladder is standard practice, as it minimizes the risk of injury to bladder during the surgery. Alternatively, some surgeons may allow the patient to void prior to the procedure and place a catheter only if needed. Catheters are discontinued as soon as safe ambulation is established to minimize patient discomfort and the risk for urinary tract infections.

Although it was once routine to shave the perineal area of women prior to a birth, either vaginal or cesarean, this practice is no longer recommended, as microabrasions created by shaving increase the chance for infection. If hair removal is necessary, clipping just prior to incision is recommended. The skin around the selected incision site is cleansed, usually with an iodine or chlorhexidine solution containing alcohol. A surgeon may instead request a solution that does not contain alcohol if immediate delivery is required, as alcohol-containing solutions are flammable and must be allowed to dry for at least 3 minutes. In addition to preparation of the skin at the surgical site, surgeons may also prepare the vagina with cleanser, particularly if the membranes are ruptured.

Drapes are placed on areas close to the surgical field. Some facilities have clear drapes available so that a woman and her birthing partner may watch the surgery. When clear drapes are not available and observation is still desired, the drapes may be positioned so the birth of the infant may be observed.

Any time a woman must assume a supine position in late pregnancy, the uterus should be displaced by at least 15°, and during a cesarean section is no exception. This tilt may be achieved by placing a rolled-up towel or wedge behind the woman's lower back, tilting the table, or other means. This practice helps avoid supine hypotension.

Anesthesia

A vast majority of cesarean deliveries are performed on women using neuraxial anesthesia. This method allows the mother to be awake for the birth and minimizes fetal exposure to medications. Maternal sedation caused by general anesthesia can inhibit early bonding with the neonate. General anesthesia may be preferred, however, if there is insufficient time to perform neuraxial anesthesia and achieve the necessary results, if an epidural was attempted and failed, if the mother refuses neuraxial anesthesia, in the case of severe hemorrhage, or in the case of contraindications to neuroaxial anesthesia, such as a spinal injury, skin infection overlying the insertion site, or a maternal clotting deficiency.

Surgery

The surgeon makes two incisions in a cesarean delivery: of the abdominal wall and of the uterus. Either may be transverse (side to side) or vertical, but transverse is the most common, specifically the Pfannenstiel incision, which is slightly curved and a few centimeters above the symphysis pubis. The middle part of the incision, which is minimally about 15 cm long, is beneath the pubic hairline. The other kind of commonly used transverse incision is the Joel-Cohen, which is straighter and higher up on the abdomen. The transverse approach is preferred generally because it results in less pain, greater wound strength, and a better aesthetic result. A vertical incision allows for faster abdominal entry, however, and may be selected if a more urgent delivery is critical (Fig. 22.13; see Fig. 17.15).

The incision of the uterus does not necessarily match the incision in the skin: a woman may have a transverse skin incision

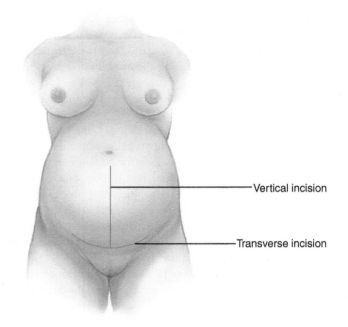

Figure 22.13. Types of abdominal incisions used for cesarean delivery. Vertical and low transverse incisions. (Reprinted with permission from Hatfield, N. T. [2014]. *Introductory maternity and pediatric nursing* [3rd ed., Fig. 11-4A]. Philadelphia, PA: Lippincott Williams & Wilkins.)

and a vertical uterine incision. This is important information to have for future pregnancies, as vertical incisions are more liable to rupture and are a contraindication to a vaginal birth after a cesarean delivery. In addition, a transverse incision is associated with less blood loss and better surgical repair (Dahlke et al., 2013). If a vertical incision of the uterus is selected, however, it may be a low vertical (in the lower uterine segment) or classical (in the upper uterine segment/fundus) incision (Fig. 22.14). Although the classical incision creates the highest risk for uterine rupture, the low vertical incision is also associated with a higher risk for rupture than a transverse incision and has the additional risk that the incision may extend into the upper uterine segment or down into the cervix, bladder, or even the vagina (Fig. 22.15).

Postoperative Care

A designated nurse and possibly other team members skilled in infant resuscitation, such as neonatologists or NICU nurses, are present to assess and care for the neonate immediately after the birth while the surgical team continues to focus on the mother. The nurse readies equipment such as a radiant warmer and equipment for neonatal resuscitation prior to the surgery. Whenever possible, the nurse should encourage the mother to hold her infant skin to skin and nurse the infant as soon after delivery as possible (see Fig. 5.8). If further support is needed, the infant may be transferred to the NICU.

After the surgery, the mother is usually moved out of the operating room and into a recovery room. The mother is now both

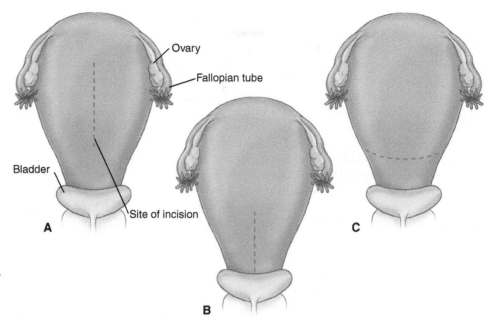

Figure 22.14. Types of uterine incisions used for cesarean delivery. (A) Classical (vertical) approach. **(B)** Low (cervical) vertical approach. **(C)** Low (cervical) transverse approach. (Reprinted with permission from Hatfield, N. T. [2014]. *Introductory maternity and pediatric nursing* [3rd ed., Fig. 11-5]. Philadelphia, PA: Lippincott Williams & Wilkins.)

a postsurgical patient and a postpartum patient, and the nurse must address both sets of needs. The nurse continues monitoring the mother's vital signs per protocol and assesses her uterine tone and vaginal and incisional bleeding at scheduled intervals (Box 22.3). A common protocol is to assess blood pressure, pulse, and respirations every 15 minutes for 2 hours following surgery, after which time assessments are done less frequently. The nurse should assess the mother's temperature twice in the first 8 hours postpartum and then once per 8-hour shift.

Frequent assessment of uterine tone and lochia are important to reduce the risk for excessive blood loss. Often, oxytocin is supplemented in the immediate postpartum period to reduce the risk for uterine atony. The nurse should keep the wound incision completely covered in the immediate postpartum period but visually inspect the dressing itself regularly for bleeding and

drainage. Nurses should be aware of abdominal and incision pain postpartum and delay fundal assessments when possible until after pain has been adequately treated.

For some women, incisional and abdominal pain can dominate the postpartum period and must be adequately addressed.

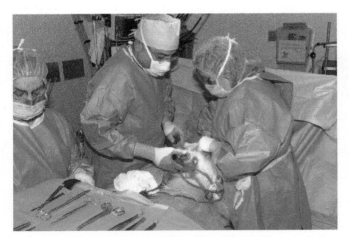

Figure 22.15. Cesarean section. (Reprinted with permission from Creason, C. [Ed.]. [2011]. *Stedman's medical terminology: Steps to success in medical language* [1st ed., Fig. 11.24]. Philadelphia, PA: Lippincott Williams & Wilkins.)

Box 22.3   Cesarean Section Postoperative Care Considerations

1. Routine monitoring per protocol
   - Systolic blood pressure should not drop below 90 mm Hg.
   - Heart rate should stay below 120 beats/min.
   - Respiratory rate should stay below 30 breaths/min.
   - Temperature
   - Oxygen saturation should remain at 95% or higher.
   - Urine output should remain at or above 30 mL/h.
   - Uterine tone and bleeding from the vagina and the incision
- Breastfeeding to be started in the delivery room
- Bladder catheter removal as soon as possible
   - Catheter is typically removed as soon as safe ambulation is established.
- Ambulation within 6 h after anesthesia effects are resolved
- Regular diet as tolerated
- Wound dressing removal from 24 to 48 h after delivery or per protocol
   - Most wounds are closed with sutures.
   - If the wound is closed with staples, anticipate removal at 4–10 d after surgery.
- Increased activity as tolerated
- Avoidance of heavy lifting and lifting from a squat position for 1–2 wk after surgery

According to institution protocol and the orders of the obstetric provider, pain in the first 24 hours or so may be managed with epidural, IV, or intramuscular opioids. Women may instead be managed with oral opioids, which, along with ibuprofen and acetaminophen, are the analgesics of choice after discontinuation of the epidural and/or IV medication. Women who experience nausea with opioids may also be provided with an antiemetic.

The nurse should encourage the patient to ambulate early and resume an oral diet as tolerated (Hsu, Hung, Chang, & Chang, 2013). If a bladder catheter was placed, the nurse removes it as soon as possible, typically once the patient can ambulate safely. Although most women are able to safely carry their infants, the nurse should discourage them from heavy lifting and lifting from a squatting position for 1 to 2 weeks to minimize stress on the healing fascia. After discharge, women may resume driving when they can do so comfortably and if they are not taking sedating medications. To drive safely, a woman must be able to complete the motions required for safe driving quickly and without hesitation.

The dressing placed on the surgical wound after the cesarean section is usually removed within 24 to 48 hours. The wound may have been closed with dissolving stitches, which do not need to be removed, or with staples, which are removed 4 to 10 days after the surgery. Women who are at a higher risk for wound complications, such as those with diabetes or who are obese, typically have their staples left in place longer.

Vaginal Birth After Cesarean

Women who underwent a cesarean section for a previous birth for reasons that are not intrinsically recurrent, such as fetal malpresentation or failure to progress, may desire to attempt a vaginal birth with a subsequent pregnancy, which is known as a trial of labor after cesarean (TOLAC).

Prevalence

Of the women who attempt a TOLAC, approximately 70% achieve a vaginal birth. The likelihood of success is far greater if labor starts naturally than if it is induced (Regan, Keup, Wolfe, Snyder, & DeFranco, 2015). The alternative to TOLAC is elective repeat cesarean delivery (ERDC). In 2000, the rate of TOLAC peaked at almost 52% with an almost 70% success rate (success being measured as a vaginal birth), but with it came an increase in reports of uterine rupture with associated maternal, fetal, and neonate mortality (Lydon-Rochelle, Holt, Easterling, & Martin, 2001; Uddin & Simon, 2013).

Indications

A TOLAC should be attempted only in settings with access to advanced obstetric care, including a ready surgical suite and an experienced team of healthcare providers, including anesthesiologists. Currently, many hospitals do not offer the option of TOLAC, at least partly because of their inability to guarantee such resources in the event of a uterine rupture. Fear of catastrophic complications, as well as liability, has discouraged some obstetric providers from encouraging or supporting TOLAC. Despite the risks associated with TOLAC and the trepidation of providers and hospitals, it is important to remember that the means of delivery is the choice of the woman and that, although TOLAC carries with it risks, ERDC does as well (Table 22.2).

The best candidates for TOLAC are women with a low risk for uterine rupture and a high likelihood for a successful vaginal birth after cesarean. Women with a low transverse incision of the uterus from a prior cesarean section are at a lower risk for rupture than women with a classic vertical incision. TOLAC with such an incision has a 60% to 80% chance of success and as low as a 0.4% risk for uterine rupture (Sabol, Denman, & Guise, 2015). Women who have successfully given birth vaginally previously, either before or after cesarean section, are more likely to have a successful TOLAC (Landon et al., 2005). As mentioned previously, spontaneous labor is also associated with superior outcomes, as well as the prior cesarean section done for a nonrecurrent indication.

Contraindications

Factors that may counter the potential for success include a close spacing of pregnancies (fewer than 6 months between the end of

Table 22.2   Incidence Rates of Pregnancy Complications in Women with TOLAC Compared With Those in Women With ERDC

Pregnancy Complication	Incidence Rate in Women With TOLAC (%)	Incidence Rate in Women With ERDC (%)
Uterine rupture	0.47	0.026
Hysterectomy	0.17	0.28
Blood transfusion	0.9	1.2
Infection	4.6	3.2
Maternal death	0.004	0.013

TOLAC, trial of labor after cesarean; ERDC, elective repeat cesarean delivery.
Adapted from Guise, J. M., Denman, M. A., Emeis, C., Marshall, N., Walker, M., Fu, R., . . . McDonagh, M. (2010). Vaginal birth after cesarean: New insights on maternal and neonatal outcomes. *Obstetrics and Gynecology, 115*(6), 1267–1278. doi:10.1097/AOG.0b013e3181df925f

one pregnancy and the beginning of the next), fetal macrosomia, advanced maternal age, maternal comorbid medical conditions, delivery at a hospital not associated with a university, more than one prior cesarean section, and a pregnancy over 40 weeks of gestation (ACOG, 2016b; Metz, Allshouse, Faucett, & Grobman, 2015). Women with contraindications to a vaginal birth or a history of uterine rupture or uterine dehiscence are poor candidates for TOLAC.

Assessment

Because of the small but real risk for uterine rupture with TOLAC, the attending obstetric provider may require, and the ACOG recommends, continuous electronic fetal monitoring (ACOG, 2017). Nurses should be aware that women who have delivered by cesarean section previously but have not delivered vaginally are likely to have a longer active phase of the first stage of labor than women who have never given birth previously. Women who have previously delivered by cesarean section and given birth vaginally can anticipate an active phase similar to that of other women who have previously given birth vaginally (Grantz et al., 2015). Although women may be induced when attempting a TOLAC, there is an increased risk of rupture. Oxytocin is considered an acceptable uterotonic for this purpose, but the use of prostaglandins is associated with uterine rupture with or without a prior cesarean section and is contraindicated for TOLAC.

Uterine Rupture

A uterine rupture is a tear in the wall of the uterus.

Prevalence

Although a uterine rupture may occur in either a scarred or unscarred uterus, it is far more prevalent in women with a uterus that is scarred, typically as a result of a previous cesarean delivery or other uterine surgery. The risk for the rupture of a uterus during labor of an unscarred uterus is about 1 in every 22,000 births. The risk of uterine rupture during labor for a woman who is attempting a TOLAC delivery is closer to 1 in 200 (Al-Zirqi, Stray-Pedersen, Forsen, Daltveit, & Vangen, 2016; Guise et al., 2010).

Etiology

In addition to the increased risk for those who have had a previous cesarean birth, the risk for uterine rupture is particularly high for women who have experienced uterine rupture in the past and women who have a vertical incision of the uterus. Labor induction, particularly with prostaglandins, but also with oxytocin, also contributes to the risk of uterine rupture in women with a history of cesarean section. Although the rate of uterine rupture is 0.5% among women with TOLAC, it is 2.45% among those with TOLAC and prostaglandin induction, an increase in risk sufficient to make the use of prostaglandins with a prior cesarean delivery a contraindication. The use of

oxytocin also contributes to the risk but is not a contraindication (ACOG, 2017).

Prognosis

Although maternal death is rare with uterine rupture, the perinatal mortality rate is as high as 6% (National Institutes of Health, 2010).

Assessment

The first signs of uterine rupture may include some of the following:

- Sudden development of a category II or III fetal heart rate pattern, often bradycardia, possibly preceded by decelerations (Fig. 22.16)
- Maternal hemodynamic instability manifested by hypotension and tachycardia
- Weakening contractions, as detected by palpation or internal monitoring (Desseauve et al., 2016)
- Loss of fetal stations (a fetus that is +3, for example, may rise to station 0)
- Abdominal pain
- Vaginal bleeding or hematuria

In some cases, a uterine rupture may not be diagnosed until the postpartum period, and the clinical presentation may be hematuria or vaginal bleeding that does not respond to uterotonics such as oxytocin. Uterine rupture is typically diagnosed definitively when a cesarean delivery is performed because of a high suspicion for rupture. In a stable couplet, however, time may be available for ultrasound imaging and the diagnosis can be made then.

Treatment

A suspicion of uterine rupture is a trigger for a cesarean section, particularly as some of the symptoms of uterine rupture—maternal hemodynamic instability, severe abdominal pain, and a persistent abnormal fetal heart tracing—are reasons in and of themselves for a cesarean delivery, regardless of the underlying cause. A patient who is hemodynamically unstable is stabilized using IV fluids and blood products prior to delivery per orders and institution protocols. If epidural or spinal anesthesia is not in place, general anesthesia is indicated because of a shorter time between administration and the achievement of results adequate for surgery. The decision to perform a hysterectomy or repair the rupture after delivery of the fetus and placenta is based on the clinical picture and, when possible, the patient's future reproductive plans.

Cord Prolapse

Cord prolapse is a condition in which the umbilical cord precedes the fetal head in the birth canal, increasing the risk of cord compression and hypoxia to the fetus. A cord prolapse may be overt or occult. With an overt prolapse, the cord slips out of the vagina ahead of the fetus (see Fig. 5.6). With an occult prolapse, the cord is descending next to the fetus and becomes entrapped between the fetus and the maternal parts.

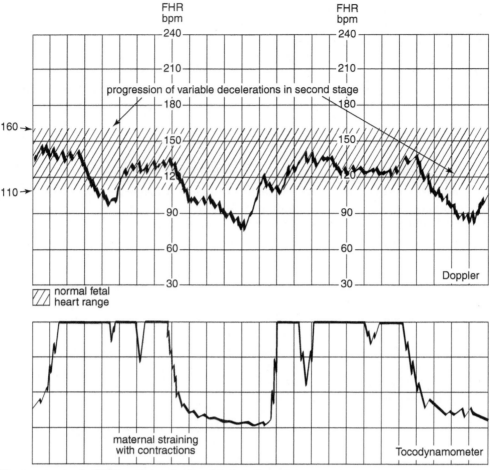

Figure 22.16. **An FHR pattern characteristic of imminent uterine rupture.** FHR, fetal heart rate; bpm, beats per minute. (Reprinted with permission from Cabaniss, M. L., & Ross, M. G. [2009]. *Fetal monitoring interpretation* [2nd ed., Fig. 7.105]. Philadelphia, PA: Lippincott Williams & Wilkins.)

In Chapter 5, Letitia experienced an overt cord prolapse. It occurred because her membranes ruptured when the fetal head was not yet engaged in the pelvis, allowing room for a loop of cord to enter the vagina ahead of the fetus.

Prevalence

Cord prolapse complicates approximately 1 out of every 150 births (Gibbons, O'Herlihy, & Murphy, 2014).

Etiology

A prolapse occurs because the presenting fetal part is not completely filling the pelvic inlet or an obstetric procedure has dislodged the presenting part, allowing passage of the cord ahead of or with the fetus (Box 22.4). The membranes are almost always ruptured at the time of prolapse.

Prognosis

Prolapse exposes the cord to the risk of compression, occlusion of the blood vessels, and vasospasm, all of which impact the gas exchange between the mother and fetus and can result in impaired fetal oxygenation.

Assessment

The first sign of a cord prolapse is generally a change in the fetal heart tracing, typically severe fetal bradycardia and variable decelerations (Fig. 22.17). Nurses should be aware that this particular change in fetal heart rate pattern may also be seen with maternal hypotension, placental abruption, uterine rupture, and uterine tachysystole. Unlike uterine rupture or placental abruption, however, cord prolapse is painless and does not cause bleeding. Rarely, the cord may be felt on vaginal examination or visualized.

Treatment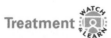

Cord prolapse is an obstetric emergency, and prompt delivery, typically by cesarean, is required to avoid fetal hypoxia and death.

Box 22.4 Risk Factors for Cord Prolapse

Maternal and Fetal

- Unengaged presenting part
- Nonvertex position (breech, transverse, etc.)
- Low birth weight
- Prematurity
- Fetal anomalies
- Uterine malformations
- Multiple pregnancy
- Polyhydramnios
- Low-lying placenta

Interventional

- Artificial rupture of membranes
- Mechanical cervical ripening with a balloon catheter
- Labor induction
- Amnioinfusion
- External cephalic version
- Internal podalic version
- Application of forceps
- Application of a vacuum extraction device
- Application of a fetal scalp electrode
- Insertion of an intrauterine pressure catheter
- Manual rotation of the fetal head

Adapted from Gabbay-Benziv, R., Maman, M., Wiznitzer, A., Linder, N., & Yogev, Y. (2014). Umbilical cord prolapse during delivery—Risk factors and pregnancy outcome: A single center experience. *Journal of Maternal-Fetal and Neonatal Medicine, 27*(1), 14–17. doi:10.3109/14767058.2013.799651

The first step for either an overt prolapse or a suspected occult prolapse is to call for help. The nurse or other provider should immediately resuscitate the fetus by moving pressure off the cord (Step-by-Step Skills 22.1). Another nurse should help prepare for an emergency delivery. If not already a component of care, the nurse should initiate continuous fetal heart rate monitoring.

Care Considerations

If the prolapse is overt, the nurse and others should handle the cord as little as possible to avoid spasm of the umbilical artery but, if possible, the obstetric provider may elect to place the cord into the vagina and cover with moist gauze (Holbrook & Phelan, 2013; Maher & Heavey, 2015). The nurse should anticipate delivery to occur immediately; if the suspected prolapse is occult and fetal heart rate abnormalities resolve with the resuscitative measures described in Step-by-Step Skills 22.1, labor may continue with expectant management, as previous to the prolapse.

Amniotic Fluid Embolism

An **amniotic fluid embolism**, also referred to as anaphylactoid syndrome of pregnancy, is a rare but devastating condition in which amniotic fluid enters the maternal circulation. It may occur during pregnancy, labor, delivery, or the immediate postpartum period.

Prevalence

Amniotic fluid embolism occurs in approximately 2 to 7 deliveries per 100,000 (Fitzpatrick, Tuffnell, Kurinczuk, & Knight, 2016; Shen, Wang, Yang, & Chen, 2016).

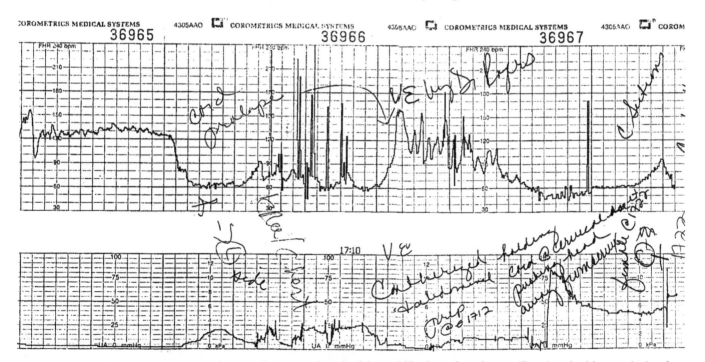

Figure 22.17. A fetal heart rate monitor tracing associated with umbilical cord prolapse. (Reprinted with permission from Scott, J. R., Gibbs, R. S., Karlan, B. Y., & Haney, A. F. [2003]. *Danforth's obstetrics and gynecology* [9th ed., Fig. 21-5]. Philadelphia, PA: Lippincott Williams & Wilkins.)

Step-by-Step Skills 22.1

Fetal Resuscitation During Cord Prolapse

1. Elevate the fetus off of the cord.
   a. Manually elevate the presenting part by reaching into the vagina with one hand and gently pushing on the fetal head, elevating it off of the cord.
   b. Position the pregnant woman face down in the knee-chest position with her buttocks elevated.
   c. Alternatively, position the mother in a steep Trendelenburg position.
   d. Fill the woman's bladder with 500–700 mL of saline via a catheter.
2. Administer a tocolytic.
3. The obstetric provider may elect to manually replace the cord into the vagina.

Etiology

Amniotic embolism occurs when amniotic fluid containing fetal and placental cells enters the maternal circulation. Although considered an unpredictable event that cannot be prevented (Shen et al., 2016), it has been associated with the following risk factors (Fitzpatrick et al., 2016):

- Labor induction
- Operative delivery
- Advanced maternal age
- Cervical lacerations
- Eclampsia
- Fetal distress
- Placenta previa
- Placental abruption
- Grand multiparity (five or more births)
- Precipitous delivery

Prognosis

Amniotic fluid embolism is associated with a maternal mortality rate of 32% (Shen et al., 2016). It can lead to respiratory failure, cardiogenic shock (inadequate blood circulation due to ineffective pumping of the heart), and an inflammatory and anaphylactoid reaction. Cardiogenic shock plays a part in most deaths associated with the condition. Respiratory failure is a feature of about half of the deaths from amniotic fluid embolism that occur in the first hour following the embolism. For survivors, permanent, severe neurologic impairment is common. For offspring, survival is also poor when the embolism occurs during pregnancy or labor and delivery, and approximately half of survivors sustain neurologic damage (Clark, 2010).

Assessment

The onset of clinical signs and symptoms of an amniotic fluid embolism is typically during labor and delivery, although it may appear as late as 48 hours after delivery. More rarely, it may present after an abortion, uterine trauma during pregnancy, or an obstetric intervention such as amniocentesis or external version. Classically, the first clinical signs and symptoms are those of respiratory failure and cardiac arrest (Box 22.5). If the patient survives, she may progress to hemorrhagic shock with disseminated intravascular coagulation (Fig. 22.18).

Treatment

There is no one treatment for a suspected amniotic fluid embolism. Rather, care is focused on correcting hypotension and hypoxemia to minimize damage to the woman and, if still pregnant, the fetus. Initial care consists of optimization of oxygen delivery to the cells, including intubation and administration of blood products, IV fluids, and vasopressor medications (Box 22.6). An emergency cesarean section may be indicated within minutes.

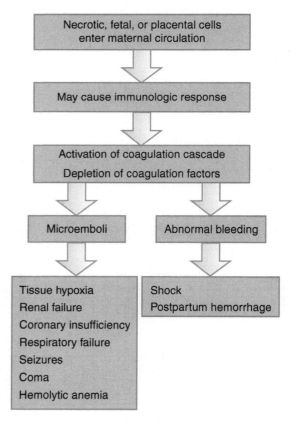

Figure 22.18. Pathogenesis of disseminated intravascular coagulation from amniotic fluid embolism. (Reprinted with permission from Nettina, S. M. [2014]. *Lippincott manual of nursing practice* [10th ed., Fig. 39-5]. Philadelphia, PA: Lippincott Williams & Wilkins.)

Box 22.5 Clinical Manifestations of Amniotic Fluid Embolism

- Cardiogenic shock
  - Hypotension
  - Tachycardia
  - Cardiac arrest
- Respiratory distress
  - Low oxygen saturation levels by pulse oximetry
  - Confusion
  - Restlessness
  - Dyspnea
  - Tachypnea
  - Cyanosis
  - Crackles and wheezing on auscultation of the lungs
  - Somnolence (sleepiness)
  - Respiratory arrest
- Coagulopathy: may occur within 10 min after cardio-pulmonary complications or may be delayed by several hours
  - Bleeding from the site of an intravenous catheter
  - Hematuria
  - Bleeding gums
  - Petechiae
  - Hemorrhage

Box 22.6 Amniotic Fluid Embolism Interventions

- Call for help.
- If prior to birth, place the woman in the side-lying position to displace the uterus.
- Continuously monitor the woman's oxygen saturation level, heart rate and rhythm, respiratory rate, and blood pressure.
- If the birth has not occurred, perform continuous fetal monitoring.
- Anticipate placement of central venous and arterial catheters for the following purposes:
  - Central venous catheter: infusion of fluids, medicine, and blood; blood draws; and monitoring of central venous pressure and central venous oxyhemoglobin saturation
  - Arterial catheter: continuous monitoring of blood pressure and monitoring of arterial blood gasses
- Administer supplemental oxygen, with the goal of keeping the PaO_2 level above 65 mm Hg, via one of the following:
  - Nonrebreather mask at a rate of 8–10 L/min
  - Resuscitation bag with 100% oxygen
  - Intubation and mechanical ventilation
- Provide hemodynamic support by administering the following, as ordered:
  - Vasopressor (i.e., norepinephrine or dopamine)
  - Intravenous fluids
  - Blood products
- Prepare for an emergent delivery, if the embolism occurs prior to birth.

Third-Stage Complications

Complications common to the third stage of labor include a retained placenta, a morbidly adherent placenta, and lacerations.

Retained Placenta

A retained placenta is one that does not detach from the uterine wall within 30 minutes after delivery of the infant.

Etiology

A retained placenta occurs because of a disruption in the normal process of the third stage of labor. A normal third stage of labor has four phases: the latent phase, the contraction phase, the detachment phase, and the expulsion phase. During the latent phase, the entire uterus contracts, with the exception of the retroplacental area directly under the placenta. During the contraction phase, the myometrium under the placenta contracts. Contractions create a sheering force that detaches the placenta from the decidua during the detachment phase. In the expulsion phase, contractions force the placenta out of the uterus.

A placenta may be retained in one of three ways:

1. It may be completely separated from the uterus but trapped behind a closing cervix (incarcerated placenta) because of the failure of the expulsion phase.
2. It may be adherent but easily separated from the wall of the uterus (placenta adherens), likely from a prolonged latent phase.
3. The villi of the placenta may have abnormally adhered to the myometrium of the uterus instead of the decidua, reducing the efficacy of the contraction phase and preventing the detachment phase (placenta accreta).

A major risk factor for retained placenta is second trimester or early third trimester delivery, with 98% of placentas requiring a full hour to pass after births in the second trimester compared with 98% of placentas being expelled in 30 minutes or less after births in the third trimester (Tuncalp, Souza, & Gulmezoglu, 2013). Other risk factors for placental retention include stillbirth, maternal age over 30 years, non-Hispanic white ethnicity, previous placental retention, velamentous cord insertion, and uterine abnormalities (Coviello, Grantz, Huang, Kelly, & Landy, 2015).

Prognosis

Failure of the placenta to detach in a timely fashion impairs both the chemical and mechanical cues that cause the uterus to contract after a birth and creates a risk for postpartum hemorrhage. Complications associated with a retained placenta include hemorrhage and endometritis postpartum. Maternal deaths from this condition are rare in high-resource facilities but may reach 1% in lower-resource settings (John, Orazulike, & Alegbeleye, 2015).

Assessment

Retained placenta is diagnosed when the placenta has not been expelled within 30 minutes after the birth of the neonate. Incarcerated placenta is diagnosed when the placenta does not pass despite indications that it has separated from the uterine wall, including lengthening of the umbilical cord, a change in the uterine shape to globular, elevation of the fundus, and a gush of blood from the vagina. Placenta adherens is diagnosed in the absence of signs of spontaneous placental separation but with easy manual detachment of the placenta from the uterine wall. The presentation of placenta accreta is similar to that of placenta adherens, but without ease of manual detachment.

Treatment

Retained placenta with severe bleeding is an obstetric emergency, and immediate manual delivery of the placenta is attempted. In the absence of severe bleeding, obstetric providers may seek to manage the patient expectantly beyond 30 minutes according to the clinical picture and institution policy. Up to half of women with retained placentas at 60 minutes go on to expel the placenta spontaneously, although the risk for hemorrhage is considerable (van Stralen, Veenhof, Holleboom, & van Roosmalen, 2013).

Traction (pulling) on the cord is a common first intervention with retained placenta. Oxytocin or a prostaglandin F2-alpha, carboprost (Hemabate), is administered if traction is unsuccessful in delivering the placenta, to mitigate hemorrhage risk. Oxytocin can also facilitate contraction of an atonic uterus, thus shortening a prolonged latent phase and facilitating detachment of an adherent placenta. In the case of a placenta entrapped behind a closing cervix, nitroglycerin can help the cervix relax, thus allowing passage of the placenta. Nitroglycerin may cause hypotension, thus blood pressure should be carefully monitored (Abdel-Aleem, Abdel-Aleem, & Shaaban, 2015).

If cord traction and medication administration fail, manual extraction of the placenta is indicated. Manual extraction is painful, and the patient should have neuraxial or general anesthesia in place, or conscious sedation. A surgical setting is preferred to optimize aseptic technique and the team's ability to successfully manage an emergency. Because of the increased risk for endometritis, an antibiotic is often administered.

The patient is generally catheterized prior to manual extraction. After sedation has been achieved, the obstetric provider reaches a hand into the uterus via the vagina while the other hand grasps the fundus of the uterus through the abdominal wall. The provider applies force back and forth directly to the placenta until it detaches from the wall of the uterus. If a manual extraction is not possible due to a constricting cervix, the provider may order nitroglycerin to be administered, as described above, or attempt to extract the placenta using forceps with or without ultrasound guidance. Note that the forceps used for such a procedure are different from the forceps used in an operative vaginal delivery. Manual or instrumental attempts should stop, however, if a **morbidly adherent placenta (MAP)** is suspected.

In Chapter 1, Bess was suspected of having a retained placenta (as had occurred in her previous birth), which was believed to be causing her immediate postpartum hemorrhage. Her birth team performed a dilation and curettage to remove any placental fragments remaining, but they found none. She ended up having to undergo an emergency hysterectomy to stop her bleeding.

Morbidly Adherent Placenta

MAP is an umbrella term that refers to placenta accreta, placenta increta, and placenta percreta (Fig. 22.19). Each is defined by the degree to which the villi of the placenta extend beyond the decidua. Placenta accreta, the attachment of the villi of the placenta to the myometrium instead of just to the decidua, accounts for a majority of the cases of MAP. The term placenta increta refers to the penetration of the placenta into the myometrium, and in placenta percreta, the chorionic villi penetrate the myometrium and may even grow into the uterine serosa and surrounding tissue.

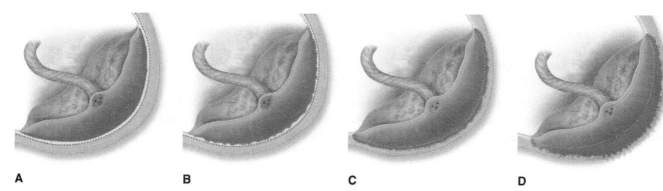

A   **B**   **C**   **D**

Figure 22.19. Classification of the placenta accreta spectrum. (A) Normal placentation. **(B)** Placenta accreta. **(C)** Placenta increta. **(D)** Placenta percreta. (Reprinted with permission from Stephenson, S. R. [2015]. *Obstetrics and Gynecology* [3rd ed., Fig. 18.12]. Philadelphia, PA: Lippincott Williams & Wilkins.)

Prevalence

MAPs were once rare, but their occurrence has increased from approximately 1 in 30,000 births to 1 in 700, a rise that has been attributed to the increase in the rate of cesarean delivery (Mehrabadi et al., 2015).

Etiology

The underlying cause for all three types of MAP appears to be defects in the decidua at the sight of implantation.

The largest risk factor for MAP is a placenta previa after a cesarean birth, with the risk increasing according to the number of cesarean deliveries. Other risks include cesarean delivery without subsequent previa (with the risk again increasing with the number of cesarean deliveries), previous uterine surgery, maternal age over 35 years, history of infertility, and pelvic radiation (Nageotte, 2014; Silver et al., 2015).

Prognosis

Because of the high risk for catastrophic bleeding, MAP is one of the most common reasons for an emergency hysterectomy in the immediate postpartum period (Mehrabadi et al., 2015). Other risks include the sequelae related to hemorrhage, including renal failure, disseminated intravascular coagulopathy, massive transfusion, and death. Nonhemorrhagic maternal risks include infection and uterine rupture.

Assessment

MAP is typically diagnosed by ultrasound antepartum. If a placenta previa is associated with the MAP, antepartum bleeding may be the first clinical sign. Otherwise, the first manifestation of MAP is hemorrhage resulting from the attempted manual extraction of the placenta.

Treatment

Because of the high risk for catastrophic bleeding, women diagnosed with MAP antepartum are delivered surgically, often from 34 to 36 weeks of gestation prior to the onset of contractions and rupture of membranes (D'Antonio et al., 2016). The preferred surgical procedure to minimize risk is a cesarean section immediately followed by a hysterectomy. Placenta percreta often invades the bladder, and a partial removal of the bladder (cystectomy) may also be necessary. Prior to delivery, the healthcare provider provides extensive patient counseling and obtains an informed consent. Optimally, an interprofessional team of physicians and nurses is assembled and a high-acuity setting is selected that is equipped to manage complications. Obstetric providers usually prefer to use general anesthesia rather than neuraxial anesthesia. Because of the potential for continued blood loss postpartum, women are often cared for in the intensive care unit postpartum.

Women who wish to preserve their fertility may instead opt for conservative management that allows her to retain her uterus. After the cesarean delivery of the neonate, the placenta is left in place and management protocols to minimize postpartum hemorrhage are initiated. The placenta is then reabsorbed, typically within three months, though subsequent surgical removal may be indicated. Many women still require a hysterectomy, however, and a majority have severe vaginal bleeding.

Because a majority of cases of MAP occur after a cesarean delivery of a prior pregnancy, MAP not detected by ultrasound but instead discovered at the time of delivery is often found during a repeat cesarean delivery. If the resources are not immediately available to manage this high-risk situation, surgery may be temporarily paused until either the necessary personnel and equipment can be gathered or the patient can be transferred. MAP identified at the time of a vaginal delivery cannot be removed manually as placenta adherens can, and an attempt to do so presents a high risk for life-threatening hemorrhage. Conversion to surgical management is required.

Care Considerations

Prior to surgery, the nurse places at least two large-bore IV lines in the patient in case a blood transfusion is required, which it is for most women with MAP (Shamshirsaz et al., 2015). The nurse also attaches pneumatic compression devices to the patient's legs to minimize the risk for postpartum venous thrombosis and places, for a majority of women, a urinary catheter.

Lacerations

Some trauma to the soft tissue is to be expected for all vaginal births. Some women may have only edema and ecchymosis, whereas others may have significant damage that requires considerable repair postpartum.

Types

Three common types of laceration that occur during vaginal birth are cervical, vaginal, and perineal.

Cervical Lacerations

Risks for cervical laceration include operative vaginal delivery, precipitous delivery, and a cerclage placed during pregnancy (Suzuki, 2015b). Although cervical lacerations are routinely assessed for in the immediate postpartum period, the first sign of a cervical laceration may be postpartum hemorrhage. A cervical laceration may be limited to the cervix or may extend into the vagina or lower uterine segment. Such damage is generally treated by surgical repair and rarely impacts future pregnancies or deliveries (Wong, Wilkes, Korgenski, Varner, & Manuck, 2016).

Perineal and Vaginal Lacerations

The perineum is the area between the vagina and the anus. Lacerations of this area are generally described as first, second, third, or fourth degree (ACOG, 2016a; Box 22.7, see Fig. 7.2). Vaginal lacerations may be deep or superficial. They may extend from perineal lacerations or occur independently. Lacerations high in the vaginal vault are associated with precipitous delivery, rapid fetal descent, and the use of forceps. Tears in the vaginal sidewall associated with third- and fourth-degree perineal lacerations represent a higher risk for injury to the pelvic floor that increase future risk for disorders of pelvic floor dysfunction, such as

Box 22.7 Perineal Lacerations

- First degree: No injury to the muscle; injury only to the skin and subcutaneous tissue of the perineum and vagina
- Second degree: Damage to the fascia and muscles of the perineum; no damage to the anal sphincter
- Third degree: As with a second-degree laceration, but additionally including damage to the external anal sphincter and possibly to the internal anal sphincter
- Fourth degree: As with a third-degree laceration, but additionally including damage to the rectal mucosa and the internal anal sphincter

incontinence and pelvic organ prolapse (Shek, Green, Hall, Guzman-Rojas, & Dietz, 2016).

In Chapter 8, Gracie had a second-degree perineal laceration following her vaginal delivery. (Hannah, in Chapter 7, experienced a first-degree perineal laceration, whereas Nancy, in Chapter 9, had a third-degree laceration, likely related to her infant's large size. Edie, in Chapter 11, experienced significant perineal lacerations and a perineal hematoma as a result of her precipitous labor and shoulder dystocia.)

Etiology

The greatest risk for damage comes from delivery that includes the use of vacuum or forceps. A longer second stage is also associated with an increased risk for severe lacerations, although the risk levels off after 3 hours. Fetal macrosomia and an OP position also increase the risk for laceration. Short maternal stature and increased maternal age also elevate risk (Simic, Cnattingius, Petersson, Sandstrom, & Stephansson, 2017). The use of an epidural, labor induction, and labor augmentation are also associated with an increased risk for severe lacerations (Pergialiotis et al., 2014). Obesity may be protective (Garretto et al., 2016).

Prognosis

Even in the absence of severe lacerations and repair, birth trauma can cause problems in the short and long term, including bowel and urinary dysfunction, pelvic organ prolapse, and sexual dysfunction.

Assessment

Immediately after all vaginal deliveries, the obstetric provider assesses the mother's perineum, vagina, cervix, and anus for bleeding and injury. This assessment should consist of both a visual assessment and a digital palpation, with special attention

paid to the anal sphincter. Injuries to the anal sphincter may go undetected without careful assessment and are a common cause of fecal incontinence postpartum.

Treatment

Although obstetric providers may repair a laceration prior to the birth of the placenta, they typically wait to do so until afterward to minimize disruption of the repair. During a repair, women are usually placed in the lithotomy position. Although a first- or second-degree laceration can usually be repaired in the delivery room, a third- or fourth-degree laceration repair may be moved to an operating room to optimize equipment, lighting, and aseptic technique. Although antibiotics are rarely given for first- and second-degree lacerations, a single dose of a broad-spectrum antibiotic is often given for more severe lacerations to minimize the risk of infection (Buppasiri, Lumbiganon, Thinkhamrop, & Thinkhamrop, 2014). The choice of anesthesia is based on the degree of injury, the requirement for relaxation for optimal repair, and the existence of a previously placed epidural. As with sutures placed during a cesarean delivery, suturing material is typically absorbable and does not need to be removed during a later procedure.

Care Considerations

To help prevent perineal lacerations, the nurse should inform women in their third trimester that perineal massage done in the 4 weeks prior to birth is associated with less need for surgical repair of lacerations postpartum (Beckmann & Stock, 2013). The nurse should explain to patients that they may perform perineal massage by moving two lubricated fingers back and forth along the posterior aspect of the vulva while applying gentle pressure toward the anus. During the second stage of labor, the nurse or another caregiver may apply warm compresses and/or massage to the perineum, which may also help minimize damage (ACOG, 2016a).

Perinatal Loss

The delivery of a fetus that has no signs of life is referred to as a **perinatal loss**, fetal demise, fetal death, stillbirth, or stillborn. Whenever possible, the term used by the mother and the partner of the pregnancy should be used. For the purposes of statistics, an intrauterine demise is referred to as a stillbirth either at or over 20 weeks of gestation or at or over 28 weeks of gestation, according to the custom of the reporting agency. Prior to this cutoff, the loss is referred to as a spontaneous abortion or miscarriage.

Prevalence

In the United States, the risk for stillbirth is approximately 6 out of every 1,000 pregnancies that reach 20 weeks. Half of these occur between 20 and 27 weeks gestation, primarily between 20 and 23 weeks (MacDorman & Gregory, 2015).

Etiology

The risk of stillbirth is higher for adolescent mothers and women over 35 years old, mothers of African descent, unmarried women, multiple gestations, and male fetuses. In developed countries such as the United States, common reasons for stillbirth include congenital anomalies, placental problems that cause intrauterine growth restriction, and maternal disease. Other causes include placental abruption, placenta previa, and cord prolapse. As many as half of stillbirths go unexplained (Aminu, Bar-Zeev, & van den Broek, 2017). Inadequate care in pregnancy, particularly during labor and delivery, may be a key factor in 10% to 60% of stillbirths (Flenady et al., 2011).

Prevention

Basic holistic strategies that promote a healthy pregnancy also reduce the risk for stillbirth. These strategies include the following (Bhutta et al., 2011):

- Taking folic acid prior to and during the pregnancy
- Routine syphilis screening and treatment
- Screening for and treatment of hypertensive disorders and maternal diabetes
- Screening for fetal growth restriction
- Close management of postterm pregnancies
- Care by skilled obstetric providers
- Access to emergency obstetric care

Antepartum monitoring with BPP and NST as well as other methods is designed to reduce stillbirth, as well as maternal monitoring for fetal movement may prevent perinatal loss. Approximately half of women report reduced fetal movement prior to stillbirth (Linde, Pettersson, & Radestad, 2015). As the rate of stillbirth goes up after 40 weeks of gestation, theoretically, induction at 40 weeks may reduce the rate of stillbirth.

The risk of stillbirth in future pregnancies is unclear. Women with a history of stillbirth often begin antepartum fetal testing 1 to 2 weeks prior to the gestational age at which the prior intrauterine demise occurred or by 32 to 34 weeks of gestation. Many obstetric providers may elect to deliver the pregnancy prior to the gestational age at which the previous demise occurred, particularly if it occurred prior to 39 weeks.

Care Considerations

After the loss of a pregnancy, the mother may experience such psychological consequences as anxiety, posttraumatic stress disorder, despair, loss of self-esteem, and depression (Mills et al., 2014). Parents who have experienced a stillbirth have identified the following as important aspects of care: support in grieving and in meeting and saying goodbye to the baby, receiving an explanation of events, organization of care, and care providers understanding the nature of grief (Saflund, Sjogren, & Wredling, 2004). Nurses should be respectful of cultural differences and of the fact that not all parents, not even parents of the same

stillbirth, grieve in the same way. Strategies to support families in their grief are itemized in Box 22.8.

Women and families experiencing a stillbirth usually want to know why it happened. Often that answer cannot be provided, although an autopsy and laboratory studies may be done. Common laboratory studies of the mother include urine toxicology, a complete blood count, fasting glucose, blood antibody screen to rule out alloimmunization, a Kleihauer–Betke test to assess for fetomaternal hemorrhage, and other testing indicated by the specific clinical picture and risk factors. An examination of the stillborn infant that includes bacterial cultures is standard. Genetic testing may also be indicated.

In the event of a stillbirth that occurs prior to and in the absence of labor, the timing of delivery must be decided. Labor starts spontaneously in most cases 1 to 2 weeks after fetal demise, and typically waiting this length of time is safe in the absence of maternal complications, although it poses a risk for developing coagulation abnormalities because of the release of thromboplastin from the placenta. Women may elect instead to be induced. A vaginal birth is usually preferred as it is typically safer than a cesarean birth with fewer risks for complications. Before 24 weeks of gestations, a dilation and evacuation may instead be selected.

At the time of the birth, the nurse and other healthcare providers should refer to the stillborn infant by its given name if one has been selected. If the reason for demise is obvious to the obstetric provider, he or she may communicate it to the family at this time. Some parents may elect to see and hold the infant, whereas others may decline. The nurse should respect and facilitate these choices.

Box 22.8 Guidelines for Supporting the Woman and Family After a Stillbirth

- Communicate warmly and genuinely.
- Avoid medical terminology; use clear lay language.
- Avoid delays in sharing information.
- Validate the emotions of the woman and family.
- Provide continuity of care when possible.
- Respect the individual needs of the mourners.
- Treat the stillborn infant with respect.
- Respect woman's preferences for seeing and/or holding the baby.
- Collect memorabilia, such as photographs and footprints.
- Refer the woman to support providers and organizations.
- Provide practical support about issues such as funeral arrangements and lactation.

Adapted from Lisy, K., Peters, M. D., Riitano, D., Jordan, Z., & Aromataris, E. (2016). Provision of meaningful care at diagnosis, birth, and after stillbirth: A qualitative synthesis of parents' experiences. *Birth, 43*(1), 6–19. doi:10.1111/birt.12217

It takes a team to manage care after a stillbirth. Social workers often help with funeral arrangements. Clergy, counselors, therapists, support groups, and psychologists may help process grief. Genetic counselors and pathologists may help provide a reason for the loss. Parents may consent to an autopsy or decline.

Women may choose to be cared for on the postpartum unit or elect for a unit that does not have healthy newborns. Stillborn infants are not issued birth certificates. They will instead be issued a Certificate of Fetal Death or a Certificate of Birth Resulting in Stillbirth. The nurse or other obstetric care provider may initiate regular contact by phone or office visits with the patient and family after discharge, which can be helpful in the first several weeks after the loss.

In Chapter 6, Rebecca experienced a fetal loss following a car accident and resulting placental abruption in her 38th week of gestation. She chose to see the body of her baby to help her process the reality of her loss.

Think Critically

1. In outline form, list the causes of dystocia according to the five Ps.
2. Explain the difference between hypertonic uterine contractions and tachysystole.
3. Shoulder dystocia has been diagnosed during a birth you are attending. As a nurse, what role do you anticipate playing with the initial interventions?
4. Explain why the mother's psyche is so critical to the success of a delivery. Brainstorm about what you, as a nurse, could do to optimize it.
5. What might make you suspect cord prolapse? What are your first actions?
6. Your patient requires an emergency cesarean section. How do you explain to her the procedure in a timely, therapeutic fashion?

References

Abdel-Aleem, H., Abdel-Aleem, M. A., & Shaaban, O. M. (2015). Nitroglycerin for management of retained placenta. *Cochrane Database of Systematic Reviews,* (11), CD007708. doi:10.1002/14651858.CD007708.pub3

Al-Zirqi, I., Stray-Pedersen, B., Forsen, L., Daltveit, A. K., & Vangen, S. (2016). Uterine rupture: Trends over 40 years. *British Journal of Obstetrics and Gynaecology, 123*(5), 780–787. doi:10.1111/1471-0528.13394

American College of Obstetricians and Gynecologists. (2015). ACOG practice bulletin no. 154: Operative vaginal delivery. *Obstetrics and Gynecology, 126*(5), e56–e65. doi:10.1097/AOG.0000000000001147

American College of Obstetricians and Gynecologists. (2016a). Practice bulletin no. 165 summary: Prevention and management of obstetric lacerations at vaginal delivery: Correction. *Obstetrics and Gynecology, 128*(2), 411. doi:10.1097/AOG.0000000000001578

American College of Obstetricians and Gynecologists. (2016b). Practice bulletin no. 173: Fetal macrosomia. *Obstetrics and Gynecology, 128*(5), e195–e209. doi:10.1097/AOG.0000000000001767

American College of Obstetricians and Gynecologists. (2017). Practice bulletin no. 184: Vaginal birth after cesarean delivery. *Obstetrics and Gynecology, 130*(5), e217–e233. doi:10.1097/AOG.0000000000002398

American College of Obstetricians and Gynecologists, & Society for Maternal-Fetal Medicine. (2014). Obstetric care consensus no. 1: Safe prevention of the primary cesarean delivery. *Obstetrics and Gynecology, 123*(3), 693–711. doi:10.1097/01.AOG.0000444441.04111.1d

Aminu, M., Bar-Zeev, S., & van den Broek, N. (2017). Cause of and factors associated with stillbirth: A systematic review of classification systems. *Acta Obstetricia et Gynecologica Scandinavica, 96*(5), 519–528. doi:10.1111/aogs.13126

Azad, M. B., Konya, T., Guttman, D. S., Field, C. J., Sears, M. R., HayGlass, K. T., . . . CHILD Study Investigators. (2015). Infant gut microbiota and food sensitization: Associations in the first year of life. *Clinical and Experimental Allergy, 45*(3), 632–643. doi:10.1111/cea.12487

Beckmann, M. M., & Stock, O. M. (2013). Antenatal perineal massage for reducing perineal trauma. *Cochrane Database of Systematic Reviews,* (4), CD005123. doi:10.1002/14651858.CD005123.pub3

Bhutta, Z. A., Yakoob, M. Y., Lawn, J. E., Rizvi, A., Friberg, I. K., Weissman, E., . . . Lancet's Stillbirths Series Steering Committee. (2011). Stillbirths: What difference can we make and at what cost? *The Lancet, 377*(9776), 1523–1538. doi:10.1016/S0140-6736(10)62269-6

Boyle, A., Reddy, U. M., Landy, H. J., Huang, C. C., Driggers, R. W., & Laughon, S. K. (2013). Primary cesarean delivery in the United States. *Obstetrics and Gynecology, 122*(1), 33–40. doi:10.1097/AOG.0b013e3182952242

Brigtsen, A. K., Jacobsen, A. F., Dedi, L., Melby, K. K., Fugelseth, D., & Whitelaw, A. (2015). Maternal colonization with group B streptococcus is associated with an increased rate of infants transferred to the neonatal intensive care unit. *Neonatology, 108*(3), 157–163. doi:10.1159/000434716

Buppasiri, P., Lumbiganon, P., Thinkhamrop, J., & Thinkhamrop, B. (2014). Antibiotic prophylaxis for third- and fourth-degree perineal tear during vaginal birth. *Cochrane Database of Systematic Reviews,* (10), CD005125. doi:10.1002/14651858.CD005125.pub4

Centers for Disease Control and Prevention. (2017). *ABCs report: Group B streptococcus, 2015.* Retrieved from https://www.cdc.gov/abcs/reports-findings/survreports/gbs15.html

Cho, C. E., & Norman, M. (2013). Cesarean section and development of the immune system in the offspring. *American Journal of Obstetrics and Gynecology, 208*(4), 249–254. doi:10.1016/j.ajog.2012.08.009

Clark, S. L. (2010). Amniotic fluid embolism. *Clinical Obstetrics and Gynecology, 53*(2), 322–328. doi:10.1097/GRF.0b013e3181e0ead2

Cluver, C., Gyte, G. M., Sinclair, M., Dowswell, T., & Hofmeyr, G. J. (2015). Interventions for helping to turn term breech babies to head first presentation when using external cephalic version. *Cochrane Database of Systematic Reviews,* (2), CD000184. doi:10.1002/14651858.CD000184.pub4

Cohen, W. R., & Friedman, E. A. (2015). Misguided guidelines for managing labor. *American Journal of Obstetrics and Gynecology, 212*(6), 753.e1–753.e3. doi:10.1016/j.ajog.2015.04.012

Coviello, E. M., Grantz, K. L., Huang, C. C., Kelly, T. E., & Landy, H. J. (2015). Risk factors for retained placenta. *American Journal of Obstetrics and Gynecology, 213*(6), 864.e1–864.e11. doi:10.1016/j.ajog.2015.07.039

Dahlke, J. D., Mendez-Figueroa, H., Rouse, D. J., Berghella, V., Baxter, J. K., & Chauhan, S. P. (2013). Evidence-based surgery for cesarean delivery: An updated systematic review. *American Journal of Obstetrics and Gynecology, 209*(4), 294–306. doi:10.1016/j.ajog.2013.02.043

D'Antonio, F., Palacios-Jaraquemada, J., Lim, P. S., Forlani, F., Lanzone, A., Timor-Tritsch, I., & Cali, G. (2016). Counseling in fetal medicine: Evidence-based answers to clinical questions on morbidly adherent placenta. *Ultrasound in Obstetrics and Gynecology, 47*(3), 290–301. doi:10.1002/uog.14950

de Hundt, M., Velzel, J., de Groot, C. J., Mol, B. W., & Kok, M. (2014). Mode of delivery after successful external cephalic version: A systematic review and meta-analysis. *Obstetrics and Gynecology, 123*(6), 1327–1334. doi:10.1097/AOG.0000000000000295

Desseauve, D., Bonifazi-Grenouilleau, M., Fritel, X., Lathelize, J., Sarreau, M., & Pierre, F. (2016). Fetal heart rate abnormalities associated with uterine rupture: A case-control study: A new time-lapse approach using a standardized classification. *European Journal of Obstetrics, Gynecology, and Reproductive Biology, 197*, 16–21. doi:10.1016/j.ejogrb.2015.10.019

Desseauve, D., Fradet, L., Lacouture, P., & Pierre, F. (2017). Position for labor and birth: State of knowledge and biomechanical perspectives. *European Journal of Obstetrics, Gynecology, and Reproductive Biology, 208*, 46–54. doi:10.1016/j.ejogrb.2016.11.006

Dodd, J. M., Crowther, C. A., Huertas, E., Guise, J. M., & Horey, D. (2013). Planned elective repeat caesarean section versus planned vaginal birth for women with a previous caesarean birth. *Cochrane Database of Systematic Reviews*, (12), CD004224. doi:10.1002/14651858.CD004224.pub3

Ebner, F., Friedl, T. W., Leinert, E., Schramm, A., Reister, F., Lato, K., . . . DeGregorio, N. (2016). Predictors for a successful external cephalic version: A single centre experience. *Archives of Gynecology and Obstetrics, 293*(4), 749–755. doi:10.1007/s00404-015-3902-z

Fitzpatrick, K. E., Tuffnell, D., Kurinczuk, J. J., & Knight, M. (2016). Incidence, risk factors, management and outcomes of amniotic-fluid embolism: A population-based cohort and nested case-control study. *British Journal of Obstetrics and Gynaecology, 123*(1), 100–109. doi:10.1111/1471-0528.13300

Flenady, V., Middleton, P., Smith, G. C., Duke, W., Erwich, J. J., Khong, T. Y., . . . Lancet's Stillbirths Series Steering Committee. (2011). Stillbirths: The way forward in high-income countries. *The Lancet, 377*(9778), 1703–1717. doi:10.1016/S0140-6736(11)60064-0

Frey, H. A., Stout, M. J., Odibo, A. O., Stamilio, D. M., Cahill, A. G., Roehl, K. A., & Macones, G. A. (2013). Risk of cesarean delivery after loop electrosurgical excision procedure. *Obstetrics and Gynecology, 121*(1), 39–45. doi:10.1097/AOG.0b013e318278f904

Friedman, A. M., Ananth, C. V., Prendergast, E., D'Alton, M. E., & Wright, J. D. (2015a). Evaluation of third-degree and fourth-degree laceration rates as quality indicators. *Obstetrics and Gynecology, 125*(4), 927–937. doi:10.1097/AOG.0000000000000720

Friedman, A. M., Ananth, C. V., Prendergast, E., D'Alton, M. E., & Wright, J. D. (2015b). Variation in and factors associated with use of episiotomy. *JAMA, 313*(2), 197–199. doi:10.1001/jama.2014.14774

Friedman, E. (1954). The graphic analysis of labor. *American Journal of Obstetrics and Gynecology, 68*(6), 1568–1575.

Fruscalzo, A., Londero, A. P., Salvador, S., Bertozzi, S., Biasioli, A., Della Martina, M., . . . Marchesoni, D. (2014). New and old predictive factors for breech presentation: Our experience in 14,433 singleton pregnancies and a literature review. *Journal of Maternal-Fetal and Neonatal Medicine, 27*(2), 167–172. doi:10.3109/14767058.2013.806891

Gardberg, M., Leonova, Y., & Laakkonen, E. (2011). Malpresentations—Impact on mode of delivery. *Acta Obstetricia et Gynecologica Scandinavica, 90*(5), 540–542. doi:10.1111/j.1600-0412.2011.01105.x

Garretto, D., Lin, B. B., Syn, H. L., Judge, N., Beckerman, K., Atallah, F., . . . Bernstein, P. S. (2016). Obesity may be protective against severe perineal lacerations. *Journal of Obesity, 2016*, 9376592. doi:10.1155/2016/9376592

Ghi, T., Youssef, A., Martelli, F., Bellussi, F., Aiello, E., Pilu, G., . . . Rizzo, G. (2016). Narrow subpubic arch angle is associated with higher risk of persistent occiput posterior position at delivery. *Ultrasound in Obstetrics and Gynecology, 48*(4), 511–515. doi:10.1002/uog.15808

Ghidini, A., Stewart, D., Pezzullo, J. C., & Locatelli, A. (2017). Neonatal complications in vacuum-assisted vaginal delivery: Are they associated with number of pulls, cup detachments, and duration of vacuum application? *Archives of Gynecology and Obstetrics, 295*(1), 67–73. doi:10.1007/s00404-016-4206-7

Gibbons, C., O'Herlihy, C., & Murphy, J. F. (2014). Umbilical cord prolapse—Changing patterns and improved outcomes: A retrospective cohort study. *British Journal of Obstetrics and Gynaecology, 121*(13), 1705–1708. doi:10.1111/1471-0528.12890

Grantz, K. L., Gonzalez-Quintero, V., Troendle, J., Reddy, U. M., Hinkle, S. N., Kominiarek, M. A., . . . Zhang, J. (2015). Labor patterns in women attempting vaginal birth after cesarean with normal neonatal outcomes. *American Journal of Obstetrics and Gynecology, 213*(2), 226.e1–226.e6. doi:10.1016/j.ajog.2015.04.033

Grootscholten, K., Kok, M., Oei, S. G., Mol, B. W., & van der Post, J. A. (2008). External cephalic version-related risks: A meta-analysis. *Obstetrics and Gynecology, 112*(5), 1143–1151. doi:10.1097/AOG.0b013e31818b4ade

Guise, J. M., Denman, M. A., Emeis, C., Marshall, N., Walker, M., Fu, R., . . . McDonagh, M. (2010). Vaginal birth after cesarean: New insights on maternal and neonatal outcomes. *Obstetrics and Gynecology, 115*(6), 1267–1278. doi:10.1097/AOG.0b013e3181df925f

Gupta, J. K., Sood, A., Hofmeyr, G. J., & Vogel, J. P. (2017). Position in the second stage of labour for women without epidural anaesthesia. *Cochrane Database of Systematic Reviews, 5*, CD002006. doi:10.1002/14651858.CD002006.pub4

Haas, D. M., Morgan, S., & Contreras, K. (2014). Vaginal preparation with antiseptic solution before cesarean section for preventing postoperative infections. *Cochrane Database of Systematic Reviews*, (12), CD007892. doi:10.1002/14651858.CD007892.pub5

Hodnett, E. D., Gates, S., Hofmeyr, G. J., & Sakala, C. (2013). Continuous support for women during childbirth. *Cochrane Database of Systematic Reviews, 7*, CD003766. doi:10.1002/14651858.CD003766.pub5

Hofmeyr, G. J., Kulier, R., & West, H. M. (2015). External cephalic version for breech presentation at term. *Cochrane Database of Systematic Reviews*, (4), CD000083. doi:10.1002/14651858.CD000083.pub3

Hofmeyr, G. J., Vogel, J. P., Cuthbert, A., & Singata, M. (2017). Fundal pressure during the second stage of labour. *Cochrane Database of Systematic Reviews, 3*, CD006067. doi:10.1002/14651858.CD006067.pub3

Holbrook, B. D., & Phelan, S. T. (2013). Umbilical cord prolapse. *Obstetrics and Gynecology Clinics of North America, 40*(1), 1–14. doi:10.1016/j.ogc.2012.11.002

Hsu, Y. Y., Hung, H. Y., Chang, S. C., & Chang, Y. J. (2013). Early oral intake and gastrointestinal function after cesarean delivery: A systematic review and meta-analysis. *Obstetrics and Gynecology, 121*(6), 1327–1334. doi:10.1097/AOG.0b013e318293698c

John, C. O., Orazulike, N., & Alegbeleye, J. (2015). An appraisal of retained placenta at the University of Port Harcourt teaching hospital: A five-year review. *Nigerian Journal of Medicine, 24*(2), 99–102.

Kominiarek, M. A., Zhang, J., Vanveldhuisen, P., Troendle, J., Beaver, J., & Hibbard, J. U. (2011). Contemporary labor patterns: The impact of maternal body mass index. *American Journal of Obstetrics and Gynecology, 205*(3), 244. e1–244.e8. doi:10.1016/j.ajog.2011.06.014

Landon, M. B., Leindecker, S., Spong, C. Y., Hauth, J. C., Bloom, S., Varner, M. W., . . . Human Development Maternal-Fetal Medicine Units Network. (2005). The MFMU cesarean registry: Factors affecting the success of trial of labor after previous cesarean delivery. *American Journal of Obstetrics and Gynecology, 193*(3 Pt. 2), 1016–1023. doi:10.1016/j.ajog.2005.05.066

Le Ray, C., Deneux-Tharaux, C., Khireddine, I., Dreyfus, M., Vardon, D., & Goffinet, F. (2013). Manual rotation to decrease operative delivery in posterior or transverse positions. *Obstetrics and Gynecology, 122*(3), 634–640. doi:10.1097/AOG.0b013e3182a10e43

Le Ray, C., Lepleux, F., De La Calle, A., Guerin, J., Sellam, N., Dreyfus, M., & Chantry, A. A. (2016). Lateral asymmetric decubitus position for the rotation of occipito-posterior positions: Multicenter randomized controlled trial EVADELA. *American Journal of Obstetrics and Gynecology, 215*(4), 511. e1–511.e7. doi:10.1016/j.ajog.2016.05.033

Lemos, A., Amorim, M. M., Dornelas de Andrade, A., de Souza, A. I., Cabral Filho, J. E., & Correia, J. B. (2017). Pushing/bearing down methods for the second stage of labour. *Cochrane Database of Systematic Reviews, 3*, CD009124. doi:10.1002/14651858.CD009124.pub3

Linde, A., Pettersson, K., & Radestad, I. (2015). Women's experiences of fetal movements before the confirmation of fetal death—Contractions misinterpreted as fetal movement. *Birth, 42*(2), 189–194. doi:10.1111/birt.12151

Lydon-Rochelle, M., Holt, V. L., Easterling, T. R., & Martin, D. P. (2001). Risk of uterine rupture during labor among women with a prior cesarean delivery. *New England Journal of Medicine, 345*(1), 3–8. doi:10.1056/NEJM200107053450101

MacDorman, M. F., & Gregory, E. C. (2015). Fetal and perinatal mortality: United States, 2013. *National Vital Statistics Reports, 64*(8), 1–24.

Mackeen, A. D., Fehnel, E., Berghella, V., & Klein, T. (2014). Morphine sleep in pregnancy. *American Journal of Perinatology, 31*(1), 85–90. doi:10.1055/s-0033-1334448

Maher, M. D., & Heavey, E. (2015). When the cord comes first: Umbilical cord prolapse. *Nursing, 45*(7), 53–56. doi:10.1097/01.NURSE.0000466449.65548.4a

Makvandi, S., Latifnejad Roudsari, R., Sadeghi, R., & Karimi, L. (2015). Effect of birth ball on labor pain relief: A systematic review and meta-analysis. *Journal of Obstetrics and Gynaecology, 41*(11), 1679–1686. doi:10.1111/jog.12802

Martin, J. A., Hamilton, B. E., Osterman, M. J., Driscoll, A. K., & Mathews, T. J. (2017). Births: Final data for 2015. *National Vital Statistics Reports, 66*(1), 1.

Mehrabadi, A., Hutcheon, J. A., Liu, S., Bartholomew, S., Kramer, M. S., Liston, R. M., . . . Maternal Health Study Group of Canadian Perinatal Surveillance System. (2015). Contribution of placenta accreta to the incidence of postpartum hemorrhage and severe postpartum hemorrhage. *Obstetrics and Gynecology, 125*(4), 814–821. doi:10.1097/AOG.0000000000000722

Metz, T. D., Allshouse, A. A., Faucett, A. M., & Grobman, W. A. (2015). Validation of a vaginal birth after cesarean delivery prediction model in women with two prior cesarean deliveries. *Obstetrics and Gynecology, 125*(4), 948–952. doi:10.1097/AOG.0000000000000744

Miller, C. M., Cohn, S., Akdagli, S., Carvalho, B., Blumenfeld, Y. J., & Butwick, A. J. (2017). Postpartum hemorrhage following vaginal delivery: Risk factors and maternal outcomes. *Journal of Perinatology, 37*(3), 243–248. doi:10.1038/jp.2016.225

Mills, T. A., Ricklesford, C., Cooke, A., Heazell, A. E., Whitworth, M., & Lavender, T. (2014). Parents' experiences and expectations of care in pregnancy after stillbirth or neonatal death: A metasynthesis. *British Journal of Obstetrics and Gynaecology, 121*(8), 943–950. doi:10.1111/1471-0528.12656

Mueller, N. T., Whyatt, R., Hoepner, L., Oberfield, S., Dominguez-Bello, M. G., Widen, E. M., . . . Rundle, A. (2015). Prenatal exposure to antibiotics, cesarean section and risk of childhood obesity. *International Journal of Obesity, 39*(4), 665–670. doi:10.1038/ijo.2014.180

Muhleman, M. A., Aly, I., Walters, A., Topale, N., Tubbs, R. S., & Loukas, M. (2017). To cut or not to cut, that is the question: A review of the anatomy, the technique, risks, and benefits of an episiotomy. *Clinical Anatomy, 30*(3), 362–372. doi:10.1002/ca.22836

Nageotte, M. P. (2014). Always be vigilant for placenta accreta. *American Journal of Obstetrics and Gynecology, 211*(2), 87–88. doi:10.1016/j.ajog.2014.04.037

National Institutes of Health. (2010). National Institutes of Health Consensus Development conference statement: Vaginal birth after cesarean: New insights March 8–10, 2010. *Obstetrics and Gynecology, 115*(6), 1279–1295. doi:10.1097/AOG.0b013e3181e459e5

National Partnership for Women and Families. (2016). *Why is the U.S. cesarean section rate so high?* Retrieved from http://www.nationalpartnership.org/research-library/maternal-health/why-is-the-c-section-rate-so-high.pdf

O'Mahony, F., Hofmeyr, G. J., & Menon, V. (2010). Choice of instruments for assisted vaginal delivery. *Cochrane Database of Systematic Reviews,* (11), CD005455. doi:10.1002/14651858.CD005455.pub2

Pattinson, R. C., Cuthbert, A., & Vannevel, V. (2017). Pelvimetry for fetal cephalic presentations at or near term for deciding on mode of delivery. *Cochrane Database of Systematic Reviews, 3,* CD000161. doi:10.1002/14651858.CD000161.pub2

Pergialiotis, V., Vlachos, D., Protopapas, A., Pappa, K., & Vlachos, G. (2014). Risk factors for severe perineal lacerations during childbirth. *International Journal of Gynecology and Obstetrics, 125*(1), 6–14. doi:10.1016/j.ijgo.2013.09.034

Regan, J., Keup, C., Wolfe, K., Snyder, C., & DeFranco, E. (2015). Vaginal birth after cesarean success in high-risk women: A population-based study. *Journal of Perinatology, 35*(4), 252–257. doi:10.1038/jp.2014.196

Roth, C., Dent, S. A., Parfitt, S. E., Hering, S. L., & Bay, R. C. (2016). Randomized controlled trial of use of the peanut ball during labor. *MCN. The American Journal of Maternal Child Nursing, 41*(3), 140–146. doi:10.1097/NMC.0000000000000232

Sabol, B., Denman, M. A., & Guise, J. M. (2015). Vaginal birth after cesarean: An effective method to reduce cesarean. *Clinical Obstetrics and Gynecology, 58*(2), 309–319. doi:10.1097/GRF.0000000000000101

Saflund, K., Sjogren, B., & Wredling, R. (2004). The role of caregivers after a stillbirth: Views and experiences of parents. *Birth, 31*(2), 132–137. doi:10.1111/j.0730-7659.2004.00291.x

Sagi-Dain, L., & Sagi, S. (2015). The role of episiotomy in prevention and management of shoulder dystocia: A systematic review. *Obstetrical and Gynecological Survey, 70*(5), 354–362. doi:10.1097/OGX.0000000000000179

Sandstrom, A., Altman, M., Cnattingius, S., Johansson, S., Ahlberg, M., & Stephansson, O. (2017). Durations of second stage of labor and pushing, and adverse neonatal outcomes: A population-based cohort study. *Journal of Perinatology, 37*(3), 236–242. doi:10.1038/jp.2016.214

Shamshirsaz, A. A., Fox, K. A., Salmanian, B., Diaz-Arrastia, C. R., Lee, W., Baker, B. W., . . . Belfort, M. A. (2015). Maternal morbidity in patients with morbidly adherent placenta treated with and without a standardized multidisciplinary approach. *American Journal of Obstetrics and Gynecology, 212*(2), 218.e1–218.e9. doi:10.1016/j.ajog.2014.08.019

Shek, K. L., Green, K., Hall, J., Guzman-Rojas, R., & Dietz, H. P. (2016). Perineal and vaginal tears are clinical markers for occult levator ani trauma: A retrospective observational study. *Ultrasound in Obstetrics and Gynecology, 47*(2), 224–227. doi:10.1002/uog.14856

Shen, F., Wang, L., Yang, W., & Chen, Y. (2016). From appearance to essence: 10 years review of atypical amniotic fluid embolism. *Archives of Gynecology and Obstetrics, 293*(2), 329–334. doi:10.1007/s00404-015-3785-z

Silver, R. M., Fox, K. A., Barton, J. R., Abuhamad, A. Z., Simhan, H., Huls, C. K., . . . Wright, J. D. (2015). Center of excellence for placenta accreta. *American Journal of Obstetrics and Gynecology, 212*(5), 561–568. doi:10.1016/j.ajog.2014.11.018

Simic, M., Cnattingius, S., Petersson, G., Sandstrom, A., & Stephansson, O. (2017). Duration of second stage of labor and instrumental delivery as risk factors for severe perineal lacerations: Population-based study. *BMC Pregnancy and Childbirth, 17*(1), 72. doi:10.1186/s12884-017-1251-6

Simpson, C. N., Chambers, C. N., Sharshiner, R., & Caughey, A. B. (2015). Effects of persistent occiput posterior position on mode of delivery. *Obstetrics and Gynecology, 125*(2015), 82S–83S.

Smaill, F. M., & Grivell, R. M. (2014). Antibiotic prophylaxis versus no prophylaxis for preventing infection after cesarean section. *Cochrane Database of Systematic Reviews,* (10), CD007482. doi:10.1002/14651858.CD007482.pub3

Smyth, R. M., Markham, C., & Dowswell, T. (2013). Amniotomy for shortening spontaneous labour. *Cochrane Database of Systematic Reviews,* (6), CD006167. doi:10.1002/14651858.CD006167.pub4

Society for Maternal-Fetal Medicine. (2016). Practice bulletin no. 169: Multifetal gestations: Twin, triplet, and higher-order multifetal pregnancies. *Obstetrics and Gynecology, 128*(4), e131–e146. doi:10.1097/AOG.0000000000001709

Spong, C. Y., Berghella, V., Wenstrom, K. D., Mercer, B. M., & Saade, G. R. (2012). Preventing the first cesarean delivery: Summary of a joint Eunice Kennedy Shriver National Institute of Child Health and Human Development, Society for Maternal-Fetal Medicine, and American College of Obstetricians and Gynecologists Workshop. *Obstetrics and Gynecology, 120*(5), 1181–1193. doi:10.1097/AOG.0b013e3182704880

Spong, C. Y., Berghella, V., Wenstrom, K. D., Mercer, B. M., & Saade, G. R. (2013). Preventing the first cesarean delivery: Summary of a joint Eunice Kennedy Shriver National Institute of Child Health and Human Development, Society for Maternal-Fetal Medicine, and American College of Obstetricians and Gynecologists workshop. In reply. *Obstetrics and Gynecology, 121*(3), 687. doi:10.1097/AOG.0b013e3182854b36

Stephansson, O., Sandstrom, A., Petersson, G., Wikstrom, A. K., & Cnattingius, S. (2016). Prolonged second stage of labour, maternal infectious disease, urinary retention and other complications in the early postpartum period. *British Journal of Obstetrics and Gynaecology, 123*(4), 608–616. doi:10.1111/1471-0528.13287

Suzuki, S. (2015a). Clinical significance of precipitous labor. *Journal of Clinical Medicine Research, 7*(3), 150–153. doi:10.14740/jocmr2058w

Suzuki, S. (2015b). Risk of intrapartum cervical lacerations in vaginal singleton deliveries in women with cerclage. *Journal of Clinical Medicine Research, 7*(9), 714–716. doi:10.14740/jocmr2227w

Tana, K. V., Rachel I. V., Kamalini, D. (2017). Risk factors for shoulder dystocia at a community-based hospital. *Obstetrics and Gynecology, PDF Only.*

Tapisiz, O. L., Aytan, H., Altinbas, S. K., Arman, F., Tuncay, G., Besli, M., . . . Danisman, N. (2014). Face presentation at term: A forgotten issue. *Journal of Obstetrics and Gynaecology, 40*(6), 1573–1577. doi:10.1111/jog.12369

Tinelli, A., Di Renzo, G. C., & Malvasi, A. (2015). The intrapartum ultrasonographic detection of the Bandl ring as a marker of dystocia. *International Journal of Gynaecology and Obstetrics, 131*(3), 310–311. doi:10.1016/j.ijgo.2015.06.030

Tolcher, M. C., Johnson, R. L., El-Nashar, S. A., & West, C. P. (2014). Decision-to-incision time and neonatal outcomes: A systematic review and meta-analysis. *Obstetrics and Gynecology, 123*(3), 536–548. doi:10.1097/AOG.0000000000000132

Truven Health Analytics. (2013). *The cost of having a baby in the United States.* http://transform.childbirthconnection.org/wp-content/uploads/2013/01/Cost-of-Having-a-Baby1.pdf.

Tuncalp, O., Souza, J. P., Gulmezoglu, M., & World Health Organization. (2013). New WHO recommendations on prevention and treatment of postpartum hemorrhage. *International Journal of Gynaecology and Obstetrics, 123*(3), 254–256. doi:10.1016/j.ijgo.2013.06.024

Tussey, C. M., Botsios, E., Gerkin, R. D., Kelly, L. A., Gamez, J., & Mensik, J. (2015). Reducing length of labor and cesarean surgery rate using a peanut ball for women laboring with an epidural. *Journal of Perinatal Education, 24*(1), 16–24. doi:10.1891/1058-1243.24.1.16

Uddin, S. F., & Simon, A. E. (2013). Rates and success rates of trial of labor after cesarean delivery in the United States, 1990–2009. *Maternal and Child Health Journal, 17*(7), 1309–1314. doi:10.1007/s10995-012-1132-6

van Stralen, G., Veenhof, M., Holleboom, C., & van Roosmalen, J. (2013). No reduction of manual removal after misoprostol for retained placenta: A double-blind, randomized trial. *Acta Obstetricia et Gynecologica Scandinavica, 92*(4), 398–403. doi:10.1111/aogs.12065

Vitner, D., Paltieli, Y., Haberman, S., Gonen, R., Ville, Y., & Nizard, J. (2015). Prospective multicenter study of ultrasound-based measurements of fetal head station and position throughout labor. *Ultrasound in Obstetrics and Gynecology, 46*(5), 611–615. doi:10.1002/uog.14821

Wei, S., Wo, B. L., Qi, H. P., Xu, H., Luo, Z. C., Roy, C., & Fraser, W. D. (2013). Early amniotomy and early oxytocin for prevention of, or therapy for, delay in first stage spontaneous labour compared with routine care. *Cochrane Database of Systematic Reviews,* (8), CD006794. doi:10.1002/14651858.CD006794.pub4

Wong, L. F., Wilkes, J., Korgenski, K., Varner, M. W., & Manuck, T. A. (2016). Intrapartum cervical laceration and subsequent pregnancy outcomes. *AJP Reports, 6*(3), e318–e323. doi:10.1055/s-0036-1592198

Zhang, J., Landy, H. J., Branch, D. W., Burkman, R., Haberman, S., Gregory, K. D., . . . Consortium on Safe Labor. (2010). Contemporary patterns of spontaneous labor with normal neonatal outcomes. *Obstetrics and Gynecology, 116*(6), 1281–1287. doi:10.1097/AOG.0b013e3181fdef6e

Zhu, B. P., Grigorescu, V., Le, T., Lin, M., Copeland, G., Barone, M., & Turabelidze, G. (2006). Labor dystocia and its association with interpregnancy interval. *American Journal of Obstetrics and Gynecology, 195*(1), 121–128. doi:10.1016/j.ajog.2005.12.016

Suggested Readings

DONA International. Retrieved from https://www.dona.org/

Simpson, K. R., & Lyndon, A. L. (2017). Consequences of delayed, unfinished, or missed nursing care during labor and birth. *Journal of Perinatal and Neonatal Nursing, 31*(1), 32–40.

Stone, S., Prater, L., & Spencer, R. (2014). Facilitating skin-to-skin contact in the operating room after cesarean birth. *Nursing for Women's Health, 18*(6), 486–499. doi:10.1111/1751-486X.12161

Sundin, C. S., & Mazac, L. B. (2017). Amniotic fluid embolism. *MCN, the American Journal of Maternal Child Nursing, 42*(1), 29–35. doi:10.1097/NMC.0000000000000292

23 Conditions Occurring After Delivery

Objectives

1. Correlate the Maternal Early Warning Criteria established by the National Partnership for Maternal Safety with postpartum conditions and their causes.
2. Identify the causes of and assessments for postpartum hemorrhage.
3. Discuss the signs and implications of hypovolemic shock, as well as the treatment and nursing care considerations for this condition.
4. Discuss the different types of thromboembolism that occur in the postpartum period and their manifestation, assessment, treatment, and care considerations.
5. Distinguish the causes and clinical manifestations of various types of infection postpartum.
6. Identify and compare the different postpartum mood disorders.

Key Terms

Atony
Coagulopathy
Endometritis
Episiotomy
Hematoma
Hypovolemic shock
Immune thrombocytopenic purpura (ITP)
Mastitis
Postpartum angiopathy

Postpartum blues
Postpartum depression
Postpartum hemorrhage (PPH)
Postpartum psychosis
Pyelonephritis
Subinvolution
Tamponade
Uterine inversion
von Willebrand disease (VWD)

Patients often think of the postpartum period as low risk, the time of healing after an altered state of health. Nurses should remember, however, that the postpartum period is still a time of altered health and that vigilance and attentive care is critical. Many of the pregnancy-related complications we have considered in previous chapters—such as preeclampsia, eclampsia, and HELLP syndrome—may also occur in the postpartum period. This chapter, however, focuses on conditions that more commonly occur during the postpartum period, such as hemorrhage.

In 2014, the National Partnership for Maternal Safety proposed criteria to help clinicians recognize postpartum early warning signs of hemorrhage, sepsis, hypertensive crisis, venous thromboembolisms, and heart failure (Box 23.1). These criteria are nonspecific but serve as helpful guidelines for nurses serving postpartum patients.

Postpartum Hemorrhage

Typical blood loss after a vaginal birth is 500 mL and after a cesarean birth is 1,000 mL. Blood loss over these values is considered postpartum hemorrhage (PPH). Nurses should be aware, however, that it is often difficult to accurately estimate the volume of blood lost, and blood loss may be hidden. Blood loss over 1,000 mL

Box 23.1   Maternal Early Warning Criteria

- Maternal agitation, confusion, or unresponsiveness
- Report of headache or shortness of breath by a patient with preeclampsia
- Systolic blood pressure <90 or >160 mm Hg
- Diastolic blood pressure > 100 mm Hg
- Heart rate <50 or >120 beats/min
- Respiratory rate <10 or >30 breaths/min
- Oxygen saturation on room air at sea level < 95%
- Oliguria for 2 or more h (<35 mL/h)

Adapted from Maguire, P. J., Power, K. A., & Turner, M. J. (2015). The maternal early warning criteria: A proposal from the National Partnership for Maternal Safety. *Obstetrics and Gynecology, 125*(2), 493–494. doi:10.1097/AOG.0000000000000660

may be classified as major and blood loss and over 2,000 mL is severe (British Journal of Obstetrics and Gynaecology, 2017). An alternate definition of PPH provides a time constraint of 24 hours of bleeding equaling more than 1,000 mL that persists despite the use of uterine massage and first-line uterotonics, such as oxytocin (The Pharmacy 23.1; Abdul-Kadir et al., 2014).

Primary or early PPH occurs within 24 hours after the birth. Delayed or secondary PPH may occur from 24 hours to 12 weeks after delivery but occurs most often within 1 to 2 weeks postpartum (Dossou, Debost-Legrand, Dechelotte, Lemery, & Vendittelli, 2015).

Prevalence

PPH occurs after approximately 3% of births in the United States (Marshall et al., 2017).

Etiology

In late pregnancy, just prior to delivery, the blood flow through the uterine artery accounts for 15% of the mother's cardiac output. After the birth of the placenta, the body normally maintains hemostasis and prevents PPH by clotting and by contraction of the myometrium of the uterus, which compresses the open blood vessels that feed the placental site. Problems with the ability of the uterus to adequately contract (as in uterine atony), or blood to clot (as in coagulopathies), or both lead to most cases of PPH (Fig. 23.1). A third cause of PPH is trauma, such as from lacerations or uterine inversion. Atony is by far the single most common cause of PPH.

Uterine Atony

Atony is failure of the uterus to sufficiently contract, thus allowing blood to seep from the site of placental implantation. In particular, uterine atony related to either infection or retained placenta or fetal membranes is the most common cause of secondary PPH. PPH resulting from atony is initially treated with firm massage of the uterus and the administration of uterotonics. It is associated with circumstances that cause greater distention of the uterus,

such as polyhydramnios, multiple pregnancies, and macrosomia (Box 23.2). Contractions that result in a prolonged or rapid labor with or without oxytocin for induction or augmentation are also a risk factor for atony. Certain medications, including magnesium sulfate (which relaxes the uterus) and some anesthesia, also contribute to risk. The related concept of subinvolution is sometimes, incorrectly, used interchangeably with atony. Subinvolution is the failure of the uterus to involute (shrink) at the anticipated rate. Atony refers to the failure of the uterine muscle to contract sufficiently to control uterine bleeding. While the term atony is specific to the muscle of the uterus, subinvolution refers to uterus as a whole.

In Chapter 2, Tati experienced late PPH because of uterine atony. The nurses on her floor worked as a team to correct the bleeding. The atony was corrected with a combination of uterine massage and methylergonovine maleate. Because her obstetric provider thought the atony might be caused by endometritis, Tati was put on an antibiotic.

Coagulopathies

A more rare cause of PPH is a **coagulopathy**, a disorder in which the blood's ability to clot is impaired. A coagulopathy may lead to PPH and, in turn, PPH results in a loss of clotting factors, thus limiting the body's ability to stop the bleeding. Coagulopathies are diagnosed by laboratory assessment and may be congenital or acquired and include immune thrombocytopenic purpura, VWD, and disseminated intravascular coagulation (DIC). See Chapter 21 for information on DIC.

von Willebrand Disease

von Willebrand Disease (VWD) is the most common inherited bleeding disorder. Its presentation is variable, however, and although up to 1.3% of the population carries the genetic tendency, the prevalence of VWD is approximately 1 in every 10,000 people (Leebeek & Eikenboom, 2016). The hallmark of VWD is a deficiency in the amount of von Willebrand factor (VWF) or in its action. When functioning correctly, VWF has a role in binding platelets to endothelial components and in fibrin clot formation. There are several different forms of VWD. Initial screening tests for the condition assess for the presence of VWF antigen, VWF activity, and factor VIII activity. Extended testing can help identify the specific etiology of the condition.

The clinical features of symptomatic VWD include bleeding from the skin, easy bruising, and extended mucosal bleeding. Women with VWD typically have a history of heavy menses. Ingesting aspirin or nonsteroidal anti-inflammatory drugs (NSAIDs) may provoke symptoms. A family history of abnormal or prolonged bleeding is common in patients with VWD, although patients with acquired VWD typically have no personal or family history. Heavy postpartum bleeding may be of acute early onset or delayed onset and may persistent for up to 3 weeks postpartum.

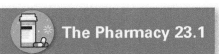

The Pharmacy 23.1 — Uterotonics for Uterine Atony and Postpartum Hemorrhage

Medication	Route and Dosing	Side Effects	Contraindications
General Medications			
Oxytocin	• 10–40 U IV in 500 mL–1 L normal saline at rate sufficient to control atony • 10 U IM	• Occasional nausea and vomiting • Rarely, water intoxication	None for postpartum hemorrhage
Tranexamic acid	1 g infused over 10–20 min	• Nausea • Vomiting • Diarrhea • Hypotension	Disseminated intravascular coagulation
15-Methylprostaglandin F_{2alpha}	• 0.25 mg IM every 15–90 min up to 8 doses • 500 µg IM up to 3 mg • 0.5 mg injected into the myometrium (uterine muscle)	• Nausea • Vomiting • Diarrhea • Headache • Fever • Chills • Tachycardia • Hypertension	• Asthma • Hypertension
Misoprostol	800–1,000 µg rectally	• Nausea • Vomiting • Diarrhea • Headache • Fever • Chills	N/A
Dinoprostone	20 mg vaginally or rectally every 2 h	• Nausea • Vomiting • Diarrhea • Headache • Fever • Chills	Caution with asthma, hypotension, or hypertension
Recombinant human factor VIIa	50–100 µg/kg every 2 h	• Fever • Headache • Joint pain • Hypertension • Hypotension • Nausea • Vomiting	N/A
Ergots			
Methylergonovine Ergometrine Ergonovine	0.2 mg IM every 2–4 h 0.5 mg IV or IM every 2 h 0.25 mg IM or IV every 2 h	• Nausea • Vomiting • Headache • Hypotension • Hypertension	Caution: Ergots should not be given to patients with cardiovascular disease or hypertension.

IV, intravenous; IM, intramuscular; N/A, not applicable.

In the case of PPH, the prolonged bleeding would be from the endometrium or from the site of a laceration or an **episiotomy**. Approximately 44% of women with VWD experience primary PPH (Govorov et al., 2016).

The treatment of VWD depends on the cause of the disease, with different etiology types responding to different treatments. The six medication categories commonly used to treat VWD include replacement therapy with VWF-containing concentrates, antifibrinolytic drugs such as tranexamic acid (particularly for bleeding from mucus membranes), topical therapy with thrombin or fibrin sealant at the site of a wound (usually used for nasal or oral bleeding), recombinant human factor VIIa, estrogen for some women, and, most commonly, desmopressin.

Desmopressin promotes the release of VWF from cell storage sites and is given intravenously (IV) or via a nasal spray. Dosing may be repeated at 12 and 24 hours. It should not be given in

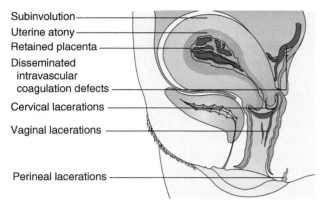

Subinvolution
Uterine atony
Retained placenta
Disseminated intravascular coagulation defects
Cervical lacerations
Vaginal lacerations
Perineal lacerations

Figure 23.1. Causes of postpartum hemorrhage. (Reprinted with permission from Willis, L. M. [Ed.]. [2017]. *Health assessment made incredibly visual* [3rd ed., unnumbered figure in Chapter 12]. Philadelphia, PA: Lippincott Williams & Wilkins.)

conjunction with antifibrinolytic agents. Patients taking desmopressin are more subject to hyponatremia if they take in excess fluids, and the medication may be less effective with successive doses (tachyphylaxis). Common side effects include facial flushing, headache, and nausea.

Immune Thrombocytopenic Purpura

Immune thrombocytopenic purpura (ITP, also called idiopathic thrombocytopenic purpura) is an acquired disorder in which autoantibodies act against platelet antigens. It can be seen in pregnancy and postpartum among women who are otherwise

---

Box 23.2 Postpartum Hemorrhage Risk Factors

Atony
- Retained placenta and/or membranes
- Failure to progress in the second stage of labor
- Adherent placenta
- Large-for-gestational-age infant
- Labor induction
- Prolonged first or second stage of labor
- High parity (having had five or more pregnancies with gestation periods of ≥20 wk)
- Uterine overdistension
- Uterine infection

Trauma
- Lacerations
- Instrumental delivery
- Large-for-gestational-age infant

Coagulopathy
- Hypertensive disorder of pregnancy
- Intrauterine fetal demise
- Fetal demise
- Sepsis
- Congenital clotting deficiency

---

healthy. Primary ITP is characterized by autoimmune platelet destruction that is not associated with any other condition. Secondary ITP is characterized by autoimmune platelet destruction that is associated with another condition, such as systemic lupus erythematosus or hepatitis C. In pregnancy, the rate of ITP is approximately 10 times that of the general population, with 1 to 3 out of 10,000 pregnant women being diagnosed with this condition (Care, Pavord, Knight, & Alfirevic, 2017).

It is likely that the autoimmune response is due to a genetic predisposition to an acquired event, such as a viral or bacterial infection, or an underlying autoimmune condition. ITP is often chronic (lasting 12 or more months).

ITP is an isolated form of thrombocytopenia. Unlike DIC, it is not associated with fever, chills, or hypotension. Unlike with severe preeclampsia or HELLP syndrome, the patient with ITP does not have elevated liver function tests. Symptoms of the condition range from mild petechiae on the extremities to severe hemorrhage, and its onset may be slow and insidious or abrupt. The worse the thrombocytopenia, the more likely the woman is to experience a dangerous bleed (Care et al., 2017).

Common findings associated with ITP include petechiae (flat, red lesions that do not blanch) and purpura, an area of discoloration on the skin caused by a coalescence of petechiae. Petechiae on the skin are sometimes called "dry petechiae" and are not considered as predictive of severe bleeding as hemorrhagic blisters of the mucosa, which are sometimes referred to as "wet petechiae." Epistaxis (nose bleed) is another common finding with ITP and may range from a minor bleed to a persistent bleed requiring packing of the nares. More severe hemorrhage is unusual, occurring in fewer than 1% of patients with ITP (Moulis et al., 2014).

Therapy for ITP is typically limited to women who are bleeding or who have a platelet count below 20,000 to 30,000/μL. Women may be treated with a transfusion of platelets. However, it is the nature of the condition that the patient's immune system destroys these, thus making this a short-term solution. Patients are treated with corticosteroids and/or IV immune globulin for a more sustained effect. A second-line agent is the thrombopoietin receptor agonist rituximab. Patients who do not respond to medication may undergo a splenectomy.

Maternal IgG may also impact the neonate, causing transient thrombocytopenia in a small minority of infants. If the neonate's blood is assessed for thrombocytopenia, blood should be taken from a cord vessel via venipuncture. Serial assessments of the neonate's platelets may be done over several days, with a rise anticipated after 2 to 5 days postpartum.

Lacerations and Birth Injuries

Another cause of PPH is trauma from incisions, uterine rupture, or lacerations obtained during labor and delivery. A uterus that is firmly contracted in the presence of continued bleeding should increase suspicion for a previously unrecognized traumatic injury. Risk factors include a rapid birth, an operative vaginal birth, abnormalities of the birth passage, maternal genital varicosities, macrosomia, and abnormalities of fetal position and presentation (see Chapter 22).

Uterine Inversion

An unusual cause of PPH is uterine inversion. **Uterine inversion** is a condition in which the uterine fundus prolapses into the endometrial cavity, turning the uterus inside out. It can result in hemorrhage and shock. A majority of inversions of the uterus occur within 24 hours after delivery (acute). An inversion that occurs from 24 hours to 4 weeks after delivery is termed subacute, and an inversion that happens 1 month or more after delivery is referred to a chronic.

Uterine inversion is described by the degree of inversion (Pauleta, Rodrigues, Melo, & Graca, 2010):

1. First degree (incomplete): Prolapse of the fundus into the uterine cavity
2. Second degree (complete): Protrusion of the fundus through the cervical os
3. Third degree (uterine prolapse): Prolapse of the fundus through the uterus to the introitus
4. Fourth degree: Complete prolapse of both the uterus and vagina (total uterine and vaginal)

The cause of uterine inversion is not completely clear, although it is often attributed to cord traction and uterine pressure during the third stage of labor. The birth of the placenta is often managed this way without uterine inversion, however, suggesting there are other contributing factors (Deneux-Tharaux et al., 2013). Risk factors for inversion include macrosomia, a short umbilical cord, first birth, uterine tumors, retained placenta, placenta accreta, and a rapid delivery. About half of the cases of uterine inversion have no risk factors (Witteveen, van Stralen, Zwart, & van Roosmalen, 2013). Uterine inversion is also described in reference to time of occurrence.

The most common presentation of uterine inversion is severe vaginal bleeding postpartum, although bleeding may also be mild. Shock can occur unrelated to the volume of blood lost because of the effect on the pelvic parasympathetic nerves. On examination, the fundus of the uterus is not palpable and, with an inversion more severe than first degree, the organ is visualized in the vagina, at the introitus, or outside the body. In the case of a first-degree inversion, blood loss is generally less severe and diagnosis may be delayed. A nonpalpable fundus is the key finding. Pain from uterine inversion may be mild or severe.

If a nurse suspects uterine inversion, she or he should call for help immediately. Any infusion with a uterotonic drug such as oxytocin should be discontinued, as the uterus must be relaxed before the obstetric provider attempts to replace it. The nurse should place two 16- or 18-gauge IV catheters and infuse fluid to adequately support blood pressure. Bradycardia resulting from parasympathetic stimulation may be corrected by 0.5 mg IV atropine given according to orders. The nurse should anticipate blood collection for a complete blood count and coagulation studies and administer blood products as ordered per protocol.

The obstetric provider typically attempts to replace the uterus immediately because this process becomes more difficult over time as the lower uterine segment and cervix involute. Uterine relaxants such as nitroglycerin and terbutaline are often required for a successful replacement. Failure of conservative replacement measures requires surgical intervention. After uterine replacement, women are usually given oxytocin to keep the uterus contracted, thus minimizing the chance of repeated inversion and atony. The obstetric provider may elect to give a single dose of an antibiotic.

Prognosis

Outcomes of PPH vary widely depending on the etiology and the volume of blood lost, and can range from mild anemia to hypovolemic shock (discussed below) and death. Also, women with PPH have three times the risk of PPH with subsequent deliveries (Oberg, Hernandez-Diaz, Palmsten, Almqvist, & Bateman, 2014).

Assessment

The symptoms of PPH depend on the volume of blood lost. The bleeding of secondary PPH is typically less acute than that of primary PPH. Moreover, blood loss from PPH may not be overtly vaginal. The woman may instead bleed into the abdomen, or the blood may be compartmentalized as a vaginal or vulvar hematoma. The nurse must be aware of status changes in a patient that suggest PPH, even in the absence of overt vaginal bleeding (Box 23.3).

Box 23.3   Postpartum Hemorrhage Blood Loss and Associated Symptoms

Loss of 500–1,000 mL
- Normal blood pressure
- Palpitations
- Lightheadedness
- Minimal increase in heart rate

Loss of 1,000–1,500 mL
- Lower blood pressure
- Weakness
- Diaphoresis
- Respiratory rate of 20–24 breaths/min
- Heart rate of 100–120 bpm

Loss of 1,500–2,000 mL
- Systolic blood pressure < 90 mm Hg
- Restlessness
- Confusion
- Pallor
- Oliguria
- Delayed capillary refill
- Heart rate of 120–140 bpm

Loss of 2,000–3,000 mL
- Blood pressure < 90 mm Hg
- Pulse pressure < 25 mm Hg
- Delayed capillary refill
- Lethargy
- Air hunger
- No urine production (anuria)
- Heart rate of >140 bpm

bpm, beats per minute.

If acute, primary PPH is suspected, the nurse should immediately assemble the team and equipment necessary to efficiently address the emergency in a timely fashion if not already present. Although PPH often occurs in the delivery room, with personnel and resources present, it may also happen on the postpartum floor when the nurse is alone. In such circumstances it is expedient to activate the emergency call system to elicit help.

After summoning help, the nurse's priority is to assess the uterus. In the case of suspected PPH with a firm uterus, the obstetric provider carefully inspects for lacerations of the perineum, vagina, and/or cervix. The obstetric provider may order laboratory studies if a clotting disorder is suspected and blood type and cross-match tests, if not on record already, in the event of a need for transfusion.

Ultrasound is a common early step to evaluate the cause of bleeding, particularly if retention of products of conception is suspected. If several weeks have passed since the birth, a positive pregnancy test suggests that the cause of bleeding is a new pregnancy, retained placental fragments or membranes, or, rarely, choriocarcinoma. If the examination of the uterus is tender and the mother has a fever and/or malodorous vaginal discharge, **endometritis** (infection of the endometrium) is suspected, and antibiotics are indicated.

Treatment

A boggy uterus requires firm massage of the fundus (Fig. 23.2). Massage of a boggy uterus often expresses clots and temporarily increases bleeding. Bladder distention can contribute to uterine atony, and a full bladder should be emptied either by the patient voiding voluntarily or by a straight or indwelling catheter as a last resort. Oxytocin is typically the first-line uterotonic medication and is given IV, 10 to 40 U in 500 mL to 1 L of normal saline at a rate sufficient to correct atony. Alternatively, 10 U may be given intramuscularly. If an IV line is not already in place, however, the nurse's priority is to establish one to facilitate medication administration and in the event of volume depletion requiring IV fluids or blood products. If the uterus remains atonic, other agents such as ergots or carboprost (The Pharmacy 23.1) are indicated.

Continued atony requires a more aggressive form of uterine massage called bimanual compression (Fig. 23.3). This is typically

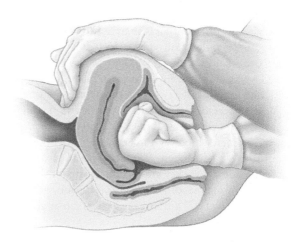

Figure 23.3. Bimanual compression of the uterus for the management of uterine atony. This technique consists of massage of the anterior wall of the uterus with a hand on the abdomen and massage through the vagina of the anterior uterine wall with the, other hand made into a fist. (Reprinted with permission from Beckmann, C. R., Herbert, W., Laube, D., Ling, F., & Smith, R. [2013]. *Obstetrics and gynecology* [7th ed., Fig. 12.1]. Philadelphia, PA: Lippincott Williams & Wilkins.)

a task for the obstetric provider and is very uncomfortable for the patient. The obstetric provider inserts a gloved fist into the vagina, pushing against the anterior wall of the vagina. With the other hand, the provider kneads the posterior wall of the uterus. The provider may also reach inside the uterus to manually remove clots or placental or membrane fragments.

If conservative methods of massage and medication are ineffective, a surgical solution is sought to stop the bleeding. A common first step is uterine **tamponade**, in which the uterus is packed or a balloon is inserted to try to occlude the blood vessels from which the bleeding is occurring by compressing the inside of the organ. The obstetric provider may perform special suturing designed to provide compression, ligation, or embolization of blood vessels feeding the uterus, or, as a last resort, a hysterectomy. In the case of retained products of conception, the obstetric provider may perform a surgical evacuation of the uterus.

In Chapter 1, Bess experienced primary PPH immediately after the birth of her baby, Milo. Because her team was unable to control her bleeding through other methods, including dilation and curettage to remove any fragments of retained placenta present (none was found) and balloon tamponade, Bess underwent an emergency hysterectomy.

Care Considerations

During treatment, the nurse may, as ordered, administer oxygen by a nonrebreather mask and, particularly if bleeding is extensive

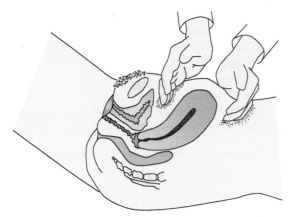

Figure 23.2. Uterine massage. (Reprinted with permission from Lippincott's Professional Development Programs February to June, 2012 releases.)

or refractory, place an indwelling catheter to facilitate urine output monitoring, as low urine output is an indication of hypovolemia. Laboratory studies at this time typically include a complete blood count and coagulation studies.

Women who have severe anemia after PPH are generally managed with oral ferrous sulfate 325 mg three times daily between meals. With successful treatment, the woman's hemoglobin level can rise within 3 weeks. Rarely, IV iron may be provided instead, and women who cannot tolerate high oral doses of iron may require a dose adjustment. Women who are weakened by anemia to the point that they are unable to care for themselves or their newborn may receive a blood transfusion, generally if the hemoglobin level is 7 g/dL or lower (Carson et al., 2016).

Hematoma

A **hematoma** is a collection of blood in the body outside of a blood vessel. Puerperal hematomas occur as a result of a birth and are an accumulation of blood in the vulva, vagina, or, rarely, the retroperitoneal space. This space is behind the peritoneum.

Prevalence

Puerperal hematomas are relatively rare, occurring with fewer than 1 out of 1,000 births. Although typically associated with birth injury, they may occasionally complicate a pregnancy (Iskender et al., 2016).

Etiology

Hematomas are most often associated with episiotomies and lacerations occurring with operative deliveries, but they can also happen with closed trauma. Risk factors include first birth, preeclampsia, prolonged first and/or second stage of labor, vulvar varicosities, multifetal pregnancy, fetal macrosomia, maternal obesity, and clotting disorders (Gurtovaya, Hanna, & Wagley, 2013; Iskender et al., 2016).

Prognosis

Although the prognosis for hematomas is generally favorable, prompt identification, thorough evaluation, and careful management are the key to positive outcomes. A retroperitoneal hematoma is an obstetric emergency with risk of death. A history of a previous hematoma is not recognized as a risk for the condition with future pregnancies (Iskender et al., 2016).

Assessment

Symptoms of a hematoma usually develop within 24 hours after the delivery. They are typically acutely painful, and the pain is often described as out of proportion to the injury because of the sensitivity of the genitalia.

A vulvar hematoma usually develops rapidly and is extremely painful. Upon examination, a purplish mass can be identified that is tense with compartmentalized bleeding.

A vaginal hematoma may exist independently or as an extension of a vulvar hematoma. A vaginal hematoma may be acutely painful but may also present as a patient report of a sensation of rectal pressure. An examination typically reveals a vaginal mass. Rarely, a vulvar hematoma may present as hypovolemic shock.

Because a larger volume of blood can accumulate in the retroperitoneal space without producing symptoms, a retroperitoneal hematoma is more likely to first present as hemodynamic instability (tachycardia and hypotension) or shock and less likely to present as pain. In some cases, it may present as a palpable abdominal mass.

If the diagnosis is uncertain, the obstetric provider may order an ultrasound or a computed tomography scan.

Treatment

The bleeding of a hematoma may be venous or arterial. Patients with a venous bleed are likely to be hemodynamically stable and receive a single large-bore IV line for fluids. Such patients are more likely to be managed conservatively. A patient who is not hemodynamically stable likely has an arterial bleed and requires two large-bore IVs for fluids and blood products, as well as immediate surgery. A complete blood count and clotting factors are ordered, particularly in the case of hemodynamic instability.

The obstetric provider may recommend treating the hematoma with surgery using local, regional, or general anesthesia, depending on the clinical situation and the provider's judgment. Alternate treatments include conservative management with observation and support and embolization of arteries. Candidates for conservative treatment must be hemodynamically stable, and the nurse must closely observe them for severe hemorrhage and hypovolemic shock. The nurse should monitor the patient's vital signs and intake and output at least hourly. The obstetric provider may order regular laboratory studies of the complete blood count and clotting factors, according to the clinical picture, and serial imaging to assess for expansion of the hematoma.

Care Considerations

Small vulvar hematomas are most likely to be managed conservatively. The nurse should provide analgesics, as ordered, and ice packs, as these hematomas are quite painful. A Foley catheter may be necessary if the hematoma interferes with urination. Small vaginal hematomas may also be managed conservatively. Retroperitoneal hematomas, however, typically do require surgery or embolization of the bleeding vessels, although conservative management may be preferred in some circumstances.

In Chapter 11, Edie was diagnosed with a vulvar hematoma after a precipitous vaginal birth and a significant perineal laceration. Her obstetric provider elected to manage her conservatively with careful observation by her nursing team.

Hypovolemic Shock

Hemorrhage, when uncontrolled, can lead to **hypovolemic shock**, a dangerous, life-threatening condition in which organs become dangerously underperfused and underoxygenated, leading to compromised function and even death.

Etiology

Hypovolemic shock is triggered when the volume of circulating blood decreases to a degree that the body's cells and organs do not have sufficient oxygen to function properly, such as a result of PPH or major trauma. Adrenal glands, sensing this hypovolemia, release catecholamines that cue arterioles and venules of organs other than the heart and brain to constrict, thus diverting blood flow to those essential organs. Low oxygenation of cells of nonessential organs causes lactic acid to accumulate, lowering the pH of the blood, resulting in acidosis. This acidosis causes the arterioles to dilate while the venules remain constricted. Because the venules are constricted while the arterioles are dilated, edema and pooling of the deoxygenated blood occurs, further decreasing perfusion and eventually leading to the death of cells.

Assessment

Nurses must be vigilant for the signs and symptoms of hypovolemic shock. Most clinical manifestations of shock are not specific to shock or sensitive, but combined they provide important clues. Although pulse oximetry is used to assess oxygen saturation, the nurse should be aware that the accuracy of this assessment is reduced in patients who are hypovolemic. An assessment of the level of consciousness can also provide information about oxygen saturation. A hypovolemic woman may have mental status changes or be restless, anxious, dizzy, or lightheaded. Confusion can be an important indicator of cerebral hypoxia.

A nurse who suspects hypovolemic shock should not delay care (Table 23.1). A rapid response is critical. Nurses should be aware that the clinical manifestations of shock may not be obvious in a postpartum woman until she has lost 40% of her blood volume.

Regular and accurate monitoring of patients diagnosed with hemorrhagic shock is essential. In some cases, hemodynamic monitoring may be ordered and a nurse may assist in the placement of a central venous pressure catheter or a pulmonary artery catheter. Both are associated with complications, such as infection, thromboembolism, damage to cardiac and vascular structures, pneumothorax, and arrhythmias. Hemodynamic monitoring measures oxygenation, flow, and pressure within the cardiovascular system. Readings include pulmonary wedge pressure, systemic and pulmonary arterial pressures, central venous pressure, the oxygen saturation of the hemoglobin of arterial blood, and mixed venous oxygen saturation. These values provide information about oxygen content of the blood and resistance of the systemic and pulmonary vasculature. Additionally, continuous electrocardiographic monitoring may be ordered. This care typically takes place in the intensive care unit.

Treatment

The management of hypovolemic shock requires restoration of circulating blood volume as well as identifying and successfully addressing the source of bleeding. Early in treatment, fluids may be simply crystalloids (usually normal saline or lactated Ringer's).

Table 23.1 Hypovolemic Shock

Clinical Presentation	Cause
Hypotension	Inadequate blood volume (a late sign of shock) Defined as any one of the following: • Systolic BP < 90 mm Hg • Decrease in systolic BP > 40 mm Hg • Decrease in systolic BP > 20 mm Hg on rising (orthostatic)
Tachycardia	A compensatory mechanism that typically occurs prior to hypotension and can also happen with hypertension
Tachypnea	A response to metabolic acidosis caused by hypoxia of the cells when the body attempts to "blow off" excess CO_2 in an attempt to compensate
Oliguria	A result of the shunting of blood away from kidneys and from the depletion of blood volume
Mental status changes	Poor perfusion, resulting in anxiety, restlessness, agitation, and apprehension that may progress to disorientation, delirium, and coma
Cool, pale, clammy, cyanotic, and/or mottled skin; poor turgor	Peripheral vasoconstriction, which redirects blood to the brain and heart; may not be present in very early or late shock
Slowed capillary refill	Poor peripheral perfusion due to the compensatory vasoconstriction promoted by the release of catecholamines

BP, blood pressure.

However, blood products are needed if bleeding continues or the patient's condition does not improve and should be infused as soon as available per institution protocols. The administration of oxygen at 10 to 12 L/min via a nonrebreather mask is standard care.

Care Considerations

If hypovolemic shock is suspected, the nurse's critical first step is to immediately call for assistance. Then, the nurse should establish two large-bore IV lines for early resuscitation with fluids and, if needed, for the administration of blood products.

Fluid Resuscitation

Initially, crystalloids are typically infused rapidly at a ratio of 3:1:3 mL of fluids introduced IV for every 1 mL of estimated blood loss.

Nurses should be vigilant for fluid overload when providing the high volume of crystalloids required for fluid resuscitation. Acute fluid overload may present as shortness of breath, pulmonary edema (crackles on auscultation), edema of the extremities or face, or ascites.

The nurse should also carefully monitor urine output using an indwelling Foley catheter, which allows for precise measurement. A urine output of less than 30 mL/h suggests continuing hypovolemia, whereas an output of 30 mL/h or greater is reassuring of restored volume. Careful regular assessment of vital signs is also crucial. Throughout the critical period of shock and resuscitation, the nurse will frequently draw blood per orders for a complete blood count and coagulation studies to evaluate the red blood cell content of the blood and to assess for DIC.

Blood Transfusion

The nurse should transfuse blood products according to institution protocols, carefully checking each unit prior to use. Typical steps include obtaining patient consent, establishing venous access, confirming patient identification, and using filtered IV tubing. The nurse should administer the blood products via a designated IV with normal saline the only other liquid. A common rate of infusion is 1 to 2 mL/min for the first 15 minutes and then titrated up as tolerated, with a total duration of infusion of 4 hours or less. The nurse may obtain an accurate new hemoglobin level reading as soon as 15 minutes after the transfusion.

Typically, the nurse should closely observe the patient for up to a half hour after the transfusion is complete. Transfusion events are itemized in Table 23.2. Important assessments associated with transfusion include inspection for bleeding suggestive of DIC (oozing from the injection sites or IV line sites, petechiae beneath the blood pressure cuff, hematuria, etc.) and auscultation of the lungs prior to, during, and just after the transfusion for crackles, which would suggest fluid overload.

Thromboembolic Disease

A venous thromboembolism (VTE) is a blood clot or multiple clots that form inside a vein.

Prevalence

A pregnancy-related VTE occurs in 1 out of every 500 to 2,000 pregnancies, and a deep vein thrombosis (DVT) is about three times as common as a pulmonary embolism (PE). In the United States, PEs account for 9.2% of maternal deaths (Centers for Disease Control and Prevention, 2017).

Etiology

In pregnancy and during the postpartum period, a woman is more likely to experience the three factors identified in Virchow's triad in 1856 as contributing to VTE: venous stasis, endothelial injury, and hypercoagulability.

- *Stasis:* The capacity of veins is expanded in pregnancy as they dilate, thus leading to slower blood flow and pooling. In addition, the pregnant uterus applies pressure to the vasculature of the lower extremities. This is particularly notable on the left side, the site of a vast majority of DVTs in pregnancy.
- *Endothelial injury:* Endothelial injury is damage to the vasculature and is particularly pertinent postpartum. Damage may occur as a laceration or from a surgical intervention. The detachment of the placenta and subsequent changes of the uteroplacental site may also contribute.
- *Hypercoagulability:* In pregnancy, several coagulation factors increase, whereas resistance to proteins that inhibit clotting decreases.

A VTE may be limited to the superficial veins or form in the deeper veins of the lower extremities. The most common location for a clot in pregnancy is the left leg. A clot that forms in the deeper veins, a DVT, can break off and travel to the pulmonary artery, where it can obstruct blood flow to the lungs. This kind of thrombosis is known as a PE.

During pregnancy, factors that increase risk for VTEs include urinary tract infections (UTIs), multiple gestations, maternal age over 34 years, obesity, diabetes, varicose veins, and inflammatory bowel disease (most commonly Crohn disease or ulcerative colitis; see Box 3.9; Abdul Sultan et al., 2013).

Postpartum, the risk for VTEs is even higher than in pregnancy: two to five times higher. This level of increased risk for VTE persists for 6 weeks postpartum, and an increased risk for VTE in general does not return to that of the general population until at least 3 months after the birth (Kamel et al., 2014). (Factors that increase risk are cesarean section, varicose veins, overweight, inflammatory bowel disease, preterm birth, hemorrhage, stillbirth, advanced maternal age, hypertension, preeclampsia, infection, and smoking; Tepper et al., 2014). Thrombophilias, including factor V Leiden or antiphospholipid syndrome, increase VTE risk for all populations.

In Chapter 3, Susan developed a DVT and a PE. Susan's risk factors included obesity and diabetes. She was treated with blood thinners and encouraged to ambulate to prevent further clotting.

Table 23.2 Transfusion Events

Reaction	Clinical Presentation*	Test Findings	Cause	Immediate Actions
Acute hemolytic reaction	• Fever • Chills • Hypotension • Back pain • DIC	• Low hemoglobin • Blood in the urine • Positive direct Coombs test • Findings of DIC (prolonged PT, prolonged aPTT, low fibrinogen, thrombocytopenia)	Usually ABO incompatibility	• Stop transfusion. • Administer IV fluids. • Administer vasopressor, as needed. • Check for clerical errors.
Anaphylactic reaction	• Hypotension • Angioedema (edema) • Wheezing • Respiratory distress	• IgA deficiency • Anti-IgA • Low oxygen saturation	Immune reaction	• Stop the transfusion. • Administer epinephrine 0.3 mL IM. • Administer IV fluids. • Prepare IV epinephrine. • Maintain the airway. • Administer oxygen. • Administer vasopressor, as needed.
Transfusion-related acute lung injury	• Respiratory distress • Hypotension	• Abnormal chest X-ray • Low oxygen saturation • Transient leukopenia • Antineutrophil or anti-HLA antibodies	Immune reaction	• Stop the transfusion.
Transfusion-associated circulatory overload	• Respiratory distress • Crackles	• Abnormal chest X-ray • Low oxygen saturation • Increased BNP or NT-proBNP	Volume overload	• Stop the transfusion. • Administer oxygen. • Administer diuretics.
Sepsis in response to a bacterial infection	• Fever > 2°C • Chills • Tachycardia • Hypotension • DIC	• Bacteremia • Leukocytosis • Findings of DIC	Contaminated blood products	• Stop the transfusion. • Resuscitate. • Culture blood from a sample taken from the opposite arm. • Seal the product and send to the laboratory.
Febrile nonhemolytic reaction	• Fever (1°C–2°C greater than normal)	None	Possible reaction to cytokines or antibodies	• Stop the transfusion. • Exclude other causes. • Administer acetaminophen.
Urticarial reaction	• Hives • No other evidence of immune reaction	N/A	Immune reaction	• Stop the transfusion. • Administer diphenhydramine.

*Signs of acute hemolytic shock occur during transfusion, within 24 hours after completion of the transfusion, or days or weeks later. Signs of anaphylactic reaction occur within seconds or minutes after the start of the transfusion. Signs of transfusion-related acute lung injury occur during or within 6 hours after the transfusion. Signs of transfusion-associated circulatory overload occur during or immediately after the transfusion. Signs of sepsis occur within 5 hours of completion of the transfusion. Signs of febrile nonhemolytic reaction occur 1 to 6 hours after the start of the transfusion. Signs of urticarial reaction occur during or just after the transfusion.

DIC, disseminated intravascular coagulation; PT, prothrombin time; aPTT, activated partial thromboplastin time; PTT, partial thromboplastin time; IV, intravenous; IgA, immunoglobulin A; BNP, brain natriuretic peptide; NT-proBNP, N-terminal pro b-type natriuretic peptide; N/A, not applicable.

Prognosis

A DVT that moves from the leg may contribute to stroke or myocardial infarction, and a PE is life-threatening.

Assessment

Deep Vein Thrombosis

The presentation of a DVT depends on its location. Pregnancy-associated DVT is almost always in the left lower extremity, although it may rarely be bilateral or in the right extremity. Iliac vein DVT is more common for women in pregnancy and postpartum than it is for the general population. The iliac vein is located in the pelvis. The entire leg can be affected, as may the buttocks, lower abdomen, and back. Typical symptoms are swelling and pain that may be diffuse, as well as localized redness, warmth, and tenderness. A proximal vein DVT is located in the leg itself, and the symptoms described are distal to the site of the clot.

A clot may also be superficial. A superficial venous thrombosis is more common than a DVT. It is generally benign and self-limiting unless larger veins are involved. Typical symptoms are pain, tenderness, induration (hardening), and erythema (redness) along the length of the vein. The vein itself may be palpable and feel cord-like. Some people may present with a low-grade fever.

A leg examination is a routine part of postpartum assessment. The nurse should examine both legs at the same time so they may be compared. Unilateral swelling, erythema, edema, and induration are particularly concerning, as are patient complaints of pain or tenderness. Bilateral edema, however, is an anticipated part of a normal postpartum course. Assessment for Homans' sign is no longer the standard of care, as it is not a sensitive or specific test.

Findings from a clinical examination alone are not sufficient to diagnose a VTE, however. The a D-dimer serum evaluation is helpful for the diagnosis of blood clots in the general population but is of limited use during pregnancy and the postpartum period because D-dimer values for this population are normally elevated even in the absence of a clot. Imaging by ultrasound is an often used diagnostic test and is highly sensitive for detecting DVT in proximal veins, although less useful for a DVT in the iliac vein. Magnetic resonance venography is superior for assessing iliac vein DVT.

Pulmonary Embolism

PEs have no specific signs or symptoms, and some of their clinical manifestations, such as dyspnea, also occur with pregnancy. Other symptoms include cough, sweating, pleuritic chest pain, and, more rarely, hemoptysis. An acute onset of any of these symptoms is concerning for a PE and should be evaluated carefully (Parilla et al., 2016).

Testing of arterial blood gases is of limited diagnostic use in detecting PEs in pregnancy because respiratory alkalosis is common to both pregnancy and PEs. As with the assessment for DVT, D-dimer use is complicated by the normal rise in levels associated with pregnancy. Echocardiography is not routinely performed to diagnose PE, although it may be used to evaluate the right ventricle in the case of a confirmed PE.

Imaging, usually a ventilation/perfusion (V/Q) scan or computed tomographic pulmonary angiography, is required for the definitive diagnosis of PE. A V/Q scan is often done in conjunction with a chest X-ray. Other less commonly used imaging methods include magnetic resonance pulmonary angiography and contrast-enhanced pulmonary artery angiography.

Treatment

Superficial and Deep Vein Thromboses

A patient with a superficial, uncomplicated thrombus is treated with supportive measures, as described in the section Care Considerations. Patients with superficial thrombi deemed higher risk due to size or location may be treated with anticoagulants or surgery (Kearon et al., 2016).

Depending on the clinical picture and the assessment of risk, patients with asymptomatic DVT of the proximal vein may be monitored with serial ultrasound and treated only if the clot grows larger or fails to resolve. Clots that are symptomatic and/or located in the iliac vein are typically treated with anticoagulants, however (Horner et al., 2014).

For postpartum patients, initial anticoagulation therapy for up to 10 days is with low-molecular-weight heparin, IV unfractionated heparin, subcutaneous heparin, or an oral factor Xa inhibitor, such as rivaroxaban or apixaban (Table 23.3). After initial therapy, the patient may continue with the original anticoagulant for a finite period of time (typically 3 months) or be switched to warfarin. Warfarin requires regular serum monitoring, with a goal of an international normalized ratio (INR) of 2.5. When switching between agents, patients should receive both heparin and warfarin for 5 days. Heparin may be stopped when the patient's INR has stayed from 2 to 3 for at least 2 consecutive days. Warfarin is considering safe with breastfeeding.

Pregnant patients are usually treated with heparin both short term and long term, as warfarin crosses the placenta and oral factor Xa inhibitors have yet to be adequately tested in pregnancy. If the timing of delivery is predictable, anticoagulation should be stopped 24 hours prior to delivery to lower the risk of hemorrhage. It should be restarted 6 hours after a vaginal birth and 12 hours after a cesarean delivery. Patients at a particularly high risk for clotting may have their anticoagulant stopped closer to delivery. Patients taking anticoagulants should not receive neuraxial anesthesia because of the high risk for a spinal hematoma. Patients reporting pain should be treated with analgesics per orders.

Pulmonary Embolism

A PE is a medical emergency. In the case of a high suspicion of PE, anticoagulant treatment should begin prior to confirmation of the diagnosis. Subcutaneous low-molecular-weight heparin, IV unfractionated heparin, or subcutaneous unfractionated heparin are generally the preferred agents. Therapy continues for approximately 6 months postpartum. After the birth, the anticoagulant may be switched from heparin to warfarin.

8

Table 23.3 Anticoagulant Monitoring

Anticoagulant Class and Drugs	Dose	Monitoring
Low-Molecular-Weight Heparin		
Dalteparin	200 U/kg/d SQ OR 100 U/kg twice daily SQ	• Titrate dose to the anti-Xa level of 0.6–1 IU/mL for twice daily administration OR 1–2 IU/mL for daily administration • First anti-Xa measured 4 h after the third or fourth dose if twice daily; OR 4 h after the second or third dose if daily; OR 4 h after the third injection with dose adjustment • Continued anti-Xa levels rarely needed in absence of further dose adjustment
Tinzaparin	175 U/kg/d SQ	
Enoxaparin	1 mg/kg twice daily SQ	
IV unfractionated heparin	• Bolus of 80 U/kg IV followed by continuous 18 U/kg/h • Titrate every 6 h until therapeutic.	• Target anti-Xa to 0.3–0.7 U. • Recheck once or twice daily.
SQ unfractionated heparin	• 17,500 U every 12 h • Titrate until therapeutic.	• Target anti-Xa to 0.3–0.7 U. • First check 6 h after the second dose. • Recheck after every second dose until target rechecked. • After target, recheck at 3 or 4 d, then every few weeks.
Oral Factor Xa		
Rivaroxaban (Xarelto)	15 mg by mouth twice daily for 3 wk, then 20 mg daily	N/A
Apixaban (Eliquis)	10 mg twice daily for 7 d, then 5 mg daily; after 6 mo, 2.5 mg twice daily	N/A
Edoxaban (Savaysa, Lixiana)	Administer after a 5-d course of heparin at 60 mg daily.	N/A
Dabigatran	Administer after a 5-d course of heparin at 150 mg twice daily.	N/A
Coumarin Anticoagulant		
Warfarin (Coumadin)	• Start the same day as heparin. • 5 mg/d for the first 2 d	• Adjust dose until the INR is 2–3 for 2 consecutive days. • Target INR: 2.5. • Discontinue heparin when INR is at the goal.

SQ, subcutaneous; IV, intravenous; N/A, not applicable; INR, international normalized ratio.

Care Considerations

Supportive measures for the care of patients with VTEs include keeping the affected leg elevated to waist level and applying warm or cold compresses for comfort. The nurse may provide NSAIDs and compression therapy with stockings or compression devices, as well, and the patient should remain ambulatory whenever possible.

Early ambulation is safe with a diagnosis of a DVT, and the nurse should encourage the patient to do it as soon and as often as possible. There is no increased risk for a PE with early ambulation. Compression stockings may be useful for patients complaining of edema or pain that limits their ability to ambulate. Limited evidence supports the use of compression stockings to prevent future DVTs, particularly when the thrombus is associated with a discrete event, such as pregnancy (Kahn, Shapiro, Ginsberg, & SOX Trial Investigators, 2014).

Postpartum Infections

Given all of the trauma and physical changes associated with both vaginal and cesarean births, as well as associated invasive interventions such as neuraxial anesthesia and urinary catheterization, it is not surprising that infections of many kinds are prevalent during the postpartum period. Determining the presence of an infection can be challenging, however, as many of the signs associated with infection are nonspecific and may occur because of other causes following delivery.

For example, shivering starting shortly after the birth and lasting for up to an hour is common and should not be viewed as evidence of fever or infection. A low-grade fever in the first 24 hours postpartum is common and typically resolves spontaneously. A fever that persists beyond this time or that has its onset from 2 to 10 days postpartum requires further investigation. Leukocytosis is a less helpful finding for women postpartum than it is for the general population, as an elevated white blood cell count is a normal finding immediately after a birth. A rise instead of a fall of white blood cells based on serial evaluations postpartum, however, does suggest infection.

Once the presence of an infection has been established, it can also be challenging to determine its cause. Common causes of fever postpartum include perineal or cesarean wound infection, endometritis, septic pelvic thrombophlebitis (inflammation of a blood vessel), mastitis, breast abscess, UTIs, and complications related to anesthesia or a reaction to another medication.

Perineal Wound Infection

An infection may occur at the site of a perineal laceration or episiotomy. Such infections are usually localized to the area of injury.

Prevalence

Infections from perineal wounds are most common when associated with third- and fourth-degree lacerations. As many as 20% of such wounds become infected (Lewicky-Gaupp, Leader-Cramer, Johnson, Kenton, & Gossett, 2015).

Etiology

Risk factors for infections from perineal wounds include an operative vaginal delivery, a long second stage, third- and fourth-degree lacerations, a mediolateral episiotomy, maternal smoking, and meconium staining of the amniotic fluid (Jallad, Steele, & Barber, 2016).

Assessment

The signs and symptoms of perineal infection include tenderness and a red and swollen appearance in the area, as well as purulent exudate from the area that is yellow and stringy.

Treatment

Treatment requires removal of sutures and opening of the wound. The obstetric provider removes any foreign material and necrotic tissue and irrigates the wound. The provider typically allows smaller wounds to heal by granulation but may suture again larger wounds when granulation is established. Antibiotics are typically unnecessary unless there is evidence of cellulitis, an infection of the dermis and subcutaneous fat. Cellulitis appears as a progressive expansion of erythema away from the wound borders.

Cesarean Wound Infection

Incision wounds from cesarean delivery are also common sites of infection postpartum.

Prevalence

The wounds of a cesarean delivery become infected after 2% to 6% of cesarean deliveries (Carter et al., 2017). Many of these cases are diagnosed after discharge, from day 4 to day 7 postpartum.

Assessment

Infections that manifest within the first 24 to 48 hours postpartum typically present with a high fever and cellulitis and are caused by group A or group B beta-hemolytic streptococcus. Other clinical signs and symptoms include induration, redness, and warmth, as well as a patient report of pain at the site of incision. The wound edges may separate, and purulent discharge and fever may be noted. Necrotizing fasciitis, an infection of the fascia that progresses rapidly and destroys skin and cutaneous tissue, may develop but is very rare. With this type of infection, drainage is thin and copious and the subcutaneous tissue bleeds easily.

Treatment

Obstetric providers open, drain, irrigate, explore, and, if necessary, debride infected cesarean incisions. Wounds are left open but kept moist and covered to protect the tissue. After granulation tissue is established, the wound can again be sutured. Wound complications are more common with unscheduled deliveries in the second stage of labor (Temming et al., 2017).

Endometritis

Endometritis is an infection of the lining of the uterus.

Etiology

Endometritis infections are caused by a mix of bacteria originating in the genital tract. Up to 27% of cesarean births are complicated by postpartum endometritis when compared with 1% to 3% of vaginal births (Mackeen, Packard, Ota, & Speer, 2015). Other, lesser risk factors include chorioamnionitis, prolonged labor, prolonged rupture of membranes, multiple cervical examinations during labor, internal monitoring during labor, meconium-stained fluid, retained placenta with manual removal, low socioeconomic status, maternal diabetes or anemia, preterm birth, operative vaginal delivery, postterm pregnancy, maternal human immunodeficiency virus infection, bacterial vaginosis in pregnancy, and group B streptococcus colonization (Mackeen et al., 2015).

Prognosis

The infection may cause the uterus to become soft and subinvoluted, which predisposes the woman to hemorrhage. Other complications may include peritonitis, thromboembolism, pelvic abscesses, and sepsis (Mackeen et al., 2015).

Assessment

Endometritis is a common cause of postpartum fever. Other signs and symptoms include a tender uterus, tachycardia, and purulent lochia. Some women may also report flu-like symptoms, such as malaise, headache, chills, and anorexia. The onset of endometritis varies, as the infection may have developed prior to delivery, during labor, or after the birth, and different bacteria provoke differences in the timing of the onset of symptoms. Although most cases of endometritis are evident in the first week, some cases are delayed until 6 weeks postpartum and may present as hemorrhage.

In most cases, endometritis is clinically diagnosed when a postpartum fever occurs on from postpartum days 2 to 10 in the absence of any other cause. Other reasons for a fever apart from endometritis include a wound infection, mastitis, aspiration pneumonia, pyelonephritis, inflammation of the spinal cord from neuraxial anesthesia, and conditions unrelated to the pregnancy, such as a viral infection.

Treatment

With uncomplicated endometritis, isolation of the causative organism is not done routinely. The condition is instead treated empirically with a broad-spectrum antibiotic, typically IV.

Lactational Mastitis

Mastitis is a condition of inflammation of the breast tissue, often associated with infection.

Etiology

Mastitis is initially provoked by engorgement of one or more milk ducts because of poor drainage caused by nipple damage or compression of a duct or ducts. Stagnation of milk can cause an overgrowth of bacteria in the milk and infection.

Factors contributing to poor drainage of one or more ducts or delayed breast emptying are risk factors for mastitis. These include consistent pressure on the breast, as from an ill-fitting bra, an oversupply of milk, infrequent feedings, nipple trauma, rapid weaning, illness of the mother or baby, maternal stress or fatigue, poor maternal position, and malpositioning of the infant during feeding. Lactating women may reduce the risk for mastitis by completely and frequently emptying their breasts of milk. People with mastitis should aim for complete emptying of the breasts at least every 2 hours, making sure to empty both breasts, beginning with the unaffected breast (because vigorous sucking initially may be very painful)

Prognosis

Women with mastitis who do not show signs of improvement within 48 to 72 hours after onset should be assessed by ultrasound for abscess. An abscess is typically tender to the touch and feels fluctuant, meaning that it can be moved or compressed when palpated. An abscess can be diagnosed by ultrasound and may be drained under ultrasound guidance. Delayed treatment with antibiotics contributes to the risk for abscess from mastitis.

Assessment

This condition causes an area of a woman's breast to become red, swollen, and painful (Fig. 23.4). It is most common in the first 3 months of lactation but can happen at any time. Symptoms that persist beyond 24 hours suggest a bacterial infection and typically include flu-like symptoms of malaise and a high fever. The breast can become quite painful.

Treatment

For the first 12 to 24 hours, mastitis may be treated conservatively with warm compresses, NSAIDS, and regular, complete emptying of the breast. Mastitis that lasts beyond this period of time is

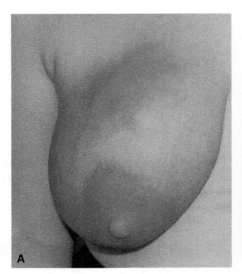 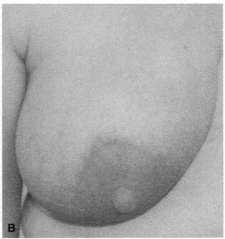

Figure 23.4. Lactational mastitis. A large abscess **(A)** was present on ultrasound which was treated by aspiration with rapid resolution **(B)**. (Reprinted with permission from Harris, J. R., Lippman, M. E., Morrow, M., & Osborne, C. K. [2010]. *Diseases of the breast* [4th ed., Fig. 6.6]. Philadelphia, PA: Lippincott Williams & Wilkins.)

considered infective and should be treated with antibiotics. A common antibiotic choice for mastitis is dicloxacillin or clindamycin for 10 to 14 days.

Urinary Tract Infection

Postpartum women are more prone to UTIs largely because of the frequency of interventions such as bladder catheterization and genital procedures such as cervical examinations and vacuum-assisted deliveries. Indwelling catheters should be removed as soon as possible to lower infection risk.

Assessment

Symptoms of a UTI limited to the bladder (cystitis) include a frequent urge to urinate, known as urinary urgency, and pain with urination. A woman with a UTI may report blood in her urine (frank hematuria) or lower abdominal discomfort. Cystitis generally does not produce systemic symptoms such as a fever or chills. The diagnosis is typically made on the basis of symptoms and laboratory test results that indicate the presence of white blood cells and/or bacteria in the urine.

Pyelonephritis is a UTI of the upper urinary tract and kidneys. Patients with pyelonephritis usually have a fever above 38°C and may report flank pain and nausea and vomiting. They also report tenderness in the area of the costovertebral angle following a light strike on the back over the kidneys. Although women with pyelonephritis typically have cystitis symptoms, some women develop pyelonephritis without them.

Treatment

UTIs are usually treated empirically with antibiotics. Clinicians may choose to have the urine cultured and tested for susceptibility to a particular antibiotic, but in the case of cystitis, this is often done only if symptoms persist after 48 to 72 hours of treatment with an empirically selected antibiotic or if an infection is recurrent. Urine is routinely cultured and tested for susceptibility in cases of pyelonephritis.

Febrile Complication of Anesthesia

General anesthesia poses a risk for aspiration pneumonia, which can cause a low-grade fever. Rarely, meningitis or an epidural abscess can result from neuraxial anesthesia.

Etiology

Aspiration pneumonia occurs with the use of general anesthesia when the patient aspirates gastric contents into the lungs, causing a chemical pneumonitis. In some cases, this bacteria of the stomach can cause a bacterial pneumonia as a result of gastric aspirates. Both chemical pneumonitis and bacterial pneumonia can cause a fever. This condition is particularly a risk when the general anesthesia is administered in emergent situations in which limited time is available to prepare the patient. An epidural abscess is more likely to occur from the placement of an epidural, whereas meningitis is more likely to result after puncture of the dura for spinal anesthesia.

Assessment

In addition to a low-grade fever, the signs and symptoms of aspiration pneumonia may include dyspnea, lung crackles, cyanosis, and hypoxemia.

The symptoms of meningitis appear within hours of the procedure and include headache and fever. The symptoms of an epidural abscess include back pain that is local and severe, progressing to "shooting" or "electric" pain along the affected nerve root. The patient may develop weakness, sensory changes, bowel and/or bladder dysfunction, and paralysis. Fever may be present or absent. The occurrence of epidural abscess or meningitis resulting from neuraxial anesthesia is rare, however (Pitkanen, Aromaa, Cozanitis, & Forster, 2013).

Treatment

Patients with aspiration pneumonia may be treated with tracheal suction and pulmonary function support, to protect the airway and improve breathing. In the case of a suspected bacterial component to the aspiration pneumonia, antibiotics are prescribed. An epidural abscess may be treated with aspiration and drainage of the abscess and antibiotics. Meningitis is treated with antibiotics.

Clostridium difficile Infection

Etiology

The use of antibiotics is common during labor and delivery and postpartum to prevent or treat bacterial infections. Ironically, however, antibiotics can contribute to bacterial infection by disrupting normal intestinal flora and facilitating colonization by the bacterium *Clostridium difficile*. Increased risk of this condition is associated with recent antibiotic administration, either current or 5 to 10 days previously.

Assessment

Symptoms associated with *C. difficile* infection include a low-grade fever, lower abdominal pain, and occurrences of watery diarrhea up to 15 times daily. The definitive diagnosis is based on laboratory testing of stool.

Treatment

Patients who are still receiving antibiotics at the time of diagnosis generally have them discontinued. Treatment with the oral antibiotic metronidazole is most often curative. For severe disease, alternate antibiotics such as vancomycin may be indicated. In the case of complications such as bowel perforation or toxic megacolon, surgery may be required.

Postpartum Headache and Associated Conditions

Women who suffered from migraine, cluster, or tension headaches previously may also experience such headaches postpartum. The occurrence of cluster and tension headaches does not typically change in pregnancy or postpartum. Migraine headaches, particularly those associated with menstruation, usually improve during pregnancy but recur postpartum. The treatment of these headaches is in keeping with what worked for the patient prior to pregnancy.

More concerning than the recurrence of chronic, primary headaches, however, is the occurrence of headaches secondary to more serious underlying conditions. For instance, a postpartum headache can be the first indication of the onset of preeclampsia or signify a worsening of previously diagnosed preeclampsia. Thus, a woman who complains of a headache postpartum should have her blood pressure checked immediately, particularly if she has an existing diagnosis of preeclampsia.

Likewise, the sudden occurrence of a "thunderclap" headache with or without neurologic symptoms should be reported immediately to the obstetric provider. Such headaches require imaging to assess for intracranial hemorrhage, vasoconstriction, and cerebral venous thrombosis.

Other types of postpartum headaches and associated conditions are discussed below.

Postpartum Stroke

Although the absolute risk of an ischemic stroke and cerebral hemorrhage associated with pregnancy is low, it can increase by as much as 3-fold in pregnancy and, particularly, in the postpartum period over that of nonpregnant women (Cheng et al., 2017). Risk factors include postpartum infection, hypertensive disorders of pregnancy, cesarean delivery, and others. A stroke can have many presentations, including neurologic deficits, severe headache, nausea and vomiting, loss of consciousness, and others. Headache is much more common with a hemorrhagic stroke than an ischemic stroke.

Postpartum Angiopathy

Postpartum angiopathy is a rare, reversible vasoconstrictive disorder. It presents as a "thunderclap" headache that is severe with a rapid onset, usually in the first week postpartum. It may include neurologic symptoms, such as one-sided weakness, visual disturbances, numbness, seizure, and speech difficulties. Blood pressure may be normal or elevated in this condition. It is usually self-limiting, although as many as 50% of women do not completely regain normal neurologic function. Death is possible in the most severe cases. There are no known effective treatments, but recurrence with future pregnancies is rare (Fugate et al., 2012).

Anesthesia-Related Headaches

The occurrence of a headache after an epidural or spinal (often called a postspinal headache or a post–dural puncture headache) is not uncommon and can be caused by leakage of the cerebrospinal fluid (CSF) and cerebral vasodilation. Such headaches are typically positional, improving with lying down and worsening with upright positions. Headaches that are not positional are unlikely to be postspinal headaches.

Postspinal headaches usually resolve within 7 to 10 days and can be cared for symptomatically using caffeine and analgesics. Alternatively, a patient may be treated with a blood patch that prevents further CSF leakage. The patch is performed by injecting the patient's blood into the epidural space to form a clot over the dura. The patches are highly effective for resolving the headache, but many patients need to have the procedure repeated if the headache returns. As noted previously, however, a headache with fever post neuraxial anesthesia is suspicious for meningitis.

Postpartum Psychiatric Disorders

There are two primary categories of depressive mood disorders associated with pregnancy: postpartum blues and postpartum depression (also called postnatal depression). Postpartum psychosis is a rare postpartum disorder that affects a woman's sense of reality. Additionally, women may also experience posttraumatic stress disorder in the postpartum period.

Postpartum Blues

Postpartum blues is a transient, self-limiting mood disorder that starts within 2 or 3 days after delivery and resolves within 2 weeks. A woman experiencing symptoms attributed to postpartum blues for longer than 2 weeks should be assessed for postpartum depression. The symptoms of postpartum blues include insomnia, fatigue, dysphoria, and impaired concentration. Such symptoms can also occur with postpartum depression. What distinguishes the two is that postpartum depression is not self-limiting and has more stringent diagnostic criteria.

Postpartum Depression

Postpartum depression is defined as major depression with an onset during pregnancy or in the first 4 weeks after the birth (American Psychiatric Association, 2013). Alternative criteria extend the diagnosis to onsets as late as 6 weeks to a year after the birth (American College of Obstetricians and Gynecologists [ACOG], 2015; Postpartum Depression: Action Towards & Treatment, 2015; Viguera et al., 2011).

Prevalence

The differing diagnostic timelines make it more challenging to assess the prevalence of the condition, although it is estimated that 10% to 16% of women experience postpartum depression, with most of those reporting the onset of symptoms within a month after the birth (Gaillard, Le Strat, Mandelbrot, Keita, & Dubertret, 2014). Approximately half of women with depression postpartum experienced the onset of symptoms before or during pregnancy (Fisher et al., 2016).

Etiology

There are many risk factors for postpartum depression (Box 23.4). Postpartum depression may have its roots in genetic factors, hormonal changes, or other changes in brain function particular to pregnancy and the postpartum period.

Box 23.4 Risk Factors for Postpartum Depression

- History of depression (two times the normal risk)
- Depression in pregnancy (five times the normal risk)
- Postpartum blues
- Stressful events during or after pregnancy
- Low socioeconomic status
- Poor social support
- Age < 25 y
- Lack of a partner
- Multiple pregnancy
- Family history of mental illness
- Physical or sexual abuse, past or present
- Unplanned pregnancy
- Poor physical health
- Anxiety disorder
- Difficult infant temperament
- Body dysphoria
- History of premenstrual syndrome or premenstrual dysphoric disorder

Adapted from Gaillard, A., Le Strat, Y., Mandelbrot, L., Keita, H., & Dubertret, C. (2014). Predictors of postpartum depression: Prospective study of 264 women followed during pregnancy and postpartum. *Psychiatry Research, 215*(2), 341–346. doi:10.1016/j.psychres.2013.10.003; American College of Obstetricians and Gynecologists. (2015). The American College of Obstetricians and Gynecologists Committee Opinion no. 630. Screening for perinatal depression. *Obstetrics and Gynecology, 125*(5), 1268–1271. doi:10.1097/01.AOG.0000465192.34779.dc

Prognosis

Postpartum depression impedes a woman's ability to fully participate in her own care and the care of her offspring (Fig. 23.5). Women with postpartum depression are less likely to breastfeed and, if they do breastfeed, do so for shorter periods of time (Dias & Figueiredo, 2015). Mothers with this condition report feeling less bonded with their babies and having fewer positive interactions, such as reading and playing games (Tikotzky, 2016). Depressed mothers are less likely to engage in protective activities, such as placing infants on their backs to sleep, baby-proofing the home, using car seats safely, and vaccinating their children (Field, 2010). Women with postpartum depression are at a higher risk for developing the condition again with future pregnancies.

Studies have shown that the children of mothers with postpartum depression are more prone to accidents and other health issues, such as asthma and diabetes (Raposa, Hammen, Brennan, & Najman, 2014). The children are more likely to be small and underweight (Stein et al., 2014). There may be a small but measureable effect on the offspring's intelligence, executive functioning, and language development (Stein et al., 2014). Maternal depression has been associated with depression, anxiety, antisocial behavior, hyperactivity, and aggression in children (Herba, 2014; Stein et al., 2014).

Postpartum depression can strain other relationships, as well, including the one with the partner. Unions strained by postpartum depression are more likely to end in separation or divorce (Reichman, Corman, & Noonan, 2015). Depression is closely tied to suicidality, and women with postpartum depression may describe thoughts of self-harm, which should always be taken seriously and addressed proactively. However, although suicide is a leading cause of death

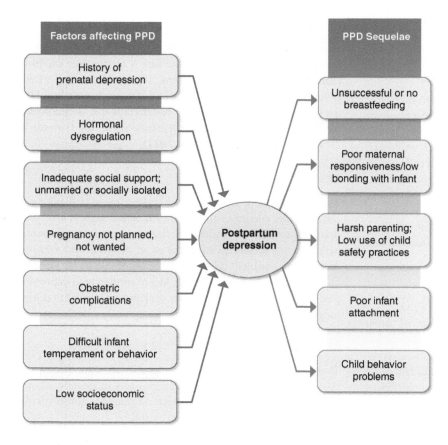

Figure 23.5. A conceptual model of postpartum depression (PPD). (Reprinted with permission from Polit, D. F., & Yang, F. M. [2016]. *Measurement and the measurement of change* [1st ed., Fig. 13.1]. Philadelphia, PA: Lippincott Williams & Wilkins.)

for women postpartum, the actual rate is approximately 1 out of 100,000 births, which amounts to a lower rate than for the general population (Khalifeh, Hunt, Appleby, & Howard, 2016).

In Chapter 12, Cara, the home health nurse caring for Loretta, suspected that Loretta might have postpartum depression. She knew that Loretta's lack of support at home could contribute to this condition. Loretta was worried that if she were diagnosed with postpartum depression, people would think that she was crazy and didn't love her baby.

Assessment

To be diagnosed with postpartum depression, a woman must meet at least five of the nine diagnostic criteria for major depressive disorder identified by the American Psychiatric Society during a 2-week period, with at least one of the symptoms being either a depressed mood or diminished pleasure in all or most activities. The reported symptoms must cause significant distress or impairment and cannot be caused by a different known condition. People with manic or hypomanic episodes are excluded from the diagnosis of a major depressive disorder (American Psychiatric Association, 2013). Somatic symptoms—such as changes in appetite, sleep, and energy level—are common in both depression and the postpartum period (ACOG, 2015).

A commonly used tool to screen for depression postpartum is the Edinburgh Postnatal Depression Scale, a 10-item survey (Cox, Holden, & Sagovsky, 1987). For this tool, clinicians may assess a score of 10, 12, or 13 as a positive screening (Wisner et al., 2013).

Routine screening for postpartum depression is done at the patient's postpartum office visit. Some pediatricians may also choose to administer screening to mothers of their pediatric patients during office visits, particularly if the mothers have declined follow-up care from their obstetric providers. Patients may be screened once or multiple times at different visits (ACOG, 2015). Evidence of the benefit of such screening, however, is limited (Thombs et al., 2014). Women who screen positive must be referred for further evaluation and treatment, ideally for services available immediately and on site. As few as 20% of women who screen positive for postpartum depression receive the recommended off-site care (Nelson, Freeman, Johnson, McIntire, & Leveno, 2013). Concerning signs for postpartum depression are summarized in Box 23.5.

Treatment

Like major depressive disorder, postpartum depression can be treated with medication and therapy.

Postpartum Psychosis

Postpartum psychosis is the disturbance of a woman's perception of reality postpartum as evidenced by hallucinations, thought disorganization, disorganized behavior, and delusions. It is a medical emergency.

Box 23.5 Warning Signs for Postpartum Depression

- Low mood for at least 2 wk
- Negative attitude toward the infant
- Little interest in the infant or infant activities
- Anxiety about the health of the infant
- Concern about the ability to care for the infant
- Use of alcohol, street drugs, drugs prescribed for others, or tobacco
- Noncompliance with recommended care
- Frequent off-schedule calls and/or visits to the healthcare provider

---

Prevalence

Postpartum psychosis diagnosis occurs in approximately 2 to 4 out of every 1,000 live births (Bergink, Rasgon, & Wisner, 2016).

Etiology

Postpartum psychosis is most common in women with bipolar disorder or who suffer from depression with schizophrenia, schizoaffective disorder, or psychosis. Fewer than 50% of women diagnosed with postpartum psychosis experience symptoms only in the postpartum period (Bergink et al., 2016; Wesseloo et al., 2016).

Prognosis

Postpartum depression is often confused with postpartum psychosis by the news media in cases of infanticide and erratic maternal behavior after a birth. Although women with postpartum depression may experience fantasies or invasive thoughts of harming their infant, they very rarely act on this impulse. In contrast, as many as 4.5% of infants born to women with postpartum psychosis are killed by their mothers either intentionally or as a result of the mother's confused and disordered behavior (Brockington, 2017). The risk for recurrence with future pregnancies is approximately 30% (Bergink et al., 2016).

Assessment

The condition may appear as soon as 48 hours after the delivery and almost always develops within the first few weeks after the birth. Psychosis manifests as bizarre behavior, confusion, hallucinations, delusions, and/or the appearance of delirium.

Treatment

The first priority in caring for a woman with postpartum psychosis is her safety and the safety of her infant. The woman is often hospitalized and isolated from the infant for its safety, which impairs bonding. The primary treatment for the disorder is antipsychotic medications as well as other treatment for underlying psychiatric disorders, such as bipolar disorder. Some women may benefit from psychotherapy in addition to medications. Women with mild or moderate disease on certain antipsychotics may be able to continue providing breast milk for their infant, either by direct nursing or by pumping.

Posttraumatic Stress Disorder

Posttraumatic stress disorder (PTSD) is a mental health disorder characterized by negative cognition and mood changes, intrusive thoughts or memories, avoidance, and a state of hyperarousal in response to a traumatic trigger (American Psychiatric Association, 2013).

Etiology

The initial trigger for PTSD may be injury, violence, or an actual or perceived threat of death or serious harm. The risk factors for PTSD after a birth include issues preceding the pregnancy, such as anxiety or sexual abuse, antepartum issues, such as poor support and pregnancy-induced illness, and delivery events, such as emergency cesarean section or severe laceration (Wilson, Sikkema, Watt, & Masenga, 2015). Women may also develop PTSD as a reaction to a spontaneous or induced pregnancy loss, particularly in the case of women who aborted electively because of fetal anomalies (Daugirdaite, van den Akker, & Purewal, 2015).

Prognosis

PTSD resulting from sexual trauma may be triggered throughout pregnancy, labor, and the postpartum period (Montgomery, Pope, & Rogers, 2015). Women with a diagnosis of PTSD are far more likely to give birth preterm spontaneously (Shaw et al., 2014). During labor and other times of high stress, women with PTSD are particularly subject to dissociation (a mental removal from the immediate reality; Lev-Wiesel, Daphna-Tekoah, & Hallak, 2009). Patients may request an elective cesarean section because of intense anxiety about birth resulting from PTSD.

Postpartum, women with PTSD may have difficulty bonding with the infant (Lev-Wiesel et al., 2009).

Assessment

A common screening tool for PTSD is the five-item Primary Care PTSD Screen for *DSM-5* (PC-PTSD-5) (https://www.ptsd.va.gov/professional/assessment/documents/pc-ptsd5-screen.pdf). Answering "yes" to any three items is considered a positive finding. Patients who screen positive are referred for further assessment and treatment.

Treatment

Treatment includes both medications and therapy.

Care Considerations

Limiting the number of care providers, examinations, and interventions can help minimize stress for women with PTSD, as can identifying each care provider's role and the purpose of each examination and procedure meticulously. Permission asking is also helpful in lessening the anxiety of a patient with PTSD. Nurses should keep in mind the four Rs of trauma when planning care (Box 23.6).

Box 23.6 The Four Rs of Providing Care After Trauma

1. *Realize* the widespread impact of trauma
2. *Recognize* the signs and symptoms of trauma
3. *Respond* by integrating knowledge about trauma into practice
4. *Resist* retraumatization

From Substance Abuse and Mental Health Services Administration. SAMHSA's efforts to address trauma and violence. Retrieved from https://www.samhsa.gov/nctic/trauma-interventions.

Think Critically

1. You are caring for a patient who gave birth an hour ago. While performing a routine assessment, you note she is bleeding heavily. What are your first steps?
2. Your patient develops a DVT postpartum. She asks you why this happened. How do you explain to her why women are more likely to get a DVT postpartum and what factors make them particularly susceptible?
3. Your patient is recovering from a recent cesarean section. She can ambulate sufficiently to use the bathroom unassisted and has had the compression devices removed from her legs. You'd like her to ambulate in the hall, but she's resistant. How would you explain to her the importance of ambulation?

4. A month after she's given birth, a patient calls the midwifery office where you work complaining of a hard, red area on one breast that appeared that morning. What diagnosis do you anticipate? What are the initial interventions? What's next if that doesn't work?
5. Your postpartum patient complains of a headache. What are some important questions to ask her? What assessments should you perform? What information could you review in her chart that might be helpful?
6. You strongly suspect that a patient you are working with is suffering from postpartum depression. She expresses a reluctance to be screened. What kinds of questions would be important to ask?

References

Abdul-Kadir, R., McLintock, C., Ducloy, A. S., El-Refaey, H., England, A., Federici, A. B., . . . Winikoff, R. (2014). Evaluation and management of postpartum hemorrhage: Consensus from an international expert panel. *Transfusion, 54*(7), 1756–1768. doi:10.1111/trf.12550

Abdul Sultan, A., West, J., Tata, L. J., Fleming, K. M., Nelson-Piercy, C., & Grainge, M. J. (2013). Risk of first venous thromboembolism in pregnant women in hospital: Population based cohort study from England. *BMJ, 347,* f6099. doi:10.1136/bmj.f6099

American College of Obstetricians and Gynecologists. (2015). The American College of Obstetricians and Gynecologists Committee Opinion no. 630. Screening for perinatal depression. *Obstetrics and Gynecology, 125*(5), 1268–1271. doi:10.1097/01.AOG.0000465192.34779.dc

American Psychiatric Association. (2013). *Diagnostic and statistical manual of mental disorders: DSM-5* (5th ed.). Arlington, VA: American Psychiatric Association.

Bergink, V., Rasgon, N., & Wisner, K. L. (2016). Postpartum psychosis: Madness, mania, and melancholia in motherhood. *American Journal of Psychiatry, 173*(12), 1179–1188. doi:10.1176/appi.ajp.2016.16040454

British Journal of Obstetrics and Gynaecology. (2017). Prevention and management of postpartum haemorrhage: Green-top guideline no. 52. *British Journal of Obstetrics and Gynaecology, 124*(5), e106–e149. doi:10.1111/1471-0528.14178

Brockington, I. (2017). Suicide and filicide in postpartum psychosis. *Archives of Women's Mental Health, 20*(1), 63–69. doi:10.1007/s00737-016-0675-8

Care, A., Pavord, S., Knight, M., & Alfirevic, Z. (2017). Severe primary autoimmune thrombocytopenia in pregnancy: A national cohort study. *British Journal of Obstetrics and Gynaecology.* doi:10.1111/1471-0528.14697

Carson, J. L., Guyatt, G., Heddle, N. M., Grossman, B. J., Cohn, C. S., Fung, M. K., . . . Tobian, A. A. (2016). Clinical practice guidelines from the AABB: Red blood cell transfusion thresholds and storage. *JAMA, 316*(19), 2025–2035. doi:10.1001/jama.2016.9185

Carter, E. B., Temming, L. A., Fowler, S., Eppes, C., Gross, G., Srinivas, S. K., . . . Tuuli, M. G. (2017). Evidence-based bundles and cesarean delivery surgical site infections: A systematic review and meta-analysis. *Obstetrics and Gynecology, 130*(4), 735–746. doi:10.1097/AOG.0000000000002249

Centers for Disease Control and Prevention. (2017). *Pregnancy mortality surveillance system.* Retrieved from https://www.cdc.gov/reproductivehealth/maternalinfanthealth/pmss.html

Cheng, C. A., Lee, J. T., Lin, H. C., Lin, H. C., Chung, C. H., Lin, F. H., . . . Chiu, H. W. (2017). Pregnancy increases stroke risk up to 1 year postpartum and reduces long-term risk. *Monthly Journal of the Association of Physicians, 110*(6), 355–360. doi:10.1093/qjmed/hcw222

Cox, J. L., Holden, J. M., & Sagovsky, R. (1987). Detection of postnatal depression. Development of the 10-item Edinburgh Postnatal Depression Scale. *British Journal of Psychiatry, 150,* 782–786.

Daugirdaite, V., van den Akker, O., & Purewal, S. (2015). Posttraumatic stress and posttraumatic stress disorder after termination of pregnancy and reproductive loss: A systematic review. *Journal of Pregnancy, 2015,* 646345. doi:10.1155/2015/646345

Deneux-Tharaux, C., Sentilhes, L., Maillard, F., Closset, E., Vardon, D., Lepercq, J., & Goffinet, F. (2013). Effect of routine controlled cord traction as part of the active management of the third stage of labour on postpartum haemorrhage: Multicentre randomised controlled trial (TRACOR). *BMJ, 346,* f1541. doi:10.1136/bmj.f1541

Dias, C. C., & Figueiredo, B. (2015). Breastfeeding and depression: A systematic review of the literature. *Journal of Affective Disorders, 171,* 142–154. doi:10.1016/j.jad.2014.09.022

Dossou, M., Debost-Legrand, A., Dechelotte, P., Lemery, D., & Vendittelli, F. (2015). Severe secondary postpartum hemorrhage: A historical cohort. *Birth, 42*(2), 149–155. doi:10.1111/birt.12164

Field, T. (2010). Postpartum depression effects on early interactions, parenting, and safety practices: A review. *Infant Behavior and Development, 33*(1), 1–6. doi:10.1016/j.infbeh.2009.10.005

Fisher, S. D., Wisner, K. L., Clark, C. T., Sit, D. K., Luther, J. F., & Wisniewski, S. (2016). Factors associated with onset timing, symptoms, and severity of depression identified in the postpartum period. *Journal of Affective Disorders, 203,* 111–120. doi:10.1016/j.jad.2016.05.063

Fugate, J. E., Ameriso, S. F., Ortiz, G., Schottlaender, L. V., Wijdicks, E. F., Flemming, K. D., & Rabinstein, A. A. (2012). Variable presentations of postpartum angiopathy. *Stroke, 43*(3), 670–676. doi:10.1161/STROKEAHA.111.639575

Gaillard, A., Le Strat, Y., Mandelbrot, L., Keita, H., & Dubertret, C. (2014). Predictors of postpartum depression: Prospective study of 264 women followed during pregnancy and postpartum. *Psychiatry Research, 215*(2), 341–346. doi:10.1016/j.psychres.2013.10.003

Govorov, I., Lofgren, S., Chaireti, R., Holmstrom, M., Bremme, K., & Mints, M. (2016). Postpartum hemorrhage in women with Von Willebrand disease—A retrospective observational study. *PLoS One, 11*(10), e0164683. doi:10.1371/journal.pone.0164683

Gurtovaya, Y., Hanna, H., & Wagley, A. (2013). Spontaneous intrapartum vulvar haematoma. *Midwives, 16*(5), 48–49.

Herba, C. M. (2014). Maternal depression and child behavioural outcomes. *Lancet Psychiatry, 1*(6), 408–409. doi:10.1016/S2215-0366(14)70375-X

Horner, D., Hogg, K., Body, R., Nash, M. J., Baglin, T., & Mackway-Jones, K. (2014). The anticoagulation of calf thrombosis (ACT) project: Results from the randomized controlled external pilot trial. *Chest, 146*(6), 1468–1477. doi:10.1378/chest.14-0235

Iskender, C., Topcu, H. O., Timur, H., Oskovi, A., Goksu, G., Sucak, A., & Danisman, N. (2016). Evaluation of risk factors in women with puerperal genital hematomas. *Journal of Maternal-Fetal and Neonatal Medicine, 29*(9), 1435–1439. doi:10.3109/14767058.2015.1051018

Jallad, K., Steele, S. E., & Barber, M. D. (2016). Breakdown of perineal laceration repair after vaginal delivery: A case-control study. *Female Pelvic Medicine and Reconstructive Surgery, 22*(4), 276–279. doi:10.1097/SPV.0000000000000274

Kahn, S. R., Shapiro, S., & Ginsberg, J. S.; SOX Trial Investigators. (2014). Compression stockings to prevent post-thrombotic syndrome—Authors' reply. *The Lancet, 384*(9938), 130–131. doi:10.1016/S0140-6736(14)61160-0

Kamel, H., Navi, B. B., Sriram, N., Hovsepian, D. A., Devereux, R. B., & Elkind, M. S. (2014). Risk of a thrombotic event after the 6-week postpartum period. *New England Journal of Medicine, 370*(14), 1307–1315. doi:10.1056/NEJMoa1311485

Kearon, C., Akl, E. A., Ornelas, J., Blaivas, A., Jimenez, D., Bounameaux, H., . . . Moores, L. (2016). Antithrombotic therapy for VTE disease: CHEST guideline and expert panel report. *Chest, 149*(2), 315–352. doi:10.1016/j.chest.2015.11.026

Khalifeh, H., Hunt, I. M., Appleby, L., & Howard, L. M. (2016). Suicide in perinatal and non-perinatal women in contact with psychiatric services: 15 year findings from a UK national inquiry. *Lancet Psychiatry, 3*(3), 233–242. doi:10.1016/S2215-0366(16)00003-1

Leebeek, F. W., & Eikenboom, J. C. (2016). Von Willebrand's disease. *New England Journal of Medicine, 375*(21), 2067–2080. doi:10.1056/NEJMra1601561

Lev-Wiesel, R., Daphna-Tekoah, S., & Hallak, M. (2009). Childhood sexual abuse as a predictor of birth-related posttraumatic stress and postpartum posttraumatic stress. *Child Abuse and Neglect, 33*(12), 877–887. doi:10.1016/j.chiabu.2009.05.004

Lewicky-Gaupp, C., Leader-Cramer, A., Johnson, L. L., Kenton, K., & Gossett, D. R. (2015). Wound complications after obstetric anal sphincter injuries. *Obstetrics and Gynecology, 125*(5), 1088–1093. doi:10.1097/AOG.0000000000000833

Mackeen, A. D., Packard, R. E., Ota, E., & Speer, L. (2015). Antibiotic regimens for postpartum endometritis. *Cochrane Database of Systematic Reviews,* (2), CD001067. doi:10.1002/14651858.CD001067.pub3

Marshall, A. L., Durani, U., Bartley, A., Hagen, C. E., Ashrani, A., Rose, C., . . . Pruthi, R. K. (2017). The impact of postpartum hemorrhage on hospital length of stay and inpatient mortality: A National Inpatient Sample-based analysis. *American Journal of Obstetrics and Gynecology, 217*(3), 344.e1–344.e6. doi:10.1016/j.ajog.2017.05.004

Montgomery, E., Pope, C., & Rogers, J. (2015). The re-enactment of childhood sexual abuse in maternity care: A qualitative study. *BMC Pregnancy and Childbirth, 15,* 194. doi:10.1186/s12884-015-0626-9

Moulis, G., Palmaro, A., Montastruc, J. L., Godeau, B., Lapeyre-Mestre, M., & Sailler, L. (2014). Epidemiology of incident immune thrombocytopenia: A nationwide population-based study in France. *Blood, 124*(22), 3308–3315. doi:10.1182/blood-2014-05-578336

Nelson, D. B., Freeman, M. P., Johnson, N. L., McIntire, D. D., & Leveno, K. J. (2013). A prospective study of postpartum depression in 17 648 parturients. *Journal of Maternal-Fetal and Neonatal Medicine, 26*(12), 1155–1161. doi:10.3109/14767058.2013.777698

Oberg, A. S., Hernandez-Diaz, S., Palmsten, K., Almqvist, C., & Bateman, B. T. (2014). Patterns of recurrence of postpartum hemorrhage in a large population-based cohort. *American Journal of Obstetrics and Gynecology, 210*(3), 229.e1–229.e8. doi:10.1016/j.ajog.2013.10.872

Parilla, B. V., Fournogerakis, R., Archer, A., Sulo, S., Laurent, L., Lee, P., . . . Kulstad, E. (2016). Diagnosing pulmonary embolism in pregnancy: Are biomarkers and clinical predictive models useful? *AJP Reports, 6*(2), e160–e164. doi:10.1055/s-0036-1582136

Pauleta, J. R., Rodrigues, R., Melo, M. A., & Graca, L. M. (2010). Ultrasonographic diagnosis of incomplete uterine inversion. *Ultrasound in Obstetrics and Gynecology, 36*(2), 260–261. doi:10.1002/uog.7735

Pitkanen, M. T., Aromaa, U., Cozanitis, D. A., & Forster, J. G. (2013). Serious complications associated with spinal and epidural anaesthesia in Finland from 2000 to 2009. *Acta Anaesthesiologica Scandinavica, 57*(5), 553–564. doi:10.1111/aas.12064

Postpartum Depression: Action Towards Causes and Treatment (PACT) Consortium. (2015). Heterogeneity of postpartum depression: A latent class analysis. *Lancet Psychiatry, 2*(1), 59–67. doi:10.1016/S2215-0366(14)00055-8

Raposa, E., Hammen, C., Brennan, P., & Najman, J. (2014). The long-term effects of maternal depression: Early childhood physical health as a pathway to offspring depression. *Journal of Adolescent Health, 54*(1), 88–93. doi:10.1016/j.jadohealth.2013.07.038

Reichman, N. E., Corman, H. & Noonan, K. (2015). Effects of maternal depression on couple relationship status. *Review of Economics of the Household, 13*, 929. doi:10.1007/s11150-013-9237-2

Shaw, J. G., Asch, S. M., Kimerling, R., Frayne, S. M., Shaw, K. A., & Phibbs, C. S. (2014). Posttraumatic stress disorder and risk of spontaneous preterm birth. *Obstetrics and Gynecology, 124*(6), 1111–1119. doi:10.1097/AOG.0000000000000542

Stein, A., Pearson, R. M., Goodman, S. H., Rapa, E., Rahman, A., McCallum, M., . . . Pariante, C. M. (2014). Effects of perinatal mental disorders on the fetus and child. *The Lancet, 384*(9956), 1800–1819. doi:10.1016/S0140-6736(14)61277-0

Temming, L. A., Raghuraman, N., Carter, E. B., Stout, M. J., Rampersad, R. M., Macones, G. A., . . . Tuuli, M. G. (2017). Impact of evidence-based interventions on wound complications after cesarean delivery. *American Journal of Obstetrics and Gynecology, 217*(4), 449.e1–449.e9. doi:10.1016/j.ajog.2017.05.070

Tepper, N. K., Boulet, S. L., Whiteman, M. K., Monsour, M., Marchbanks, P. A., Hooper, W. C., & Curtis, K. M. (2014). Postpartum venous thromboembolism: Incidence and risk factors. *Obstetrics and Gynecology, 123*(5), 987–996. doi:10.1097/AOG.0000000000000230

Thombs, B. D., Arthurs, E., Coronado-Montoya, S., Roseman, M., Delisle, V. C., Leavens, A., . . . Zelkowitz, P. (2014). Depression screening and patient outcomes in pregnancy or postpartum: A systematic review. *Journal of Psychosomatic Research, 76*(6), 433–446. doi:10.1016/j.jpsychores.2014.01.006

Tikotzky, L. (2016). Postpartum maternal sleep, maternal depressive symptoms and self-perceived mother-infant emotional relationship. *Behavioral Sleep Medicine, 14*(1), 5–22. doi:10.1080/15402002.2014.940111

Viguera, A. C., Tondo, L., Koukopoulos, A. E., Reginaldi, D., Lepri, B., & Baldessarini, R. J. (2011). Episodes of mood disorders in 2,252 pregnancies and postpartum periods. *American Journal of Psychiatry, 168*(11), 1179–1185. doi:10.1176/appi.ajp.2011.11010148

Wesseloo, R., Kamperman, A. M., Munk-Olsen, T., Pop, V. J., Kushner, S. A., & Bergink, V. (2016). Risk of postpartum relapse in bipolar disorder and postpartum psychosis: A systematic review and meta-analysis. *American Journal of Psychiatry, 173*(2), 117–127. doi:10.1176/appi.ajp.2015.15010124

Wilson, S. M., Sikkema, K. J., Watt, M. H., & Masenga, G. G. (2015). Psychological symptoms among obstetric fistula patients compared to gynecology outpatients in Tanzania. *International Journal of Behavioral Medicine, 22*(5), 605–613. doi:10.1007/s12529-015-9466-2

Wisner, K. L., Sit, D. K., McShea, M. C., Rizzo, D. M., Zoretich, R. A., Hughes, C. L., . . . Hanusa, B. H. (2013). Onset timing, thoughts of self-harm, and diagnoses in postpartum women with screen-positive depression findings. *JAMA Psychiatry, 70*(5), 490–498. doi:10.1001/jamapsychiatry.2013.87

Witteveen, T., van Stralen, G., Zwart, J., & van Roosmalen, J. (2013). Puerperal uterine inversion in the Netherlands: A nationwide cohort study. *Acta Obstetricia et Gynecologica Scandinavica, 92*(3), 334–337. doi:10.1111/j.1600-0412.2012.01514.x

Suggested Readings

PTSD: National Center for PTSD. Retrieved from http://www.ptsd.va.gov

Suplee, P. D., Kleppel, L., Santa-Donato, A., & Bingham, D. (2017). Improving postpartum education about warning signs of maternal morbidity and mortality. *Nursing for Women's Health, 20*(6), 552–567. doi:10.1016/j.nwh.2016.10.009

The Postpartum Hemorrhage Project. Retrieved from https://www.awhonn.org/?page=PPH

24

Conditions in the Newborn Related to Gestational Age, Size, Injury, and Pain

Objectives

1. Describe the purpose and placement of the different tubes, catheters, and other lines used to provide intensive care to neonates.
2. Identify the physiologic differences in preterm infants compared with term infants and the corresponding variations in care that are required.
3. Compare the different methods of feeding of the neonate and discuss the indications and considerations for each method.
4. Explain the potential implications and care considerations for late preterm and postterm infants, particularly related to fetal growth restriction and macrosomia.
5. Identify the causes and implications of select birth injuries.
6. Discuss the different causes of neonatal pain and how to identify, prevent, and treat this pain.

Key Terms

Apnea
Circumoral
Continuous positive airway pressure (CPAP)
Enteral tube feeding
Extracorporeal membrane oxygenation (ECMO)
Fetal growth restriction (FGR)
Germinal matrix
Impedance pneumography
Infant mortality rate
Intraventricular hemorrhage (IVH)
Large for gestational age (LGA)
Macrosomia

Neonatal death
Nonnutritive sucking (NNS)
Parenteral feeding
Patent ductus arteriosus (PDA)
Periventricular leukomalacia
Persistent pulmonary hypertension of the neonate (PPHN)
Postneonatal death
Postterm infant
Preterm infant
Respiratory distress syndrome (RDS)
Small for gestational age (SGA)

Conditions in the newborn related to gestational age can have a significant impact on mortality. The United States ranks 30th worldwide in terms of lowest infant mortality rate, largely because of the high rate of infants born prematurely. In contrast to Japan's infant mortality rate of 2.2 deaths per 1,000 live births, the rate in the United States was 6.2 deaths per 1,000 live births in 2012,

down from 9 deaths per 1,000 live births in 1990. Notably, the infant mortality rate is 2.3 times higher for African American infants than for American infants of European descent (Osterman, Kochanek, MacDorman, Strobino, & Guyer, 2015).

Infant mortality rate refers to the number of infants per 1,000 born live who die within the first year of life. A **neonatal death**

refers to the death of an infant within the first 28 days after birth. Postneonatal death refers to the death of an infant that occurs from 29 days to 1 year after birth. In the United States, complications of low birth weight or prematurity accounts for 18% of infant deaths (Osterman et al., 2015). Among infants born at term, the leading causes of death are asphyxia and infection in the first 28 days after birth (neonatal deaths) and sudden infant death syndrome in the postneonatal period. In the United States, only 2% of infants are born prior to 32 weeks of gestation, but these infants account for up to one half of infant deaths (Osterman et al., 2015).

Note that the term "postmenstrual age" is often used to describe the age of a preterm infant in relation to gestational age. For example, a 2-week-old infant born at 32 weeks of gestation would have a postmenstrual age of 34 weeks. A 4-week-old infant born at 26 weeks would have a postmenstrual age of 30 weeks.

Birth size also significantly affects infant mortality. Infants born weighing less than 500 g have a 15% chance of surviving their first year (Matthews, MacDorman, & Thoma, 2015), and low birth weight is the single greatest cause of infant, child, and adolescent mortality worldwide (Watkins, Kotecha, & Kotecha, 2016).

After presenting tubes, vents, and other equipment used to manage the care of preterm and critically ill newborns, this chapter covers conditions in the newborn and associated care considerations related to gestational age, size, injury, and pain.

Tubes, Vents, and Environment

The neonatal intensive care unit (NICU) can be an intimidating place for healthcare providers and for parents. Nurses can help allay the anxiety of those new to the unit by explaining what all of the machinery does and what the lines, tubes, and vents are for. In addition, oxygenation for neonates is often improved when they are in the prone position, so children may be positioned lying on their fronts (prone) rather than their backs (supine; Gillies, Wells, & Bhandari, 2012). Because contemporary infant care guidelines warn caregivers to place infants on their backs to sleep to reduce the risk for sudden infant death syndrome, this prone positioning for ventilation may seem to them like irresponsible care. The nurse should reassure families that infant respirations, oxygenation, and blood oxygen levels are carefully monitored during hospitalization, thereby reducing the risk for sudden infant death syndrome. However, the nurse should also instruct families after discharge to place infants in the supine position for sleep unless otherwise indicated.

In Chapter 10, recall that a neonatal nurse practitioner, Eric, was careful to explain to Lexi and Joe Cowslip about the lines, tubes, and other equipment that would be used to care for their preterm newborn in the NICU.

Environment

The NICU is often organized as a single room, an open bay. Such a design allows for a rapid response to crisis and facilitates

collaboration and communication. Unfortunately, when the NICU is filled with many monitors, care providers, patients, and families, this design also contributes to increased light and noise (Meredith, Jnah, & Newberry, 2017). A newer organization of the NICU, often called the single-family unit (SFU), allows for care of each neonate and family in a room isolated from the cumulative sound and lights required by others. The SFU model is associated with better weight gain, fewer medical procedures, better feeding, less sepsis, better infant engagement, less physiologic stress, less lethargy, and less pain. Nurses report a better working environment and more positive staff attitudes with the SFU model (Lester et al., 2014).

Although not well studied, sound reduction by the use of earplugs in infants in the NICU may improve weight gain and mental development for infants (Almadhoob & Ohlsson, 2015). Likewise, on the basis of some small studies, diurnal cycling of the light in the unit, rather than keeping it continuously dimmed or bright, is associated with improved weight gain, less retinopathy of prematurity (ROP), and less crying (Morag & Ohlsson, 2016).

Nasogastric Tube

The nasogastric (NG) tube is used for feeding as well as for suction of the gastric contents. The tube is inserted through one of the nares and into the stomach. Because a misplaced NG tube poses a risk of aspiration, the nurse should measure the anticipated length of the tube necessary to reach the stomach prior to placing it and then advance the tube to that mark (Fig. 24.1). The nurse should then verify the mark in relation to the nares prior to each feeding. The nurse may also verify placement by aspirating fluids and checking for color and pH. Gastric aspirate has an anticipated pH of 1 to 4. NG tube placement is sometimes verified by forcing air into the tube while auscultating the stomach, although this is not a particularly accurate method. Imaging to confirm NG tube placement remains the most accurate method but is also the most expensive. Usually, multiple means of confirmation are used. The nurse should verify NG tube placement prior to each feeding or administration of medication and check it at least every 8 hours if in continuous use. However, some providers

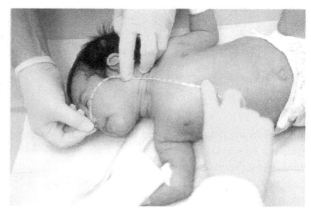

Figure 24.1. Measurement of a nasogastric tube prior to placement. (Reprinted with permission from Lippincott's Nursing Procedures and Skills 2009.)

prefer orogastric tubes, which start in the mouth rather than the nose, to avoid occlusion of the nares and to allow for nasal respiratory support. Some infants may tolerate a gastric tube in one location but not another.

Umbilical Artery Catheter

The umbilical artery catheter (UAC) is placed directly into the stump of the umbilical cord (Fig. 24.2). It is threaded through one of the two umbilical arteries and into the aorta. The UAC is used to monitor the arterial blood pressure and arterial blood gases and for angiography (examination of blood vessels). It can also provide ready access to the circulation for blood sampling and fluid and medication administration. It may be used for exchange transfusion when the blood of the neonate must be removed and replaced by donor blood. It is rarely left in place past the first week after birth. Placement of the line is confirmed by radiology.

Umbilical Vein Catheter

The umbilical vein catheter is placed in the vein of the umbilical stump and progressed through the ductus venosus, into the hepatic

vein, and finally into the inferior caval vein (Fig. 24.2). The tip of the catheter should be at the level of the diaphragm, as confirmed by radiology. Like the umbilical vein catheter, it can remain in place for about a week after the birth. It can be used for fluid and medication administration and exchange transfusion. It may also be used for central pressure monitoring.

Peripherally Inserted Central Catheter

A peripherally inserted central catheter (PICC) is used when intermediate-term intravenous (IV) access is required. This type of catheter also allows for central pressure monitoring. The PICC is typically placed in the cephalic vein of the arm or in the saphenous vein of the leg, and ports can be accessed at these locations. The terminal tip is located in a large central vein, as confirmed by imaging.

Nasal Cannula

Low-flow continuous oxygenation can be obtained by nasal cannula (Fig. 24.3). This method of oxygenation support is more common for the older infant. The cannula may remain in place

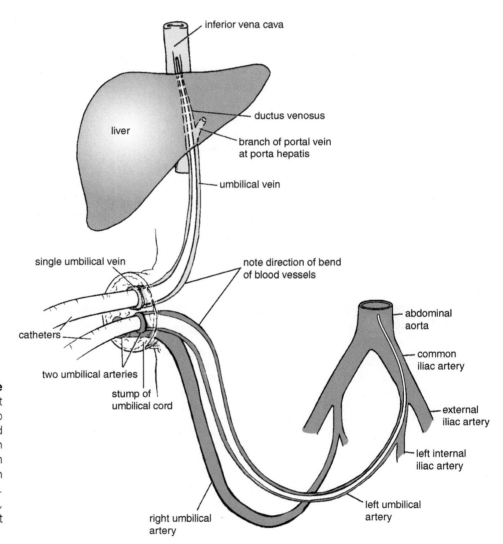

Figure 24.2. Catheterization of the umbilical blood vessels. Arrangement of the single umbilical vein and the two umbilical arteries in the umbilical cord and the paths taken by the catheter in the umbilical vein and the catheter in the umbilical artery. (Reprinted with permission from Snell, R. S. [2012]. *Clinical anatomy by regions* [9th ed., Fig. 4-39]. Philadelphia, PA: Lippincott Williams & Wilkins.)

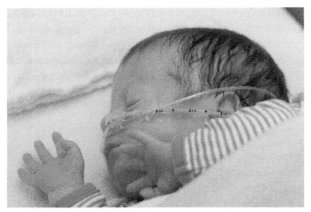

Figure 24.3. Nasal cannula. (Reprinted with permission from Evans, R. J., Brown, Y. M., & Evans, M. K. [2014]. *Canadian maternity, newborn, and women's health nursing* [2nd ed., Fig. 22.2]. Philadelphia, PA: Lippincott Williams & Wilkins.)

through feedings and allows for superior visualization of the baby's face when compared with other methods. Nasal cannulas may be occluded by secretions and should be inspected and cleaned regularly. Nasal cannulas are available in different sizes, and optimal sizing is important.

Continuous Positive Airway Pressure Therapy

Continuous positive airway pressure (CPAP) therapy is useful for infants unable to obtain adequate oxygenation by nasal cannula alone. CPAP for infants may be delivered by nasal prongs or by a mask that covers the nose. The constant airflow provided by the device helps keep the alveoli open, improving functional residual capacity. This also helps reduce pulmonary shunting, a condition in which the alveoli are well perfused with blood on one side but poorly ventilated on the other side, inhibiting gas exchange. CPAP is associated with less treatment harm than mechanical ventilation (Ho, Subramaniam, & Davis, 2015).

Endotracheal Tube

The endotracheal tube (ET) may be placed through one of the nares or the mouth of the infant. The process of tube placement

is referred to as intubation. The ET tube provides direct oxygen support to the lungs but is associated with a greater risk of treatment damage than less invasive methods. The ET is attached by tubing to a ventilator. The ventilator is set according to the needs of the infant. It may provide full breathing in the absence of spontaneous respiration or oxygen and pressure support in the event of spontaneous respirations (Table 24.1).

Oxygen Hood

An oxygen hood is an appropriate choice for infants who do not require supplemental pressure support (Fig. 24.4). The oxygen enters the hood through a gas inlet. The nurse should check the oxygen levels of the neonate hourly or according to orders and institution protocols. If the infant is removed from the hood for feeding or other care, oxygen should be provided by an alternate method, such as nasal cannula.

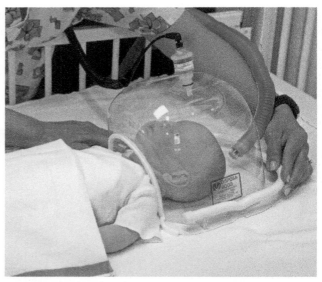

Figure 24.4. Oxygen hood. (Reprinted with permission from Lynn, P. [2015]. *Taylor's clinical nursing skills: A nursing process approach* [4th ed., unnumbered figure in Skill Variation box in Chapter 14]. Philadelphia, PA: Lippincott Williams & Wilkins.)

Table 24.1 Assisted Ventilation by Intubation Methods

Method	Description
Synchronized (patient-triggered) intermittent mandatory ventilation	• Ventilator-delivered breaths synchronized with spontaneous breathing • May improve comfort • May be set for full or partial synchronization
Pressure-limited ventilation	Inspiratory time and pressure preset by the clinician
Volume-targeted ventilation	Volume delivered varies per breath to achieve a particular tidal volume set by the clinician
High-frequency ventilation	Small volumes of gas delivered at 300–1,500 breaths/min to maintain lung expansion while contributing to the tidal volumes

Preterm Infants

A **preterm infant** is an infant born prior to 37 weeks of gestation. In the United States, approximately 11.6% of births occur prior to 37 weeks of gestation and 3.4% occur prior to 34 weeks (Osterman et al., 2015). Since 1990, there has been a 21% increase on average in the birth weight of preterm neonates, although the overall rate has dropped from a peak of 12.8% in 2006. Multiple gestation pregnancies resulting from artificial reproductive technology and advanced maternal age are thought to be important reasons for the high rate of preterm births, as half of twin pregnancies and over 90% of triplet pregnancies are born prematurely (Osterman et al., 2015).

You probably recall that Lexi Cowslip, in Chapter 10, was considered to be of advanced maternal age. Her age was likely a factor contributing to her preterm birth.

Birth weight and gestation age are often related, but each factor independently plays an important predictive role. The mortality rate is 2.1 per 1,000 live births for infants weighing over 2,500 g (5.5 lb) compared with 853 per 1,000 live births for those weighing under 500 g (1.1 lb). The mortality rate is 1.75 per 1,000 live births for infants born at 40 weeks and 374.74 per 1,000 live births for infants born before 28 weeks of gestation (Matthews et al., 2015).

Nursing care is carried out according to the specific needs of the infant, although classification by gestation age and size can be predictive (Table 24.2; see Fig. 1.16). Infants born prior to term are at particular risk for breathing problems, including **respiratory distress syndrome (RDS)** and bronchopulmonary dysplasia (BPD), as well as necrotizing enterocolitis (NEC), ROP, and **intraventricular hemorrhage (IVH)** and periventricular hemorrhage. Infants may be smaller because of gestational age or genetics, but also because of intrauterine growth restriction, reflecting placental insufficiency or maternal illness, malnutrition, or drug use.

Table 24.2 Terminology Related to Gestational Age and Size

Term	Meaning
Gestational Age at Birth	
Preterm (or premature)	Birth prior to 37 wk of gestation
Extremely preterm	Birth prior to 28 wk of gestation
Very preterm	Birth from 28 to 31 6/7 wk of gestation
Moderate-to-late preterm	Birth from 32 to 36 6/7 wk of gestation
Late preterm*	Birth from 34 to 36 6/7 wk of gestation
Early term	Birth from 37 to 38 6/7 wk of gestation
Full term	Birth from 39 to 40 6/7 wk of gestation
Late term	Birth from 41 to 41 6/7 wk of gestation
Postterm (or postmature)	Birth at 42 wk of gestation or later
Birth Weight, Regardless of Gestational Age at Birth	
Low	Birth weight less than 2,500 g (5.5 lb)
Very low	Birth weight less than 1,500 g (3.3 lb)
Extremely low	Birth weight less than 1,000 g (2.2 lb)
Size for Gestational Age (see Fig. 1.16)	
Appropriate	Weight from 10% to 90% on a growth chart
Small	Weight less than 10% on a growth chart
Large	Weight greater than 90% on a growth chart

(continued)

Table 24.2 Terminology Related to Gestational Age and Size (continued)	
Term	**Meaning**
IUGR	
Symmetric	• IUGR that is global: the head, torso, and extremities are symmetrically undersized • Also called global growth restriction • Indicates that growth has been slow throughout pregnancy • Associated with a higher incidence of permanent neurologic problems
Asymmetric	• IUGR in which the head grows normally but the body grows slowly • Slowed growth of the body typically occurs in the third trimester, after normal growth in the first two

*Term use varies among organizations.
IUGR, intrauterine growth restriction.
Adapted from Hamilton, B. E., Martin, J. A., Osterman, M. J., Curtin, S. C., & Matthews, T. J. (2015). Births: Final data for 2014. *National Vital Statistics Reports, 64*(12), 1–64.

Over time, the survivability of prematurity has improved because of modifications in care provided. The first infant incubators went into regular use at the turn of the 20th century (Perry, 2017). Since then, maternal perinatal steroid treatment, oxygen therapy, surfactant, and nutrition therapy have all helped revolutionize the care of preterm newborns. The care is not without a price, however. NICU costs for infants born prematurely add up to billions of dollars annually. Complications relating to prematurity can be lifelong.

Variations in Physiologic Function and Care Considerations

Preterm infants experience variations in physiologic function because of their lack of development, which require special care, as is discussed in this section.

Respiratory

The final stage of lung development in the fetus is the saccular stage, during which the alveoli form and mature. Primitive alveoli begin to appear at approximately 24 weeks of gestation, and mature, functional alveoli are not present until after 32 weeks of gestation. A term infant is born with approximately 50 to 150 million alveoli, whereas the preterm infant has fewer in accordance with the degree of prematurity.

Pulmonary surfactant lines the alveoli and reduces surface tension, thus making it less possible for the alveoli to collapse and facilitating alveoli expansion and gas exchange. Surfactant is created starting at approximately 20 weeks of gestation. In premature infants, both the amount and the quality of surfactant are decreased.

Additional aspects of prematurity that may contribute to inadequate respiratory function are lumen size and the lack of a gag reflex. The smaller lumens of the respiratory system (trachea, bronchi, bronchioles) characteristic of preterm infants lead to diminished gas exchange and a greater susceptibility to collapse. Because of immaturity of the central nervous system, most preterm infants do not have a gag reflex, putting them at a greater risk for aspiration and aspiration pneumonia.

Infants normally breathe very rapidly, at a rate from 30 to 60 breaths per minute. Normal infant breathing includes a simultaneous rise of the chest and the abdomen, and an irregular pattern is not abnormal. Periodic breathing is normal for preterm infants. With periodic breathing, an infant may not breathe for up to 10 seconds and then take several rapid breaths over the following 10 to 15 seconds to compensate. Periodic breathing is not concerning, although apnea, stopping breathing for 20 seconds or more, is.

In addition to apnea, nurses must be alert for other signs of respiratory distress. Common early signs are nasal flaring and grunting with expiration. Other signs can include intercostal, suprasternal, or subcostal retractions, circumoral (around the mouth) or general cyanosis, and seesaw breathing, during which the infant chest rises while the abdomen falls, and vice versa.

Apnea of Prematurity

Apnea of prematurity occurs because of immaturity of the respiratory control system.

Prevalence. Apnea is relatively rare in healthy term infants but occurs in half of neonates born from 33 to 34 6/7 weeks of gestation and almost all infants born prior to 28 weeks.

Etiology. The lower the gestational age and birth weight at the time of birth, the more likely the infant is to have apnea. Apnea is classified as central (an absence of respiratory effort), obstructive (there are respiratory efforts, but the upper airway is obstructed), or mixed (both central and obstructive). In prematurity, most apnea is either central or mixed.

Signs and Symptoms. Apnea is clinically significant if breathing activity stops for 20 or more seconds or if breathing stops for shorter periods of time but is associated with bradycardia (a heart rate equal to or less than 70 or 80 beats per minute) or hypoxemia (oxygen saturation below 80% or 85%).

Prognosis. It is not uncommon for apneic episodes to become more frequent a few weeks after the birth and for this increased frequency to persist for several weeks. Very preterm infants often continue to have apnea beyond what would have been 38 weeks of gestation. This usually resolves by 44 weeks postmenstrual age and may prolong the time in the hospital.

Assessment. To assess for apnea and the resultant hypoxemia and bradycardia, nurses continuously monitor infants in the NICU by pulse oximetry, cardiac monitors (Fig. 24.5), and **impedance pneumography**. Impedance pneumography is used to monitor the activity of breathing. In infants breathing without

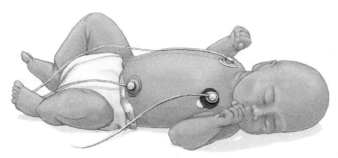

Figure 24.5. Placement of cardiac apnea monitor leads. The white lead is placed on the right upper chest, the black on the left upper chest, and the green or red on the abdomen (not over bone). (Reprinted with permission from Kyle, T., & Carman, S. [2013]. *Essentials of pediatric nursing* [2nd ed., Fig. 10.14]. Philadelphia, PA: Lippincott Williams & Wilkins.)

respiratory support or with CPAP, apnea is generally evident within a few days after birth and usually occurs with bradycardia and hypoxemia. In infants receiving mechanical ventilation, hypoxemia and bradycardia may still occur.

Prevention. Infants born prior to 35 weeks of gestation are all considered at risk for apnea, and preventative measures may reduce their risk for apnea and the damage from hypoxemia that can result. A stable environmental temperature may help reduce or prevent apnea. Infants should be positioned with their necks in a neutral position, neither flexed nor extended, thus reducing obstructive apnea risk. The baseline oxygen saturation goal is from 90% to 95% so that, in the event of apnea, severe oxygen desaturation is less likely. The healthcare team must evaluate for and treat the underlying causes of apnea, such as sepsis.

Treatment. Occasional apnea may be treated with tactile stimulation of the infant. Frequent apnea or apnea that includes hypoxemia and bradycardia, however, is treated more aggressively with respiratory and/or medication support.

CPAP can be a helpful intervention for mixed and obstructive apnea as the continuous pressure can "splint" open the airways. It is not likely a helpful intervention for central apnea, however. Pharmaceutical therapy with a methylxanthine typically stimulates the breathing center of the brain and treats central apnea. Caffeine and theophylline may both be used for this purpose, although caffeine is generally the preferred agent due to a superior safety profile and lower risk of side effects (The Pharmacy 24.1; Doyle

The Pharmacy 24.1	Caffeine Citrate
Overview	• A central nervous system stimulant, a methylxanthine
Route and dosing	• Oral or intravenous • Loading dose: 20–80 mg/kg • Maintenance dose: 5–10 mg/kg/d once daily starting 24 h after the loading dose; may be titrated up by 5 mg/kg/d to a maximum of 20 mg/kg/d in refractory patients on the basis of clinical response and serum caffeine concentrations
Care considerations	• The dose listed here is of caffeine citrate, which is 50% caffeine. Thus, the loading dose of 20 mg/kg of caffeine citrate contains 10 mg/kg of caffeine. Take care to note how the dose is written prior to administration. • Neonates should be given only caffeine citrate, *not* caffeine sodium benzoate.
Warning signs	Signs of necrotizing enterocolitis, an adverse effect: • Tachycardia • Feeding intolerance • Temperature instability • Abdominal distention • Bloody stools Signs of "gasping syndrome," an adverse effect of toxicity: • Respiratory distress • Metabolic acidosis • Gasping • Seizures • Hypotension

et al., 2016). The prophylactic administration of a methylxanthine prior to a diagnosis of apnea is gaining popularity and is associated with a small reduction in infant mortality, BPD, and **patent ductus arteriosus** (**PDA**; Abu Jawdeh et al., 2013). The side effects of methylxanthine include tachycardia and feeding intolerance.

Care Considerations. Many institutions do not discharge an infant with apnea until the episodes of apnea and the administration of apnea medication have stopped. Other institutions may allow the infant to be discharged home with cardiorespiratory monitoring (Fig. 24.6) and possibly caffeine therapy. As with any discharge of a patient who will require home use of medical equipment, caregivers must demonstrate proficiency in its use and an ability to interpret results and implement treatment, including cardiopulmonary resuscitation. Monitoring can generally be discontinued by 44 weeks postmenstrual age unless apneic episodes continue.

Respiratory Distress Syndrome

RDS, formerly known as hyaline membrane disease, is a condition caused by insufficient surfactant in immature lungs. It is a serious condition common to prematurity. The condition typically begins to resolve within 72 hours after the birth, although care in this time is critical.

Remember Gracie Munez in Chapter 8? Her baby was diagnosed with RDS.

Prevalence. The risk for RDS reduces as the gestational age increases. RDS is present in almost all infants born prior to 28 weeks. It occurs in approximately 10% of infants born at 34 weeks of gestation and very few born at or after 38 weeks (Hibbard et al., 2010).

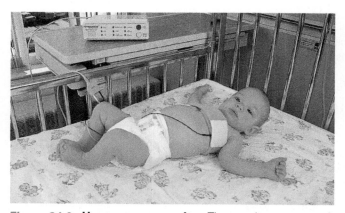

Figure 24.6. Home apnea monitor. The monitor uses a soft belt with a Velcro attachment to hold two leads in the appropriate position on the chest. (Reprinted with permission from Kyle, T., & Carman, S. [2013]. *Essentials of pediatric nursing* [2nd ed., Fig. 18.15]. Philadelphia, PA: Lippincott Williams & Wilkins.)

Etiology. Too little surfactant of low quality causes the alveoli to collapse with expiration, resulting in low lung volume and reduced lung compliance (the ability of the lung to expand). This leads to hypoxemia. In addition, the lack of surfactant causes inflammation, which results in pulmonary edema, which further decreases gas exchange. The reduced oxygenation causes respiratory acidosis and may also lead to metabolic acidosis. The acidosis causes constriction of the pulmonary vasculature (pulmonary vascular resistance), which can lead to reopening of or failure to close the ductus arteriosus and/or foramen ovale and right-to-left shunting of the blood in the heart, which worsens hypoxemia.

Male infants of European ancestry are at a highest risk for RDS, whereas infants of Asian, African, and Hispanic ancestry are at lower risk (Anadkat, Kuzniewicz, Chaudhari, Cole, & Hamvas, 2012). Maternal corticosteroid injections given in anticipation of a preterm birth enhance lung maturity and surfactant production, reducing RDS risk (see The Pharmacy 8.2).

As you'll recall, Lexi Cowslip in Chapter 10 was given a corticosteroid injection before her anticipated preterm labor and delivery. Her baby still developed RDS, however.

Signs and Symptoms. The clinical signs of RDS may be evident immediately after the birth or within 6 hours. Poor air exchange is evidenced by low oxygen saturation. On examination, the infant may be pale or cyanotic. Decreased lung sounds may be auscultated, or crackles if pulmonary edema is present. The nurse may note retractions and nasal flaring upon inspection, indicating the use of the accessory muscles of breathing. The infant is typically tachypneic. Expiratory grunting indicates exhalation against a partially closed glottis, an adaptation that slows the decrease in lung volume. Chest radiography reveals low lung volume and a ground glass appearance (Fig. 24.7).

Prognosis. Blood oxygen saturation levels below and above the optimal range of 90% to 95% are associated with worse outcomes. High oxygen levels increase the risk for vasoconstriction, increasing the risk for ROP, and low oxygen levels increase the risk of neurodevelopmental impairment and death (Manja, Lakshminrusimha, & Cook, 2015).

Leakage of air from the lungs resulting from spontaneous alveolus rupture or from mechanical ventilation occurs in RDS patients and is a common acute problem associated with RDS, although it may also happen with other underlying lung problems, including meconium aspiration syndrome (MAS). Air that leaks into the pleural space produces a pneumothorax, whereas air that leaks into the mediastinum causes a pneumomediastinum. Air may leak into the lung tissue (pulmonary interstitial emphysema), reducing lung compliance. Air may also rarely leak into the peritoneal space, the pericardial space, or the subcutaneous tissue.

Infants with a pneumothorax exhibit signs of respiratory distress. On examination the chest is asymmetrical, with decreased breath sounds on the affected side. In the case of a large pneumothorax, the

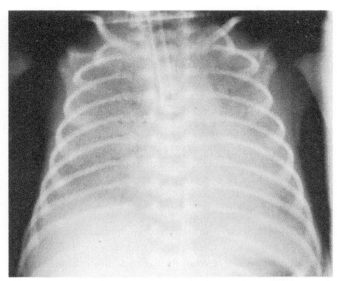

Figure 24.7. Radiographic image of the chest of an infant with respiratory distress syndrome. Note the diffusely opaque lung fields and the indistinct cardiac outline. (Reprinted with permission from McMillan, J. A., Feigin R. D., DeAngelis, C., & Jones, M. D. [Eds.]. [2007]. *Oski's solution: Oski's pediatrics: Principles and practice* [4th ed., Fig. 42.2]. Philadelphia, PA: Lippincott Williams & Wilkins.)

nurse should observe for hypotension, hypoxemia, and bradycardia that may occur because of an increase in pressure inside the thorax, which, in turn, leads to decreased cardiac output. The nurse should assess for a pneumothorax in cases of abrupt onset respiratory distress and changes in cardiovascular status or a drop in oxygenation in an infant who is mechanically ventilated. Imaging may be used to confirm the diagnosis. Depending on the degree of pneumothorax, it may either resolve spontaneously in a few days under careful observation or require placement of a chest tube or thoracentesis.

The most common chronic complication of RDS is BPD, discussed in Chapter 25.

Assessment. Assessment includes physical examination, observing for the signs and symptoms described above, and continuous monitoring of blood oxygen saturation and laboratory testing of blood gases as ordered. The target partial pressure of carbon dioxide for this population is typically 45 to 60 mm Hg (Thome et al., 2015). Blood samples for the monitoring of blood gases and acid–base balance should be done from arterial samples. Chest radiography may also be indicated.

Treatment. All infants at risk for RDS should receive respiratory support by way of nasal CPAP or nasal intermittent ventilation to provide positive end expiratory pressure (PEEP) to prevent the alveoli from collapsing. Although more aggressive ventilation was once the standard of care, less invasive methods are effective and pose less risk of harm from intubation and ventilation. Some infants who are not adequately supported by nasal CPAP, however, may still require intubation and ventilation along with the administration of surfactant (American Academy of Pediatrics, 2014; Sakonidou & Dhaliwal, 2015).

Respiratory acidosis, hypoxemia, and severe apnea are indications for intubation and ventilation. Failure of CPAP therapy alone occurs with 43% of infants born from 25 to 28 weeks of gestation and 21% of those born from 29 to 32 weeks of gestation (Dargaville et al., 2016).

Surfactant therapy, if necessary, is usually started within 30 to 60 minutes after birth after a trial of CPAP. Surfactant is either bovine or porcine, and consideration of a family's culture may be necessary when the surfactant is selected. Individuals who identify as Jewish or Muslim may object to porcine surfactant, whereas families that identify as Hindu may object to a bovine preparation. Although synthetic surfactant has been created, it is no longer commercially available in the United States at the time of this writing. Surfactant may be administered via the ET or by less invasive methods such as aerosolization, intratracheal catheter, or mask (Rigo, Lefebvre, & Broux, 2016).

Nitrous oxide was once used commonly to improve pulmonary vasodilation. It was used as a routine or rescue therapy either alone or in conjunction with other therapies. More recent research indicates it is not beneficial for reducing mortality in the neonate and does not reduce the risk for developing BPD. Current guidelines recommend against its use for RDS (Kumar & American Academy of Pediatrics, 2014; Sakonidou & Dhaliwal, 2015).

Care Considerations. Supportive care of newborns with RDS is critical to outcomes. Reducing stress reduces oxygen consumption and caloric needs. Fluid management and nutrition are also important. Below are some key aspects of nursing care for newborns with RDS.

- A critical part of reducing stress in the neonate is thermoregulation. The nurse may place an abdominal sensor on the infant set to 36.5°C to 37°C, which acts a thermostat to regulate the temperature control of the incubator or radiant warmer.
- Diuretics are rarely indicated. However, excessive fluids increase the risk for serious complications such as BPD, a PDA, and NEC (Bell & Acarregui, 2014). Therefore, the nurse should monitor and manage the infant's fluid intake and output per orders.
- Hypotension is a common finding with RDS, and thus the nurse should monitor for it. Intervention is not required, however, unless the infant is poorly perfused.
- Adequate nutrition to maintain metabolic processes, growth, and development is important to care and is discussed later in this chapter.

Cardiovascular

Common cardiovascular issues in the preterm neonate, particularly those who are very low birth weight (VLBW) or extremely low birth weight (ELBW), are a PDA and low blood pressure.

Patent Ductus Arteriosus

The ductus arteriosus is a blood vessel that connects the pulmonary artery to the proximal descending aorta, allowing blood to bypass the fetal lungs. The ductus arteriosus is typically significantly narrowed within the first 24 hours of life and completely sealed within 3 weeks. In some infants, however, the ductus arteriosus remains open for longer after birth, which can pose problems.

Prevalence. Almost all infants born at term have complete closure of the ductus arteriosus at 72 hours after the birth. In healthy infants born at 30 weeks, the ductus arteriosus closes most often within 96 hours. Infants born under 30 weeks of gestation have a high probability of having a delayed closure, particularly in the presence of RDS.

Signs and Symptoms. Symptoms depend on the degree of the PDA. A small PDA may present as a systolic murmur in the neonate or a continuous murmur in older infants. A moderate PDA can create a left-to-right shunt, which increases the workload of the left atrium and ventricle, causing ventricular dilation and dysfunction. A large PDA can lead to increased pulmonary vascular resistance, a right-to-left shunt, and cyanotic heart disease, as well as changes to the pulmonary vasculature. In an infant, a large PDA may present as respiratory distress, poor feeding, and failure to thrive.

Clinical signs usually develop within 2 to 3 days after birth. A murmur is a common sign but may be absent within the first 3 days after the birth. Infants with a clinically significant PDA typically have an exaggerated ventricular impulse and bounding pulses because of an increase in cardiac output. The pulse pressure with a clinically significant PDA is wider, with more than 25 mm Hg between systolic and diastolic pressures. Apnea and tachypnea may also be evident. Pulse oximetry assessed from the right thumb and a great toe usually reveals at least a 10% difference in oxygen saturation.

Prognosis. The infants are at a higher risk for NEC and IVH.

Assessment. The diagnosis of PDA is usually confirmed by echocardiography, although an electrocardiogram or chest X-ray may also be ordered.

Treatment. Cyclooxygenase inhibitors, such as ibuprofen and indomethacin, which are contraindicated in late pregnancy because of the risk for premature closure of the ductus arteriosus of the fetus, are often used to encourage closure of a PDA in preterm infants. Ibuprofen is the current drug of choice, as its use is associated with a lower risk of NEC, a shorter duration of mechanical ventilation, and a lower risk for renal insufficiency than the use of indomethacin. Typical IV dosing of ibuprofen for closure of PDA is an initial dose of 10 mg/kg and then two further doses of 5 mg/kg at 24-hour intervals (Ohlsson, Walia, & Shah, 2015). Multiple doses may be required, particularly for infants born at earlier gestational ages and infants not exposed to corticosteroid therapy in utero. Infants with severe respiratory distress may also require repeat dosing to achieve PDA closure.

Loop diuretics are contraindicated in the first few weeks of life as they cause the renal synthesis of prostaglandin E2 and may inhibit closure of the ductus arteriosus. Diuretics are sometimes given during early infancy to preterm infants to avoid fluid overload

and pulmonary edema, but in such cases, loop diuretics such as furosemide, which are often the first diuretic of choice for adults with fluid overload, should be avoided. Rather, thiazide diuretics are typically the first-line diuretic choice for this population.

Infants who do not respond to pharmaceutical treatment for PDA closure may require surgery to close the ductus arteriosus. These infants are at a greater risk for cardiovascular compromise and hypoperfusion postoperatively and must be carefully monitored. The use of inotropic agents as well as blood volume support may be required to maintain blood pressure and tissue perfusion (El-Khuffash, Jain, & McNamara, 2013).

Care Considerations. Supportive therapies include maintaining a thermal neutral environment and adequate oxygenation to avoid taxing the heart more than is necessary. Infants who are experiencing respiratory compromise in addition to or because of PDA should receive PEEP.

Low Blood Pressure

Infants born prematurely, particularly those who are ELBW, are more prone to low blood pressure, even in the absence of shock. Low blood pressure creates a risk for hypoperfusion of the tissues. Expansion of the blood volume with normal saline or with blood products such as albumin or fresh frozen plasma may be used to increase blood pressure. Inotropic agents such as dopamine, dobutamine, and/or epinephrine may be trialed if volume expansion is insufficient for increasing blood pressure.

Hematologic

For infants born prior to 32 weeks of gestation, anemia is typically evident from 3 to 12 weeks after birth and resolves by 6 months of age.

Etiology

Erythropoiesis is decreased after birth due to increased tissue oxygenation and a reduction in erythropoietin from the kidneys and liver, where most fetal red blood cells are produced. In prematurity, the newborn cannot adequately maintain erythropoietin production to increase the number of mature red blood cells. Also contributing to anemia is the frequent need for blood testing, as numerous samples are drawn, and even the relatively small volumes drawn for phlebotomy are significant when the overall volume of blood in a preterm neonate is so small (Lemyre, Sample, Lacaze-Masmonteil, Canadian Paediatric Society & Fetus and Newborn Committee, 2015). Another factor contributing to anemia is the relatively short life span of the red blood cell in preterm infants. Although the typical life span of a red blood cell is 100 to 120 days in an adult and 60 to 80 days in a term newborn, it is only 45 to 50 days in an ELBW infant.

Signs and Symptoms

As with all humans, the preterm neonate may experience an increase in heart rate and stroke volume in response to anemia, which helps compensate for the low oxygen-carrying capacity of the blood. Respiratory disease and the higher oxygen affinity of fetal hemoglobin, however, mean that these compensatory strategies are less effective for maintaining oxygen delivery. For some infants who are able to compensate successfully, however, hemoglobin levels may drop as low as 7 g/dL without symptoms. The other signs of anemia of prematurity include poor weight gain, increased supplemental oxygen requirements, bradycardia, and apnea.

Assessment

Assessment includes observation for signs and symptoms discussed above, as well as laboratory testing of a complete blood count at least weekly.

Treatment

The iron stores of preterm infants do not typically last for more than 2 to 3 months after the birth. Infants who are formula fed may not need additional iron supplementation, although infants who are breastfed or are fed using a low-iron formula need supplementation in the case of anemia. Supplementation at a rate of 2 to 4 mg/kg daily with a maximum dose of 15 mg total is recommended (Baker, Greer, & Committee on Nutrition American Academy of Pediatrics, 2010).

A transfusion of red blood cells may be indicated for infants who are symptomatic. Transfusions are not risk-free, however, and the temporary improvement in oxygenation inhibits erythropoiesis production. The use of a erythropoiesis-stimulating agent may be of limited benefit for reducing the need for transfusion, although it does not improve outcomes overall (Aher & Ohlsson, 2014).

Care Considerations

Nurses should be aware that blood transfusion may not be acceptable to all families for religious and/or cultural reasons. Some families may elect to give directed donor blood, in which the related donor with a compatible blood type gives blood for use by the specified infant.

Neurologic

The **germinal matrix**, adjacent to the lateral ventricles, is a highly vascular area of the brain of the fetus and preterm neonate that is active in cell differentiation. The vasculature of the germinal matrix is thin-walled, increasing the risk of bleeding. The germinal matrix starts to involute at 28 weeks of gestation and is typically resolved by 35 to 36 weeks of gestation.

The germinal matrix is susceptible to fluctuations in the cerebral blood flow. The immaturity and thus impaired autoregulation of preterm infants create these dangerous fluctuations, and it's important that healthcare providers provide as stable an environment as possible to minimize fluctuations in blood flow. Hypotension, respiratory distress, interventions causing either hypoxic or hyperoxic episodes, acidosis, unpleasant stimuli such as suctioning, and cardiopulmonary resuscitation can all cause dangerous fluctuations in the cerebral blood flow (Handley, Sun, Wyckoff, & Lee, 2015; Thome et al., 2015).

Two neurologic conditions of particular concern in the preterm infant are IVH and **periventricular leukomalacia**.

Intraventricular Hemorrhage

IVH is bleeding into the lateral ventricles of the brain and is one of the most common and dangerous causes of brain injury, with short- and long-term consequences for the preterm infant. In preterm infants, the bleeding typically originates in the germinal matrix.

Prevalence. IVH occurs in 20% of VLBW infants and 45% of ELBW infants (Stoll et al., 2010). It is far more common in infants born prior to 30 weeks of gestation, although up to 6% of infants born from 30 to 34 weeks develop IVH (Bhat et al., 2012). IVH is rare in term infants, and when it occurs, a minority of the bleeding originates from the germinal matrix, 35% comes from the choroid plexus, and the remainder comes from either a different brain structure or unknown source.

Etiology. The ventricles are cavities within the brain filled with cerebrospinal fluid (CSF). They are lined by the choroid plexus, which produces the CSF. In preterm infants, bleeding into the ventricles generally comes from the germinal matrix.

In addition to the risks for germinal matrix bleeding cited previously, maternal preeclampsia, fetal asphyxia prior to birth, and maternal chorioamnionitis are risk factors for IVH (Mendola et al., 2015). Antenatal steroid therapy is protective and is associated with drops in the rate of IVH. During the birth, a breech delivery and intrapartum asphyxia increase the risk for IVH. Theoretically, compression of the head during vaginal birth increases intracranial pressure and the risk for IVH. There is insufficient evidence that a cesarean section is protective, however (Alfirevic, Milan, & Livio, 2013). Delayed cord clamping is protective (Chiruvolu et al., 2015).

Signs and Symptoms. Most cases of IVH occur within the first 5 days after birth, with half occurring in the first 6 hours (Al-Abdi & Al-Aamri, 2014). Manifestations of the condition are varied. As many as half the cases of IVH occur without clinical signs and are diagnosed only with routine ultrasonography. The rarest presentation is catastrophic deterioration. When clinical signs do appear, they are more frequently nonspecific and saltatory (progressing in bursts instead of gradually; Box 24.1).

Prognosis. The severity of IVH is a major determinant of outcomes. Death occurs in 4% of infants with a grade I IVH, 10% with a grade II IVH, 18% with a grade III IVH, and 40% with a grade IV IVH. More severe IVH is also associated with an increased risk for IVH-related complications (Christian et al., 2016). Cerebral palsy is diagnosed in more than half of children with IVH as neonates. Higher-grade IVH is associated with a higher risk for the condition than lower-grade IVH (Kitai, Hirai, Ohmura, Ogura, & Arai, 2015).

Posthemorrhagic hydrocephalus (PHH), which involves progressive dilation of the ventricles, is a major complication of IVH and occurs in approximately 25% of infants diagnosed with IVH (Klinger et al., 2016). It typically occurs after severe IVH, although it may also occur after mild IVH, and usually begins within 3 weeks after the IVH. The risk of PHH is higher with

Box 24.1 Clinical Manifestations of Intraventricular Hemorrhage

Saltatory manifestations, appearing over hours or days

- Reduced movement
- Disturbed respirations
- Altered level of consciousness
- Hypotonia

Catastrophic manifestations, appearing over minutes or hours

- Flaccidity
- Fixed pupils and other abnormalities of cranial nerves from pressure on cranial nerves
- Seizures
- Hypoventilation and/or apnea
- Coma
- Metabolic acidosis from poor oxygen profusion
- Decreased hematocrit levels due to bleeding
- Hypotension
- Bradycardia
- Bulging of the anterior fontanelle

Box 24.2 Grading of Intraventricular Hemorrhage

Mild

- Grade I: Bleeding is confined to the germinal matrix.
- Grade II: Blood occupies 50% or less of the lateral ventricle volume.

Severe

- Grade III: Blood occupies more than 50% of the lateral ventricle volume.
- Grade IV: Bleeding extends to the white matter adjacent to the ventricle.

larger IVH and lower gestational age at birth (Radic, Vincer, & McNeely, 2015). Assessment for the condition includes daily head measurements and weekly ultrasounds, although an increase in head circumference is a late sign of PHH. Many cases of PHH resolve spontaneously, whereas some require direct drainage of the ventricles either episodically or continuously by shunt.

Periventricular hemorrhagic infarction (PVHI) is synonymous with a grade IV IVH and involves a disruption of the blood supply to particular areas of the brain. Most often, portions of the parietal and frontal lobes are affected, either unilaterally or bilaterally. Patients with PVHI typically have muscle weakness of all four limbs (quadriparesis) or weakness on one side of the body (hemiparesis), as well as lifelong intellectual deficits.

Assessment. IVH is diagnosed by ultrasound. Many institutions routinely screen for IVH by ultrasound, as 50% of cases are silent in presentation. Often, infants born before 30 weeks of gestation are screened at 1 or 2 weeks after birth and then again from 36 to 40 weeks postmenstrual age. Infants born at a later gestational age may not be screened but should be evaluated according to risk and symptoms. A grading system is used to define the bleeding originating from the germinal matrix on a scale from I to IV (Box 24.2).

Care Considerations. Care of the infant after a diagnosis of IVH is supportive, with attention to avoiding triggers similar to those that can contribute to the development of IVH, such as hypertension and hypotension. Other measures include providing adequate oxygenation and optimized nutritional, fluid, and metabolic support. Seizures are treated to avoid alterations to cerebral blood flow and blood pressure.

Periventricular Leukomalacia

Periventricular leukomalacia is injury to the white matter of the brain and is the most common cause of cerebral palsy.

Prevalence. Periventricular leukomalacia is most common in infants born prior to 32 weeks of gestation, although it may also occur in late preterm and term infants.

Etiology. It is caused by ischemia or infection.

Prognosis. Periventricular leukomalacia is associated with impairments of vision and intellect, cerebral palsy, epilepsy, and/or paralysis in children, with diagnosis typically in early infancy. Deficits are dependent on associated damage and may be minor or significant.

More extensive injury is associated with worse outcomes (Imamura et al., 2013). An ischemic form may occur prenatally and is associated with stillbirth and death shortly after birth. It occurs more often in the presence of maternal infections, such as chorioamnionitis. Other risk factors are similar to those for IVH and are associated with immature autoregulation of the preterm neonate.

Assessment. It is diagnosed by imaging.

Treatment. No particular management is recommended beyond standard supportive care.

Renal

The kidneys are critical for maintaining fluid and electrolyte balance and for the excretion of waste and the production of erythropoietin for red blood cell production. The kidney has a full complement of nephrons by 36 weeks of gestation, but even in a term neonate, renal function is still immature. In the first weeks after the birth, the kidneys of both term and preterm infants mature rapidly. Prior to this time, however, particularly for very preterm and low birth weight infants, overhydration, dehydration, and electrolyte balance have little margin for error. Because of a decreased glomerular filtration rate, many drugs given to the neonate have a longer half-life and the nurse must carefully monitor their levels by laboratory testing as ordered.

Immune

Maternal immunoglobulin G (IgG) is transferred to the fetus via the placenta after 32 weeks of gestation. Infants born prematurely have less IgG than infants born at term, impairing their ability to fight infection. In addition, the ability of the premature neonate's system to identify targets for IgG (opsonization) is immature, as is the complement system. (IgG triggers the complement system, which produces the immune proteins that eliminate pathogens). IgM and IgA take time after birth to reach effective levels. The skin and mucus membranes of the preterm neonate are thin and immature and have poor tissue integrity, and thus provide less of a barrier to infection than they do in a term neonate. In addition, invasive procedures and devices, such as venous and arterial catheters and feeding tubes, which are used more commonly in infants of lower gestational age and size, increase risk for infection. Evidence of maternal infection intrapartum, premature rupture of membranes, and maternal group B streptococcus (GBS) colonization all increase the likelihood of infection in the neonate.

You may recall that Hannah Wilder in Chapter 7 was GBS-positive with chorioamnionitis, raising concerns for neonatal sepsis.

Sepsis is a critical condition in which the body's immune response to an infection causes systemic inflammation and damage to body tissues. This condition is discussed in detail in the remainder of this section.

Prevalence

Although early-onset sepsis (onset in the first 3 days after birth) occurs in only 3.5% or fewer of preterm infants, late-onset sepsis (onset 72 hours or more after the birth) is very common, occurring in up to 43% of infants born prematurely (Stoll et al., 2015).

Etiology

Early sepsis is a result of vertical transmission from the mother via either the placenta or the amniotic fluid. Late sepsis may result from colonization from maternal transmission that develops into a later infection or from horizontal transmission from an environmental source, an invasive procedure, or contact with healthcare providers. Lower birth weights and earlier gestations are risk factors for sepsis.

Signs and Symptoms

The signs of neonatal sepsis are nonspecific and subtle. Even small changes in the activity and feeding of the neonate are possible evidence of infection (Box 24.3). It is critical that sepsis be recognized early. Aseptic technique and careful handwashing are critical in providing care to minimize infection risk.

Box 24.3 Signs of Neonatal Infection

Respiratory distress
- Tachypnea
- Apnea
- Retraction
- Nasal flaring
- Expiratory grunting
- Increased need for ventilatory support
- Acidosis

Lethargy (late sign)
Irritability (late sign)
Hypotonia
Feeding intolerance
Vomiting
Diarrhea
Glucose instability
- Hypoglycemia
- Hyperglycemia

Cardiovascular changes
- Tachycardia
- Bradycardia (late sign)
- Hypotension (late sign)
- Poor perfusion
  - Cyanosis
  - Pallor (late sign)
  - Poor capillary refill

Jaundice
Temperature instability
Oliguria (late sign)
Metabolic acidosis
Thrombocytopenia
- Petechiae

Neutropenia

Adapted from Bekhof, J., Reitsma, J. B., Kok, J. H., & Van Straaten, I. H. (2013). Clinical signs to identify late-onset sepsis in preterm infants. *European Journal of Pediatrics, 172*(4), 501–508. doi:10.1007/s00431-012-1910-6

Prognosis

Sepsis increases the mortality rate of the infants and results in longer hospital stays and an increased risk of complications and interventions. It is also associated with growth impairment and poor neurodevelopmental outcomes (Stoll et al., 2015). Because of the immaturity of the immune system and epithelial protections, preterm infants are also more likely to develop a yeast infection in the blood, candidemia. Such infections in preterm and low birth weight infants have a particularly poor prognosis.

Severe complications associated with sepsis include septic shock and systemic inflammatory response syndrome. Septic shock refers to sepsis with cardiovascular dysfunction. Septic shock results in poor tissue perfusion and typically manifests as hypotension, pallor, initial tachycardia followed by bradycardia, oliguria, and neurologic changes. When a patient is severely septic, as evidenced by respiratory distress, cardiovascular dysfunction, and multiorgan failure, an inflammatory response termed systemic inflammatory response syndrome is launched.

Assessment

Because the signs of sepsis are so vague and nonspecific, diagnosis must be made by laboratory evaluation. Blood culture provides the definitive diagnosis. Blood may be obtained by sampling from an indwelling umbilical or vascular access catheter or by venipuncture or arterial culture. In VLBW infants, however, the volume obtained may be insufficient for an adequate culture because a minimum of 0.5 mL of blood is required. Antibiotics given to the mother prior to birth also impact the accuracy of the culture. Ideally, more than one sample should be obtained, as sample contamination is not uncommon, and two or more positive cultures confirm the diagnosis. Taking too few blood cultures increases the risk for false negatives, and it takes considerable time (2 to 3 days for some bacteria, 10 days for others, and as long as 30 days for fungi) to get culture results. Thus, antibiotics are often given with a diagnosis of "probable sepsis."

A lumbar puncture may be performed in infants at the same time as the blood culture as neonates often do not manifest signs of meningitis. Laboratory testing includes a CSF culture, Gram stain, cell count with differential, and protein and glucose concentrations. A urine culture is generally not done in neonates prior to 6 days of age. In infants with late-onset infection, cultures should be obtained from other potential foci of infection, such as skin lesions.

Absolute neutrophil count and the ratio of immature to total neutrophils are not sensitive measures for diagnosing neonatal sepsis in preterm or term infants (Hornik et al., 2012). A C-reactive protein (CRP) level is sensitive for predicting sepsis but is not specific, as it may also be elevated with noninfectious causes of inflammation, such as fetal distress or maternal fever, regardless of gestational age at birth (Lacaze-Masmonteil, Rosychuk, & Robinson, 2014). Serial tests of CRP level are useful, however, for following the course of the infection and determining the efficacy of antibiotic therapy. Molecular techniques such as polymerase chain reaction to test for ribosomal RNA are a highly accurate, rapid means of assessing for infection, require a smaller amount of blood, and are not affected by the maternal use of antibiotics. They are more costly, however, and often require sending specimens to large outside laboratories for evaluation.

Treatment

Antibiotics are the primary treatment for sepsis. Another critical intervention is IV fluid resuscitation with isotonic saline to ensure adequate perfusion, accompanied by regular evaluation of both fluid and electrolyte balance. Patients who fail to respond to IV fluid resuscitation for perfusion may require inotropic therapy, typically with dopamine.

A select group of patients over 34 weeks of gestation may require **extracorporeal membrane oxygenation (ECMO)**. This intervention is not used in infants younger than 34 weeks because it must be used in conjunction with an anticoagulant, which is contraindicated in younger infants because of an increased risk for IVH with these agents. ECMO provides both cardiac and respiratory support to optimize gas exchange (Dellinger et al., 2013). ECMO is used for hypoxemia because of cardiac or respiratory

insufficiency when there is no adequate response to other treatments. Only nurses specially trained in its use may administer ECMO. A typical ECMO setup is illustrated in Figure 24.8.

Care Considerations

As with all newborns, particularly preterm newborns, a thermoneutral environment is important to minimize stress. The administration and monitoring of antibiotics used to treat sepsis is a nursing responsibility. Supportive care includes maximizing oxygenation, including the use of supplemental oxygenation and ventilation as needed.

Infection Prevention

Careful hand hygiene is one of the most effective means of minimizing care-associated infections. In 2009, the World Health Organization released guidelines for optimal hand hygiene (Box 24.4; Pittet, Allegranzi, Boyce, & World Health Organization World Alliance for Patient Safety First Global Patient Safety Challenge Core Group of Experts, 2009). Central line sites should be monitored daily, as well as cleaned and redressed each week or according to institution protocol. Tubes such as catheters should be removed as soon as possible to reduce infection risk. Early feeding with breast milk reduces the need for central venous lines and parenteral nutrition. Colostrum and breast milk also contain important immune components such as IgA and lactoferrin and have been shown to reduce the risk of sepsis (Pammi & Abrams, 2015). Breast milk may also have properties important to the long- and short-term development of the neonatal immune system (Turfkruyer & Verhasselt, 2015).

Temperature

Hypothermia

Preterm and low birth weight infants are at an increased risk for hypothermia, or low body temperature, from the moment of birth.

Prevalence. A 2016 study found that over half of preterm infants were hypothermic at the time of admission, with a corresponding increased risk of neonatal death (Wilson et al., 2016). Another study found that over 40% of neonates born at 33 weeks of gestation or less have a temperature of 36.5°C or less on admission to the NICU (Laptook et al., 2018).

Etiology. Several factors related to immaturity increase the risk of hypothermia in preterm neonates. Because the accumulation of subcutaneous fat and brown fat, which provide heat insulation in the body, is a physical developmental task of later pregnancy, preterm infants have less fat reserve, increasing their risk for hypothermia. Moreover, whereas a healthy term infant maintains a flexed position, which helps maintain body heat, a premature infant does not have the muscle tone to maintain the flexed position and thus exposes greater body surface area. Finally, the temperature center of the brain in preterm infants is immature and less able to perform the function of thermoregulation.

Signs and Symptoms. Because of continuous temperature monitoring, hypothermia is relatively rare after the temperature has been stabilized in the NICU. If hypothermia is present,

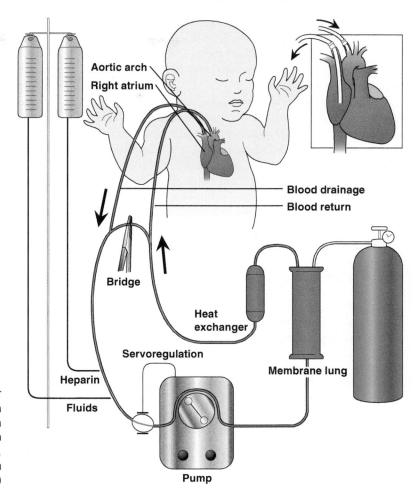

Figure 24.8. ECMO setup. ECMO is a process for removing blood from the heart, filtering out carbon dioxide from it, and oxygenating it, thus serving as an artificial heart and lung machine. It is used in preterm neonates with respiratory distress syndrome. ECMO, extracorporeal membrane oxygenation. (Reprinted with permission from Lippincott's Nursing Advisor 2013.)

Box 24.4 The World Health Organization's Guidelines on Hand Hygiene in Healthcare

- Wash hands that are visibly soiled with soap and water.
- If hands are not visibly soiled, you may use an alcohol-based hand rub instead of soap and water.
- Keep sleeves above the elbows during handwashing.
- Remove rings and bracelets prior to handwashing and replace them after the end of the shift.
- Designate a stethoscope to use with each neonate and clean it prior to and after each use.
- Wash hands prior to and after each contact with the infant, regardless of glove use.
- Wear gloves if you anticipate having contact with mucus membranes, blood products or body fluids, or a site vulnerable to infection.
- Replace gloves between separate incidences of contact with different potentially contaminated parts of the body.
- Keep nails short and do not wear artificial nails.

Adapted from Pittet, D., Allegranzi, B., Boyce, J., & World Health Organization World Alliance for Patient Safety First Global Patient Safety Challenge Core Group of Experts. (2009). The World Health Organization Guidelines on Hand Hygiene in Health Care and their consensus recommendations. *Infection Control and Hospital Epidemiology, 30*(7), 611–622. doi:10.1086/600379

---

though, the infant may appear pale, mottled, or cyanotic and be cool to the touch.

Prognosis. The increased effort of the preterm neonate to achieve temperature stabilization in a cold environment can lead to hypoglycemia and acidosis, which can, in turn, increase the risk for IVH and pulmonary hemorrhage.

Assessment. Assessment of temperature in the NICU is often continuous by a sensor placed on the abdomen, as described earlier in this chapter. Alternatively, axillary or rectal temperature may be assessed periodically.

Treatment. Traditionally, mild hypothermia is treated with slow rewarming to avoid cardiac arrhythmias and apnea, whereas more severe hypothermia (body temperatures below 35°C [95°F]) is treated with more rapid rewarming. There is little evidence to support one pace of rewarming over another, however, and current guidelines do not recommend one over the other (Wyckoff et al., 2015). Rewarming is typically achieved by radiant warmer and/or warming mattress.

Care Considerations. Nurses must be aware that heat loss may happen by evaporation, conduction, convection, and/or radiation (see Table 18.2). Standard practice after any delivery to reduce the risk of neonatal hypothermia is to maintain a warm delivery room, dry the newborn immediately after birth, replace any wet blankets with dry ones, and perform assessments and interventions with the newborn either skin-to-skin with the mother or under a prewarmed radiant heater.

Additional measures are often used to maintain the body heat in a preterm infant. The use of warmed, humidified gases for resuscitation may minimize hypothermia (de Almeida et al., 2014). Thermal mattresses can aid in maintaining optimal temperatures. In addition, preterm infants are often placed in polyurethane or polyethylene wraps or bags and hats with excellent results (see Fig. 10.5). Nurses should be aware, however, that this practice may increase the risk of hyperthermia, particularly when used in conjunction with a warming mattress (McCarthy, Molloy, Twomey, Murphy, & O'Donnell, 2013). Infants cannot sweat, and overheating may contribute to apnea. Once in the NICU, preterm babies are most often kept inside an incubator or under a radiant warmer.

Cold Stress

Regardless of gestational age and condition, a neonate with uncorrected hypothermia is at risk for cold stress.

Etiology. As the infant's temperature drops, blood vessels constrict to maintain heat. The metabolic rate of the newborn increases, as does oxygen consumption. To support the increased metabolism, more energy is recruited, decreasing glycogen stores and creating a risk for hypoglycemia and metabolic acidosis. Surfactant production is compromised as metabolic resources are diverted to thermogenesis. The infant becomes tachypneic as the increased metabolism creates an increased need for oxygen.

In addition to a drop in skin temperature and a change in skin color, vasoconstriction directly impacts pulmonary perfusion. Although there is greater ventilation due to an increased breathing rate, there is less perfusion of the lungs and thus overall a decrease in circulating oxygen and a drop in the pH of the blood, causing respiratory acidosis. This, in combination with the reduced surfactant production, may cause respiratory distress and exacerbate any other respiratory disease.

In addition, the increase in cardiac output coupled with the vasoconstriction in the pulmonary bed creates a pulmonary hypertension that may maintain or reopen the ductus arteriosus.

Signs and Symptoms. Vasoconstriction causes the skin to feel cool and appear pale or mottled. Respiratory distress is evident.

Prognosis. Prolonged cold stress can lead to respiratory distress, acidosis, hypoglycemia, and reopening of, or failure to close, the ductus arteriosus.

Care Considerations. Assessment, treatment, and care considerations for cold stress are the same as for hypothermia, as discussed above.

Growth and Development

For the purposes of growth and development assessment of preterm infants, a corrected age is used. An infant born 8 weeks prematurely, for example, is at 32 weeks of gestation at birth. At 8 weeks of chronological age (time since birth), this same infant is at 40 weeks of postmenstrual age and is assessed according to the expectations of that gestation. An infant born 8 weeks prematurely, therefore, at 6 months of chronological age is assessed according to the developmental and growth expectations of a 4-month-old who was born at 40 weeks of gestation.

Optimal weight gain of a preterm neonate is almost twice that of a term infant, as significant growth normally occurs in the third trimester of pregnancy. Target weight gain for a preterm infant is a minimum of 18 g/kg/d and then 20 to 30 g/kg/d once the infant weighs 2 kg. Growth progress as measured by weight is corrected for the first 2 years of life. Progress as measured by height is corrected for the first 40 months of age, and head circumference is corrected for the first 18 months. Developmental milestones such as walking, talking, and fine motor skills are corrected until about the age of 2 and a half years.

Weight is the standard measurement used to assess growth in the NICU, as it reflects day-to-day changes better than length and head measurements can. The weight gain goal for infants born preterm is from 18 to 30 g/kg/d, depending on weight. The nutrition goal is intake of 160 mL/kg/d of fortified breast milk or formula specially designed for preterm infants.

Growth for infants in the NICU is compromised by both stress, which increases metabolic needs and diverts nutrition away from growth, and inadequate intake. Infants born prematurely can tolerate only limited enteral feedings and/or parenteral nutrition. As a result, many low birth weight infants are below the 10th percentile for weight at the time of discharge. Discharge at a weight below the 10th percentile is classified as postnatal growth failure (Horbar et al., 2015).

Infants with BPD are at particular risk for postnatal growth failure, both in the NICU and after discharge, due to chronic hypoxia, increased energy expenditure, and poor tolerance for feeding, as well as a weak suck. Infants who are intubated often experience challenges with feeding because of a disruption in the development of feeding rhythms.

Growth is carefully followed after discharge either weekly or every other week for up to 6 months and then every month or 2 months. The average height and weight of infants born prematurely remain shorter and lighter beyond infancy and into adulthood (Horemuzova, Amark, Jacobson, Soder, & Hagenas, 2014).

Nutrition

Preterm infants have high energy needs, both because they are in a high-needs stage of growth and because of an increase in metabolic needs due to conditions such as infection and respiratory illness. Complicating the clinical picture is the physiologic immaturity that makes adequate intake and the use of nutrients challenging. The ability of the neonate to suck, swallow, and gag and to coordinate the movement of sucking and breathing is inhibited by immature reflexes and muscle development. Gastric motility is decreased when compared with a term newborn, and enzyme activity is immature, limiting the neonate's ability to digest efficiently.

Beyond the high energy needs and immature ability to take in and process nutrition is the further complication of feeding risks. Incorrect feeding can cause feeding intolerance or, potentially catastrophically, NEC. Some infants for medical or developmental reasons may not be able to obtain sufficient nutrition by enteral (gastrointestinal) feeding and may instead require that all or part of their nutritional needs be met by **parenteral feeding**.

Recall that Kylie, Lexi Cowslip's preterm infant in Chapter 10, initially received parenteral feeding and then was gradually introduced to enteral (tube) feeding. Once she could tolerate receiving enteral feedings large enough to sustain her, she was weaned off of parenteral feeding.

Fluid intake and the intake of calories, protein, and nutrients as specified are monitored daily, as well as weight. Length and head circumference are monitored weekly. Once full-volume enteric feeding is established, hemoglobin, hematocrit, calcium, phosphorus, alkaline phosphatase, and blood urea nitrogen (BUN) levels are monitored every 2 to 3 weeks. Measurement of calcium, phosphorus, and alkaline phosphatase aid in the assessment of the bone mineral status, as low levels suggest the risk of rickets. A BUN level over 10 reflects sufficient protein intake. Infants may also have electrolytes checked at this time, particularly those on diuretic therapy or with growth slower than anticipated (see Fig. 1.16).

Nonnutritive Sucking and Mouth Swabbing
Nonnutritive sucking (NNS) shortens the time of transition from tube feeding to oral feeding in preterm infants and shortens the total duration of their hospital stay. Although NNS does not improve weight gain, it is thought to improve digestion and is known to have a calming effect. NNS facilitates the development of feeding skills and a positive association between sucking, swallowing, and satiety. NNS may be provided at the breast during kangaroo care or with a pacifier or gloved finger. NNS has a soothing effect for infants generally (Foster, Psaila, & Patterson, 2016).

Regardless of feeding method, infants who cannot receive nutrition by direct oral intake may still benefit from colostrum. Starting shortly after the birth, when possible, the mouths of infants should be swabbed with colostrum expressed from the mother every 3 hours. This promotes the growth of beneficial bacteria and provides immune benefits (Sohn, Kalanetra, Mills, & Underwood, 2016). Swabbing of the mouth can also be a way for new parents to help care for delicate infants who may be too fragile to even withstand the stimulation of being held.

Parenteral Feeding
Often, older infants can rely on enteric feeding orally or by tube alone, but most VLBW infants and other infants who cannot receive sufficient nutrition enterally require parenteral nutrition to optimize outcomes. Poor nutrition in the first few weeks after birth for these infants can lead to detrimental outcomes that

may be irreversible. The use of parenteral nutrition can improve neurodevelopmental outcomes and growth while reducing the risk of infant mortality, BPD, and NEC.

If needed, parenteral nutrition is generally started within 24 hours after the birth. It can be infused through peripheral or central veins, and infection is the most serious potential complication of the treatment. The calorie goal for an infant fed parenterally is lower than for an infant receiving enteral feedings because of less fecal energy loss, less activity, and less cold stress. The calorie goal for an infant receiving parenteral feedings is 80 to 100 kcal/d when compared with the 120 kcal/d for the enterally fed infant. Individual infant requirements may vary, however, according to specific metabolic needs. Early infusions typically include glucose, amino acids, and lipids. Supplementation with calcium and vitamins is standard, and electrolytes are provided on the basis of laboratory results. Infants receiving long-term ongoing parenteral nutrition require the addition of trace elements. Regular laboratory work is required to assess treatment (Table 24.3).

Enteral Tube Feeding
Infants too immature to coordinate sucking, swallowing, and breathing often require **enteral tube feeding**, as Lexi Cowslip's infant did in Chapter 10. Infants easily fatigued by suckling and infants in respiratory distress also benefit from this feeding method. Infants weighing under 1,800 g at birth (usually less than 32 weeks of gestation at birth) usually require their initial feeding by tube, as well. The tube for infants who are simply premature and are expected to be able to suckle in the future is typically an NG or orogastric tube. Although an orogastric tube may be the preferred tube for infants with nasal respiratory support, NG tubes are often better tolerated.

Infants with major neurologic or congenital problems not expected to successfully suckle in the short term may require a gastrostomy. After the gastronomy site has healed, the infant receives small feedings by gravity over 20 to 30 minutes to avoid abdominal distention, which can lead to reflux into the esophagus and aspiration of gastric contents. As with all indwelling lines, meticulous skin care is critical to reducing infection risk.

Initial tube feedings are often small to "prime" the gastrointestinal tract and are called trophic feedings (Morgan, Young, & McGuire, 2014). The typical trophic feeding is 15 to 25 mL/kg/d in volume and may be done with preterm infant formula or unfortified expressed breast milk. Undiluted breast milk when available from the infant's mother or from a breast milk bank is generally preferred, as full enteral feeds are achieved more rapidly with breast milk and intestinal motility is better.

The volume of feedings increases according to infant tolerance of feedings as well as size and current postmenstrual age. Volume titrations vary between institutions, although an increase of 15 to 25 mL/kg/d is typical for infants who are tolerating feedings. As the volume of enteral feedings increases, the volume of parenteral feedings decreases, and parenteral feeding is typically stopped altogether when the infant is tolerating 100 mL/kg/d of enteral feeding. At a volume of 80 mL/kg/d, less calorically dense formula is traded for 24 kcal/oz formula, which is designed for preterm infants; infants fed breast milk have the milk fortified. The target

Table 24.3 Laboratory Tests Associated With Parenteral Feeding

Laboratory Test	Reason	Timing
Urine glucose	To detect glucose in the urine (glycosuria), which indicates high glucose serum levels, beyond the renal reabsorption threshold	Daily until stable and then as indicated
Serum triglyceride	To adjust lipid dosing	As indicated
Blood urea nitrogen	To adjust amino acid dosing	After the first week and then on alternate weeks
Electrolytes (sodium, potassium, chloride, bicarbonate)	To adjust electrolyte supplementation	Daily until stable and then as indicated
Calcium	To evaluate the sufficiency of calcium and phosphorous intake • Hypocalcemia indicates inadequate calcium intake • Hypercalcemia can indicate phosphorus insufficiency	After the first week and then on alternate weeks
Phosphorus	To evaluate the sufficiency of phosphorus intake and renal function • High phosphorus may indicate renal insufficiency • Low phosphorus indicates the need for supplementation	After the first week and then on alternate weeks
Magnesium	To evaluate the sufficiency of magnesium intake • May be initially elevated • Typically declines within 1 wk after birth and should then be supplemented	After the first week and then on alternate weeks
Alkaline phosphatase	To evaluate the sufficiency of calcium and phosphorous intake and the rate of growth	After the first week and then on alternate weeks
Liver function tests	To assess for cholestasis (a complication of parenteral nutrition) and liver function	After the first week and then on alternate weeks
Creatinine	To assess creatinine level • Elevation may indicate renal dysfunction that could cause excretion of nutrients	After the first week and then on alternate weeks

volume for enteric feeding is 160 mL/kg/d of fortified breast milk or calorically dense formula.

Tube feedings administered by syringe are typically scheduled every 2 to 3 hours. Infants fed more frequently tend to tolerate greater volumes of milk or formula, gain weight more quickly, and receive parenteral nutrition less frequently. Alternatively, infants may be fed continuously by infusion pump.

Tolerating enteral feedings is a significant issue for preterm infants, particularly those less than 28 weeks of postmenstrual age. Feeding intolerance is the primary factor in decisions about feeding volume and discontinuation. There are four major assessments to consider for feeding intolerance: vomiting, abdominal examination, gastric fluid residual, and stool output (Box 24.5). In addition, changes in clinical status such as bradycardia, apnea, or lethargy may be signs of feeding intolerance.

Box 24.5 Assessment Findings Concerning for Feeding Intolerance

• Abdominal examination findings
  ○ Decreased or absent bowel sounds
  ○ Abdominal tenderness or distention
• Vomiting
• Gastric residual fluid findings
  ○ Increased volume of fluid
  ○ Green fluid
  ○ Red fluid
• Stool-related findings
  ○ Change in frequency of defecation
  ○ Presence of blood

The gastric residual volume is an indirect measure of bowel motility and is typically checked just prior to any enteric tube feeding. Infants fed continuously should have their gastric residual checked every 2 to 4 hours or according to protocol. The infant stomach generally empties fairly rapidly. A residual volume greater than 50% of the volume fed in the last 3 hours *or* a volume of greater than 2 mL/kg is considered abnormal. Aspirates under this volume may be refed to the infant. There is normal variation between infants, however, and residuals should be considered in this context. Additionally, some infants may have better gastric emptying in one position than another. Delayed gastric emptying may also be evidence of a different, systemic problem. Green residual may indicate stomach overdistension or a bowel obstruction. Red residual is blood and may reflect an inflammatory process or mechanical injury to the mucosa from the tube. Gross blood in the stool can be a sign of feeding intolerance but may also indicate NEC.

Feeding intolerance may be addressed by delaying feedings and by reducing the starting volume. However, prolonged withholding of feeding may contribute to intestinal atrophy and the need for a longer course of parenteral nutrition.

Oral Feeding

Oral feeding without a tube can usually start in infants who are 32 to 34 weeks of gestational age. Infants who are at 34 weeks of gestation or greater at birth often do not require tube feeding at all, although some may require supplemental nutrition by this method for a period of time. Feeding may be by breast, bottle, cup, spoon, or syringe. Sucking for nonnutritive purposes, or "practice" sucking, may be encouraged in any infant who is medically stable.

The nurse should encourage mothers who cannot directly feed their infants or whose infants can sustain only partial feeds to pump and store their breast milk. Hospital-grade pumps work best for most women in terms of optimizing milk extraction. Regardless of whether they are pumping their breast milk or feeding their infants directly, mothers providing nutrition to preterm infants need a great deal of support and encouragement.

Assessing feeding is just as important for infants fed orally as for those fed by other methods. Infants who fail to gain adequate weight, are unable to consume at least 180 mL/kg/d, or have abnormal laboratory test findings indicating poor bone growth or inadequate protein intake may require fortified breast milk or feeding with formula at 30 cal/oz. Infants who are gaining weight well and have normal laboratory test results, however, may have unfortified breast milk or 20 kcal/oz infant formula.

Late Preterm Infants: Common Conditions and Care Considerations

An infant born from 34 0/7 to 36 6/7 weeks of gestation is considered late preterm. Although they are often the same size as some term infants, late preterm infants have higher morbidity and mortality rates than term infants because of physiologic and metabolic immaturity. Approximately a quarter of a million late preterm births occur annually, and the rise in preterm births over the last 30 years

is primarily due to an increase in births from 34 0/7 to 36 6/7 weeks of gestation (Hamilton, Martin, & Osterman, 2016). The rise in late preterm births is attributed to increased surveillance of pregnancy conditions of the mother, fetus, and/or placenta that indicate an earlier birth by induction or cesarean section. An increase in the rate of multiple pregnancies is also a factor, as is the increase in maternal age over the last 30 years, inaccurate pregnancy dating, and the increase in maternal obesity (Martin, Hamilton, Osterman, Curtin, & Matthews, 2015).

If you'll recall, Gracie Munez in Chapter 8 delivered her baby at 34 weeks of gestation, after experiencing preterm premature rupture of membranes. So, her baby, Eddie, was considered late preterm.

Late preterm infants have a rate of neonatal complications many times higher than that of term neonates. They are more likely to experience apnea, feeding difficulties, hyperbilirubinemia, hypoglycemia, hypothermia, low Apgar scores, and respiratory distress (Seikku et al., 2016). Although certainly some neonates may experience these complications as a result of the gestational complications that indicated an early delivery, birth from 34 0/7 to 36 6/7 weeks of gestation is an independent risk factor for complications.

Letitia Richford's baby, in Chapter 5, was a late preterm infant and therefore had to be monitored closely for hyperbilirubinemia and hypoglycemia.

Hypothermia

Late preterm infants are more at risk for hypothermia because of reasons of anatomic immaturity. Term infants generally gain adipose tissue in the final weeks of pregnancy. Late preterm infants have had less time to build up these fat stores. Their stores of brown fat, which generate heat in early infancy, are also smaller and deplete more rapidly. Their ratio of surface area to weight is larger, putting them at a greater risk for heat loss. Because of these differences, late preterm infants are at a greater risk for hypothermia and cold stress, as discussed earlier in this chapter. Late preterm infants benefit particularly from skin-to-skin contact for temperature regulation. The nurse should regularly monitor the newborn's temperature and keep the newborn swaddled when not being held for warmth and protection from drafts.

Hypoglycemia

Late preterm infants are far more likely to develop hypoglycemia than term infants. It occurs because of failure of the immature metabolic system of the neonate to respond adequately to the loss of the maternal glucose supply. When caring for neonates with hypoglycemia, the nurse should follow the institution's protocol for blood glucose monitoring until the infant is feeding well and the blood glucose level has stabilized. Hypoglycemia is generally treated when blood glucose levels drop below 40 or 45 mg/dL or with symptoms of hypoglycemia (see Box 3.10). Asymptomatic infants are usually treated with oral feedings with breast milk or formula. Symptomatic patients may be treated with IV dextrose.

Respiratory Distress

Late preterm infants are at a higher risk for respiratory distress stemming from a number of causes, including RDS. They are more likely to experience respiratory failure and require ventilator support than term infants. Development of the terminal respiratory sacs and alveoli continue through week 36 of gestation, and a surfactant surge occurs around week 34, right at the beginning of the late preterm period. The result for a late preterm infant is underdevelopment of the respiratory system when compared with a term infant. The incidence of apnea is also many times higher in late preterm infants than term infants, and the occurrence of sudden infant death syndrome, an apneic event, is also higher (King, Gazmararian, & Shapiro-Mendoza, 2014). The nurse should carefully monitor respiratory status in the late preterm infant, who may go home with an apnea monitor. The nurse should also perform a car seat challenge prior to discharge (see Box 5.8).

Jaundice

Late preterm infants are twice as likely to develop prolonged hyperbilirubinemia because of immaturity of the hepatic bilirubin conjugation pathways. In addition, challenges with feeding slow the passage of meconium, thus increasing bilirubin levels in the system. Because of immaturity of the blood–brain barrier and lower concentrations of albumin, which binds to bilirubin, late preterm infants are more likely than term infants to experience brain injury from high bilirubin concentrations. Bilirubin levels tend to peak at the end of the first week of life, and high bilirubin levels are the most common reason for late preterm infants to be readmitted. Early follow-up with the neonate's pediatric provider after discharge is important to monitor bilirubin levels.

Feeding Difficulties

Orobuccal strength and the ability to coordinate sucking, swallowing, and breathing are not fully developed in the late preterm infant, leading to feeding challenges. Late preterm infants are also more likely to become sleepy, fatigued, and difficult to rouse adequately to feed. Although breastfeeding remains the feeding method of choice, mothers may need to express milk to encourage supply and supplement the infant with breast milk from a cup, spoon, syringe, or artificial nipple until the infant can adequately feed and the milk supply is established. Skin-to-skin contact is helpful for encouraging feeding as well as for thermoregulation. The nurse should review the use of the breast pump and safe handling and storage of the milk with the mother (see Box 18.9). Parents may be advised to chart and record infant input and output. Failure to feed and dehydration create risks for readmission and IV hydration.

Long-Term Morbidity

The brain of a late preterm infant is about 65% of the size of a term infant. Brain immaturity and gestational factors that necessitated early birth likely contribute to the increased risk for cerebral palsy and cognitive delay in this population. Late preterm birth is also associated with developmental and academic delays. Infants born late preterm are less likely to graduate from high school and college (Shah, Kaciroti, Richards, Oh, & Lumeng, 2016).

Postterm Infants

A **postterm infant** is an infant born at a gestational age beyond 42 weeks. The rate of postterm births over the past 30 years has approximately halved because of a more thorough understanding of the risks of postmaturity and, as a result, earlier labor inductions and cesarean sections (Hamilton, Martin, Osterman, Curtin, & Matthews, 2015). A postterm pregnancy is more likely than a term pregnancy to result in a higher birth weight infant and even macrosomia. Conversely, a postterm pregnancy may also result in **fetal growth restriction (FGR)** because of insufficiency of an aging placenta, with the result of an infant who is **small for gestational age (SGA)**. Macrosomic infants generally appear large but otherwise normal. A postterm FGR infant, however, is more concerning because the smaller size is due to the inadequate transfer of nutrition and oxygen from the placenta. The FGR infant appears long and thin, often with meconium-stained skin. The skin appears loose and the creases at the joints are prominent. There is generally more scalp hair on a postterm infant but an absence of vernix caseosa and little to no lanugo. The nails are long and the infant appears alert. The postterm FGR infant is sometimes referred to as having dysmaturity syndrome.

The risk for perinatal mortality is significantly increased in a postterm pregnancy when compared with a term pregnancy. The placental insufficiency that contributes to FGR may also result in fetal asphyxia and an increased mortality rate.

Complications are more common in infants of postterm pregnancies, and the type of complication depends on the fetal presentation: macrosomia or dysmaturity syndrome. For macrosomic infants, greater size puts them at a higher risk for birth injuries resulting from shoulder dystocia, prolonged labor, and cephalopelvic disproportion. They may have more desquamation of their skin, which peaks at about a week after the birth (Fig. 24.9).

Because of placental insufficiency, oligohydramnios may occur in FGR infants, creating a greater risk for cord compression. Complications common to other SGA infants can occur with dysmaturity syndrome, as well, including polycythemia, hypoglycemia, impaired thermoregulation, impaired immune function, and hypocalcemia.

Regardless of classification as macrosomic or FGR, postterm infants are at an increased risk for perinatal asphyxia, as evidenced by lower Apgar scores. Postterm infants are more likely to be admitted to the NICU and to be diagnosed with a respiratory or infectious condition (Linder et al., 2017).

Children born post term are more likely to develop cerebral palsy. They are more likely to have epilepsy in the first year of life but not beyond. There may be a modest increased risk for

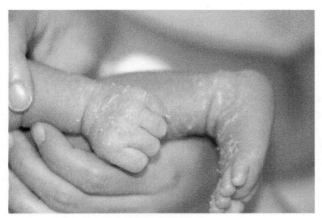

Figure 24.9. **Peeling of the skin.** Desquamation, or peeling of the skin, is rare in premature infants but quite common in full-term and, especially, postmature infants. (Reprinted with permission from Salimpour, R. R., Salimpour, P., & Salimpour, P. [2014]. *Photographic atlas of pediatric disorders and diagnosis* [1st ed., unnumbered figure]. Philadelphia, PA: Lippincott Williams & Wilkins.)

intellectual disability (Figlio, Guryan, Karbownik, & Roth, 2016; Seikku et al., 2016).

Women with postterm births most often have had antepartum screening for fetal well-being. They may have had a harrowing labor and birth with a macrosomic infant. These infants often appear different from their mothers' impressions of the typical newborn, with peeling skin, and possible meconium staining. The nurse should inform parents that this appearance is normal for this gestation. Baths with mild soap are useful for washing away meconium, and peeling resolves after a few weeks.

Fetal Growth Restriction

SGA is generally conceptualized as below the 10th percentile on growth charts. It should be noted, however, that this criteria does not consider nonpathologic factors that may contribute to small size, including the height and weight of parents and ethnicity. FGR refers only to SGA infants who are small due to environmental or pathologic genetic reasons.

Etiology

FGR infants did not achieve full growth potential in utero because of factors pertaining either to the intrauterine environment or to a genetic pathology. The remainder of this section refers to FGR infants who are SGA due to compromise of the intrauterine environment.

FGR infants are small because their supply of nutrients from the placenta in utero was low. FGR fetuses compensate for the reduced supply of nutrients by slowing growth of the body while diverting nutrients to brain growth and lung maturation. The supply of red blood cells is increased to optimize oxygen-carrying capacity (Tudehope, Vento, Bhutta, & Pachi, 2013). Less energy is expended to grow lean body mass and fat and for energy reserves.

FGR is divided into symmetric and asymmetric. The onset of symmetric FGR is earlier in the pregnancy. All organ systems,

including the brain, are affected equally, so the head and body are proportionate. Symmetric FGR is typically caused by a chromosomal abnormality or a congenital infection, although it may also occur with early onset of a poor supply of intrauterine nutrients. Unlike symmetric FGR, asymmetric FGR has a later onset in the third trimester or the late second trimester. It is a result of a low nutrient supply. Growth of the body is asymmetric with the brain growth, and thus head circumference is preserved, but the weight and length are compromised.

Signs and Symptoms

The face of an FGR infant typically has a shrunken appearance. The cranial sutures may appear unusually wide, with abnormally large fontanelles. The umbilical cord may be thinner than usual, and meconium staining of the infant, cord, fluid, and placenta may be present. The head appears abnormally large with asymmetric FGR. Classically, the skin of infants with FGR appears loose and peeling and muscle mass and subcutaneous fat are diminished.

Prognosis

FGR fetuses are at a greater risk for prematurity, and delivery is often induced if FGR is strongly suspected during pregnancy and the risks of prematurity are deemed less than the risks of an insufficient intrauterine environment. Premature FGR infants are at a greater risk for complications of prematurity, including RDS and NEC, than preterm infants who are appropriate for gestational age (AGA; De Jesus et al., 2013).

FGR infants are at an increased risk for asphyxia, poor immune function, polycythemia, hypoglycemia, poor thermoregulation, MAS, Persistent pulmonary hypertension of the neonate (PPHN), and death (Liu, Wang, Wang, Wang, & Liu, 2014). Some of these complications are described earlier in this chapter or in the next chapter, and others are reviewed below.

FGR infants are more likely to be shorter and weigh less into adulthood. They are also at an increased risk for neurodevelopmental abnormalities and reduced cognitive performance (Levine et al., 2015).

Perinatal Asphyxia

FGR from impaired placental function is worsened by uterine contractions. This impaired function can result in hypoxia of the infant that, in turn, causes metabolic acidosis. This puts FGR infants at a higher risk for NEC, pulmonary edema, RDS, MAS, PPHN, myocardial dysfunction, and injury to the kidneys and gastrointestinal tract (Christensen, Baer, & Yaish, 2015). Thermoregulation by use of a skin-to-skin contact, an isolette, or a radiant warmer is critical to avoiding cold stress, which can exacerbate problems related to perinatal asphyxia.

Hypoglycemia

Because infants with FGR are at a known risk for hypoglycemia, glucose screening is indicated after the first feed, which ideally occurs within an hour after the birth. Prefeed glucose screening is then recommended every 3 to 6 hours for the first 24 to 48 hours after birth. Testing is usually with a point-of-care heel stick (see Step-by-Step Skills 3.1). Institutions may require a confirmatory laboratory test for the diagnosis of hypoglycemia.

A newborn identified as hypoglycemic by institution standards may require regular monitoring for an extended period of time. A common goal for symptomatic infants are serum glucose levels is greater than 50 mg/dL for newborns younger than 48 hours and greater than 60 mg/dL for older infants (Stanley et al., 2015). Lower glucose levels are generally tolerated for infants who are asymptomatic. These infants may not be treated unless symptoms occur or their serum glucose level drops below the following values: less than 25 mg/dL for infants less than 4 hours old; less than 35 mg/dL for infants 4 to 24 hours old; less than 50 mg/dL for infants 24 to 48 hours old; and less than 60 mg/dL for infants older than 48 hours (Stanley et al., 2015).

Symptoms of hypoglycemia can be classified as neurogenic (autonomic symptoms from hypoglycemia) or neuroglycopenic (caused by dysfunction of the brain due to a deficient glucose supply; Box 24.6). Newborn infants may also experience hypothermia, cyanosis, bradycardia, and apnea as a result of hypoglycemia.

Because symptomatic hypoglycemia can result in injury to the brain, it is usually treated aggressively with IV dextrose. Typical initial dosing for dextrose is a bolus of 2 mL/kg of 10% dextrose in water over 5 minutes followed by a continuous infusion at a rate of 6 to 8 mg/kg/min (Stanley et al., 2015). Infants who are asymptomatic and above the minimum targets identified above may be fed orally instead.

Polycythemia

Polycythemia is common in FGR infants. Polycythemia is a condition in which an infant has a large number of circulating red blood cells that were produced because of fetal hypoxia stimulating increased erythropoietin and thus red blood cell production. A hematocrit or hemoglobin concentration more than two standard deviations above normal for gestational age measured from capillary blood is considered diagnostic for polycythemia. Hyperviscosity of the blood may occur in infants with a hematocrit above 65%.

Approximately half of infants with polycythemia have no signs. It is not clear whether signs develop as a result of polycythemia or are simply associated with other complications that often co-occur. In infants who are symptomatic, poor feeding, vomiting, hypoglycemia, cyanosis, and apnea are the most commonly associated signs and usually occur within 2 hours after the birth. Other associated signs include tachypnea, oliguria, and jitteriness. Infants with polycythemia tend to have lengthier stays in the NICU. Infants who do not develop signs of polycythemia within 77 hours after birth are unlikely to do so, as the hematocrit peaks at 2.8 hours of age before dropping slowly until 77 hours and then dropping more precipitously. Many infants develop hyperbilirubinemia as the circulating red blood cells begin to break down, releasing bilirubin. Screening for polycythemia is not generally recommended for infants who appear well. Indicated treatment includes close observation, IV hydration, and, rarely, partial exchange transfusion of the blood (Alsafadi et al., 2014).

Other infants at risk for polycythemia include those born at term with delayed cord clamping at birth; monochorionic twins who undergo a twin-to-twin blood transfusion; infants of diabetic mothers; infants who are **large for gestational age (LGA)**; infants with adrenal hyperplasia, hypothyroidism, or hyperthyroidism; and infants with certain chromosomal abnormalities.

Hypocalcemia

Hypocalcemia occurs in the first 2 to 3 days after birth and happens more frequency in infants with FGR, infants with perinatal asphyxia or hypoparathyroidism, and infants of mothers with diabetes. In the case of FGR, reduced passage of calcium across the placenta is thought to be the cause. Perinatal asphyxia is more common in FGR infants and may also play a part.

Most infants with hypocalcemia do not have symptoms. When symptoms do occur, they are a result of neuromuscular irritability. These signs include jitteriness, muscle jerking in response to stimuli, seizure activity, laryngospasm resulting in stridor, bronchospasm causing wheezing, and vomiting from spasm of the pylorus. At-risk infants are generally screened at 12, 24, and 48 hours after birth. Hypocalcemic infants who are asymptomatic are monitored regularly until regular, calcium-rich feeding is established. Healthy, feeding infants weighing over 1,500 g and healthy infants of mothers with diabetes are generally not screened in the absence of symptoms. Nutritional therapy is usually sufficient to treat asymptomatic infants, whereas symptomatic infants may require IV supplementation of calcium gluconate.

Late hypoglycemia, which occurs after day 2 or 3 of life and usually in the first week, is associated with bicarbonate and lipid infusions, as well as acute renal failure and phototherapy for the treatment of hyperbilirubinemia.

Box 24.6 Clinical Signs of Hypoglycemia

Neurogenic
- Irritability
- Jitteriness/tremors
- Pallor
- Sweating
- Tachypnea

Neuroglycopenic
- Change in level of consciousness (coma, lethargy)
- Hypotonia
- Poor feeding and/or poor suck
- Seizures
- Weak or high-pitched cry

Assessment

Moderate FGR is defined as weight in the 3rd to 10th percentiles, whereas severe FGR is defined as weight below the 3rd percentile. Confirmation of the diagnosis of FGR, however, requires that other factors be considered, including the size of the parents, ethnicity, and the appearance of the infant beyond weight. The ponderal index (PI) is a useful tool for detecting asymmetric FGR. The PI is the ratio of body weight to length: (weight [in g] × 100) ÷ (length [in cm])^3. A PI below the 10th percentile indicates poor intrauterine nutrition.

Macrosomia

LGA is defined as an infant who is above the 90th percentile for weight, and the larger the infant, the greater the risk for harm to the mother and the neonate at the time of birth. The term **macrosomia** is based on weight regardless of gestational age. It is defined as a birth weight greater than 4,000 g or 4,500 g. For context, a term infant weighing from 2,500 to 3,999 g is considered AGA.

Recall that Susan Rockwell's baby, Winston, in Chapter 3, was macrosomic, weighing 9 lb and 3 oz (over 4,100 g). Susan was obese, and developed gestational diabetes, which likely contributed.

Etiology

Macrosomia is more common in infants of mothers with obesity, diabetes, and excessive weight gain in pregnancy. It is also more common in some ethnic groups and in infants whose mothers were macrosomic at birth. Some genetic syndromes can also contribute to macrosomia. Higher birth weights are more common with postterm pregnancies, advanced maternal age, male infants, and women who have given birth previously (Araujo Junior, Peixoto, Zamarian, Elito Junior, & Tonni, 2017).

Recall that Nancy Ng's baby, Jonathan, in Chapter 9, was macrosomic, weighing 4,400 g, or about 9 lb and 7 oz. Nancy developed gestational diabetes in pregnancy (like Susan in Chapter 3).

Prognosis

Macrosomic infants are at a higher risk for RDS, mechanical ventilation, a low Apgar score, MAS, hypoglycemia, polycythemia, perinatal asphyxia, and death when compared with infants assessed as AGA. They are also at an increased risk for birth injury due to shoulder dystocia (brachial plexus injury and clavicular injury).

Shoulder dystocia occurs after the birth of the head and requires additional obstetric maneuvers for the birth of the shoulders. Although macrosomia is not the only risk factor for shoulder dystocia, the two are often associated (see Box 11.6). The most common associated injuries to the newborn include temporary brachial plexus injury, fracture of the clavicle, fracture of the humerus, permanent brachial plexus injury, and, more rarely, death. Injuries may be related to the labor and dystocia itself, delivery interventions, or compression of the umbilical cord or blood vessels in the fetal neck. For further details on these and other birth injuries in the newborn, see the section "Birth Trauma".

Assessment

Polycythemia and hypoglycemia related to macrosomia should be assessed for and managed as described previously.

Birth Trauma

Birth trauma or birth injury is any compromise of a newborn's function or structure as a result of a birth-associated event. Injury may occur during labor or during or immediately after delivery. In addition to macrosomia, factors that increase the risk for birth injury are maternal obesity, any fetal presentation other than vertex, operative vaginal delivery, and cesarean delivery. Discussed below are integumentary, musculoskeletal, and neurologic injuries to the newborn associated with birth. Also, see Chapter 18 for descriptions and a comparison of caput succedaneum, cephalohematoma, and subgaleal hemorrhage.

Integumentary Injuries

Bruising

Bruising is typically found on the presenting part of the infant. Bruising of the genitals, for example, is a finding typical of a breach delivery, whereas petechiae of the face and head may be seen in an infant born vertex. These petechiae usually resolve within a few days. Progressive petechiae, particularly when associated with other bleeding, is concerning for thrombocytopenia. Although bruising itself is generally self-limiting, breakdown of red blood cells as the bruising resolves can develop into pathologic hyperbilirubinemia. Earlier postdischarge follow-up to assess for jaundice may be indicated for infants with severe bruising.

Fat Necrosis

Subcutaneous fat necrosis presents as indurated plaques or erythematous nodules on the body or face of the infant in the first 6 weeks after the birth. Hypercalcemia may develop as a consequence of the condition, so although it is self-limiting, it is important that it be recognized. Approximately 63% of infants with subcutaneous fat necrosis develop hypercalcemia (Del Pozzo-Magana & Ho, 2016). The plaques and induration or erythematous nodules typically resolve over the course of weeks or months. All but one of the recorded cases have resolved completely by 9 months of age

(Beuzeboc Gerard et al., 2014). Scarring is rare. Infants who develop subcutaneous fat necrosis are usually born at term. Risk factors include hypoxia, the use of therapeutic hypothermia, maternal diabetes or hypertension, placental abruption, and preeclampsia (Del Pozzo-Magana & Ho, 2016).

Lacerations

Lacerations are the most common birth injury associated with cesarean section. They occur most often with emergency deliveries and are typically superficial. Most injuries of this sort occur to the face or scalp, and a small number are serious enough to require plastic surgery. Most can be repaired with adhesive strips. Lacerations may also occur during a vaginal delivery, typically to the presenting part at the time of an episiotomy.

Musculoskeletal Injuries

Nasal Septal Dislocation

Dislocation of the nasal septum occurs with a small number of births because of compression of the nose during passage through the birth canal. The infant's nose appears to deviate from the midline position. The nares are asymmetric, with one appearing flattened. An otolaryngologist usually diagnoses the condition and corrects it within 3 days of the birth to avoid deformity. Severe dislocation can result in obstruction of the airway, resulting in respiratory distress.

Fractures

Parents of an infant with a fracture are often worried they may hurt their infant while handling him or her. Nursing staff can provide guidance for safe handling of the infant and support of the injury.

Clavicle

The clavicle is the most commonly fractured bone of the neonate. Although shoulder dystocia is often associated with clavicle fracture, it is not the only risk factor. Fractures of the clavicle have also been recorded in otherwise uncomplicated births of macrosomic infants, infants born to women of advanced maternal age, and infants with an unusually low head-to-chest circumference ratio and a vacuum delivery (Ahn et al., 2015). Infants are usually asymptomatic and the diagnosis is made by radiology. Such injuries heal spontaneously with no long-term consequences. Infants signaling pain may be treated with analgesics. The arm on that side may be placed in a long sleeve and pinned at 90-degree flexion to the chest.

Humerus

Fracture of the humerus is rare in the newborn. Like the clavicle fracture, it's associated with shoulder dystocia and macrosomia. Other risks for humeral fracture include breech delivery, cesarean delivery, and low birth weight. The cesarean delivery, in fact, poses a greater risk for long bone fracture than vaginal birth (Basha, Amarin, & Abu-Hassan, 2013).

An infant with a fracture of the humerus has a muted Moro reflex and reduced movement of the arm. Palpation of the arm reveals a pain response, as well as swelling and crepitus. Diagnosis is by imaging. Treatment includes immobilization of the arm at 90° of flexion with a shirt, as described above, or an elastic wrap.

Femur

The femur fracture is rarer than the humeral fracture and tends to occur at the proximal end of the femur, closer to the hip. It occurs more often with twin pregnancies, breech births, and prematurity. Swelling may be present or absent. Diagnosis is by imaging. A Pavlik harness is typically used to stabilize the injury (Fig. 24.10).

Skull

Most skull fractures of neonates are depressed skull fractures. A depressed skull fracture is caused by the inward buckling of the skull. It can happen spontaneously during a vaginal birth as the fetal head is pushed against the bones of the maternal pelvis and spine. A skull fracture may also result from a forceps delivery. Spontaneous depressed skull fractures that occur in the absence of forceps intervention are rarely associated with neurologic damage. A depressed skull fracture that occurs as a result of forceps, however, presents an increased risk for cephalohematoma (see Figs. 9.11 and 18.6) and intracranial bleeding. Although the spontaneous skull fracture can be typically assessed by a simple

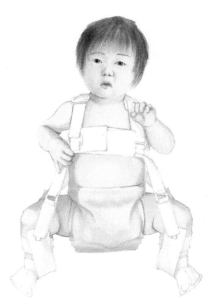

Figure 24.10. A Pavlik harness for the treatment of congenital hip dysplasia and femur fracture. The harness is composed of shoulder straps, stirrups, and a chest strap. It is placed on both legs, even if only one hip is dislocated or broken. (Reprinted with permission from Hatfield, N. T. [2014]. *Introductory maternity and pediatric nursing* [3rd ed., Fig. 21-25]. Philadelphia, PA: Lippincott Williams & Wilkins.)

X-ray, the increased likelihood of bleeding with a forceps-induced fracture requires evaluation by computed tomography (CT) and evaluation by a neurologist.

Neurologic Injuries

Ocular Injuries

Subconjunctival hemorrhages look alarming but are very common in neonates, along with retinal hemorrhages (Fig. 24.11). They resolve spontaneously within 2 weeks, however. More severe eye injuries, such as blood in the vitreous or anterior chamber, orbital fracture, or damage to a lacrimal gland, are rare and more often associated with forceps delivery. These require management by an ophthalmologist.

Intracranial Hemorrhage

Although intracranial hemorrhage (ICH) is rare, its risk of occurrence increases with forceps and vacuum-assisted delivery. Although IVH is a form of ICH, it occurs only rarely as a birth injury associated with term infants. In term infants, most cases of IVH are grade 1 and resolve spontaneously with no long-term consequences (Sirgiovanni et al., 2014). The other forms of ICH include subdural hemorrhage, subarachnoid hemorrhage (SAH), and epidural hemorrhage (EDH). An infant may be diagnosed with multiple kinds of ICH. The diagnosis of ICH is best made by CT or magnetic resonance imaging.

Subdural Hemorrhage

A subdural hemorrhage occurs because of the tearing of veins between the dura mater and the arachnoid membrane. There is typically no evidence on the scalp suggesting injury. Infants may be asymptomatic. If symptoms do occur, they usually appear within the first 48 hours after injury, as seizures and/or apnea and respiratory distress. Infants may also display altered tone or level of consciousness or appear irritable.

Most neonates can be managed without surgical intervention and are monitored regularly with vital signs and serial hematocrits. The collection of blood generally resolves within the first few months of life. Occasionally, surgical intervention is necessary to reduce intracranial pressure and brainstem compression. Infants experiencing seizure activity may be treated with antiepileptics,

often phenobarbital. Approximately 80% of infants recover without disability (Shah & Wusthoff, 2016).

Subarachnoid Hemorrhage

An SAH is venous bleeding into the subarachnoid space. The presentation is similar to that of a subdural hemorrhage. Treatment is typically conservative. Occasionally, a large SAH may interfere with the normal reabsorption of CSF, leading to hydrocephalus. The prognosis is usually good, although an SAH located in the frontal lobe or in multiple areas is associated with inferior outcomes (Shah & Wusthoff, 2016).

Epidural Hemorrhage

The rare EDH occurs because of the tearing of an artery between the dura and the skull and is often associated with a linear fracture of the skull in the peritemporal area. It occurs more frequently with operative first-time vaginal deliveries and frequently co-occurs with cephalohematoma. Because the source of the bleed is arterial rather than venous, the condition of the neonate may deteriorate quickly.

Symptoms typical of EDH include seizures and hypotonia. As bleeding progresses and the intracranial pressure rises, the fontanelles bulge and alterations are noted in the neonate's vital signs and level of consciousness. Although a clinically stable neonate with a small EDH may be managed conservatively with close observation, a larger EDH and increased intracranial pressure require surgical intervention.

Brachial Plexus Injury

The brachial plexus is a network of nerves that innervate the muscles and skin of the arms and shoulders. They emerge bilaterally at the level of the cervical and upper thoracic vertebrae. Stretching and traction on the brachial plexus is the most common cause of injury; the compression of the nerves, hemorrhage, and oxygen deprivation of the neonate may also contribute. Stretching and traction applied by the obstetric provider in an effort to manage shoulder dystocia may be contributory, but labor and pushing alone without intervention may also provide force sufficient to cause injury, particularly in the presence of uterine abnormalities such as fibroids (Ouzounian, 2014).

A brachial plexus injury is typically unilateral but may on occasion present bilaterally. How a brachial plexus injury manifests depends on the level of the injury. Injury at vertebrae C5 and C6 accounts for about half of cases and is referred to as Erb palsy. Infants with Erb palsy have an upper arm that is adducted and internally rotated. The forearm is extended and movement of the wrist and hand are normal. Injury at this level is associated with injury to the phrenic nerve, which can cause diaphragmatic paralysis. The diagnosis of phrenic nerve damage is supported by asymmetric expansion of the chest with breathing and impaired oxygenation and/or feeding. These infants usually require mechanical ventilation in the short term and may require corrective surgery.

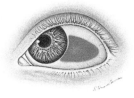

Figure 24.11. Subconjunctival hemorrhage. (Reprinted with permission from Bickley, L. S., & Szilagyi, P. [2003]. *Bates' guide to physical examination and history taking* [8th ed., unnumbered figure]. Philadelphia, PA: Lippincott Williams & Wilkins.)

Recall that Edie Wilson in Chapter 11 went into precipitous labor and experienced shoulder dystocia. As a result of the shoulder dystocia, her baby sustained a brachial plexus injury, resulting in Erb palsy and a limp left arm, which the pediatrician anticipated would resolve spontaneously with time.

Injury at vertebrae C5, C6, and C7 is referred to as Erb palsy plus and accounts for 35% of injuries. As with Erb palsy, the upper arm is adducted and internally rotated. Unlike Erb palsy, however, the forearm is extended and pronated and there is flexion of the wrists and fingers (waiter's tip posture). Injury from vertebrae C5 to T1 typically presents as arm paralysis with some finger flexion, although a more severe manifestation is a flail arm (a complete lack of mobility and sensation of the arm) and Horner syndrome, which affects the nerve activity of one side of the face, including the eye. Klumpke palsy occurs because of damage between vertebrae C8 and T1 and manifests as hand paralysis and Horner syndrome (Ouzounian, 2014).

Although most infants with a brachial plexus injury recover over a few months, up to half continue to experience some functional impairment. More extensive injury is associated with a less complete recovery. Early improvement in the first weeks after birth, recovery of upper arm strength before 5 months, and elbow strength and flexion by 3 months are all associated with better outcomes. A lack of spontaneous progress is associated with a less hopeful outcome (American College of Obstetricians and Gynecologists, 2014). Surgery for nerve repair and contractures may be considered in some cases.

Physical therapy is the first-line treatment for brachial plexus injuries and typically starts at the end of the first week after birth. Physical therapy is used to promote muscle strength and function. Splints may be used to prevent contractures of the elbow and fingers (Yang, 2014).

Facial Nerve Trauma

Birth trauma to the facial nerve (cranial nerve VII) may occur because of prolonged pressure against the bones of the maternal pelvis but is more often associated with a forceps delivery. The neonate has reduced movement on the side of the injury, as evidenced by incomplete closure of the eye and flattening of the nasolabial fold. The neonate's forehead does not wrinkle, and the mouth draws over to the undamaged side when the newborn cries (Fig. 24.12). The paralysis is usually temporary and begins to resolve over hours, although complete recovery may take months.

Feeding may be particularly challenging for these infants because of an inability to form a seal around the nipple with one side of the mouth. Because the eye cannot close completely, it may need to be taped shut, with artificial tears used to protect the cornea.

Spinal Cord Injury

Injury to the spinal cord due to birth trauma is rare and occurs most commonly at the level of the cervical spine because of

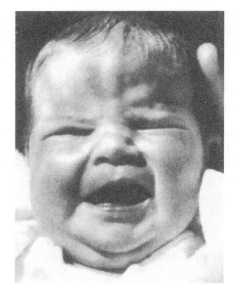

Figure 24.12. Facial nerve paralysis. Notice the asymmetry of the mouth during crying. (Reprinted with permission from Simpson, K. R., & Creehan, P. A. [2008]. *AWHONN's perinatal nursing* [3rd ed., Fig. 12.11]. Philadelphia, PA: Lippincott Williams & Wilkins.)

traction and rotation. The use of forceps and a breech delivery pose the greatest risk, although the occurrence remains low. Manifestations and prognosis depend on the location of the injury and its severity. Damage to the lower spinal cord may result in paraplegia. Upper lesions, particularly those of the brainstem, have a high mortality rate. Infants may appear well initially but experience deterioration over the course of days, with worsening respiratory function, paralysis, flaccid extremities, and death. Infants may alternatively be stillborn or die soon after birth.

Neonatal Pain

Infants admitted to the NICU experience on average 5 to 15 painful procedures every day, including needlesticks, suctioning, and other diagnostic and therapeutic activities (Schiavenato & Holsti, 2017). The other sources of pain include surgery, birth trauma, and severe disease, such as NEC, and the sequelae of severe disease. Although it was historically believed that neonates did not experience pain or require assessment or pain intervention, we now know this to be false. By the middle of the second trimester of pregnancy, the fetus has a functional sensory system.

Not treating pain adequately can have a long-term effect on how the neonate responds to pain throughout his or her lifetime. Neonates exposed to pain repeatedly in the first days of life have a heightened risk for developing chronic pain and an increased sensitivity to pain later in life. Repeated pain exposure can cause neurodevelopmental changes that result in cognitive delay, hormonal dysregulation, and neuroprocessing deficits (Doesburg et al., 2013).

Box 24.7 Parameters for Neonatal Pain Assessment

Physiologic

- Vital signs
  - Change in heart rate
  - Change in respiratory rate
  - Change in blood pressure
- Respiratory
  - Change in breathing pattern
  - Change in oxygen saturation
- Integumentary
  - Sweating of palms
  - Change in skin color
- Other
  - Increased intracranial pressure
  - Change in heart rate variability
  - Change in pupil size

Behavioral responses

- Crying
  - Change in crying pattern
  - Change in acoustic features of cry
  - Changes in consolability
- Movement
  - Change in facial expression
    - Brow bulge, eye squeeze, nasolabial furrow, open mouth
  - Hand and body movements
  - Changes in muscle tone

Assessment

Adequately assessing pain in the neonate is essential for appropriate treatment. Pain assessment for neonates can be quite challenging, however. Pain is subjective, as is the assessment of neonatal pain. There can be significant variability among observers evaluating behavioral responses to assess pain. Most pain scales are developed and validated with healthy infants who are either term or near term. Nurses assessing neonatal pain in ill infants and very preterm infants should be aware of more subtle signs of distress, as this cohort may have a more muted behavioral response to pain because they lack the strength, energy, and vigor for a more robust response. Parameters to consider in neonatal pain assessment are itemized in Box 24.7.

As is true for older children and adults experiencing prolonged or chronic pain, the behavioral and physiologic responses to the noxious stimuli are blunted. Infants experiencing persistent pain after surgery, for example, may appear passive, with a reduced respiratory rate and reduced variability in heart rate. Body movements and facial expressions are limited. These variables limit the usefulness of assessment tools used to detect acute pain (American Academy of Pediatrics, 2016). There is not at this time a well-validated tool for the evaluation of prolonged pain in the neonate (Gibbins et al., 2014). Only 10% of neonates are assessed daily for prolonged pain (Anand et al., 2017).

Institutions often select one or more tools to use in the NICU to standardize evaluation. Examples include the following:

- Premature Infant Pain Profile
- Neonatal Pain Agitation and Sedation Scale
- Neonatal Infant Pain Scale
- Crying, Requires Oxygen Saturation, Increased Vital Signs, Expression, Sleeplessness
- Neonatal Facial Coding System
- Douleur Aiguë Nouveau-né scale
- Behavioral Infant Pain Profile
- Comfort neo scale

A different approach, which has not been validated, is the "pain detection method," which considers the body region stimulation and the type of noxious stimuli present to determine the presence of pain (Bellieni, Tei, & Buonocore, 2015).

Prevention and Treatment

We know that pain control has long-term as well as short-term benefits for newborns. Better than relieving pain, however, is avoiding or minimizing pain. We know that certain procedures, such as tube placement, catheterization, suctioning, and circumcision, are painful. The postoperative period is painful, as are diseases such as NEC. Reducing the number of painful procedures is a goal for all care providers. Pain should be treated preemptively when possible. When pain is recognized during assessment, it should be treated proactively. Measures of pain relief may be pharmacologic or nonpharmacologic (Box 24.8).

Parents can often actively participate in relieving pain for the neonate. Providing skin-to-skin contact is a role for either parent. Oral sucrose and NNS can be provided by a parent, as can cuddling and rocking, when appropriate. Nurses should assure parents that their infant's pain is actively monitored and addressed, and that the nurse is advocating for the newborn's optimal comfort. Parents should be informed that pain may not be completely avoidable but that it will be minimized as much as possible. In some circumstances, parents may be taught to assess pain according to the tool used by the NICU, thus taking an active and important role in care of the infant.

Box 24.8 Pain Management for the Neonate

- Nonpharmacologic
  - Breastfeeding
  - Nonnutritive sucking (pacifier)
  - Swaddling
  - Skin-to-skin contact
  - Oral sucrose
- Pharmacologic
  - Topical anesthesia
  - Acetaminophen (oral, intravenous, or rectal)
  - Opioids (intravenous fentanyl or morphine)
  - Nerve block with lidocaine
  - Deep sedation

Think Critically

1. You are caring for a neonate with umbilical catheters. How do you explain their function to the parents of the infant?
2. Describe different methods of oxygen support for neonates and when each method is most appropriate.
3. How does apnea differ from normal breathing in the neonate?
4. How does the immune system differ in a preterm infant?
5. What is cold stress?
6. What would make you think a neonate is experiencing feeding intolerance?
7. Your patient was born prematurely and is not yet ready for enteral feedings. You would like the parents to participate in swabbing the inside of the infant's mouth with colostrum. How do you explain the purpose and importance of this practice?
8. Your patient was delivered at 42 weeks of gestation and is small for gestational age. What are the potential health implications for this neonate?
9. A forceps delivery should be attempted only by a trained and experienced healthcare provider. What birth injuries are associated with this method of birth?
10. How would a neonate in chronic pain look different from a neonate experiencing pain acutely?

References

Abu Jawdeh, E. G., O'Riordan, M., Limrungsikul, A., Bandyopadhyay, A., Argus, B. M., Nakad, P. E., . . . Martin, R. J. (2013). Methylxanthine use for apnea of prematurity among an international cohort of neonatologists. *Journal of Neonatal-Perinatal Medicine, 6*(3), 251–256. doi:10.3233/NPM-1371013

Aher, S. M., & Ohlsson, A. (2014). Late erythropoietin for preventing red blood cell transfusion in preterm and/or low birth weight infants. *Cochrane Database of Systematic Reviews,* (4), CD004868. doi:10.1002/14651858. CD004868.pub4

Ahn, E. S., Jung, M. S., Lee, Y. K., Ko, S. Y., Shin, S. M., & Hahn, M. H. (2015). Neonatal clavicular fracture: Recent 10 year study. *Pediatrics International, 57*(1), 60–63. doi:10.1111/ped.12497

Al-Abdi, S. Y., & Al-Aamri, M. A. (2014). A systematic review and meta-analysis of the timing of early intraventricular hemorrhage in preterm neonates: Clinical and research implications. *Journal of Clinical Neonatology, 3*(2), 76–88. doi:10.4103/2249-4847.134674

Alfirevic, Z., Milan, S. J., & Livio, S. (2013). Caesarean section versus vaginal delivery for preterm birth in singletons. *Cochrane Database of Systematic Reviews,* (9), CD000078. doi:10.1002/14651858.CD000078.pub3

Almadhoob, A., & Ohlsson, A. (2015). Sound reduction management in the neonatal intensive care unit for preterm or very low birth weight infants. *Cochrane Database of Systematic Reviews, 1,* CD010333. doi:10.1002/14651858. CD010333.pub2

Alsafadi, T. R., Hashmi, S. M., Youssef, H. A., Suliman, A. K., Abbas, H. M., & Albaloushi, M. H. (2014). Polycythemia in neonatal intensive care unit, risk factors, symptoms, pattern, and management controversy. *Journal of Clinical Neonatology, 3*(2), 93–98. doi:10.4103/2249-4847.134683

American Academy of Pediatrics. (2014). Respiratory support in preterm infants at birth. *Pediatrics, 133*(1), 171–174. doi:10.1542/peds.2013-3442

American Academy of Pediatrics. (2016). Prevention and management of procedural pain in the neonate: An update. *Pediatrics, 137*(2), e20154271. doi:10.1542/peds.2015-4271

American College of Obstetricians and Gynecologists. (2014). Executive summary: Neonatal brachial plexus palsy. Report of the American College of Obstetricians and Gynecologists' Task Force on Neonatal Brachial Plexus Palsy. *Obstetrics and Gynecology, 123*(4), 902–904. doi:10.1097/01.AOG.0000445582.43112.9a

Anadkat, J. S., Kuzniewicz, M. W., Chaudhari, B. P., Cole, F. S., & Hamvas, A. (2012). Increased risk for respiratory distress among white, male, late preterm and term infants. *Journal of Perinatology, 32*(10), 780–785. doi:10.1038/jp.2011.191

Anand, K. J. S., Eriksson, M., Boyle, E. M., Avila-Alvarez, A., Andersen, R. D., Sarafidis, K., . . . Carbajal, R.; EUROPAIN Survey Working Group of the NeoOpioid Consortium. (2017). Assessment of continuous pain in newborns admitted to NICUs in 18 European countries. *Acta Paediatrica, 106*(8), 1248–1259. doi:10.1111/apa.13810

Araujo Junior, E., Peixoto, A. B., Zamarian, A. C., Elito Junior, J., & Tonni, G. (2017). Macrosomia. *Best Practice and Research. Clinical Obstetrics and Gynaecology, 38,* 83–96. doi:10.1016/j.bpobgyn.2016.08.003

Baker, R. D., Greer, F. R., & Committee on Nutrition American Academy of Pediatrics. (2010). Diagnosis and prevention of iron deficiency and iron-deficiency anemia in infants and young children (0–3 years of age). *Pediatrics, 126*(5), 1040–1050. doi:10.1542/peds.2010-2576

Basha, A., Amarin, Z., & Abu-Hassan, F. (2013). Birth-associated long-bone fractures. *International Journal of Gynaecology and Obstetrics, 123*(2), 127–130. doi:10.1016/j.ijgo.2013.05.013

Bell, E. F., & Acarregui, M. J. (2014). Restricted versus liberal water intake for preventing morbidity and mortality in preterm infants. *Cochrane Database of Systematic Reviews,* (12), CD000503. doi:10.1002/14651858.CD000503.pub3

Bellieni, C. V., Tei, M., & Buonocore, G. (2015). Should we assess pain in newborn infants using a scoring system or just a detection method? *Acta Paediatrica, 104*(3), 221–224. doi:10.1111/apa.12882

Beuzeboc Gerard, M., Aillet, S., Bertheuil, N., Delliere, V., Thienot, S., & Watier, E. (2014). Surgical management of subcutaneous fat necrosis of the newborn required due to a lack of improvement: A very rare case. *British Journal of Dermatology, 171*(1), 183–185. doi:10.1111/bjd.12798

Bhat, V., Karam, M., Saslow, J., Taylor, H., Pyon, K., Kemble, N., . . . Aghai, Z. H. (2012). Utility of performing routine head ultrasounds in preterm infants with gestational age 30–34 weeks. *Journal of Maternal-Fetal and Neonatal Medicine, 25*(2), 116–119. doi:10.3109/14767058.2011.557755

Chiruvolu, A., Tolia, V. N., Qin, H., Stone, G. L., Rich, D., Conant, R. J., & Inzer, R. W. (2015). Effect of delayed cord clamping on very preterm infants. *American Journal of Obstetrics and Gynecology, 213*(5), 676.e1–676. e7. doi:10.1016/j.ajog.2015.07.016

Christensen, R. D., Baer, V. L., & Yaish, H. M. (2015). Thrombocytopenia in late preterm and term neonates after perinatal asphyxia. *Transfusion, 55*(1), 187–196. doi:10.1111/trf.12777

Christian, E. A., Jin, D. L., Attenello, F., Wen, T., Cen, S., Mack, W. J., . . . McComb, J. G. (2016). Trends in hospitalization of preterm infants with intraventricular hemorrhage and hydrocephalus in the United States, 2000–2010. *Journal of Neurosurgery. Pediatrics, 17*(3), 260–269. doi:10.3171/2015.7.PEDS15140

Dargaville, P. A., Gerber, A., Johansson, S., De Paoli, A. G., Kamlin, C. O., Orsini, F., & Davis, P. G.; Australian and New Zealand Neonatal Network. (2016). Incidence and outcome of CPAP failure in preterm infants. *Pediatrics, 138*(1). doi:10.1542/peds.2015-3985

de Almeida, M. F., Guinsburg, R., Sancho, G. A., Rosa, I. R., Lamy, Z. C., Martinez, F. E., . . . Silveira Rde, C.; Brazilian Network on Neonatal Research. (2014). Hypothermia and early neonatal mortality in preterm infants. *Journal of Pediatrics, 164*(2), 271.e1–275.e1. doi:10.1016/j.jpeds.2013.09.049

De Jesus, L. C., Pappas, A., Shankaran, S., Li, L., Das, A., Bell, E. F., . . . Higgins, R. D.; Eunice Kennedy Shriver National Institute of Health and Human Development Neonatal Research Network. (2013). Outcomes of small for gestational age infants born at <27 weeks' gestation. *Journal of Pediatrics, 163*(1), 55.e1–60.e3. doi:10.1016/j.jpeds.2012.12.097

Dellinger, R. P., Levy, M. M., Rhodes, A., Annane, D., Gerlach, H., Opal, S. M., . . . Moreno, R.; Surviving Sepsis Campaign Guidelines Committee Including the Pediatric Subgroup. (2013). Surviving sepsis campaign: International guidelines for management of severe sepsis and septic shock: 2012. *Critical Care Medicine, 41*(2), 580–637. doi:10.1097/CCM.0b013e31827e83af

Del Pozzo-Magana, B. R., & Ho, N. (2016). Subcutaneous fat necrosis of the newborn: A 20-year retrospective study. *Pediatric Dermatology, 33*(6), e353–e355. doi:10.1111/pde.12973

Doesburg, S. M., Chau, C. M., Cheung, T. P., Moiseev, A., Ribary, U., Herdman, A. T., . . . Grunau, R. E. (2013). Neonatal pain-related stress, functional cortical activity and visual-perceptual abilities in school-age children born at extremely low gestational age. *Pain, 154*(10), 1946–1952. doi:10.1016/j.pain.2013.04.009

Doyle, J., Davidson, D., Katz, S., Varela, M., Demeglio, D., & DeCristofaro, J. (2016). Apnea of prematurity and caffeine pharmacokinetics: Potential impact on hospital discharge. *Journal of Perinatology, 36*(2), 141–144. doi:10.1038/jp.2015.167

El-Khuffash, A. F., Jain, A., & McNamara, P. J. (2013). Ligation of the patent ductus arteriosus in preterm infants: Understanding the physiology. *Journal of Pediatrics, 162*(6), 1100–1106. doi:10.1016/j.jpeds.2012.12.094

Figlio, D. N., Guryan, J., Karbownik, K., & Roth, J. (2016). Long-term cognitive and health outcomes of school-aged children who were born late-term vs full-term. *JAMA Pediatrics, 170*(8), 758–764. doi:10.1001/jamapediatrics.2016.0238

Foster, J. P., Psaila, K., & Patterson, T. (2016). Non-nutritive sucking for increasing physiologic stability and nutrition in preterm infants. *Cochrane Database of Systematic Reviews, 10*, CD001071. doi:10.1002/14651858.CD001071.pub3

Gibbins, S., Stevens, B. J., Yamada, J., Dionne, K., Campbell-Yeo, M., Lee, G., . . . Taddio, A. (2014). Validation of the premature infant pain profile-revised (PIPP-R). *Early Human Development, 90*(4), 189–193. doi:10.1016/j.earlhumdev.2014.01.005

Gillies, D., Wells, D., & Bhandari, A. P. (2012). Positioning for acute respiratory distress in hospitalised infants and children. *Cochrane Database of Systematic Reviews,* (7), CD003645. doi:10.1002/14651858.CD003645.pub3

Hamilton, B. E., Martin, J. A., & Osterman, M. J. (2016). Births: Preliminary data for 2015. *National Vital Statistics Reports, 65*(3), 1–15.

Hamilton, B. E., Martin, J. A., Osterman, M. J., Curtin, S. C., & Matthews, T. J. (2015). Births: Final data for 2014. *National Vital Statistics Reports, 64*(12), 1–64.

Handley, S. C., Sun, Y., Wyckoff, M. H., & Lee, H. C. (2015). Outcomes of extremely preterm infants after delivery room cardiopulmonary resuscitation in a population-based cohort. *Journal of Perinatology, 35*(5), 379–383. doi:10.1038/jp.2014.222

Hibbard, J. U., Wilkins, I., Sun, L., Gregory, K., Haberman, S., . . . Zhang, J.; Consortium on Safe Labor. (2010). Respiratory morbidity in late preterm births. *JAMA, 304*(4), 419–425. doi:10.1001/jama.2010.1015

Ho, J. J., Subramaniam, P., & Davis, P. G. (2015). Continuous distending pressure for respiratory distress in preterm infants. *Cochrane Database of Systematic Reviews,* (7), CD002271. doi:10.1002/14651858.CD002271.pub2

Horbar, J. D., Ehrenkranz, R. A., Badger, G. J., Edwards, E. M., Morrow, K. A., Soll, R. F., . . . Bellu, R. (2015). Weight growth velocity and postnatal growth failure in infants 501 to 1500 grams: 2000–2013. *Pediatrics, 136*(1), e84–e92. doi:10.1542/peds.2015-0129

Horemuzova, E., Amark, P., Jacobson, L., Soder, O., & Hagenas, L. (2014). Growth charts and long-term sequelae in extreme preterm infants—From full-term age to 10 years. *Acta Paediatrica, 103*(1), 38–47. doi:10.1111/apa.12451

Hornik, C. P., Benjamin, D. K., Becker, K. C., Benjamin, D. K., Jr., Li, J., Clark, R. H., . . . Smith, P. B. (2012). Use of the complete blood cell count in late-onset neonatal sepsis. *Pediatric Infectious Disease Journal, 31*(8), 803–807. doi:10.1097/INF.0b013e31825691e4

Imamura, T., Ariga, H., Kaneko, M., Watanabe, M., Shibukawa, Y., Fukuda, Y., . . . Fujiki, T. (2013). Neurodevelopmental outcomes of children with periventricular leukomalacia. *Pediatrics and Neonatology, 54*(6), 367–372. doi:10.1016/j.pedneo.2013.04.006

King, J. P., Gazmararian, J. A., & Shapiro-Mendoza, C. K. (2014). Disparities in mortality rates among US infants born late preterm or early term, 2003–2005. *Maternal and Child Health Journal, 18*(1), 233–241. doi:10.1007/s10995-013-1259-0

Kitai, Y., Hirai, S., Ohmura, K., Ogura, K., & Arai, H. (2015). Cerebellar injury in preterm children with cerebral palsy after intraventricular hemorrhage: Prevalence and relationship to functional outcomes. *Brain and Development, 37*(8), 758–763. doi:10.1016/j.braindev.2014.12.009

Klinger, G., Osovsky, M., Boyko, V., Sokolover, N., Sirota, L., Lerner-Geva, L., & Reichman, B. (2016). Risk factors associated with post-hemorrhagic hydrocephalus among very low birth weight infants of 24–28 weeks gestation. *Journal of Perinatology, 36*(7), 557–563. doi:10.1038/jp.2016.18

Kumar, P.; & American Academy of Pediatrics. (2014). Use of inhaled nitric oxide in preterm infants. *Pediatrics, 133*(1), 164–170. doi:10.1542/peds.2013-3444

Lacaze-Masmonteil, T., Rosychuk, R. J., & Robinson, J. L. (2014). Value of a single C-reactive protein measurement at 18 h of age. *Archives of Disease in Childhood. Fetal and Neonatal Edition, 99*(1), F76–F79. doi:10.1136/archdischild-2013-303984

Laptook, A. R., Bell, E. F., Shankaran, S., Boghossian, N. S., Wyckoff, M. H., Kandefer, S., . . . Higgins, R.; Generic and Moderate Preterm Subcommittees of the NICHD Neonatal Research Network. (2018). Admission temperature and associated mortality and morbidity among moderately and extremely preterm infants. *Journal of Pediatrics, 192*, 53.e2–59.e2. doi:10.1016/j.jpeds.2017.09.021

Lemyre, B., Sample, M., & Lacaze-Masmonteil, T.; Canadian Paediatric Society; Fetus and Newborn Committee. (2015). Minimizing blood loss and the need for transfusions in very premature infants. *Pediatrics and Child Health, 20*(8), 451–462.

Lester, B. M., Hawes, K., Abar, B., Sullivan, M., Miller, R., Bigsby, R., . . . Padbury, J. F. (2014). Single-family room care and neurobehavioral and medical outcomes in preterm infants. *Pediatrics, 134*(4), 754–760. doi:10.1542/peds.2013-4252

Levine, T. A., Grunau, R. E., McAuliffe, F. M., Pinnamaneni, R., Foran, A., & Alderdice, F. A. (2015). Early childhood neurodevelopment after intrauterine growth restriction: A systematic review. *Pediatrics, 135*(1), 126–141. doi:10.1542/peds.2014-1143

Linder, N., Hiersch, L., Fridman, E., Klinger, G., Lubin, D., Kouadio, F., & Melamed, N. (2017). Post-term pregnancy is an independent risk factor for neonatal morbidity even in low-risk singleton pregnancies. *Archives of Disease in Childhood. Fetal and Neonatal Edition, 102*(4), F286–F290. doi:10.1136/archdischild-2015-308553

Liu, J., Wang, X. F., Wang, Y., Wang, H. W., & Liu, Y. (2014). The incidence rate, high-risk factors, and short- and long-term adverse outcomes of fetal growth restriction: A report from Mainland China. *Medicine (Baltimore), 93*(27), e210. doi:10.1097/MD.0000000000000210

Manja, V., Lakshminrusimha, S., & Cook, D. J. (2015). Oxygen saturation target range for extremely preterm infants: A systematic review and meta-analysis. *JAMA Pediatrics, 169*(4), 332–340. doi:10.1001/jamapediatrics.2014.3307

Martin, J. A., Hamilton, B. E., Osterman, M. J., Curtin, S. C., & Matthews, T. J. (2015). Births: Final data for 2013. *National Vital Statistics Reports, 64*(1), 1–65.

Matthews, T. J., MacDorman, M. F., & Thoma, M. E. (2015). Infant mortality statistics from the 2013 period linked birth/infant death data set. *National Vital Statistics Reports, 64*(9), 1–30.

McCarthy, L. K., Molloy, E. J., Twomey, A. R., Murphy, J. F., & O'Donnell, C. P. (2013). A randomized trial of exothermic mattresses for preterm newborns in polyethylene bags. *Pediatrics, 132*(1), e135–e141. doi:10.1542/peds.2013-0279

Mendola, P., Mumford, S. L., Mannisto, T. I., Holston, A., Reddy, U. M., & Laughon, S. K. (2015). Controlled direct effects of preeclampsia on neonatal health after accounting for mediation by preterm birth. *Epidemiology, 26*(1), 17–26. doi:10.1097/EDE.0000000000000213

Meredith, J. L., Jnah, A., & Newberry, D. (2017). The NICU environment: Infusing single-family room benefits into the open-bay setting. *Neonatal Network, 36*(2), 69–76. doi:10.1891/0730-0832.36.2.69

Morag, I., & Ohlsson, A. (2016). Cycled light in the intensive care unit for preterm and low birth weight infants. *Cochrane Database of Systematic Reviews,* (8), CD006982. doi:10.1002/14651858.CD006982.pub4

Morgan, J., Young, L., & McGuire, W. (2014). Delayed introduction of progressive enteral feeds to prevent necrotising enterocolitis in very low birth weight infants. *Cochrane Database of Systematic Reviews,* (12), CD001970. doi:10.1002/14651858.CD001970.pub5

Ohlsson, A., Walia, R., & Shah, S. S. (2015). Ibuprofen for the treatment of patent ductus arteriosus in preterm or low birth weight (or both) infants. *Cochrane Database of Systematic Reviews,* (2), CD003481. doi:10.1002/14651858.CD003481.pub6

Osterman, M. J., Kochanek, K. D., MacDorman, M. F., Strobino, D. M., & Guyer, B. (2015). Annual summary of vital statistics: 2012–2013. *Pediatrics, 135*(6), 1115–1125. doi:10.1542/peds.2015-0434

Ouzounian, J. G. (2014). Risk factors for neonatal brachial plexus palsy. *Seminars in Perinatology, 38*(4), 219–221. doi:10.1053/j.semperi.2014.04.008

Pammi, M., & Abrams, S. A. (2015). Oral lactoferrin for the prevention of sepsis and necrotizing enterocolitis in preterm infants. *Cochrane Database of Systematic Reviews,* (2), CD007137. doi:10.1002/14651858.CD007137.pub4

Perry, S. E. (2017). A historical perspective on the transport of premature infants. *Journal of Obstetric, Gynecologic, and Neonatal Nursing, 46*(4), 647–656. doi:10.1016/j.jogn.2016.09.007

Pittet, D., Allegranzi, B., Boyce, J., & World Health Organization World Alliance for Patient Safety First Global Patient Safety Challenge Core Group of Experts. (2009). The World Health Organization Guidelines on Hand Hygiene in Health Care and their consensus recommendations. *Infection Control and Hospital Epidemiology, 30*(7), 611–622. doi:10.1086/600379

Radic, J. A., Vincer, M., & McNeely, P. D. (2015). Temporal trends of intraventricular hemorrhage of prematurity in Nova Scotia from 1993 to 2012. *Journal of Neurosurgery. Pediatrics, 15*(6), 573–579. doi:10.3171/2014.11.PEDS14363

Rigo, V., Lefebvre, C., & Broux, I. (2016). Surfactant instillation in spontaneously breathing preterm infants: A systematic review and meta-analysis. *European Journal of Pediatrics, 175*(12), 1933–1942. doi:10.1007/s00431-016-2789-4

Sakonidou, S., & Dhaliwal, J. (2015). The management of neonatal respiratory distress syndrome in preterm infants (European Consensus Guidelines—2013 update). *Archives of Disease in Childhood. Education and Practice Edition, 100*(5), 257–259. doi:10.1136/archdischild-2014-306642

Schiavenato, M., & Holsti, L. (2017). Defining procedural distress in the NICU and what can be done about it. *Neonatal Network, 36*(1), 12–17. doi:10.1891/0730-0832.36.1.12

Seikku, L., Gissler, M., Andersson, S., Rahkonen, P., Stefanovic, V., Tikkanen, M., ... Rahkonen, L. (2016). Asphyxia, neurologic morbidity, and perinatal mortality in early-term and postterm birth. *Pediatrics, 137*(6). doi:10.1542/peds.2015-3334

Shah, N. A., & Wusthoff, C. J. (2016). Intracranial hemorrhage in the neonate. *Neonatal Network, 35*(2), 67–71. doi:10.1891/0730-0832.35.2.67

Shah, P., Kaciroti, N., Richards, B., Oh, W., & Lumeng, J. C. (2016). Developmental outcomes of late preterm infants from infancy to kindergarten. *Pediatrics, 138*(2). doi:10.1542/peds.2015-3496

Sirgiovanni, I., Avignone, S., Groppo, M., Bassi, L., Passera, S., Schiavolin, P., ... Mosca, F. (2014). Intracranial haemorrhage: An incidental finding at magnetic resonance imaging in a cohort of late preterm and term infants. *Pediatric Radiology, 44*(3), 289–296. doi:10.1007/s00247-013-2826-7

Sohn, K., Kalanetra, K. M., Mills, D. A., & Underwood, M. A. (2016). Buccal administration of human colostrum: Impact on the oral microbiota of premature infants. *Journal of Perinatology, 36*(2), 106–111. doi:10.1038/jp.2015.157

Stanley, C. A., Rozance, P. J., Thornton, P. S., De Leon, D. D., Harris, D., Haymond, M. W., ... Wolfsdorf, J. I. (2015). Re-evaluating "transitional neonatal hypoglycemia": Mechanism and implications for management. *Journal of Pediatrics, 166*(6), 1520.e1–1525.e1. doi:10.1016/j.jpeds.2015.02.045

Stoll, B. J., Hansen, N. I., Bell, E. F., Shankaran, S., Laptook, A. R., Walsh, M. C., ... Higgins, R. D.; Eunice Kennedy Shriver National Institute of Child Health and Human Development Neonatal Research Network. (2010). Neonatal outcomes of extremely preterm infants from the NICHD Neonatal Research Network. *Pediatrics, 126*(3), 443–456. doi:10.1542/peds.2009-2959

Stoll, B. J., Hansen, N. I., Bell, E. F., Walsh, M. C., Carlo, W. A., Shankaran, S., ... Higgins, R. D.; Eunice Kennedy Shriver National Institute of Child Health and Human Development Neonatal Research Network. (2015). Trends in care practices, morbidity, and mortality of extremely preterm neonates, 1993–2012. *JAMA, 314*(10), 1039–1051. doi:10.1001/jama.2015.10244

Thome, U. H., Genzel-Boroviczeny, O., Bohnhorst, B., Schmid, M., Fuchs, H., Rohde, O., ... Hummler, H. D.; PHELBI Study Group. (2015). Permissive hypercapnia in extremely low birthweight infants (PHELBI): A randomised controlled multicentre trial. *The Lancet. Respiratory Medicine, 3*(7), 534–543. doi:10.1016/S2213-2600(15)00204-0

Tudehope, D., Vento, M., Bhutta, Z., & Pachi, P. (2013). Nutritional requirements and feeding recommendations for small for gestational age infants. *Journal of Pediatrics, 162*(3 Suppl.), S81–S89. doi:10.1016/j.jpeds.2012.11.057

Turfkruyer, M., & Verhasselt, V. (2015). Breast milk and its impact on maturation of the neonatal immune system. *Current Opinion in Infectious Diseases, 28*(3), 199–206. doi:10.1097/QCO.0000000000000165

Watkins, W. J., Kotecha, S. J., & Kotecha, S. (2016). All-cause mortality of low birthweight infants in infancy, childhood, and adolescence: Population study of England and Wales. *PLoS Medicine, 13*(5), e1002018. doi:10.1371/journal.pmed.1002018

Wilson, E., Maier, R. F., Norman, M., Misselwitz, B., Howell, E. A., Zeitlin, J., & Bonamy, A. K.; Effective Perinatal Intensive Care in Europe (EPICE) Research Group. (2016). Admission hypothermia in very preterm infants and neonatal mortality and morbidity. *Journal of Pediatrics, 175*, 61.e4–67. e4. doi:10.1016/j.jpeds.2016.04.016

Wyckoff, M. H., Aziz, K., Escobedo, M. B., Kapadia, V. S., Kattwinkel, J., Perlman, J. M., ... Zaichkin, J. G. (2015). Part 13: Neonatal Resuscitation: 2015 American Heart Association Guidelines Update for Cardiopulmonary Resuscitation and Emergency Cardiovascular Care (Reprint). *Pediatrics, 136* Suppl. 2, S196–S218. doi:10.1542/peds.2015-3373G

Yang, L. J. (2014). Neonatal brachial plexus palsy—Management and prognostic factors. *Seminars in Perinatology, 38*(4), 222–234. doi:10.1053/j.semperi.2014.04.009

Suggested Readings

Galarza-Winton, M. E., Dicky, T., O'Leary, L., Lee, S. K., & O'Brien, K. (2013). Implementing family-integrated care in the NICU: Educating nurses. *Advances in Neonatal Care, 13*(5), 335–340. doi:10.1097/ANC.0b013e3182a14cde

Kristoffersen, L., Stoen, R., Hansen, L. F., Wilhelmsen, J., & Bergseng, H. (2016). Skin-to-skin care after birth for moderately preterm infants. *Journal of Obstetric, Gynecologic, and Neonatal Nursing, 45*(3), 339–345. doi:10.1016/j.jogn.2016.02.007

Lawn, J. E., Davidge, R., Paul, V. K., von Xylander, S., de Graft Johnson, J., Costello, A., ... Molyneux, L. (2013). Born too soon: Care for the preterm baby. *Reproductive Health, 10* Suppl. 1, S5. doi:10.1186/1742-4755-10-S1-S5

Orsi, K. C., Avena, M. J., Lurdes de Cacia Pradella-Hallinan, M., da Luz Goncalves Pedreira, M., Tsunemi, M. H., Machado Avelar, A. F., & Pinheiro, E. M. (2017). Effects of handling and environment on preterm newborns sleeping in incubators. *Journal of Obstetric, Gynecologic, and Neonatal Nursing, 46*(2), 238–247. doi:10.1016/j.jogn.2016.09.005

25 Acquired Conditions and Congenital Abnormalities in the Newborn

Objectives

1. Identify the causes of jaundice and assessments and interventions to address it.
2. Describe pulmonary conditions that are specific to neonates, as well as assessment and care considerations.
3. Discuss the factors that contribute to retinopathy of prematurity and the pertinent assessments and potential complications.
4. Identify the risk factors, signs, and interventions pertinent to necrotizing enterocolitis.
5. Discuss the risk factors and assessments for neurologic injury of the newborn.
6. Explain the impact of maternal substance use and abuse on the neonate and pertinent interventions.
7. Identify maternal and nosocomial infections that can impact the neonate.
8. Differentiate congenital defects that occur in different body systems from one another.

Key Terms

Acute bilirubin encephalopathy (ABE)
Aliquots
Bilirubin-induced neurologic dysfunction (BIND)
Chancre
Choanal atresia
Chorioretinitis
Congenital diaphragmatic hernia
Hydrops
Hyperbilirubinemia
Ileostomy
Kernicterus
Laryngeal atresia
Laryngeal webs
Laryngomalacia
Nikolsky's sign
Pneumatosis intestinalis
Pneumoperitoneum
Reanastomosis
Tracheal atresia
Tracheomalacia

The neonatal period is a particularly vulnerable time. Some conditions discussed in this chapter, such as hyperbilirubinemia, are sequelae of other, underlying problems. Other conditions, such as ambiguous genitalia, may have intense psychosocial implications but, depending on etiology, may not be immediately life threatening. Other conditions, such as tracheal atresia, are almost always incompatible with life.

For a new learner, these myriad conditions and consequences can be overwhelming. A careful understanding, for example, of how bilirubin is created makes it easier to predict which infants may develop pathologic hyperbilirubinemia. An understanding of fetal lung development and both fetal and newborn circulations makes it easier to differentiate between various conditions while understanding the underlying etiologies and predicting suitable interventions.

Conditions of Hyperbilirubinemia in the Newborn

Hyperbilirubinemia is a greater-than-normal blood level of bilirubin. The upper limit of normal for an adult for serum bilirubin level is 1 mg/dL. Most newborn infants, however, exceed this level. In most cases, this is considered physiologic—a normal and expected examination finding—and is known as physiologic jaundice. In some cases, however, hyperbilirubinemia is pathologic and can have serious implications for the newborn.

Etiology

When hemoglobin from red blood cells breaks down, bilirubin is produced. This process of heme catabolism accounts for a majority of bilirubin. Bilirubin binds to the protein albumin and is transported to the liver. In the liver, the bilirubin is detached from the albumin molecule, taken up by hepatocytes, and conjugated. Conjugated bilirubin is then excreted in bile into the digestive tract. Conjugated bilirubin cannot be reabsorbed by the epithelial cells of the intestine.

Physiologic Jaundice

Physiologic jaundice is expected in the newborn and results from the increased production of bilirubin, decreased clearance of bilirubin, and increased enterohepatic circulation.

- Physiologic increased bilirubin production: Fetal red blood cells have a life span of approximately 85 days, as opposed to 100 to 120 days for an adult, resulting in more rapid turnover of the cells and thus increased production of bilirubin. In addition, the hematocrit of a newborn is 50% to 60%, as opposed to 36% to 54% for adults.
- Physiologic changes in bilirubin clearance: The level of an enzyme critical to bilirubin clearance does not reach adult levels until more than 3 months after the birth.
- Enterohepatic circulation of bilirubin: The adult gut has bacteria that break down conjugated bilirubin for excretion. The gut of the newborn, however, is initially sterile, precluding the breakdown of the conjugated bilirubin into another compound, urobilin, which is excreted. Instead, a different enzyme in the gut deconjugates the bilirubin. This unconjugated bilirubin, unlike conjugated bilirubin, can be absorbed by the epithelium of the gut and deposited back into the circulation, increasing serum levels of bilirubin. This process is called the "enterohepatic circulation of bilirubin."

Pathologic Hyperbilirubinemia

Severe hyperbilirubinemia, which results from pathologic causes, is defined as a serum bilirubin level above the 95th percentile, according to the Bhutani nomogram (see Fig. 5.10). Other indications of severe hyperbilirubinemia include jaundice that develops in the first 24 hours, a rise in serum bilirubin faster than 0.2 mg/dL/h, and jaundice that persists for longer than 2 weeks in a term infant. High blood levels of conjugated bilirubin suggest cholestasis (stopped or slow transit of bile from the liver). Pathologic causes of hyperbilirubinemia are discussed below.

- Pathologic increased bilirubin production: The most common cause of pathologic hyperbilirubinemia is a disease process that includes hemolysis and leads to an increase in bilirubin production. Examples of such disease processes are as follows:
  - Incompatibility of ABO or Rh(D) blood type between mother and newborn: This occurs when the mother is sensitized to the incompatible blood type and maternal antigens cross the placenta and attack fetal red blood cells, leading to isoimmune-mediated hemolysis.
  - Increased breakdown of red blood cells from a cephalhematoma or other collection of blood, or from polycythemia
  - Sepsis of the newborn
  - Defects of the cell membrane or enzymes of the red blood cells
- Pathologic decreased clearance: Hyperbilirubinemia can also be caused by decreased clearance of bilirubin due to the following:
  - The genetic defects that disrupt conjugation of bilirubin and reduce hepatic bilirubin clearance
  - Maternal diabetes
  - Congenital hypothyroidism
  - Galactosemia (a disorder in the metabolism of the simple sugar galactose from an enzyme deficiency or liver impairment)
- Pathologic enterohepatic circulation: Disruption of circulation from the liver to the bile can also cause hyperbilirubinemia. Associated factors include the following:
  - Breast milk jaundice: Not truly pathologic, it is a pattern of jaundice starting 3 to 5 days after the birth and peaking within 2 weeks. Normal bilirubin levels are reached between 3 weeks and 3 months later (Maisels et al., 2014). Serum bilirubin is generally mildly elevated, above 5 mg/dL for several weeks. The nurse should monitor such infants closely. Rising levels of unconjugated bilirubin suggest a different cause of the jaundice, whereas increased levels of conjugated bilirubin suggest cholestasis.
  - Breastfeeding failure jaundice: This is jaundice that appears within the first week of birth, with weight and fluid loss in excess of the norm. Decreased intake slows the passage of stool and bilirubin elimination via the digestive system, increasing exposure time to deconjugating enzymes, and the reuptake of deconjugated bilirubin by the fetal circulation. Because of a clear increased risk of developing pathologic jaundice for breastfed infants, the nurse should thoroughly assess newborns feeding prior to discharge and provide assistance as necessary both in the hospital and at home.

- Intestinal obstruction: Slowed or stopped bowel transit due to an ileus or other anatomic reason exposes conjugated bilirubin to the deconjugating enzyme for a longer period of time, increasing the likelihood of bilirubin being reintroduced to the infant's circulation.

Signs and Symptoms

Clinical manifestations of hyperbilirubinemia include yellowing of the skin that starts in the face and moves down to the torso and extremities as bilirubin levels rise. The white sclera of the eye also appears yellowed as the overlying conjunctival membranes take on the pigment.

Prognosis

Bilirubin is a neurotoxin that can cause cell death and necrosis. Severe hyperbilirubinemia is classified as a serum bilirubin level above 25 mg/dL. At this level, neonates are at risk for **bilirubin-induced neurologic dysfunction (BIND)**, which occurs when serum bilirubin crosses the blood–brain barrier and binds to brain tissue, causing symptoms. The term **acute bilirubin encephalopathy (ABE)** refers to the acute clinical manifestations of BIND (Box 25.1). ABE may be permanent or reversible. Infants presenting with BIND and ABE are treated with an exchange transfusion regardless of bilirubin levels. **Kernicterus** refers to the permanent, irreversible effects of BIND (Box 25.2). Most but not all infants who develop kernicterus first have signs of ABE. The risk for kernicterus for infants with a serum bilirubin level over 25 mg/dL is 6%. If serum levels are over 30 mg/dL, the risk is 14% to 25%. Nearly all infants with a serum bilirubin level over 35 mg/dL are diagnosed with kernicterus (Bhutani & Johnson, 2009). Since the advent of the routine use of Rh_o (D) immune globulin for Rh(D)-negative women in pregnancy, kernicterus has become exceedingly rare and is reported for fewer than 1 out of every 200,000 live births (Brooks, Fisher-Owens, Wu, Strauss, & Newman, 2011).

Assessment

Term and Late Preterm Infants

In infants of European or African descent, serum bilirubin level normally peaks from 48 to 96 hours after birth at 7 to 9 mg/dL. In infants of Asian descent, the level may peak later, from 72 to 120 hours after birth, at 10 to 14 mg/dL. Late preterm infants may also experience a later peak. Physiologic jaundice usually resolves within a few weeks.

The nurse should assess all infants after birth for jaundice by visual inspection every 8 to 12 hours. Infants who are jaundiced prior to 24 hours are at particular risk for severe hyperbilirubinemia, most often due to ABO or Rh(D) incompatibility. The nurse should quantitatively assess infants who are jaundiced prior to 24 hours with direct measurement of serum bilirubin levels by blood draw or by transcutaneous measurement of bilirubin (TcB) per institution protocol (see Fig. 5.9). Infants who develop jaundice later than 24 hours after birth should have a quantitative evaluation of bilirubin done if the jaundice spreads below the level of the umbilicus. Many institutions now have a policy to universally screen all infants quantitatively prior to discharge, usually by TcB. Nurses should be aware, however, that TcB may underestimate bilirubin levels. High or borderline levels must be confirmed by serum testing. Institutions protocols vary, and some may mandate screening be done only on infants deemed high risk. Risk factors for developing severe hyperbilirubinemia are summarized in Box 25.3. The pediatric care provider again assesses infants for jaundice after discharge.

Letitia Richford's baby, in Chapter 5, was a late preterm infant (born at about 36 weeks of gestation) and underwent monitoring by TcB for hyperbilirubinemia. She was not found to have hyperbilirubinemia, however.

Preterm Infants

There is no consensus for treatment thresholds for infants born before 35 weeks of gestation, and different providers and institutions may base screening and treatment protocols on weight or gestational age at birth. Preterm infants are likely more susceptible to neurologic dysfunction from bilirubin at lower levels than are term and late preterm infants. To complicate the picture, the manifestations of neurologic dysfunction caused by elevated bilirubin levels are similar to other complications of the preterm neonate.

Box 25.1 Acute Bilirubin Encephalopathy Clinical Presentation

- Lethargy
- Fever
- Irritability
- Jitteriness
- Hypotonia (arching of the neck and back with stimulation)
- Poor feeding
- Apnea
- Seizures
- High-pitched cry

Box 25.2 Kernicterus Clinical Presentation

- Cerebral palsy
- Sensorineural hearing loss
- Gaze abnormalities
- Dental enamel dysplasia

Box 25.3 Risk Factors for the Development of Severe Hyperbilirubinemia in Term and Late Preterm Infants

High Risk

- High bilirubin levels prior to discharge
- Jaundice onset in the first 24 h after birth
- Maternal/infant blood group incompatibility with positive direct Coombs' test result
- Known hemolytic disease of the newborn
- Birth from 35–36 wk of gestation
- Treatment of a sibling for hyperbilirubinemia
- Cephalohematoma
- Extensive bruising
- Poor breastfeeding
- Mother of East Asian ethnicity

Moderate Risk

- Intermediate bilirubin levels prior to discharge
- Birth from 37–38 wk of gestation
- Jaundice prior to discharge
- Sibling with a discharge following suspected hyperbilirubinemia
- Macrosomic infant of a diabetic mother
- Maternal age of 25 y or more
- Male infant

Factors That Reduce Risk

- Predischarge bilirubin level in the low-risk zone
- Birth at or after 41 wk of gestation
- Bottle-feeding exclusively
- African ethnicity
- Discharge from the hospital at or after 72 h postpartum

Adapted from American Academy of Pediatrics Subcommittee on Hyperbilirubinemia. (2004). Management of hyperbilirubinemia in the newborn infant 35 or more weeks of gestation. *Pediatrics*, *114*(1), 297–316.

Treatment

The goal of treating elevated bilirubin levels is to avoid kernicterus. Adequate reduction can usually be achieved by phototherapy, although an exchange transfusion may be indicated for very high levels of bilirubin that do not decrease adequately with phototherapy. Generally, the care provider's decision to monitor, treat with phototherapy, or treat with an exchange transfusion is informed by a calculation that includes the age in hours since birth, total serum bilirubin value, and gestational age at birth. In addition, factors that may make an infant more susceptible to damage from hyperbilirubinemia are considered. These factors include ABO or Rh(D) incompatibility, asphyxia, lethargy, sepsis, acidosis, temperature instability, and G6PD deficiency (G6PD deficiency is a genetic condition that causes hemolysis in reaction to infections, some medications, and other stressors). The care provider may also use the ratio of serum bilirubin to albumin to help guide decision-making.

Phototherapy

Phototherapy has been used for nearly 60 years now and is considered a safe intervention. It reduces serum bilirubin levels and thus the risk of needing an exchange transfusion.

Infants receiving phototherapy are generally treated in the hospital. Low-risk infants may remain in the regular nursery, whereas high-risk infants may instead be admitted to the neonatal intensive care unit (NICU). Some low-risk infants may have the option of phototherapy at home. Infants requiring intense phototherapy, sometimes called "crash cart phototherapy," who are at particular risk for requiring a transfusion, may lie on a phototherapy mattress as well as receiving the more typical overhead lights.

Phototherapy requires exposure of the infant's skin to a particular wavelength of light. The primary mechanism of action is the conversion of bilirubin to lumirubin when exposed to light set at 460 to 490 nm (blue light). Unlike conjugation of bilirubin, the conversion of bilirubin to lumirubin is not reversible. Lumirubin does not require conjugation in the liver as it is more soluble than bilirubin, and it can be excreted directly into the bile and the urine, thus lowering serum bilirubin levels.

A measurable difference in bilirubin levels can occur within 2 hours of initiation of phototherapy treatment, and the bilirubin level is reduced by at least 2 mg/dL within 6 hours. Intensive phototherapy (lights over and under the infant) can reduce bilirubin levels by up to 40% in 24 hours, whereas the more conventional overhead-only phototherapy can result in an up to 20% reduction in the first 18 hours. The higher the bilirubin levels, the faster levels decline. In addition, the greater the surface area of the infant exposed to phototherapy, the faster the rate of bilirubin reduction (American Academy of Pediatrics Subcommittee on Hyperbilirubinemia, 2004).

Technique

The larger the surface area of the body exposed, the more effective phototherapy is. Thus, the nurse should minimize the body surface covered by a diaper. The nurse places a blindfold over the infant's eyes to protect them and must position it to avoid covering the nares. The nurse should position the infant on his or her back in an open bassinet or warmer. Incubators are avoided whenever possible as they prevent optimal positioning of the light close to the infant. The use of white, reflective material or foil on surfaces around the infant increases the efficacy of the therapy.

The dosing of phototherapy is referred to as irradiance. Higher irradiance is more effective. Irradiance levels depend on the light used, the exposed surface area of the infant, and the distance between the light and the infant. Irradiance is expressed as $\mu W/cm^2/nm$ (microwatts per centimeter squared of exposed body surface area per nanometer of wavelength from 425 to 475 nm). The usual irradiance for conventional phototherapy is 6 to 12 $\mu W/cm^2/nm$.

Intensive therapy requires over twice that irradiance, more than 30 $\mu W/cm^2/nm$. This goal can be reached by moving the light closer to the infant and adding a phototherapy pad or mattress.

In low-resource settings, filtered sunlight has been shown to be a safe and effective means of treating hyperbilirubinemia (Slusher et al., 2014).

Infants with serum bilirubin levels exceeding 20 mg/dL should be under lights continuously. After bilirubin levels have dropped below 20 mg/dL, phototherapy may be temporarily discontinued for feeding and bonding activities.

Monitoring

During phototherapy, the infant's temperature, serum bilirubin level, hydration status, and exposure time must be closely monitored. More modern light-emitting diode phototherapy emits little heat, which reduces hyperthermia and fluid loss. However, infants requiring continuous phototherapy may have less oral intake, which increases the risk for dehydration and weight loss. The frequency of bilirubin monitoring depends on the clinical presentation. When the bilirubin level is rising during initial hospitalization, serum levels are usually monitored within 4 to 6 hours after the initiation of phototherapy and then again within 8 to 12 hours. If an infant is readmitted after discharge with a serum bilirubin level exceeding the 95th percentile, a serum bilirubin level is checked early, after 2 to 3 hours, to assess for adequate response. Hydration is generally achieved with oral feedings, although intravenous (IV) hydration may be required if oral intake is insufficient.

Discontinuation depends on the circumstances under which phototherapy was started. If an infant is admitted with severe hyperbilirubinemia after discharge, the goal serum bilirubin level is 12 to 14 mg/dL. If phototherapy was started during initial hospitalization to avoid severe hyperbilirubinemia, phototherapy is discontinued when the serum bilirubin has dropped to or below the level it was at the start of therapy. Serum bilirubin level is rechecked at 18 to 24 hours after cessation of phototherapy to assess for rebound, particularly if treatment was begun during hospitalization to avoid severe hyperbilirubinemia. Rebound occurs less frequently in those readmitted after discharge. Rebound hyperbilirubinemia is rarely clinically significant enough to require further treatment (Chang, Kuzniewicz, McCulloch, & Newman, 2017).

Infants with hyperbilirubinemia and cholestasis (defined as a conjugated serum bilirubin level over 2 mg/dL) occasionally develop bronze baby syndrome. Bronze baby syndrome involves a gray-brown discoloration of the skin, urine, and serum of the infant. Note that phototherapy is not an effective treatment for jaundice with conjugated serum bilirubin.

Adverse Effects

Apart from the risks for dehydration, interrupted breastfeeding, and hyperthermia previously mentioned, adverse short-term effects of phototherapy are rare and few. Newborns may occasionally develop a benign erythematous rash that resolves without intervention.

There is, however, a correlation between the development of cancer and phototherapy that suggests a causal relationship, highlighting the importance of using phototherapy sparingly and only when needed (Chang et al., 2017).

Exchange Transfusion

Although exchange transfusion is the most effective means of rapidly removing bilirubin from the circulation, it is expensive and time-consuming and requires clinical expertise, and thus is done rarely. As with phototherapy, the decision to initiate an exchange transfusion is informed by a calculation of gestational age, hours since birth, and serum bilirubin values. Infants with a serum bilirubin level over 25 mg/dL, the cutoff for severe hyperbilirubinemia, are usually treated with an exchange transfusion immediately if they have neurologic symptoms. In the absence of neurologic symptoms, intensive phototherapy may be trialed first. Time is required to implement an exchange transfusion, and intensive phototherapy is administered during setup.

An exchange transfusion removes bilirubin from the circulation. It is particularly effective in the case of isoimmune hemolysis (hemolysis caused by ABO or Rh(D) incompatibility), as the exchange transfusion also removes the maternal antibodies that are continuing to destroy red blood cells. The procedure approximately halves the level of serum bilirubin immediately, although the level rises to approximately two thirds of preexchange levels as extravascular and vascular bilirubin reequilibrates after approximately 4 hours.

An exchange transfusion is done via a central catheter over about 1 to 2 hours. The patient receives an infusion of albumin at 1 g/kg 1 to 2 hours prior to the procedure to draw more bilirubin out of the extravascular circulation. The blood is removed and then replaced at 10% of total volume at a time. These units are called **aliquots**, which means sample or portion. The total circulating blood volume of a neonate is 80 to 90 mL/kg, and a "double volume exchange" is standard, meaning that the total volume is replaced twice (160 to 180 mL/kg). This results in the exchange of approximately 85% of total blood volume.

Complications of High-Risk Newborns

Pulmonary Conditions

Respiratory distress syndrome (RDS) is the respiratory condition most associated with prematurity. Bronchopulmonary dysplasia (BPD) is a treatment complication of artificial respiratory support. Persistent pulmonary hypertension of the neonate (PPHN) is most common among late preterm infants, and transient tachypnea (TTN) occurs in term or preterm infants. Meconium aspiration syndrome (MAS) is respiratory distress of infants that is associated with meconium staining of the amniotic fluid in the absence of a different explanation for symptoms. All five conditions present as respiratory distress and can be challenging for new learners to differentiate (Table 25.1). BPD, PPHN, MAS, and TTN are discussed in this section. RDS is discussed in Chapter 24.

Bronchopulmonary Dysplasia

BPD is also known as neonatal chronic lung disease.

Etiology

BPD is a disorder that results from the administration of oxygen and mechanical ventilation for the treatment of RDS. Infection may also be a contributing factor for some infants. Very low birth weight (VLBW) and extremely low birth weight (ELBW)

Table 25.1 Conditions Causing Neonatal Respiratory Distress

Condition	Symptoms	Cause	Care
Respiratory distress syndrome	• Tachypnea • Nasal flaring • Expiratory grunting • Retractions • Cyanosis • Pallor	• Surfactant insufficiency • Immature lungs • Prematurity	• Assisted ventilation • Surfactant • Supportive therapy • Typically progresses for 48–72 h and resolves within a week
Bronchopulmonary dysplasia	• Tachypnea • Retractions • Rales • Wheezing	Lung damage resulting from artificial respiratory support in premature infants	• Respiratory support • Most improve over 2–4 mo. Some require persistent support.
Persistent pulmonary hypertension	• Most common in term infants • Usually presents within 24 h after birth as respiratory distress • Cyanosis • Prominent apical impulse • Split S2 heart sound • Systolic murmur	• Persistence of pulmonary vascular resistance that causes right-to-left shunting and hypoxemia • Underdeveloped pulmonary vasculature • Abnormal pulmonary vasculature • Lung disease	• Supportive care • Nitric oxide • ECMO • Treatment of underlying respiratory disease
Transient tachypnea	• Most common in late preterm, term, and postterm infants • Onset within 2 h after birth • Tachypnea • Nasal flaring • Expiratory grunting • Retractions • Cyanosis	Failure to clear fluid from the lungs	• Supportive care • Typically resolves within 24–72 h • Oxygen supplementation as needed to keep oxygen saturation >90%
Meconium aspiration syndrome	• Meconium-stained fluid • Respiratory or neurologic depression at birth • Postmature or small for gestational age • Respiratory distress • Cyanosis • Symptoms develop within 15 min after birth • Rales and rhonchi • Increased AP diameter • Pneumothorax or pneumomediastinum • PPHN	Chronic asphyxia and infection can lead to meconium staining of the amniotic fluid, which is then aspirated by the fetus resulting in: • Airway obstruction • Inflammation and chemical irritation • Infection • Inactivation of surfactant	• Supportive care • Antibiotics • Surfactant • Nitric oxide • ECMO

ECMO, extracorporeal membrane oxygenation; AP, anteroposterior; PPHN, persistent pulmonary hypertension of the neonate.

infants are at greater risk, and risk increases with the duration of mechanical ventilation and oxygen supplementation. Less aggressive ventilation that does not overdistend air spaces appears to result in a milder form of BPD. High concentrations of oxygen further contribute to the development of BPD (Wai et al., 2016). Sepsis can contribute to the development of BPD, as can chorioamnionitis.

Signs and Symptoms

Infants with BPD typically have pulmonary edema and/or atelectasis and are tachypneic as a result. They may also exhibit other signs of respiratory distress, such as severe retractions. Narrowed airways caused by scarring, edema, or other causes may result in expiratory wheezing. Functionally, patients have decreased tidal volume and lung compliance and increased airway resistance. Gas trapping from airway obstruction can result in hyperinflation of the lungs. BPD is categorized as either "classic BPD" or "new BPD".

- Classic BPD: This type is associated with airway injury, inflammation, and scarring of the alveoli from oxygen toxicity, barotrauma (injury from increased pressure), and infection. It is rarer today than new BPD. As adults, patients with this condition may have emphysema-like changes as seen in imaging studies (Greenough, 2013).
- New BPD: This type is associated with impaired alveolar development due to prematurity and low birth weight, fewer, larger alveoli, and abnormalities of pulmonary vasculature.

Prognosis

Most infants diagnosed with BPD improve over the course of 2 to 4 months, although some may require support by ventilator or supplemental oxygen for longer than 4 months. Lifelong abnormalities of pulmonary function tests are common in these patients, indicating obstructive lung disease. Many also have reactive airway disease (asthma-like symptoms). Infants with BPD and individuals with a history of BPD may also have abnormalities in their ability to increase or decrease ventilation in response to hypoxemia and hyperoxia. Individuals with a history of BPD are at an increased risk for neurodevelopmental delay and cerebral palsy.

Infants with severe BPD may experience acute episodes of pulmonary decompensation that may occur for a number of reasons, including an air leak (pneumothorax or pneumomediastinum), pulmonary edema, reactive airway, infection, and others.

Assessment

Evaluation may include a complete blood count, assessment of blood gasses, infection assessment, chest radiography, lung examination, and evaluation for fluid retention. Continuous pulse oximetry and periodic blood gas sampling are performed.

Treatment

Respiratory care for infants diagnosed with BPD is supportive, and small tidal volumes are used with mechanical ventilation to minimize injury when possible. Some infants may require more aggressive care, however, to splint open airways and minimize atelectasis. Ventilation is weaned as tolerated, and suctioning is minimized as much as possible. A tracheostomy may be performed for patients who require prolonged ventilation. Supplemental oxygen is used for adequate oxygen perfusion but also to avoid increases in pulmonary vascular resistance, which could lead to hypertrophy of the right ventricle (cor pulmonale) as it must pump harder to move blood through the vascular beds of the lungs in the case of increased pulmonary vascular resistance. High concentrations of oxygen, however, can contribute to pulmonary edema and inflammation, as well as risking the development of retinopathy of prematurity (ROP). An ophthalmologic examination can determine when mature retinal vascularization has been reached, at which time an oxygen target above 90% to 95% is no longer considered an ROP risk.

Bronchodilators and corticosteroids may be helpful for some infants but are not used routinely.

Infants with BPD have a higher nutritional requirement than those without BPD. The total energy needs can increase to 150 kcal/kg/d, with a total required protein intake of 3.5 to 4 g/kg/d. To complicate matters, infants with BPD are often fluid-restricted because of pulmonary edema, so the required nutrients must be delivered in a lower volume of liquid. Human milk fortifier is typically used for infants fed with human milk, and a more calorically dense formula is used for infants not receiving human milk. The fluid intake allowed may be as little as 100 to 120 mL/kg/d for severely ill infants and as much as 140 to 150 mL/kg/d for infants with milder disease. Rarely, a diuretic may be used for infants with severe disease who do not adequately respond to fluid restriction. The nurse should monitor serum electrolytes per orders with the use of diuretics starting on day 2 and then at least weekly.

Care Considerations

Infants with BPD should have a car seat challenge prior to discharge, as the condition increases the risk for oxygen desaturation, bradycardia, and apnea while sitting (see Box 5.8). Vaccinations for respiratory disease are particularly important for this population, as is the avoidance of tobacco smoke. All infants with BPD should have follow-up scheduled with a pulmonologist after discharge.

Transient Tachypnea of the Newborn

TTN is a self-limiting form of pulmonary edema resulting from delayed clearance and reabsorption of fetal alveolar fluid.

Etiology

When delayed reabsorption of lung fluid occurs, the fluid fills the air spaces and must be cleared by the lymphatic system. Decreased compliance of the lungs due to extra fluid causes tachypnea, and excess fluid can lead to air trapping. This combination of factors means the alveoli are poorly ventilated, leading to hypoxemia and occasionally hypercapnia.

Infants born by cesarean section and preterm infants are at a higher risk for TTN than infants born vaginally and at term. The infants of diabetic mothers are also at a higher risk for TTN, as are infants born to women with asthma.

Signs and Symptoms

TTN manifests within 2 hours after birth with symptoms of respiratory distress. Tachypnea is most common, although newborns may also have nasal flaring, expiratory grunting, retractions, and cyanosis. Breath sounds are usually clear, and symptoms typically clear in 24 to 48 hours but may persist for up to 72 hours.

Assessment

TTN is self-limited and benign and can be diagnosed clinically. Other more serious problems, however, may have a similar presentation, and thus further evaluation may be indicated.

Infants with TTN usually do not require oxygen supplementation at greater than 40% to maintain an oxygen saturation above 90%. A greater need for respiratory support may make the infant's team suspicious of a different respiratory disorder, such as RDS. Cardiac disease should also be ruled out. Infants who do not improve within 24 hours may be evaluated for pneumonia and sepsis. Abnormalities of the complete blood count and differential may prompt an earlier evaluation for infection.

Treatment

The goals of TTN treatment are supportive. If oxygen therapy is required, oxygen saturation is kept above 90%, usually by use of a hood or nasal cannula. As is standard when hypothermia is not an indicated treatment, infants are kept in a thermal-neutral environment. Infants with tachypnea may not be able to feed orally and may instead be fed by orogastric or nasogastric tube. Providers may elect to restrict fluids for the first 24 hours of life for infants with severe TTN (40 mL/kg/d for term infants, 60 mL/kg/d for preterm infants). Diuretics have not been shown to improve outcomes for this population (Kassab, Khriesat, & Anabrees, 2015).

Meconium Aspiration Syndrome

MAS is respiratory distress of the neonate in the presence of meconium-stained fluid without other explanation.

Prevalence

Meconium stained amniotic fluid (MSAF) occurs in 5% to 24% of pregnancies, but only 5% of infants born through MSAF develop MAS (Nair & Lakshminrusimha, 2014). The risk of MAS and MSAF is greatest in infants small for gestational age (SGA) and in infants born post term (after 42 weeks).

Etiology

MAS results from the passage of meconium in utero followed by an aspiration of MSAF, which leads to respiratory disease and hypoxemia and acidosis (Fig. 25.1). The condition is sometimes complicated by PPHN. Although MSAF can be a benign finding associated with maturity, MSAF can also result from intrauterine

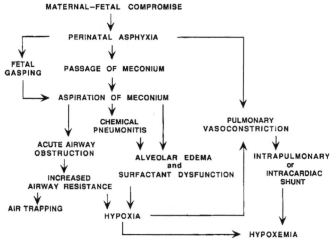

Figure 25.1. Pathophysiology of meconium aspiration. (Reprinted with permission from MacDonald, M. G., & Seshia, M. M. K. [2016]. *Avery's neonatology* [7th ed., Fig. 26.7]. Philadelphia, PA: Lippincott Williams & Wilkins.)

stress that causes both passage of meconium and the gasping reflex that results in aspiration. Many neonates born with MSAF have neurologic and/or respiratory depression, likely because of hypoxia and shock. Aspiration of MSAF can lead to physical obstruction of the airway, chemical irritation causing lung inflammation, infection, and the inactivation of pulmonary surfactant.

Signs and Symptoms

Infants with MAS show signs of respiratory distress within 15 minutes after birth and typically require ventilator support. Although newborn infants usually have an increased anterior-or-posterior diameter when compared with adults, this is even more pronounced in infants with MAS due to trapping of the air. On auscultation, rales and rhonchi are heard. Because of air trapping, pneumothorax and pneumomediastinum are common.

Assessment

Healthcare providers often use a chest radiograph to confirm the clinical diagnosis, and arterial blood gasses are evaluated to assess respiratory status and plan interventions. Continuous pulse oximetry should be expected. Echocardiography is done to diagnose PPHN, if suspected.

Treatment

Some MAS can be prevented by limiting the duration of a pregnancy to 41 weeks to avoid postmaturity. Amniotic fluid infusion has not been found to reduce the risk of MAS in the case of identified MSAF (Hofmeyr, Xu, & Eke, 2014). Although it was once standard practice to suction the airways of all infants born with MSAF, this practice is not supported by the evidence (Wyckoff et al., 2015).

Care focuses on the maintenance of adequate ventilation and perfusion, the correction of metabolic abnormalities such as acidosis and hypoglycemia, and providing antibiotics as indicated. A thermal-neutral environment is promoted. Respiratory interventions may include oxygen supplementation, mechanical ventilation, surfactant therapy, nitric oxide, and extracorporeal membrane oxygenation (ECMO).

Persistent Pulmonary Hypertension of the Newborn

Although the name makes PPHN sound like a pulmonary issue, it is in truth both a heart and lung issue.

Prevalence

PPHN is relatively rare, occurring with approximately 0.2% of live births (Steurer et al., 2017).

Etiology

Immediately after birth, the fetal circulation normally transitions to extrauterine circulation, and this transition includes closure of the ductus arteriosus and foramen ovale. A reduction in pulmonary vascular resistance occurs as air spaces open and oxygenation improves. Simultaneously, the systemic vascular resistance increases. If the pulmonary vascular resistance remains high in relation to the systemic vascular resistance, it is called PPHN. With PPHN, the force required of the right side of the heart to force blood through the pulmonary vascular exceeds the force required of the left side of the heart to pump blood through the body. When the right side of the heart pumps harder than the left side of the heart, a right-to-left shunt is created. A right-to-left shunt means that deoxygenated blood bypasses the lungs, causing severe hypoxemia. PPHN primarily occurs in infants born at 34 weeks of gestation or later. There are three causes: underdevelopment of the pulmonary vasculature, abnormal development of the pulmonary vasculature, and maladaptation to a perinatal condition that leads to pulmonary vasoconstriction.

- Underdevelopment of the lungs: The underdevelopment of the lungs, can happen with a number of conditions. Neonates born with renal agenesis, congenital pulmonary malformation, congenital diaphragmatic hernia, and intrauterine growth restriction (IUGR) are all at a higher risk for the underdevelopment of the lungs (Sharma, Berkelhamer, & Lakshminrusimha, 2015).
- Maldevelopment of the Lungs: In the case of maldevelopment, the lungs are completely developed, but the muscle layer around the pulmonary arterioles is abnormally thick. In the weeks after the birth, however, this muscle layer remodels, creating a drop in pulmonary vascular resistance. Postterm infants and infants with MAS are more likely to have maldevelopment of the lung vasculature. Abnormalities of the fetal circulation, such as premature closure of the foramen ovale or ductus arteriosus or high placental vascular resistance, can also contribute to maldevelopment.
- Maladaptation: In the case of maladaptation, the pulmonary vascular bed is anatomically normal, but a condition of the neonate has caused vasoconstriction of the pulmonary vasculature. The pulmonary vascular bed is particularly sensitive to low oxygen and constricts when hypoxia and acidosis are present. This constriction causes the pulmonary vascular resistance to increase. Conditions leading to maladaptation include bacterial infections and lung disease.

Risk factors for PPHN include a gestational age from 34 to 37 weeks, being small or large for gestational age, maternal diabetes and obesity, advanced maternal age, and African descent. Neonates are more likely to develop the condition if they experienced any of the following in utero: tachycardia or bradycardia, MASF, preterm premature rupture of membranes (PPROM), or exposure to selective serotonin reuptake inhibitors (SSRIs). A majority of infants diagnosed with PPHN have an additional pulmonary diagnosis, such as RDS, MAS, pneumonia, diaphragmatic hernia, or pulmonary hypoplasia. MAS is the most common cause of PPHN (Nair & Lakshminrusimha, 2014; Steurer et al., 2017).

Signs and Symptoms

PPHN typically manifests within 24 hours after birth as cyanosis and respiratory distress (tachypnea, grunting, retractions, and nasal flaring). Because MAS and PPHN often co-occur, infants with PPHN often have meconium staining of the nails and skin. Most infants who go on to be diagnosed with PPHN received a respiratory intervention at the time of delivery, such as exogenous oxygen administration or endotracheal intubation. Infants may have an abnormally prominent apical pulse, a split of the S2 heart sound, or a systolic murmur at the left lower sternal border over the tricuspid valve.

Prognosis

PPHN is associated with an overall mortality rate of approximately 10%. Survivors of severe disease are at an increased risk for hearing deficits, developmental delay, and cerebral palsy (Bendapudi, Rao, & Greenough, 2015).

Assessment

Diagnosis of PPHN is generally made by echocardiography, including Doppler studies that reveal a right-to-left shunt. Pulse oximetry at pre- and postductal locations, such as the right thumb and a great toe, usually show a difference in oxygen saturation of more than 10%, indicating patent ductus arteriosus (PDA). The difference may not be evident if shunting is instead through the foramen ovale, however. Arterial blood gasses vary according to the underlying cause of the PPHN.

Treatment

Care of the infant with PPHN is generally supportive, with maintenance of the following: adequate oxygenation, nutrition, circulatory support, acidosis correction, and temperature. Acidosis is generally corrected by the administration of IV sodium acetate. In severe cases of PPHN that do not respond to supportive measures, a vasodilatory agent such as inhaled nitrous oxide may be used. ECMO may be required until correction of the pulmonary vascular resistance. Underlying causes of PPHN should be addressed simultaneously. For example, in the case of RDS and MAS, surfactant administration may be required. Handling of the neonate should be limited, as it can cause and worsen hypoxemia (Bendapudi et al., 2015).

Because oxygen dilates the pulmonary vasculature, it is often given at 100% briefly in an attempt to reverse the vasoconstriction of the pulmonary blood vessels. The oxygen saturation goal is typically set from 90% to 95%, and failure to meet this standard is an indication for advanced treatment such as nitrous oxide and ECMO.

Care Considerations

Because of the high risk for hearing deficits, cerebral palsy, and developmental delay in infants with severe PPHN requiring nitrous oxide or ECMO, children who experienced PPHN should be assessed regularly for deficits during infancy early childhood.

Retinopathy of Prematurity

ROP is a leading cause of blindness in children in the United States.

Etiology

ROP occurs because of abnormal vascular growth of the blood vessels of the retina in infants born prematurely. The abnormal blood vessels are more permeable and leak, leading to edema and hemorrhage of the retina. This causes scarring that pulls on the retina, leading to distortion or even detachment. In most cases, however, the abnormal vasculature and tissue regress without permanent damage.

Lower gestational age is associated with a higher risk for ROP and worse outcomes. ROP is rare in high-resource settings for infants born after 32 weeks of gestation (Fielder, Blencowe, O'Connor, & Gilbert, 2015). A 2015 report put the risk of ROP for infants in high-resource settings who are under 1,500 g at 12.5% (Painter, Wilkinson, Desai, Goldacre, & Patel, 2015).

The primary risk factors for ROP are low gestational age and weight. Other risk factors relate to comorbidities and to care. The use of artificial ventilation for more than a week and surfactant therapy are the most prominent intervention-related risk factors, although hyperglycemia, insulin therapy, poor caloric intake, early use of erythropoietin for anemia, and high-volume blood transfusion can also contribute. Additional comorbidities that may contribute to the development of ROP include intraventricular hemorrhage, sepsis, and BPD. Increased oxygenation also plays a role in the development of ROP. The target blood oxygen saturation level for a preterm infant to meet the metabolic needs while minimizing the risk for ROP and lung injury is 90% (Stoltz Sjostrom et al., 2016). Breast milk may be protective (Bharwani et al., 2016).

Signs and Symptoms

The signs of ROP include edema and hemorrhage of the retina, scarring of the retina, and retinal distortion or even detachment. ROP changes usually start around 34 weeks postmenstrual age and advance until week 40 to 45 postmenstrual age before it begins to resolve spontaneously.

Prognosis

Although ROP regresses and resolves spontaneously in a majority of infants, others require treatment. If left untreated, a small number with advanced disease lose some or all visual acuity.

Assessment

Screening for ROP is done by an ophthalmologist, usually beginning at approximately 4 weeks after birth for at-risk infants. Examinations are repeated every 1 to 3 weeks thereafter. Screenings are ended when the risk for ROP ends (typically from 45 to 50 weeks of postmenstrual age), ROP is regressing, the retina is fully vascularized, or treatment is needed.

Treatment

ROP treatment is required only for severe disease. Treatment is generally by laser photocoagulation and/or one of the anti–vascular endothelial growth factor monoclonal antibodies, bevacizumab or ranibizumab (Hwang, Hubbard, Hutchinson, & Lambert, 2015).

Necrotizing Enterocolitis

Necrotizing enterocolitis (NEC) is ischemic necrosis of the intestines and is a gastrointestinal emergency. Almost all NEC occurs in preterm infants, particularly those weighing under 1,500 g at birth.

Prevalence

Younger, smaller infants are more susceptible, and the overall rate for infants born prior to 33 weeks of gestation is approximately 5% (Yee et al., 2012).

Etiology

It is believed that the mucosa of the intestines of preterm infants may be permeable to bacteria, whereas defenses such as immunoglobulin A and mucosal enzymes are immature and are unable to launch an adequate response, predisposing them to NEC. Delayed transit time from bowel immaturity may also allow for a greater proliferation of harmful bacteria. Failure of colonization of "good" commensal gut bacteria may also contribute (Warner et al., 2016). Antenatal corticosteroid therapy is protective against NEC. In term infants, the development of NEC is associated with comorbidities such as sepsis and congenital heart disease (Short et al., 2014).

Recall that Kylie, Lexi Cowslip's preterm infant in Chapter 10, was born at 29 weeks of gestation and developed NEC after receiving enteral tube feedings of expressed breast milk. She was given several antibiotics and placed on total parenteral nutrition, and did not require surgery.

Although a small number of infants who have never been fed enterally develop NEC, a majority have begun oral feedings, which contribute to the development of NEC because they provide the nutrients that feed the growth of the bacteria in the gut as well as nourishing the neonate. Development of NEC does not seem to be associated with the rate of feeding advancement or timing of initial feedings. Trophic feedings do not appear to reduce the chances of developing NEC, although they remain the standard for feeding initiation in many institutions (Morgan, Young, & McGuire, 2014).

The development of NEC is significantly less likely with human breast milk feedings than with formula feedings (Quigley & McGuire, 2014). Probiotics may provide some benefit, although data is as yet inconsistent and no standardized dosing or optimal strain has been identified (Billimoria, Pandya, Bhatt, & Pandya, 2016). Histamine-2 blockers such as ranitidine and famotidine are sometimes given for reflux in infants but should be avoided if possible because they lower the gastric acidity, thus increasing the risk for NEC. Antibiotic use is also associated with NEC and empirical therapy should be avoided when possible (Greenwood et al., 2014).

Signs and Symptoms

Most preterm infants with NEC appear initially healthy. NEC onset tends to be earlier in older infants and may not manifest for over a month after birth in preterm infants. The first sign of a problem is typically feeding intolerance (see Box 24.5). Systemic signs are nonspecific and include respiratory failure, apnea, hypotension, and temperature instability.

Prognosis

Short-term complications are often related to infection, including abscess formation and sepsis; disseminated intravascular coagulation; respiratory failure, hypotension, and shock; and metabolic complications, such as hypoglycemia and metabolic acidosis. Up to a quarter of patients diagnosed with NEC may experience intestinal strictures (intestinal narrowing), which usually develop in the first 3 months after the NEC diagnosis but may take as long as 20 months to be detected (Heida et al., 2016). Strictures can result in slower stool transit and bacterial overgrowth, which may result in bowel obstruction, failure to thrive, infection, and bloody stools. Strictures may resolve spontaneously or require surgical correction.

Infants who require removal of necrotic sections of bowel may have short bowel syndrome, resulting in malabsorption. This malabsorption results in a chronic need for total parenteral nutrition (TPN), which puts them at considerable risk for sepsis and liver failure. For these infants, intestinal and even liver transplantation may be required. In general, the infants who do best after a diagnosis of NEC are of higher birth weight and do not require surgical intervention. The mortality rate for ELBW infants requiring surgical intervention, however, is high.

Assessment

NEC is graded on the basis of systemic, intestinal, and radiographic findings according to the Bell staging criteria (Table 25.2). Infants are treated according to clinical presentation rather than staging. Stage I is unconfirmed NEC but often progresses to Stage II and/or III. Alternatively, Stage I may regress over time. Stages II and III are confirmed NEC.

Although systemic and abdominal signs may suggest NEC, abdominal imaging is used to confirm the diagnosis. Imaging can reveal an abnormal gas pattern and dilated intestines with early NEC. In Stages II and III, **pneumatosis intestinalis** is seen in almost all patients. Pneumatosis intestinalis is the collection of gasses within the wall of the small bowel and is considered the hallmark of NEC. **Pneumoperitoneum**, the collection of air in the abdominal cavity, is seen with bowel perforation. Fixed loops of bowel are called sentinel loops and suggest necrosis of the bowel and/or perforation of the bowel. Commonly drawn laboratory tests include a complete blood count, coagulation studies, and serum chemistries (Box 25.4). Sepsis often occurs with NEC, so a blood culture and, if indicated, a CSF culture are often done at the time of diagnosis to guide therapy (Bizzarro, Ehrenkranz, & Gallagher, 2014).

Treatment

Antibiotic therapy is standard for treating NEC. A broad-spectrum regimen is typically used that includes two or more agents over a period of 10 to 14 days. Laboratory monitoring to determine the success of treatment is generally done every 12 to 24 hours and includes a complete blood count with differential, electrolytes, blood urea nitrogen and creatinine, and acid–base studies. Radiographic monitoring is initially obtained every 6 to 12 hours and then as indicated by disease progression or regression.

A pediatric surgeon sees all infants with suspected or confirmed NEC, evaluates the clinical situation, and assesses if and when a surgical intervention is required. Many infants improve with supportive care and antibiotics, whereas others progress in the disease. Perforation of the bowel by necrosis requires surgical intervention. Continued clinical deterioration, ascites, and/or an abdominal mass or intestinal obstruction are also indications for surgery.

Surgery may consist of removal of necrotic sections of the bowel or primary peritoneal drainage. Primary peritoneal drainage can be performed at the bedside using local anesthesia. A Penrose drain is placed in the abdomen and left in place until drainage ceases. Resection of the bowel may require placement of an **ileostomy** (diversion of the bowel through an opening in the abdomen). **Reanastomosis** (reversal of the ileostomy) is typically performed 2 to 3 months later. Removal of a short section of bowel may not require an ileostomy.

Care Considerations

The nurse should initiate supportive care for all patients with NEC. This care includes bowel rest with discontinuation of enteric feedings and nasogastric suctioning for gastrointestinal decompression. TPN is started for adequate nutritional support as well as fluid replacement, as necessary. Cardiovascular support may require an inotropic medication such as dopamine to correct hypotension, in addition to the fluid replacement. Some neonates may require respiratory support by way of oxygen supplementation and/or ventilator.

Neonatal Encephalopathy

Neonatal encephalopathy (NE) is a term applied to infants born at or after 35 weeks of gestation who demonstrate disturbed neurologic function as manifested by seizure or a reduced level of consciousness.

Prevalence

A 2013 survey found an occurrence rate for NE of 8.5 per 1,000 live births (Lee et al., 2013).

Etiology

The underlying cause of the brain injury causing the disturbed neurologic function is often unknown, although perinatal asphyxia is a common cause. When NE is caused by perinatal asphyxia, it is called hypoxic-ischemic encephalopathy (HIE).

Signs and Symptoms

In addition to seizure and reduced level of consciousness, infants with NE may also exhibit diminished reflexes and muscle tone and have difficulty maintaining respiratory function. A low Apgar score, a weak or absent cry, and feeding difficulties are common findings with NE (American College of Obstetricians and Gynecologists [ACOG], 2014). Signs consistent with HIE include a 5-minute and a 10-minute Apgar score below five, fetal umbilical

Table 25.2 Bell Staging Criteria for Necrotizing Enterocolitis

Condition	Stage					
	IA	IB	IIA	IIB	IIIA	IIIB
Temperature instability	X	X	X	X	X	X
Apnea	X	X	X	X	X	X
Lethargy	X	X	X	X	X	X
Bradycardia	X	X	X	X	X	X
Metabolic acidosis				X	X	X
Thrombocytopenia				X	X	X
Hypotension					X	X
Bradycardia					X	X
Severe apnea					X	X
Respiratory acidosis					X	X
Neutropenia					X	X
Increased gastric residual	X	X	X	X	X	X
Abdominal distention	X	X	X	X	X	X
Heme-positive stool	X					
Emesis	X	X	X	X	X	X
Bloody stool		X	X	X	X	X
Absent bowel sounds			X	X	X	X
Abdominal tenderness			X/O	X	X	X
Abdominal cellulitis				X/O	X/O	X/O
Right lower quadrant mass				X/O	X/O	X/O
Intestinal dilation, mild ileus	X/O	X/O	X	X	X	X
Pneumatosis intestinalis			X	X	X	X
Ascites				X	X	X
Pneumoperitoneum						X

Pneumoperitoneum: abnormal presence of gas in the abdominal cavity.
Pneumatosis intestinalis: presence of gas within the wall of the intestine.
X, present; X/O, present or absent.
Adapted from Bell, M. J., Ternberg, J. L., Feigin, R. D., Keating, J. P., Marshall, R., Barton, L., & Brotherton, T. (1978). Neonatal necrotizing enterocolitis. Therapeutic decisions based upon clinical staging. *Annals of Surgery, 187*(1), 1–7.

artery acidemia, evidence of acute brain injury by neuroimaging, and multisystem organ failure (ACOG, 2014).

Prognosis

The severity of the condition is classified as mild, moderate, or severe according to specific clinical findings, and this classification is highly predictive of long-term outcomes.

- Mild: Absent seizure activity, normal muscle tone; the neonate is hyperexcitable and hyperalert
- Moderate: Seizure activity often present; hypotonia and decreased movement
- Severe: Seizures usually present; primitive reflexes, flaccid muscles, stuporous

A term infant with mild NE has a high probability of normal function during follow-up in early childhood, whereas the

Box 25.4 Interpretation of Laboratory Test Results Associated With Necrotizing Enterocolitis

- Absolute neutrophil count <1,500/μL: Common with necrotizing enterocolitis, associated with poor outcome
- Declining platelet levels: Necrotic bowel, worsening disease
- Rising platelet levels: Improved condition
- Low platelet levels + prolonged prothrombin time and partial thromboplastin time + decreased serum factor V and fibrinogen levels + increased D-dimer level: Disseminated intravascular coagulation
- Hyponatremia + elevated glucose level + metabolic acidosis: Sepsis and/or bowel necrosis

prognosis is less optimistic for neonates with a moderate or severe presentation (Sarnat & Sarnat, 1976).

Assessment

Neuroimaging by magnetic resonance imaging (MRI) or magnetic resonance spectroscopy can be very helpful for predicting long-term outcomes, as can electroencephalography (Massaro, 2015; Awal, Lai, Azemi, Boashash, & Colditz, 2016).

Treatment

Treatment goals for NE include the following: maintaining physiologic homeostasis by avoiding hypoxemia or hyperoxia by maintaining ventilation and by avoiding hypotension or hypertension to ensure organ and brain perfusion; seizure control; and controlling brain edema by avoiding fluid overload. Therapeutic hypothermia starting within 6 hours after the birth and lasting for 72 hours is an effective neuroprotective therapy for infants of at least 36 weeks of gestation. For therapeutic hypothermia, the neonate's core temperature is kept from 33°C to 35°C (91.4°F to 95°F; Fig. 25.2; Papile et al., 2014, Wyckoff et al., 2015).

Maternal Diabetes

The impact of maternal diabetes on the fetus and neonate largely depends on the time of onset of diabetes, the type of diabetes, and the level of glycemic control. As discussed previously, poor glycemic control with preexisting diabetes in the first trimester increases the risk for birth defects and spontaneous abortion as compared with the nondiabetic population. Fetal hyperglycemia,

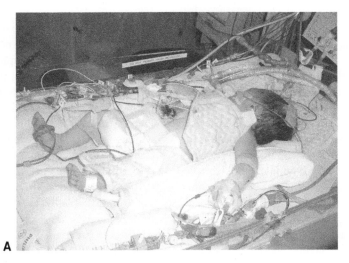

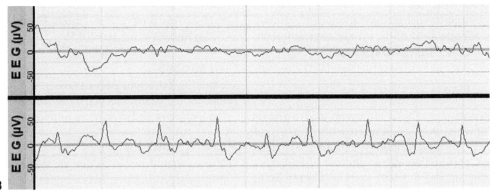

Figure 25.2. Therapeutic hypothermia. (A) A term infant with hypoxic-ischemic encephalopathy receiving therapeutic hypothermia via a cooling wrap around the trunk and thighs and being monitored by EEG. **(B)** The upper EEG trace shows normal brain activity. The lower EEG trace shows a seizure, with rhythmic sharp waves. EEG, electroencephalography. (Reprinted with permission from MacDonald, M. G., & Seshia, M. M. K. [2016]. *Avery's neonatology* [7th ed., Fig. 46.10]. Philadelphia, PA: Lippincott Williams & Wilkins.)

hyperinsulinemia, and macrosomia can occur in the second and third trimesters of pregnancy.

Maternal glucose passes the placenta, but maternal insulin does not. The fetus must produce an excessive amount of insulin to compensate for the excess maternal glucose, which, in turn, leads to increased oxygen consumption and possible hypoxia. Hypoxia increases the risk for stillbirth and metabolic acidosis and cues the kidneys to produce more erythropoietin, which leads to polycythemia. The excess recruitment of iron to produce red blood cells diverts the nutrient from the heart and brain, which may result in altered development. The stress of hypoxia increases catecholamine production, which may also contribute to cardiomyopathy, as well as stillbirth. High levels of insulin production are thought to delay lung maturity. The excess maternal glucose, coupled with excess fetal insulin, a growth hormone, causes macrosomia.

Thus, common complications of maternal diabetes include macrosomia, prematurity, respiratory distress, and hyperbilirubinemia. Other potential complications include perinatal asphyxia, hypoglycemia, hypocalcemia, polycythemia, low iron stores, and cardiomyopathy (Mitanchez et al., 2015).

Recall that Nancy Ng in Chapter 9 developed gestational diabetes and that her baby, Jonathan, was macrosomic, weighing 4,400 g, or about 9 lb and 7 oz.

The risk for major congenital anomalies is higher for women with preexisting diabetes than women without diabetes, and poorer glycemic control is associated with worse outcomes, regardless of the type of preexisting diabetes. The risk for congenital defects in a well-controlled diabetic pregnancy is about twice what it is in a nondiabetic pregnancy. In a poorly controlled diabetic pregnancy, the risk can be over 12 times that of a nondiabetic pregnancy (Al-Agha et al., 2012). Such anomalies account for more than 75% perinatal deaths associated with diabetes (Mitanchez et al., 2015). In infants of mothers diagnosed with gestational diabetes, the risk for anomalies is also increased, although to a much lesser degree (Leirgul et al., 2016). Congenital anomalies associated with diabetes include structural coronary defects, neural tube defects (NTDs), gastrointestinal malformations, limb contractures, cleft palate, abnormalities of the vertebrae, genitourinary malformations, and caudal regression syndrome.

Maternal Drug Use

Neonatal abstinence syndrome (NAS) is the term used to describe the constellation of withdrawal symptoms that occurs as a result of in utero exposure to opioids, including methadone, buprenorphine, oxycodone, and hydrocodone. The use of additional substances, including nicotine and some psychiatric medications, may compound NAS symptoms. Other substances, however, may cause symptoms that mimic NAS, including antidepressants, antipsychotics, alcohol, nicotine, and benzodiazepines.

The use of opioids during pregnancy has increased, as has neonatal admission for the treatment of NAS. Between 2004 and 2013, NAS diagnoses have increased from 7 of every 1,000 NICU admissions to 27 out of every NICU admissions. The current median duration of the NICU stay for an infant with NAS is 19 days (Tolia et al., 2015).

Careful questioning is essential for discovering the last use of substances to plan care. Alcohol withdrawal, for example, occurs within 3 to 12 hours of the birth because of a short half-life. Opioid withdrawal, on the other hand, may not start for 48 to 72 hours or more after birth, and withdrawal from barbiturates may not begin for a week.

Tobacco

Etiology
Smoking exposes the mother and fetus to thousands of chemicals and causes vasoconstriction, making it difficult to narrow down the exact cause of complications (Leite, Albieri, Kjaer, & Jensen, 2014).

Signs and Symptoms
Neonates of mothers who smoke may display more irritability and hypertonicity and less ability to self-soothe when compared with infants not exposed to tobacco in utero.

Prognosis
Women who smoke tobacco or use snuff are approximately twice as likely to deliver preterm either spontaneously or induced in response to pregnancy complications that are more frequent in women who smoke, such as placental abruption, chorioamnionitis, preeclampsia, and PPROM. Infants are also more likely to be SGA (Ko et al., 2014). Although the overall rate of congenital malformations is not higher overall in the pregnancies of women who use tobacco, cardiac and gastrointestinal defects, as well as clubfoot, are all more common in this population (Holbrook, 2016).

Smoking may contribute to sudden infant death syndrome (SIDS) and the development of type 2 diabetes later in life. Behavioral problems, including attention deficit hyperactivity disorder, may be more common. The offspring of women who smoked in pregnancy are more likely to develop asthma in childhood. Offspring may also be at a greater risk for neurologic disorders such as schizophrenia and Tourette syndrome (Bauer et al., 2016; Browne et al., 2016, Cornelius, 2014; Holbrook, 2016; Rubens & Sarnat, 2013).

Treatment
Smoking cessation, particularly in the first trimester, greatly reduces the chances of pregnancy complications and improves the long-term and short-term outlook for offspring.

Care Considerations
Nurses should be aware that smoking can negatively impact milk production, taste, and composition, leading to poor weight gain and earlier cessation of breastfeeding. Infants of mothers who smoke shortly before nursing tend to sleep poorly and for a shorter duration (Napierala, Mazela, Merritt, & Florek, 2016).

Opioids

Opioids are a class of substances that have morphine-like activities, including heroin, methadone, buprenorphine, fentanyl, hydromorphone, and oxycodone.

Etiology

A fetus may be chronically exposed to opioids during pregnancy because the mother has a substance use disorder, is undergoing maintenance therapy for addiction with methadone or buprenorphine, or is treated with an opioid throughout pregnancy for chronic pain. Nearly all infants born to mothers using opioids either by prescription or illicitly develop NAS as they withdraw from opioids that crossed the placenta. The amount and type of opioid exposure in utero, concurrent tobacco use, and the use of SSRIs in pregnancy increase the risk for NAS (Patrick et al., 2015).

Signs and Symptoms

NAS due to opioids usually first manifests from 48 to 72 hours after birth, although it may take as long as 5 days for the first signs to appear. NAS is typically described as dysfunction in four domains: state control and attention, motor and tone control, sensory integration, and autonomic functioning (Box 25.5). Infants with NAS are also at a higher risk for respiratory complications, SGA, and seizures.

There is wide variability in the timing of symptom presentation as well as the types of symptoms and severity displayed by a particular infant. Preterm infants often have a muted expression of NAS. Infants withdrawing from heroin, which has a shorter half-life, usually begin to withdraw within 24 hours after birth. The opioid replacement medications, methadone and buprenorphine, have longer half-lives, and thus withdrawal from them does not typically occur until 24 to 72 hours after the birth and may be delayed until as long as 5 days or more after the birth. Because of this uncertainly, neonates at risk for NAS are usually not discharged until 4 to 5 days after the birth with a clear follow-up plan with the outpatient pediatrics department (Kocherlakota, 2014).

Prognosis

Long-term outcomes are difficult to tease out in this population because of confounders. A confounder is a variable other than the one being studied that makes a conclusion less evident. However, treatment for trauma, abuse, and mental and behavioral disorders does appear to be more common for children who were treated for NAS as neonates (Uebel et al., 2015). Intelligence quotient may be measurably lower in such children, as well (Nygaard, Moe, Slinning, & Walhovd, 2015).

Treatment

The goal of pharmacologic therapy is to reduce the symptoms of NAS. Most neonates do not require pharmacologic therapy but can instead receive supportive care until they are done withdrawing. Although infants with NAS who are not treated with medications for withdrawal can usually be cared for in the regular nursery, those receiving medications for withdrawal are usually transferred to the NICU.

The first-line pharmacologic therapy for infants whose NAS scores exceed the threshold set by the institution and neonatology provider is an opioid. Morphine, methadone, and buprenorphine are all used for this purpose and are well studied. Recent data, however, suggest that treatment with buprenorphine may require a shorter duration of therapy (Kraft et al., 2017). Infants who receive insufficient relief with the maximum dose of the selected first-line medication are treated with a second medication, often clonidine or phenobarbital.

Once the patient responds sufficiently to medication as evidenced by NAS scoring and is gaining weight, the patient is weaned off of the medication. The infant may be discharged after being weaned from the medication with a stable condition for at least 24 hours. Planning for discharge must include social work and an evaluation of the home environment and maternal substance abuse status. SIDS (Box 25.6) is more common in this population, and the nurse should take special care to educate caregivers about safe sleep practices (Cohen, Morley, & Coombs, 2015). The nurse should arrange follow-up with the outpatient pediatrics department prior to discharge.

Care Considerations

Compassionate, collaborative nursing care is critical when caring for a couplet coping with NAS. Other important team members include those from neonatology and social services. Plans should be in place for follow-up care, including continuing maintenance therapy for mothers on methadone or buprenorphine.

Box 25.5 Signs of Neonatal Abstinence Syndrome

General
- Irritability
- High-pitched cry
- Sleep/wake disturbance
- Failure to thrive

Alterations in Movement
- Hypertonia
- Hyperactive reflexes
- Tremors
- Skin excoriation

Gastrointestinal
- Disorganized feeding
- Vomiting
- Frequent loose stool

Autonomic Dysfunction
- Sweating
- Sneezing
- Mottled skin
- Fever
- Nasal stuffiness
- Yawning

Management of the neonate includes supportive nonpharmacologic care and pharmacologic care as needed with a goal of adequate nutrition, sleep, and weight gain. Supportive, infant-specific care is essential regardless of the clinical presentation. Infants with tremors often prefer to be swaddled and laid on their side or gently rocked to help them better organize behavior. Swaddling also minimizes the risk for excoriation due to excessive rubbing. Minimizing auditory, tactile, and visual stimuli is also helpful for most NAS infants. Caregivers should avoid eye contact with infants who display a worsening of symptoms such as irritability or hypertonia with eye contact. Infants often find the use of a pacifier helpful for self-regulation, although caregivers should avoid excoriating the chin. Caregivers should change diapers promptly and use a barrier cream to avoid skin breakdown from frequent stooling. The nurse should inform parents of the strategies used in caring for the infant and the reasoning behind them so they may use them in their own provision of care.

Small, frequent feedings are often most appropriate to minimize regurgitation and maximize weight gain. Breastfeeding is encouraged for many mothers who are maintained with opium-replacement therapy. Both methadone and buprenorphine pass into the breast milk in low concentrations that appear to be safe. The low concentration of opioid replacement medications in breast milk appears to reduce the severity of NAS, although it is not a replacement for pharmaceutical treatment if needed. Women using opioid replacement medications often have an abundant milk supply, and the nurse should instruct them in the use of a pump and optimal breast milk storage (Box 18.9) (Welle-Strand et al., 2013).

The decision to initiate medication therapy for infants for the treatment of NAS is based on the severity of clinical manifestations, typically as scored according to the institution's preferred tool and protocol. Scoring is begun at birth and repeated every 3 to 4 hours during the infant's hospitalization. The mother and other caregivers may also be recruited to observe the baby for signs of NAS. For example, the nurse might not be present to observe the infant sneeze or yawn, making the report of the caregivers important for accurate scoring.

Alcohol

Exposure to alcohol in utero is the number one cause of preventable birth defects and developmental disabilities. Prenatal alcohol exposure can result in fetal alcohol spectrum disorder (FASD), which expresses as a wide range of physical, mental, cognitive, and behavioral clinical manifestations with high cost to the individual and society. FASD is not in itself a diagnosis but refers rather to a collection of disorders associated with maternal alcohol consumption in pregnancy (Table 25.3).

Prevalence

Worldwide, the prevalence of FASD is estimated at 23 per 1,000 live births (Roozen et al., 2016).

Etiology

There is no recognized safe amount of alcohol consumption in pregnancy. Alcohol is a central nervous system (CNS) teratogen that is eliminated inefficiently from the fetal environment, meaning that even a small amount ingested infrequently may lead to prolonged exposure by the fetus (Heller & Burd, 2014). There is also no safe time in pregnancy for the mother to consume alcohol. The CNS develops throughout pregnancy and is thus always vulnerable. In addition, first trimester exposure is associated with major structural defects, second trimester exposure is associated with spontaneous abortion and early stillbirth, and third trimester exposure is associated with poor growth (Muggli et al., 2017).

Signs and Symptoms

The characteristic facial features of a thin upper lip, short palpebral fissures (small eyes), and a smooth philtrum must be present for a diagnosis of fetal alcohol syndrome or partial fetal alcohol syndrome but may or may not be present for the diagnosis of neurobehavioral disorder associated with prenatal alcohol exposure (Fig. 25.3). Various other minor anomalies of the face and other structures are common but not necessary for diagnosis (Hoyme et al., 2016).

CNS involvement is often classified as structural, neurologic, or functional, and the manifestations vary with age. Structural

Table 25.3 Conditions of Fetal Alcohol Spectrum Disorder

Condition	Description
Fetal alcohol syndrome	• Growth restriction (10th percentile or less) • Evidence of brain involvement • Neurobehavioral impairment • Two or more characteristic facial features: short palpebral fissures (eye openings), thin upper lip, or smooth philtrum
Partial fetal alcohol syndrome	With documented alcohol exposure: • Evidence of brain involvement • At least two characteristic facial features Without documented alcohol exposure: • Neurobehavioral impairment • At least two characteristic facial features • Growth restriction (10th percentile or less) *or* neurologic involvement
Alcohol-related neurodevelopmental disorder	• Documented exposure to alcohol in utero • Neurobehavioral impairment • Must be diagnosed at age 3 y or older
Neurobehavioral disorder associated with prenatal alcohol exposure	• Documented alcohol exposure in utero • Neurobehavioral impairment • A diagnosis of exclusion (i.e., no other exposure or condition is explanatory)
Alcohol-related birth defects	• Documented exposure to alcohol in utero • At least one malformation associated with alcohol exposure

Evidence of brain involvement (one or more of the following):
• Head circumference at or below the 10th percentile (at or below the 3rd percentile if height and weight are below the 10th percentile)
• Structural abnormalities of the brain as evidenced by imaging
• Recurrent seizures not attributed to another cause
• Hard or soft neurologic signs
  ○ Hard signs: abnormal reflexes or tone, cranial nerve deficits
  ○ Soft signs: poor balance, right-left confusion, difficulty with motor sequencing, difficulty with rapid successive movements, motor-visual difficulties

Evidence of neurobehavioral impairment (one or more of the following):
• Significant intellectual or cognitive defects
• Motor delays
• Executive functioning delays
• Attention or hyperactivity disorder
• Poor social skills
• Poor self-regulation
• Memory deficits
• Language problems

Adapted from Hoyme, H. E., Kalberg, W. O., Elliott, A. J., Blankenship, J., Buckley, D., Marais, A. S., ... May, P. A. (2016). Updated clinical guidelines for diagnosing fetal alcohol spectrum disorders. *Pediatrics, 138*(2). doi:10.1542/peds.2015-4256; Hagan, J. F., Jr., Balachova, T., Bertrand, J., Chasnoff, I., Dang, E., Fernandez-Baca, D., ... American Academy of Pediatrics. (2016). Neurobehavioral disorder associated with prenatal alcohol exposure. *Pediatrics, 138*(4). doi:10.1542/peds.2015-1553.

abnormalities include a head circumference below the 10th percentile (below the 3rd percentile for individuals below the 10th percentile by height and weight) and abnormalities noted by neuroimaging. Functional abnormalities include cognitive impairment, slow processing speed, impaired planning and decision-making, hyperactivity, impaired motor function, poor impulse control, and poor social skills (Hoyme et al., 2016;

Lucas et al., 2014; Weyrauch, Schwartz, Hart, Klug, & Burd, 2017).

Prognosis

Major structural defects associated with prenatal alcohol exposure may be cardiac, renal, or skeletal. Structural defects causing hearing loss may be sensorineural or conductive and occur in

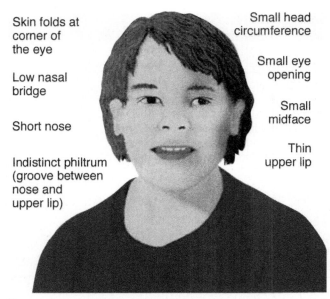

Skin folds at
corner of
the eye

Low nasal
bridge

Short nose

Indistinct philtrum
(groove between
nose and
upper lip)

Small head
circumference

Small eye
opening

Small
midface

Thin
upper lip

Figure 25.3. Facial features of fetal alcohol syndrome. A child presenting with the characteristic pattern of abnormal facial features diagnostic c for fetal alcohol spectrum disorder, including short palpebral fissure lengths (distance from A to B), smooth philtrum, and thin upper lip. (Reprinted from the United States Department of Health and Human Services, National Institute on Alcohol Abuse and Alcoholism. [2004]. *Alcohol alert number 63: Alcohol and the developing brain* (5 p.). Bethesda, MD: Author.)

18% of those diagnosed with FASD. Structural ocular defects that result in vision impairment occur in 28% of those diagnosed with FASD (Hoyme et al., 2016; Popova et al., 2016).

The long-term prognosis for individuals diagnosed with FASD is discouraging, with high rates of HIV infection, substance abuse, car accidents, suicide, and homicide (Rangmar et al., 2015). In one cohort of 415 individuals diagnosed with FASD, more than half got in trouble with the law and 50% were incarcerated. Nearly half displayed inappropriate sexual behavior (Streissguth et al., 2004).

Care Considerations

Individuals with FASD and their caregivers benefit from an interprofessional approach that may include social work, occupational therapy, physical therapy, and speech therapy, as well as nursing, medicine, and psychology as indicated. Several parent training programs are available to help families learn to care for children with the diagnosis, including Families Moving Forward, which is a program for families with children diagnosed with FASD with behavioral issues, and Strongest Families FASD Parenting Program, which is a program to help reduce behavioral problems and caregiver distress (Bertrand & Interventions for Children with Fetal Alcohol Spectrum Disorders Research, 2009; Turner et al., 2015).

Cocaine

Maternal cocaine use during pregnancy can result in IUGR, preterm birth, and structural deficits in the brain of offspring (Cain, Bornick, & Whiteman, 2013; Grewen et al., 2014).

Neurobehavioral abnormalities, including irritability, tremors, excess suck, hyper-alertness, tachypnea, apnea, and a high-pitched cry often present 48 to 72 hours after the birth. Because of cocaine's long half-life, these clinical manifestations are likely due to the drug itself rather than withdrawal (Hudak & Tan, 2012). There are likely no long-term direct effects of maternal cocaine use, although earlier studies suggested that offspring may have more difficulty with tasks requiring sustained attention (Williams & Ross, 2007).

Marijuana

Marijuana is the most commonly used illicit drug in pregnancy (Ko, Farr, Tong, Creanga, & Callaghan, 2015). It may be smoked, inhaled in vaporized form, drunk in tea form, or eaten as an ingredient in food, often baked goods. Marijuana use in pregnancy is not associated with prematurity, low birth weight, congenital abnormalities, NICU admission, or perinatal mortality (Mark, Desai, & Terplan, 2016). Infants may be more jittery and irritable when compared with infants not exposed to marijuana in utero.

Maternal marijuana use in pregnancy, particularly heavy use, may impact the child's intelligence, attention span, visual memory, and executive function. Offspring may be more susceptible to anxiety and depression and have deficits in memory, learning, and impulse control (Behnke & Smith, 2013). Marijuana use is discouraged when breastfeeding (ACOG, 2017).

Amphetamines

Amphetamines are stimulants, such as those used to treat attention deficit hyperactivity disorder and narcolepsy. They are addictive and are also used illicitly. Common illicit forms include methylenedioxymethamphetamine (MDMA, Molly, ecstasy), methamphetamine (ice, meth, crystal meth), 3,4-methylenedioxyamphetamine (MDA, love drug), and 3,4-Methylenedioxy-*N*-ethylamphetamine (MDEA, Eve). It is associated with IUGR, prematurity, and perinatal death (Wright, Schuetter, Tellei, & Sauvage, 2015). Motor and cognitive impairment of offspring is associated with frequent use in pregnancy (Eze et al., 2016). It is unclear whether amphetamines cause withdrawal symptoms in the neonate.

Barbiturates

Barbiturates are used therapeutically to treat seizures and cluster and migraine headaches as well as para-operative sedatives. They are used recreationally to achieve a feeling of contentment and euphoria and are addictive. They are associated with various congenital malformations both mild and severe (Tomson et al., 2011). Maternal use of barbiturates during pregnancy is not associated with a greater risk for prematurity or growth restriction in the fetus, but the neonate may experience withdrawal symptoms beginning 2 to 14 days after the birth.

Withdrawal occurs in an acute stage and a subacute stage. During the acute stage, the infant may cry constantly. The infant may be irritable and display hiccups, tremors, mouthing motions, and sleeplessness. During the subacute stage, which may last as long as 2 to 4 months, the infant is likely to remain irritable, with sleep disturbance and sensitivity to sound, and to eat voraciously, with frequent regurgitation.

Care for infants withdrawing from barbiturates includes reducing stimuli by swaddling, keeping lights dim, and keeping noise levels low. If supportive care is insufficient, phenobarbital is used to ease withdrawal symptoms.

Caffeine

Low-to-moderate caffeine consumption in pregnancy is unlikely to result in poor pregnancy outcomes. There may be a small increased risk for spontaneous abortion in early pregnancy with a consumption of more than the equivalent of one cup of coffee per day (Hahn et al., 2015). There may be a small increased risk for birth defects even with minimal caffeine consumption (Chen et al., 2012). Other analyses, however, have found no correlation between caffeine consumption and birth defects (Brent, Christian, & Diener, 2011). Fetal growth restriction is unlikely with moderate caffeine consumption (two to three cups of coffee a day; Doepker et al., 2016). There does not appear to be an increased risk for preterm birth with any level of caffeine consumption (Maslova, Bhattacharya, Lin, & Michels, 2010).

Caffeine withdrawal in the neonate of a mother with heavy, prolonged caffeine consumption may be observed shortly after the birth as irritability, jitteriness, and vomiting that typically resolve within 84 hours. Caffeine use in pregnancy does not appear to be associated with long-term neurologic or developmental consequences (Klebanoff & Keim, 2015). Caffeine is safe with breastfeeding.

Selective Serotonin Reuptake Inhibitors and Serotonin-Norepinephrine Reuptake Inhibitors

SSRIs and serotonin-norepinephrine reuptake inhibitors (SNRIs) are first- and second-line medications used to treat multiple mental health conditions, including depression, anxiety, and posttraumatic stress disorder. SSRIs and SNRIs are used by about 8% of pregnant and lactating mothers (Huybrechts et al., 2013). These medications are likely not teratogenic (Furu et al., 2015; Malm et al., 2015). SSRIs and SNRIs do not pose an increased risk for spontaneous abortion (Andersen, Andersen, Horwitz, Poulsen, & Jimenez-Solem, 2014). The use of these medications in pregnancy likely does not contribute to the risk for preterm birth (Malm et al., 2015).

The risk of an Apgar score lower than 7 at 5 minutes is higher for infants born to women taking SSRIs or SNRIs (Malm et al., 2015). The use of SSRIs and SNRIs in pregnancy is not, however, associated with an increase in the rate of perinatal death (Stephansson et al., 2013).

Newborns of mothers who took SSRIs and SNRIs in the third trimester of pregnancy may develop poor neonatal adjustment syndrome (Box 25.7). The condition is reported in 5% to 85% of births to women taking SNRIs or SSRIs and is usually mild, although it may at times require medical intervention (Grigoriadis et al., 2013). The wide range of reporting is due to variations in

Box 25.7 Signs of Poor Neonatal Adjustment Syndrome

- Irritability
- Continuous crying
- Agitation
- Restlessness
- Respiratory distress
- Seizures
- Sleep difficulties
  - Insomnia
  - Somnolence
- Feeding difficulties
  - Poor feeding
  - Vomiting
  - Diarrhea
- Altered muscle tone
- Hyperreflexia
- Jitteriness
- Shivering
- Tremors

Adapted from Salisbury, A. L., O'Grady, K. E., Battle, C. L., Wisner, K. L., Anderson, G. M., Stroud, L. R., ... Lester, B. M. (2016). The roles of maternal depression, serotonin reuptake inhibitor treatment, and concomitant benzodiazepine use on infant neurobehavioral functioning over the first postnatal month. *American Journal of Psychiatry, 173*(2), 147–157. doi:10.1176/appi.ajp.2015.14080989.

defining the syndrome. Preterm infants and infants exposed to other medications in addition to an SSRI or SNRI in pregnancy are more likely to develop the syndrome and to have a more severe presentation (Salisbury et al., 2016). The syndrome is self-limiting, although signs may persist for 2 to 4 weeks (Salisbury et al., 2016).

Breastfeeding is not contraindicated for women using SSRIs or SNRIs and it may help ease the clinical manifestations of poor neonatal adjustment syndrome (Kieviet et al., 2015). Fetal exposure to SSRIs or SNRIs appears to have little to no impact on growth, intelligence, behavior, or the language or motor skills of offspring (Grzeskowiak et al., 2016; Siminerio, Venkataramanan, & Caritis, 2016; Wisner et al., 2013).

Neonatal Infection

Neonatal infections may be acquired in utero or during or after the birth. The infectious agent may be viral, fungal, or bacterial. Newborns have an immature immune system, making them particularly susceptible to infection and severe consequences resulting from infection.

Sepsis

Neonatal sepsis is the presence of a bacterium, fungus, or virus in the blood, as confirmed by blood culture and manifested by systemic signs of infection. Early-onset sepsis occurs in the first 7 days after the birth, and late-onset sepsis occurs after the first week.

Prevalence

Sepsis occurs in just 1 or 2 out of every 1,000 live births, although the rate is higher for preterm infants. Although rare in newborns, it is an important cause of morbidity and mortality.

Etiology

Early-onset sepsis is usually due to exposure to bacteria from contaminated amniotic fluid or from the mother's lower genital tract during the birth. Chorioamnionitis is an important risk factor for early-onset sepsis, as is group B streptococcus (GBS) colonization. Late-onset sepsis may also be from vertical transmission (from mother to infant) or may result from an exposure to an environmental source or care provider, as can occur with the placement of an IV or other invasive procedure.

GBS and *Escherichia coli* infections account for approximately 75% of cases of neonatal sepsis, and the remainder are attributed to various other bacteria, including *Listeria monocytogenes, Staphylococcus aureus, Enterococcus,* and others. Other more rare causes are herpes simplex virus (HSV), enterovirus, parechovirus, and *Candida.* Because so many infections are vertically transmitted, it's important to consider the maternal risk factors (Box 25.8).

Signs and Symptoms

The signs of neonatal septic shock are often subtle and nonspecific (see Box 7.12). Nurses should be alert for changes in the infant's usual feeding or activity pattern in infants at risk for sepsis, as that may be an early indication of distress.

Prognosis

In most cases, treated symptomatic infants with sepsis improve within 48 hours, and cultures repeated after this time are negative.

Box 25.8 Risk Factors for Neonatal Sepsis

Prenatal
- Chorioamnionitis
- Maternal intrapartum temperature of 100.4°F or greater
- Delivery prior to 37 wk of gestation
- Maternal group B streptococcus colonization
- Prolonged rupture of membranes of 18 h or more

Intrapartum
- Fetal tachycardia
- Meconium-stained fluid
- Use of a fetal scalp electrode
- Use of forceps

Neonatal
- Apgar score of 6 or less

Adapted from Polin, R. A.; Committee on Fetus and Newborn. (2012). Management of neonates with suspected or proven early-onset bacterial sepsis. *Pediatrics, 129*(5), 1006–1015. doi:10.1542/peds.2012-0541.

A culture that continues to grow bacteria suggests the need for a change in antibiotic therapy.

Assessment

Infants who are at risk but are not symptomatic are generally observed for at least 2 days and may receive a limited diagnostic evaluation on the basis of risk. Infants presenting with suspected late-onset sepsis also have cultures gathered from urine and potential infection site (tracheal aspirates, IV site, etc.).

Sepsis may be confirmed only by culture. When the culture does not isolate a pathogen but the neonate continues to manifest signs concerning for sepsis, the condition is referred to as probable sepsis. Sepsis is considered unlikely if signs of infection resolve and cultures are negative after 48 hours.

Treatment

Infants deemed symptomatic receive empiric treatment with antibiotics simultaneous to a full diagnostic evaluation (Boxes 25.9 and 25.10). If signs and symptoms resolve and cultures are negative, empiric antibiotic treatment is stopped in this population.

Box 25.9 Diagnostic Evaluation for Suspected Sepsis in a Symptomatic Neonate

Standard Tests
- Blood culture
  - From venipuncture, arterial puncture, or newly inserted venous or arterial catheter
  - One to two samples
  - Minimum volume of 1 mL per sample
  - Results in 24–36 h
- Lumbar puncture (if stable)
  - Infants often asymptomatic with meningitis
  - Performed prior to antibiotic start
  - Gram stain, culture, cell count with differential, protein, glucose
  - Over one third of infants with meningitis have a negative blood culture (Polin et al., 2012)
- Complete blood count with differential and platelet count
  - Obtain 6–12 h after birth
  - More useful for ruling out sepsis than ruling it in
    - A normal immature-to-total neutrophil ratio can help rule out sepsis.
    - A low neutrophil count is more indicative of sepsis than a high count.
- Chest X-ray if respiratory symptoms are present
- If intubated, cultures of tracheal aspirates

Additional Tests for Late-Onset Sepsis
- Urine culture: Obtained by catheter or bladder tap
- Foci culture

Box 25.10 Indications for Empiric Treatment With Antibiotics for Suspected Sepsis in Symptomatic Neonate

- Ill appearance of neonate
- Concerning symptoms
  - Temperature instability
  - Irritability
  - Lethargy
  - Respiratory symptoms
  - Poor feeding
  - Tachycardia
  - Poor perfusion
  - Hypotension
- Cerebrospinal fluid pleocytosis (white blood cell count of >20–30 cells/μL)
- Suspected or confirmed chorioamnionitis
- Positive culture of blood, cerebrospinal fluid, or urine

Care Considerations

Supportive care includes monitoring and maintaining adequate perfusion and oxygenation, preventing metabolic acidosis and hypoglycemia, and maintaining fluid and electrolyte balance.

Group B Streptococcus

As discussed in earlier chapters (Chapters 7 and 22), GBS is a significant cause of neonatal sepsis, although the risk of vertical transmission from mother to infant at the time of birth has reduced since routine antibiotic administration during labor became the standard of care.

Prevalence

Overall, a decline of early-onset GBS has been attributed to universal GBS screening for pregnant women in late pregnancy and the routine use of intrapartum antibiotic prophylaxis for those who are colonized with the bacteria. That number has now plateaued, however, despite widespread screening and prophylaxis. Approximately half of cases are identified in preterm neonates.

Etiology

Neonatal GBS acquired by the fetus after the rupture of membranes is responsible for early-onset disease. Disease of later onset is more likely caused by encounters with colonized individuals. Early-onset GBS infection of the neonate usually presents before 24 hours postpartum but may occur at any time in the first week after birth. Late-onset GBS usually presents 4 to 5 weeks after the birth but can occur between 1 week and 89 days. Late, late–onset GBS occurs in infants older than 3 months and is associated with immaturity and a depressed immune system (American Academy of Pediatrics, 2015c).

You may recall that Hannah Wilder in Chapter 7 was GBS-positive with chorioamnionitis, raising concerns for neonatal sepsis.

Although approximately half of cases of GBS are in infants born to mothers who did not receive antibiotic prophylaxis, only a very few infants born to untreated mothers develop early-onset GBS disease. Several factors have been associated with an increased likelihood for the development of early-onset GBS (Box 25.11). Intrapartum antibiotic prophylaxis has no effect on the incidence of late-onset or late, late–onset GBS, thus making it unlikely that late-onset and late, late–onset GBS are caused by vertical transmission. The diagnosis and management of GBS disease are similar to that discussed in the Sepsis section previously.

Signs and Symptoms

Early-Onset GBS Presentation

Early-onset GBS disease may manifest as sepsis, pneumonia, or meningitis, with most displaying symptoms within 24 hours after the birth. Sepsis without foci is the most common presentation, occurring in 80% to 85% of neonates diagnosed with the disease (see Sepsis in earlier section). Pneumonia occurs with or without sepsis in 10% of cases. Pneumonia presents as increased work of breathing that may include grunting, nasal flaring, and retractions, as well as tachypnea and hypoxia. Pneumonia is confirmed by chest X-ray. Meningitis occurs in approximately 7% of cases of early-onset GBS disease. It typically, like pneumonia, manifests as respiratory abnormalities rather that signs consistent with CNS inflammation (Phares et al., 2008).

Box 25.11 Risk Factors for Early-Onset Group B Streptococcus Disease

- Gestational age less than 37 wk at delivery
- Premature rupture of membranes
- Rupture of membranes 18 or more hr prior to delivery
- Chorioamnionitis
- Group B streptococcus in urine during the current pregnancy
- Prior delivery of an infant with group B streptococcus disease
- Temperature of 100.4°F or greater during labor
- Heavy maternal colonization
- Insufficient maternal immunoglobulin G at term

Adapted from Polin, R. A.; Committee on Fetus and Newborn. (2012). Management of neonates with suspected or proven early-onset bacterial sepsis. *Pediatrics, 129*(5), 1006–1015. doi:10.1542/peds.2012-0541; Baker, C. J., Carey, V. J., Rench, M. A., Edwards, M. S., Hillier, S. L., Kasper, D. L., & Platt, R. (2014). Maternal antibody at delivery protects neonates from early onset group B streptococcal disease. *Journal of Infectious Diseases, 209*(5), 781–788. doi:10.1093/infdis/jit549.

Late-Onset GBS Presentation

Late-onset GBS presents as sepsis in about 65% of cases and as meningitis or a focal infection in up to 40% of cases. The common sites of focal infection include bones and joints, and cellulitis often occurs. The most common presentation is a fever of 38°C or higher with a current or recent history of a respiratory infection. The infant may also be irritable or lethargic with poor feeding with respiratory signs such as grunting, tachypnea, and apnea. With late-onset GBS, infants are less likely to exhibit signs of shock. Late-onset GBS meningitis is more likely to present with classic meningitis signs, such as nuchal rigidity, neurologic findings, and seizure, than is early-onset GBS (Berardi et al., 2013).

Late, late–onset GBS is typically sepsis without a focus. If there is a focus, the locations may include bones, joints, the CNS, or intravascular catheter sites. GBS infection after 6 months of age is associated with a compromised immune system.

Skin and Soft Tissue Bacterial Infection

Etiology

Most skin and soft tissue infections of the neonate are caused by *S. aureus*, although, as mentioned previously, GBS can also cause cellulitis. Group A streptococcus, *L. monocytogenes*, *Pseudomonas aeruginosa*, *Treponema pallidum*, and *Haemophilus influenzae type B* are less common causes.

Signs and Symptoms

Infections may present as vesiculobullous or pustular lesions. *S. aureus* can cause pyoderma, which appears as erythematous papules and pustules with a honey-colored crust, often in the areas of skin trauma.

Prognosis

S. aureus produces toxins that can cause the skin to slough, called staphylococcal scalded skin syndrome (SSSS, also called Ritter disease; Fig. 25.4). Usually seen at day 3 to 7 after birth, SSSS initially presents as bullae that break down easily. Infants are typically irritable and febrile. Gentle pressure is applied to the skin, causing separation and sloughing of the epidermis (Nikolsky's sign). Conjunctivitis is common, although the mucus membranes are not involved. Because the dermis is not involved, scarring does not result from the condition.

Assessment

The etiology of the infection can be discerned by cultures. Depending on presentation, cultures may be taken from multiple areas, including the blood, overt area of infection, umbilicus, urine, and the nasopharynx.

Treatment

IV antibiotics are administered, often nafcillin, oxacillin, or, in areas with a high methicillin-resistant *S. aureus* prevalence, vancomycin. Supportive therapy includes the application of creams and ointments and the maintenance of fluid and electrolyte balance.

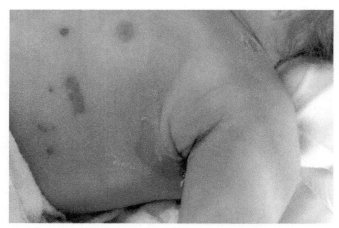

Figure 25.4. Staphylococcal scalded skin syndrome. Note the scalded appearance of the skin under the ruptured bullae of the chest and axilla in this child with staphylococcal scalded skin syndrome. (Reprinted with permission from *Lippincott Nursing Advisor February 2014 release*. Philadelphia, PA: Lippincott Williams & Wilkins.)

Congenital Syphilis

Syphilis transmitted vertically from mother to fetus is referred to as congenital syphilis. It can result in stillbirth, prematurity, low birth weight, hydrops fetalis, or fetal damage that may or may not be clinically obvious at the time of birth (Centers for Disease Control and Prevention, 2016). Screening of the mother for syphilis is a standard part of prenatal care.

Prevalence

Between 2005 and 2014, the rate of reported cases of congenital syphilis ranged between 8 and 12 cases per 100,000 live births. In 2014, the rate of congenital syphilis was the highest it had been since 2001. Among reported cases, a quarter of mothers had received no prenatal care. Of the remaining cases, 43% had received no treatment for syphilis in pregnancy and 30% had been inadequately treated (Bowen, Su, Torrone, Kidd, & Weinstock, 2015).

Etiology

The bacterium responsible for syphilis, *T. pallidum*, passes the placenta to infect the fetus. Occasionally, the bacteria may instead pass to the fetus at the time of birth from an infectious chancre (a lesion that is an early and transient manifestation of the infection). The disease of syphilis has a primary, secondary, and tertiary stage, as well as a latency period (see Chapter 28). Vertical transmission is possible when the disease is in the primary or secondary stage or in early latency. Syphilis is not transmitted via breast milk, although transmission could occur via a chancre on the breast.

Signs and Symptoms

Up to 90% of infants born with congenital syphilis will have no symptoms at birth, and symptoms, when they do occur, are highly variable (Bowen et al., 2015). For those who are symptomatic, clinical manifestations can range broadly from enlargement of the liver to rhinitis to sepsis. The umbilical cord may take on a stark "barber pole" appearance with red and blue stripes coupled with white streaks with areas of necrosis. The placenta itself may appear unusually large and pale. The liver of nearly all infants with syphilis will be enlarged, although this may not be immediately obvious clinically (Lago, Vaccari, & Fiori, 2013).

Rhinitis of syphilis, if it occurs, will generally appear in the first week although rarely after the third month. The discharge may be white, purulent, or bloody and is of larger volume and for longer duration than would be expected for a common viral rhinitis. The nasal discharge is highly infectious.

In infants, the rash of syphilis is usually most prominent over the buttocks, back, back of thighs, and soles of feet (Fig. 25.5). The rash is maculopapular with red or pink color initially that fades to a darker red or copper color following desquamation and crusting of the lesions. The rash may be present at birth or appear a few weeks after rhinitis. When present at birth, it may be bullous or ulcerative instead of maculopapular. Skin manifestations may alternately be fissures, flat and wart-like lesions, or patches on mucosal tissue.

Other nonspecific manifestations of syphilis in the neonate include generalized lymphadenopathy, fetal **hydrops** (abnormal fluid accumulation), fever, myocarditis, pneumonia, limb pain that results in limited movement, sepsis, lack of eyebrows, glaucoma, cataracts, uveitis, rectal bleeding, NEC, malabsorption, and renal complications (Lago et al., 2013). CNS manifestations may occur anytime in the first year and may present as meningitis, pituitary dysfunction, neurodevelopmental regression, or other. CNS involvement may also be asymptomatic.

Prognosis

A small percentage of infants diagnosed with congenital syphilis do not survive even with treatment. Even despite adequate treatment, some infants and older children will develop persistent keratitis and skeletal abnormalities because of inflammation and scarring that occurred prior to successful treatment.

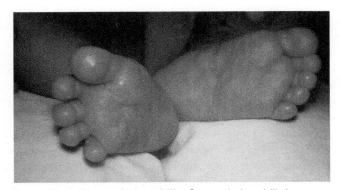

Figure 25.5. Congenital syphilis. Congenital syphilis has many manifestations, including pigmented lesions on the soles, as seen in this infant. (Reprinted with permission from Fleisher, G. R., Ludwig, S., & Baskin, M. N. [2004]. *Atlas of pediatric emergency medicine* [1st ed., Fig. 14.24]. Philadelphia, PA: Lippincott Williams & Wilkins.)

Manifestations of congenital syphilis that start 2 or more years after birth are referred to as late and may occur in infants born to mothers who were not treated in pregnancy and who were not treated themselves within 3 months of birth. Clinical manifestations may be of the facial features, eyes, ears, oropharynx, skin, mucous membranes, brain, skeleton, or blood.

Assessment

A blood test may reveal the presence of the causative bacteria, anemia, thrombocytopenia, and either a low or high white blood cell count. An evaluation of the cerebrospinal fluid (CSF) may be ordered to identify the causative bacteria and to assess the levels of white blood cells and protein. Chest X-rays may be ordered to identify pneumonia (Workowski & Bolan, 2015).

Treatment

Syphilis is treated with penicillin G. The route and dosing of the medication depend on the results of the blood work, long-bone imaging, and lumbar puncture. The infant is followed with an antibody titer every 2 to 3 months. Additional treatment with antibiotics may be indicated.

Gonorrhea

Ophthalmia neonatorum (newborn conjunctivitis) caused by *Neisseria gonorrhoeae* was once the leading cause of blindness. It is a primary reason that newborns are treated routinely with an antibiotic eye ointment (usually erythromycin or tetracycline) at the time of birth.

Prevalence

In developed countries, the incidence of gonorrhea in pregnancy is rare, with transmission to the neonate occurring in approximately a third of cases. Coinfection with *Chlamydia trachomatis* is common (Workowski & Bolan, 2015).

Etiology

Infection of the neonate typically happens at the time of delivery, although it may happen at any point after the rupture of membranes. The bacterium does not pass the placenta, although a maternal infection increases the risk for preterm birth (Workowski & Bolan, 2015).

Signs and Symptoms

The most common site of infection is the eye of the neonate, ophthalmia neonatorum. The conjunctivitis manifests 2 to 5 days after birth as profuse exudate and eyelid swelling.

Prognosis

Left untreated, scarring of the structures of the eye and permanent visual impairment can result.

Assessment

The cause can be diagnosed by a culture of the exudate.

Treatment

Presumptive treatment with antibiotics, particularly a single dose of ceftriaxone or cefotaxime IV or IM, is typically curative. Infants are also treated if the mother carries the diagnosis and was not adequately treated. Occasionally, alternate infection sites may be identified, including the mucosa. The infection may disseminate to the blood, joints, or CSF if left untreated (Workowski & Bolan, 2015).

Chlamydia

Chlamydia is the most common sexually transmitted bacterial infection in the United States.

Prevalence

The occurrence rate in pregnancy is as low as 2% and as high as 20% depending on the population evaluated. The rate of transmission to the neonate born vaginally to an infected mother is from 50% to 70%. Conjunctivitis and pneumonia are the most common manifestations (American Academy of Pediatrics, 2015b).

Etiology

As with gonorrhea, transmission of chlamydia to the neonate occurs during a vaginal birth, although there are some case reports of transmission to infants born by cesarean section with or without rupture of membranes, suggesting the causative bacterium, *C. trachomatis*, may pass the membranes or placenta.

Signs and Symptoms

The conjunctivitis of chlamydia normally manifests from 5 to 14 days after the delivery and appears as swelling and discharge.

Prognosis

Treatment typically results in healing without complications. An infection left untreated can cause scarring of the cornea and conjunctiva, leading to vision deficits.

Approximately half of infants who develop pneumonia because of *C. trachomatis* have a history of conjunctivitis. The pneumonia usually appears later, from 4 to 12 weeks postpartum. There is often no fever with the pneumonia.

Assessment

Diagnosis is by culture or nucleic acid amplification tests. Infants under a month of age who develop conjunctivitis, as well as infants under 3 months of age who develop pneumonia, should be tested.

Treatment

Oral treatment with azithromycin daily for 3 days is the preferred treatment and is usually effective for eradicating the infection. In a minority of patients, additional dosing with erythromycin may be indicated (Workowski & Bolan, 2015).

Herpes

Prevalence

Infection of the neonate with the HSV occurs in up to 1 out of every 3,200 births and accounts for 0.6% of neonatal death in the hospital (Flagg & Weinstock, 2011).

Etiology

It is most common for neonates with HSV to have been exposed perinatally from the genital tract of the mother at the time of delivery, although women with a history of HSV outbreaks are typically instructed to take acyclovir from 36 weeks on to suppress outbreaks and viral shedding. About 10% of cases are acquired postnatally from a caregiver with an active lesion (as with herpes labialis—a cold sore). Only 1 out of every 250,000 live births is thought to involve an intrauterine transmission of HSV (Marquez, Levy, Munoz, & Palazzi, 2011).

When the HSV infection is intrauterine, it is usually a result of a primary infection of the mother during pregnancy. Perinatal infections are due to active shedding of the HSV virus during labor and delivery. A longer duration of rupture of membranes, use of fetal scalp monitor, active outbreak, and maternal fever are all risk factors for transmission.

Signs and Symptoms

Neonatal HSV is categorized as localized to the skin, eye, and mouth (SEM); CNS involvement with or without SEM; or disseminated disease.

Nearly half of neonatal HSV presents as SEM, typically within the first 2 to 6 weeks of birth (Jones, Raynes-Greenow, & Isaacs, 2014). The usual skin manifestations are clustered vesicles, most commonly over the presenting part. An affected eye may appear red and excessively watery, with or without surrounding skin vesicles. Ulcerative lesions may appear anywhere on the mucosa. Neonates must undergo evaluation for CNS and disseminated disease.

Neonatal HSV CNS disease may occur independently, with SEM, or with disseminated disease, usually within the first 2 to 6 weeks of the birth. Manifestations include seizures, irritability, lethargy, tremors, temperature instability, a bulging anterior fontanel, and/or poor feeding, similar to what is seen with other causes of meningitis. Without the presence of SEM or CSF studies that include HSV testing, the disease may not be recognized.

Approximately a quarter of infants with neonatal HSV develop disseminated disease. Like HSV CNS, disseminate disease may be difficult to recognize without SEM manifestations. Affected organs can include the liver, lungs, CNS, heart, adrenal glands, bone marrow, kidneys, gastrointestinal tract, skin, and mucous membranes. Clinical signs usually appear within the first week and include temperature dysregulation, respiratory distress and apnea, lethargy and irritability, abdominal distention, ascites, and an enlarged liver.

Prognosis

Intrauterine HSV infection is associated with damage to the placenta and umbilical cord as well as hydrops fetalis and fetal demise. Infants who survive may have severe CNS damage, damage to the eyes, pneumonitis, and skin vesicles, ulcerations, and scarring.

If caught early, neonatal HSV limited to SEM has a favorable prognosis. Death in the first year of life is rare with SEM. Treated infants have a 4% mortality rate in the first year and a 30% chance of normal neurologic development. Recurrence of SEM occurs in most children and is a lifelong risk. Long-term suppressive therapy with acyclovir reduces risk (Cantey et al., 2012).

The mortality rate for infants with disseminated neonatal HSV disease who are treated is close to 30%. If left untreated due to a clinical assumption of bacterial sepsis, however, disseminated disease is associated with a higher mortality rate (Cantey et al., 2012).

Assessment

HSV may be diagnosed by testing samples of lesions, CSF, blood, or plasma. Additional testing may include a complete blood count with differential and platelet count, and liver and kidney function tests. An electroencephalogram is a sensitive test for detecting HSV CNS disease. All infants diagnosed with HSV should have an ophthalmologic evaluation and neuroimaging (American Academy of Pediatrics, 2015d).

Treatment

The antiviral medication acyclovir by IV is used to treat all forms of neonatal HSV. The use of acyclovir stops disease progression of HSV to CNS and disseminated involvement and reduces the mortality rate. A typical acyclovir dosing is 60 mg/kg/d in a divided dose every 8 hours. Therapy is continued for 14 days for SEM and for 21 days with CNS and disseminated disease. Renal and neutrophil monitoring is done regularly during therapy. Nurses should be aware that infiltration of acyclovir into the soft tissue can cause extensive damage. Careful maintenance of the infusion site is critical. After the initial treatment, neonates are given acyclovir at a suppressive dose three times daily for 6 months to reduce recurrences and improve neurologic outcomes. In the case of ocular involvement, a topical ophthalmic solution may be used in addition to systemic therapy.

Toxoplasmosis

Toxoplasma gondii is a common protozoan parasite that rarely causes symptoms in a mature, immunocompetent host.

Prevalence

In the United States, the rate of congenital toxoplasmosis is approximately 0.5 in 10,000 live births (Peyron et al., 2017).

Etiology

Pregnant women may come in contact with *T. gondii* via cat feces, contaminated soil, and the ingestion of undercooked meat. *T. gondii* passes the placenta most frequently if the first maternal exposure to the pathogen is during pregnancy. Rarely, the disease may be reactivated from an earlier exposure if the woman is immunocompromised.

Signs and Symptoms

Clinically significant toxoplasmosis is identified, in 10% to 30% of infected infants at birth. Manifestations may include inflammation of the retina, CSF abnormalities, anemia, seizure activity, calcifications of the brain, jaundice, fever, enlargement of the spleen or liver, lymphadenopathy, lung inflammation, hydrocephalus, vomiting, rash, bleeding, thrombocytopenia, abnormally small eyeballs, and/or an increase of the eosinophil count (American Academy of Pediatrics, 2015e).

Prognosis

The risk to the fetus depends on the gestation of the pregnancy at the time of maternal infection. Generally, the more progressed the pregnancy, the lower the severity of the disease in the fetus. An untreated infection in early pregnancy can lead to fetal demise, or severe ophthalmologic or neurologic consequences. Infection from the second trimester onward results in subclinical or milder disease.

Newborns who had little or no evidence of disease at birth are still at risk for late manifestations if left untreated. By far the most common late manifestation is chorioretinitis, an inflammation of the eye that can lead to vision loss. Other potential late complications of the infection include intellectual disability, loss of hearing and vision, motor deficits, seizures, microcephaly, and hydrocephalus and abnormalities of growth and development. Although the prognosis is good for infants who are treated, caregivers should be aware that *T. gondii* cannot be effectively eradicated from the eye and CNS. Late relapses are not uncommon and may manifest as retinal or neurologic complications (Wallon et al., 2014).

Assessment

The diagnosis of toxoplasmosis can be made by blood test. Blood testing can be complicated and will need to be repeated in the event of equivocal results. Other initial testing may include CSF evaluation, a complete blood count with differential and platelet count, liver and kidney function tests, antibody testing, and urine testing.

Treatment

Infants are generally treated with a combination of pyrimethamine, sulfadiazine, and folinic acid for 1 to 2 years. Folinic acid helps counteract the toxicity of pyrimethamine. The main side effect of the pyrimethamine is neutropenia, which may require a decrease of the dose of pyrimethamine or an increase in the dose of folinic acid. A complete blood count is monitored regularly throughout treatment. Serum follow-up is performed regularly to isolate the pathogen for the first 18 months, and clinical follow-up with routine neurologic and ophthalmologic exams is done throughout childhood. A glucocorticoid may also be administered if the inflammation of the retina threatens the vision of the infant.

Hepatitis B

Hepatitis B infection of the neonate occurs because of perinatal exposure. The use of an antiviral such as tenofovir disoproxil fumarate can greatly reduce the risk of transmission of the virus to the neonate (Terrault et al., 2016). After the birth, newborns who test positive for HBsAG should receive the first dose of the three-dose hepatitis B vaccine series and a dose of the HBIG within 12 hours of birth for passive-active immunization. This use of active–passive immunization can reduce transmission by 95%. Without this prophylaxis, the risk for infection is up to 90% (Schillie et al., 2015).

Neonates rarely show signs of disease. Elevated liver enzymes may be detected in the first 6 months after birth, and some infants will develop acute hepatitis. Most infants not treated with active–passive immunization will develop a chronic infection that can lead to cirrhosis and liver cancer. Maternal hepatitis B is not a contraindication to breastfeeding.

Human Immunodeficiency Virus

Etiology

Approximately two thirds of cases of mother-to-child transmission occur intrapartum (Burgard et al., 2012). Women with a HIV RNA plasma load of 1,000 copies/mL who are taking antiretroviral treatment (ART) are at a low risk for transmitting the virus at the time of delivery, regardless of the method of delivery or the duration of membrane rupture. Women with a higher viral load, however, are at a higher risk of transmitting the virus to the newborn. Obstetric providers in this case may recommend a cesarean delivery at 38 weeks to reduce transmission risk. Women should continue taking their ART medications through labor and delivery. In general, fetal exposure to maternal fluids, including blood, is minimized intrapartum, and monitoring with fetal scalp electrode is avoided when possible.

Prognosis

When treated, the mortality rate for children infected with the HIV virus is under 1 per 100 (Mirani et al., 2015). Without treatment, about half of children with congenital HIV die within 2 years after birth (Joint United Nations Programme on HIV and AIDS, 2016).

Without treatment, the HIV virus causes progressive immunosuppression, leaving patients open to opportunistic infections. AIDS is defined as either a CD4$^+$ T cell count below 200 cells/μL or the occurrence of specific diseases associated with HIV infection. Besides *Pneumocystis carinii* pneumonia (also referred to as *Pneumocystis jirovecii* pneumonia), oral candidiasis, failure to thrive, developmental delay, hepatosplenomegaly, and lymphadenopathy are common manifestations of HIV infection infants, particularly those who are not undergoing ART. In addition to *P. carinii* pneumonia, other opportunistic infections associated with HIV in children include recurrent bacterial infections, extra-ocular cytomegalovirus, disseminated nontuberculous mycobacterium, esophageal candidiasis, and HSV.

Children may also develop wasting syndrome, which can impact normal growth and development and is associated with a high risk for disease progression, and HIV encephalopathy, which causes developmental and cognitive disorders. The course of the disease may be rapid, with clinical manifestations and severe immune compromise happening in the first year. The more common slower course develops over 5 to 6 years or more.

Long-term morbidities for those undergoing ART may be attributed to the disease, the treatment, or the strain of living with a chronic and possibly terminal condition. These morbidities include anxiety and mood disorders, substance abuse, dyslipidemia, cardiomyopathy, atherosclerosis, insulin resistance, diabetes, decreased mineral density, and renal disease (Berti et al., 2015; Fortuny et al., 2015).

Assessment

The tests used to detect HIV in the wider population isolate antibodies. In infants, the maternal antibodies may persist, although the child is not in fact infected. Different testing is required to isolate the viral components.

DNA PCR testing of the infant is 55% accurate at the time of birth, 90% accurate at 2 to 4 weeks, and 100% accurate by 6 months (Burgard et al., 2012). RNA testing is likely equally sensitive and specific and may be better for detecting the virus at the time of birth. Testing is generally recommended between 2 and 3 weeks of age, at 1 to 2 months, and then again at 4 to 6 months. Confirmatory testing is required for diagnosis. Infants of mothers who did not receive appropriate ART or who were diagnosed acutely during pregnancy should be tested at birth and in accordance with the schedule detailed for lower risk infants. Some experts recommend follow-up antibody testing at 12 to 18 months as a majority of neonates will clear the maternal antibodies within 10 months or birth (Kourtis, King, Nelson, Jamieson, & van der Horst, 2015; Panel on Antiretroviral Therapy and Medical Management of HIV-Infected Children, 2017).

Treatment

In high-resource settings, optimal treatment to minimize transmission of the HIV virus from the mother to the neonate includes ART during pregnancy and intrapartum for the mother and then postpartum for the infant. ART reduces the risk of transmission of HIV as well as suppressing HIV RNA and thus reducing HIV-related complications. Breastfeeding by mothers who are HIV positive is contraindicated in high-resource settings because of the risk of virus transmission to the infant. In low-resource settings with limited access to formula and clean water, breastfeeding improves infant survival and is not contraindicated.

Many newly pregnancy women will already be taking ART. For those who are not, early initiation of treatment is associated with superior viral suppression and a reduced likelihood of transmission. Women who are receiving ART prior to conception have a 0.2% chance of transmission to offspring, and a 0.4% chance of transmission if ART is started in the first trimester. The risk rises to 0.9% if ART is not started until the second trimester and 2.2% if ART is started in the third trimester (Mandelbrot et al.,

2015). Some women may choose to delay ART, however, until after the first trimester when the risk of teratogenic effects of the medication is highest.

Infant ART prophylaxis is begun within the first 6 to 12 hours after birth. Infants born to mothers with an HIV RNA load of 1,000 copies/mL or less may require only a 4- to 6-week course of zidovudine. The infants of mothers with less viral suppression or who did not receive ART during pregnancy or only received it near the time of delivery will likely be given nevirapine and/or lamivudine as well. The additional two drugs may be discontinued after 2 weeks, with only the zidovudine continued for the full 6 weeks. Infants who are at risk for HIV are treated with trimethoprim-sulfamethoxazole prophylactically because the risk for *P. carinii* pneumonia, a complication of HIV, is so common in this population. The medication may be discontinued if and when the child is found clear of HIV infection.

Cytomegalovirus

Congenital cytomegalovirus (CMV) is the leading cause of nonhereditary sensorineural hearing loss and is responsible for a range of other long-term neurodevelopmental disabilities. Infants are classified as asymptomatic or symptomatic with a failed hearing screen.

Prevalence

Approximately 40,000 infants (0.6% of all live births) in the United States are infected by congenital CMV (Manicklal, Emery, Lazzarotto, Boppana, & Gupta, 2013).

Etiology

CMV is a herpes virus, and like other herpes viruses, it has periods of latency and reactivation. CMV infection of the mother is exceedingly common and offspring have approximately a 1% to 5% chance of contracting the infection. Most infections of the mother and the infant are, however, asymptomatic. Approximately half of women of childbearing age in developed countries have acquired the virus. In such countries, the main risk for infection is frequent contact with children under the age of 3. If the virus is contracted during pregnancy, the chance of vertical transmission to the fetus is almost 40% in the first trimester and 65% in the third trimester. Women may also pass the virus onto the fetus with reactivation of the latent virus as may happen with immunocompromise, or during reinfection from a different strain. The chance of transmission in the case of a previously existing infection is under 2% (Manicklal et al., 2013; Picone et al., 2013).

Signs and Symptoms

Approximately 90% of infants infected congenitally are asymptomatic. The remaining infected infants may experience sensorineural hearing loss, ocular abnormalities that rarely threaten vision, and/or mild abnormalities of neural imaging. These infants are born on average at a slightly earlier gestation and are of lower birth weight (Goderis et al., 2014). In some cases hearing loss may be delayed. Hearing loss may be in one or both ears and may

be progressive or may fluctuate through adolescence. Of infants who fail the universal newborn hearing screening program, 6% have congenital CMV. As many as 20% of children with hearing loss can attribute that loss to the virus (Goderis et al., 2014).

Other findings with neonatal CMV may include petechiae, jaundice at birth, hepatosplenomegaly, SGA, microcephaly, lethargy, hypotonia, poor suck, chorioretinitis, seizures, hemolytic anemia, and/or pneumonia (Fig. 25.6; Dreher et al., 2014). Chorioretinitis is correlated with poor neurodevelopmental outcomes (Ghekiere et al., 2012).

Prognosis

As many as 10% of infants with symptomatic congenital CMV infection will have life-threatening disease, and approximately 4% to 8% will die in the first year. The cause of death is generally severe end organ damage or hemophagocytic disease (a syndrome of excessive immune response). Survivors of such fulminant disease typically have long-term neurologic impairment (Lopez, Ortega-Sanchez, & Bialek, 2014). Long-term outcomes may include hearing loss, intellectual disability, cerebral palsy, seizures, eye disease, dental disease, and liver disease.

Assessment

Infants who are SGA, or who have microcephaly, thrombocytopenia, hepatosplenomegaly, jaundice at birth, a compromised immune system, hearing loss, neuroimaging consistent with CMV, an ultrasound in pregnancy consistent with CMV, or a mother with known or suspected CMV infection in pregnancy should be tested for the virus. Testing may be done from samples of urine or saliva within the first 3 weeks of life (a positive result after 3 weeks may indicate infection after the birth. Postnatal infection is typically benign). If in utero testing is desired, the sample may be taken from the amniotic fluid or cord blood.

After diagnosis, common assessment includes a complete physical exam, a complete blood count with differential and platelet count, coagulation studies, liver function test, hearing function test, hearing test, evaluation by ophthalmology, and neuroimaging.

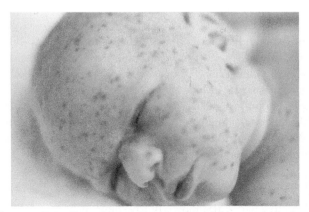

Figure 25.6. Petechiae associated with congenital cytomegalovirus infection. (Reprinted with permission from Stocker, J. T., Dehner, L. P., & Husain, A. N. [2011]. *Stocker and Dehner's pediatric pathology* [3rd ed., Fig. 6.2B]. Philadelphia, PA: Lippincott Williams & Wilkins.)

Treatment

The first-line treatment for symptomatic neonates is IV ganciclovir or valganciclovir, antiviral medications. Antiviral medications have not been found effective for reducing perinatal transmission, nor do they significantly improve hearing outcomes for newborns who pass their newborn hearing screening (Kimberlin et al., 2015). Mild-to-moderate neutropenia is a common side effect with the use of these medications (Kimberlin et al., 2015). Thrombocytopenia, liver toxicity, and renal toxicity are also possible. As with acyclovir, the IV site should be carefully managed as extravasation can result in soft tissue damage and scarring. The treatment duration is up to 6 months for life-threatening disease.

Rubella

The term "congenital rubella syndrome" (CRS) refers to birth defects that result from exposure to the rubella virus in utero.

Prevalence

CRS is rare in countries with high immunization rates. Today, in the United States only a few cases are reported annually, and these cases typically arise from mothers born in countries with less robust immunization programs (McLean et al., 2013). In 2015, Rubella was declared to have been eliminated in the Americas. Globally, reported (Eurosurveillance Editorial Team, 2015) cases of rubella declined by 95% between 2000 and 2014.

Etiology

Maternal-fetal transmission generally occurs 5 to 7 days after the mother is infected. The virus infects to placenta, damaging blood vessels and causing ischemia. Clinical manifestations vary according to the gestational age at time of infection. The highest risk time for infection is the first 10 weeks. The classic triad of CRS is cardiac disease, cataracts, and deafness, although rubella can impact almost every organ system. The infection is chronic, and manifestations of the virus may appear throughout the life span.

Signs and Symptoms

A congenital rubella infection is subclinical for a majority of neonates, although most will develop clinical manifestations within the first 5 years of life. For neonates that present with disease, manifestations may include growth restriction, large anterior fontanelle, hearing loss, cataracts, glaucoma, retinopathy, pneumonia, cardiac defects, jaundice, hepatitis, hepatosplenomegaly, bone lesions, petechiae (blueberry muffin rash; Fig. 25.7), hemolytic anemia, and thrombocytopenia.

Prognosis

Of children with CRS, most will have permanent deafness and heart disease. The most common heart defects in this population are PDA and pulmonary artery stenosis, although other associated defects have been reported. Cataracts are the most common ocular manifestation, with glaucoma occurring less frequently. Microcephaly is the most common CNS abnormality, although

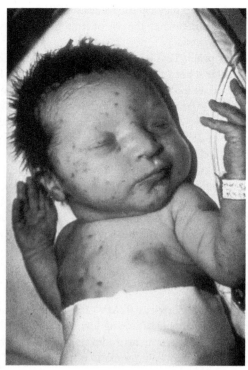

Figure 25.7. Congenital rubella. Blueberry muffin rash of congenital rubella. (Photo courtesy of the Centers for Disease Control and Prevention.)

intellectual disability, behavioral and psychiatric disorders, autism, and motor delay have also been reported. These and other manifestations may occur after the neonatal period.

Assessment

Infection should be suspected in any infant born to a mother with documented or suspected rubella infection in pregnancy and in any infant with clinical manifestations consistent with infection, including hearing loss. The virus can be isolated from nasopharyngeal secretions, blood, urine, or CSF in children under a year old.

Care Considerations

Confirmed cases must be reported to the Centers for Disease Control and Prevention.

Varicella

Like HSV and CMV, varicella is a member of the herpesvirus family. It is the virus responsible for chickenpox and herpes zoster (shingles).

Etiology

Neonatal varicella is different from congenital varicella syndrome. Neonatal varicella is most often found in infants whose mothers were exposed to varicella or exhibited symptoms of chickenpox or shingles in the final 2 weeks of pregnancy. Congenital varicella is rare and results from exposure earlier in pregnancy. The neonate may also acquire the virus postnatally, although this tends to be milder.

Signs and Symptoms

Congenital varicella syndrome may cause skin lesions, ocular defections, limb abnormalities, and CNS abnormalities that include intellectual disability and seizures.

The signs of neonatal varicella may be mild as with chicken-pox, with lesions that resolve within 10 days. Alternatively, the more dangerous disseminated form of the infection can include pneumonia, hepatitis, and meningoencephalitis.

Prognosis

Neonatal varicella is particularly dangerous to the neonate if the symptoms of infection occur within 5 days of delivery. The risk may be somewhat mitigated by the administration of varicella-zoster immune globulin to the infant within a day of the birth.

Assessment

The diagnosis is usually made clinically on the basis of the lesions (Fig. 25.8). Cultures can take several weeks to grow. PCR testing from cultures of lesions and fluid can also be helpful diagnostically (American Academy of Pediatrics, 2015f).

Treatment

As with HSV, acyclovir can help mitigate the course of severe disease and should be started as soon as possible after symptom onset. Fevers are rare with neonatal varicella infection. Breast-feeding is not contraindicated and may provide protection from the virus via maternal antibodies.

Care Considerations

Mothers and infants with active disease must be isolated. If the mother's active disease resolved 21 days prior to delivery, she does not need to be isolated, although her infant should not come in contact with other infants. If the mother was exposed 6 to 21 days prior to delivery, she and her infant should be isolated from other patients. If exposure was 6 or fewer days prior to delivery, isolation is not necessary as this would be too early in the disease course for varicella to manifest.

Candidiasis

Candida albicans is the third most common cause of late onset neonatal sepsis (occurring after the first 72 hours of life), although other *Candida* species are also responsible for infections of the neonate.

Etiology

Candida infections are most common in ELBW and VLBW infants. The bloodstream is the most common site for a *Candida* infection, but the meningitis, urinary tract, and other infections are possible. The infection may be primary or secondary to a bacterial infection. *Candida* may be transferred from the mother or from hospital staff or the environment.

Signs and Symptoms

Candida infections of the neonate can be broken into four categories: mucocutaneous candidiasis, which includes diaper dermatitis and oral thrush (Fig. 25.9); systemic candidiasis that progresses from a localized infection to a disseminated infection; catheter-related infections that do not disseminate to multiple organs; and invasive focal infections such as meningitis, peritonitis, and infections of the urinary tract (Hundalani & Pammi, 2013).

Prognosis

Asymptomatic colonization by *Candida* of the skin, the lower genital tract, and the gastrointestinal tract is exceedingly common and can be localized in most new mothers. At birth, the

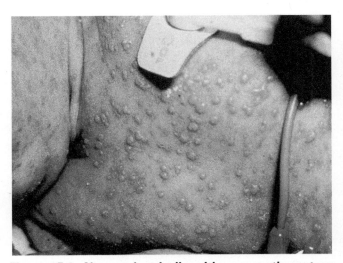

Figure 25.8. Neonatal varicella with very erythematous vesicles on the chest and more crusts on the face. (Reprinted with permission from Burkhart, C., Morrell, D., Goldsmith, L. A., Papier, A., Green, B., Dasher, D., & Gomathy, S. [Eds.]. [2010]. *VisualDx: Essential pediatric dermatology* [1st ed., Fig. 4.265]. Philadelphia, PA: Lippincott Williams & Wilkins.)

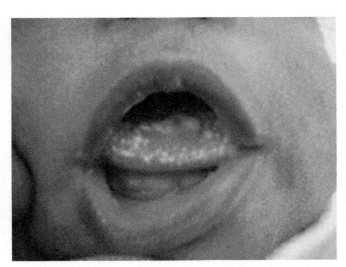

Figure 25.9. Thick white patches in the infant with oral candidiasis (thrush). (Reprinted with permission from Ricci, S. S., Kyle, T., & Carman, S. [2017]. *Maternity and pediatric nursing* [3rd ed., Fig. 42.8]. Philadelphia, PA: Lippincott Williams & Wilkins.)

neonate often becomes colonized as well. Colonization of itself is not harmful, but an invasive fungal infection resulting from colonization can be devastating. The factors that increase the risk for a colonization becoming an invasive include a compromised immune system, breakage of the skin (such as from the placement of an IV or surgery), dense colonization, and multiple colonization sites. Reported mortality rates for *Candida* infection vary but may be as high as 50% for invasive infections (Adams-Chapman et al., 2013).

Assessment

Candida can be diagnosed by culture. Multiple blood cultures may be required to achieve an accurate result. Nurses should be aware that it can take as long as 4 days to achieve culture growth and a diagnosis. In the case of oral thrush and diaper dermatitis, the diagnosis is usually clinical and culture may be necessary only in the case of treatment failure.

Treatment

Infants with a systemic infection should have any medical hardware such as IV or urinary catheters removed immediately. The most commonly used antifungal in the neonate is amphotericin B. Because there are some infections that do not respond to this medication, however, antifungal sensitivity is usually done in the lab and a different medication may be more suitable. Because of the potential adverse effects of amphotericin B, infants administered this medication are regularly assessed by complete blood count, serum potassium, magnesium, creatinine, and liver enzymes. Mucocutaneous infections can generally be treated topically. Rarely, infections that do not respond adequately to medication will require surgical intervention (American Academy of Pediatrics, 2015a).

Zika

Zika is a mosquito-borne virus that can result in severe congenital anomalies if the mother is exposed during pregnancy or prior to conception. Men are instructed to wait at least 6 months from the time of possible exposure before attempting conception, and women are instructed to wait at least 8 weeks (Petersen et al., 2016).

Etiology

Although the virus is most frequently transmitted by mosquito bite, it can also be transmitted sexually, vertically, or by blood or organ transmission. Zika outbreaks have occurred in Africa, Southeast Asia, the Pacific Islands, the Caribbean, and the Americas. In the United States, transmission has occurred in Florida and Texas (Lee et al., 2016). Maternal infection leads to infection of the placenta and transmission of the virus to the fetus.

Signs and Symptoms

The virus is associated with microcephaly, craniofacial disproportion related to microcephaly (face appears large compared

with head), cutis gyrata (wrinkling of scalp as it exceeds scull growth), craniosynostosis (premature fusion of sutures of skull), hypertonia, spasticity, seizures, hearing loss, abnormalities of the eye, irritability, hyperreflexia, SGA, cardiac anomalies, and contractures (Meneses et al., 2017). It should be noted, however, that the study of congenital Zika is still fairly new, and other common manifestations may be noted as neonates and children are studied over time (Costello et al., 2016).

Prognosis

The estimated risk of congenital anomalies in infants born to women infected with Zika ranges from 10% to 42% (Honein et al., 2017; Reynolds et al., 2017).

Assessment

Evaluation of infants with physical findings consistent with congenital Zika or born to mothers with laboratory evidence of Zika include a thorough physical exam, testing for Zika, neuroimaging, a hearing test, and additional exams as indicated by clinical presentation.

Treatment

There is no treatment specific to Zika. Supportive care is indicated to address seizures, hearing loss, spasticity, feeding difficulties, and other presenting problems. There is currently no vaccine available.

Congenital Abnormalities in the Newborn

Congenital anomalies of the newborn, which occur in approximately 3% of live births, account for approximately 20% of deaths in infancy (Osterman, Kochanek, MacDorman, Strobino, & Guyer, 2015).

Congenital Heart Disease

Heart disease is the leading cause of infant death from a congenital defect, and occurs with up to 1% of births (Liu et al., 2013). Structural cardiovascular malformations identified in neonates include transposition of the great arteries, double outlet right ventricle, ventricular septal defect, truncus arteriosus, tricuspid atresia, truncus arteriosus, Tetralogy of Fallot, atrioventricular septum defect, anomalous pulmonary venous return, coarctation of the aorta, and atrial septum defect (Oyen et al., 2016; Table 25.4). Defects may be identified by fetal echocardiography prior to birth.

Etiology

Risk factors include a family history of congenital heart disease, certain genetic syndromes, the use of assisted reproductive technology, prematurity, and certain in utero infections. Maternal conditions may increase the risk for congenital heart disease, including diabetes, obesity, hypothyroidism, hypertension,

Table 25.4 Structural Congenital Defects of the Heart

Name and Description	Image

Transposition of the great arteries: A "swap" of the aorta and the pulmonary artery. Thus, oxygen-poor blood is cycled through the body, bypassing the heart, whereas oxygen-rich blood is cycled through the lungs.

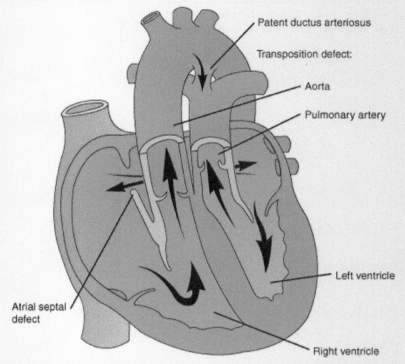

Reprinted with permission from Kline-Tilford, A. M., & Haut, C. (2016). *Lippincott certification review: Pediatric acute care nurse practitioner* (1st ed., Fig. 5.13). Philadelphia, PA: Lippincott Williams & Wilkins.

Double outlet right ventricle: Both the pulmonary artery and the aorta rise from the right ventricle. This defect has several variations and co-occurs with ventricular septal defect. LA, left atrium; RA, right atrium; LV, left ventricle; RV, right ventricle; Ao, aorta; PA, pulmonary artery; VSD, ventricular septal defect.

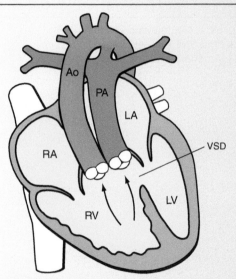

Reprinted with permission from Abuhamad, A. Z., & Chaoui, R. (2016). *A practical guide to fetal echocardiography: Normal and abnormal hearts* (1st ed., Fig. 27.1). Philadelphia, PA: Lippincott Williams & Wilkins.

(continued)

Table 25.4 Structural Congenital Defects of the Heart (continued)

Name and Description	Image

Ventricular septal defect: An opening in the wall between the left and right ventricles.

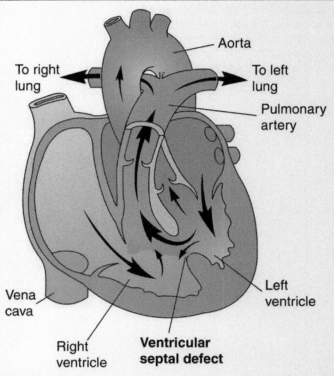

Reprinted with permission from Kline-Tilford, A. M., & Haut, C. (2016). *Lippincott certification review: Pediatric acute care nurse practitioner* (1st ed., Fig. 5.6). Philadelphia, PA: Lippincott Williams & Wilkins.

Truncus arteriosus: A single blood vessel rises out of the right and left ventricles instead of the pulmonary artery and aorta.

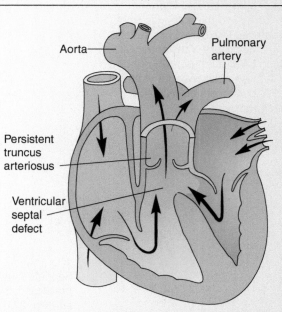

Reprinted with permission from Pillitteri, A. (2002). *Maternal and child health nursing: Care of the childbearing and childrearing family* (4th ed., Fig. 41-17). Philadelphia, PA: Lippincott Williams & Wilkins.

Table 25.4 Structural Congenital Defects of the Heart (continued)

Name and Description	Image

Tricuspid atresia: The tricuspid valve between the right atrium and the right ventricle is abnormally developed or absent. It co-occurs with atrial septal defect, ventricular septal defect, and patent ductus arteriosus.

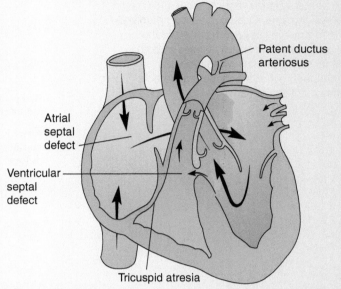

Reprinted with permission from Pillitteri, A. (2002). *Maternal and child health nursing: Care of the childbearing and childrearing family* (4th ed., Fig. 41-18). Philadelphia, PA: Lippincott Williams & Wilkins.

Tetralogy of Fallot: "Tetra" means "four." Tetralogy of Fallot combines four defects: a stenotic pulmonary artery that leads to hypertrophy of the right ventricle; ventricular septal defect, which, with hypertrophy of the right ventricle, creates a right-to-left shunt; and an aorta that overrides both ventricles, thus carrying both oxygenated and deoxygenated blood to the systemic circulation.

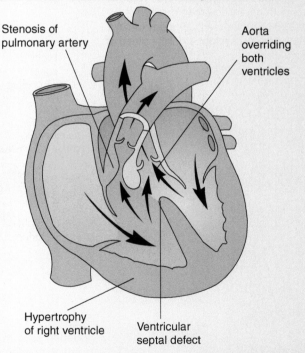

Reprinted with permission from Pillitteri, A. (2014). *Maternal and child health nursing: Care of the childbearing and childrearing family* (7th ed., Fig. 41-19). Philadelphia, PA: Lippincott Williams & Wilkins.

(continued)

Table 25.4 Structural Congenital Defects of the Heart (continued)

Name and Description	Image

Atrial septal defect: A hole in the wall between the atria. Occurs most commonly at the foramen ovale, which is part of the fetal circulation that usually closes at birth. An atrial septal defect, when it occurs independently of other congenital defects, creates a left-to-right shunt.

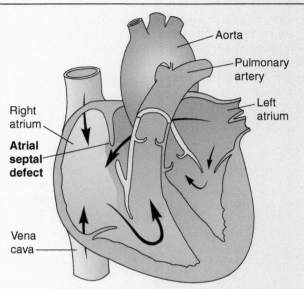

Reprinted with permission from Rosdahl, C. B., & Kowalski, M. T. (2016). *Textbook of basic nursing* (10th ed., Fig. 72.9B). Philadelphia, PA: Lippincott Williams & Wilkins.

Total anomalous pulmonary venous return: Coexists with patent foramen ovale or another atrial septal defect. Blood returns from the lungs to the right atrium instead of the left atrium.

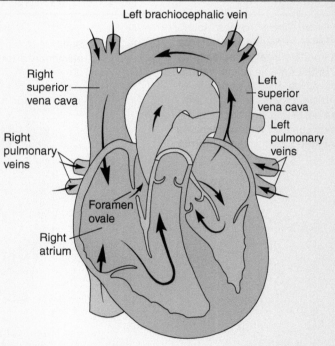

Reprinted with permission from Pillitteri, A. (2014). *Maternal and child health nursing: Care of the childbearing and childrearing family* (7th ed., Fig. 41-16). Philadelphia, PA: Lippincott Williams & Wilkins.

Table 25.4 Structural Congenital Defects of the Heart (continued)

Name and Description	Image
Atrioventricular canal defect: Incomplete fusion of the cardiac cushions between the two sides of the heart. Blood flows freely through all four chambers of the heart. As the left side of the heart is more muscular, flow is generally from left to right.	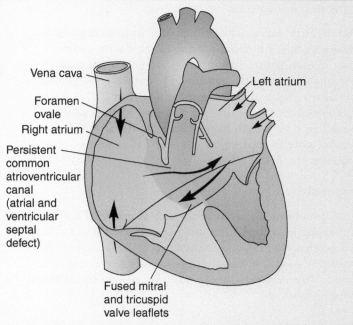 Vena cava Foramen ovale Right atrium Persistent common atrioventricular canal (atrial and ventricular septal defect) Left atrium Fused mitral and tricuspid valve leaflets Reprinted with permission from Pillitteri, A. (2014). *Maternal and child health nursing: Care of the childbearing and childrearing family* (7th ed., Fig. 41-10). Philadelphia, PA: Lippincott Williams & Wilkins.
Coarctation of the aorta: Narrowing of the aorta, usually near the site of the ductus arteriosus.	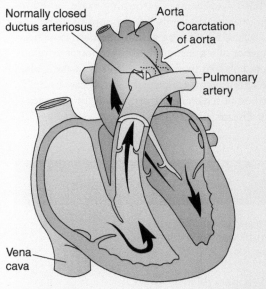 Normally closed ductus arteriosus Aorta Coarctation of aorta Pulmonary artery Vena cava Reprinted with permission from Pillitteri, A. (2014). *Maternal and child health nursing: Care of the childbearing and childrearing family* (7th ed., Fig. 41-14). Philadelphia, PA: Lippincott Williams & Wilkins.

and epilepsy. Maternal alcohol use, smoking, and the use of some medications are also associated with a higher risk for congenital heart disease.

Signs and Symptoms

After the birth, many infants will appear normal during routine assessment but will decompensate as the ductus arteriosus closes. Other infants may manifest symptoms immediately after birth. Acute early signs include cyanosis, tachypnea, pulmonary edema, and cardiogenic shock (Box 25.12). Later signs can occur after discharge and may include excessive irritability, poor weight gain, a delay in motor milestones, excessive sweating, central cyanosis or pallor, and excessive sleepiness or reduced activity.

Prognosis

Congenital heart disease is referred to as critical if surgical intervention is required in the first year. It is referred to as ductal-dependent if a PDA is necessary to maintain pulmonary and circulatory blood flow. Congenital heart disease is referred to as cyanotic if it reintroduces deoxygenated blood to the circulation, bypassing the lungs.

Assessment

Nurses should be aware that the presentation of congenital heart disease is often late and subtle and frequently missed during a routine newborn assessment. Concerning exam variations include an abnormal heart rate (below 90 bpm or above 160 consistently), a lack of S2 splitting with inspiration, extra heart sounds, the presence of a murmur, diminished lower extremity pulses, and/or an enlarged liver. Many hospitals in the United States mandate screening for congenital heart disease by SpO_2, an effective method of screening for many, but not all, types of congenital heart disease (Box 25.13).

Box 25.12   Signs of Cardiogenic Shock

- Inadequate perfusion of tissue
  - Cool extremities
  - Acrocyanosis
  - Pallor
  - Delayed capillary refill
- Abnormal heart rate
  - Tachycardia common
  - Bradycardia, late
  - Bradycardia, early (typically in preterm infants)
- Metabolic acidosis
- Lethargy, irritability, coma, hypotonia, diminished or absent reflexes
- Oliguria
- Apnea
- Hypotension (late finding)

Box 25.13   Screening for Congenital Heart Disease by Pulse Oximetry

Guidelines

- Screening should be done 24 h or more after birth.
- Blood oxygen saturation (SpO_2) should be measured from the right hand *and* either foot.

Diagnostic Criteria for a Positive Screen

- SpO_2 below 90% in either location
- SpO_2 below 95% in *both* locations in three different readings, each separated by 1 h
- A difference in SpO_2 of more than 3% between extremities in three different readings, each separated by 1 h

Adapted from Mahle, W. T., Martin, G. R., Beekman, R. H., III, & Morrow, W. R., Section on Cardiology and Cardiac Surgery Executive Committee. (2012). Endorsement of Health and Human Services recommendation for pulse oximetry screening for critical congenital heart disease. *Pediatrics, 129*(1), 190–192. doi:10.1542/peds.2011-3211.

Neurologic Abnormalities

Neural Tube Defects

NTDs include anencephaly, encephalocele, and spina bifida. Low levels of maternal folic acid in very early pregnancy and medications that are folic acids antagonists, including some antiepileptics, are the major risk factors, as is maternal diabetes. Some genetic syndromes are associated with NTDs. There is likely a yet-to-be recognized genetic component as NTDs tend to recur in families, and females are more susceptible (Ross, Mason, & Finnell, 2017). Elevation of the maternal temperature in the first trimester of pregnancy due to fever, sauna, hot tub, or other causes is a known teratogen associated with clef palate and heart disease, as well as NTDs (Dreier, Andersen, & Berg-Beckhoff, 2014). Maternal obesity significantly increases the risk of NTDs (Khoshnood et al., 2015).

The prevalence of NTDs in the United States is low, occurring in 5.3 per every 10,000 births (Zaganjor et al., 2016).

Anencephaly

Anencephaly is an open defect in which the cranial neural tube is exposed. It results from failure of the anterior neural tube to close at day-25 post conception. This failure to close results in the destruction of the brain tissue, and portions of the brain are missing, whereas other parts of the nervous system may be malformed, including the brainstem, optic nerves, spinal cord, and cerebellum. Large portions of the cranium are missing. The neonates often have some brainstem function, including spontaneous breathing and reflexes. Up to 75% are stillborn. Those who survive typically live for only a few days or weeks.

Anencephaly is routinely screened for prenatally with maternal serum alpha-fetoprotein (AFP) levels and ultrasound. Most cases of prenatal detection are followed by pregnancy termination. Other congenital malformations of various organ systems, including cardiac and skeletal, frequently coexist. There is no treatment available for anencephaly. It is considered incompatible with life. There is a small risk of recurrence if anencephaly was diagnosed with a previous pregnancy.

Encephalocele

Encephalocele is an NTD in which the brain and/or meninges protrudes through a skull defect called a cranium bifidum. The protrusion is covered with skin. Like anencephaly, it involves failure of the anterior neural tube to close. An encephalocele most commonly occurs at the back of the head at the level of the occiput and is usually overt. Sincipital encephaloceles occur in the frontal bone and may be occult or overt, causing facial deformity. Basal encephaloceles occur mid-facially. Like the sincipital encephalocele, it may be occult or cause overt midfacial deformity. Alternatively, it may cause symptoms such as impaired breathing, meningitis, nasal discharge, and related complications. The protruding tissue may be nonfunctional or include neural tissue. Other cerebral malformation and genetic syndromes are often associated with encephalocele, although it may also arise spontaneously.

As with anencephaly, routine prenatal screening maternal serum AFP levels and ultrasonography identifies a majority of cases of encephalocele. Overt diagnosis is made at the time of birth. A nonovert clinical presentation can be confirmed by computed tomography (CT) or MRI. Infants with large encephaloceles may require a cesarean delivery. Surgical correction is routine. Neurodevelopmental outcomes are dependent on the size and location of the encephalocele.

Spina Bifida

The term spina bifida refers to the incomplete closure of the vertebrae around the spinal cord. It results from failure of the spinal neural tube to close by 28 days after fertilization. The three types include spina bifida occulta, meningocele, and myelomeningocele (Fig. 25.10). The most common site for spina bifida is the lower spine, although it may occur higher as well.

Spina Bifida Occulta. Spina bifida occulta is the most benign of the three types. Although the vertebrae have not fused normally, the neural tissue is not exposed and the skin remains intact. Imaging of the spine is diagnostic. It typically affects the 5th lumbar and 1st sacral vertebrae and does not generally have any consequences or require any treatment. People with spina bifida occulta may have indications of the underlying problem in the skin over the vertebral opening, including a deep dimple or sinus, a hairy patch, a birth mark or hypopigmented spot, or a fatty lump.

The most commonly associated complication with spina bifida occulta is tethered cord syndrome (TCS). TCS involves a malattachment of the caudal spinal cord that causes stretching of the cord. This stretch can cause motor and sensory dysfunction that may present as loss of bladder control or gait abnormalities. Older children are more likely to complain of pain of the lower back, perineum, and legs. Progressive scoliosis is common (Shin et al., 2013).

Meningocele. As with spina bifida occulta, skin still covers the spinal defect of a meningocele; however, the meninges (the membrane surrounding the spinal cord) protrudes through the opening in the spine. The nervous system remains undamaged, although tethered cord may occur with this defect as well. It can typically be repaired with no long-lasting nerve damage.

Myelomeningocele. Myelomeningocele is by far the most common type of spina bifida. Both the meninges and the nerve tissue come through the opening in the spine, resulting in damage to both. Neurologic manifestations of the myelomeningocele depend on the level of the lesion, and typically involve complete paralysis and absence of sensation. In almost all cases, patients will have fecal and urinary function compromise.

Most patients will have brainstem dysfunction because of the Chiari II malformation (brain tissue extending into the spinal cord). With the Chiari II malformation, swallowing, apnea, strabismus, and stridor caused by paresis of the vocal cords is common. Often, the breathing center of the brain is compromised, causing an abnormal respiratory response to alkalosis and acidosis.

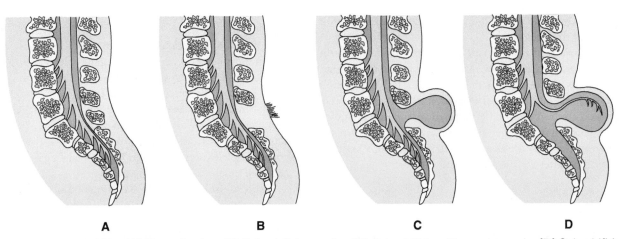

A   **B**   **C**   **D**

Figure 25.10. Spina bifida. (A) Normal spine. **(B)** Spina bifida occulta. **(C)** Spina bifida with meningocele. **(D)** Spina bifida with myelomeningocele. (Reprinted with permission from Rosdahl, C. B., & Kowalski, M. T. [2016]. *Textbook of basic nursing* [10th ed., Fig. 72.4]. Philadelphia, PA: Lippincott Williams & Wilkins.)

Hydrocephalus is also common with a Chiari II malformation (Moldenhauer et al., 2015).

In as many as 70% of cases of prenatal diagnosis of myelomeningocele, the pregnancy ends in elective or spontaneous abortion (Wilson, & SOGC Genetics Committee; Special Contributor, 2014). Fetal surgery between 18 and 25 weeks gestation is becoming an increasingly common intervention for women seeking to continue the pregnancy. Fetal surgery stops the leakage of the spinal fluid from the spina bifida, thus preventing or reversing the Chiari II malformation and is performed at a specialized fetal surgery center (Cohen et al., 2014). Surgery, however, carries a risk of preterm delivery, placental abruption, and uterine dehiscence at the surgical site.

In the case of fetuses that have not had successful intrauterine surgery, hydrocephalus leading to macrocephaly may indicate an earlier birth, although a term birth is still preferred. Immediately after the birth, an assessment is performed to determine the nature of the myelomeningocele but also to assess for common associated problems, including contractures of the lower extremities, club feet, kyphosis, and other congenital defects.

Surgical closure of the defect is performed within the first 3 days of the birth for infants who have not had an intrauterine operation. Earlier surgery and routine use of antibiotics for this population lower the risk for a CNS infection. Once the myelomeningocele has been repaired, many infants who did not have it previously will develop hydrocephalus. The head should be measured according to a regular schedule to assess for growth and the rate of growth. A shunt may be placed to drain fluid from the ventricles of the brain to the abdomen in the case of rapid growth of hydrocephalus that causes clinical instability. Baseline CT, MRI, and muscle testing is standard for all infants, so that progress or deterioration may be assessed.

Hydrocephalus

Hydrocephalus is the accumulation of CSF in the ventricles of the brain and the subarachnoid space that leads to dilation of the ventricles. The two kinds are obstructive and communicating. Obstructive hydrocephalus is due to a blockage in the ventricular system, as with the Chiari II malformation common to myelomeningocele. Communicating hydrocephalus results from impaired absorption of the CSF.

Hydrocephalus in the neonate occurs prior to fusion of the suture of the skulls, except in rare cases of premature suture closure. Because of this, increased intracranial pressure (ICP) is generally not a feature or is mild. Instead, an enlarging head circumference is the most common feature. Other physical findings, including headache, behavioral changes, developmental delay, nausea and vomiting, and lethargy are closely tied to increased ICP and thus more common after closure of the skull sutures.

Microcephaly

Infants are considered microcephalic according to the definition of a occipitofrontal circumference (OFC) that is two standard deviations below the mean for gestation, age, and sex. Microencephaly, on the other hand, is an abnormally small brain as diagnosed by neuroimaging. Microencephaly may be present without microcephaly, but microcephaly is almost always associated with microencephaly. Congenital microcephaly is present by 36 weeks gestation or at birth. Postnatal microcephaly refers to abnormally slow growth after birth. Microcephaly may be isolated or part of a syndrome or associated with other anomalies apart from a recognized syndrome.

Etiology

In a 2014 study, 29% of cases of microcephaly were caused by genetic aberrations, 27% were caused by prenatal or perinatal injury (maternal disease, exposure to a teratogen, birth injury), 2% were caused by premature fusion of skull sutures (carniosynostosis), 2% were caused by postnatal injury, and 41% were from unknown causes (von der Hagen et al., 2014). Approximately 1% to 4% of infants exposed to the Zika virus in utero will be diagnosed with microcephaly (Honein et al., 2017).

Prognosis

Of children diagnosed with microcephaly, 65% will be developmentally delayed or have an intellectual disability, and 43% will be diagnosed with epilepsy (von der Hagen et al., 2014). The prognosis is generally worse when the microcephaly is postnatal, caused by an infection, or is associated with other malformations (Deloison, Chalouhi, Bernard, Ville, & Salomon, 2012).

Assessment

Microcephaly may be diagnosed by ultrasound prior to birth or by OFC measurement after birth. Subsequent evaluation will include a thorough history and exam. Genetic studies and testing for congenital disease is often ordered. Metabolic disorders may co-occur and tests for these conditions may be ordered. Neuroimaging may be helpful for identifying the structural abnormalities of the brain.

Orofacial Cleft

An orofacial cleft is the most common craniofacial malformation and consists of a cleft lip with or without a cleft palate or a cleft palate independent of a cleft lip.

Etiology

Most of the orofacial clefts occur as part of a genetic syndrome. Maternal exposure to certain teratogenic medications such as valproate and methotrexate are also associated with orofacial clefts (Jackson, Bromley, Morrow, Irwin, & Clayton-Smith, 2016). Smoking has been associated with oral facial clefting as has maternal alcohol use in pregnancy (Butali et al., 2013). Both maternal diabetes and maternal obesity increase the risk for an orofacial cleft (Kutbi et al., 2017). Orofacial clefts are usually identified by ultrasound during pregnancy.

Failure of the lip to close by day 35 post conception produces a cleft that may split the upper lip or extend to cleft the palate or impact other facial elements, such as eyes, nose, and forehead. When just the palate is cleft, the lack of fusion of the palate occurs prior to 56 to 58 days post conception, after closure of the lip. Additional malformations are common, particularly if the cleft is midline. Affected systems include cardiovascular, skeletal, and the

CNS. Chromosomal abnormalities and malformations occurring in other systems are more common when the infant has both a cleft lip and cleft palate and rare with an isolated cleft lip or palate.

Treatment

Surgical repair for a cleft lip is usually performed at 3 months of age, and palate repair is performed at 6 months. Multiple surgeries may be required for severe malformations. Additional support may be required from specialists such as speech-language pathologists, plastic surgeons, and orthodontists. Speech difficulties are common later in life even with repair, as are dental problems.

Care Considerations

Depending on the type and degree of malformation, infants may require additional support for breathing and feeding after birth (Fig. 25.11). Infants with a cleft lip may be unable to form a seal around the nipple. With a cleft palate, infants are unable to create the suction necessary to extract milk. Some infants who have only a cleft lip may breastfeed successfully, whereas others, including those with cleft palates, can bottle-feed with the use of special nipples and devices.

Gastrointestinal Abnormalities

Gastrointestinal anomalies may be overt and immediately apparent with routine prenatal screening or at the time of birth, or they may become apparent over time. They may occur anywhere along the gastrointestinal tract, from mouth to anus.

Hypoplastic Left Colon Syndrome

Hypoplastic left colon syndrome (HLCS) is the most common cause of bowel obstruction in the neonates of diabetic mothers. Approximately half of the cases of HLCS are in this population. Maternal use of psychotropic drugs in the third trimester is also a risk factor as are other sources of neonatal stress, including preeclampsia and eclampsia. With HLCS, transit of meconium stops in the last third of the colon at or near the splenic flexure. The condition is diagnosed by contrast enema.

Patients with HLCS do not pass meconium in the first 36 hours after birth. Their abdomens become distended and they may have bilious vomiting. For a small number of infants, the colon will perforate within the first 36 hours of life, particularly if an enema is not performed within the first 24 hours of presenting symptoms. HLCS will most often resolve spontaneously.

Tracheoesophageal Fistula and Esophageal Atresia

A tracheoesophageal fistula (TEF) is an abnormal passage joining the trachea and the esophagus (Fig. 25.12). TEF almost always co-occurs with esophageal atresia (EA). The formation of the fistula is thought to derive from an error in embryonic lung formation. Approximately half of the cases of TEF and EA occur with other malformations, particularly those of the heart and the genitourinary system (Cassina et al., 2016).

Polyhydramnios occurs in most pregnancies complicated by TEF and EA. Infants will become symptomatic shortly after the birth. Symptoms include the production of excess secretions that interfere with feedings and cause choking, drooling, and respiratory distress. Depending on the morphology of the defect and the passage of air from the trachea to the esophagus, gastric distention occurs. Reflux into the esophagus, through the fistula and into the trachea, causes aspiration pneumonia. Patients with a more mild form of the malformation may have diagnosis delayed for weeks or even years, even into adulthood. For these individuals the primary sign may be recurrent pneumonia or respiratory distress with feeding. Treatment is typically surgical. Although the prognosis is usually good, some respiratory and gastrointestinal complications may be long term (Krishnan et al., 2016).

Intestinal Atresia

Intestinal atresia is complete obstruction of the lumen of the intestine caused by a congenital defect. It can occur at any point in the gastrointestinal tract, but the small intestine is affected most commonly. Regardless of the location of the obstruction, the typical symptoms of vomiting and abdominal distention usually

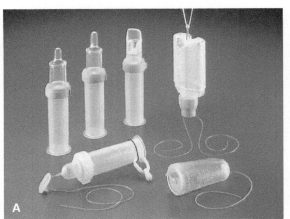

Figure 25.11. Feeding a newborn with congenital cleft lip or palate. (A) Special nipples and feeding devices. **(B)** Correct positioning for feeding. (Reprinted with permission from Evans, R. J., Brown, Y. M., & Evans, M. K. [2014]. *Canadian maternity, newborn, and women's health nursing* [2nd ed., Fig. 22.12]. Philadelphia, PA: Lippincott Williams & Wilkins.)

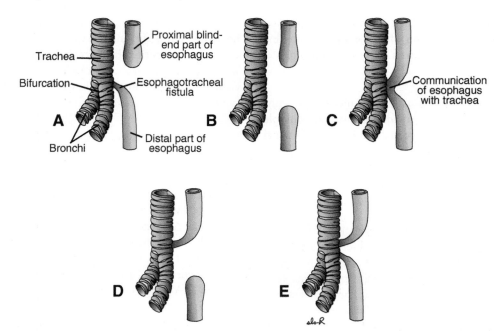

Figure 25.12. Types of tracheoesophageal anomalies. (A) The most frequent abnormality (90% of cases) occurs with the upper esophagus ending in a blind pouch and the lower segment forming a fistula with the trachea. **(B)** Isolated esophageal atresia (4% of cases). **(C)** H-type tracheoesophageal fistula (4% of cases). **(D and E)** Other variations (each 1% of cases). (Reprinted with permission from Sadler, T. W. [2003]. *Langman's medical embryology* [9th ed.]. Baltimore, MD: Lippincott Williams & Wilkins.)

occur within the first 48 hours. If the obstruction is incomplete, a diagnosis may be delayed for days or weeks. Because of the delayed or suspended passage of meconium, infants with intestinal atresia are at a higher risk for hyperbilirubinemia. Treatment is surgical.

Duodenal Atresia

Duodenal atresia is an absence or closure of part of the duodenum. Infants with duodenal atresia will often be able to pass meconium but also have gastric distension and vomiting. Vomiting usually begins within 48 hours of the birth. It is often associated with cardiac, renal, and vertebral malformations and Down syndrome.

On prenatal ultrasound, polyhydramnios may be noted, as well as dilation of the fetal stomach. After birth, the diagnosis is confirmed by X-rays performed to assess abdominal distention and vomiting. Surgery is necessary to correct duodenal atresia.

Jejunal and Ileal Atresia

Jejunal and ileal atresia has been classified into four types on the basis of the characteristics of the atresia. Type I is the least common form, and type III is the most common form (Box 25.14). Regardless of type, the cause is thought to be disruption of blood supply to parts of the fetal gut. Risk factors include maternal use of medications that cause vasoconstriction and cigarette smoking. In some cases there may be a genetic component (Chen et al., 2013; Filges et al., 2016).

As with other forms of intestinal atresia, vomiting and abdominal distention usually occur within days of birth with or without the passage of meconium. Most cases of jejunal and ileal atresia occur independently without other malformations. A form of jejunal and ileal atresia that occurs with a meconium ileus, however, is almost always due to cystic fibrosis.

Colonic Atresia

The causes and risk factors for colon atresia are believed to be the same as those for jejunal and ileal atresia (Adams & Stanton, 2014). There may be an association, however, between colonic atresia and congenital varicella syndrome. It may occur along with Hirschsprung disease, gastroschisis, skeletal abnormalities, and other intestinal atresias.

Because colonic atresia occurs in the distal bowel, symptoms may be of later onset but still typically occur within 3 days of birth. The symptoms of intestinal atresia occur with colonic atresia as well: abdominal distention, vomiting, and failure to pass meconium. Treatment is surgical.

Anorectal Malformations

Anorectal malformations include congenital defects of the anus, rectum, and genitourinary system ranging from an

---

Box 25.14 Classification of Jejunal and Ileal Atresia

- Type I: The lumen is obstructed by a membrane but remains intact; there is no external evidence of obstruction.
- Type II: The lumen of the bowel is split, and the segments are connected by a fibrous band.
- Type IIIA: Similar to Type II, but the ends are not connected.
- Type IIIB: A section of bowel is absent. The distal segment is short and takes on a spiral appearance.
- Type IV: Multiple Type II and IIIA atresias are present.

imperforate anus to a persistent cloaca. A cloaca is a single orifice that serves reproductive function and is also the terminal end of the urinary and digestive tracts (Fig. 25.13). A cloaca is a structure typically seen only in birds, fish, and monotremes. Marsupials have a version of a cloaca, although the genital tract and anus are separate. Mammals, including humans, have an embryonic cloaca that differentiates according to function: an anus for both sexes, a urethra and vagina in females, and the penile urethra in men. Failure of the cloaca to differentiate between 7 and 8 weeks post conception results in anorectal malformation.

A malformation is considered high if it occurs above the muscles of the pelvic floor and low if it occurs below the level of the pelvic floor muscles. High lesions are usually fistulas from the bowel to the bladder or perineum. Low lesions generally do not include fistulas. A high lesion with a fistulous tract may be difficult to tell from a cloaca on visual exam. Surgical intervention is necessary for optimal function. Low lesions typically have good outcomes, whereas patients with repairs of high lesions most often have persistent fecal incontinence. Other anomalies of different body systems occur in about half the cases of anorectal malformation. They are more frequently seen in infants with trisomy 21 (Down syndrome).

Hirschsprung Disease

Hirschsprung disease is a disorder of the enervation of the colon that causes a functional obstruction.

Prevalence

It occurs more often in males and is diagnosed in approximately 1 out of every 5,000 live births (Best et al., 2014).

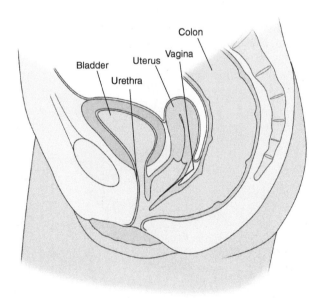

Figure 25.13. Cloaca. Cloaca is a high-level anomaly with the vagina, urethra, and rectum sharing a single perineal opening. (Reprinted with permission from Baskin, L. S. [2018]. *Handbook of pediatric urology* [3rd ed., Fig. 16.4]. Philadelphia, PA: Lippincott Williams & Wilkins.)

Etiology

The defect is believed to occur between weeks 4 and 7 of gestation (McKeown, Stamp, Hao, & Young, 2013). All or part of the colon may be affected; short-affected segments are associated with less serious disease, and longer-affected segments are associated with more serious disease. Hirschsprung disease has a strong genetic component, with at least 12 mutations identified as contributory with numerous associated genetic syndromes, including Down syndrome (Goldstein, Hofstra, & Burns, 2013). Up to a quarter of those diagnosed will also have anomalies of the kidneys, urinary tract, vision, hearing, heart, and/or anorectal malformations (Hofmann & Puri, 2013; Pini Prato et al., 2013).

Signs and Symptoms

As with intestinal atresia, most infants are diagnosed as neonates and first present with abdominal distention, vomiting of bile, and failure to pass meconium within the first 48 hour of the birth. Infants may present with enterocolitis (bowel inflammation), which looks similar to sepsis, with abdominal distention, diarrhea, vomiting, and fever.

Patients with less severe disease may not be diagnosed until later in childhood or into adulthood. Symptoms in this case often include abdominal distention and constipation that do not respond well to treatment.

Prognosis

Long-term outcomes are good, although fecal incontinence, constipation, and enterocolitis are common complications.

Assessment

Diagnosis may be confirmed by biopsy, barium enema, and imaging.

Treatment

Surgery is the mainstay of treatment, with removal of the abnormal section of bowel.

Supportive care, IV antibiotics, and rectal irrigation are helpful in such cases, and a colostomy may be required.

Omphalocele

An omphalocele is a defect of the abdominal wall. The defect is an opening at the level of the umbilical cord that contains abdominal contents. The defect is covered by the peritoneum and a membrane of amnion with Wharton's jelly between the two layers. The umbilical cord itself inserts atop the translucent sac containing the abdominal contents (Fig. 25.14).

Prevalence

An omphalocele occurs in approximately 3 out of every 10,000 pregnancies (Kirby et al., 2013).

Etiology

An omphalocele is a developmental defect that occurs between approximately the 11th and 12 postmenstrual week in utero. Pregnancies to women younger than 20 and older than 40 have about twice the risk as pregnancies to women between the ages

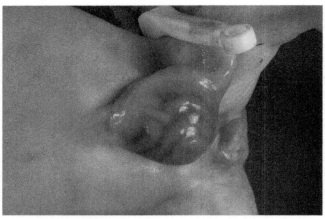

Figure 25.14. Omphalocele. A translucent membrane covers the abdominal organs, which are protruding through an abdominal wall defect in this newborn. Note the insertion of the umbilicus into the center of the omphalocele sac. (Reprinted with permission from Husain, A. N., Stocker, J. T., & Dehner, L. P. [2016]. *Stocker and Dehner's pediatric pathology* [4th ed., Fig. 14.14]. Philadelphia, PA: Lippincott Williams & Wilkins.)

of 20 and 40. Male fetuses and fetuses of multiple pregnancies are at higher risk (Marshall et al., 2015).

Prognosis

Over 80% of infants with an omphalocele will have additional structural abnormalities that are gastrointestinal, cardiac, genitourinary, orofacial clefts, and/or NTDs. SGA, polyhydramnios, and defects of the diaphragm are also more common (Fleurke-Rozema et al., 2017; Marshall et al., 2015). Several genetic syndromes are associated with omphalocele.

Over 90% of neonates born with omphalocele will survive to be discharged. Just under 10% will develop PPH, which is more common with large defects. Of those who develop PPH with omphalocele, nearly half will not survive (Corey et al., 2014).

Assessment

An omphalocele can be identified by ultrasound as early as the late first trimester of the pregnancy. Maternal serum AFP is elevated in most pregnancies complicated by omphalocele, and an increased nuchal translucency is common (see Fig. 1.5).

Because of the strong association between omphalocele and genetic abnormalities, genetic studies are commonly offered when the diagnosis is made prenatally. A fetal echocardiogram is often done because of the increased risk for cardiac malformation. Serial ultrasounds are generally done every 3 to 4 weeks to assess fetal growth. NSTs and/or BPPs are started at 32 weeks as late fetal demise is more common in this population (Deng et al., 2014).

Treatment

A spontaneous vaginal delivery is generally preferred in the absence of other complications that may indicate an early induced or cesarean delivery.

In the delivery room, the omphalocele is wrapped in a sterile dressing to prevent heat and fluid loss. The stomach is decompressed with an orogastric or nasogastric tube. A peripheral IV line is established. If the infant appears to have vascular compromise as indicated by tachycardia, cyanosis, or low blood pressure, it may be positioned on its left side. A thermoneutral environment is maintained, and the infant receives IV fluids and antibiotics per orders. Multiple surgeries may be required depending on the nature of the omphalocele.

Gastroschisis

Unlike omphalocele, gastroschisis is an abdominal wall defect that is typically associated with the bowel herniation (Fig. 25.15) with no containing overlying membrane.

Prevalence

Gastroschisis occurs in 3 or 4 out of every 10,000 pregnancies (Friedman, Ananth, Siddiq, D'Alton, & Wright, 2016). Gastroschisis is far more common in pregnancies to women under the age of 20 (Friedman et al., 2016).

Etiology

Gastroschisis typically occurs to the right of midline of the abdomen and is under 4 cm in diameter and, unlike omphalocele, the umbilical cord is adjacent but separate from the defect. Omphalocele often includes the liver, but typically only the bowel has herniated in the case of gastroschisis. Gastroschisis occurs due to a defect in the formation of the abdominal wall in the embryonic period. Gastroschisis is not associated with poor maternal nutrition, but smoking, maternal immune response, and exposure to agricultural chemicals may contribute (Shaw et al., 2014).

Prognosis

Simple gastroschisis is not associated with other issues, and complex gastroschisis is associated with intestinal abnormalities. Bowel dilation and thickening are common with the condition, likely due to prolonged exposure to amniotic fluid,

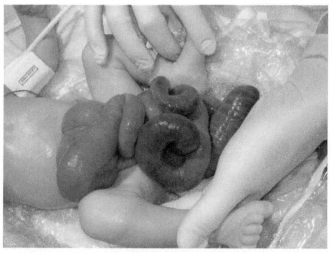

Figure 25.15. Gastroschisis with thick and matted bowel. (Reprinted with permission from MacDonald, M. G., & Seshia, M. M. K. [2016]. *Avery's neonatology* [7th ed., Fig. 41.22]. Philadelphia, PA: Lippincott Williams & Wilkins.)

but the effect of these changes on overall prognosis is unclear (Martillotti et al., 2016). Gastroschisis is not usually associated with defects in other systems. Although omphalocele is often associated with chromosomal abnormalities, gastroschisis is not, and genetic testing is generally not indicated when the condition is diagnosed.

Assessment

Gastroschisis is usually diagnosed prenatally by ultrasound. After diagnosis, ultrasounds are generally performed every 3 to 4 weeks to assess fetal growth and amniotic fluid volume, as growth restriction, oligohydramnios, and polyhydramnios are all common. At 32 weeks, a schedule of regular evaluation by NST and BPP is generally recommended (Perry et al., 2017).

Treatment

Gastroschisis is not an indication for a cesarean delivery or preterm induction in the absence of other complications. Delivery room procedures are similar to those for infants with omphalocele. The condition is treated surgically, with 70% of infants requiring one surgery and the remaining requiring multiple procedures. The overall survival rate is over 90% (Corey et al., 2014). Possible complications include adhesions and short bowel syndrome (van Manen et al., 2013).

Respiratory Abnormalities

Respiratory distress at the time of birth is most often from lung immaturity or MAS, but it may also result from a congenital lung anomaly. Common anomalies include laryngeal web, choanal atresia, congenital diaphragmatic hernia, and tracheoesophageal fistula.

Laryngomalacia

Laryngomalacia is an overly compliant larynx that collapses with inspiration. The collapse of the larynx causes a stridor that is heard on inspiration during the neonatal period and through infancy. It typically resolves between 12 and 18 months of age. The stridor is most pronounced when the infant is supine and less so when the infant is prone. The stridor is often most obvious when the infant is sleeping or feeding and less so when the infant is crying. The stridor is at its loudest with crying with a severe form of the condition, however. Many infants with laryngomalacia will also have gastric reflux, feeding difficulties, and disordered breathing while sleeping. The diagnosis can be confirmed by laryngoscopy. Although infants with a mild form of the disease generally do not require treatment, some infants with more severe disease may require surgery (Carter et al., 2016).

Tracheomalacia

Similarly, **tracheomalacia** is an overly compliant trachea that collapses with breathing. Most defects are intrathoracic, resulting in collapse of the airway during expiration. If the defect is higher, out of the thorax, collapse will happen with inspiration. It may be caused by a defect in the cartilage of the trachea, by compression of the trachea by other structures such as an enlarged heart, or

as a result of interventions such as positive pressure ventilation or by inflammation. If the tracheomalacia is within the chest, the presentation is usually a harsh cough. If the tracheomalacia is higher, the presentation is stridor. Bronchoscopy is diagnostic. Spontaneous resolution over 6 months to a year is expected, although a minority will require a tracheal stent or other surgical intervention (Hysinger & Panitch, 2016).

Laryngeal Atresia

Laryngeal atresia is a complete blockage of the larynx by cartilage or other tissue. An immediate tracheotomy at birth is imperative to infant survival. It is usually recognized by ultrasound antepartum. If it is not, the diagnosis is quickly suspected if the infant cannot breathe or cry. In some cases, an ex utero intrapartum tracheotomy is performed. This procedure is a modified cesarean section that allows for the procedure to be performed prior to the removal of the uteroplacental blood flow. Later in life airway reconstruction may be attempted (Elliott et al., 2013).

Similarly, **choanal atresia** is complete blockage of the nose and occurs in approximately 1 in 7,000 births. Choanal atresia may impact one or both nares. It may occur in isolation or with abnormalities. Unilateral choanal atresia usually presents later in life, whereas bilateral atresia is usually suspected in infancy because of noisy breathing, airway obstruction, and cyanosis that worsens with feeding and improves with crying. The inability to pass a nasogastric catheter through the nares is telling, and a CT confirms the condition. Supportive treatment with the placement of an airway and gavage feedings is necessary until the choanal atresia can be surgically corrected and the infant has recovered.

Laryngeal Webs

Laryngeal webs are a failure of the two sides of the larynx to separate. They are most often congenital but can also result from trauma, such as intubation or surgery. Approximately 10% of patients with congenital laryngeal webs have other upper respiratory abnormalities or cardiac defects. Laryngeal webs often present as respiratory distress or an abnormal cry. Laryngeal webs are treated surgically (de Trey, Lambercy, Monnier, & Sandu, 2016).

Tracheal Atresia

Tracheal atresia, unlike laryngeal atresia, is usually fatal as there is a complete or partial absence of the trachea below the larynx. It can be diagnosed by prenatal ultrasound. At the time of the birth the infant cannot cry or breathe. Tracheal atresia almost always co-occurs with other respiratory anomalies, gastrointestinal abnormalities, and congenital heart defects (Mohammed, West, Bewick, & Wickstead, 2016).

Congenital Diaphragmatic Hernia

Congenital diaphragmatic hernia is a condition in which the abdominal contents herniate through the diaphragm and into the chest.

Prevalence

This condition occurs in 1 to 4 out of every 10,000 live births. The pressure of the herniated viscera interferes with lung development, causing pulmonary hypoplasia (loss of lung mass) and pulmonary hypertension. The development of cardiac structures may be impacted by impinging visceral mass. Surfactant development may also be affected (Leeuwen & Fitzgerald, 2014).

Etiology

The hernia is typically on the left side of the diaphragm, although it may also be on the right or, rarely, bilateral. When the hernia occurs on the left, the stomach is often involved, when on the right, the liver. Regardless of the location, the bowel is involved. The severity of the disease is typically higher with right-sided liver herniation. Pulmonary changes are almost always bilateral but most pronounced on the ipsilateral (same) side.

Diaphragmatic hernia is more likely to be identified prenatally by ultrasound if it is associated with other congenital abnormalities, although up to 70% of cases are isolated with no other abnormalities detected. An underlying chromosomal syndrome is identified with a minority of cases.

Signs and Symptoms

After birth, the typical presentation of diaphragmatic hernia is respiratory distress consistent with the degree of herniation and the development of PPHN. On inspection, the infant will have a barrel-shaped chest and a depressed abdomen because of the passage of abdominal contents into the chest. The heartbeat may be displaced to the side contralateral (opposite) of the herniation as the mediastinum is shifted. Breath sounds may be diminished or absent.

Assessment

When a diaphragmatic hernia is suspected, prenatal evaluation includes an MRI to estimate the impact on lung volume, echocardiography to detect cardiac abnormalities, and genetic studies from the samples of amniotic fluid of the fetus to identify congenital abnormalities. Antepartum testing includes serial NSTs or BPPs and ultrasound examinations to assess growth and amniotic fluid volume.

Diagnosis in the neonate is by chest X-ray.

Treatment

Prenatal intrauterine repair may be attempted. Labor is often induced so the fetus may be closely monitored from the beginning. ECMO may be required for survival after delivery to maintain oxygenation.

Postnatal management includes stabilization of the neonate's blood pressure, oxygenation, and acid–base balance followed by surgical repair. When born in a care facility with ECMO capability, survivability is up to 92% (Burgos, Modee, Ost, & Frenckner, 2017).

Genitourinary Abnormalities

Hypospadias and Epispadias

Hypospadias is the malplacement of the urethra on the ventral aspect of the penis (Fig. 25.16). Epispadias is the abnormal placement of the urethra on the dorsal aspect of the penis. Urethral

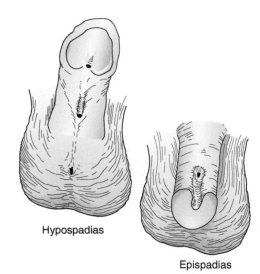

Figure 25.16. Hypospadias and epispadias. (Reprinted with permission from Porth, C. M. [2015]. *Essentials of pathophysiology: Concepts of altered health states* [4th ed., Fig. 39-13]. Philadelphia, PA: Lippincott Williams & Wilkins.)

placement may be anywhere along the glands or shaft of the penis. In the case of hypospadias, the placement may also be on the scrotum or perineum. Hypospadias occurs in approximately 1 out of every 200 male births and may occur independently or as part of a genetic syndrome (Schneuer, Holland, Pereira, Bower, & Nassar, 2015). Risk factors include maternal diabetes, advanced maternal age, preterm birth, exposure to smoking and pesticides, and placental insufficiency (van der Horst & de Wall, 2017). Epispadias is usually associated with bladder exstrophy.

Exstrophy–Epispadias Complex

Exstrophy–epispadias complex includes three different categories of anomalies: epispadias, bladder exstrophy, and cloacal exstrophy.

Prevalence

Epispadias is typically associated with exstrophy and occurs independently in only 1 out of every 200,000 to 400,000 live births. Bladder exstrophy is more common in males and is reported in 1 out of every 20,000 to 33,000 births (Reinfeldt Engberg, Mantel, Fossum, & Nordenskjold, 2016).

Etiology

Epispadias is the failure of the urethra to close, so that it lies flat and open on the dorsum of the penis. Bladder exstrophy is an "inside out" bladder that sits atop of instead of inside of the abdomen. Cloacal exstrophy includes exstrophy of both the bladder and large intestine and abnormalities of the gastrointestinal tract and genitalia (Reinfeldt Engberg et al., 2016).

Prognosis

Bladder exstrophy may be isolated or may occur with other abnormalities. Commonly associated malformations include a low-set umbilicus, pelvic malformation, hip dysplasia, anterior displacement of the anus, and inguinal hernia. Penile anomalies can include epispadias, dorsal curvature of the shaft of the penis, absence of the dorsal foreskin, exposure of the prostate gland, and foreshortening of the penis. Females too may have epispadias, as well as bifurcation of the clitoris, lateral displacement of the labia minora, and shortening of the vagina (Reinfeldt Engberg et al., 2016).

Short-term complications may include dehiscence of the bladder, urinary tract infections, bladder stone, perforation of the bladder, fistula formation, and injury to the penis. Long-term complications can include epididymitis (inflammation of the epididymis) or vaginal or rectal prolapse. The risk for bladder and colon cancer may be higher in this population.

Assessment

Diagnosis is often made prenatally by ultrasound. It is also diagnosed clinically by inspection at the time of delivery. Laboratory evaluations include a complete blood count, serum electrolytes, and renal function tests. Imaging studies evaluate the kidneys, abdomen, and pelvis.

Treatment

At the time of delivery after the routine clamping of the cord, the usual plastic clamp is replaced by a cloth ligature to minimize trauma to the adjacent bladder. The bladder itself is covered with a protective dressing and may be irrigated periodically with sterile saline.

Surgery is curative and is usually performed within days of the birth or between 6 and 12 weeks dependent on the clinical picture.

Care Considerations

Although urinary continence is achieved for most patients, some may experience poor body image as a result of the appearance of their genitalia. This can result in restricted sexual activity, anxiety, depression, and an increase in suicide and suicidal ideation (Ellison, Shnorhavorian, Willihnganz-Lawson, Grady, & Merguerian, 2016).

Ambiguous Genitalia

Conditions, including ambiguous genitalia, are often called disorders of sex development (DSD).

Prevalence

Ambiguous genitalia is identified in approximately 1 in 5,000 births, whereas atypical genitalia is recognized in 1 in 300 infants. Both are considered DSD, but whereas atypical genitalia is still consistent with male or female, ambiguous genitalia is less easily categorized (Davies & Cheetham, 2017).

Etiology

Variations may be due to genetic, hormonal, or embryonic abnormalities. Ambiguous genitalia in virilized XX and undervirilized XY infants is most often caused by congenital adrenal hyperplasia, which can lead to a life-threatening adrenal crisis.

Signs and Symptoms

Manifestations include bilateral cryptorchidism (undescended testicles), hypospadias that occurs on the scrotum or perineum, clitoromegaly (enlarged clitoris), fusion of the posterior labia, and female appearance but with palpable gonad with or without inguinal hernia. The presentation depends on the particular etiology.

Prognosis

Ambiguous genitalia resulting from congenital adrenal hyperplasia can become a life-threatening adrenal crisis and must be managed acutely. Other outcomes depend on the etiology and selected treatment.

Assessment

Initial evaluation includes a thorough history and physical, genetic evaluation, ultrasound of the abdomen and pelvis, and a hormonal study, including adrenal function. From this evaluation infants are categorized as virilized XX, undervirilized XY, or mixed sex chromosome pattern.

Urgent studies related to congenital adrenal hyperplasia include 17-hydroxyprogesterone, plasma glucose, and serum and urine electrolytes. An adrenal crisis causes salt-wasting crisis. Hypercalcemia with or without hyponatremia, metabolic acidosis, and hypoglycemia suggest this condition.

Care Considerations

Less life-threatening than adrenal hyperplasia but no less acute is the distress that can be felt by the family. The plan made for the infant will require evaluation and consultation with endocrinologists, geneticists, and surgeons potentially creating a period of intense uncertainty and complicated decision-making. Families need psychological and educational support at this time. Birth certificates can be delayed until the family, informed by their healthcare team, has determined how they intend to address their child's sex.

Guidance given to families regarding the rearing of the child as regarding their sex is based on the most probable gender identity to optimize psychosocial and psychosexual functioning. The judgment about probable gender identity is based on the specific diagnosis and degree of androgen exposure in utero as well as the potential for sexual function and fertility in adulthood.

Some etiologies of ambiguous genitalia provide a more predictable gender identity outcome, whereas others are more variable. Flexibility of the family to allow the child to identify their own gender over time may be advised. The family must be included in these discussions and the sociocultural background taken into account. Ultimately the family has the responsibility of caring for the children and making decisions about upbringing and surgery if indicated and should be supported whenever possible (Gonzalez & Ludwikowski, 2016).

Advocacy groups recommend that surgery not be performed until after the child is mature enough to confirm its own gender identity and make its own informed decision. This, however, removes the parents' choice to do what they think best for the child and requires them to raise a child of an ambiguous sex, which many might find is beyond what they can do (Diamond & Garland, 2014). There are no controlled studies comparing the advantages and disadvantages of early versus later genital surgery (Eckoldt-Wolke, 2014). Long-term management should consider medical, psychosocial, and psychosexual concerns.

Musculoskeletal Abnormalities

Hip Dysplasia

Hip dysplasia may be evident at birth or become evident during infancy and childhood. What appears initially to be hip dysplasia in the infant may simply be laxity in the hips that corrects over time. Risk factors include a breech position at or after 34 weeks gestation, a family history of hip dysplasia, oligohydramnios, female sex, first birth, and large birth weight.

Prevalence

Approximately 1% of neonates are diagnosed with hip dysplasia by clinical examination. The prevalence is two to four times as high when screening is by ultrasound rather than clinical assessment (Kolb et al., 2016).

Etiology

Hip dysplasia may occur as part of a syndrome but more often is an isolated occurrence. Variations include dislocation (no contact between acetabulum and femoral head), subluxation (only partial contact between acetabulum and femoral head), dislocatable (femoral head is within acetabulum at rest but can be dislocated), sublucable (femoral head is within acetabulum at rest but can be partially dislocated), reducable (hip is dislocated at rest but can the femoral head can be manipulated into the acetabulum), and dysplasia (abnormality in the anatomy of the joint itself, most commonly a shallow acetabulum). About a third of cases involve both hips. When only one hip is affected, it's more often the left hip.

Prognosis

Although most newborn hip stability corrects within the first year without intervention, hip dysplasia that does not correct and a lack of intervention may result in pain, osteoarthritis, and functional disability in adolescence and early adulthood. Alternatively, for women, pain may start during pregnancy or

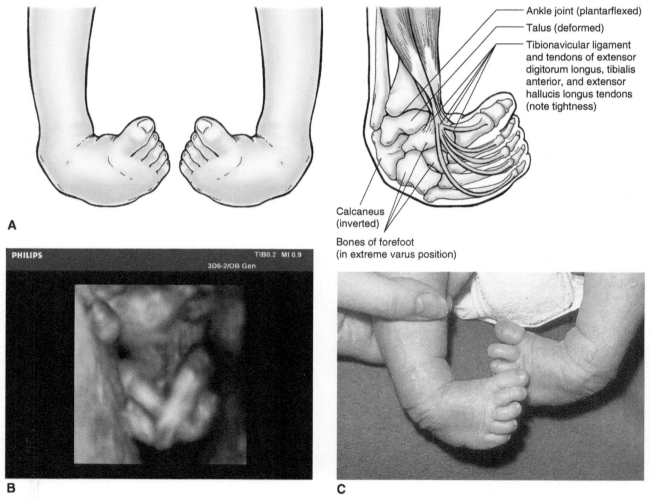

Figure 25.17. Clubfoot. (A) Artist's rendering of a clubfoot. **(B)** Three-dimensional image of a clubfoot. **(C)** Postnatal image of a fetus with bilateral clubfoot. (Reprinted with permission from Stephenson, S. R. [2015]. *Obstetrics and gynecology* [3rd ed., Fig. 23.25]. Philadelphia, PA: Lippincott Williams & Wilkins.)

menopause. Osteoarthritis presenting in the fourth through sixth decade of life is often associated with minor uncorrected hip dysplasia.

Assessment

Examinations for hip dysplasia typically start shortly after birth and continue until the child is walking independently. For infants, the exam assesses hip stability, and for older infants and children, the important factor is range of motion (Shaw & Segal, 2016). Until 4 to 6 months, ultrasound is the preferred method of imaging following an abnormal exam.

The American Academy of Orthopedic Surgeons and the United States Preventative Services Task Force recommends against universal screening of infants for hip dysplasia because of the risk for overdiagnosis and overtreatment. The Pediatric Orthopedic Society of North America advocates for regular clinical assessment for all infants until they are walking, and imaging for those with risk factors (Mulpuri, Song, Goldberg, & Sevarino, 2015; Schwend et al., 2007; U.S. Preventive Services Task Force, 2006).

Treatment

The goal of treatment is to facilitate the alignment of the acetabulum and the femoral head. Laxity and mild instability in infants younger than a month is a common finding for which routine follow-up assessments are sufficient. A hip that is dislocated or dislocatable, however, should be managed in conjunction with an orthopedic surgeon. Treatment is generally not initiated until after 4 weeks of age to allow time for spontaneous resolution (Larson, Patel, Weatherford, & Janicki, 2017).

The most common intervention when clinical correction of dysplasia is deemed necessary is a Pavlik harness, which limits adduction and extension of the hip and stabilizes it hip. Use of the harness is discontinued if the dysplasia is not corrected in the first 3 weeks of use and replaced with a rigid device that does not allow movement. Failure of both methods is an indication for surgical correction (Omeroglu, Kose, & Akceylan, 2016). Parents of children in a harness should be instructed to keep skin as clean and dry as possible to avoid skin breakdown.

Clubfoot

Clubfoot is a deformity in which the foot or feet is sharply plantar flexed with the sole facing inward (Fig. 25.17). The deformity affects all structures of the foot, including the bones, muscles, tendons, and blood vessels. Although it may be associated with chromosomal or genetic abnormalities, it is often an isolated anomaly. A positional form is associated with a restricted intrauterine environment as may occur with oligohydramnios. In this case, the clubfoot is not rigid and the foot may be easily manually reduced to a neutral position to improve spontaneously over time. In the case of a clubfoot that is not positional, the primary abnormality is a deformity of the talus. This causes joint subluxation and abnormal development of the soft tissues. The foot, calf, and leg are undersized. Management includes casting and bracing.

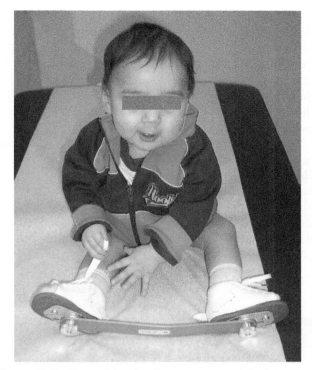

Figure 25.18. Foot-abduction brace worn at night for several years after clubfoot deformity correction using the Ponseti method. (Reprinted with permission from Mosca, V. S. [2014]. *Principles and management of pediatric foot and ankle deformities and malformations* [1st ed., Fig. 4.2]. Philadelphia, PA: Lippincott Williams & Wilkins.)

Treatment begins almost immediately after birth and involves frequent repositioning of the foot for several months followed by a program of maintenance (Fig. 25.18). The most commonly used method of correction is called the Ponseti method. Surgical intervention may be required.

Syndactyly and Polydactyly

Syndactyly is the fusion of the digits of the hands or feet and polydactyly is extra digits (Fig. 25.19). Either may occur as independent anomalies or as part of a syndrome.

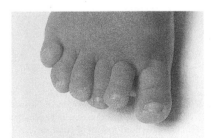

Figure 25.19. Polydactyly. An infant with trisomy 13 has supernumerary digits (polydactyly). (Reprinted with permission from Ricci, S. S. [2009]. *Essentials of maternity, newborn, & women's health nursing* [2nd ed., Fig. 10.19]. Philadelphia, PA: Lippincott Williams & Wilkins.)

Polydactyly is usually soft tissue that can be removed, although occasionally it may contain a bone or even joints. Very rarely polydactyly manifests as a complete functional digit. Because of the association with genetic syndromes, genetic testing of the newborn may be advised. In some cases, parents may elect to allow the children to make a decision about their extra digit(s) when they are mature (Samra, Bourne, Beckett, Matthew, & Thomson, 2016).

Simple syndactyly involves fusion of the soft tissues of adjacent digits, whereas complex syndactyly includes fusion of the bones (Fig. 25.20). Complex syndactyly occurs as part of a syndrome. Incomplete syndactyly does not include fusion of the tips of the digits although complete syndactyly does. Syndactyly is usually treated surgically between the ages of 6 and 24 months depending on location. Depending on the clinical picture, genetic testing may be advised.

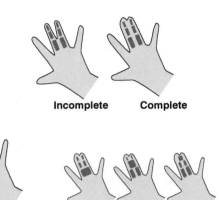

Figure 25.20. Classification of syndactyly. Syndactyly may be complete or incomplete, simple or complex. (Reprinted with permission from Staheli, L. T. [2016]. *Fundamentals of pediatric orthopedics* [5th ed., Fig. 13.119]. Philadelphia, PA: Lippincott Williams & Wilkins.)

Think Critically

1. You are caring for a family with an infant with severe hyperbilirubinemia undergoing "crash cart" phototherapy. What do you see as your nursing responsibilities to the infant's family? How would you explain the situation and facilitate bonding?

2. You are caring for an infant who is being cared for with hypothermia. How do you explain to the parent why this is an appropriate treatment for the newborn?

3. You suspect that a new mother used an illicit substance during pregnancy that is now impacting her neonate. What signs in the neonate have raised your suspicion, and for which substance? What is your next step?

4. You are caring for a newborn with neonatal abstinence syndrome. How do you include infant-specific interventions in the care of this newborn?

5. You are caring for an infant with staphylococcal scalded skin syndrome. You explain to the worried parents that the condition will not cause scarring. Why is that?

6. Look at Table 25.4. Consider each structural congenital heart anomaly and the impact it would have on the neonate's circulation. In which direction would the blood shunt? Would it change? What kind of blood is sent into the systemic circulation? Oxygenated? Deoxygenated? What are the differences in the demands on the heart due to the circulatory change?

7. You are screening a newborn for congenital heart disease. The blood oxygen saturation between sites differs by 4%. What do you do next?

8. An infant with a repaired neural tube defect is being monitored for hydrocephalus. Why is this monitoring critical at this time?

9. What is the difference between an omphalocele and gastroschisis? How do their prognoses differ?

10. You are caring for a family of an infant with ambiguous genitalia. When discussing the infant, what does therapeutic communication sound like to you?

References

Adams, S. D., & Stanton, M. P. (2014). Malrotation and intestinal atresias. *Early Human Development, 90*(12), 921–925. doi:10.1016/j.earlhumdev.2014.09.017

Adams-Chapman, I., Bann, C. M., Das, A., Goldberg, R. N., Stoll, B. J., Walsh, M. C., … Benjamin, D. K.; Human Development Neonatal Research Network. (2013). Neurodevelopmental outcome of extremely low birth weight infants with Candida infection. *Journal of Pediatrics, 163*(4), 961.e3–967.e3. doi:10.1016/j.jpeds.2013.04.034

Al-Agha, R., Firth, R. G., Byrne, M., Murray, S., Daly, S., Foley, M., … Kinsley, B. T. (2012). Outcome of pregnancy in type 1 diabetes mellitus (T1DMP): Results from combined diabetes-obstetrical clinics in Dublin in three university teaching hospitals (1995–2006). *Irish Journal of Medical Science, 181*(1), 105–109. doi:10.1007/s11845-011-0781-6

American Academy of Pediatrics. (2015a). Candidiasis. In D. W. Kimberlin (Ed.), *Red book: 2015 Report of the committee on infectious diseases* (30th ed.). Elk Grove Village, IL: Author.

American Academy of Pediatrics. (2015b). Chlamydia trachomatis. In D. W. Kimberlin (Ed.), *Red book: 2015 Report of the committee on infectious diseases.* Elk Grove Village, IL: Author.

American Academy of Pediatrics. (2015c). Group B streptococcal infections. In D. W. Kimberlin (Ed.), *Red book: 2015 Report of the committee on infectious diseases* (30th ed., pp. 745). Elk Grove Village, IL: Author.

American Academy of Pediatrics. (2015d). Herpes simplex. In D. W. Kimberlin (Ed.), *Red book: 2015 Report of the committee on infectious diseases* (pp. 432). Elk Grove Village, IL: Author.

American Academy of Pediatrics. (2015e). Toxoplasma gondii infections (Toxoplasmosis). In D. W. Kimberlin (Ed.), *Red book: 2015 Report of the committee on infectious diseases* (30th ed., pp. 787). Elk Grove Village, IL: Author.

American Academy of Pediatrics. (2015f). Varicella-zoster virus infections. In D. W. Kimberlin (Ed.), *Red book: 2015 Report of the committee on infectious diseases* (30th ed.). Elk Grove Village, IL: Author.

American Academy of Pediatrics Subcommittee on Hyperbilirubinemia. (2004). Management of hyperbilirubinemia in the newborn infant 35 or more weeks of gestation. *Pediatrics, 114*(1), 297–316.

American College of Obstetricians and Gynecologists. (2014). Executive summary: Neonatal encephalopathy and neurologic outcome, second edition. Report of the American College of Obstetricians and Gynecologists' Task Force on Neonatal Encephalopathy. *Obstetrics and Gynecology, 123*(4), 896–901. doi:10.1097/01.AOG.0000445580.65983.d2

American College of Obstetricians and Gynecologists. (2017). Committee opinion no. 722: Marijuana use during pregnancy and lactation. *Obstetrics and Gynecology, 130*(4), e205–e209. doi:10.1097/AOG .0000000000002354

Andersen, J. T., Andersen, N. L., Horwitz, H., Poulsen, H. E., & Jimenez-Solem, E. (2014). Exposure to selective serotonin reuptake inhibitors in early pregnancy and the risk of miscarriage. *Obstetrics and Gynecology, 124*(4), 655–661. doi:10.1097/AOG.0000000000000447

Awal, M. A., Lai, M. M., Azemi, G., Boashash, B., & Colditz, P. B. (2016). EEG background features that predict outcome in term neonates with hypoxic ischaemic encephalopathy: A structured review. *Clinical Neurophysiology, 127*(1), 285–296. doi:10.1016/j.clinph.2015.05.018

Bauer, T., Trump, S., Ishaque, N., Thurmann, L., Gu, L., Bauer, M., ... Lehmann, I. (2016). Environment-induced epigenetic reprogramming in genomic regulatory elements in smoking mothers and their children. *Molecular Systems Biology, 12*(3), 861. doi:10.15252/msb.20156520

Behnke, M., & Smith, V. C.; Committee on Substance Abuse; Committee on Fetus and Newborn. (2013). Prenatal substance abuse: Short- and long-term effects on the exposed fetus. *Pediatrics, 131*(3), e1009–e1024. doi:10.1542/peds.2012-3931

Bendapudi, P., Rao, G. G., & Greenough, A. (2015). Diagnosis and management of persistent pulmonary hypertension of the newborn. *Paediatric Respiratory Reviews, 16*(3), 157–161. doi:10.1016/j.prrv.2015.02.001

Berardi, A., Rossi, C., Lugli, L., Creti, R., Bacchi Reggiani, M. L., Lanari, M., ... Ferrari, F.; Gbs Prevention Working Group Emilia-Romagna. (2013). Group B streptococcus late-onset disease: 2003–2010. *Pediatrics, 131*(2), e361–e368. doi:10.1542/peds.2012-1231

Berti, E., Thorne, C., Noguera-Julian, A., Rojo, P., Galli, L., de Martino, M., & Chiappini, E. (2015). The new face of the pediatric HIV epidemic in Western countries: Demographic characteristics, morbidity and mortality of the pediatric HIV-infected population. *Pediatric Infectious Disease Journal, 34*(5 Suppl. 1), S7–S13. doi:10.1097/INF.0000000000000660

Bertrand, J., & Interventions for Children with Fetal Alcohol Spectrum Disorders Research Consortium. (2009). Interventions for children with fetal alcohol spectrum disorders (FASDs): Overview of findings for five innovative research projects. *Research in Developmental Disabilities, 30*(5), 986–1006. doi:10.1016/j.ridd.2009.02.003

Best, K. E., Addor, M. C., Arriola, L., Balku, E., Barisic, I., Bianchi, F., ... Rankin, J. (2014). Hirschsprung's disease prevalence in Europe: A register based study. *Birth Defects Research. Part A, Clinical and Molecular Teratology, 100*(9), 695–702. doi:10.1002/bdra.23269

Bharwani, S. K., Green, B. F., Pezzullo, J. C., Bharwani, S. S., Bharwani, S. S., & Dhanireddy, R. (2016). Systematic review and meta-analysis of human milk intake and retinopathy of prematurity: A significant update. *Journal of Perinatology, 36*(11), 913–920. doi:10.1038/jp.2016.98

Bhutani, V. K., & Johnson, L. (2009). A proposal to prevent severe neonatal hyperbilirubinemia and kernicterus. *J Perinatol, 29 Suppl 1*, S61–67. doi:10.1038/jp.2008.213

Billimoria, Z. C., Pandya, S., Bhatt, P., & Pandya, B. (2016). Probiotics-to use, or not to use? An updated meta-analysis. *Clinical Pediatrics, 55*(13), 1242–1244. doi:10.1177/0009922816664067

Bizzarro, M. J., Ehrenkranz, R. A., & Gallagher, P. G. (2014). Concurrent bloodstream infections in infants with necrotizing enterocolitis. *Journal of Pediatrics, 164*(1), 61–66. doi:10.1016/j.jpeds.2013.09.020

Bowen, V., Su, J., Torrone, E., Kidd, S., & Weinstock, H. (2015). Increase in incidence of congenital syphilis—United States, 2012–2014. *MMWR Morbidity and Mortality Weekly Report, 64*(44), 1241–1245. doi:10.15585/mmwr.mm6444a3

Brent, R. L., Christian, M. S., & Diener, R. M. (2011). Evaluation of the reproductive and developmental risks of caffeine. *Birth Defects Research. Part B, Developmental and Reproductive Toxicology, 92*(2), 152–187. doi:10.1002/bdrb.20288

Brooks, J. C., Fisher-Owens, S. A., Wu, Y. W., Strauss, D. J., & Newman, T. B. (2011). Evidence suggests there was not a "resurgence" of kernicterus in the 1990s. *Pediatrics, 127*(4), 672–679. doi:10.1542/peds.2010-2476

Browne, H. A., Modabbernia, A., Buxbaum, J. D., Hansen, S. N., Schendel, D. E., Parner, E. T., ... Grice, D. E. (2016). Prenatal maternal smoking and increased risk for Tourette syndrome and chronic tic disorders. *Journal of the American Academy of Child and Adolescent Psychiatry, 55*(9), 784–791. doi:10.1016/j.jaac.2016.06.010

Burgard, M., Blanche, S., Jasseron, C., Descamps, P., Allemon, M. C., Ciraru-Vigneron, N., ... Rouzioux, C.; Agence Nationale de Recherche sur le SIDA et les Hepatites virales French Perinatal Cohort. (2012). Performance of HIV-1 DNA or HIV-1 RNA tests for early diagnosis of perinatal HIV-1 infection during anti-retroviral prophylaxis. *Journal of Pediatrics, 160*(1), 60.e1–66. e1. doi:10.1016/j.jpeds.2011.06.053

Burgos, C. M., Modee, A., Ost, E., & Frenckner, B. (2017). Addressing the causes of late mortality in infants with congenital diaphragmatic hernia. *Journal of Pediatric Surgery, 52*(4), 526–529. doi:10.1016/j.jpedsurg.2016.08.028

Butali, A., Little, J., Chevrier, C., Cordier, S., Steegers-Theunissen, R., Jugessur, A., ... Mossey, P. A. (2013). Folic acid supplementation use and the MTHFR C677T polymorphism in orofacial clefts etiology: An individual participant data pooled-analysis. *Birth Defects Research. Part A, Clinical and Molecular Teratology, 97*(8), 509–514. doi:10.1002/bdra.23133

Cain, M. A., Bornick, P., & Whiteman, V. (2013). The maternal, fetal, and neonatal effects of cocaine exposure in pregnancy. *Clinical Obstetrics and Gynecology, 56*(1), 124–132. doi:10.1097/GRF.0b013e31827ae167

Cantey, J. B., Mejias, A., Wallihan, R., Doern, C., Brock, E., Salamon, D., ... Sanchez, P. J. (2012). Use of blood polymerase chain reaction testing for diagnosis of herpes simplex virus infection. *Journal of Pediatrics, 161*(2), 357–361. doi:10.1016/j.jpeds.2012.04.009

Carter, J., Rahbar, R., Brigger, M., Chan, K., Cheng, A., Daniel, S. J., ... Thompson, D. (2016). International Pediatric ORL Group (IPOG) laryngomalacia consensus recommendations. *International Journal of Pediatric Otorhinolaryngology, 86*, 256–261. doi:10.1016/j.ijporl.2016.04.007

Cassina, M., Ruol, M., Pertile, R., Midrio, P., Piffer, S., Vicenzi, V., ... Clementi, M. (2016). Prevalence, characteristics, and survival of children with esophageal atresia: A 32-year population-based study including 1,417,724 consecutive newborns. *Birth Defects Research. Part A, Clinical and Molecular Teratology, 106*(7), 542–548. doi:10.1002/bdra.23493

Centers for Disease Control and Prevention. (2016, October 18). *Appendix C. STD surveillance case definitions.* Retrieved from https://www.cdc.gov/std/stats16/appendix-c.htm

Chang, P. W., Kuzniewicz, M. W., McCulloch, C. E., & Newman, T. B. (2017). A clinical prediction rule for rebound hyperbilirubinemia following inpatient phototherapy. *Pediatrics, 139*(3). doi:10.1542/peds.2016-2896

Chen, L., Bell, E. M., Browne, M. L., Druschel, C. M., Romitti, P. A., Schmidt, R. J., ... Olney, R. S.; National Birth Defects Prevention Study. (2012). Maternal caffeine consumption and risk of congenital limb deficiencies. *Birth Defects Research. Part A, Clinical and Molecular Teratology, 94*(12), 1033–1043. doi:10.1002/bdra.23050

Chen, R., Giliani, S., Lanzi, G., Mias, G. I., Lonardi, S., Dobbs, K., ... Notarangelo, L. D. (2013). Whole-exome sequencing identifies tetratricopeptide repeat domain 7A (TTC7A) mutations for combined immunodeficiency with intestinal atresias. *Journal of Allergy and Clinical Immunology, 132*(3), 656.e17–664.e17. doi:10.1016/j.jaci.2013.06.013

Cohen, A. R., Couto, J., Cummings, J. J., Johnson, A., Joseph, G., Kaufman, B. A., ... Wax, J. R.; MMC Maternal-Fetal Management Task Force. (2014). Position statement on fetal myelomeningocele repair. *American Journal of Obstetrics and Gynecology, 210*(2), 107–111. doi:10.1016/j.ajog.2013.09.016

Cohen, M. C., Morley, S. R., & Coombs, R. C. (2015). Maternal use of methadone and risk of sudden neonatal death. *Acta Paediatrica, 104*(9), 883–887. doi:10.1111/apa.13046

Corey, K. M., Hornik, C. P., Laughon, M. M., McHutchison, K., Clark, R. H., & Smith, P. B. (2014). Frequency of anomalies and hospital outcomes in infants with gastroschisis and omphalocele. *Early Human Development, 90*(8), 421–424. doi:10.1016/j.earlhumdev.2014.05.006

Cornelius, M. D. (2014). People with schizophrenia are more likely to have a mother who smoked during pregnancy than people without the condition. *Evidence Based Nursing, 17*(3), 80. doi:10.1136/eb-2013-101549

Costello, A., Dua, T., Duran, P., Gulmezoglu, M., Oladapo, O. T., Perea, W., ... Saxena, S. (2016). Defining the syndrome associated with congenital Zika virus infection. *Bulletin of the World Health Organization, 94*(6), 406-406A. doi:10.2471/BLT.16.176990

Davies, J. H., & Cheetham, T. (2017). Recognition and assessment of atypical and ambiguous genitalia in the newborn. *Archives of Disease in Childhood, 102*(10), 968–974. doi:10.1136/archdischild-2016-311270

Deloison, B., Chalouhi, G. E., Bernard, J. P., Ville, Y., & Salomon, L. J. (2012). Outcomes of fetuses with small head circumference on second-trimester ultrasonography. *Prenatal Diagnosis, 32*(9), 869–874. doi:10.1002/pd.3923

Deng, K., Qiu, J., Dai, L., Yi, L., Deng, C., Mu, Y., & Zhu, J. (2014). Perinatal mortality in pregnancies with omphalocele: Data from the Chinese national birth defects monitoring network, 1996–2006. *BMC Pediatrics, 14*, 160. doi:10.1186/1471-2431-14-160 de Trey, L. A., Lambercy, K., Monnier, P., & Sandu, K. (2016). Management of severe congenital laryngeal webs — A 12 year review. *International Journal of Pediatric Otorhinolaryngology, 86*, 82–86. doi:10.1016/j.ijporl.2016.04.006

Diamond, M., & Garland, J. (2014). Evidence regarding cosmetic and medically unnecessary surgery on infants. *Journal of Pediatric Urology, 10*(1), 2–6. doi:10.1016/j.jpurol.2013.10.021

Doepker, C., Lieberman, H. R., Smith, A. P., Peck, J. D., El-Sohemy, A., & Welsh, B. T. (2016). Caffeine: Friend or foe? *Annual Review of Food Science and Technology, 7*, 117–137. doi:10.1146/annurev-food-041715-033243

Dreher, A. M., Arora, N., Fowler, K. B., Novak, Z., Britt, W. J., Boppana, S. B., & Ross, S. A. (2014). Spectrum of disease and outcome in children with symptomatic congenital cytomegalovirus infection. *Journal of Pediatrics, 164*(4), 855–859. doi:10.1016/j.jpeds.2013.12.007

Dreier, J. W., Andersen, A. M., & Berg-Beckhoff, G. (2014). Systematic review and meta-analyses: Fever in pregnancy and health impacts in the offspring. *Pediatrics, 133*(3), e674–e688. doi:10.1542/peds.2013-3205

Eckoldt-Wolke, F. (2014). Timing of surgery for feminizing genitoplasty in patients suffering from congenital adrenal hyperplasia. *Endocrine Development, 27*, 203–209. doi:10.1159/000363664

Elliott, R., Vallera, C., Heitmiller, E. S., Isaac, G., Lee, M., Crino, J., ... Ishman, S. L. (2013). Ex utero intrapartum treatment procedure for management of congenital high airway obstruction syndrome in a vertex/breech twin gestation. *International Journal of Pediatric Otorhinolaryngology, 77*(3), 439–442. doi:10.1016/j.ijporl.2012.11.023

Ellison, J. S., Shnorhavorian, M., Willihnganz-Lawson, K., Grady, R., & Merguerian, P. A. (2016). A critical appraisal of continence in bladder exstrophy: Long-term outcomes of the complete primary repair. *Journal of Pediatric Urology, 12*(4), 205.e1–207.e1. doi:10.1016/j.jpurol.2016.04.005

Eurosurveillance Editorial Team. (2015). The Americas region declares that rubella has been eliminated. *Euro Surveillance, 20*(18).

Eze, N., Smith, L. M., LaGasse, L. L., Derauf, C., Newman, E., Arria, A., ... Lester, B. M. (2016). School-aged outcomes following prenatal methamphetamine exposure: 7.5-year follow-up from the infant development, environment, and lifestyle study. *Journal of Pediatrics, 170*, 34.e1–38.e1. doi:10.1016/j.jpeds.2015.11.070

Fielder, A., Blencowe, H., O'Connor, A., & Gilbert, C. (2015). Impact of retinopathy of prematurity on ocular structures and visual functions. *Archives of Disease in Childhood. Fetal and Neonatal Edition, 100*(2), F179–F184. doi:10.1136/archdischild-2014-306207

Filges, I., Bruder, E., Brandal, K., Meier, S., Undlien, D. E., Waage, T. R., ... Stromme, P. (2016). Stromme syndrome is a ciliary disorder caused by mutations in CENPF. *Human Mutation, 37*(4), 359–363. doi:10.1002/humu.22960

Flagg, E. W., & Weinstock, H. (2011). Incidence of neonatal herpes simplex virus infections in the United States, 2006. *Pediatrics, 127*(1), e1–e8. doi:10.1542/peds.2010-0134

Fleurke-Rozema, H., van de Kamp, K., Bakker, M., Pajkrt, E., Bilardo, C., & Snijders, R. (2017). Prevalence, timing of diagnosis and pregnancy outcome of abdominal wall defects after the introduction of a national prenatal screening program. *Prenatal Diagnosis, 37*(4), 383–388. doi:10.1002/pd.5023

Fortuny, C., Deya-Martinez, A., Chiappini, E., Galli, L., de Martino, M., & Noguera-Julian, A. (2015). Metabolic and renal adverse effects of antiretroviral therapy in HIV-infected children and adolescents. *Pediatric Infectious Disease Journal, 34*(5 Suppl. 1), S36–S43. doi:10.1097/INF.0000000000000663

Friedman, A. M., Ananth, C. V., Siddiq, Z., D'Alton, M. E., & Wright, J. D. (2016). Gastroschisis: Epidemiology and mode of delivery, 2005–2013. *American Journal of Obstetrics and Gynecology, 215*(3), 348.e1–349.e1. doi:10.1016/j.ajog.2016.03.039

Furu, K., Kieler, H., Haglund, B., Engeland, A., Selmer, R., Stephansson, O., ... Norgaard, M. (2015). Selective serotonin reuptake inhibitors and venlafaxine in early pregnancy and risk of birth defects: Population based cohort study and sibling design. *BMJ, 350*, h1798. doi:10.1136/bmj.h1798

Ghekiere, S., Allegaert, K., Cossey, V., Van Ranst, M., Cassiman, C., & Casteels, I. (2012). Ophthalmological findings in congenital cytomegalovirus infection: When to screen, when to treat? *Journal of Pediatric Ophthalmology and Strabismus, 49*(5), 274–282. doi:10.3928/01913913-20120710-03

Goderis, J., De Leenheer, E., Smets, K., Van Hoecke, H., Keymeulen, A., & Dhooge, I. (2014). Hearing loss and congenital CMV infection: A systematic review. *Pediatrics, 134*(5), 972–982. doi:10.1542/peds.2014-1173

Goldstein, A. M., Hofstra, R. M., & Burns, A. J. (2013). Building a brain in the gut: Development of the enteric nervous system. *Clinical Genetics, 83*(4), 307–316. doi:10.1111/cge.12054

Gonzalez, R., & Ludwikowski, B. M. (2016). Should CAH in females be classified as DSD? *Frontiers in Pediatrics, 4*, 48. doi:10.3389/fped.2016.00048

Greenough, A. (2013). Long-term respiratory consequences of premature birth at less than 32 weeks of gestation. *Early Human Development, 89* Suppl. 2, S25–S27. doi:10.1016/j.earlhumdev.2013.07.004

Greenwood, C., Morrow, A. L., Lagomarcino, A. J., Altaye, M., Taft, D. H., Yu, Z., ... Schibler, K. R. (2014). Early empiric antibiotic use in preterm infants is associated with lower bacterial diversity and higher relative abundance of Enterobacter. *Journal of Pediatrics, 165*(1), 23–29. doi:10.1016/j.jpeds.2014.01.010

Grewen, K., Burchinal, M., Vachet, C., Gouttard, S., Gilmore, J. H., Lin, W., ... Gerig, G. (2014). Prenatal cocaine effects on brain structure in early infancy. *Neuroimage, 101*, 114–123. doi:10.1016/j.neuroimage.2014.06.070

Grigoriadis, S., VonderPorten, E. H., Mamisashvili, L., Eady, A., Tomlinson, G., Dennis, C. L., ... Ross, L. E. (2013). The effect of prenatal antidepressant exposure on neonatal adaptation: A systematic review and meta-analysis. *Journal of Clinical Psychiatry, 74*(4), e309–e320. doi:10.4088/JCP.12r07967

Grzeskowiak, L. E., Morrison, J. L., Henriksen, T. B., Bech, B. H., Obel, C., Olsen, J., & Pedersen, L. H. (2016). Prenatal antidepressant exposure and child behavioural outcomes at 7 years of age: A study within the Danish National Birth Cohort. *British Journal of Obstetrics and Gynaecology, 123*(12), 1919–1928. doi:10.1111/1471-0528.13611

Hahn, K. A., Wise, L. A., Rothman, K. J., Mikkelsen, E. M., Brogly, S. B., Sorensen, H. T., ... Hatch, E. E. (2015). Caffeine and caffeinated beverage consumption and risk of spontaneous abortion. *Human Reproduction, 30*(5), 1246–1255. doi:10.1093/humrep/dev063

Heida, F. H., Loos, M. H., Stolwijk, L., Te Kiefte, B. J., van den Ende, S. J., Onland, W., ... Bakx, R. (2016). Risk factors associated with postnecrotizing enterocolitis strictures in infants. *Journal of Pediatric Surgery, 51*(7), 1126–1130. doi:10.1016/j.jpedsurg.2015.09.015

Heller, M., & Burd, L. (2014). Review of ethanol dispersion, distribution, and elimination from the fetal compartment. *Birth Defects Research. Part A, Clinical and Molecular Teratology, 100*(4), 277–283. doi:10.1002/bdra.23232

Hofmann, A. D., & Puri, P. (2013). Association of Hirschsprung's disease and anorectal malformation: A systematic review. *Pediatric Surgery International, 29*(9), 913–917. doi:10.1007/s00383-013-3352-2

Hofmeyr, G. J., Xu, H., & Eke, A. C. (2014). Amnioinfusion for meconium-stained liquor in labour. *Cochrane Database of Systematic Reviews, (1)*, CD000014. doi:10.1002/14651858.CD000014.pub4

Holbrook, B. D. (2016). The effects of nicotine on human fetal development. *Birth Defects Research. Part C, Embryo Today, 108*(2), 181–192. doi:10.1002/bdrc.21128

Honein, M. A., Dawson, A. L., Petersen, E. E., Jones, A. M., Lee, E. H., Yazdy, M. M., ... Jamieson, D. J.; US Zika Pregnancy Registry Collaboration. (2017). Birth defects among fetuses and infants of US women with evidence of possible zika virus infection during pregnancy. *JAMA, 317*(1), 59–68. doi:10.1001/jama.2016.19006

Hoyme, H. E., Kalberg, W. O., Elliott, A. J., Blankenship, J., Buckley, D., Marais, A. S., ... May, P. A. (2016). Updated clinical guidelines for diagnosing fetal alcohol spectrum disorders. *Pediatrics, 138*(2). doi:10.1542/peds.2015-4256

Hudak, M. L., & Tan, R. C., Committee On Drugs; Committee On Fetus and Newborn; American Academy of Pediatrics. (2012). Neonatal drug withdrawal. *Pediatrics, 129*(2), e540–e560. doi:10.1542/peds.2011-3212

Hundalani, S., & Pammi, M. (2013). Invasive fungal infections in newborns and current management strategies. *Expert Review of Anti-Infective Therapy, 11*(7), 709–721. doi:10.1586/14787210.2013.811925

Huybrechts, K. F., Palmsten, K., Mogun, H., Kowal, M., Avorn, J., Setoguchi-Iwata, S., & Hernandez-Diaz, S. (2013). National trends in antidepressant medication treatment among publicly insured pregnant women. *General Hospital Psychiatry, 35*(3), 265–271. doi:10.1016/j.genhosppsych.2012.12.010

Hwang, C. K., Hubbard, G. B., Hutchinson, A. K., & Lambert, S. R. (2015). Outcomes after intravitreal bevacizumab versus laser photocoagulation for retinopathy of prematurity: A 5-year retrospective analysis. *Ophthalmology, 122*(5), 1008–1015. doi:10.1016/j.ophtha.2014.12.017

Hysinger, E. B., & Panitch, H. B. (2016). Paediatric tracheomalacia. *Paediatric Respiratory Reviews, 17*, 9–15. doi:10.1016/j.prrv.2015.03.002

Jackson, A., Bromley, R., Morrow, J., Irwin, B., & Clayton-Smith, J. (2016). In utero exposure to valproate increases the risk of isolated cleft palate. *Archives of Disease in Childhood. Fetal and Neonatal Edition, 101*(3), F207–F211. doi:10.1136/archdischild-2015-308278

Joint United Nations Programme on HIV and AIDS. (2016). *On the fast-track to an aids-free generation.* Retrieved from http://www.unaids.org/sites/default/files/media_asset/GlobalPlan2016_en.pdf

Jones, C. A., Raynes-Greenow, C., & Isaacs, D. (2014). Population-based surveillance of neonatal herpes simplex virus infection in Australia, 1997–2011. *Clinical Infectious Diseases, 59*(4), 525–531. doi:10.1093/cid/ciu381

Kassab, M., Khriesat, W. M., & Anabrees, J. (2015). Diuretics for transient tachypnoea of the newborn. *Cochrane Database of Systematic Reviews*, (11), CD003064. doi:10.1002/14651858.CD003064.pub3

Khoshnood, B., Loane, M., de Walle, H., Arriola, L., Addor, M. C., Barisic, I., ... Dolk, H. (2015). Long term trends in prevalence of neural tube defects in Europe: Population based study. *BMJ, 351*, h5949. doi:10.1136/bmj.h5949

Kieviet, N., Hoppenbrouwers, C., Dolman, K. M., Berkhof, J., Wennink, H., & Honig, A. (2015). Risk factors for poor neonatal adaptation after exposure to antidepressants in utero. *Acta Paediatrica, 104*(4), 384–391. doi:10.1111/apa.12921

Kimberlin, D. W., Jester, P. M., Sanchez, P. J., Ahmed, A., Arav-Boger, R., Michaels, M. G., ... Whitley, R. J.; Infectious Diseases Collaborative Antiviral Study Group. (2015). Valganciclovir for symptomatic congenital cytomegalovirus disease. *New England Journal of Medicine, 372*(10), 933–943. doi:10.1056/NEJMoa1404599

Kirby, R. S., Marshall, J., Tanner, J. P., Salemi, J. L., Feldkamp, M. L., Marengo, L., ... Kucik, J. E.; National Birth Defects Prevention Network. (2013). Prevalence and correlates of gastroschisis in 15 states, 1995 to 2005. *Obstetrics and Gynecology, 122*(2 Pt 1), 275–281. doi:10.1097/AOG.0b013e31829cbbb4

Klebanoff, M. A., & Keim, S. A. (2015). Maternal caffeine intake during pregnancy and child cognition and behavior at 4 and 7 years of age. *American Journal of Epidemiology, 182*(12), 1023–1032. doi:10.1093/aje/kwv136

Ko, J. Y., Farr, S. L., Tong, V. T., Creanga, A. A., & Callaghan, W. M. (2015). Prevalence and patterns of marijuana use among pregnant and nonpregnant women of reproductive age. *American Journal of Obstetrics and Gynecology, 213*(2), 201.e1–201.e10. doi:10.1016/j.ajog.2015.03.021

Ko, T. J., Tsai, L. Y., Chu, L. C., Yeh, S. J., Leung, C., Chen, C. Y., ... Hsieh, W. S. (2014). Parental smoking during pregnancy and its association with low birth weight, small for gestational age, and preterm birth offspring: A birth cohort study. *Pediatrics and Neonatology, 55*(1), 20–27. doi:10.1016/j.pedneo.2013.05.005

Kocherlakota, P. (2014). Neonatal abstinence syndrome. *Pediatrics, 134*(2), e547–e561. doi:10.1542/peds.2013-3524

Kolb, A., Schweiger, N., Mailath-Pokorny, M., Kaider, A., Hobusch, G., Chiari, C., & Windhager, R. (2016). Low incidence of early developmental dysplasia of the hip in universal ultrasonographic screening of newborns: Analysis and evaluation of risk factors. *International Orthopaedics, 40*(1), 123–127. doi:10.1007/s00264-015-2799-2

Kourtis, A. P., King, C. C., Nelson, J., Jamieson, D. J., & van der Horst, C. (2015). Time of HIV diagnosis in infants after weaning from breast milk. *AIDS, 29*(14), 1897–1898. doi:10.1097/QAD.0000000000000796

Kraft, W. K., Adeniyi-Jones, S. C., Chervoneva, I., Greenspan, J. S., Abatemarco, D., Kaltenbach, K., & Ehrlich, M. E. (2017). Buprenorphine for the treatment of the neonatal abstinence syndrome. *New England Journal of Medicine, 376*(24), 2341–2348. doi:10.1056/NEJMoa1614835

Krishnan, U., Mousa, H., Dall'Oglio, L., Homaira, N., Rosen, R., Faure, C., & Gottrand, F. (2016). ESPGHAN-NASPGHAN guidelines for the evaluation and treatment of gastrointestinal and nutritional complications in children with esophageal atresia-tracheoesophageal fistula. *Journal of Pediatric Gastroenterology and Nutrition, 63*(5), 550–570. doi:10.1097/MPG.0000000000001401

Kutbi, H., Wehby, G. L., Moreno Uribe, L. M., Romitti, P. A., Carmichael, S., Shaw, G. M., ... Munger, R. G. (2017). Maternal underweight and obesity and risk of orofacial clefts in a large international consortium of population-based studies. *International Journal of Epidemiology, 46*(1), 190–199. doi:10.1093/ije/dyw035

Lago, E. G., Vaccari, A., & Fiori, R. M. (2013). Clinical features and follow-up of congenital syphilis. *Sexually Transmitted Diseases, 40*(2), 85–94. doi:10.1097/OLQ.0b013e31827bd688

Larson, J. E., Patel, A. R., Weatherford, B., & Janicki, J. A. (2017). Timing of pavlik harness initiation: Can we wait? *Journal of Pediatric Orthopedics.* doi:10.1097/BPO.0000000000000930

Lee, A. C., Kozuki, N., Blencowe, H., Vos, T., Bahalim, A., Darmstadt, G. L., ... Lawn, J. E. (2013). Intrapartum-related neonatal encephalopathy incidence and impairment at regional and global levels for 2010 with trends from 1990. *Pediatric Research, 74* Suppl. 1, 50–72. doi:10.1038/pr.2013.206

Lee, C. T., Vora, N. M., Bajwa, W., Boyd, L., Harper, S., Kass, D., ... Varma, J. K.; NYC Zika Response Team. (2016). Zika virus surveillance and preparedness—New York City, 2015–2016. *MMWR Morbidity and Mortality Weekly Report, 65*(24), 629–635. doi:10.15585/mmwr.mm6524e3

Leeuwen, L., & Fitzgerald, D. A. (2014). Congenital diaphragmatic hernia. *Journal of Paediatrics and Child Health, 50*(9), 667–673. doi:10.1111/jpc.12508

Leirgul, E., Brodwall, K., Greve, G., Vollset, S. E., Holmstrom, H., Tell, G. S., & Oyen, N. (2016). Maternal diabetes, birth weight, and neonatal risk of congenital heart defects in Norway, 1994–2009. *Obstetrics and Gynecology, 128*(5), 1116–1125. doi:10.1097/AOG.0000000000001694

Leite, M., Albieri, V., Kjaer, S. K., & Jensen, A. (2014). Maternal smoking in pregnancy and risk for congenital malformations: Results of a Danish register-based cohort study. *Acta obstetricia et gynecologica Scandinavica, 93*(8), 825–834. doi:10.1111/aogs.12433

Liu, S., Joseph, K. S., Lisonkova, S., Rouleau, J., Van den Hof, M., Sauve, R., ... Kramer, M. S.; Canadian Perinatal Surveillance System. (2013). Association between maternal chronic conditions and congenital heart defects: A population-based cohort study. *Circulation, 128*(6), 583–589. doi:10.1161/CIRCULATIONAHA.112.001054

Lopez, A. S., Ortega-Sanchez, I. R., & Bialek, S. R. (2014). Congenital cytomegalovirus-related hospitalizations in infants <1 year of age, United States, 1997–2009. *Pediatric Infectious Disease Journal, 33*(11), 1119–1123. doi:10.1097/INF.0000000000000421

Lucas, B. R., Latimer, J., Pinto, R. Z., Ferreira, M. L., Doney, R., Lau, M., ... Elliott, E. J. (2014). Gross motor deficits in children prenatally exposed to alcohol: A meta-analysis. *Pediatrics, 134*(1), e192–e209. doi:10.1542/peds.2013-3733

Maisels, M. J., Clune, S., Coleman, K., Gendelman, B., Kendall, A., McManus, S., & Smyth, M. (2014). The natural history of jaundice in predominantly breastfed infants. *Pediatrics, 134*(2), e340–e345. doi:10.1542/peds.2013-4299

Malm, H., Sourander, A., Gissler, M., Gyllenberg, D., Hinkka-Yli-Salomaki, S., McKeague, I. W., ... Brown, A. S. (2015). Pregnancy complications following prenatal exposure to SSRIs or maternal psychiatric disorders: Results from population-based national register data. *American Journal of Psychiatry, 172*(12), 1224–1232. doi:10.1176/appi.ajp.2015.14121575

Mandelbrot, L., Tubiana, R., Le Chenadec, J., Dollfus, C., Faye, A., Pannier, E., ... Blanche, S.; ANRS-EPF Study Group. (2015). No perinatal HIV-1 transmission from women with effective antiretroviral therapy starting before conception. *Clinical Infectious Diseases, 61*(11), 1715–1725. doi:10.1093/cid/civ578

Manicklal, S., Emery, V. C., Lazzarotto, T., Boppana, S. B., & Gupta, R. K. (2013). The "silent" global burden of congenital cytomegalovirus. *Clinical Microbiology Reviews, 26*(1), 86–102. doi:10.1128/CMR.00062-12

Mark, K., Desai, A., & Terplan, M. (2016). Marijuana use and pregnancy: Prevalence, associated characteristics, and birth outcomes. *Archives of Women's Mental Health, 19*(1), 105–111. doi:10.1007/s00737-015-0529-9

Marquez, L., Levy, M. L., Munoz, F. M., & Palazzi, D. L. (2011). A report of three cases and review of intrauterine herpes simplex virus infection. *Pediatric Infectious Disease Journal, 30*(2), 153–157. doi:10.1097/INF.0b013e3181f55a5c

Marshall, J., Salemi, J. L., Tanner, J. P., Ramakrishnan, R., Feldkamp, M. L., Marengo, L. K., ... Kirby, R. S.; National Birth Defects Prevention Network. (2015). Prevalence, correlates, and outcomes of omphalocele in the United States, 1995–2005. *Obstetrics and Gynecology, 126*(2), 284–293. doi:10.1097/AOG.0000000000000920

Martillotti, G., Boucoiran, I., Damphousse, A., Grignon, A., Dube, E., Moussa, A., ... Morin, L. (2016). Predicting perinatal outcome from prenatal ultrasound characteristics in pregnancies complicated by gastroschisis. *Fetal Diagnosis and Therapy, 39*(4), 279–286. doi:10.1159/000440699

Maslova, E., Bhattacharya, S., Lin, S. W., & Michels, K. B. (2010). Caffeine consumption during pregnancy and risk of preterm birth: A meta-analysis. *American Journal of Clinical Nutrition, 92*(5), 1120–1132. doi:10.3945/ajcn.2010.29789

Massaro, A. N. (2015). MRI for neurodevelopmental prognostication in the high-risk term infant. *Seminars in Perinatology, 39*(2), 159–167. doi:10.1053/j.semperi.2015.01.009

McKeown, S. J., Stamp, L., Hao, M. M., & Young, H. M. (2013). Hirschsprung disease: A developmental disorder of the enteric nervous system. *Wiley Interdisciplinary Reviews. Developmental Biology, 2*(1), 113–129. doi:10.1002/wdev.57

McLean, H. Q., Fiebelkorn, A. P., Temte, J. L., Wallace, G. S., Centers for Disease Control and Prevention. (2013). Prevention of measles, rubella, congenital rubella syndrome, and mumps, 2013: Summary recommendations of the Advisory Committee on Immunization Practices (ACIP). *MMWR Recommendations and Reports, 62*(RR-04), 1–34.

Meneses, J. D. A., Ishigami, A. C., de Mello, L. M., de Albuquerque, L. L., de Brito, C. A. A., Cordeiro, M. T., & Pena, L. J. (2017). Lessons learned at the epicenter of Brazil's congenital zika epidemic: Evidence from 87 confirmed cases. *Clinical Infectious Diseases, 64*(10), 1302–1308. doi:10.1093/cid/cix166

Mirani, G., Williams, P. L., Chernoff, M., Abzug, M. J., Levin, M. J., Seage, G. R., III, ... Van Dyke, R. B.; IMPAACT P1074 Study Team. (2015). Changing trends in complications and mortality rates among US youth and young adults with HIV infection in the era of combination antiretroviral therapy. *Clinical Infectious Diseases, 61*(12), 1850–1861. doi:10.1093/cid/civ687

Mitanchez, D., Yzydorczyk, C., Siddeek, B., Boubred, F., Benahmed, M., & Simeoni, U. (2015). The offspring of the diabetic mother—Short- and long-term implications. *Best Practice and Research. Clinical Obstetrics and Gynaecology, 29*(2), 256–269. doi:10.1016/j.bpobgyn.2014.08.004

Mohammed, H., West, K., Bewick, J., & Wickstead, M. (2016). Tracheal agenesis, a frightening scenario. *Journal of Laryngology and Otology, 130*(3), 314–317. doi:10.1017/S0022215115003515

Moldenhauer, J. S., Soni, S., Rintoul, N. E., Spinner, S. S., Khalek, N., Martinez-Poyer, J., ... Adzick, N. S. (2015). Fetal myelomeningocele repair: The post-MOMS experience at the Children's Hospital of Philadelphia. *Fetal Diagnosis and Therapy, 37*(3), 235–240. doi:10.1159/000365353

Morgan, J., Young, L., & McGuire, W. (2014). Delayed introduction of progressive enteral feeds to prevent necrotising enterocolitis in very low birth weight infants. *Cochrane Database of Systematic Reviews, (12),* CD001970. doi:10.1002/14651858.CD001970.pub5

Muggli, E., Matthews, H., Penington, A., Claes, P., O'Leary, C., Forster, D., ... Halliday, J. (2017). Association between prenatal alcohol exposure and craniofacial shape of children at 12 months of age. *JAMA Pediatrics, 171*(8), 771–780. doi:10.1001/jamapediatrics.2017.0778

Mulpuri, K., Song, K. M., Goldberg, M. J., & Sevarino, K. (2015). Detection and nonoperative management of pediatric developmental dysplasia of the hip in infants up to six months of age. *Journal of the American Academy of Orthopaedic Surgeons, 23*(3), 202–205. doi:10.5435/JAAOS-D-15-00006

Nair, J., & Lakshminrusimha, S. (2014). Update on PPHN: Mechanisms and treatment. *Seminars in Perinatology, 38*(2), 78–91. doi:10.1053/j.semperi.2013.11.004

Napierala, M., Mazela, J., Merritt, T. A., & Florek, E. (2016). Tobacco smoking and breastfeeding: Effect on the lactation process, breast milk composition and infant development. A critical review. *Environmental Research, 151,* 321–338. doi:10.1016/j.envres.2016.08.002

Nygaard, E., Moe, V., Slinning, K., & Walhovd, K. B. (2015). Longitudinal cognitive development of children born to mothers with opioid and polysubstance use. *Pediatric Research, 78*(3), 330–335. doi:10.1038/pr.2015.95

Omeroglu, H., Kose, N., & Akceylan, A. (2016). Success of pavlik harness treatment decreases in patients >/= 4 months and in ultrasonographically dislocated hips in developmental dysplasia of the hip. *Clinical Orthopaedics and Related Research, 474*(5), 1146–1152. doi:10.1007/s11999-015-4388-5

Osterman, M. J., Kochanek, K. D., MacDorman, M. F., Strobino, D. M., & Guyer, B. (2015). Annual summary of vital statistics: 2012–2013. *Pediatrics, 135*(6), 1115–1125. doi:10.1542/peds.2015-0434

Oyen, N., Diaz, L. J., Leirgul, E., Boyd, H. A., Priest, J., Mathiesen, E. R., ... Melbye, M. (2016). Prepregnancy diabetes and offspring risk of congenital heart disease: A nationwide cohort study. *Circulation, 133*(23), 2243–2253. doi:10.1161/CIRCULATIONAHA.115.017465

Painter, S. L., Wilkinson, A. R., Desai, P., Goldacre, M. J., & Patel, C. K. (2015). Incidence and treatment of retinopathy of prematurity in England between 1990 and 2011: Database study. *British Journal of Ophthalmology, 99*(6), 807–811. doi:10.1136/bjophthalmol-2014-305561

Panel on Antiretroviral Therapy and Medical Management of HIV-Infected Children. (2017, April 27). *Guidelines for the use of antiretroviral agents in pediatric HIV infection.* Retrieved from http://aidsinfo.nih.gov/contentfiles/lvguidelines/pediatricguidelines.pdf

Papile, L. A., Baley, J. E., Benitz, W., Cummings, J., Carlo, W. A., Eichenwald, E., ... Wang, K. S. (2014). Hypothermia and neonatal encephalopathy. *Pediatrics, 133*(6), 1146–1150. doi:10.1542/peds.2014-0899

Patrick, S. W., Dudley, J., Martin, P. R., Harrell, F. E., Warren, M. D., Hartmann, K. E., ... Cooper, W. O. (2015). Prescription opioid epidemic and infant outcomes. *Pediatrics, 135*(5), 842–850. doi:10.1542/peds.2014-3299

Perry, H., Healy, C., Wellesley, D., Hall, N. J., Drewett, M., Burge, D. M., & Howe, D. T. (2017). Intrauterine death rate in gastroschisis following the introduction of an antenatal surveillance program: Retrospective observational study. *Journal of Obstetrics and Gynaecology Research, 43*(3), 492–497. doi:10.1111/jog.13245

Petersen, E. E., Meaney-Delman, D., Neblett-Fanfair, R., Havers, F., Oduyebo, T., Hills, S. L., ... Brooks, J. T. (2016). Update: Interim guidance for preconception counseling and prevention of sexual transmission of zika virus for persons with possible zika virus exposure—United States, September 2016. *MMWR Morbidity and Mortality Weekly Report, 65*(39), 1077–1081. doi:10.15585/mmwr.mm6539e1

Peyron, F., Mc Leod, R., Ajzenberg, D., Contopoulos-Ioannidis, D., Kieffer, F., Mandelbrot, L., ... Montoya, J. G. (2017). Congenital toxoplasmosis in France and the United States: One parasite, two diverging approaches. *PLoS Neglected Tropical Diseases, 11*(2), e0005222. doi:10.1371/journal.pntd.0005222

Phares, C. R., Lynfield, R., Farley, M. M., Mohle-Boetani, J., Harrison, L. H., Petit, S., ... Schrag, S. J.; Active Bacterial Core Surveillance/Emerging Infections Program Network. (2008). Epidemiology of invasive group B streptococcal disease in the United States, 1999–2005. *JAMA, 299*(17), 2056–2065. doi:10.1001/jama.299.17.2056

Picone, O., Vauloup-Fellous, C., Cordier, A. G., Guitton, S., Senat, M. V., Fuchs, F., ... Benachi, A. (2013). A series of 238 cytomegalovirus primary infections during pregnancy: Description and outcome. *Prenatal Diagnosis, 33*(8), 751–758. doi:10.1002/pd.4118

Pini Prato, A., Rossi, V., Mosconi, M., Holm, C., Lantieri, F., Griseri, P., ... Mattioli, G. (2013). A prospective observational study of associated anomalies in Hirschsprung's disease. *Orphanet Journal of Rare Diseases, 8,* 184. doi:10.1186/1750-1172-8-184

Polin, R. A., Committee on Fetus and Newborn. (2012). Management of neonates with suspected or proven early-onset bacterial sepsis. *Pediatrics, 129*(5), 1006–1015. doi:10.1542/peds.2012-0541

Popova, S., Lange, S., Shield, K., Mihic, A., Chudley, A. E., Mukherjee, R. A., ... Rehm, J. (2016). Comorbidity of fetal alcohol spectrum disorder: A systematic review and meta-analysis. *The Lancet, 387*(10022), 978–987. doi:10.1016/S0140-6736(15)01345-8

Quigley, M., & McGuire, W. (2014). Formula versus donor breast milk for feeding preterm or low birth weight infants. *Cochrane Database of Systematic Reviews, (4),* CD002971. doi:10.1002/14651858.CD002971.pub3

Rangmar, J., Hjern, A., Vinnerljung, B., Stromland, K., Aronson, M., & Fahlke, C. (2015). Psychosocial outcomes of fetal alcohol syndrome in adulthood. *Pediatrics, 135*(1), e52–e58. doi:10.1542/peds.2014-1915

Reinfeldt Engberg, G., Mantel, A., Fossum, M., & Nordenskjold, A. (2016). Maternal and fetal risk factors for bladder exstrophy: A nationwide Swedish case-control study. *Journal of Pediatric Urology, 12*(5), 304.e1–304.e7. doi:10.1016/j.jpurol.2016.05.035

Reynolds, M. R., Jones, A. M., Petersen, E. E., Lee, E. H., Rice, M. E., Bingham, A., ... Honein, M. A.; U.S. Zika Pregnancy Registry Collaboration. (2017). Vital signs: Update on zika virus-associated birth defects and evaluation of all U.S. infants with congenital zika virus exposure—U.S. zika pregnancy registry, 2016. *MMWR Morbidity and Mortality Weekly Report, 66*(13), 366–373. doi:10.15585/mmwr.mm6613e1

Roozen, S., Peters, G. J., Kok, G., Townend, D., Nijhuis, J., & Curfs, L. (2016). Worldwide prevalence of fetal alcohol spectrum disorders: A systematic literature review including meta-analysis. *Alcoholism, Clinical and Experimental Research, 40*(1), 18–32. doi:10.1111/acer.12939

Ross, M. E., Mason, C. E., & Finnell, R. H. (2017). Genomic approaches to the assessment of human spina bifida risk. *Birth Defects Research, 109*(2), 120–128. doi:10.1002/bdra.23592

Rubens, D., & Sarnat, H. B. (2013). Sudden infant death syndrome: An update and new perspectives of etiology. *Handbook of Clinical Neurology, 112,* 867–874. doi:10.1016/B978-0-444-52910-7.00008-8

Salisbury, A. L., O'Grady, K. E., Battle, C. L., Wisner, K. L., Anderson, G. M., Stroud, L. R., ... Lester, B. M. (2016). The roles of maternal depression, serotonin reuptake inhibitor treatment, and concomitant benzodiazepine use on infant neurobehavioral functioning over the first postnatal month. *American Journal of Psychiatry, 173*(2), 147–157. doi:10.1176/appi.ajp.2015.14080989

Samra, S., Bourne, D., Beckett, J., Matthew, M., & Thomson, J. G. (2016). Decision-making and management of ulnar polydactyly of the newborn: Outcomes and satisfaction. *journal of Hand Surgery Asian-Pacific Volume, 21*(3), 313–320. doi:10.1142/S2424835516500272

Sarnat, H. B., & Sarnat, M. S. (1976). Neonatal encephalopathy following fetal distress. A clinical and electroencephalographic study. *Archives of Neurology, 33*(10), 696–705.

Schillie, S., Walker, T., Veselsky, S., Crowley, S., Dusek, C., Lazaroff, J., ... Murphy, T. V. (2015). Outcomes of infants born to women infected with hepatitis B. *Pediatrics, 135*(5), e1141–e1147. doi:10.1542/peds.2014-3213

Schneuer, F. J., Holland, A. J., Pereira, G., Bower, C., & Nassar, N. (2015). Prevalence, repairs and complications of hypospadias: An Australian population-based study. *Archives of Disease in Childhood, 100*(11), 1038–1043. doi:10.1136/archdischild-2015-308809

Schwend, R. M., Schoenecker, P., Richards, B. S., Flynn, J. M., Vitale, M., & Pediatric Orthopaedic Society of North America. (2007). Screening the newborn for developmental dysplasia of the hip: Now what do we do? *Journal of Pediatric Orthopedics, 27*(6), 607–610. doi:10.1097/BPO.0b013e318142551e

Sharma, V., Berkelhamer, S., & Lakshminrusimha, S. (2015). Persistent pulmonary hypertension of the newborn. *Maternal Health, Neonatology and Perinatology, 1,* 14. doi:10.1186/s40748-015-0015-4

Shaw, B. A., & Segal, L. S. (2016). Evaluation and referral for developmental dysplasia of the hip in infants. *Pediatrics, 138*(6). doi:10.1542/peds.2016-3107

Shaw, G. M., Yang, W., Roberts, E., Kegley, S. E., Padula, A., English, P. B., & Carmichael, S. L. (2014). Early pregnancy agricultural pesticide exposures and risk of gastroschisis among offspring in the San Joaquin Valley of California. *Birth Defects Research. Part A, Clinical and Molecular Teratology, 100*(9), 686–694. doi:10.1002/bdra.23263

Shin, S. H., Im, Y. J., Lee, M. J., Lee, Y. S., Choi, E. K., & Han, S. W. (2013). Spina bifida occulta: Not to be overlooked in children with nocturnal enuresis. *International Journal of Urology, 20*(8), 831–835. doi:10.1111/iju.12054

Short, S. S., Papillon, S., Berel, D., Ford, H. R., Frykman, P. K., & Kawaguchi, A. (2014). Late onset of necrotizing enterocolitis in the full-term infant is associated with increased mortality: Results from a two-center analysis. *Journal of Pediatric Surgery, 49*(6), 950–953. doi:10.1016/j.jpedsurg.2014.01.028

Siminerio, L., Venkataramanan, R., & Caritis, S. (2016). Selective serotonin reuptake inhibitors and childhood motor skill impairment-what can be concluded? *British Journal of Obstetrics and Gynaecology, 123*(12), 1918. doi:10.1111/1471-0528.13581

Slusher, T. M., Vreman, H. J., Olusanya, B. O., Wong, R. J., Brearley, A. M., Vaucher, Y. E., & Stevenson, D. K. (2014). Safety and efficacy of filtered sunlight in treatment of jaundice in African neonates. *Pediatrics, 133*(6), e1568–e1574. doi:10.1542/peds.2013-3500

Stephansson, O., Kieler, H., Haglund, B., Artama, M., Engeland, A., Furu, K., ... Valdimarsdottir, U. (2013). Selective serotonin reuptake inhibitors during pregnancy and risk of stillbirth and infant mortality. *JAMA, 309*(1), 48–54. doi:10.1001/jama.2012.153812

Steurer, M. A., Jelliffe-Pawlowski, L. L., Baer, R. J., Partridge, J. C., Rogers, E. E., & Keller, R. L. (2017). Persistent pulmonary hypertension of the newborn in late preterm and term infants in California. *Pediatrics, 139*(1). doi:10.1542/peds.2016-1165

Stoltz Sjostrom, E., Lundgren, P., Ohlund, I., Holmstrom, G., Hellstrom, A., & Domellof, M. (2016). Low energy intake during the first 4 weeks of life increases the risk for severe retinopathy of prematurity in extremely preterm infants. *Archives of Disease in Childhood. Fetal and Neonatal Edition, 101*(2), F108–F113. doi:10.1136/archdischild-2014-306816

Streissguth, A. P., Bookstein, F. L., Barr, H. M., Sampson, P. D., O'Malley, K., & Young, J. K. (2004). Risk factors for adverse life outcomes in fetal alcohol syndrome and fetal alcohol effects. *Journal of Developmental and Behavioral Pediatrics, 25*(4), 228–238.

Terrault, N. A., Bzowej, N. H., Chang, K. M., Hwang, J. P., Jonas, M. M., & Murad, M. H.; American Association for the Study of Liver Diseases. (2016). AASLD guidelines for treatment of chronic hepatitis B. *Hepatology, 63*(1), 261–283. doi:10.1002/hep.28156

Tolia, V. N., Patrick, S. W., Bennett, M. M., Murthy, K., Sousa, J., Smith, P. B., ... Spitzer, A. R. (2015). Increasing incidence of the neonatal abstinence syndrome in U.S. neonatal ICUs. *New England Journal of Medicine, 372*(22), 2118–2126. doi:10.1056/NEJMsa1500439

Tomson, T., Battino, D., Bonizzoni, E., Craig, J., Lindhout, D., Sabers, A., ... Vajda, F.; EURAP Study Group. (2011). Dose-dependent risk of malformations with antiepileptic drugs: An analysis of data from the EURAP epilepsy and pregnancy registry. *The Lancet. Neurology, 10*(7), 609–617. doi:10.1016/S1474-4422(11)70107-7

Turner, K., Reynolds, J. N., McGrath, P., Lingley-Pottie, P., Huguet, A., Hewitt, A., ... Roane, J. (2015). Guided internet-based parent training for challenging behavior in children with fetal alcohol spectrum disorder (strongest families FASD): Study protocol for a randomized controlled trial. *JMIR Research Protocols, 4*(4), e112. doi:10.2196/resprot.4723

Uebel, H., Wright, I. M., Burns, L., Hilder, L., Bajuk, B., Breen, C., ... Oei, J. L. (2015). Reasons for rehospitalization in children who had neonatal abstinence syndrome. *Pediatrics, 136*(4), e811–e820. doi:10.1542/peds.2014-2767

U.S. Preventive Services Task Force. (2006). Screening for developmental dysplasia of the hip: Recommendation statement. *Pediatrics, 117*(3), 898–902. doi:10.1542/peds.2005-1995

von der Hagen, M., Pivarcsi, M., Liebe, J., von Bernuth, H., Didonato, N., Hennermann, J. B., ... Kaindl, A. M. (2014). Diagnostic approach to microcephaly in childhood: A two-center study and review of the literature. *Developmental Medicine and Child Neurology, 56*(8), 732–741. doi:10.1111/dmcn.12425

van der Horst, H. J., & de Wall, L. L. (2017). Hypospadias, all there is to know. *European Journal of Pediatrics, 176*(4), 435–441. doi:10.1007/s00431-017-2864-5

van Manen, M., Hendson, L., Wiley, M., Evans, M., Taghaddos, S., & Dinu, I. (2013). Early childhood outcomes of infants born with gastroschisis. *Journal of Pediatric Surgery, 48*(8), 1682–1687. doi:10.1016/j.jpedsurg.2013.01.021

Wai, K. C., Kohn, M. A., Ballard, R. A., Truog, W. E., Black, D. M., Asselin, J. M., ... Trial of Late Surfactant Study Group. (2016). Early cumulative supplemental oxygen predicts bronchopulmonary dysplasia in high risk extremely low gestational age newborns. *Journal of Pediatrics, 177*, 97.e2–102.e2. doi:10.1016/j.jpeds.2016.06.079

Wallon, M., Garweg, J. G., Abrahamowicz, M., Cornu, C., Vinault, S., Quantin, C., ... Binquet, C. (2014). Ophthalmic outcomes of congenital toxoplasmosis followed until adolescence. *Pediatrics, 133*(3), e601–e608. doi:10.1542/peds.2013-2153

Warner, B. B., Deych, E., Zhou, Y., Hall-Moore, C., Weinstock, G. M., Sodergren, E., ... Tarr, P. I. (2016). Gut bacteria dysbiosis and necrotising enterocolitis in very low birthweight infants: A prospective case-control study. *The Lancet, 387*(10031), 1928–1936. doi:10.1016/S0140-6736(16)00081-7

Welle-Strand, G. K., Skurtveit, S., Jansson, L. M., Bakstad, B., Bjarko, L., & Ravndal, E. (2013). Breastfeeding reduces the need for withdrawal treatment in opioid-exposed infants. *Acta Paediatrica, 102*(11), 1060–1066. doi:10.1111/apa.12378

Weyrauch, D., Schwartz, M., Hart, B., Klug, M. G., & Burd, L. (2017). Comorbid mental disorders in fetal alcohol spectrum disorders: A systematic review. *Journal of Developmental and Behavioral Pediatrics, 38*(4), 283–291. doi:10.1097/DBP.0000000000000440

Williams, J. H., & Ross, L. (2007). Consequences of prenatal toxin exposure for mental health in children and adolescents: A systematic review. *European Child and Adolescent Psychiatry, 16*(4), 243–253. doi:10.1007/s00787-006-0596-6

Wilson, R. D., & SOGC Genetics Committee; Special Contributor. (2014). Prenatal screening, diagnosis, and pregnancy management of fetal neural tube defects. *Journal of Obstetrics and Gynaecology Canada, 36*(10), 927–939. doi:10.1016/S1701-2163(15)30444-8

Wisner, K. L., Bogen, D. L., Sit, D., McShea, M., Hughes, C., Rizzo, D., ... Wisniewski, S. W. (2013). Does fetal exposure to SSRIs or maternal depression impact infant growth? *American Journal of Psychiatry, 170*(5), 485–493. doi:10.1176/appi.ajp.2012.11121873

Workowski, K. A., & Bolan, G. A.; Centers for Disease Control and Prevention. (2015). Sexually transmitted diseases treatment guidelines, 2015. *MMWR Recommendations and Reports, 64*(RR-03), 1–137.

Wright, T. E., Schuetter, R., Tellei, J., & Sauvage, L. (2015). Methamphetamines and pregnancy outcomes. *Journal of Addiction Medicine, 9*(2), 111–117. doi:10.1097/ADM.0000000000000101

Wyckoff, M. H., Aziz, K., Escobedo, M. B., Kapadia, V. S., Kattwinkel, J., Perlman, J. M., ... Zaichkin, J. G. (2015). Part 13: Neonatal resuscitation: 2015 American Heart Association guidelines update for cardiopulmonary resuscitation and emergency cardiovascular care. *Circulation, 132*(18 Suppl. 2), S543–S560. doi:10.1161/CIR.0000000000000267

Yee, W. H., Soraisham, A. S., Shah, V. S., Aziz, K., Yoon, W., Lee, S. K., & Canadian Neonatal Network. (2012). Incidence and timing of presentation of necrotizing enterocolitis in preterm infants. *Pediatrics, 129*(2), e298–e304. doi:10.1542/peds.2011-2022

Zaganjor, I., Sekkarie, A., Tsang, B. L., Williams, J., Razzaghi, H., Mulinare, J., ... Rosenthal, J. (2016). Describing the prevalence of neural tube defects worldwide: A systematic literature review. *PLoS One, 11*(4), e0151586. doi:10.1371/journal.pone.0151586

Suggested Readings

Boettiger, M., Tyer-Viola, L., & Hagan, J. (2017). Nurses' early recognition of neonatal sepsis. *Journal of Obstetric, Gynecologic, and Neonatal Nursing, 46*(6), 834–845. doi:10.1016/j.jogn.2017.08.007

Cleft Lip and Palate Association. Retrieved from www.clapa.com

Craig, A., James, C., Bainter, J., Lucas, F. L., Evans, S., & Glazer, J. (2017). Survey of neonatal intensive care unit nurse attitudes toward therapeutic hypothermia treatment. *Advances in Neonatal Care, 17*(2), 123–130. doi:10.1097/ANC.0000000000000339

Disorders of Sex Development Guidelines. Retrieved from http://www.dsd-guidelines.org

MacMullen, N. J., Dulski, L. A., & Blobaum, P. (2014). Evidence-based interventions for neonatal abstinence syndrome. *Pediatric Nursing, 40*(4), 165–172, 203.

Unit 4
Women's and Gendered Health

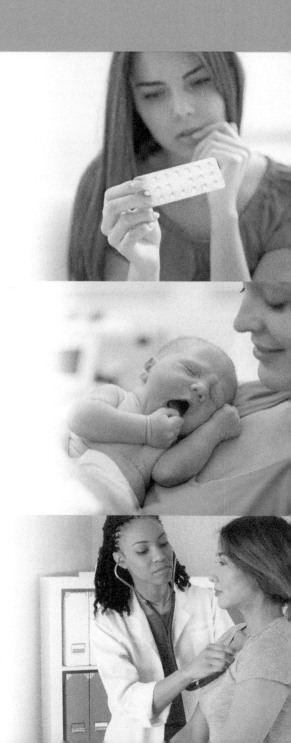

26 Wellness and Health Promotion

Objectives

1. Describe the guidelines, rationale, and process for cervical cancer screening.
2. Identify risk factors for breast cancer, discuss recommendations for routine screening, and explain the procedure for breast examination.
3. Identify several tools used in intimate partner violence screening.
4. List and describe the roles of macronutrients and micronutrients in the body.
5. Discuss options for nutrition assessment and how each is used.
6. Describe the benefits of physical activity to women, the recommended type and amount of physical activity, and the nurse's role in promoting physical activity in women.
7. Define and explain the differences between sex, gender, and sexual orientation.
8. Discuss recommendations for the screening of sexually transmitted infections.

Key Terms

Breast awareness
Calorie
Cisgender
Colposcopy
Eating disorder
Exercise
Gender
Gender dysphoria
Gender expression
Gender identity
Gender role
Genderqueer
Glycemic index
Human papillomavirus (HPV)
Intimate partner violence (IPV)

Macronutrients
Metaplasia
Micronutrients
Natal sex
Pap test
Physical activity
Screening
Sexual assault
Sexual orientation
Squamocolumnar junction (SCJ)
Transformation zone
Transgender
Transman
Transwoman

Wellness is the concept of making choices to enhance and maintain health, such as regular exercise, stress reduction, and a well-balanced diet. Health promotion is the enabling of wellness activities by education, facilitation, and encouragement. Nurses have an important part to play in health promotion to enhance wellness. Preventative care is care provided to prevent and detect disease or to optimize wellness. Preventative care is often conceptualized as the three levels of prevention:

- Primary prevention: An intervention to prevent or deter illness, injury, or disease. Examples include vaccinations, exercise, and a healthy diet.
- Secondary prevention: Screening and interventions designed to mitigate disease, most often prior to the onset of symptoms. Examples include the Pap test, cholesterol screening, and screening for sexually transmitted infections (STI).
- Tertiary prevention: Interventions meant to modify the disease process and the experience of disease after it has progressed beyond its early stages. The goal of tertiary prevention is not to prevent disease but rather to minimize the complications and disability associated with disease. Examples include physical therapy, cardiac rehabilitation, and chemotherapy.

An important part of secondary prevention is screening. **Screening** is a type of early, routine evaluation designed to identify the presence of conditions in individuals in the general population or in a subgroup at increased risk for developing the condition, with a goal of altering the course of the condition or avoiding transmission to others. Screening for chlamydia, for example, leads to treatment of the infection to reduce the risk for long-term harm and transmission to partners. As we will see in this chapter, some screening, such as breast self-examinations for the identification of breast cancer, is no longer generally supported by professional organizations because it fails to change the course of disease, and breast cancer, of course, is not contagious. In addition, such screening can lead to unnecessary diagnostic testing, false positives, and unnecessary treatment.

Guidelines for screening change frequently in healthcare, and women's healthcare is no exception. Such changes may be uncomfortable for patients who question whether the care they are getting is appropriate. Nurses and other healthcare providers must know the current evidence for best practice and guidelines for care, so that they can provide the best care for patients and inform them of current practice, which helps build and keep patient trust.

Cervical Cancer Screening, Assessment, and Management

More than half of women who develop cervical cancer have not been adequately screened, highlighting the importance of screening (Ponka & Dickinson, 2014). Cervical cancer screening detects precancerous lesions as well as early disease when it can still be managed. Screening is associated with a reduction in the rate of invasive cancer and a higher rate of cure.

Pap Test

Cervical cancer screening is done primarily with the **Pap test**, also known as the Pap smear. This test allows clinicians to identify abnormalities that can lead to cervical cancer before cancer develops, allowing patients to be treated in advance of the disease. The Pap test was first presented by Georgios Papanikolaou, a Greek physician, in 1928. It went into general use as a screening examination for cervical cancer in the 1950s.

Since the time when the Pap test first became standard screening, the rates of cervical cancer occurrence and associated death have gone down significantly. Cervical cancer, once one of the most common cancers in women, now ranks number 14. Still, efforts continue to reduce its occurrence and mortality even more. In the United States, reducing the rate of death from cervical cancer from 2.4 per 100,000 females to 2.2 per 100,000 females is a goal of Healthy People 2020 (Healthy People 2020, 2017).

In developing nations, however, the statistics are much grimmer. Today, 80% of cervical cancers happen in the developing world. In many countries it remains the leading cause of death for women (National Institutes of Health, 2013).

Etiology of Cervical Cancer

The primary cause of cervical cancer is infection with certain types of the **human papillomavirus (HPV)**. HPV is the most common STI in the United States. It is detected in 99.7% cases of cervical cancer (Van Kriekinge, Castellsague, Cibula, & Demarteau, 2014). Most people who are sexually active become infected with at least one form of HPV during their lifetime (Centers for Disease Control and Prevention [CDC], 2017). There are over 40 types of HPV that infect the genitals. High-risk types are associated with cervical changes that can lead to cervical cancer, and low-risk types are associated with genital warts, which rarely become cancerous. Types 16 and 18 are associated with a majority of cervical cancers. Other cancers associated with HPV infection are anal, penile, vulvar, vaginal, and head and neck cancers.

Most HPV infections resolve in 6 to 12 months. However, infections with forms that pose a high risk for cancer, including 16 and 18, are more likely to persist. These persistent infections are associated with changes to the cells of the cervix that can lead to cancer. It typically takes 5 to 10 years from the time of initial exposure to HPV for such precancerous changes of the cervix to develop; in 90% of the cases of infection, however, HPV regresses without causing changes (Van Kriekinge et al., 2014).

Risks of Overdiagnosis and Unnecessary Treatment With Screening

Because HPV and HPV-induced lesions usually clear spontaneously without intervention, screening may lead to overdiagnosis and unnecessary treatment. This is particularly true in younger women, in whom HPV infections tend to be transient and any lesions have a higher likelihood for spontaneous regression. Treatment for concerning changes to cervical cells and cervical cancer includes the removal of the cervical tissue. Such treatment can have long-term implications for future childbearing, including pregnancy loss in the second trimester, preterm premature rupture of membranes, preterm delivery, and cervical stenosis that may impair conception and menstruation (Kyrgiou et al., 2014). In addition, further testing and treatment have psychological and monetary costs.

Screening Process

Screening for cervical cancer includes a Pap test, HPV testing, or both. For a Pap test, the examiner collects a small sample of cells from the **transformation zone** and the **squamocolumnar junction (SCJ)** of the cervix (Fig. 26.1). The SCJ is an area where the squamous cells of the ectocervix meet the columnar epithelium of the endocervix. The columnar cells transform into squamous cells by a process called **metaplasia** in the transformation zone, which surrounds the SCJ. It is in the transformation zone that abnormal cells develop. The collected cells are then sent to a laboratory to be examined microscopically. Most modern Pap tests are performed by adding the collected cells to a liquid medium (Fig. 26.2), although some examiners may still perform the traditional slide

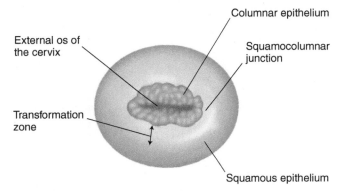

Figure 26.1. Transformation zone of the external cervical os. The transformation zone comprises the area distal to the squamocolumnar junction and is the site of squamous metaplasia. (Reprinted with permission from Bickley, L. S., & Szilagyi, P. [2003]. *Bates' guide to physical examination and history taking* [8th ed., unnumbered figure]. Philadelphia, PA: Lippincott Williams & Wilkins.)

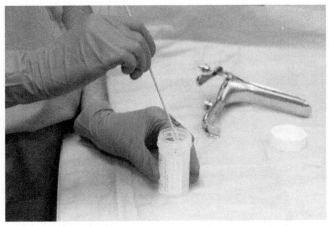

Figure 26.2. Collection of cells in a solution during liquid-based Pap testing. (Reprinted with permission from Jensen, S. [2011]. *Nursing health assessment: A best practice approach* [1st ed., Fig. 17.25]. Philadelphia, PA: Lippincott Williams & Wilkins.)

Pap test. Testing for HPV may also be performed from a liquid sample but not from a slide sample. Sample collection for HPV screening is otherwise the same as for a Pap smear.

Timing of Screening

In the United States, screening for cervical cancer by Pap test alone begins at the age of 21 in immunocompetent women who are asymptomatic, regardless of sexual activity (when testing is done for someone who is symptomatic, it is no longer screening but rather diagnostic; American College of Obstetricians and Gynecologists [ACOG], 2016; Moyer & U.S. Preventive Services Task Force, 2012a; Saslow et al., 2012). Even women who do not report sexual activity should be screened at the age of 21, as women may not disclose their sexual history for many reasons.

The harms outweigh any benefits of screening in women under 21 years old, as HPV infection and cervical changes tend to resolve spontaneously in this age group. In addition, the slow rate of progression from HPV infection to observable changes of the cervix makes it unlikely that a dangerous progression would occur before the age of 21 (ACOG, 2010). The incidence of cervical cancer among young women 15 to 19 years old in the United States is one out of every million. The most common time for a precancerous cervical lesion related to HPV to be identified by a Pap smear is 10 years after the age at which the woman became sexually active (Castle et al., 2009). The chances of regression of low-grade lesions are from 90% to 95%, and high-grade lesions also often regress spontaneously, as well (Szarewski & Sasieni, 2004). From 21 to 30 years of age, women should be screened with a Pap test every 3 years. Between the ages of 25 and 29, a pap with a low grade abnormality referred to as ASC-US should also be tested for HPV. This is referred to as reflex testing.

After the age of 30, women may continue to be screened with the Pap test alone every 3 years. Alternatively, they may be screened with a combination of a Pap test and HPV testing every 5 years (often referred to as co-testing). Women younger than 30 years are more likely than older women to have transient HPV infections, which could lead to extensive and unnecessary follow-up, were co-testing the norm for younger women (Moyer & U.S. Preventive Services Task Force, 2012a). HPV is more likely to be persistent in women over 30 years old.

Screening for women may end at the age of 65, provided they are not at an increased risk for cervical cancer, have had at least two consecutive negative co-tests or three negative Pap tests in the past 10 years, and have no history of high-grade abnormalities or cancer of the cervix (Saslow et al., 2012). Women older than 65 years are unlikely to benefit from screening because of age and the slowness of HPV-related changes. High-grade lesions are rare in this population (Saad et al., 2006).

In Chapter 1, Bess had a normal Pap test that was negative for HPV 2 years ago. Because of this, she did not need another screening for 3 years and was not screened for cervical changes during her first prenatal visit.

Screening Exceptions

Women who have had a hysterectomy that included removal of the cervix with no history of cervical cancer or cervical intraepithelial neoplasia (CIN) grade 2 or 3 have a very small risk for cervical and vaginal cancer and should not be screened. Women with a history of hysterectomy with an intact cervix should continue to be screened according to age and history. Women with a history of cervical cancer or CIN 2 or 3 should continue to be screened for 20 years after completion of treatment for cancer or CIN.

The daughters of mothers who took diethylstilbestrol in pregnancy are at a higher risk for a clear-cell adenocarcinoma of the cervix and/or vagina that is unrelated to HPV. Cervical cancer screening for this population is often more frequent, although the risk for this cancer in this population is approximately 1 out of 1,000 women exposed in utero (Huo, Anderson, Palmer, & Herbst, 2017).

Management of Abnormal Results

Follow-up care for an abnormal Pap test and/or positive HPV test is based on the specific result of the Pap test, the age of the patient, and the type of HPV discovered (Table 26.1). A previous history of abnormal results and follow-up are also important to creating a follow-up plan. It is important to note that cervical cancer is not congenital, and therefore, a family history of cervical cancer does not increase risk.

Table 26.1   Cervical Cytology (Pap Test) Management

| | | Screening Recommendations by Age | | | | |
| | | | | 30 y and Older | | |
Result	Meaning	21–24 y	25–29 y	HPV⁻	HPV⁺	HPV?
Normal	No abnormalities	Pap every 3 y	Pap every 3 y	Co-test every 5 y OR Pap only every 3 y	Co-test in 12 mo OR HPV genotyping	Co-test or Pap only in 3 y
ASC-US	Atypical cells of undetermined significance	Repeat cytology in 1 y OR HPV testing	HPV testing OR repeat cytology in 1 y	Repeat co-test in 3 y	Colpo	HPV testing OR repeat cytology in 1 y
ASC-H	Changes in cervical cells have been seen, cannot rule out HSIL	Colpo	Colpo	Colpo	Colpo	Colpo
LSIL	Low-grade squamous intraepithelial lesion	Repeat cytology in 1 y	Colpo	Colpo OR co-test in 1 y	Colpo	Colpo
HSIL	High-grade intraepithelial lesion	Colpo OR treatment	Colpo OR treatment	Colpo OR treatment	Colpo OR treatment	Colpo OR treatment
AGC	Atypical glandular cells*	Colpo	Colpo	Colpo	Colpo	Colpo
NILM but EC/TZ absent/ insufficient	Negative Pap, but the endocervical transition zone is absent	Pap every 3 y	Pap every 3 y	Co-test every 5 y OR Pap only every 3 y	Co-test in 1 y OR HPV genotyping	HPV testing OR repeat cytology in 3 y
Unsatisfactory	Sufficient cells not submitted	Repeat in 2–4 mo	Repeat in 2–4 mo	Repeat in 2–4 mo	Colpo	

*AGC that is atypical endometrial cells require sampling of the endometrium and endocervix.
Colpo, colposcopy; HPV, human papillomavirus; HPV−, human papillomavirus–negative; HPV+, human papillomavirus–positive; HPV?, human papillomavirus status unknown.
Adapted from Massad, L. S., Einstein, M. H., Huh, W. K., Katki, H. A., Kinney, W. K., Schiffman, M., . . . Lawson, H. W.; 2012 ASCCP Consensus Guidelines Conference. (2013). 2012 updated consensus guidelines for the management of abnormal cervical cancer screening tests and cancer precursors. *Obstetrics and Gynecology, 121*(4), 829–846. doi:10.1097/AOG.0b013e3182883a34

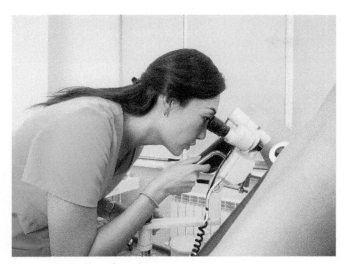

Figure 26.3. Use of a colposcope.

Common next steps after an abnormal Pap include more frequent testing with a Pap and/or HPV test and colposcopy. **Colposcopy** is an examination of the cervix with a microscope (Fig. 26.3). The examiner applies acetic acid (vinegar) to the cervix, which turns abnormal cells white. An iodine-based solution called Lugol's iodine is often also used to further highlight and differentiate abnormal cells from normal cells. On the basis of these observations, small biopsies of the cervix are gathered and sent to a pathologist for evaluation. Note that results from a Pap test are referred to as cytology results and results from a biopsy are histology results. Cytology is considered screening, whereas histology is diagnostic.

Human Papillomavirus Vaccination

Effectiveness

Although it is anticipated that the advent of the HPV vaccine will dramatically reduce the incidence of cervical abnormalities and cancer, the available vaccines do not protect against all forms of HPV. In addition, many young women may already have been exposed to HPV prior to vaccine administration. The vaccine is effective in protecting individuals from select strains of HPV, but it does not treat HPV infections that were acquired previously. At this time, no alteration in the screening schedule is recommended for women who have been vaccinated (ACOG, 2016).

Approximately 70% of cervical cancers are caused by HPV 16 and 18 and an additional 20% are caused by HPV 31, 33, 45, 52, and 58. HPV 9 and 11 cause 90% of anogenital warts. Of the three HPV vaccinations available, Gardasil, Gardasil 9, and Cervarix, only Gardasil 9, which provides protection against all of the HPV types mentioned in this paragraph, is marketed in the United States. Approximately 90% of anal cancers are also caused by HPV 16 and 18, as are a large portion of cancers of the head and neck, vulva, penis, and vagina. Since the start of routine vaccination, the prevalence of HPV among teens has decreased by 64% (Markowitz et al., 2016). The Healthy People 2020 HPV vaccination completion goal for teens of any gender aged 13 to 15 is 80% (Healthy People 2020, 2017).

Timing

Optimally, individuals should be vaccinated before they become sexually active. Vaccination of females is recommended from 11 to 12 years old but can be started as early as 9 years old and as late as 26 years old. Males similarly are advised to receive the vaccination from 11 to 12 years old and may have it as early as 9 years old. Catchup for males, however, is recommended by the age of 21. Men who have sex with men are still recommended for vaccination up until the age of 26. Although other men may have the vaccination until this age, as well, it is not considered a high enough priority to include on routine vaccine schedules and may not be covered by health insurance.

Although vaccination would still be effective in individuals older than 26 years, it is believed that this cohort likely already has had exposure to one or more HPV types covered by the vaccine and is less likely to encounter additional types than a younger person is. Although a blood test does exist to test for prior HPV exposure, it is expensive, unreliable, and, in the United States, used only in research settings, thus making it impossible to confirm HPV exposure that is not current and detected by direct cervical HPV testing. It may still be worthwhile to vaccinate, however, for individuals who are not involved in a lifelong monogamous relationship. HPV vaccination after the age of 26 is generally not covered by insurance.

Individuals vaccinated before the age of 15 need only two inoculations, with the second given 6 to 12 months after the first. Vaccination after the age of 15 requires a series of three injections, with the second 1 to 2 months after the first and the third 6 months after the first. If a second or third dose is missed, the next injection may be given without restarting the series.

Risks

As with all vaccinations, there is a small risk for syncope immediately after administration. The nurse should instruct patients who have received an HPV vaccination to wait for 15 minutes prior to leaving the office. Also in keeping with other vaccinations, mild injection site pain, erythema, and edema are not uncommon. Other adverse events attributed to vaccination for HPV have not been substantiated by research (CDC, 2013; Moreira et al., 2016; Scheller et al., 2015). Vaccination against HPV has not been associated in studies with an increase in sexual risk-taking (Jena, Goldman, & Seabury, 2015; Smith, Kaufman, Strumpf, & Levesque, 2015).

Barriers to Vaccination

Despite the HPV vaccine having a strong record of safety and efficacy, its rate of use is poor, with 54% of eligible females receiving one dose and only a third receiving a second dose. Overall, just 42% of girls and 22% of boys from 11 to 13 years old have been fully vaccinated. Reasons given for this low rate of use include a perceived lack of need, concerns about safety, a lack of knowledge about the vaccination, current lack of sexual activity of the child, and failure of care providers to recommend the vaccination (CDC, 2013; Markowitz et al., 2016). Research has shown that healthcare providers often fail to offer the vaccination if they perceive the parents do not want to discuss it, if they believe their patients are at low risk, or if they are uncomfortable discussing sex. The least likely to receive advice to vaccinate were young males from ethnic minorities. This weak and mixed messaging is thought to have inhibited the use of the vaccination. A robust provider recommendation is the most important factor associated with improved vaccine use (Gilkey & McRee, 2016).

Breast Cancer Screening

Breast cancer, the most frequent cause of cancer-related deaths worldwide, is far more survivable than it once was. This increased survivability is primarily due to improvements in breast cancer treatment rather than the routine adoption of mammography for breast cancer screening. In fact, as many as a third of new diagnoses of breast cancer may be erroneous as a direct result of screening (Bleyer & Welch, 2012; Welch, Prorok, O'Malley, & Kramer, 2016). For every 2,000 women with an average risk for breast cancer who are screened over 10 years, it is estimated that one death due to breast cancer is avoided and 10 healthy women are overdiagnosed and unnecessarily treated (Marmot et al., 2013; Pace & Keating, 2014). Critical to finding the balance between underdiagnosis from a lack of screening and overdiagnosis from unnecessary screening is determining which patients are most at risk for developing breast cancer and would benefit most from earlier rather than later treatment. Healthy People 2020 breast cancer goals include reducing the rate of death from female breast cancer, reducing late-stage female breast cancer, and increasing the proportion of women who receive breast cancer screening on the basis of the most recent guidelines (Healthy People 2020, 2017).

Risk Assessment

Many tools exist to predict a woman's lifetime risk for developing breast cancer, with varying degrees of accuracy. They cannot, however, predict a woman's lifetime risk of dying of breast cancer. This is an important distinction, as not all cancers are aggressive and life-threatening.

Women without known risks based on personal or family history have an average risk for developing breast cancer, with a lifetime risk of about 12.4% (Siu & U.S. Preventive Services Task Force, 2016). Factors that contribute to a woman having a moderate or high risk of developing breast cancer are itemized in Box 26.1.

Risk Prediction Models

The Gail model (https://www.cancer.gov/bcrisktool/), which is used frequently in primary care to calculate risk, also takes into account the personal history of breast biopsy, *BRCA* gene mutation, age, age at first menses, age at birth of first child, and ethnicity. It provides a risk percentage of developing breast cancer before the age of 90 and within the next 5 years when compared with women with an average risk. Other risk prediction models, such as the Ontario Family History Risk Assessment Tool, the Manchester Scoring System, the Referral Screening Tool, the Pedigree Assessment Tool, and the Family History Screen (FHS-7), focus solely on a family history of breast, ovarian, fallopian tube, and/or peritoneal cancer.

Women deemed high risk according to risk screening tools may have different recommendations for screening, including

---

Box 26.1   Risk Factors for Developing Breast Cancer

- Personal or family history of breast, ovarian, or peritoneal cancer
- Genetic predisposition (*BRCA* mutation–positive)
- Radiation to the chest from ages 10 to 30
- First birth after the age of 30
- Never given birth
- Dense breasts
- History of benign biopsy
- Use of exogenous estrogen

Adapted from Ashur, M. L. (1993). Asking about domestic violence: SAFE questions. *JAMA, 269*(18), 2367; Alpert, E. (2015). *Intimate partner violence: A clinician's guide to identification, assessment, intervention, and prevention.* Retrieved from http://www.massmed.org/partnerviolence; McFarlane, J., Parker, B., Soeken, K., & Bullock, L. (1992). Assessing for abuse during pregnancy. Severity and frequency of injuries and associated entry into prenatal care. *JAMA, 267*(23), 3176–3178; Sherin, K. M., Sinacore, J. M., Li, X. Q., Zitter, R. E., & Shakil, A. (1998). HITS: A short domestic violence screening tool for use in a family practice setting. *Family Medicine, 30*(7), 508–512; Feldhaus, K. M., Koziol-McLain, J., Amsbury, H. L., Norton, I. M., Lowenstein, S. R., & Abbott, J. T. (1997). Accuracy of 3 brief screening questions for detecting partner violence in the emergency department. *JAMA, 277*(17), 1357–1361.

---

earlier and more frequent mammograms and routine magnetic resonance imaging (MRI).

BRCA Gene Mutation

Most women who develop breast cancer do so spontaneously without a genetic predisposition to the disease. Only 5% to 10% of women who develop breast cancer have a hereditary form of the disease. Of these women, the most commonly identified cause is a mutation of the breast cancer susceptibility gene 1 or 2 (*BRCA1* or *BRCA2*; Couch, Nathanson, & Offit, 2014). Numerous other mutations can also contribute to breast cancer risk but are individually less significant.

The *BRCA* mutations are autosomal dominant, meaning that a parent with the mutation has a 50/50 chance of passing the gene and the greater susceptibility to breast cancer on to offspring. In families with the *BRCA* mutation, breast cancer is often common, with onset prior to menopause. Other cancers associated with the *BRCA* mutation are ovarian cancer, prostate cancer, pancreatic cancer, and male breast cancer. The risk is particularly pronounced for those of Ashkenazi Jewish ethnicity.

The risk of developing breast cancer by the age of 70 for women with the *BRCA1* or *BRCA2* gene mutation is 60% and 55%, respectively. The risk for developing ovarian cancer in this cohort is 59% for women carrying the *BRCA1* mutation and 16% for women with the *BRCA2* mutation (Mavaddat et al., 2013). The average age of diagnosis of breast cancer for women with the *BRCA1* mutation is 43 years and for those with the *BRCA2* mutation is 47 years (van der Kolk et al., 2010).

Because of this elevated risk, recommended screening for women carrying a *BRCA* mutation is very different from that for the general population. These women are encouraged to perform breast self-exams from the age of 18 and to undergo clinical breast examinations every 6 to 12 months beginning at the age of 25. Women with *BRCA* mutations are advised to have annual breast MRIs from 25 to 29 years of age, and both annual breast MRIs and annual mammograms starting at the age of 30. They are presented with the option of a mastectomy and medications to reduce risk without a diagnosis of breast cancer. Bilateral salpingo-oophorectomy to remove the fallopian tubes and ovaries is a treatment option recommended for this population and, if chosen, should be performed when the woman is 35 to 40 years of age or finished with childbearing (National Comprehensive Cancer Network, 2016).

Screening Imaging

Mammogram is currently the standard imaging method for breast cancer screening. It is a low-energy X-ray of the breast. During a mammogram, the breast is compressed between two plates to improve image quality and reduce the amount of radiation needed for adequate imaging (Fig. 26.4). This compression can be uncomfortable, particularly for women with small breasts and around the time of menses for women who have not yet gone through menopause. Routine mammograms usually include two views of each breast, one vertical (craniocaudal) and

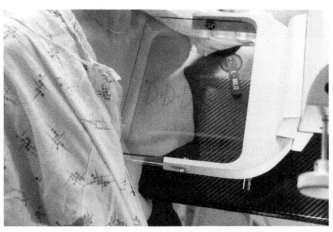

Figure 26.4. A woman undergoing a mammogram. Note the compression of the breast. (Reprinted with permission from McGreer, M. A., & Carter, P. J. [2011]. *Workbook for Lippincott's textbook for personal support workers: A humanistic approach to caregiving* [Workbook ed., Fig. 33.6]. Philadelphia, PA: Lippincott Williams & Wilkins.)

one horizontal (mediolateral oblique). A radiologist assesses the images and assigns a Breast Imaging Reporting and Data System (BI-RADS) category to the findings (Table 26.2).

Table 26.2 Mammogram BI-RADS Findings Categories

BI-RADS Category	Finding	Description
0	Incomplete assessment	This finding indicates the need for additional imaging evaluation (usually ultrasound or another mammogram) and/or prior mammograms for comparison.
1	Negative	This finding indicates a completely negative examination. Routine follow-up is recommended.
2	Benign findings	This finding indicates the presence of benign nodules, such as fibroadenomas, cysts, or calcifications, with no concern for malignancy and no further action needed. Routine follow-up is recommended.
3	Probably benign finding	This finding indicates a lack of characteristically benign features but a likelihood of malignancy of less than 2%. These types of findings are followed at shorter intervals than 1 y to assess for stability. The lesion is usually followed with mammography and/or ultrasound at 6-mo intervals for 1 y and annually for an additional 2 y or every 6 mo for a total of 2 y. Follow-up may be at shorter intervals. At any of the interval follow-ups, the lesion could be downgraded or upgraded on the basis of new imaging.
4	Suspicious abnormality	This finding indicates the presence of a lesion with features suspicious for malignancy and thus the need for biopsy. The chance that the finding is a cancer is from 2%–94%.
5	Highly suggestive of malignancy; biopsy indicated	This finding indicates a suspicion for malignancy of 95%–100%.
6	Further imaging required	This finding indicates a patient with an established biopsy-proven cancer who requires further imaging.

BI-RADS, Breast Imaging Reporting and Data System.
Adapted from American College of Radiology. (2013). *BI-RADS®—Mammography*. Retrieved from https://www.acr.org/Quality-Safety/Resources/BIRADS/Mammography

Table 26.3 Breast Cancer Screening Recommendations for Women of Average Risk

Organization	Mammogram Screening				Clinical Breast Exam Screening	Breast Self-Exam Screening
	Frequency	40–49 y	50–69 y	>70 y		
US Preventive Services Task Force	Every 2 y	SDM with patient	Yes	Yes until age 74	Insufficient evidence	Breast awareness
Canadian Task Force on Preventive Health Care	Every 2–3 y	No	Yes	Yes until age 74	Not recommended	Not recommended
National Health Service, United Kingdom	Every 3 y	Start at age 47	Yes	Yes until age 73	Not recommended	Breast awareness
Royal Australian College of General Practitioners	Every 2 y	No	Yes	No	Not recommended	Breast awareness
American College of Obstetricians and Gynecologists	Every 1–2 y	SDM with patient	Yes	Stop at age 75 ; ages ≥75, SDM with patient	Every 1–3 y ages 29–39; annually ages ≥40	Breast awareness
American College of Physicians	Every 1–2 y	SDM with patient	Yes	Yes	Insufficient evidence	Breast awareness
American Academy of Family Physicians	Every 2 y	SDM with patient	Yes	Yes until age 74	Insufficient evidence	Not recommended
American Cancer Society	Annually ages 45–54; every 2 y ages ≥55	Start at age 45	Yes	Yes	Not recommended	Not recommended
American College of Radiology	Annually	Yes	Yes	Yes	N/A	N/A
National Comprehensive Cancer Network	Annually	Yes	Yes	Yes	Every 1–3 y ages 25–39; annually ages ≥40	Breast awareness

N/A, not applicable; SDM, shared decision-making.

Adapted from U.S. Preventive Services Task Force. (2014). *Final recommendation statement: Breast cancer: Screening.* Retrieved from https://www.uspreventiveservicestaskforce.org/Page/Document/RecommendationStatementFinal/breast-cancer-screening; Gotzsche, P. C. (2011). Time to stop mammography screening? *Canadian Medical Association Journal, 183*(17), 1957–1958. doi:10.1503/cmaj.111721; Public Health England. (2016). *NHS Breast Screening Programme: Clinical guidance for breast cancer screening assessment.* Retrieved from https://associationofbreastsurgery.org.uk/media/1414/nhs-bsp-clinical-guidance-for-breast-cancer-screening-assessment.pdf; Royal Australian College of General Practitioners. (2016). Breast cancer. In *Guidelines for preventive activities in general practice* (9th ed., pp. 109–112). East Melbourne, Victoria: Author; Wilt, T. J., Harris, R. P., Qaseem, A., & High Value Care Task Force of the American College of Physicians. (2015). Screening for cancer: Advice for high-value care from the American College of Physicians. *Annals of Internal Medicine, 162*(10), 718–725. doi:10.7326/M14-2326; American Academy of Family Physicians. (2017). *Summary of recommendations for clinical preventive services.* Retrieved from https://www.aafp.org/dam/AAFP/documents/patient_care/clinical_recommendations/cps-recommendations.pdf; Oeffinger, K. C., Fontham, E. T., Etzioni, R., Herzig, A., Michaelson, J. S., Shih, Y. C., . . . Wender, R.; American Cancer Society. (2015). Breast cancer screening for women at average risk: 2015 guideline update from the American Cancer Society. *JAMA, 314*(15), 1599–1614. doi:10.1001/jama.2015.12783; American College of Radiology. (2015). *ACR and SBI continue to recommend regular mammography starting at age 40.* Retrieved from https://www.acr.org/About-Us/Media-Center/Press-Releases/2015-Press-Releases/20151020-ACR-SBI-Recommend-Mammography-at-Age-40; National Comprehensive Cancer Network. (2017). *National comprehensive cancer network.* Retrieved from https://www.nccn.org/professionals/physician_gls/pdf/breast-screening.pdf; American College of Obstetricians and Gynecologists. (2017). Practice bulletin number 179: Breast cancer risk assessment and screening in average-risk women. *Obstetrics and Gynecology, 130*(1), e1–e16. doi:10.1097/AOG.0000000000002158.

Table 26.4 BI-RADS Breast Density Categories

BI-RADS Breast Density Category	Description
A	Almost entirely fatty
B	Scattered areas of fibroglandular density
C	Heterogeneously dense (may obscure small masses)
D	Extremely dense (lowers the sensitivity of mammography)

BI-RADS, Breast Imaging Reporting and Data System.

Ultrasound may be used for follow-up imaging if a suspicious lesion is noted on mammogram, but it is not a primary screening method. MRI may be indicated for women who are at a particularly high risk for developing cancer. Other imaging techniques, such as molecular imaging and tomosynthesis, are emerging but are not yet recommended for routine use. Tomosynthesis, sometimes referred to as three-dimensional, or 3-D, mammography, may be most helpful for women with particularly dense breast tissue.

Younger women have denser breasts, which make mammograms less sensitive. Breast cancer is quite rare in women under 40 years old, after which time the risk of a breast cancer diagnosis rises. Screening recommendations vary according to expert group and professional organization (Table 26.3).

Several states have passed laws mandating reporting of dense breasts on mammogram reports. Breasts are composed of fat, which appears black on a mammogram, and other tissue, which appears white. Breasts are considered dense when the amount of tissue that appears white on the mammogram is high in proportion to the amount of tissue that appears black. This is a radiologic diagnosis, however, and does not correlate with breast clinical examination. The danger of high breast density is that the large areas of white seen on the mammogram may obscure or hide masses, making the mammogram less sensitive for detecting breast cancer in women with dense breasts, such as younger women. The most common means of communicating information about breast density is an additional four-point scale BI-RADS designation (Table 26.4). Breasts categorized as C or D are generally considered dense. Not only are dense breasts more difficult to assess for breast cancer lesions, but they are also an independent risk for developing breast cancer, although not for dying from it (Gierach et al., 2012). Recommended supplemental screening for women with dense breasts may include whole-breast ultrasound, tomosynthesis, or MRI.

Clinical Breast Examination

Although clinical breast examinations (CBEs) were once a mainstay of breast cancer screening, few organizations now recommend them for routine screening. There is a lack of data regarding the efficacy of CBE used either independently or in conjunction with

mammogram and some evidence of harm or potential harm from overdiagnosis associated with it (U.S. Preventive Services Task Force, 2014). A thorough CBE takes a minimum of 3 minutes per breast to perform, a standard rarely met in clinical practice, which greatly reduces the sensitivity of the examination (Miller et al., 2014). The effectiveness of CBE has yet to be confirmed in a large standardized study (U.S. Preventive Services Task Force, 2014). The CBE is still, however, an important evaluation tool for women presenting with breast complaints such as pain, nipple discharge, or a palpable mass.

Some clinicians may still offer routine CBE, however, and patients may request it. The nurse should inform patients of the low sensitivity of the examination and, as with any screening, the risk for false positives, which require further testing. No major professional organization has endorsed routine CBE for women under the age of 25.

Breast Self-Examination

Another former mainstay of breast cancer screening, breast self-examination (BSE), is also no longer routinely recommended for screening. BSE is a practice in which the patient thoroughly examines her breasts monthly for changes that could indicate breast cancer. Although there are few randomized trials of BSE, 1 study of 266,064 women found that performing BSE over the course of 10 years did not decrease the number of breast cancer deaths but did increase the discovery of benign lesions that then required further evaluation (Thomas et al., 2002).

Approximately 80% of cancers not discovered by mammogram are discovered by a woman, but during her regular routine (showering, dressing, etc.) rather than by BSE (National Breast Cancer Coalition, 2011). The current recommendation from many organizations is for women to develop breast awareness. **Breast awareness** is a familiarity with one's breasts for the purpose of being able to detect any changes that occur in them that might indicate breast cancer. This approach requires a woman to know what her breasts look and feel like and to report any concerning changes to a healthcare provider (Siu & U.S. Preventive Services Task Force, 2016).

Intimate Partner Violence Screening

The term **intimate partner violence (IPV)**, sometimes called domestic violence or spousal abuse, refers to an actual or threatened physical, sexual, or psychological harm caused by a current or former intimate partner (Fig. 26.5). Victims of IPV may be of any gender identity, age, socioeconomic class, ethnicity, or sexual preference. Risk factors for IPV are included in Box 12.1. Victims of IPV are often reluctant to disclose the abuse for various reasons, including shame, a desire to protect their partner, or fear that disclosing the abuse will lead to retaliatory action by their abuser, among other reasons. Victims of IPV often have multiple encounters with healthcare providers before they choose to disclose the abuse. Healthy People 2020 goals pertaining to IPV include reducing physical, sexual, and psychological violence as well as stalking by current or former intimate partners (Healthy People 2020, 2017).

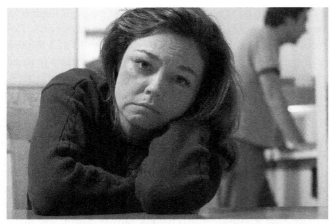

Figure 26.5. Intimate partner violence has physical, psychological, and social ramifications. Many victims do not know where to turn or how to receive help. Nurses and other healthcare providers must offer frontline assistance through regular screening, teaching, and treatment efforts. (Reprinted with permission from Mohr, W. K. [2013]. *Psychiatric-mental health nursing: Evidence-based concepts, skills, and practices* [8th ed., Fig. 33.4]. Philadelphia, PA: Lippincott Williams & Wilkins.)

When patients are assessed for IPV because of a clinical suspicion, the screening is considered diagnostic. Generalized screening in the absence of clinical suspicion, however, increases the identification of IPV (O'Doherty et al., 2015). What is less clear is whether screening improves health outcomes. It seems likely, however, that screening provides some benefit to women during pregnancy and unlikely that it causes harm (Moyer & U. S. Preventive Services Task Force, 2013; Taft et al., 2013). The victims themselves are the ones most likely to be uncomfortable with routine screening, because they are concerned about being judged by the interviewer, provoking more abuse, and being disappointed by the provider's response to the disclosure (Zeitler et al., 2006).

In Chapter 12, a nurse named Julia asked Loretta whether she felt safe in her home and in her relationship. Loretta said that she had already answered that question on paper, but Julia explained that, at her practice, they ask once on paper and once in person. Still, Loretta didn't talk to anyone about it until she got to know a home health nurse, Cara. Even then, she had a hard time thinking of her relationship as abusive.

Different organizations have different policies about IPV screening. Some may choose to screen at a woman's first visit or at visits during each trimester of pregnancy. Others may screen annually. Still others may elect not to screen but instead to assess for IPV only in certain clinical situations, such as pregnancy, trauma, or a positive screening for an STI.

Healthcare providers may also be uncomfortable with IPV screening, creating a barrier to implementation. Additionally,

screening for IPV can be time-consuming, particularly in the case of a positive screening. Healthcare providers may be uncertain about how to act on the information in a way that is productive and therapeutic. A systemic approach that includes training and integration of IPV screening into workflows can aid in regular implementation.

Many different clinical tools exist to screen for IPV. Although longer surveys may provide a more complex and nuanced picture, nurses and other healthcare providers often prefer shorter surveys for clinical practice (Ashur, 1993; Alpert, 2015; Feldhaus et al., 1997; McFarlane, Parker, Soeken, & Bullock, 1992; Sherin, Sinacore, Li, Zitter, & Shakil, 1998). The nurse must use care when delivering the questions, which may feel invasive to the patient and trigger shame or anxiety. Normalizing the questioning by making it routine instead of targeted to the individual can be helpful. An example of a normalizing statement is, "Violence in relationships is really common. We like to screen all of our patients for safety in their relationships so we can offer help as needed." The nurse should then ask the questions without hesitation or judgment. Alternatively, the nurse may administer the questionnaires on paper or by computer. Regardless of the method of screening used, it is essential that the partner of the patient is not present during the screening.

Nutrition

Our understanding of the components of a healthy diet has evolved over time. Although dietary guidelines vary among different organizations, there is consensus about the nutrition topics reviewed here, including caloric balance, macronutrients, and micronutrients. Healthy People 2020 goals for nutrition and weight status are itemized in Box 26.2.

Calories

A **calorie** is a unit of energy. Our bodies need a particular amount of energy, as measured in calories, to function. The amount varies according to age, sex, weight, and activity level. Overnutrition can lead to overweight and obesity, whereas undernutrition can lead to weight loss over time (Fig. 26.6). For people who are a healthy weight, calorie intake optimally should match the energy expended. Many people incorrectly estimate their calorie intake by erroneously perceiving portion size, meal composition, and the number of calories consumed. Calculators such as the one available on the United States Department of Agriculture website can be helpful for calculating daily calorie requirements and for goal planning: https://www.supertracker.usda.gov/bwp/index.html.

Macronutrients

Macronutrients are nutrients that the body needs to function properly and include fats, carbohydrates, and protein. According to current guidelines put forward by the United States Department of Health and Human Services, 45% to 65% of calories should come from carbohydrates, 10% to 35% from protein, and 20% to 35% from fat. Added sugars, such as those found in drinks,

Box 26.2 Healthy People 2020 Goals for Nutrition and Weight Status

- Increase the number of states with nutrition standards for foods and beverages provided to preschool-aged children in child care
- Increase the proportion of schools that offer nutritious foods and beverages outside of school meals
- Increase the number of states that have state-level policies that incentivize food retail outlets to provide foods that are encouraged by the Dietary Guidelines for Americans
- Increase the proportion of Americans who have access to a food retail outlet that sells a variety of foods that are encouraged by the Dietary Guidelines for Americans
- Increase the proportion of primary care physicians who regularly measure the body mass index of their patients
- Increase the proportion of physician office visits that include counseling or education related to nutrition or weight
- Increase the proportion of worksites that offer nutrition or weight management classes or counseling
- Reduce the proportion of adults who are obese
- Reduce the proportion of children and adolescents who are considered obese
- Prevent inappropriate weight gain in youth and adults
- Eliminate very low food security among children
- Reduce household food insecurity and in doing so reduce hunger
- Increase the contribution of fruits to the diets of the population aged 2 and older
- Increase the variety and contribution of vegetables to the diets of the population aged 2 and older
- Increase the contribution of whole grains to the diets of the population aged 2 and older
- Reduce the consumption of calories from solid fats and added sugars in the population aged 2 and older
- Reduce the consumption of saturated fat in the population aged 2 and older
- Reduce the consumption of sodium in the population aged 2 and older
- Increase the consumption of calcium in the population aged 2 and older
- Reduce iron deficiency among young children and females of childbearing age
- Reduce iron deficiency among pregnant females

Adapted from Healthy People 2020. (2017). *2020 topics and objectives*. Retrieved from https://www.healthypeople.gov/2020/topics-objectives.

should be limited to 10% or less of daily calories consumed (Fig. 26.7; U.S. Department of Health and Human Services & U.S. Department of Agriculture, 2015).

In Chapter 3, Susan was obese and worked with a nutritionist throughout her pregnancy to establish healthy eating habits. Susan tried hard to minimize her consumption of simple carbohydrates while eating more vegetables and lean proteins.

Carbohydrates

Not all sources of carbohydrates are equally good. Whole-grain carbohydrates, such as oatmeal, fruits, and whole-grain bread, are believed to be healthier than simple carbohydrates, such as sugar and white flour. Simple carbohydrates can lead to short-term spikes in blood glucose level and have a higher glycemic index. The **glycemic index** is a measure of the effect of a food on blood glucose level, with the value of 100 equaling pure glucose. An apple, for example, has a glycemic index of 39, whereas pure glucose has a glycemic index of 100 (Fig. 26.8).

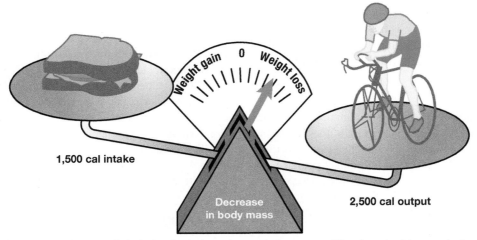

Figure 26.6. A negative energy balance. Calorie intake is less than calorie output. (Reprinted with permission from Dudek, S. G. [2014]. *Nutrition essentials for nursing practice* [7th ed., Fig. 7.5]. Philadelphia, PA: Lippincott Williams & Wilkins.)

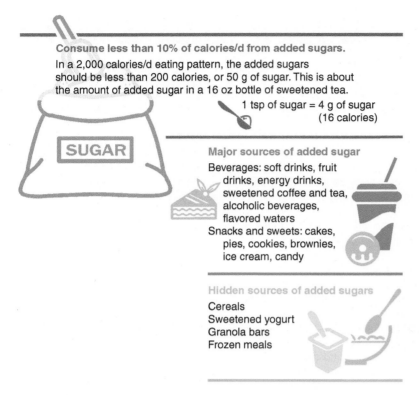

Consume less than 10% of calories/d from added sugars.

In a 2,000 calories/d eating pattern, the added sugars should be less than 200 calories, or 50 g of sugar. This is about the amount of added sugar in a 16 oz bottle of sweetened tea.

1 tsp of sugar = 4 g of sugar (16 calories)

Major sources of added sugar

Beverages: soft drinks, fruit drinks, energy drinks, sweetened coffee and tea, alcoholic beverages, flavored waters
Snacks and sweets: cakes, pies, cookies, brownies, ice cream, candy

Hidden sources of added sugars

Cereals
Sweetened yogurt
Granola bars
Frozen meals

Figure 26.7. Sources of added sugar consumed by the U.S. population ages 2 years and older. (Reprinted with permission from Dudek, S. G. [2018]. *Nutrition essentials for nursing practice* [8th ed., Fig. 2.8]. Philadelphia, PA: Lippincott Williams & Wilkins.)

Frequent consumption of foods with a high glycemic index is associated with coronary heart disease, type 2 diabetes, and other health problems (Bhupathiraju et al., 2014; Mirrahimi et al., 2014; Schwingshackl & Hoffmann, 2013; Turati et al., 2015).

Protein

Protein sources may be plant or animal in origin. Examples include fish, poultry, soy products, beans, pork, beef, milk products, nuts, and seeds. Lean proteins, such as poultry, fish, beans, and soy products, are generally preferred to red meat, such as steak and hamburgers. Consumption of red meat is associated with increased mortality from all causes, whereas consumption of other proteins correlates with lower risk (Etemadi et al., 2017). Processed red meat is particularly associated with poor health outcomes (Bellavia, Larsson, Bottai, Wolk, & Orsini, 2014). On the other hand, consumption of oily fish such as salmon four or more times a week is associated with a reduced risk of an acute coronary event (Leung Yinko, Stark, Thanassoulis, & Pilote, 2014).

Fat

The type of fat consumed is likely more important than the amount of fat. Although some trans-fats occur naturally, most are found in processed foods and appear to be harmful to the cardiovascular system (Chowdhury et al., 2014). Consumption of saturated fats, which are primarily derived from animal products, is associated with increased blood cholesterol levels. Decreasing the intake of saturated fats, and particularly replacing saturated fats with polyunsaturated fats, may reduce the risk for coronary heart disease (Zong et al., 2016). Monounsaturated fats may have a plant or animal origin. Examples of plant-sourced monounsaturated fats

are olive and canola oils. Monounsaturated fats do not appear to contribute to coronary heart disease (Chowdhury et al., 2014). The U.S. Dietary Guidelines recommend diets rich in omega-6 (n-6) and omega-3 (n-3) polyunsaturated fatty acids, which may be derived from plants and fish. Consumption of n-6 and n-3 polyunsaturated fatty acids reduces the risk for coronary heart disease and type 2 diabetes (Farvid et al., 2014; Imamura et al., 2016). The nurse should instruct patients to replace solid fats with liquid fats when possible, to keep trans-fatty acid consumption low, and to consume less than 10% of their calories from fat in saturated form (U.S. Department of Health and Human Services & U.S. Department of Agriculture, 2015).

Fiber

Although fiber is not a macronutrient in the traditional sense (it does not provide calories), fiber consumption in the amount of 14 g per 1,000 calories consumed is recommended (U.S. Department of Health and Human Services & U.S. Department of Agriculture, 2015). Fiber may be consumed as a supplement, such as psyllium seed, or as a food source, such as whole-grain bread and brown rice. Refined carbohydrates, such as white bread or white rice, have far less fiber. Diets high in fiber are associated with a significant reduction in coronary heart disease, type 2 diabetes, colon cancer, and all-cause mortality (Hartley, May, Loveman, Colquitt, & Rees, 2016; Kim & Je, 2014; Li et al., 2014).

Micronutrients

Micronutrients are nutrients that the body needs in small quantities to function properly and include vitamins and

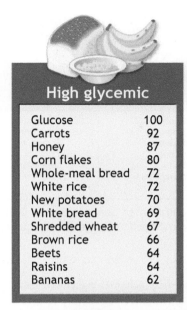
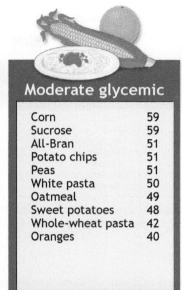

High glycemic		Moderate glycemic		Low glycemic	
Glucose	100	Corn	59	Apples	39
Carrots	92	Sucrose	59	Fish sticks	38
Honey	87	All-Bran	51	Butter beans	36
Corn flakes	80	Potato chips	51	Navy beans	31
Whole-meal bread	72	Peas	51	Kidney beans	29
White rice	72	White pasta	50	Lentils	29
New potatoes	70	Oatmeal	49	Sausage	28
White bread	69	Sweet potatoes	48	Fructose	20
Shredded wheat	67	Whole-wheat pasta	42	Peanuts	13
Brown rice	66	Oranges	40		
Beets	64				
Raisins	64				
Bananas	62				

High GI Diet			Low GI Diet		
	CHO (g)	Contribution to Total GI		CHO (g)	Contribution to Total GI
Breakfast			**Breakfast**		
30 g corn flakes	25	9.9	30 g All-Bran	24	4.7
1 banana	30	7.8	1 diced peach	8	1.1
1 slice whole-meal bread	12	3.8	1 slice grain bread	14	2.2
1 tsp margarine			1 tsp margarine		
			1 tsp jelly		
Snack			**Snack**		
1 crumpet	20	6.4	1 slice grain fruit loaf	20	4.1
1 tsp margarine			1 tsp margarine		
Lunch			**Lunch**		
2 slices whole-meal bread	23.5	7.6	2 slices grain bread	28	4.5
2 tsp margarine			2 tsp margarine		
25 g cheese			25 g cheese		
1 cup diced cantaloupe	8	10.4	1 apple	20	3.6
Snack			**Snack**		
4 plain sweet biscuits	28	10.4	200 g low-fat fruit yogurt	26	4.1
Dinner			**Dinner**		
120 g lean steak			120 g lean minced beef		
1 cup of mashed potatoes	32	12.1	1 cup boiled pasta	34	6.4
1/2 cup of carrots	4	1.7	1 cup of tomato and onion sauce	8	2.5
1/2 cup of green beans	2	0.6	Green salad with vinaigrette	1	0.6
50 g broccoli					
Snack			**Snack**		
290 g watermelon	15	5.1	1 orange	10	2.1
1 cup of reduced-fat milk throughout day	14	1.9	1 cup of reduced-fat milk throughout day	14	1.9
Total	212	69.8	**Total**	212	39.0

For each diet, the carbohydrate choices are maximized for differences between the two diets.

Figure 26.8. **Common food sources of carbohydrates categorized by the level of glycemic index** (GI). (Reprinted with permission from Brand-Miller, J., & Foster-Powell, K. [1999]. Diets with a low glycemic index: From theory to practice. *Nutrition Today, 34*, 64.)

minerals that we consume as part of our diet (Figs. 26.9 and 26.10). With the exception of vitamin D, humans cannot create micronutrients. With a balanced diet, micronutrient deficiencies are unlikely in the absence of a condition that causes malabsorption, such as ulcerative colitis or gastric bypass.

Older adults are more likely to have micronutrient deficiencies that are related to diet and changes in the gastrointestinal system. Vegans may require vitamin B supplementation. People with little sun exposure may need supplementation with vitamin D.

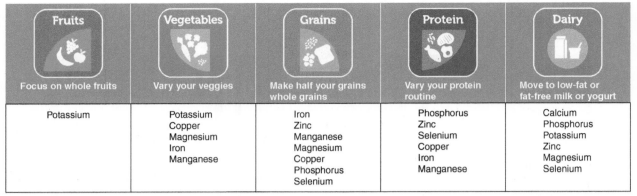

| Fruits | Vegetables | Grains | Protein | Dairy |
Focus on whole fruits	Vary your veggies	Make half your grains whole grains	Vary your protein routine	Move to low-fat or fat-free milk or yogurt
Potassium	Potassium Copper Magnesium Iron Manganese	Iron Zinc Manganese Magnesium Copper Phosphorus Selenium	Phosphorus Zinc Selenium Copper Iron Manganese	Calcium Phosphorus Potassium Zinc Magnesium Selenium

Figure 26.9. Key mineral contributions of food groups. (U.S. Department of Health and Human Services & U.S. Department of Agriculture. [2015]. *2015–2020 Dietary guidelines for Americans* [8th ed.]. Retrieved from https://health.gov/dietaryguidelines/2015)

Women who are pregnant require increased levels of folic acid and may require iron supplementation (see Chapter 15). People who consume large quantities of alcohol often require supplementation with thiamine. Routine vitamin supplementation without risk factors or evidence of deficiency is not generally recommended (Guallar, Stranges, Mulrow, Appel, & Miller, 2013). The optimal means of taking in adequate micronutrients is a balanced diet of macronutrients that includes at least 2.5 servings of vegetables, 2 servings of fruit daily, and 5.5 oz of protein (U.S. Department of Health and Human Services & U.S. Department of Agriculture, 2015).

Diet Assessment

The goal of a dietary evaluation is to identify areas in which a patient needs education or other interventions to improve nutrition. Although a professional dietician may need to manage patients with complex conditions or situations, nurses and other healthcare providers may perform the initial assessment of all patients and manage patients with less complex conditions or situations in a primary care setting. In some settings, nurses may take a lead role in guiding patients' dietary and lifestyle changes. A complete assessment evaluates the patient for weight loss or gain, food allergies and intolerances, alterations in the ability to digest food, eating disorders, changes in appetite, the ability to chew and swallow, and the skills and readiness of the patient to implement change.

An assessment of the patient's diet can identify the components that may contribute to or lessen health risks. An evaluation should include questions about portion size, food-related behaviors, and foods consumed.

Portion Sizes

Many people have difficulty estimating portion size and tend to underestimate the quantity of food they consume. Helpful visualizations of portion size are included in Table 26.5.

Portion size is also included, among other helpful information, on the Nutrition Facts label on food products (Fig. 26.11). Several changes to the label were implemented in 2016 to encourage consumers to make better-informed food choices. Critical changes include improved visibility of serving size and calorie information. The nurse should tell patients that information on the label is based on a 2,000 calorie diet, which is appropriate for some but not all patients. Many patients require far fewer calories and others require more.

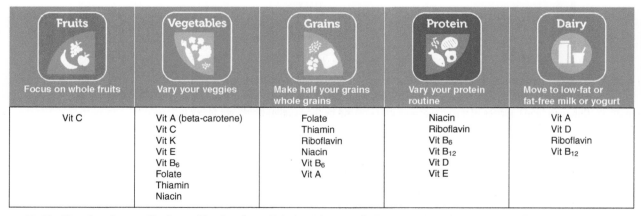

| Fruits | Vegetables | Grains | Protein | Dairy |
Focus on whole fruits	Vary your veggies	Make half your grains whole grains	Vary your protein routine	Move to low-fat or fat-free milk or yogurt
Vit C	Vit A (beta-carotene) Vit C Vit K Vit E Vit B_6 Folate Thiamin Niacin	Folate Thiamin Riboflavin Niacin Vit B_6 Vit A	Niacin Riboflavin Vit B_6 Vit B_{12} Vit D Vit E	Vit A Vit D Riboflavin Vit B_{12}

Figure 26.10. Key vitamin contributions of food groups. (Adapted from U.S. Department of Agriculture, Center for Nutrition Policy and Promotion. [2016]. Available at www.choosemyplate.gov. Accessed 2/13/16.)

Table 26.5 Portion Size Estimator

Measured Amount	Equivalent
1 Cup	Fist
½ Cup	Rounded handful
¼ Cup	Golf ball
3 Oz	Deck of cards
1 ½ Oz	Six dice
1 Teaspoon	Tip of the thumb

method depends on the setting, clinical presentation, and clinician preference. In certain circumstances, environmental and behavioral assessments and screening for eating disorders may be appropriate to conduct.

Unstructured Interview

The unstructured interview allows the patient to guide information sharing and to reflect on her own diet with guidance from the nurse. Such an interview often starts with the question, "What changes do you think you should make to your diet?" or "What can you do to improve your diet?" An advantage of this approach is that it helps the nurse quickly home in on areas the patient may be more willing to address and strengths that may be built on. The nurse may then negotiate change with the patient by asking questions such as, "What changes can you see yourself making now?" and "What barriers do you see to making a change?" The nurse should follow up with the patient on changes the patient has agreed to make at future visits.

Assessment Options

A nurse may assess an individual's diet with a simple, unstructured interview, a 24-hour diet recall interview, a food diary or online food tracker, or a formal questionnaire. The choice of assessment

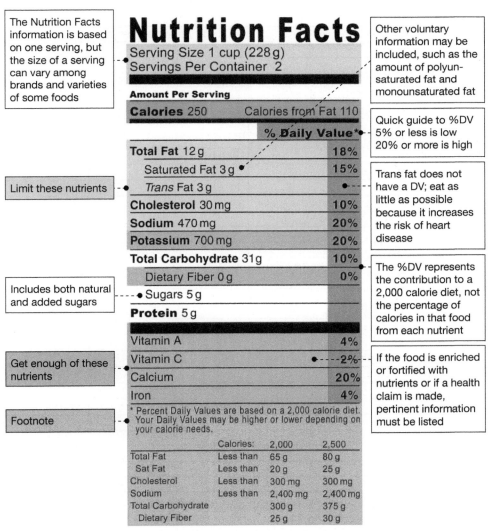

Figure 26.11. "Nutrition Facts" label. (From U.S. Food and Drug Administration.)

Changes may be small. For example, patients may agree to cut back on sugary beverages or to limit the number of times they eat dessert in a single week. A patient may agree to integrate an additional portion of fruits or vegetables into her diet daily or to refer to the Nutrition Facts label prior to preparing or eating a meal or snack. Although these changes may be insignificant alone, combined they can lead to significant health changes. Successful changes over time can help a patient feel more confident in her ability to implement change and more motivated to attempt larger dietary and lifestyle changes.

24-Hour Diet Recall

During a 24-hour diet recall interview, the nurse asks the patient to report what the patient ate and drank, portion size, and the method of food preparation over the course of the past 24 hours. Such interviews are typically guided by clusters of questions about eating such as, "What did you have to eat first yesterday?" and "What did you eat next?" rather than a generalized question such as, "What did you eat yesterday?" This systemic approach may be helpful for guiding recall. As with any patient interaction,

FOOD DIARY

NAME_____ TEL_____

AGE_____ SEX_____ Height _____ Weight_____ BMI____

Type of Foods/Beverages		Quantity Eaten (cup, oz, tbsp, tsp, etc.)	Preparation Method
BREAKFAST			
7:30 AM:	Orange juice	½ cup	Bagel Shop
	Bagel	Whole	
	Cream cheese	2 tablespoons	
	Coffee	2 cups	
	Milk and sugar	½ cup , 2 packets	
SNACK			
10:00 AM	Chocolate cookies	2	
	Orange soda	12 oz can	
LUNCH			
1:00 PM	Mushroom Pizza	2 slices	School Cafeteria
	Orange soda	12 oz can	
	Cheese cake	1 slice	
SNACK			
4:00 PM	Whole-wheat pretzels	1 bag	Vending machine
DINNER			
7:00 PM	Turkey	6 oz	Roasted
	Potato	1 medium	Baked
	Sour Cream	2 Tablespoons	
	Broccoli	1 cup	Sauteed
	Oil	2 Tablespoons	
	Gravy	½ cup	Canned
SNACK			
9:30 PM	Popcorn	3 cups	Microwave

Figure 26.12. Food diary. Shown is a sample-completed food diary, which is a form on which patients may record their daily intake of foods. A single form may be used for the 24-hour recall, or multiple forms may be used in the 3- to 7-day food diary. (Reprinted with permission from Wilkins, E. M. [2013]. *Clinical practice of the dental hygienist* [11th ed., Fig. 34.5]. Philadelphia, PA: Lippincott Williams & Wilkins.)

the nurse should avoid using leading questions when possible. If a nurse wants to know whether a patient buttered her bread, the nurse should ask whether the patient had anything with her bread rather than whether she put butter on her bread.

Food Diary

A food diary, similar to a 24-hour recall, involves tracking food consumption episodically. Unlike with a 24-hour recall, however, the individual records information about food, drink, portion size, and preparation method as it occurs rather than depending on recall. Nurses often provide patients with a take-home form for this purpose (this form may also be used for the retrospective 24-hour food recall; Fig. 26.12). An alternative to the written record is the use of websites and phone applications designed for food tracking (Box 26.3).

Food Frequency Questionnaire

A food frequency questionnaire includes questions about the consumption of particular foods or particular food groups, such as fruits or vegetables. This approach can be particularly helpful when assessing for foods that have a clearly delineated category, such as fruit or red meat, but is less helpful for assessing something like processed foods, which occur in every category of food. The questions about food frequency relate to particular discrete periods of time, such as, "How many times do you eat fruit in a day?" or "How many servings of red meat did you consume in the past month?" Food frequency questionnaires are more focused than food diaries, as they are typically used to assess for a particular eating behavior that may be reflected by a particular health outcome. A person with high cholesterol, for example, may be questioned about the intake of sources of saturated fats, which may contribute to high cholesterol, and sources of fiber, which may help decrease cholesterol.

Environmental and Behavioral Assessments

We eat to nourish our bodies, but eating can also be a means of socializing, bonding, and comfort. Our access to food and, in particular, to quality food can be impacted by location, income, and time. Time can also influence our ability and motivation to prepare foods instead of consuming processed foods or eating in a restaurant. People may be more inclined to eat, or to overeat, at particular times of day. In households with more than one member, the food preferences of multiple individuals need to be accounted for, which may result in more or less healthy food choices. A woman in a household with children, for example, may have limited time for food preparation as well as meal options limited by finances and juvenile food preferences. Cultural and religious practices, such as fasts and food prohibitions, also impact food consumption. It is important when evaluating a person's diet and nutrition to be aware of these elements and factor them into both assessment and proposed interventions.

Because food is so woven into our lives and food habits so ingrained, it can be challenging at times for individuals to recognize behaviors that may lead to poor food choices. An individual, for example, may habitually grab a bag of chips and a sugary drink on the way home from work each evening. Although doing this occasionally over time is unlikely to cause harm, as a daily ritual it may lead to unexpected weight gain. In such a case, the nurse could encourage the patient to instead keep healthful snacks, such as fruit, at work to eat on the way home, which could be a small healthy change that may lead to others.

Screening for Eating Disorders

An **eating disorder** is a pattern of eating that impairs psychological or physical functioning. The best-known eating disorders are anorexia nervosa and bulimia nervosa. Other eating disorders include binge eating disorder, avoidant/restrictive food intake disorder, rumination disorder, and pica (Box 26.4). This section

---

Box 26.3 Examples of Popular Food-Tracking Websites and Applications

Phone Applications
- Lose It! By FitNow
- My Plate Calorie Tracker by LiveStrong
- Calorie Counter and Diet Tracker by MyFitnessPal
- Calorie Counter and Food Diary by MyNetDiary

Websites
- www.myfitnesspal.com
- www.sparkpeople.com
- http://www.livestrong.com/myplate/
- https://www.supertracker.usda.gov/

Box 26.4 Categories of Eating Disorders

- *Anorexia nervosa:* an intense fear of weight gain, abnormally low weight, calorie restriction, and a distorted perception of one's body
- *Bulimia nervosa:* episodes of binge eating with compensatory behaviors such as vomiting, inappropriate use of laxatives or diuretics, excessive exercise, or fasting
- *Binge eating disorder:* binge eating and a sense of not being in control of eating but without the compensatory actions typical of bulimia nervosa
- *Avoidant/restrictive food intake disorder:* avoidance or restriction of food without body perception distortion resulting in impaired psychosocial functioning, enteral feedings or nutritional supplements for adequate intake, substantial weight loss, and/or a nutritional deficiency
- *Rumination disorder:* regurgitation of food that is then spit out or reconsumed
- *Pica:* consumption of nonnutritive substances, such as cloth, soap, chalk, dirt, pebbles, hair, clay, paper, or coal

Adapted from Cotton, M. A., Ball, C., & Robinson, P. (2003). Four simple questions can help screen for eating disorders. *Journal of General Internal Medicine, 18*(1), 53–56.

provides an overview of screening for disordered eating. Screening may be routine for a particular patient population in some clinical settings or may be cued by clinical manifestations, such as weight fluctuation, teeth erosion, disruption of menstruation, chronic constipation, dehydration, gastric reflux, syncope, and others. See Chapter 30 for more about eating disorders.

Commonly used clinical tools for assessing disordered eating include the Eating Attitudes Test (EAT), the SCOFF questionnaire, and the Eating Disorder Screen for Primary Care. Both the SCOFF questionnaire (Morgan, Reid, & Lacey, 1999) and the Eating Disorder Screen for Primary Care (Cotton, Ball, & Robinson, 2003) include five brief questions and may be completed quickly and routinely. The EAT is more extensive, with 26 questions (Mintz & O'Halloran, 2000).

Physical Activity

Questions about physical activity, including those related to duration, intensity, type, and frequency, should be a part of any wellness screening. **Physical activity** is contraction of the skeletal muscles that increase the energy expended by the individual above the level of the basal metabolism. Physical activity may be associated with any task, whereas **exercise** refers specifically to any activity designed to increase or maintain physical fitness.

Physical fitness refers to cardiovascular endurance as well as the state of the skeletal muscles themselves (strength, endurance, flexibility, speed, etc.). Current physical activity guidelines recommend a minimum of 2.5 hours of moderate-intensity aerobic activity or 1 hour and 15 minutes of vigorous-intensity aerobic activity per week (Box 26.5; U.S. Department of Health and Human Services, 2008). In addition, adults should perform moderate- or high-intensity muscle-strengthening activities on 2 or more days a week (U.S. Department of Health and Human Services, 2008). Healthy People 2020 goals are detailed in Box 26.6.

Physical inactivity was estimated to account for 5.3 million deaths worldwide in 2008 (Lee et al., 2012). In contrast, the health benefits of physical activity are numerous (Box 26.7). In addition, prolonged sitting is associated with an increased risk for cardiovascular disease, type 2 diabetes, and cancer that may or may not be mitigated by concentrated periods of physical activity at other times (Ekelund et al., 2016).

However, increased physical activity is associated with its own risks, including the following: injury, arrhythmias in individuals with prior arrhythmia or underlying cardiac disease, sudden cardiac death, myocardial infarction, rhabdomyolysis, bronchoconstriction, hyperthermia, hypothermia, and dehydration. Therefore,

---

Box 26.5 Examples of Moderate- and Vigorous-Intensity Activities

Moderate Intensity

- Walking briskly (3 miles/h or faster, but not race-walking)
- Water aerobics
- Bicycling slower than 10 miles/h
- Tennis (doubles)
- Ballroom dancing
- General gardening

Vigorous Intensity

- Race-walking, jogging, or running
- Swimming laps
- Tennis (singles)
- Aerobic dancing
- Bicycling 10 miles/h or faster
- Jumping rope
- Heavy gardening (continuous digging or hoeing, with heart rate increases)
- Hiking uphill or with a heavy backpack

Adapted from U.S. Department of Health and Human Services. (2008). *2008 physical activity guidelines for Americans.* Retrieved from www.health.gov/paguidelines.

Box 26.6 Healthy People 2020 Physical Activity Goals

- Reduce the proportion of adults who engage in no leisure-time physical activity
- Increase the proportion of adults who meet current Federal physical activity guidelines for aerobic physical activity and for muscle-strengthening activity
- Increase the proportion of adolescents who meet current Federal physical activity guidelines for aerobic physical activity and for muscle-strengthening activity
- Increase the proportion of the nation's public and private schools that require daily physical education for all students
- Increase regularly scheduled elementary school recess in the United States
- Increase the proportion of children and adolescents who do not exceed recommended limits for screen time
- Increase the number of states with licensing regulations for physical activity provided in child care
- Increase the proportion of the nation's public and private schools that provide access to their physical activity spaces and facilities for all persons outside of normal school hours (i.e., before and after the school day, on weekends, and during summer and other vacations)
- Increase the proportion of physician office visits that include counseling or education related to physical activity
- Increase the proportion of employed adults who have access to and participate in employer-based exercise facilities and exercise programs
- Increase the proportion of trips made by walking
- Increase the proportion of trips made by bicycling
- Increase legislative policies for the built environment that enhance access to and availability of physical activity opportunities

Adapted from Healthy People 2020. (2017). *2020 topics and objectives.* Retrieved from https://www.healthypeople.gov/2020/topics-objectives.

Box 26.7 Benefits of Physical Activity

Strong Evidence

- Lower risk of early death
- Lower risk of coronary heart disease
- Lower risk of stroke
- Lower risk of high blood pressure
- Lower risk of adverse blood lipid profile
- Lower risk of type 2 diabetes
- Lower risk of metabolic syndrome
- Lower risk of colon cancer
- Lower risk of breast cancer
- Prevention of weight gain
- Weight loss, particularly when combined with reduced calorie intake
- Improved cardiorespiratory and muscular fitness
- Prevention of falls
- Reduced depression
- Better cognitive function (for older adults)

Moderate-to-Strong Evidence

- Better functional health (for older adults)
- Reduced abdominal obesity

Moderate Evidence

- Lower risk of hip fracture
- Lower risk of lung cancer
- Lower risk of endometrial cancer
- Weight maintenance after weight loss
- Increased bone density
- Improved sleep quality

Adapted from U.S. Department of Health and Human Services. (2008). *2008 physical activity guidelines for Americans*. Retrieved from www.health.gov/paguidelines.

individuals with underlying health conditions, particularly cardiac issues, should undergo screening by a clinician prior to starting an exercise program. Evaluation of such individuals may include an electrocardiogram and a thorough review of the person's health history (Whitfield, Pettee Gabriel, Rahbar, & Kohl, 2014).

Counseling about the benefits of exercise may help encourage patients to start or continue increased physical activity, particularly patients who exhibit a willingness to make changes (Lin et al., 2014; Moyer & U.S. Preventive Services Task Force, 2012b). Exercising within a social structure, such as planned classes or an "exercise buddy" system, may also help encourage regular, sustained activity. Higher-intensity activity may have greater benefits overall, but a sedentary person is more likely to benefit from starting with lower-intensity activities and gradually increasing intensity and duration. Even small changes, such as taking the stairs and parking at the further end of the parking lot, can make incremental differences to patient fitness. Patients should aim to experience breathlessness, sweating, and fatigue as markers of adequate exercise. A goal heart rate is not necessary. People with little to no experience with exercise may benefit from a fitness consultation with a personal trainer or similar exercise professional.

Sexual Health and Gender Identity

Sexual health is an essential health domain that is often disregarded. Screening that pertains to sexual behavior, sexual preference, and gender identity can help the nurse identify areas for risk reduction and help facilitate better access to services and appropriate screening and treatment as needed.

It is essential that a patient feel safe, particularly when communicating about sex and sexuality. Patients may be embarrassed and wary of disclosing deeply personal information, and it is important that the nurse remain neutral and nonjudgmental, normalizing the conversation as much as possible. The nurse must keep in mind that sex is a normal and essential aspect of the human experience and that responsible sexual behavior is fundamental to public health (Healthy People 2020 goals related to sex are itemized in Box 26.8). Confidentiality is critical, and the nurse may need to remind the patient of the nurse's discretion. As with any patient interaction, the nurse should communicate respect to

Box 26.8 Healthy People 2020 Goals Pertaining to Sex and Gender Identity

- Reduce the proportion of adolescents and young adults with *Chlamydia trachomatis* infections
- Increase the proportion of sexually active females aged 24 and under enrolled in Medicaid plans who are screened for genital Chlamydia infections during the measurement year
- Increase the proportion of sexually active females aged 16–20 enrolled in Medicaid plans who are screened for genital Chlamydia infections during the measurement year
- Increase the proportion of sexually active females aged 24 and under enrolled in commercial health insurance plans who are screened for genital Chlamydia infections during the measurement year
- Reduce the proportion of females aged 15–44 who have ever required treatment for PID
- Reduce gonorrhea rates
- Reduce sustained domestic transmission of primary and secondary syphilis
- Reduce congenital syphilis
- Reduce the proportion of females with HPV infection
- Reduce the proportion of young adults with genital herpes infection due to herpes simplex type 2
- Increase the proportion of middle and high schools that prohibit harassment on the basis of a student's sexual orientation or gender identity

(continued)

Box 26.8 Healthy People 2020 Goals Pertaining to Sex and Gender Identity (continued)

- Increase the proportion of pregnancies that are intended
- Reduce the proportion of females experiencing pregnancy despite use of a reversible contraceptive method
- Increase the proportion of publicly funded family planning clinics that offer the full range of FDA-approved methods of contraception, including emergency contraception, onsite
- Increase the proportion of health insurance plans that cover contraceptive supplies and services
- Reduce the proportion of pregnancies conceived within 18 mo of a previous birth
- Increase the proportion of females at risk for unintended pregnancy or their partners who used contraception at most recent sexual intercourse
- Increase the proportion of sexually experienced persons who received reproductive health services
- Reduce pregnancies among adolescent females
- Increase the proportion of adolescents aged 17 and under who have never had sexual intercourse
- Increase the proportion of sexually active persons aged 15–19 who use condoms to both prevent pregnancy and provide barrier protection against disease
- Increase the proportion of sexually active persons aged 15–19 who use condoms and hormonal or intrauterine contraception to both prevent pregnancy and provide barrier protection against disease
- Increase the proportion of adolescents who received formal instruction on reproductive health topics before they were 18 y old
- Increase the proportion of adolescents who talked to a parent or guardian about reproductive health topics before they were 18 y old
- Increase the number of states that set the income eligibility level for Medicaid-covered family planning services to at least the same level used to determine eligibility for Medicaid-covered, pregnancy-related care
- Increase the percentage of women aged 15–44 y who adopt or continue to use the most effective or moderately effective methods of contraception
- Increase the vaccination coverage level of 3 doses of HPV vaccine for females by age 13–15
- Increase the vaccination coverage level of 3 doses of HPV vaccine for males by age 13–15
- Reduce sexual violence
- Reduce the number of new HIV diagnoses
- Reduce the number of new HIV infections among adolescents and adults
- Reduce the percentage of young gay and bisexual males in grades 9 through 12 who engage in HIV-risk behaviors
- Reduce the proportion of persons with a diagnosis of Stage 3 HIV (AIDS) within 3 mo of diagnosis of HIV infection
- Increase the proportion of persons living with HIV who know their serostatus
- Increase the proportion of adolescents and adults who have been tested for HIV in the past 12 mo
- Increase the proportion of substance abuse treatment facilities that offer HIV/AIDS education, counseling, and support
- Increase the proportion of sexually active persons who use condoms
- Reduce the proportion of men who have sex with men who reported unprotected anal intercourse with a partner of discordant or unknown status during their last sexual encounter
- Reduce deaths from HIV infection
- Increase the proportion of persons who are linked to HIV medical care (had a routine HIV medical visit) within 3 mo of HIV diagnosis
- Increase the proportion of persons with an HIV diagnosis who had at least one HIV medical care visit in each 6-mo period of the 24-mo measurement period, with a minimum of 60 d between medical visits
- Increase the proportion of persons with an HIV diagnosis in medical care who were prescribed antiretroviral therapy for the treatment of HIV infection at any time in the 12-mo measurement period
- Increase the percentage of persons with diagnosed HIV infection who are virally suppressed
- Increase the number of population-based data systems used to monitor Healthy People 2020 objectives that include in their core a standardized set of questions that identify lesbian, gay, bisexual, and transgender populations
- Increase the number of states, territories, and the District of Columbia that include questions that identify sexual orientation and gender identity on state-level surveys or data systems

AIDS, acquired immune deficiency syndrome; FDA, Food and Drug Administration; HIV, human immunodeficiency virus; HPV, human papillomavirus; PID, pelvic inflammatory disease.
Adapted from Healthy People 2020. (2017). *2020 topics and objectives*. Retrieved from https://www.healthypeople.gov/2020/topics-objectives.

the patient, avoid making assumptions and using medical jargon, and listen carefully to the patient's responses. The nurse should ask questions that are specific and nonleading.

Distinguishing Sex From Gender

Genetics, hormone expression, and anatomic characteristics determine an individual's natal, biologic, or anatomic sex. A child is generally reared according to the natal sex identified at birth. As discussed in Chapter 25, for some individuals, the identification of natal sex may be challenging.

Sex, however, is different from gender, although the two terms are often used synonymously. **Gender** is a construct informed by culture and by an individual's perception of self as pertains to aspects of femaleness or maleness. **Gender role** is the set of societal expectations placed on individuals on the basis of gender, typically either male or female. **Gender identity** is a person's innate sense of being male, female, or neither male nor female. **Gender expression** is how a person presents to the world (male, female, or neither male nor female), which does not necessarily correlate with the person's gender identity. A person may present as female, for example, but internally identify as male.

The term **transgender** is used to refer to individuals whose gender identity is not the same as their assigned natal sex. A person whose gender identity does align with the assigned natal sex may be referred to as **cisgender**. The term transgender man or **transman** describes a person with a male gender identity who was assigned female at birth. The term transgender woman or **transwoman** describes a person with a female gender identity who was assigned male at birth. **Genderqueer** and gender non-conforming are terms often used to refer to individuals assigned either sex at birth who identify as neither male nor female but as a fluid combination of the two. In many Western societies, gender is understood as male or female and failure to conform to one or the other is considered abnormal. **Gender dysphoria** and gender incongruence are terms used to describe the distress or discomfort an individual experiences as a result of that individual's gender identity and assigned sex not aligning. The failure of an individual's gender expression to match assigned sex may cause the individual to be stigmatized and ostracized (Wylie et al., 2016). Approximately 0.5% to 2% of adolescents and adults identify as transgender, with an approximately even distribution between those assigned male or female at birth (Winter et al., 2016).

The Diagnostic and Statistical Manual of Mental Disorders previously referred to the experience of a gender identity not aligned with natal sex as "gender identity disorder." The fifth edition of this manual, which is the most recent, instead refers to "gender dysphoria," which, rather than referring to being transgendered and gender nonconformity as pathologic, captures the distress caused by the mismatch between a person's natal sex/assigned gender and gender identity, as well as the interference with normal functioning caused by that distress (American Psychiatric Association, 2013).

Teens and adults whose gender identity does not conform to their natal sex are at high risk for risk-taking behavior, including unsafe sex and substance abuse. They are more likely to be victimized verbally and physically or to be sexually exploited. They are at a greater risk for social isolation, homelessness, depression, anxiety, unemployment, self-harm, and suicide (Aitken, VanderLaan, Wasserman, Stojanovski, & Zucker, 2016; Reisner, Biello, et al., 2016; Reisner, Katz-Wise, Gordon, Corliss, & Austin, 2016).

The nurse should take care to refer to the patient by the latter's preferred pronoun. The gender indicated in a person's insurance coverage documentation and other legal documents may be discordant with the person's gender identity, and many electronic health records do not allow space for gender identity as opposed to natal sex, making correctly addressing the patient more challenging. Building a trusting relationship with all patients is a critical step. In the case of a patient whose gender expression does not match their documented sex, the person's not revealing natal sex may have real health consequences. A transman with a cervix, for example, still requires routine screening for cervical cancer. For more about care for lesbian, gay, bisexual, transgender, and queer or questioning (LGBTQ) patients, see Chapter 30.

Sexual Orientation

Although gender refers to who a person is, **sexual orientation** refers to whom a person is attracted to sexually. However, a person may identify as heterosexual or homosexual and still engage in sexual activity with people of different gender identities. Some individuals may decline to identify as homosexual, heterosexual, or bisexual, and it is important for the nurse to inquire about sexual behavior as opposed to sexual orientation (Fig. 26.13). Different STI screening is recommended for men who have sex with men, for example.

In the context of gender identity (Fig. 26.13), sexual orientation is based on the gender with which the person identifies. A transman who is sexually attracted to other men may identify as a homosexual man. A transwoman who is sexually attracted to men may identify as a heterosexual woman (for more about

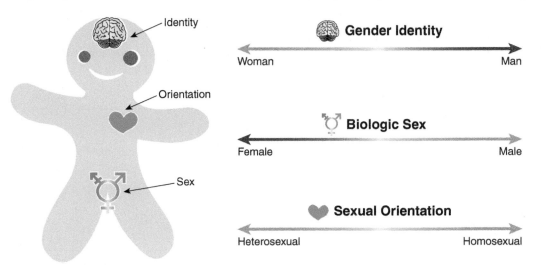

Figure 26.13. The genderbread person. The genderbread person is an educational tool used to explain the distinctions between experienced gender (termed gender identity here), gender assigned at birth (termed biologic sex here), and sexual or romantic orientation. (Adapted from itspronouncedmetrosexual.com.)

Table 26.6 Centers for Disease Control and Prevention STI Screening Recommendations

Infection	Recommended Screening
Chlamydia	• Annual screening for sexually active women <25 y old • Women ≥25 y old with new sex partners, more than one sex partner, a sex partner with multiple sex partners, or a sex partner with a known STI • Pregnant women <25 y old and women with new sexual partners, more than one sex partner, a sex partner with multiple sex partners, or a sex partner with a known STI, at the first visit and during the third trimester • Incarcerated women ≤35 y old • Incarcerated men <30 y old • Urethral testing annually for men who have insertive intercourse • Rectal testing annually for men who have anal-receptive intercourse • Pharyngeal testing annually for men who have oral-receptive intercourse • Initial examination after a sexual assault • 1–2 wk after a sexual assault
Gonorrhea	• Annual screening for sexually active women <25 y old • Women ≥25 y old with new sex partners, more than one sex partner, a sex partner with multiple sex partners, or a sex partner with a known STI • Pregnant women <25 y old and women with new sexual partners, more than one sex partner, a sex partner with multiple sex partners, or a sex partner with a known STI, at the first visit and during the third trimester • Incarcerated women <35 y old • Incarcerated men <30 y old • Urethral testing at least annually for men who have insertive intercourse • Rectal testing at least annually for men who have anal-receptive intercourse • Pharyngeal testing at least annually for men who have oral-receptive intercourse • Initial examination after a sexual assault • 1–2 wk after a sexual assault
Trichomoniasis	• Not indicated in the general population • At the first visit for HIV-positive women who are pregnant • Annual screening for women who are HIV-positive • Initial examination after a sexual assault • 1–2 wk after a sexual assault
Herpes simplex virus	• Not indicated in the general population
Syphilis	• Pregnant women at the first visit • At least annually for men who have sex with men • Universal screening of persons in correctional facilities, based on prevalence in the facility and local area • Initial examination after a sexual assault • 4–6 wk after a sexual assault
HIV	• All adolescents • Pregnant women at the first visit • At least annually for men who have sex with men if he or his partner has had more than one partner and HIV status is unknown • All people seeking STI treatment • All people 13–64 y old • Initial examination after a sexual assault • 6 wk after a sexual assault • 3–6 mo after a sexual assault
HPV	• See the cervical cancer screening section earlier in the chapter for information about high-risk HPV screening. • Visual examination for warts from low-risk HPV 1–2 mo after a sexual assault

Table 26.6 Centers for Disease Control and Prevention STI Screening Recommendations (continued)

Infection	Recommended Screening
Hepatitis B virus	• All pregnant women (for HBsAg) at the first visit, regardless of past testing or vaccination • Past and current drug users • Unvaccinated sex partners and household and needle-sharing partners of people who test positive for hepatitis B virus • Initial examination after a sexual assault
Hepatitis C virus	• All pregnant women with current or past injection drug use, a blood transfusion or organ transplantation prior to 1992, an unregulated tattoo, long-term hemodialysis, or intranasal drug use, at the first visit • Past and current drug users • Blood transfusions and/or organ transplantations prior to 1992 • Long-term hemodialysis • Born to a mother with hepatitis C virus • Intranasal drug use • Unregulated tattoo • All persons born from 1945 to 1965 • Individuals who test positive for HIV

STI, sexually transmitted infection; HIV, human immunodeficiency virus; HPV, human papillomavirus; HBsAg, hepatitis B virus surface antigen.
Adapted from Workowski, K. A. (2015). Centers for Disease Control and Prevention sexually transmitted diseases treatment guidelines. *Clinical Infectious Diseases, 61* Suppl. 8, S759–S762. doi:10.1093/cid/civ771.

care for LGBTQ patients, see Chapter 30). Note that people may also identify as asexual, meaning they are not interested in having sex with anyone.

Sexual Assault

An unwelcome sexual act performed on one person by another person is **sexual assault**. In the United States, 18% to 19% of women are sexually assaulted during their lifetime (Breiding et al., 2014). Acute evaluation and treatment of women after sexual assault is detailed in Chapter 30. Nurses should be aware that victims of sexual assault are at a higher risk for posttraumatic stress disorder, anxiety, depression, and suicide. They are more likely to misuse prescription medications. They are at an increased risk for pelvic pain, dyspareunia (pain with sex), urinary tract infections, and cervical cancer. Pelvic examinations may trigger anxiety and posttraumatic stress disorder in victims of sexual assault, putting them at a higher risk for inadequate screening for cervical cancer (Jina & Thomas, 2013). For more about sexual assault, see Chapter 30.

Screening for STIs

Screening for STIs is based on risk in accordance with sexual activity and sex. All individuals should be screened according to their sexual activity and anatomy present. Table 26.6 reviews screening guidelines put forth by the Centers for Disease Control and Prevention (Workowski, 2015). For more information about STIs, including prevention, assessment, clinical presentation, and treatment, see Chapter 28.

Think Critically

1. You have a patient who is accustomed to having a yearly Pap test, despite never having had an abnormal result. She is surprised when you tell her she only needs a Pap smear with human papillomavirus (HPV) testing every 5 years. How do you explain the change in guidelines to her?
2. You are on the phone with a patient who has a new diagnosis of HPV but a normal Pap test. How do you explain these findings to her?
3. You have a patient who calls you, concerned that her mammogram report includes information about her breasts being dense. How do you explain to her the significance of this finding?
4. Why would it be important to know if a patient was a victim of sexual assault?
5. How would you explain the difference between a macronutrient and a micronutrient?
6. Why is it important to know someone's natal sex and gender identity?
7. Brainstorm three different things you can do as a nurse to be more inclusive of individuals who identify as transgender.

References

American College of Obstetricians and Gynecologists. (2010). ACOG committee opinion no. 463: Cervical cancer in adolescents: Screening, evaluation, and management. *Obstetrics and Gynecology, 116*(2 Pt 1), 469–472. doi:10.1097/AOG.0b013e3181eeb30f

American College of Obstetricians and Gynecologists. (2016). Practice bulletin no. 168: Cervical cancer screening and prevention. *Obstetrics and Gynecology, 128*(4), e111–e130. doi:10.1097/AOG.0000000000001708

Aitken, M., VanderLaan, D. P., Wasserman, L., Stojanovski, S., & Zucker, K. J. (2016). Self-harm and suicidality in children referred for gender dysphoria. *Journal of the American Academy of Child and Adolescent Psychiatry, 55*(6), 513–520. doi:10.1016/j.jaac.2016.04.001

Alpert, E. (2015). *Intimate partner violence: A clinician's guide to identification, assessment, intervention, and prevention.* Retrieved from http://www.massmed.org/partnerviolence/

American Psychiatric Association. (2013). Gender dysphoria. In *Diagnostic and statistical manual of mental disorders* (5th ed., p. 451). Arlington, VA: Author.

Ashur, M. L. (1993). Asking about domestic violence: SAFE questions. *JAMA, 269*(18), 2367.

Bellavia, A., Larsson, S. C., Bottai, M., Wolk, A., & Orsini, N. (2014). Differences in survival associated with processed and with nonprocessed red meat consumption. *American Journal of Clinical Nutrition, 100*(3), 924–929. doi:10.3945/ajcn.114.086249

Bhupathiraju, S. N., Tobias, D. K., Malik, V. S., Pan, A., Hruby, A., Manson, J. E., . . . Hu, F. B. (2014). Glycemic index, glycemic load, and risk of type 2 diabetes: Results from 3 large US cohorts and an updated meta-analysis. *American Journal of Clinical Nutrition, 100*(1), 218–232. doi:10.3945/ajcn.113.079533

Bleyer, A., & Welch, H. G. (2012). Effect of three decades of screening mammography on breast-cancer incidence. *New England Journal of Medicine, 367*(21), 1998–2005. doi:10.1056/NEJMoa1206809

Breiding, M. J., Smith, S. G., Basile, K. C., Walters, M. L., Chen, J., & Merrick, M. T. (2014). Prevalence and characteristics of sexual violence, stalking, and intimate partner violence victimization—National intimate partner and sexual violence survey, United States, 2011. *MMWR Surveillance Summaries, 63*(8), 1–18.

Castle, P. E., Fetterman, B., Akhtar, I., Husain, M., Gold, M. A., Guido, R., . . . Kinney, W. (2009). Age-appropriate use of human papillomavirus vaccines in the U.S. *Gynecologic Oncology, 114*(2), 365–369. doi:10.1016/j.ygyno.2009.04.035

Centers for Disease Control and Prevention. (2013). Human papillomavirus vaccination coverage among adolescent girls, 2007–2012, and postlicensure vaccine safety monitoring, 2006–2013—United States. *Morbidity and Mortality Weekly Report (MMWR), 62*(29), 591–595.

Centers for Disease Control and Prevention. (2017). *Human papillomavirus (HPV).* Retrieved from https://www.cdc.gov/std/hpv/stdfact-hpv.htm

Chowdhury, R., Warnakula, S., Kunutsor, S., Crowe, F., Ward, H. A., Johnson, L., . . . Di Angelantonio, E. (2014). Association of dietary, circulating, and supplement fatty acids with coronary risk: A systematic review and meta-analysis. *Annals of Internal Medicine, 160*(6), 398–406. doi:10.7326/M13-1788

Cotton, M. A., Ball, C., & Robinson, P. (2003). Four simple questions can help screen for eating disorders. *Journal of General Internal Medicine, 18*(1), 53–56.

Couch, F. J., Nathanson, K. L., & Offit, K. (2014). Two decades after BRCA: Setting paradigms in personalized cancer care and prevention. *Science, 343*(6178), 1466–1470. doi:10.1126/science.1251827

Ekelund, U., Steene-Johannessen, J., Brown, W. J., Fagerland, M. W., Owen, N., Powell, K. E., . . . Lee, I. M.; Lancet Sedentary Behaviour Working Group. (2016). Does physical activity attenuate, or even eliminate, the detrimental association of sitting time with mortality? A harmonised meta-analysis of data from more than 1 million men and women. *The Lancet, 388*(10051), 1302–1310. doi:10.1016/S0140-6736(16)30370-1

Etemadi, A., Sinha, R., Ward, M. H., Graubard, B. I., Inoue-Choi, M., Dawsey, S. M., & Abnet, C. C. (2017). Mortality from different causes associated with meat, heme iron, nitrates, and nitrites in the NIH-AARP Diet and Health Study: Population based cohort study. *BMJ, 357*, j1957. doi:10.1136/bmj.j1957

Farvid, M. S., Ding, M., Pan, A., Sun, Q., Chiuve, S. E., Steffen, L. M., . . . Hu, F. B. (2014). Dietary linoleic acid and risk of coronary heart disease: A systematic review and meta-analysis of prospective cohort studies. *Circulation, 130*(18), 1568–1578. doi:10.1161/CIRCULATIONAHA.114.010236

Feldhaus, K. M., Koziol-McLain, J., Amsbury, H. L., Norton, I. M., Lowenstein, S. R., & Abbott, J. T. (1997). Accuracy of 3 brief screening questions for detecting partner violence in the emergency department. *JAMA, 277*(17), 1357–1361.

Gierach, G. L., Ichikawa, L., Kerlikowske, K., Brinton, L. A., Farhat, G. N., Vacek, P. M., . . . Sherman, M. E. (2012). Relationship between mammographic density and breast cancer death in the Breast Cancer Surveillance Consortium. *Journal of the National Cancer Institute, 104*(16), 1218–1227. doi:10.1093/jnci/djs327

Gilkey, M. B., & McRee, A. L. (2016). Provider communication about HPV vaccination: A systematic review. *Human Vaccines and Immunotherapeutics, 12*(6), 1454–1468. doi:10.1080/21645515.2015.1129090

Guallar, E., Stranges, S., Mulrow, C., Appel, L. J., & Miller, E. R., III. (2013). Enough is enough: Stop wasting money on vitamin and mineral supplements. *Annals of Internal Medicine, 159*(12), 850–851. doi:10.7326/0003-4819-159-12-201312170-00011

Hartley, L., May, M. D., Loveman, E., Colquitt, J. L., & Rees, K. (2016). Dietary fibre for the primary prevention of cardiovascular disease. *Cochrane Database of Systematic Reviews*, (1), CD011472. doi:10.1002/14651858.CD011472.pub2

Healthy People 2020. (2017). *2020 topics and objectives.* Retrieved from https://www.healthypeople.gov/2020/topics-objectives

Huo, D., Anderson, D., Palmer, J. R., & Herbst, A. L. (2017). Incidence rates and risks of diethylstilbestrol-related clear-cell adenocarcinoma of the vagina and cervix: Update after 40-year follow-up. *Gynecologic Oncology, 146*(3), 566–571. doi:10.1016/j.ygyno.2017.06.028

Imamura, F., Micha, R., Wu, J. H., de Oliveira Otto, M. C., Otite, F. O., Abioye, A. I., & Mozaffarian, D. (2016). Effects of saturated fat, polyunsaturated fat, monounsaturated fat, and carbohydrate on glucose-insulin homeostasis: A systematic review and meta-analysis of randomised controlled feeding trials. *PLoS Medicine, 13*(7), e1002087. doi:10.1371/journal.pmed.1002087

Jena, A. B., Goldman, D. P., & Seabury, S. A. (2015). Incidence of sexually transmitted infections after human papillomavirus vaccination among adolescent females. *JAMA Internal Medicine, 175*(4), 617–623. doi:10.1001/jamainternmed.2014.7886

Jina, R., & Thomas, L. S. (2013). Health consequences of sexual violence against women. *Best Practice and Research. Clinical Obstetrics and Gynaecology, 27*(1), 15–26. doi:10.1016/j.bpobgyn.2012.08.012

Kim, Y., & Je, Y. (2014). Dietary fiber intake and total mortality: A meta-analysis of prospective cohort studies. *American Journal of Epidemiology, 180*(6), 565–573. doi:10.1093/aje/kwu174

Kyrgiou, M., Mitra, A., Arbyn, M., Stasinou, S. M., Martin-Hirsch, P., Bennett, P., & Paraskevaidis, E. (2014). Fertility and early pregnancy outcomes after treatment for cervical intraepithelial neoplasia: Systematic review and meta-analysis. *BMJ, 349*, g6192. doi:10.1136/bmj.g6192

Lee, I. M., Shiroma, E. J., Lobelo, F., Puska, P., Blair, S. N., Katzmarzyk, P. T., & Lancet Physical Activity Series Working Group. (2012). Effect of physical inactivity on major non-communicable diseases worldwide: An analysis of burden of disease and life expectancy. *The Lancet, 380*(9838), 219–229. doi:10.1016/S0140-6736(12)61031-9

Leung Yinko, S. S., Stark, K. D., Thanassoulis, G., & Pilote, L. (2014). Fish consumption and acute coronary syndrome: A meta-analysis. *American Journal of Medicine, 127*(9), 848.e2–857.e2. doi:10.1016/j.amjmed.2014.04.016

Li, S., Flint, A., Pai, J. K., Forman, J. P., Hu, F. B., Willett, W. C., . . . Rimm, E. B. (2014). Dietary fiber intake and mortality among survivors of myocardial infarction: Prospective cohort study. *BMJ, 348*, g2659. doi:10.1136/bmj.g2659

Lin, J. S., O'Connor, E., Evans, C. V., Senger, C. A., Rowland, M. G., & Groom, H. C. (2014). Behavioral counseling to promote a healthy lifestyle in persons with cardiovascular risk factors: A systematic review for the U.S. Preventive Services Task Force. *Annals of Internal Medicine, 161*(8), 568–578. doi:10.7326/M14-0130

Markowitz, L. E., Liu, G., Hariri, S., Steinau, M., Dunne, E. F., & Unger, E. R. (2016). Prevalence of HPV after introduction of the vaccination program in the United States. *Pediatrics, 137*(3), e20151968. doi:10.1542/peds.2015-1968

Marmot, M. G., Altman, D. G., Cameron, D. A., Dewar, J. A., Thompson, S. G., & Wilcox, M. (2013). The benefits and harms of breast cancer screening: An independent review. *British Journal of Cancer, 108*(11), 2205–2240. doi:10.1038/bjc.2013.177

Mavaddat, N., Peock, S., Frost, D., Ellis, S., Platte, R., Fineberg, E., . . . Easton, D. F.; EMBRACE. (2013). Cancer risks for BRCA1 and BRCA2 mutation carriers: Results from prospective analysis of EMBRACE. *Journal of the National Cancer Institute, 105*(11), 812–822. doi:10.1093/jnci/djt095

McFarlane, J., Parker, B., Soeken, K., & Bullock, L. (1992). Assessing for abuse during pregnancy. Severity and frequency of injuries and associated entry into prenatal care. *JAMA, 267*(23), 3176–3178.

Miller, A. B., Wall, C., Baines, C. J., Sun, P., To, T., & Narod, S. A. (2014). Twenty five year follow-up for breast cancer incidence and mortality of the Canadian National Breast Screening Study: Randomised screening trial. *BMJ, 348*, g366. doi:10.1136/bmj.g366

Mintz, L. B., & O'Halloran, M. S. (2000). The Eating Attitudes Test: Validation with DSM-IV eating disorder criteria. *Journal of Personality Assessment, 74*(3), 489–503. doi:10.1207/S15327752JPA7403_11

Mirrahimi, A., Chiavaroli, L., Srichaikul, K., Augustin, L. S., Sievenpiper, J. L., Kendall, C. W., & Jenkins, D. J. (2014). The role of glycemic index and glycemic load in cardiovascular disease and its risk factors: A review of the recent literature. *Current Atherosclerosis Reports, 16*(1), 381. doi:10.1007/s11883-013-0381-1

Moreira, E. D., Jr., Block, S. L., Ferris, D., Giuliano, A. R., Iversen, O. E., Joura, E. A., . . . Luxembourg, A. (2016). Safety profile of the 9-valent HPV vaccine: A combined analysis of 7 phase III clinical trials. *Pediatrics, 138*(2). doi:10.1542/peds.2015-4387

Morgan, J. F., Reid, F., & Lacey, J. H. (1999). The SCOFF questionnaire: Assessment of a new screening tool for eating disorders. *BMJ, 319*(7223), 1467–1468.

Moyer, V. A., & U.S. Preventive Services Task Force. (2012a). Behavioral counseling interventions to promote a healthful diet and physical activity for cardiovascular disease prevention in adults: U.S. Preventive Services Task Force recommendation statement. *Annals of Internal Medicine, 157*(5), 367–371. doi:10.7326/0003-4819-157-5-201209040-00486

Moyer, V. A., & U.S. Preventive Services Task Force. (2012b). Screening for cervical cancer: U.S. Preventive Services Task Force recommendation statement. *Annals of Internal Medicine, 156*(12), 880–891, W312. doi:10.7326/0003-4819-156-12-201206190-00424

Moyer, V. A., & U.S. Preventive Services Task Force. (2013). Screening for intimate partner violence and abuse of elderly and vulnerable adults: U.S. Preventive Services Task Force recommendation statement. *Annals of Internal Medicine, 158*(6), 478–486. doi:10.7326/0003-4819-158-6-201303190-00588

National Breast Cancer Coalition. (2011). *Breast self-exam: Position statement.* Retrieved from http://www.breastcancerdeadline2020.org/breast-cancer-information/breast-cancer-information-and-positions/bse-position.pdf

National Comprehensive Cancer Network. (2016). *Genetic/familial high-risk assessment: Breast and ovarian. NCCN Guidelines for detection, prevention, & risk reduction. Version 2.* Retrieved from www.nccn.org/professionals/physician_gls/pdf/genetics_screening.pdf

National Institutes of Health. (2013). *Cervical cancer.* Retrieved from https://report.nih.gov/nihfactsheets/viewfactsheet.aspx?csid=76

O'Doherty, L., Hegarty, K., Ramsay, J., Davidson, L. L., Feder, G., & Taft, A. (2015). Screening women for intimate partner violence in healthcare settings. *Cochrane Database of Systematic Reviews,* (7), CD007007. doi:10.1002/14651858.CD007007.pub3

Pace, L. E., & Keating, N. L. (2014). A systematic assessment of benefits and risks to guide breast cancer screening decisions. *JAMA, 311*(13), 1327–1335. doi:10.1001/jama.2014.1398

Ponka, D., & Dickinson, J. (2014). Screening with the Pap test. *Canadian Medical Association Journal, 186*(18), 1394. doi:10.1503/cmaj.141199

Reisner, S. L., Biello, K. B., White Hughto, J. M., Kuhns, L., Mayer, K. H., Garofalo, R., & Mimiaga, M. J. (2016). Psychiatric diagnoses and comorbidities in a diverse, multicity cohort of young transgender women: Baseline findings from project LifeSkills. *JAMA Pediatrics, 170*(5), 481–486. doi:10.1001/jamapediatrics.2016.0067

Reisner, S. L., Katz-Wise, S. L., Gordon, A. R., Corliss, H. L., & Austin, S. B. (2016). Social epidemiology of depression and anxiety by gender identity. *Journal of Adolescent Health, 59*(2), 203–208. doi:10.1016/j.jadohealth.2016.04.006

Saad, R. S., Dabbs, D. J., Kordunsky, L., Kanbour-Shakir, A., Silverman, J. F., Liu, Y., & Kanbour, A. (2006). Clinical significance of cytologic diagnosis of atypical squamous cells, cannot exclude high grade, in perimenopausal and postmenopausal women. *American Journal of Clinical Pathology, 126*(3), 381–388. doi:10.1309/XVB01JQYQNM7MJXU

Saslow, D., Solomon, D., Lawson, H. W., Killackey, M., Kulasingam, S. L., Cain, J., . . . Myers, E. R.; ACS-ASCCP-ASCP Cervical Cancer Guideline Committee. (2012). American Cancer Society, American Society for Colposcopy and Cervical Pathology, and American Society for Clinical Pathology screening guidelines for the prevention and early detection of cervical cancer. *CA: A Cancer Journal for Clinicians, 62*(3), 147–172. doi:10.3322/caac.21139

Scheller, N. M., Svanstrom, H., Pasternak, B., Arnheim-Dahlstrom, L., Sundstrom, K., Fink, K., & Hviid, A. (2015). Quadrivalent HPV vaccination and risk of multiple sclerosis and other demyelinating diseases of the central nervous system. *JAMA, 313*(1), 54–61. doi:10.1001/jama.2014.16946

Schwingshackl, L., & Hoffmann, G. (2013). Long-term effects of low glycemic index/load vs. high glycemic index/load diets on parameters of obesity and obesity-associated risks: A systematic review and meta-analysis. *Nutrition, Metabolism, and Cardiovascular Diseases, 23*(8), 699–706. doi:10.1016/j.numecd.2013.04.008

Sherin, K. M., Sinacore, J. M., Li, X. Q., Zitter, R. E., & Shakil, A. (1998). HITS: A short domestic violence screening tool for use in a family practice setting. *Family Medicine, 30*(7), 508–512.

Siu, A. L., & U.S. Preventive Services Task Force. (2016). Screening for breast cancer: U.S. Preventive Services Task Force Recommendation Statement. *Annals of Internal Medicine, 164*(4), 279–296. doi:10.7326/M15-2886

Smith, L. M., Kaufman, J. S., Strumpf, E. C., & Levesque, L. E. (2015). Effect of human papillomavirus (HPV) vaccination on clinical indicators of sexual behaviour among adolescent girls: The Ontario Grade 8 HPV Vaccine Cohort Study. *Canadian Medical Association Journal, 187*(2), E74–E81. doi:10.1503/cmaj.140900

Szarewski, A., & Sasieni, P. (2004). Cervical screening in adolescents—At least do no harm. *The Lancet, 364*(9446), 1642–1644. doi:10.1016/S0140-6736(04)17366-2

Taft, A., O'Doherty, L., Hegarty, K., Ramsay, J., Davidson, L., & Feder, G. (2013). Screening women for intimate partner violence in healthcare settings. *Cochrane Database of Systematic Reviews,* (4), CD007007. doi:10.1002/14651858.CD007007.pub2

Thomas, D. B., Gao, D. L., Ray, R. M., Wang, W. W., Allison, C. J., Chen, F. L., . . . Self, S. G. (2002). Randomized trial of breast self-examination in Shanghai: Final results. *Journal of the National Cancer Institute, 94*(19), 1445–1457.

Turati, F., Galeone, C., Gandini, S., Augustin, L. S., Jenkins, D. J., Pelucchi, C., & La Vecchia, C. (2015). High glycemic index and glycemic load are associated with moderately increased cancer risk. *Molecular Nutrition and Food Research, 59*(7), 1384–1394. doi:10.1002/mnfr.201400594

U.S. Department of Health and Human Services. (2008). *2008 physical activity guidelines for Americans.* Retrieved from www.health.gov/paguidelines

U.S. Department of Health and Human Services & U.S. Department of Agriculture. (2015). *2015–2020 dietary guidelines for Americans. 8th ed.* Retrieved from https://health.gov/dietaryguidelines/2015/resources/2015-2020_Dietary_Guidelines.pdf

U.S. Preventive Services Task Force. (2014). *Final recommendation statement: Breast cancer: Screening*. Retrieved from https://www.uspreventiveservicestaskforce.org/Page/Document/RecommendationStatementFinal/breast-cancer-screening

van der Kolk, D. M., de Bock, G. H., Leegte, B. K., Schaapveld, M., Mourits, M. J., de Vries, J., . . . Oosterwijk, J. C. (2010). Penetrance of breast cancer, ovarian cancer and contralateral breast cancer in BRCA1 and BRCA2 families: High cancer incidence at older age. *Breast Cancer Research and Treatment, 124*(3), 643–651. doi:10.1007/s10549-010-0805-3

Van Kriekinge, G., Castellsague, X., Cibula, D., & Demarteau, N. (2014). Estimation of the potential overall impact of human papillomavirus vaccination on cervical cancer cases and deaths. *Vaccine, 32*(6), 733–739. doi:10.1016/j.vaccine.2013.11.049

Welch, H. G., Prorok, P. C., O'Malley, A. J., & Kramer, B. S. (2016). Breast-cancer tumor size, overdiagnosis, and mammography screening effectiveness. *New England Journal of Medicine, 375*(15), 1438–1447. doi:10.1056/NEJMoa1600249

Whitfield, G. P., Pettee Gabriel, K. K., Rahbar, M. H., & Kohl, H. W., III. (2014). Application of the American Heart Association/American College of Sports Medicine Adult Preparticipation Screening Checklist to a nationally representative sample of US adults aged >=40 years from the National Health and Nutrition Examination Survey 2001 to 2004. *Circulation, 129*(10), 1113–1120. doi:10.1161/CIRCULATIONAHA.113.004160

Winter, S., Diamond, M., Green, J., Karasic, D., Reed, T., Whittle, S., & Wylie, K. (2016). Transgender people: Health at the margins of society. *The Lancet, 388*(10042), 390–400. doi:10.1016/S0140-6736(16)00683-8

Workowski, K. A. (2015). Centers for Disease Control and Prevention sexually transmitted diseases treatment guidelines. *Clinical Infectious Diseases, 61* Suppl. 8, S759–S762. doi:10.1093/cid/civ771

Wylie, K., Knudson, G., Khan, S. I., Bonierbale, M., Watanyusakul, S., & Baral, S. (2016). Serving transgender people: Clinical care considerations and service delivery models in transgender health. *The Lancet, 388*(10042), 401–411. doi:10.1016/S0140-6736(16)00682-6

Zeitler, M. S., Paine, A. D., Breitbart, V., Rickert, V. I., Olson, C., Stevens, L., . . . Davidson, L. L. (2006). Attitudes about intimate partner violence screening among an ethnically diverse sample of young women. *Journal of Adolescent Health, 39*(1), 119.e1–119.e8. doi:10.1016/j.jadohealth.2005.09.004

Zong, G., Li, Y., Wanders, A. J., Alssema, M., Zock, P. L., Willett, W. C., . . . Sun, Q. (2016). Intake of individual saturated fatty acids and risk of coronary heart disease in US men and women: Two prospective longitudinal cohort studies. *BMJ, 355*, i5796. doi:10.1136/bmj.i5796

Suggested Readings

The Fenway Institute. (2017). *The National LGBT health education center*. Retrieved from http://fenwayhealth.org/the-fenway-institute/education/the-national-lgbt-health-education-center/

U.S. Preventive Services Task Force. (2018). *Published recommendations*. Retrieved from https://www.uspreventiveservicestaskforce.org/BrowseRec/Index

Workowski, K. A., & Bolan, G. A. (2015). Sexually transmitted diseases treatment guidelines, 2015. *MMWR Recommendations and Reports, 64*, 1–137.

27

Common Gynecologic Conditions

Gynecology is the practice of healthcare that is particular to the female anatomy: the breasts, vulva, vagina, cervix, uterus, and ovaries. Often, issues of female urology, such as urinary incontinence, are also accounted for in this category. Although screening such as that detailed in the previous chapter can identify early and mitigate the effects of common gynecologic problems such as cervical cancer or breast cancer, other congenital or acquired problems cannot be screened for and may even be a normal part of the aging process.

Many women seek care from a gynecologist only if they suspect a problem, and it is not unusual for women to delay care because of fear or embarrassment. This problem is most acute for obese women, who may perceive that their weight is stigmatized by their healthcare providers. It is an important role of the nurse to treat all patients with respect and to encourage good self-care. It is also a nursing responsibility to act as an advocate for patients who may be reluctant to seek care or to advocate for themselves.

Abnormal Uterine Bleeding

To understand abnormal uterine bleeding (AUB), it is important to understand what kind of bleeding is normal. The length of a woman's menstrual cycle is defined as the number of days from the first day of one menstrual period to the first day of the next menstrual period. Normal menstrual bleeding starts every 24 to 38 days. A woman's period is considered regular if the difference between her shortest cycle and her longest cycle is no more than 7 to 9 days. For example, if there are 24 days between one period and the next, and then 30 days between the next two starts of menses, this would be considered regular. A bleeding duration of 8 days or less for a single menstrual period is considered normal. The volume of blood loss varies between women and is considered normal when it does not interfere with physical or emotional health or quality of life.

Abnormalities of Frequency

A menstrual period that starts more frequently than every 24 days is referred to as frequent uterine bleeding. A period that starts less frequently than every 38 days is referred to as infrequent uterine bleeding (note that some healthcare providers may refer to this as oligomenorrhea).

Primary amenorrhea is the lack of any period by the age of 15. Secondary amenorrhea is a condition in which a woman who previously had regular menstrual cycles has no bleeding for 3 months or longer. Amenorrhea has various causes (Fig. 27.1). Primary amenorrhea may be caused by anatomic, genetic, or hormonal abnormalities, low weight, or a delay in puberty caused by illness and is evaluated by physical examination, imaging, and laboratory studies.

The most common cause of secondary amenorrhea in women who are sexually active is pregnancy. Other causes include Asherman syndrome (uterine adhesions, usually from instrumentation): hormonal dysfunction of the thyroid, hypothalamus, pituitary gland, or ovaries; polycystic ovarian syndrome (PCOS); low body fat; excessive exercise; sudden weight loss; and severe emotional distress. Systemic illnesses, such as type 1 diabetes and celiac disease, may also cause amenorrhea.

Abnormalities of Regularity

Variation in the length of a menstrual cycle (starting with day 1 of one menses and ending with day 1 of the next menses) of 7 to 9 days is considered normal. Greater variation is more common in women at either the beginning or end of their reproductive life span. Women may also sometimes have very long or very short cycles. Long cycles may be associated with ovulatory dysfunction. A majority of the variation in cycle length occurs in the time between the beginning of menstruation and the beginning of ovulation. The time between ovulation and menstruation is approximately 14 days. Thus, very long cycles suggest delayed or absent ovulation. Shorter cycles, particularly those occurring later in a woman's reproductive life span, often occur during the transition to menopause and is more associated with a shortened luteal phase (the time between ovulation and the start of the next menses).

Abnormalities of Duration

Menstrual bleeding that consistently lasts longer than 8 days per period is referred to as prolonged menstrual bleeding, which often co-occurs with heavy menstrual bleeding. Brief menstrual bleeding is not considered pathologic; there is no lower limit on how little bleeding is considered normal beyond amenorrhea.

Abnormalities of Volume

What defines heavy menstrual bleeding is largely subjective and often reported by the patient as a volume of bleeding that interferes with physical or emotional well-being or quality of life. Women with heavy bleeding may complain of fatigue and menstrual pain (dysmenorrhea). Light menstrual bleeding is a rare clinical complaint. When perceived by the patient as a change, it may be associated with hormonal contraception. In some cases, light menstrual bleeding may be caused by cervical stenosis (failure of the cervix to open) or Asherman syndrome. Nurses should be aware that that the blood component of menstrual discharge makes up only 30% to 50% of the total volume and that blood in the toilet may appear to be higher in volume than it actually is, because of being diluted by water.

Bleeding Between Periods

Bleeding between periods is referred to as intermenstrual bleeding and may be difficult to differentiate from frequent menstrual bleeding. Bleeding may also be from a site other than the endometrium, such as lesions of the cervix or the vaginal walls. For some women, intermenstrual bleeding may be regular and predictable and occur at a certain point in the menstrual cycle; in this case, it is referred to as cyclic intermenstrual bleeding. Some women, for example, may experience scant bleeding with ovulation. For other women, intermenstrual bleeding may be irregular, in which case it is referred to as acyclic bleeding. Both cyclic and acyclic intermenstrual bleeding may be caused by benign or malignant lesions of the cervix or endometrium. Acyclic intermenstrual bleeding may also be caused by genital tract infections such as chlamydia.

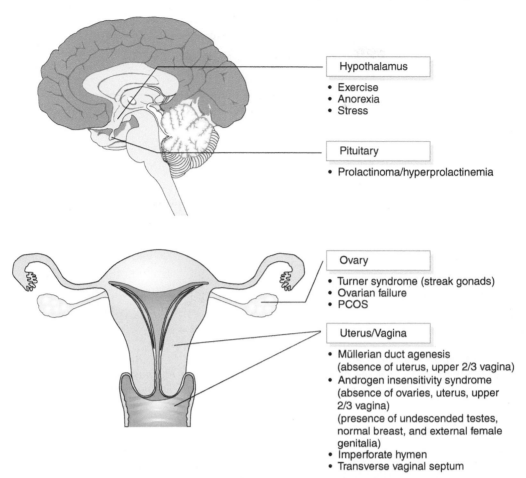

Figure 27.1. Causes of amenorrhea within the hypothalamic–pituitary–ovarian–uterine framework. Stress, exercise, and anorexia act at the level of the hypothalamus to stop the menstrual cycle. Prolactin tumors at the pituitary level disrupt the neuroendocrine regulation of gonadotropin-releasing hormone, resulting in an abnormal menstrual function. At the ovarian level, ovarian failure, polycystic ovary syndrome, and streak gonads of Turner syndrome result in menstrual dysfunction. Müllerian duct agenesis, imperforate hymen, and androgen insensitivity syndrome are abnormalities at the uterine and vaginal level. PCOS, polycystic ovary syndrome. (Reprinted with permission from McInnis, M. [2015]. *Step-up to USMLE step 1 2015* [7th ed., Fig. 8-8]. Philadelphia, PA: Lippincott Williams & Wilkins.)

Causes of AUB: PALM-COEIN Classification System

AUB that consists of heavy menstrual bleeding or bleeding between periods (intermenstrual bleeding) is summarized in the PALM-COEIN classification system (Fig. 27.2; American College of Obstetricians and Gynecologists [ACOG], 2013a). The cause of bleeding may be structural (polyp, adenomyosis, leiomyoma, or malignancy or hyperplasia) or nonstructural (coagulopathy, ovulatory dysfunction, endometrial causes, iatrogenic causes, or causes not yet classified). Note that the PALM-COEIN classification system applies only to women who are not pregnant and are of reproductive age.

Polyps (AUB-P)

Polyps that cause AUB are benign tumors of the cervix or the endometrium (Fig. 27.3). Cervical polyps are typically readily visualized during a speculum examination. Endometrial polyps may prolapse through the cervical os and also be visualized during a speculum examination, although imaging of the uterus may be required for identification.

Cervical polyps are more common in women over the age of 40 and are usually less than 3 cm in diameter. They are typically removed in the office if they are causing symptoms such as bleeding and discharge or if they appear abnormal, and removal is painless. Although polyps are rarely malignant, they are typically sent to the laboratory for confirmation.

Endometrial polyps are most common in women of later reproductive age and occur less frequently after menopause. Risk factors include obesity and hormonal replacement post menopause. Endometrial polyps are usually identified during assessment for AUB or infertility but may be found incidentally. Most women with symptomatic polyps complain of intermenstrual or postmenstrual bleeding. Endometrial polyps are diagnosed by a pathologist after an endometrial biopsy or polypectomy (removal of a polyp or polyps). A vast majority are benign. However, endometrial polyps must also be evaluated by a pathologist to confirm the diagnosis.

> **Abnormal uterine bleeding:**
> - Heavy menstrual bleeding (AUB/HMB)
> - Intermenstrual bleeding (AUB/IMB)

> **PALM—structural causes:**
> **P**olyp (AUB-P)
> **A**denomyosis (AUB-A)
> **L**eiomyoma (AUB-L)
>   Submucosal leiomyoma (AUB-LSM)
>   Other leiomyoma (AUB-LO)
> **M**alignancy and hyperplasia (AUB-M)

> **COEIN—nonstructural causes:**
> **C**oagulopathy (AUB-C)
> **O**vulatory dysfunction (AUB-O)
> **E**ndometrial (AUB-E)
> **I**atrogenic (AUB-I)
> **N**ot yet classified (AUB-N)

Figure 27.2. FIGO classification system. (Data from Munro, M. G., Critchley, H. O., Broder, M. S., et al. [2011]. FIGO classification system (PALM-COEIN) for the causes of abnormal uterine bleeding in nongravid women of reproductive age. FIGO, Federation of Obstetricians and Gynecologists. FIGO Working Group on Menstrual Disorders. *International Journal of Gynecology and Obstetrics, 113*, 3–13.)

Adenomyosis (AUB-A)

Adenomyosis is the presence of endometrial-type tissue within the myometrium (the muscle of the uterus; Fig. 27.4). This tissue causes hypertrophy (enlargement of cells) and hyperplasia (new cell growth) in the surrounding myometrium, which results in a uterus that is concentrically enlarged up to the size of a 12-week pregnancy. Women with adenomyosis may have heavy menstrual bleeding and dysmenorrhea (pain with menses). Some women may experience chronic pelvic pain related to adenomyosis. Although adenomyosis may occur in women at any time during their reproductive life span, it is most commonly reported in women aged 40 to 50 years and often co-occurs with uterine fibroids.

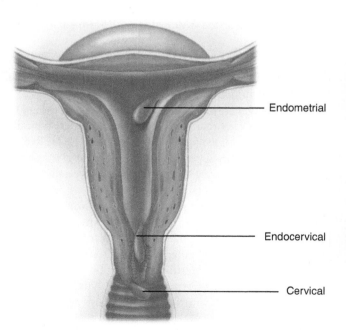

Figure 27.3. Cervical, endocervical, and endometrial polyps. (Reprinted with permission from Ricci, S. S. [2013]. *Essentials of maternity, newborn, & women's health nursing* [3rd ed., Fig. 7.3]. Philadelphia, PA: Lippincott Williams & Wilkins.)

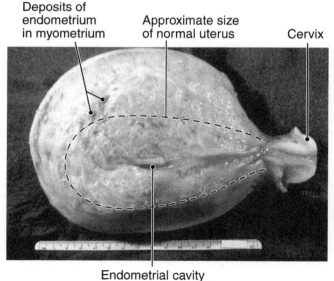

Figure 27.4. Adenomyosis. The enlargement of this uterus is caused by endometrial implants in the myometrium. Dotted lines indicate the normal size of the uterus. (Reprinted with permission from McConnell, T. H. [2014]. *The nature of disease: Pathology for the health professions* [2nd ed., Fig. 17.23]. Philadelphia, PA: Lippincott Williams & Wilkins.)

Although a definitive diagnosis of adenomyosis is made by a pathologist, heavy menstrual bleeding with dysmenorrhea and a uniformly enlarged uterus is highly suggestive of the condition. Further information may be gained by imaging of the uterus. Adenomyosis may be treated conservatively with hormonal contraceptives, such as the combined oral contraceptive or a levonorgestrel intrauterine device, or surgically with uterine artery embolization or hysterectomy.

Leiomyomas (AUB-L)

Leiomyomas are benign tumors of the uterus. They are also referred to as uterine fibroids or uterine myomas. Fibroids arise in women of reproductive age from the muscular layer of the uterus, the myometrium. When symptomatic, leiomyomas manifest as abnormal, often very heavy, uterine bleeding and pelvic pain or pressure. They may also contribute to subfertility and pregnancy complications. They have no malignant potential.

Leiomyomas are described in four main categories according to location: submucosal, intramural, subserosal, and cervical (Fig. 27.5). Submucosal leiomyomas occur just below the endometrium and protrude into the uterine cavity. Submucosal leiomyomas are a major source of abnormally heavy bleeding, particularly for women in perimenopause. Intramural leiomyomas are located within the wall of the uterus and can become so large as to distort the uterus. Subserosal leiomyomas arise just below the serosal surface (the outer lining of the uterus). Subserosal leiomyomas, just like some submucosal leiomyomas, may be pedunculated and move freely within the abdominal cavity within the limits of their stalks. Cervical leiomyomas arise from the cervix rather than the body of the uterus.

Leiomyomas become increasingly common with age and are typically asymptomatic. Although 70% or more of women develop fibroids during their lifetime, only a minority of those who do develop them report associated symptoms such as bleeding and pelvic pain or pressure. Leiomyomas typically regress with menopause. Although most leiomyomas are small and asymptomatic, they are clinically apparent by symptoms, uterine enlargement, or ultrasound in nearly 50% of perimenopausal women of African descent and 35% of perimenopausal women of European descent (Butt, Jeffery, & Van der Spuy, 2012). Various genetic, hormonal, and nutritional factors may reduce or increase the risk for clinically significant fibroids.

Abnormal bleeding and menstrual cramps are the most common symptoms from leiomyomas, although abdominal pain and a sensation of tightness or pressure may also be reported. The abnormal bleeding associated with leiomyomas is typically heavy and prolonged menses. Bleeding and menstrual cramping may be significant enough to lead to anemia, embarrassment from bleeding through clothing, and lost productivity due to temporary incapacitation. Although submucosal fibroids (the ones immediately adjacent to the endometrium) are most frequently associated with heavy menses, intramural and cervical leiomyomas may also be a cause, and subserosal leiomyomas are less likely to contribute.

The sensation of pelvic pressure and pain and leiomyoma-related issues of the urinary tract and bowel, including urinary frequency and constipation, are due to the bulk of large fibroids. A very large leiomyoma may even enlarge the uterus enough that it compresses the vena cava and increases the risk of a thromboembolism (Rosenfeld & Byard, 2012). Rarely, pain may be caused by degeneration of the fibroid or twisting and torsion of a pedunculated fibroid.

Leiomyomas that distort the uterine cavity can result in miscarriage and subfertility. Despite the perception that leiomyomas grow in pregnancy, they generally remain stable in size (Ciavattini et al., 2016). Pain is the most common fibroid symptom in pregnancy, particularly for women with fibroids that are 5 cm or larger. Pain is more likely to appear in the first half of pregnancy. There is also a small increased risk of preterm labor and birth. The risk of

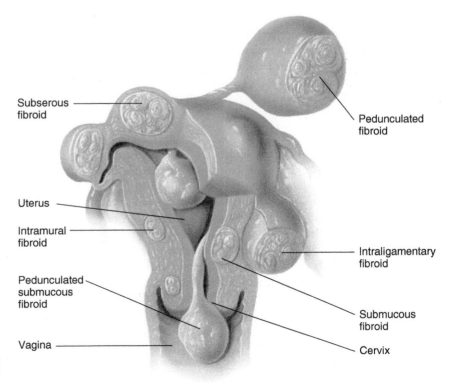

Figure 27.5. Varieties of uterine leiomyomas. (Reprinted with permission from Anatomical Chart Company.)

Subserous fibroid

Pedunculated fibroid

Uterus

Intramural fibroid

Intraligamentary fibroid

Pedunculated submucous fibroid

Submucous fibroid

Vagina

Cervix

antepartum bleeding and placental abruption is also higher for women with leiomyomas, particularly if the placenta overlies a submucosal fibroid. A leiomyoma that distorts the uterine cavity may lead to malpresentation of the fetus. Dysfunctional labor and uterine tachysystole are also more common among women with leiomyomas. Such factors lead to an increased rate of cesarean delivery, particularly for women in whom the leiomyoma or leiomyomas are located in the lower uterine segment (Michels, Velez Edwards, Baird, Savitz, & Hartmann, 2014).

The diagnosis of a leiomyoma or leiomyomas is usually made by pelvic and abdominal examination and pelvic imaging after a patient report of heavy and prolonged menses, a sensation of pelvic pain or pressure, or infertility. The size of the leiomyoma is typically reported in reference to uterine distortion and uterine size at pregnancy. Thus, a uterus enlarged such that the fundus is at the umbilicus would be referred to as 20-week size.

Although uterine leiomyomas typically shrink and become asymptomatic with menopause, earlier treatment may be indicated when the presence of leiomyomas has a significant impact on health and/or quality of life. Estrogen–progestin contraceptives, progestin implants, and progesterone-releasing intrauterine contraceptive devices are often used as a first-line treatment of fibroids. Gonadotropin-releasing hormone (GnRH) agonists are a more effective treatment but have significant hypoestrogenic side effects, including hot flashes, vaginal dryness, joint and muscle pain, and sleep disturbance as well as significant bone loss when used for a year or more. Because of this, GnRH agonists are primarily used in the short term preoperatively to correct anemia and reduce the size of the leiomyoma.

Hysterectomy is the most common type of surgery used to treat leiomyomas and is particularly preferred by women who do not wish to preserve fertility. Myomectomy, removal of fibroids alone, is another surgical option for women who have not completed childbearing or who wish to retain their uterus. Endometrial ablation, which may be done in the hospital or on an outpatient basis with heat or cryotherapy, is another option for women who wish to retain their uterus but have completed childbearing. Other procedures that allow for localized destruction of the leiomyomas or occlusion of blood flow to leiomyomas may be alternatively proposed.

Malignancy and Hyperplasia (AUB-M)

Postmenstrual bleeding and intermenstrual or heavy menstrual bleeding that are otherwise unexplained are suspicious for hyperplasia and malignancy of the endometrium. Up to 15% of women with postmenopausal bleeding are diagnosed with endometrial hyperplasia, and up to 5% to 10% are diagnosed with endometrial cancer (Cote et al., 2014).

Hyperplasia (abnormal proliferation of endometrial glands) can be identified by ultrasound. Hyperplasia may occur without atypia (nonneoplastic) or with atypia (endometrial intraepithelial neoplasm; Emons, Beckmann, Schmidt, Mallmann, & Uterus Commission of the Gynecological Oncology Working, 2015). Differentiating between the two types requires a biopsy of the endometrium. Endometrial biopsy is done by passing a curettage through the cervix to collect a sample (Fig. 27.6). Hyperplasia may coexist with endometrial carcinoma or progress to endometrial

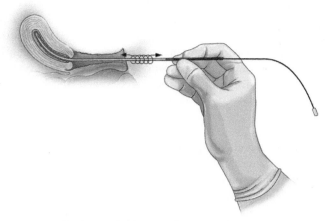

Figure 27.6. Endometrial biopsy. The practitioner uses a combination of rotating and in-and-out movements of the sampling device to obtain an endometrial biopsy specimen. (Reprinted with permission from Mayeaux, E. J. [2009]. Endometrial biopsy. In E. J. Mayeaux [Ed.], *The essential guide to primary care procedures.* Philadelphia, PA: Lippincott Williams & Wilkins.)

carcinoma. Hyperplasia with atypia is more likely to progress to carcinoma than hyperplasia without atypia. The main risk factor for hyperplasia is exposure to continuous estrogen unopposed by progestin. Obesity is a common source of unopposed estrogen.

A majority of women with cancer of the endometrium present with AUB (Fig. 27.7). Approximately 17% of endometrial carcinomas occur in women aged 45 years to menopausal, and 5% occur in women aged 35 to 44 years, with the remainder occurring

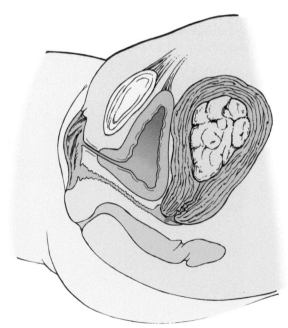

Figure 27.7. Uterine enlargement and bleeding due to uterine cancer (cancer of the endometrium). The uterus may be enlarged with a malignant mass. Irregular bleeding, bleeding between periods, or postmenopausal bleeding may be the first sign of a problem. (Reprinted with permission from Weber, J. R., & Kelley, J. H. [2003]. *Health assessment in nursing with case studies on bonus CD-ROM* [2nd ed., Fig. 20.8]. Philadelphia, PA: Lippincott Williams & Wilkins.)

in women who are postmenopausal (National Cancer Institute). Bleeding is the cardinal sign of endometrial cancer in women who are postmenopausal. Endometrial cancer should be suspected for women younger than 45 years with persistent AUB with unopposed estrogen exposure (due most often to obesity or chronic anovulation) or for whom medical management of AUB has failed. Women aged 45 years to menopausal with AUB should also be assessed for endometrial cancer, particularly those with frequent menses, intermenstrual bleeding, or heavy or prolonged flow. Occasionally, endometrial cancer may be identified by Papanicolaou (Pap) test. Nurses should be aware that a Pap test is not considered sensitive for detecting endometrial cancer and that an endometrial biopsy is still required with AUB suspicious for endometrial cancer.

Although most cancers of the uterus arise from the endometrium and are adenocarcinomas (glandular cancers), a small minority are sarcomas (cancer arising from connective tissue such as muscle or fat). Uterine sarcomas are more common in women over 60 years old, women of African descent, and women who received pelvic radiation or used the drug tamoxifen for 5 or more years. Up to 56% of women over 40 years old with uterine sarcomas present with AUB (Prat & Mbatani, 2015). See the Gynecologic Cancers section for more about cancers of the uterus.

Coagulopathy (AUB-C)

Up to a quarter of women with heavy menstrual bleeding have a coagulopathy, usually von Willebrand disease (ACOG, 2013b). Von Willebrand disease is a common clotting disorder that is usually hereditary but may also be acquired. It is a deficiency of the von Willebrand factor, which is required for the adhesion of platelets (Fig. 27.8). In addition to heavy menses, women with von Willebrand disease may experience excessive blood loss with childbirth, easy bruising, bleeding of the gums, and nose bleeds. Some types of von Willebrand disease may be treated with desmopressin at a time of anticipated bleeding, such as prior to surgery or dental work. Hormonal contraceptives are often used to treat heavy menses. Diagnosis is by careful history taking and laboratory assessment.

Ovulatory Dysfunction (AUB-O)

AUB from ovulatory disorders includes a cycle length that varies by more than 7 days over the course of at least 1 full year. Women with ovulatory dysfunction usually experience irregular bleeding of different volumes, from light to heavy. Ovulatory dysfunction includes anovulation (not ovulating), infrequent ovulation, and luteal out-of-phase events. Luteal out-of-phase events happen

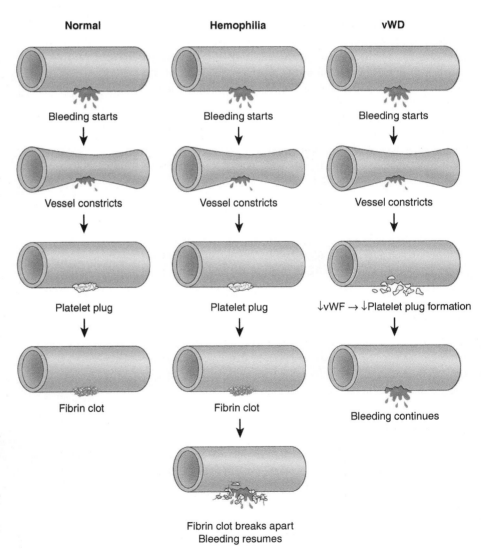

Figure 27.8. Differences in bleeding: Normal, hemophilia, and von Willebrand disease. vWD, von Willebrand disease; vWF, von Willebrand factor. (Reprinted with permission from Farrell, M. [2017]. *Smeltzer & Bare's textbook of medical-surgical nursing* [4th ed., Fig. 28.8]. Philadelphia, PA: Lippincott Williams & Wilkins.)

Box 27.1 Medications That May Cause Ovulatory Disorders

- Antidepressants
- Antipsychotics
- Corticosteroids
- Chemotherapy
- Hormonal contraceptives

more frequently in later reproductive years and are a hormonal mistiming that results in heavy menstrual bleeding.

The cause of ovulatory dysfunction often cannot be identified. Potential contributors include weight loss or gain, excessive exercise, low body fat, eating disorders, stress, some medications (Box 27.1), and endocrine abnormalities, such as hypothyroidism, hyperprolactinemia, and PCOS (see below). A careful history and evaluation that includes laboratory testing is often helpful in isolating a cause.

Endometrial Causes (AUB-E)

Women with regular menses usually ovulate normally. For women with regular menses who have heavy menstrual bleeding and sometimes intermenstrual bleeding in whom no other cause, such as coagulopathy, can be discovered, AUB-E is diagnosed. This is a diagnosis of exclusion that assumes a disorder of the endometrium to achieve hemostasis. There is no diagnostic test available (Maybin & Critchley, 2015).

Also included in the category of AUB-E is inflammation of the endometrium, such as may occur with some sexually transmitted infections such as chlamydia and gonorrhea.

Iatrogenic Causes (AUB-I)

The term iatrogenic refers to a condition that is caused by a medical examination or treatment. There is some overlap between AUB-I and AUB-O causes, as medications that cause ovulatory dysfunction can also be considered an iatrogenic cause of AUB. Other iatrogenic causes of AUB include anticoagulants and intrauterine devices.

Not Otherwise Classified (AUB-N)

The AUB-N category is reserved for causes of AUB that are poorly understood or defined, very rare, or that do not easily fit into a different category. AUB caused by malformation of the vasculature would be included in this category.

Dysmenorrhea

Dysmenorrhea is pain with menstruation that can be so severe as to limit daily activities such as work, exercise, self-care, and other responsibilities. A majority of women of reproductive age worldwide report dysmenorrhea at some point in their lives. The two categories of dysmenorrhea are primary and secondary. Primary dysmenorrhea refers to dysmenorrhea that occurs in the absence of another cause that could account for the recurrent lower abdominal pain and cramping. Primary dysmenorrhea usually begins in adolescence after the establishment of ovulation, which usually begins within 2 to 5 years after menarche (first menses). Secondary dysmenorrhea has similar symptoms but with a recognized underlying cause, such as endometriosis or adenomyosis. Dysmenorrhea occurs only in women of reproductive age and is more common in younger women (Fig. 27.9).

During menses, prostaglandins are released that induce uterine contractions that can result in a high intrauterine pressure. When the intrauterine pressures exceed arterial pressure, blood cannot reach the uterus, causing painful ischemia. Pain may begin as early as 48 hours prior to the start of menstrual bleeding, lasts for 12 to 72 hours, and occurs with all or most menses. For most women, dysmenorrhea is crampy, intermittent, and localized to the lower abdomen. For some women, however, the pain may be a continuous ache and may also refer to the back or thighs. Pain may be mild to severe and associated symptoms can include fatigue, headache, diarrhea, nausea, and malaise. For most women, primary dysmenorrhea improves after childbirth and with age.

First-line medications for the treatment of primary dysmenorrhea include nonsteroidal anti-inflammatory drugs (NSAIDs) such as ibuprofen, and hormonal contraceptives. Self-care measures

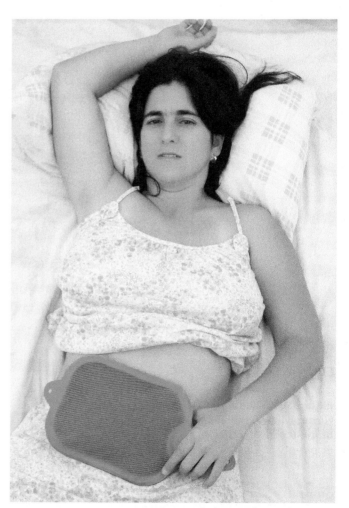

Figure 27.9. A young woman experiencing dysmenorrhea.

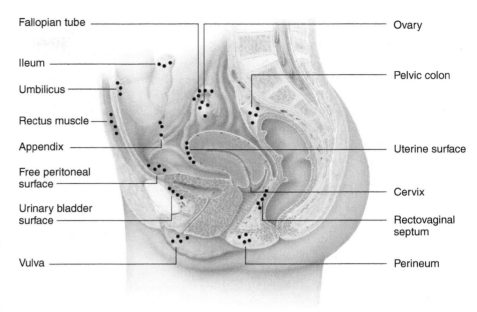

Figure 27.10. Common sites of endometriosis. Although endometriosis is most commonly found in the pelvic area, it can occur in any organ system. (Reprinted with permission from Lippincott's Nursing Advisor, 2012.)

that may offer relief include the application of heat to the lower abdomen, exercise, and orgasm. Some women may find supplementation with vitamin B_1, fish oil, vitamin B_6, and/or vitamin E helpful. Adherence to a low-fat, vegetarian diet is associated with an improvement in dysmenorrhea, as is a high intake of dairy products (three to four daily; Lee et al., 2015).

Endometriosis

Endometriosis is the presence of endometrial tissue outside of the uterus. The lesions of endometriosis are found most often in the pelvis but can be found in any organ system (Fig. 27.10). Presentation is variable but may include dysmenorrhea, dyspareunia, infertility, a pelvic mass, or other pain. It may also be an incidental finding identified at the time of surgery for an unrelated problem. Endometriosis is rarely identified prior to menarche or after menopause. The peak age for the diagnosis of endometriosis is 25 to 35 years old. Because women are often asymptomatic, it is challenging to know how prevalent the condition is. In addition, endometriosis can be definitively diagnosed only by surgery (Hickey, Ballard, & Farquhar, 2014). In one study, endometriosis was diagnosed surgically in 21% of women with pelvic pain reported prior to surgery, 57% of women with endometriosis suspected prior to surgery, and 8% of women who reported no pelvic pain prior to surgery (Mowers et al., 2016). Women with endometriosis are far less likely to report dysmenorrhea, heavy menses, or abdominopelvic pain when compared with women without endometriosis.

The cause of endometriosis is not well understood. Although endometriosis is often explained as retrograde menstruation (the exiting of menstrual products from the uterus by the fallopian tubes rather than the cervix), 10% of women with endometriosis do not have retrograde menstruation, and the presence of endometriosis in girls prior to menarche and even the occasional

person with male anatomy makes this explanation insufficient (Mowers et al., 2016). Pain caused by endometriosis is related to inflammatory changes. Infertility and subfertility related to endometriosis are caused by anatomic distortions of the structures of the pelvis and products of inflammation, including overproduction of prostaglandins and macrophages, that interfere with the function of the ovaries, fallopian tubes, and endometrium.

The findings on physical examination of women with endometriosis are often normal but may include nodules palpated during a bimanual examination (Fig. 27.11). Rarely, lesions may be seen on the cervix or vaginal wall. Laboratory testing is generally not helpful for making the diagnosis or following the course of treatment. Imaging may be useful for identifying endometriosis, but the condition is definitively diagnosed by the examination by a pathologist of tissue retrieved during surgery.

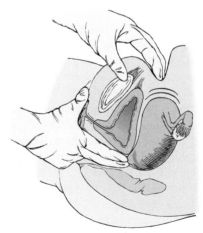

Figure 27.11. Palpating the uterus during a bimanual examination. (Reprinted with permission from Weber, J. R., & Kelley, J. H. [2014]. *Health assessment in nursing* [5th ed., Fig. 27.14]. Philadelphia, PA: Lippincott Williams & Wilkins.)

Instead of seeking a definitive diagnosis, which requires a highly invasive procedure, many women receive a presumptive diagnosis and are treated with well-tolerated, low-risk methods. Failure to respond to such treatment is an indication to exclude the diagnosis or seek a definitive surgical diagnosis prior to pursuing treatments with a higher likelihood of adverse effects (Barcellos, Lasmar, & Lasmar, 2016). Some experts in endometriosis, however, may instead diagnose endometriosis on the basis of a combination of imaging, examination, and biopsy involving less invasive routes (Vercellini et al., 2016).

First-line treatment for women with pelvic pain and a presumptive diagnosis of endometriosis is a combined oral contraceptive and an NSAID such as ibuprofen. Women for whom estrogen is contraindicated may be prescribed a progestin-only pill and an NSAID, instead. Symptoms are anticipated to improve within 3 to 4 months. Women who do not respond to treatment may be treated with a GnRH agonist, which produces a hypoestrogenic effect, which can be limited by treating simultaneously with supplemental progestin. Other options include the levonorgestrel intrauterine system, a medroxyprogesterone injection, and a contraceptive implant (see Chapter 29 for more information about the methods of contraception).

Failure of medical treatment is an indication for laparoscopy for definitive diagnosis and treatment. At the time of surgery, endometriosis lesions are removed, as are endometriomas (cysts that form on the ovaries and that arise from endometriosis lesions; also referred to as chocolate cysts). Adhesions are web-like sheets of scar tissue that can develop in the abdomen as part of the inflammatory process. They are a common result of the inflammation typical of endometriosis and are usually removed at the time of surgery but may also develop in response to other inflammation triggers, including such surgery. Because of this, adhesions that are removed during surgery often recur because of surgery. Women not wishing to preserve fertility may instead opt for the more definitive hysterectomy and bilateral oophorectomy. After surgery, hormonal contraceptives are usually started immediately to suppress recurrence in women not seeking pregnancy.

Dyspareunia

Dyspareunia (female sexual pain) is pain of the vulva, vagina, or pelvis that is either caused or made worse by sexual activity. It can impact a woman's relationship with her sexual partner, self-esteem, and quality of life. Dyspareunia has many different causes, and it is not always possible to determine the cause of a particular woman's pain. A woman may also have more than one cause of dyspareunia. Dyspareunia may range from mild to severe and may be localized or generalized. It may be temporary and fleeting or lifelong. Causes may be physical, psychological, or a combination of both. See Box 27.2 for the classifications of dyspareunia offered by the Fourth International Consultation on Sexual Medicine (McCabe et al., 2016).

Risk factors for dyspareunia include a history of sexual abuse, anxiety, depression, and pelvic inflammatory disease. Risk factors for vulvodynia (persistent vulvar pain without a known cause) include anxiety and depression. Childhood sexual abuse may also be a risk factor (Khandker, Brady, Stewart, & Harlow, 2014). The causes of female sexual pain are itemized in Box 27.3.

Box 27.2 Classifications of Dyspareunia

- Pain with vaginal penetration during intercourse
- Marked vulvovaginal or pelvic pain during genital contact (i.e., genital sexual pain)
- Marked fear or anxiety about vulvovaginal or pelvic pain in anticipation of, during, or as a result of genital contact
- Marked hypertonicity or overactivity of pelvic floor muscles with or without genital contact (i.e., vaginismus)

Box 27.3 Causes of Dyspareunia

- *Infections:* Pelvic inflammatory disease, candidiasis, bacterial vaginosis, gonorrhea, chlamydia, herpes simplex virus, or a urinary tract infection (see Chapter 28)
- *Poor lubrication and vaginal dryness:* Insufficient arousal or a side effect of hormonal contraception, breastfeeding, or menopause
- *Menopause:* Reduced elasticity of the vulva and vagina from the low estrogen state, causing a reduced capacity for the vagina to expand and elongate
- *Endometriosis:* Sexual pain that tends to be deep and may be an episodic worsening of chronic pelvic pain
- *Physical trauma:* Often from obstetrical or gynecologic surgery but may also be a result of accidental injury or sexual abuse
- *Inflammatory disorders:* Vulva—lichen sclerosus and lichen planus; bowel—inflammatory bowel disease; general—endometriosis or infection
- *Neurologic disorders:* Fibromyalgia, Parkinson disease, and multiple sclerosis
- *Psychosocial causes:* An experience of sexual pain during intercourse, as from sexual abuse, resulting in anxiety that may cause involuntary or voluntary contraction of the pelvic muscles, which can make penetration painful or even impossible (vaginismus); fear of sexual pain, inhibiting arousal, which in turn inhibits lubrication, leading to sexual pain; depression and anxiety in the absence of poor lubrication and vaginismus
- *Relationship stress*
- *Malignancy:* A malignancy of the gastrointestinal, reproductive, or urinary tract (rarely); treatments for cancer, such as radiation and surgery
- *Anatomic causes:* Pelvic pain from pelvic floor prolapse, congenital anomalies, and myofascial pelvic pain syndrome (caused by contracted bands of the skeletal muscle; pain may be episodic or continuous)

Adapted from Boomershine, C. S. (2015). Fibromyalgia: The prototypical central sensitivity syndrome. *Current Rheumatology Reviews, 11*(2), 131–145; Graziottin, A., Gambini, D., & Bertolasi, L. (2015). Genital and sexual pain in women. *Handbook of Clinical Neurology, 130,* 395–412. doi:10.1016/B978-0-444-63247-0.00023-7; Levin, R. J., Both, S., Georgiadis, J., Kukkonen, T., Park, K., & Yang, C. C. (2016). The physiology of female sexual function and the pathophysiology of female sexual dysfunction (committee 13A). *Journal of Sexual Medicine, 13*(5), 733–759. doi:10.1016/j.jsxm.2016.02.172.

An evaluation of dyspareunia includes a careful history that evaluates the timing of pain (with genital touching, with penetration, with deep thrusting, or after sex), location (vulva, perineum, introitus, or pelvis), onset, pain characteristics, pattern of pain, pain at other times besides intercourse, and pain relief measures attempted. The nurse should obtain a careful sexual history, including the patient's current sexual relationship and safety within the relationship. The nurse should ask the patient about associated symptoms, such as pain with urination, bowel changes, and vaginal odor, itching, or discharge. A thorough genital examination is performed. A laboratory testing of lesions, vaginal discharge, and urine may be ordered according to history and examination results. Imaging studies may also be indicated, particularly for deep pelvic pain. Treatment is according to the suspected or known underlying cause of dyspareunia.

Pelvic Floor Dysfunction

The pelvic organs are held in place by a combination of connective tissue and the muscles of the pelvic floor. The primary supports of the pelvic organs are the muscles of the levator ani complex, which form a kind of sling upon which the pelvic organs rest. Relaxation of or damage to the levator ani complex or the connective tissue can cause pelvic organ prolapse, in which the pelvic organs prolapse into or beyond the vagina.

Pelvic organ prolapse may involve prolapse of the bladder (cystocele), rectum (rectocele), bowel (enterocele), or uterus. Uterine prolapse is the descent of the uterus into the lower vagina or even through the introitus (Fig. 27.12). The alternate terms "anterior wall prolapse and posterior wall prolapse" are often used in place of cystocele or rectocele. The term "apical compartment

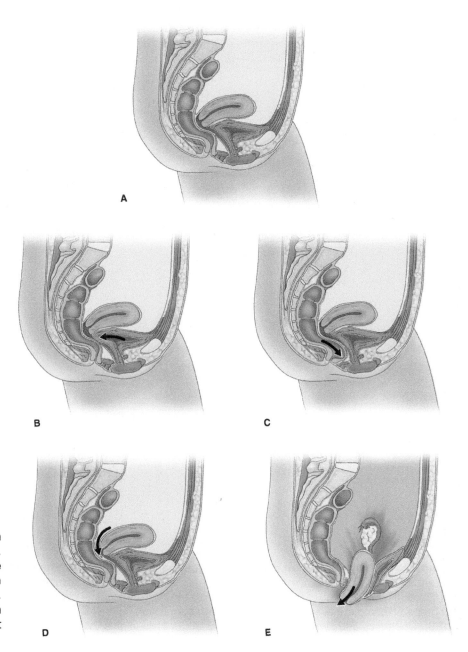

Figure 27.12. Types of pelvic organ prolapse. (A) No prolapse. **(B)** Cystocele. **(C)** Rectocele. **(D)** Enterocele. **(E)** Uterine prolapse. (Reprinted with permission from Timby, B. K., & Smith, N. E. [2018]. *Introductory medical-surgical nursing* [12th ed., Fig. 53.6]. Philadelphia, PA: Lippincott Williams & Wilkins.)

prolapse" may be used instead of uterine prolapse. Herniation of all three compartments (anterior, posterior, and apical) through the vaginal introitus is known as a uterine procidentia. Prolapse is classified according to stages, from 0 (no prolapse) to IV (complete eversion; Fig. 27.13).

The risk for pelvic floor prolapse increases with the number of births, and vaginal births are associated with a higher risk than cesarean births (Glazener et al., 2013). Prolapse is sometimes referred to as a "late complication of pregnancy," as it becomes increasingly common as women age. Obese women are as much as twice as likely to develop pelvic organ prolapse (Giri, Hartmann, Hellwege, Velez Edwards, & Edwards, 2017). Hysterectomy is associated with a higher risk of apical prolapse, as after a hysterectomy, the apex of the vagina descends toward or beyond the introitus (Grigoriadis, Valla, Zacharakis, Protopapas, & Athanasiou, 2015).

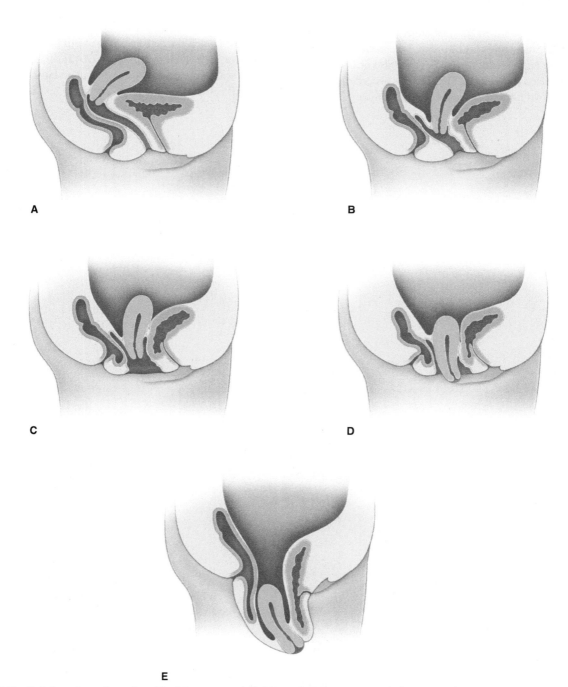

Figure 27.13. Pelvic relaxation classified by stage. (A) Stage 0 (no prolapse). **(B)** Stage I (leading edge of the prolapse is more than 1 cm above the hymen). **(C)** Stage II (leading edge of the prolapse is less than or equal to 1 cm below the hymen). **(D)** Stage III (leading edge of the prolapse is more than 1 cm beyond the hymen, but less than or equal to the total vaginal length). **(E)** Stage IV (complete eversion). (Reprinted with permission from Beckmann, C. R., Herbert, W., Laube, D., Ling, F., & Smith, R. [2013]. *Obstetrics and gynecology* [7th ed., Fig. 30.2]. Philadelphia, PA: Lippincott Williams & Wilkins.)

The clinical manifestations of organ prolapse depend on the nature of the prolapse but may be experienced as vaginal pressure, pelvic pain, a bulge at the opening of the vagina, problems with defecation or urination, or sexual dysfunction. Women may find that the symptoms worsen throughout the day as they remain upright. Up to 19% of women in the United States have surgery for urinary incontinence or other complications of pelvic floor prolapse, with 30% requiring repeat surgeries (Kurkijarvi, Aaltonen, Gissler, & Makinen, 2017).

Treatment is indicated when women express distressing symptoms, particularly obstructed urination resulting from a urethra kinked from an anterior wall prolapse or obstructed defecation resulting from a posterior wall prolapse. Conservative treatments include vaginal pessaries (space-filling devices of various shapes and sizes placed within the vagina to assist pelvic organ support; see Fig. 17.11) and pelvic floor physical therapy. Surgery may be appropriate when conservative treatments fail or are declined. The risk for recurrence of prolapse is up to 19% after surgery (Lavelle, Christie, Alhalabi, & Zimmern, 2016).

A form of pelvic floor dysfunction unrelated to pelvic organ prolapse is myofascial pain syndrome (MPPS). MPPS may occur in men or women and is characterized by tight, short pelvic floor muscles with trigger points that can cause pain that refers to the vagina, perineum, vulva, rectum, thighs, buttocks, bladder, and lower abdomen. The patient may also experience sensations of burning, itching, urinary urgency, and pain. Symptoms may be continuous or episodic, as with dyspareunia. It is a clinical diagnosis that is made after a physical examination. Initial treatment is pelvic floor physical therapy (Jafri, 2014).

Urinary Incontinence

Urinary incontinence falls into three broad categories: stress incontinence, urge incontinence, and overflow incontinence. When stress and urge incontinence co-occur, it is referred to as mixed incontinence. Incontinence can contribute to irritation and infections of the perineum related to moisture and skin breakdown. Urinary frequency, urinary urgency, and nocturia (awakening with the urge to urinate, which is typically urge and overflow incontinence) increase the risk for falls. Incontinence can contribute to sexual dysfunction because of fear or anxiety about involuntary loss of urine during sexual activity. Incontinence diminishes overall quality of life and contributes to anxiety, depression, and social isolation. Incontinence increases the burden of care giving for individuals who require assistance with the activities of daily living.

Incontinence is quite common with pregnancy. Approximately 17% of women 20 years and older experience involuntary loss of urine, with the incidence increasing as women age (Wu et al., 2014). Other risk factors include past pregnancy, obesity, vaginal birth, family history, aging, smoking, vaginal atrophy, radiation therapy, high caffeine intake, high-impact activities, fecal incontinence, and depression (Al-Mukhtar Othman, Akervall, Milsom, & Gyhagen, 2017; Matthews, Whitehead, Townsend, & Grodstein, 2013; Wu et al., 2014).

Women may be hesitant to report urinary incontinence because they are embarrassed by the condition or believe incontinence to be a normal consequence of aging. Alternatively, they may not find the involuntary loss of urine distressing. The nurse should ask women with increased risk, such as those who are obese, have pelvic organ prolapse, or are over 65 years old, about symptoms specifically. A careful history and voiding diary are important for identifying the type of incontinence and helpful interventions (Fig. 27.14). A physical examination can identify pelvic floor dysfunction as the cause, and a simple urine test can identify a urinary tract infection as the cause. Other advanced testing includes a bladder stress test, postvoid residual test, urodynamic testing, and an assessment of urethral mobility.

Stress Incontinence

Stress incontinence is the involuntary leakage of urine that occurs as a result of an increase in intraabdominal pressure. Such pressure may be from sneezing, laughing, coughing, exercise, or other exertion. The two causes are anatomic: urethral hypermobility caused by insufficient pelvic floor musculature and resulting from childbirth or the chronic pressure from obesity chronic cough, and other sources of intraabdominal pressure and the loss of urethral tone (intrinsic sphincteric deficiency), also a result of a chronic increase in intraabdominal pressure.

Urgency Incontinence

Urgency incontinence, also called "urge incontinence," includes a sudden strong urge to void prior to the involuntary loss of urine. Loss of urine may be minimal or enough to soak clothing. When the sudden strong urge to void occurs without loss of urine, it is referred to as overactive bladder. The cause is overactivity of the muscle of the bladder, the detrusor muscle, as the bladder fills.

Overflow Incontinence

Overflow incontinence is caused by detrusor underactivity rather than overactivity. It may also be caused by an obstruction of the bladder outlet. People with overflow incontinence complain of a continuous leakage of urine, weak stream, urinary frequency and hesitancy, and frequent awakening to urinate (nocturia). Causes of outlet obstruction include uterine fibroids, pelvic organ prolapse, and surgery.

Treatment

Treatment of urinary incontinence depends on the type of incontinence and contributing factors. Lifestyle interventions such as weight loss and limiting alcoholic and caffeinated beverages can be helpful, although fluid restriction is typically not recommended, to avoid dehydration. Women, particularly those who complain of nocturia, should limit fluid intake prior to going to bed, however. Correcting constipation may improve symptoms. Pelvic floor exercises are often the first-line treatment. As these muscles can be challenging to localize, working with a physical therapist

This form is meant to be completed by the patient.

This voiding diary records your amount of fluid intake, amount you void and if there is any leakage of urine. It should be completed for an entire 24-hr period. For the most useful results, it should be done over 2 or 3 separate 24-hr periods. You must measure and complete this form every time you void or experience urinary leakage. Please bring these voiding diary records to your next Urology office visit. Copy additional pages if needed.

How to complete this form:
1. Begin the record with your first morning void after you wake up for the day.
2. Measure all fluid intake and the amount voided in mL or ounces. Ladies can measure the amount of urine by placing a plastic bowl or collection container that we can provide to you on the toilet seat. Men can void into a suitable collection jar or other container.
3. If you experience sudden leakage of urine, note the activity you were doing at the time of leakage (laughing, coughing, sneezing, lifting, etc.).
4. If you experience urinary leakage, use the following scale to estimate the amount of urine that you leaked:

      1 = Dampness
      2 = Wet underwear or pad
      3 = Soaked through or emptied bladder

5. Indicate by **Yes/No** if when you leaked you had an urge to void. FVC

Your Name: _____Date:_____

Your Physician's Name: _____

Time (AM or PM)	Fluid Intake (Type and amount in ounces or mL)	Amount Voided (In ounces or mL)	Leak Volume (See above for estimate)	Did you have an urge with leakage? (Yes/No)	Physical activity at time of leakage

Figure 27.14. Voiding diary. (Reprinted with permission from Gomella, L. G. [2015]. *The 5-minute urology consult* [3rd ed.]. Philadelphia, PA: Lippincott Williams & Wilkins.)

who specializes in the pelvic floor can be helpful (Dumoulin, Hay-Smith, & Mac Habee-Seguin, 2014; see Patient Teaching 15.1). Women who are perimenopausal or postmenopausal may find an improvement in symptoms over the course of 3 months with vaginal estrogen therapy.

Pessaries may be helpful for women with stress incontinence, and surgery has a high cure rate (Labrie et al., 2013). Women with urgency incontinence may benefit from treatment with an antimuscarinic or a beta-3 agonist. Nurses should be aware that the side effects of antimuscarinics include oral dryness and constipation.

Genital Tract Fistulas

Genital tract fistulas are abnormal passages that develop between the vagina, uterus, or cervix and the bladder, urethra, rectum, abdominal cavity, or perineum (Fig. 27.15). In the United States, they are rare complications of gynecologic surgery and are less commonly associated with childbirth, radiation therapy, and other pelvic pathology. In developing countries, they are a common complication of labor dystocia.

The clinical manifestations of a fistula vary according to site. A vesicovaginal fistula, which occurs between the bladder and the vagina, can cause leakage of urine from the vagina, for example. A rectovaginal fistula can cause the passage of stool or flatus through the vagina. Diagnosis is usually by physical examination.

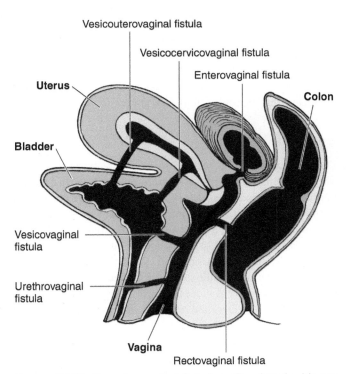

Figure 27.15. Female genital fistulas. (Reprinted with permission from Beckmann, C. R. B., Ling, F. W., Smith, R. P., Barzansky, B. M., & Herbert, W. N. P. [2006]. *Obstetrics and gynecology* [5th ed., Fig. 29.3]. Philadelphia, PA: Lippincott Williams & Wilkins.)

Successful repair is possible in most patients, although repeat procedures may be required (Barone et al., 2015).

Nurses should be aware that genital fistulas may be a source of great distress. A woman with a fistula may feel unclean, unhygienic, and out of control of her own bodily functions. She may no longer consider herself a sexual being, or she may be rejected by her partner or partners. Short- and long-term strategies to improve cleanliness may include deodorizing, douching, enemas, perineal irrigation, sitz baths, and protective pads or panties.

Menopause

Natural menopause is achieved when a woman has not menstruated for a full 12 months in the absence of any other reason. Humans are among only a handful of species that go through menopause, and the reason for this transition remains unclear. Surgical menopause occurs with removal of the ovaries. On average, women reach natural menopause at the age of approximately 51 or 52 years. Menopause prior to the age of 40 years is considered premature ovarian failure but has the same clinical signs and outcomes as typically timed menopause. Along with cessation of menses, menopause includes ovarian follicular depletion, low estrogen levels, and high levels of follicle-stimulating hormone. The time prior to menopause is referred to as perimenopause or the menopausal transition and typically lasts approximately 4 years, although hot flashes may last as long as 10 years or more. Perimenopause is characterized by menstrual irregularities, endocrine changes, and the onset of symptoms we commonly associate with menopause, including hot flashes, vaginal dryness, disturbed sleep, and mood symptoms.

A majority of women in perimenopause experience hot flashes, and most have them for more than 1 year but less than 5 years, although some may continue to have occasional symptoms well into their seventh decade. The sleep of women in perimenopause can be disturbed by night sweats (hot flashes while sleeping) as well as an increase in anxiety, depression, restless leg syndrome, sleep apnea, and insomnia. Depression is far more common in perimenopause than it is after menopause. Many women describe having issues with concentration and cognitive function during perimenopause, although a causal link between the two has not been substantiated by research. Depression and anxiety, however, have a recognized role in compromised cognition.

As estrogen levels drop during perimenopause, vaginal lubrication diminishes and the vaginal mucosa becomes progressively more dry and less elastic. The opening of the vagina (the introitus) narrows, and the labia minora flatten. The skin of the vulva and vagina becomes pale over time, and pubic hair sparse. Continuing sexual activity may help maintain the size and shape of the vagina.

More than half of women describe joint pain at midlife, with women who are depressed or obese more likely to do so. More women report joint pain when perimenopausal or postmenopausal than when premenopausal, and treatment with a combination of estrogen and progestin appears to be effective for relieving symptoms, suggesting a hormonal role in joint pain (Blumel et al., 2013; Chlebowski et al., 2013).

Long-term consequences of the loss of ovarian estrogen include bone loss, increased risk for cardiovascular disease, and increased falls. The role of low estrogen levels in skin changes, changes in body composition, osteoarthritis, and the development of dementia is less clear (Gleason et al., 2015).

Estrogen replacement was once a routine strategy for reducing the short- and long-term consequences of low estrogen levels. Concerns about the association between exogenous hormone use and breast cancer and between exogenous hormone use and cardiovascular disease, however, have greatly reduced this practice. Long-term use of estrogen is no longer recommended for disease prevention, although it was once thought to be a viable strategy for systemic reducing the risk for cardiovascular disease, osteoporosis, and dementia.

Women who do elect for the short-term use of estrogen and have an intact uterus must use the estrogen in conjunction with progestin. Failure to use progestin with estrogen in this population can result in endometrial hyperplasia and cancer. Indications for the short-term use of hormone replacement include hot flashes, night sweats, vaginal atrophy, mood disturbances, and joint pain. Vaginal symptoms of low estrogen levels may be treated with topical vaginal estrogen instead. A common recommendation for therapy duration is no more than 5 years and not beyond the age of 60 years, although some women with persistent symptoms may elect to use hormone therapy longer in consultation with their healthcare provider.

Benign Ovarian Cysts

Ovarian cysts may be functional or nonfunctional. The functional cysts of the ovary are a part of ovulatory function. Cyst formation is a normal part of follicle recruitment. The recruited follicle matures and then ruptures, releasing the ovum. The location of the follicle is the site of the corpus luteum. The corpus luteum then resolves spontaneously as a normal part of the menstrual cycle if pregnancy does not occur. Failure of these cysts to resolve creates functional cysts called luteal cysts, or corpus luteum cysts. Another kind of functional cyst, a follicular cyst, occurs when a follicle forms and either fails to rupture or ruptures but fails to drain completely. Nonfunctional benign cysts include dermoid cysts and ovarian fibromas.

Follicular Cysts

Follicular cysts occur when the rupture of the recruited follicle does not occur. On ultrasound they appear simple, in that they are thin walled with only one fluid-filled chamber. There are generally no symptoms associated with the follicular cyst unless it becomes quite large, ruptures, becomes hemorrhagic, or ovarian torsion occurs. Intervention is rarely required for identified large cysts, although some providers may recommend regular ultrasounds to follow the progress of the cyst. Cystectomy, removal of the cyst, may be recommended. There are no medications known to help with cyst resolution. Hormonal contraceptives that limit follicle recruitment, particularly those that contain estrogen and progestin, prevent ovarian cysts. The ovarian cysts of PCOS are follicular.

Rupture of a large follicular cyst can cause severe pelvic pain for 24 to 48 hours. The pain is due to leakage of fluid or blood from the cyst, which is irritating to the perineum. Pain typically presents as unilateral pelvic pain, often after sex. Pain from noncomplicated cysts is self-limiting and may be managed by observation. Rarely, rupture of a cyst can lead to hemorrhage with significant blood loss that requires fluid replacement, transfusion, or even surgery. Ovarian torsion is the twisting of the ovary, which results in twisting of the fallopian tube and occlusion of blood flow, which, in turn, can lead to ischemia and necrosis. It is considered a medical emergency. Ovarian torsion is most often associated with large cysts that distort the size and shape of the ovary, causing it to rotate.

Corpus Luteum Cysts

Corpus luteal cysts occur when the corpus luteum fails to involute. On ultrasound they may appear simple, similar to the follicular cyst, or complex, with multiple chambers or debris within the cyst and thick walls. Like a follicular cyst, a corpus luteal cyst typically resolves within a few weeks or months without symptoms in the absence of hemorrhage, rupture, or torsion.

Theca Lutein Cysts

Theca lutein cysts are an uncommon form of functional ovarian cyst that are most often associated with a hydatidiform mole but may also occur with a large placenta, as occurs with a multiple pregnancy, diabetes, or isoimmunization with pregnancy. They may also occur with ovarian hyperstimulation, as with fertility treatments. The root cause is exposure to high levels of human chorionic gonadotropin (hCG) or an abnormal sensitivity to hCG. Theca lutein cysts are usually bilateral and often cause a sense of pelvic fullness and pressure. Such cysts can contribute to preeclampsia, hyperemesis gravidarum, thyroid dysfunction, and maternal virilization, including hirsutism. The cysts resolve gradually after the source of hCG is gone.

Dermoid Cysts

Dermoid cysts are also referred to as mature cystic teratomas. They are benign ovarian tumors containing ectodermal, mesodermal, and endodermal tissue. They usually occur unilaterally but may be bilateral. They commonly contain teeth, hair, skin, nails, cartilage, blood, thyroid tissue, ocular tissue, blood, and sebum (Fig. 27.16). Most women with dermoid cysts are asymptomatic, although torsion and cyst rupture are possible. A definitive diagnosis is made surgically. Cystectomy is commonly recommended to avoid complications. Rarely, these cysts may become malignant. Dermoid cysts may also occur near the lateral aspect of the eyebrow (periorbital dermoid cysts) or along the spine (spinal dermoid cysts).

Ovarian Fibromas

An ovarian fibroma is a sex cord–stromal tumor. A sex cord–stromal tumor arises from the germ cells of the ovaries or testes. In women they occur most often postmenopausally, are benign, and

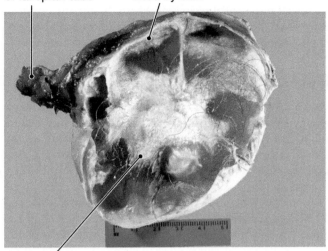

Fimbriated end of fallopian tube

Wall of cyst lined by skin

Mass of hair and sebaceous material

Figure 27.16. Benign dermoid cyst. Note the hair and sebaceous material. (Reprinted with permission from McConnell, T. H. [2007]. *The nature of disease: Pathology for the health professions* [1st ed., Fig. 21.28]. Philadelphia, PA: Lippincott Williams & Wilkins.)

are not hormonally active. They can be identified by ultrasound and may co-occur with ascites and an elevated level of cancer antigen 125 (CA-125), mimicking epithelial ovarian cancer. They are typically treated surgically.

Polycystic Ovarian Syndrome

The most common cause of infertility and subfertility in women is PCOS. PCOS is an endocrine disorder characterized by ovulatory dysfunction and hyperandrogenism that most often first appears in adolescence and persists throughout the reproductive life span. It is associated with a higher risk for other endocrine disorders, such as type 2 diabetes and metabolic syndrome, as well as cardiovascular disease and endometrial cancer. PCOS is a syndrome rather than a disease, which means it may have multiple causes. Approximately a quarter of women with PCOS have a mother who has also been diagnosed with PCOS. A wide variety of genes have been identified that may contribute to the syndrome (Rosenfield & Ehrmann, 2016). Other factors associated with the syndrome, such as obesity and insulin resistance, may be causative, a result of the syndrome, or both.

In Chapter 2, Tatiana was diagnosed with PCOS as a teenager. The nurse practitioner caring for her, Elsa, initially suspected the condition because of Tati's irregular periods and signs of hyperandrogenism, including hirsutism and oily skin.

Clinical features typical of PCOS include the following: menstrual irregularities (ovulatory dysfunction); hyperandrogenism, often manifesting as moderate-to-severe acne, hirsutism, multiple cysts on the ovaries (polycystic ovaries), obesity, insulin resistance, and thinning scalp hair; weight gain; ovarian cysts; and mental health problems (National Institutes of Health, 2012). Patients often manifest only some of these features, which can make diagnosis challenging.

Different presentations of PCOS, or phenotypes, include classic PCOS, hyperandrogenic anovulation, ovulatory PCOS, and nonhyperandrogenic PCOS, listed in order of severity (Box 27.4). A different version of the diagnostic criteria for PCOS has been proposed for adolescents because of variations in ovulation, hyperandrogenism, and ovarian cysts that are typical in adolescence (Box 27.5; Rosenfield, 2015).

Obesity and insulin resistance (prediabetes and type 2 diabetes) are frequently associated with PCOS but are not part of the diagnostic criteria. In fact, approximately half of individuals with PCOS are not obese and do not have insulin resistance. However, about 10% of women diagnosed with PCOS develop type 2 diabetes by the age of 40 (Joham, Ranasinha, Zoungas, Moran, & Teede, 2014). Women with PCOS are approximately twice as likely to develop metabolic syndrome as are women who do not carry the diagnosis. Metabolic syndrome is diagnostically defined as having at least three of the following five conditions: elevated blood pressure, elevated fasting plasma glucose level, high triglycerides level, low high-density lipoprotein level, and abdominal obesity. Patients with metabolic syndrome are at a high risk for type 2 diabetes and cardiovascular disease.

Box 27.4 Polycystic Ovarian Syndrome Phenotypes

Phenotype 1 (Classic PCOS)
- Ultrasonic evidence of a polycystic ovary
- Evidence of oligoanovulation
- Clinical or laboratory evidence of hyperandrogenism

Phenotype 2 (Hyperandrogenic Anovulation)
- Evidence of oligoanovulation
- Clinical or laboratory evidence of hyperandrogenism

Phenotype 3 (Ovulatory PCOS)
- Ultrasonic evidence of a polycystic ovary
- Clinical or laboratory evidence of hyperandrogenism

Phenotype 4 (Nonandrogenic PCOS)
- Ultrasonic evidence of a polycystic ovary
- Evidence of oligoanovulation

PCOS, polycystic ovarian syndrome.
Adapted from National Institutes of Health. (2012). *Evidence-based methodology workshop on polycystic ovary syndrome.* Retrieved from https://www.nichd.nih.gov/news/resources/spotlight/112112-pcos; Rotterdam Eshre Asrm-Sponsored PCOS Consensus Workshop Group. (2004). Revised 2003 consensus on diagnostic criteria and long-term health risks related to polycystic ovary syndrome. *Fertility and Sterility, 81*(1), 19–25.

Box 27.5 Polycystic Ovarian Syndrome Diagnostic Criteria for Adolescents

Diagnosis requires at least one indication from the category of abnormal uterine bleeding and one indication from the category of evidence of hyperandrogenism.

Abnormal Uterine Bleeding Pattern

- Abnormal for age or for time since first menses
- Symptoms persist for 1 or 2 y

Evidence of Hyperandrogenism

- Moderate-to-severe hirsutism
- Moderate-to-severe acne
- Persistent laboratory elevation of testosterone

Adapted from Legro, R. S., Arslanian, S. A., Ehrmann, D. A., Hoeger, K. M., Murad, M. H., Pasquali, R., & Welt, C. K.; Endocrine Society. (2013). Diagnosis and treatment of polycystic ovary syndrome: An Endocrine Society clinical practice guideline. *Journal of Clinical Endocrinology and Metabolism, 98*(12), 4565–4592. doi:10.1210/jc.2013-2350; Rosenfield, R. L. (2015). The diagnosis of polycystic ovary syndrome in adolescents. *Pediatrics, 136*(6), 1154–1165. doi:10.1542/peds.2015-1430.

Women with PCOS, particularly those with insulin resistance, are far more likely to develop obstructive sleep apnea than women without PCOS. Sleep apnea often first presents as excessive daytime sleepiness. An abnormal lipid profile is another common finding associated with PCOS. Women with PCOS are more likely to suffer from anxiety and depression than women of a similar body mass index without PCOS. They are also more likely report a lower quality of life (Legro et al., 2013).

Treatment goals for PCOS are based on the specific clinical manifestations of a particular patient as well as any associated health issues such as obesity and insulin resistance and mood disorders. Chronic anovulation and lack of menses can cause endometrial hyperplasia and cancer; thus, prevention of endometrial hyperplasia is a priority. Women with PCOS who do not regularly menstruate often make the mistake of thinking they do not ovulate. They may still ovulate intermittently, however, so contraception remains a priority if they do not wish to get pregnant. Women seeking pregnancy, however, may require ovulation induction to achieve a more predictable window of fertility and thus to achieve pregnancy.

For women who are overweight or obese, lifestyle changes that lead to weight loss can be effective for reducing hyperandrogenism and insulin resistance as well as regulating ovulation and increasing fertility. The use of an estrogen–progestin contraceptive can help manage hyperandrogenism, address menstrual irregularities, and prevent endometrial hyperplasia. For women for whom estrogen is contraindicated, a progestin method can help reduce the risk of endometrial hyperplasia, although it does not address the hyperandrogenism. As an alternative, the medication metformin can restore menstrual regularity in up to 50% of women (Morley, Tang, & Balen, 2017). Women may also take the diuretic spironolactone, which has antiandrogenic properties, to counteract hyperandrogenism but must use contraception while taking it because of its potential teratogenic effects. Spironolactone does not, however, regulate menses. Women seeking pregnancy may need additional treatment to induce ovulation (see Chapter 29).

Gynecologic Cancers

There are five primary types of cancer that are collectively referred to as gynecologic cancers: uterine, cervical, ovarian, vaginal, and vulvar. The risk for gynecologic cancers increases with age. As with all cancers, they are named for the body part in which they start regardless of metastases, and they are most treatable when discovered early.

A common method of staging cancer is referred to as the TNM staging system. The T refers to the size and extent of the primary tumor, N refers to the number of lymph nodes to which the cancer has spread, and M refers to metastasis (spread to other body parts; Box 27.6). Additional specific staging criteria for gynecologic cancers are provided by the International Federation of Obstetricians and Gynecologists (FIGO; Figo Committee on Gynecologic Oncology, 2014; Mutch & Prat, 2014).

A tumor that is well differentiated is more similar to normal tissue and is likely to grow and spread more slowly. Tumors described as poorly differentiated or undifferentiated have less in common with normal tissue and are likely to grow and spread more quickly. Tumors are graded according to the degree of cell abnormality. Tumors are typically graded 0 through 4 unless a different grading system is specified (Box 27.7).

Box 27.6 TNM Staging System for Cancer

Primary Tumor (T)

- *TX:* Main tumor cannot be measured.
- *T0:* Main tumor cannot be found.
- *T1, T2, T3, T4:* Refers to the size and/or extent of the main tumor. The higher the number after the T, the larger the tumor or the more it has grown into nearby tissues. Ts may be further divided to provide more detail, such as T3a and T3b.

Regional Lymph Nodes (N)

- *NX:* Cancer in nearby lymph nodes cannot be measured.
- *N0:* There is no cancer in nearby lymph nodes.
- *N1, N2, N3:* Refers to the number and location of lymph nodes that contain cancer. The higher the number after the N, the more lymph nodes that contain cancer.

Distant Metastasis (M)

- *MX:* Metastasis cannot be measured.
- *M0:* Cancer has not spread to other parts of the body.
- *M1:* Cancer has spread to other parts of the body.

Box 27.7 Tumor Grading

- *GX:* Grade cannot be assessed (undetermined grade)
- *G1:* Well differentiated (low grade)
- *G2:* Moderately differentiated (intermediate grade)
- *G3:* Poorly differentiated (high grade)
- *G4:* Undifferentiated (high grade)

Uterine Cancer

The incidence of uterine cancer is almost 15 per 100,000 women, making it the most commonly diagnosed gynecologic malignancy in the developed world (Torre et al., 2015). Cancer of the uterus includes two main types: uterine sarcoma and endometrial adenocarcinoma. As mentioned earlier in the chapter, most cancers of the uterus arise from the glandular structures of the endometrium and are thus adenocarcinomas. Much more rare are uterine sarcomas (tumors arising from bones and soft tissue), which account for only 3% to 9% of uterine cancers (Trope, Abeler, & Kristensen, 2012). Staging of uterine cancer is in accordance with the TNM and FIGO staging systems.

Uterine Sarcoma

Uterine sarcomas are more aggressive than the more common endometrial adeno carcinomas and have a poorer prognosis. There are several different types and subtypes that are classified according to histopathology, which is the examination of tissue samples by a pathologist. The average age of the patient at diagnosis is 60 years, and women of African descent are at a greater risk for developing this type of cancer than women of European descent and have a poorer prognosis. The use of tamoxifen, a medication to prevent breast cancer, for 5 or more years also increases risk somewhat, although the absolute risk remains low. Uterine sarcomas are also associated with some hereditary risk.

On examination and imaging, a uterine sarcoma can appear identical to a benign leiomyoma (fibroid), and often diagnosis cannot be made until after the surgery to remove the tumor or tumors. The first step in treatment is often surgery for removal of the uterus (hysterectomy), with or without a bilateral salpingo-oophorectomy (removal of the fallopian tubes and ovaries). Staging of the cancer is performed at this time. If the cancer is already beyond the confines of the uterus, however, the decision may be made to defer surgery in favor of medical treatment. Lymph nodes may be removed and examined by a pathologist for staging purposes at the discretion of the surgeon.

Adjuvant therapy is treatment designed to help eliminate a disease and prevent its recurrence. Decisions about adjuvant therapy are made on the basis of the clinical situation, including the stage and grade of the tumor. Patients with uterine sarcomas may benefit from chemotherapy. Radiation therapy may reduce local recurrence of disease but creates a risk for scar tissue that can cause later problems with strictures and fistulas, as well as a risk for secondary malignancies resulting directly from radiation.

The prognosis for women with uterine sarcomas depends on the type and stage of sarcoma. Women with endometrial stromal sarcoma discovered in stage I, for example, have a 90% 5-year survival rate. Women with undifferentiated endometrial sarcoma, however, survive only 12 months, on average, from the time of diagnosis, regardless of staging (Tanner, Garg, Leitao, Soslow, & Hensley, 2012).

Follow-up for all patients with uterine sarcomas is generally with a physical examination every 3 months for 2 years and then every 6 to 12 months. A computed tomography (CT) scan of the pelvis, chest, and abdomen every 6 to 12 months for the first 5 years after surgery is common practice (NCCN Clinical Practice Guidelines in Oncology, 2017). Recurrence may be treated with endocrine agents, chemotherapy, or additional surgery.

Endometrial Adenocarcinoma

Endometrial adenocarcinomas are far more common than uterine sarcomas, accounting for 90% to 97% of uterine malignancies. The identification and risk factors of endometrial cancer are discussed earlier in the chapter. There are two types of endometrial adenocarcinomas: type 1 and type 2. Both are diagnosed on the basis of examination by a pathologist of a tissue sample.

Type 1

Type 1 endometrial carcinomas, also referred to as low-grade endometrioid endometrial carcinomas, account for most endometrial adenocarcinomas. Risk factors include excess exposure to endogenous estrogen (sources include obesity, anovulation with infrequent menses, and estrogen-secreting tumors) and exogenous estrogen (such as from postmenopausal estrogen replacement therapy without progestin). Reduced risk is associated with the hormonal methods of contraception, the older age of childbearing, breastfeeding, physical activity, and the consumption of green tea and coffee (Iversen, Sivasubramaniam, Lee, Fielding, & Hannaford, 2017; Jordan et al., 2017; Schmid et al., 2015).

Type 1 neoplasms of the endometrium are low grade and usually present at an early stage, resulting in a generally good prognosis. Although women diagnosed with early-stage disease (stage I or II) can generally be treated with surgery alone, women with late-stage disease (stage III or IV) typically require chemotherapy and radiation in addition to surgery.

Type 2

Type 2 endometrial carcinomas include grade 3 endometrioid carcinomas as well as serous, clear-cell, mixed-cell, and undifferentiated neoplasms. The high-grade endometrioid carcinomas are estrogen sensitive, but the other neoplasm types are not. The cause of these cancers is not as clear, but there is likely a strong genetic component. Type 2 carcinomas are more aggressive and generally have a worse prognosis. Obesity, a prime risk factor for type 1 endometrial carcinomas, is a less significant risk factor for type 2 endometrial carcinomas. Unlike type 1 carcinomas, which are usually identified in stage I or II, type 2 endometrial neoplasms are usually diagnosed in stage III or IV.

Surgical treatment to remove as much of the cancer as possible is the first-line treatment. Recurrence with distant metastasis is more common with type II than type I. Chemotherapy and radiation are recommended adjuvant therapy for many if not most women with type 2 endometrial carcinomas.

Posttreatment Care

The goal of surveillance after treatment is early detection of recurrence, which typically occurs, if at all, within the first 3 years after treatment. The disease most commonly recurs in the pelvis, abdomen, lung, and vagina. Clinical manifestations of recurrence include pelvic or abdominal pain, vaginal bleeding, unintentional weight loss, and a persistent cough. Asymptomatic screening for recurrence includes a careful history and physical examination. Other assessments may include abdominal and pelvic ultrasound or CT, chest X-ray, a serum CA-125 test, and/or a Pap test of the vaginal vault.

Sexual dysfunction is a common complaint of women after treatment for endometrial cancer. Women who have had abdominal lymph nodes removed for disease staging and treatment may complain of significant lymphedema, which usually presents as edema of the lower extremities. Radiation therapy to the pelvis can cause chronic changes to bowel and bladder function. Neuropathy and fatigue are common effects of chemotherapy and may persist after treatment has ended.

Cervical Cancer

Cervical cancer develops from abnormal changes in the cells of the cervix, most commonly as a result of infection with the human papillomavirus (HPV). For more information on cervical cancer etiology and screening, see Chapter 26.

These abnormal changes manifest initially as precancerous lesions. Biopsies taken of the cervix at the time of colposcopy and assessed by a pathologist may return a result of no pathology, cervical intraepithelial neoplasia (CIN), or adenocarcinoma in situ (AIS). CIN refers to abnormalities in the squamous cells of the cervix, which occur commonly and can develop into squamous cell carcinoma of the cervix. AIS refers to abnormalities in the glandular cells of the cervix, which occur less commonly and can develop into adenocarcinoma of the cervix. Squamous cell carcinoma and adenocarcinoma are the two types of invasive cervical cancer.

Cervical Intraepithelial Neoplasia

CIN is graded 1, 2, or 3, with CIN 1 indicating low-grade abnormalities and 2 and 3 high-grade abnormalities. CIN 1 is more likely to regress and less likely to progress to cervical cancer, whereas higher-grade lesions present a higher risk for progression to invasive cancer.

Women with CIN 1 are usually assessed regularly with Pap and HPV co-testing in accordance with the results of prior Pap and HPV results. In some cases, such as in findings of high-grade abnormalities on the Pap test or a history of repeat CIN 1 on multiple biopsies over 2 years, follow-up may be continued or the patient may elect for treatment.

High-grade CIN treatment options include excision of the transformation zone of the cervix or ablation. Women with recurrence may be offered a hysterectomy. In the United States, excision is most often done by a loop electrosurgical excision procedure (LEEP), which has the advantage of providing a sample for study by the pathologist. This sample can be used to determine whether the entire lesion was excised or abnormal tissue was left in place. In contrast, ablation does not provide a sample for examination. Both can be performed in the office setting.

The LEEP procedure is usually done such that a cone-shaped specimen is removed that includes the transformation zone of the cervix and a portion of the endocervix. Although LEEP is now the most commonly used method, a cone biopsy may also be done with a scalpel (Fig. 27.17). Such a procedure is referred to as a cold-knife conization. A laser may also be used to excise the specimen. Ablation may be done with either a laser or cryotherapy. Both excision and ablation are 90% to 95% curative (Martin-Hirsch, Paraskevaidis, Bryant, & Dickinson, 2013).

After treatment for CIN 2 or 3, co-testing with Pap and HPV is indicated at 12 and 24 months. If test findings at both time points are negative, a third co-testing is indicated after 3 years. If the result from this co-testing is negative, the patient may resume routine screening. Abnormal findings from co-testing during this period (Pap and/or HPV) are an indication for a colposcopy and biopsy of the endocervix. Even in the absence of abnormal findings from the Pap or HPV test, routine screening should continue for at least 20 years, even if the patient is beyond the age recommended for routine screening. If, however, examination of the biopsy reveals positive margins, suggesting that not all abnormal cells have been removed, earlier co-testing or a repeat excision may be recommended (Massad et al., 2013).

Adenocarcinoma In Situ

AIS is a premalignant condition of the glandular cells of the cervix and a precursor to adenocarcinoma of the cervix. Adenocarcinoma of the cervix is, as mentioned previously, far less common than squamous cell cervical cancer. Risk factors are the same for both. AIS is almost always detected because of abnormalities discovered by a Pap test, but may very rarely present as a complaint of vaginal bleeding. As for squamous abnormalities, a colposcopy is indicated and a sampling from the endocervix is obtained. A negative sample of the endocervix is an indication for an endometrial biopsy and conization.

AIS often has "skip lesions," meaning that negative margins from a cone specimen do not necessarily indicate the absence of disease. Although the limits of a particular lesion may have been obtained, an additional lesion may start after a "skip." The risk of residual AIS after a conization with positive margins is 52.8% and with negative margins is 20.3%. The risk for invasive adenocarcinoma within 5 years after diagnosis of AIS is 5.2% for women with positive margins and 0.1% for women with negative margins (Salani, Puri, & Bristow, 2009). Because of this, hysterectomy is the standard treatment for a diagnosis of AIS. After hysterectomy, a Pap test and HPV testing of the vagina are done at 6 and 12 months and then annually if normal. Abnormalities

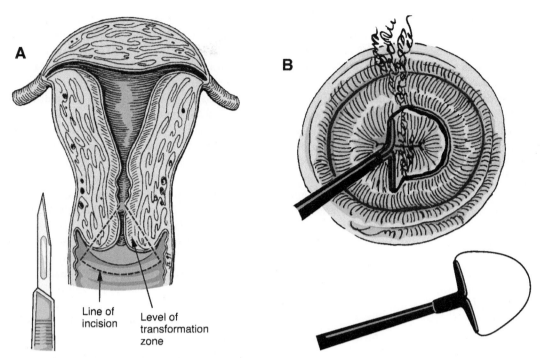

Figure 27.17. Conization of the cervix. (A) Cold-knife technique. **(B)** Loop electrosurgical excision procedure technique. (Reprinted with permission from Beckmann, C. R. B., Ling, F. W., Smith, R. P., Barzansky, B. M., & Herbert, W. N. P. [2006]. *Obstetrics and gynecology* [5th ed., Fig. 29.3]. Philadelphia, PA: Lippincott Williams & Wilkins.)

are followed by colposcopy and ablation or excision, as indicated (Massad et al., 2013).

Women who wish to retain fertility, however, may elect instead for surveillance following conization in the case of negative margins. In this case, a Pap smear and HPV testing are done every 6 months for 2 years and then annually. Abnormalities are followed by colposcopy and endocervical biopsy and treated with repeat cervical conization or hysterectomy, as indicated. After childbearing, a hysterectomy is recommended (Massad et al., 2013).

Invasive Cervical Cancer

Cervical cancer is now the third-most common gynecologic cancer and cause of death from gynecologic cancer in the United States and other developed countries (Torre et al., 2015). It can spread by extension to the uterus, vagina, abdominal cavity, bladder, or rectum or by the lymphatic system, usually to the lungs, liver, bones, bowel, spleen, and/or adrenal glands. Early cervical cancer is generally asymptomatic, whereas later cervical cancer can present as AUB, postcoital bleeding (bleeding after sex), vaginal discharge, back pain, or bowel or urinary symptoms. Initial assessment of a patient with suspected cervical cancer includes a physical examination, Pap test, and HPV testing. In the case of a high index of suspicion, a colposcopy may be done and biopsies collected prior to the return of the results of the Pap and HPV tests.

Cervical cancer is considered early stage when it is confined to the uterus. Women with microscopic disease may elect for treatment with a cone biopsy or hysterectomy. Women who wish to bear children in the future may elect for cone biopsy or a

trachelectomy (removal of cervix while keeping uterus). Women who are not good surgical candidates should receive radiation and may also be treated with chemotherapy (NCCN Clinical Practice Guidelines in Oncology, 2016). Women with more advanced disease may be treated surgically, with radiation, and/or with chemotherapy, depending on staging, health status, and shared decision-making between the patient and the healthcare team.

After treatment, those deemed high risk are assessed every 3 months for the first 2 years, every 6 months until 5 years after treatment, and then annually. Patients with a low risk of recurrence are assessed every 6 months for the first 2 years and then annually. Follow-up assessment includes a careful history and physical examination and an annual Pap test of the cervix and/or vagina. The symptoms of vaginal bleeding, bowel or bladder changes, or a sensation of pelvic pressure are concerning for recurrence. Most recurrences are identified within 2 years after initial treatment.

As with other patients who have received radiation to the pelvis and abdomen, bowel and bladder dysfunction and sexual dysfunction and fatigue are common sequelae of treatment. Compared with survivors of other gynecologic cancers, people with a history of cervical cancer are more subject to mood disturbances, particularly anxiety, dysphoria, anger, and confusion (Mantegna et al., 2013).

Ovarian Cancer

High-grade epithelial ovarian, fallopian tube, and peritoneal cancers are all considered a single disease with an identical prognosis and treatment plan. For the purpose of this section, the term "ovarian cancer" will be used to describe all high-grade epithelial ovarian, fallopian tube, and peritoneal cancers. Other forms of ovarian malignancy, including epithelial borderline neoplasm, malignant ovarian germ cell tumor, and malignant sex cord–stromal tumor, are rare and beyond the scope of this text.

Ovarian cancer is the leading cause of death from gynecologic cancer in the United States, with 22,000 new cases and 14,000 deaths annually (Siegel, Miller, & Jemal, 2017). Survival is vastly better when ovarian cancer is identified in an early stage, although this is rarely the case. Most ovarian cancers are identified at stage III or IV. Currently, no reliable screening is offered for women at an average risk for ovarian cancer. Women with a known familial syndrome for ovarian cancer are offered prophylactic surgery to remove the ovaries and fallopian tubes (and, in the case of a breast cancer [BRCA] gene mutation, the breasts), to reduce risk. Women who decline surgery can be followed by ultrasound and measurement of the serum tumor marker CA-125 every 6 months beginning at the age of 30 years, or 5 to 10 years prior to the age of the earliest diagnosis of ovarian cancer in the family.

Approximately 10% to 15% of women who develop ovarian cancer have a strong family history of ovarian cancer. Women with one first- or second-degree family member with ovarian cancer have an up to 5% greater risk of developing breast cancer. Women with a known hereditary ovarian syndrome, such as the Lynch syndrome II or a breast cancer susceptibility gene 1 or 2 (BRCA1 or BRCA2) mutation, have a 15% to 40% chance of developing ovarian cancer (Mavaddat et al., 2013). The risk for ovarian cancer is increased for women with endometriosis or PCOS and those who use hormone replacement therapy during perimenopause and postmenopause. Infertility is a risk factor, but the treatment for infertility is not. The use of hormonal contraception reduces risk, as does a history of pregnancy and breastfeeding. Surgical removal of the ovaries and fallopian tubes also reduces risk (Soini et al., 2014).

Ovarian cancer is particularly lethal because it is so often caught late because of few and vague early symptoms. The most common early symptoms experienced are abdominal pain and bloating and an increase in abdominal girth. Later signs are associated with ascites and metastases to the bowel or omentum and include nausea, anorexia, and early satiety. Physical examination findings suggestive of ovarian cancer are abdominal ascites, masses of the adnexa and mid or left upper abdomen, pleural effusion, and lymphadenopathy of the groin or supraclavicular chain. An abnormal finding on examination is typically followed by imaging with ultrasound and possibly a CT scan. The serum CA-125 tumor marker is nonspecific and not particularly sensitive: women with early disease often have a normal value, and other conditions, including endometriosis, fibroids, and cirrhosis of the liver, can cause elevated levels. CA-125 is most useful for tracking the course of the disease and treatment. The diagnosis of ovarian cancer and disease staging is ultimately done surgically and by pathology. At the time of surgery, as much of the cancer is removed as possible, a process called "cytoreduction." This process may include resection of the bowel or bladder, lymphadenectomy, removal of the omentum, appendectomy, splenectomy, or liver resection.

Treatment with either intravenous or peritoneal chemotherapy typically starts soon after surgery. Following treatment, office visits that include testing for CA-125, a thorough history, and a physical and pelvic examination are indicated every 3 to 6 months for 5 years and then annually.

Patients diagnosed very early in the disease have an overall survival rate of almost 90% after 5 years. Patients diagnosed at stage III or IV have a 17% to 59% survival rate at 5 years (American Cancer Society, 2016b). Collectively, 46% of women diagnosed with ovarian cancer live for 5 years and 33% live for 10 years or more. There are about 200,000 survivors of ovarian cancer in the United States, most of whom are living with the disease. The rate of recurrence is 25% when caught early and 80% when found at an advanced stage (DeSantis et al., 2014).

Survivors of ovarian cancer often have lifetime issues associated with treatment. Chemotherapy is neurotoxic, and complaints of ringing in the ears, hearing loss, neuropathy of the feet, neuropathy of the hands, ambulation difficulties, and muscle cramps are common. These effects are associated with an overall reduction in quality of life (Ezendam et al., 2014). Many women who undergo chemotherapy with the agents used to treat ovarian cancer complain of long-term cognitive dysfunction, or "chemo brain" (Jung et al., 2017). Also common are fatigue, gastrointestinal distress, and surgical complications. Most report that ovarian cancer has a negative effect on their sex life. Most experience ongoing psychological distress to some degree throughout the course of their disease in the form of depression, anxiety, fear, guilt, or poor body image (Heo, Chun, Oh, Noh, & Kim, 2017).

Vaginal Cancer

Vaginal cancer is rare, accounting for 4,000 cancer diagnoses and 900 deaths in the United States annually (Siegel, Miller, & Jemal, 2015). The most common age for a diagnosis of squamous cell carcinoma of the vulva, the most common type, is approximately 60 years, although cases have been recorded in much younger women. Vaginal cancer is associated with HPV and thus has the same risk factors as those of cervical cancer: smoking, early initiation of sexual activity, and multiple sex partners. In addition, a previous history of a different gynecologic cancer, particularly cervical cancer and high-grade CIN, presents a risk for vaginal cancer.

A minority of women diagnosed with vaginal cancer are asymptomatic, and their cancer is discovered incidentally at the time of examination or cytology screening of the cervix. A majority present with vaginal bleeding, usually postcoital or postmenopausal. Alternatively, the patient may note a vaginal mass. Rarely, symptoms noted are those related to extension to the bladder, bowel, or other reproductive organs. Vaginal cancer is a histologic diagnosis made from biopsies taken from the vagina.

Treatment is similar to that used for cervical cancer. Complications include the formation of fistulas and strictures and other effects of surgery and radiation. Recurrence is generally treated by surgery or chemotherapy. For those deemed low risk, follow-up after treatment is every 6 months for the first 2 years and then annually. For women with high-risk disease, follow-up is every

3 months for the first 2 years, then every 6 months until 5 years, and then annually. Cytology of the vagina and cervix, if needed, is done annually. The most important predictor of prognosis is the stage of the tumor at the time of discovery.

Vulvar Cancer

Cancer of the vulva is the fourth-most common gynecologic cancer in developed countries, accounting for 5% to 6% of cases. In the United States, there are approximately 6,000 cases diagnosed annually and 1,000 deaths (Siegel et al., 2017). The average age at the time of diagnosis is 68. The overall survival rate after 5 years is 72%. Women with localized disease have an over 86% chance of survival to 5 years, whereas women diagnosed at a late stage have a 17% chance of survival (National Cancer Institute). Risk factors include the following: a history of CIN, cervical cancer, or vulvar intraepithelial neoplasia (VIN); smoking; lichen sclerosis of the vulva (a benign, plaque-like atrophy; Fig. 27.18); compromised immunity; and northern European descent (Brinton, Thistle, Liao, & Trabert, 2017). The HPV

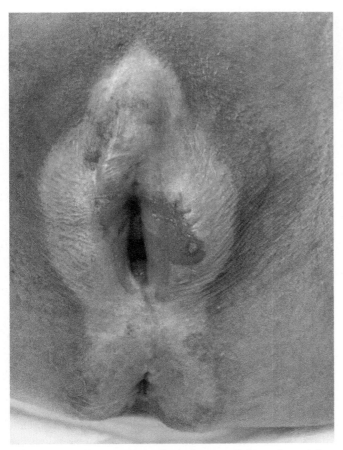

Figure 27.18. Squamous cell carcinoma of the vulva arising in a patient with long-standing lichen sclerosus. Note the butterfly distribution of the lichen sclerosus, the flattening of the vulvar structures, and the early invasive cancer on the left. (Reprinted with permission from Berek, J. S., & Hacker, N. F. [2015]. *Berek and Hacker's gynecologic oncology* [6th ed., Fig. 13.2]. Philadelphia, PA: Lippincott Williams & Wilkins.)

virus is discovered in almost 87% of VIN and 29% of invasive vulvar cancer (de Sanjose et al., 2013).

Vulvar cancer may appear as a plaque, ulcer, or mass. The most common site is the labia majora, although lesions may also be found on the labia minora, the perineum, the clitoris, or the mons (Fig. 27.19). Pruritus is a common-associated complaint. Some women may complain of vulvar or rectal bleeding, dysuria (pain with urination), dyschezia (pain with defecation), edema of the lower extremities, or enlarged lymph nodes of the groin. Diagnosis is based on the histologic results of vulvar biopsy.

Of the several histologic types of vulvar cancer, squamous cell carcinoma is by far the most common. Other types include basal cell carcinoma, melanoma, sarcoma, Paget disease (a kind of adenocarcinoma), and cancers of the Bartholin glands. Treatment is according to type and stage. Surgery is by vulvar excision and may involve partial or complete removal of the vulva (vulvectomy), lymph node biopsy, and lymph node removal. Chemotherapy and radiation therapy may be indicated.

After treatment, women with early-stage disease are followed every 6 months for 2 years and then annually. Women with advanced-stage disease should be followed every 3 months for the first 2 years, then every 6 months until year 5, and then annually. At the time of follow-up, a thorough physical examination is indicated. A cervical Pap test should be done annually, or a vaginal Pap should be done if the cervix is absent. Recurrence may be vulvar, inguinal, pelvic, or distant. Sexual dysfunction after treatment is common.

Conditions of the Breasts

The breasts are attached to the muscles of the chest between the second and sixth ribs by connective tissue. Most women have breasts that are roughly symmetric, although variations in size and shape between breasts are common. Breast asymmetry is particularly common among adolescents and is considered normal. Each breast is made up of lobes lined with acini cells that produce milk and colostrum, ducts that carry milk and colostrum to the nipple, and fat. The ducts converge at the nipple (also called the mammary papilla) in a "shower head" configuration, with 4 to 20 openings to the surface. The nipple itself is surrounded by an areola of a similar color. For most women, the nipple is elevated, but many women have flat nipples that elevate only with cold or stimulation.

The term **micromastia** refers to underdevelopment of the breast tissue, the appearance of which may be reversed with breast augmentation. Micromastia with normal sexual development is not considered pathologic. Conditions that may contribute to micromastia include ovarian failure, androgen excess, hypothyroidism, mitral valve prolapse, chest radiation, and connective tissue disorders. A variation of micromastia, **tuberous breast** development, refers to underdevelopment of the breast and the comparative overdevelopment of the nipple and areola.

Macromastia, also referred to as juvenile breast hypertrophy or virginal breast hypertrophy, is hyperplasia of the breasts resulting in very large breasts. Growth may be either symmetric or

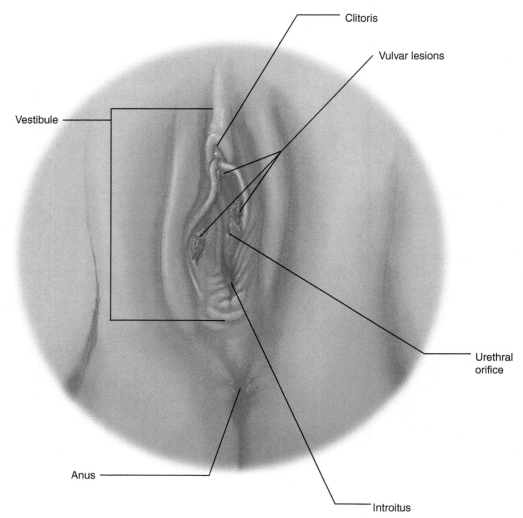

Clitoris

Vulvar lesions

Vestibule

Urethral orifice

Anus

Introitus

Figure 27.19. Vulvar cancer. (Reprinted with permission from Anatomical Chart Company.)

asymmetric. Very large breasts can result in significant back and neck pain. Breast reduction surgery usually does not impact a woman's ability to breastfeed in the future (Nguyen, Palladino, Sonnema, & Petty, 2013). Breast reduction should be done after it is reasonable to expect that full breast development has been achieved.

Accessory breast tissue refers to any breast tissue beyond the two breasts typical for humans and occurs in approximately 1% of the population. **Polymastia** refers to the presence of any accessory breast tissue, and **polythelia** refers to the presence of additional nipples (also referred to as supernumerary nipples). Accessory breast tissue most often refers to polythelia, consisting of a small nipple and areola, although glandular tissue may be present. Accessory breast tissue occurs along the "milk line" (Fig. 27.20), with the lower axilla being the most common site. Rarely, polymastia may cause painful swelling during pregnancy or develop a benign or malignant tumor.

The term **athelia** refers to the absence of a nipple, and **amastia** refers to the absence of breast tissue.

Breast Cancer

In the United States in 2017, it is expected that 252,710 new cases of invasive breast cancer will be diagnosed in women and 40,610 will die from their disease. Approximately 1 in 8 women in the United States will be diagnosed with breast cancer during her lifetime, 85% of whom have no family history of the disease. African American women are disproportionately more likely to die of the disease than women of other ethnicities (Breastcancer. org, 2017). Approximately 5% of women with a diagnosis of breast cancer have metastatic disease, and 30% diagnosed with nonmetastatic disease will develop later metastases. Metastatic disease is not considered curable, although interventions can significantly improve the duration of survival.

Imaging

A majority of cases of breast cancer are discovered by mammogram and may not be palpable with examination. (See Chapter 26 for information on breast cancer screening.)

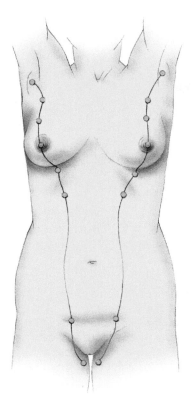

Figure 27.20. Mammary milk line. (Reprinted with permission from Jones, H. W., & Rock, J. A. [2015]. *Te Linde's operative gynecology* [11th ed., Fig. 45.1]. Philadelphia, PA: Lippincott Williams & Wilkins.)

After an abnormality is discovered on mammogram, additional imaging is generally performed, as well as ultrasound if indicated prior to biopsy. Some breast cancers present clinically between mammograms and are referred to as interval cancers. Approximately 15% of breast cancers fall into this category. These too require diagnostic imaging and possibly ultrasound prior to biopsy.

Suspicious findings by mammogram include soft tissue masses and calcifications. Soft tissue masses may be spiculated, irregular, round, or ovoid. Calcifications are classified as microcalcifications or macrocalcifications. Microcalcifications are 1 mm or less and number more than 4 or 5 per cubic centimeter. They are seen in a majority of cancers detected by mammogram. Macrocalcifications are larger and have a much lower association with malignancy. Abnormal mammograms are categorized using the Breast Imaging Reporting and Data System, which helps define the abnormality and guide follow-up (see Table 26.2).

Magnetic resonance imaging (MRI) as a screening modality is recommended for some women at a high risk for breast cancer (see Chapter 26) and is also sometimes used to help guide surgical interventions, particularly in the case of clinical examination findings discordant with the mammogram, cancers contiguous with the chest wall, axillary node metastases in the absence of a recognized primary tumor, Paget disease, and for those at a high risk for bilateral disease.

Diagnosis, Grading, and Staging

The diagnosis of breast cancer is done by needle biopsy from the core of the lesion. If a mass is readily palpable and superficial, the biopsy may be done without imaging. For lesions that are deeper and more difficult to localize, a biopsy is generally done with ultrasound guidance. A stereotactic breast biopsy allows for precision sampling by using two mammogram images to guide sampling (Fig. 27.21). Rarely, an open biopsy is done via an incision.

Biopsy results are often available within a day after sampling. The report can confirm or rule out a cancer but also provide information about the grade of the cancer. The grade helps the treatment team discern how aggressive the cancer is. The sample is also examined for the presence of estrogen or progesterone receptors. The presence of one or both of these receptors means that the tumor responds to hormones and helps guide both surgical and medical treatment. Women with tumors that overexpress human epidermal growth factor receptor 2 (HER2) are treated with therapies that target this tumor type. Tumors that are negative for estrogen and progesterone receptors and HER2 are more aggressive and challenging to treat and carry a poorer prognosis. Approximately 80% of tumors are positive for estrogen and/or progesterone receptors, 23% overexpress HER2, and 13% are triple negative (negative for estrogen, progesterone, and HER2).

The staging of cancer requires knowledge of the extent of the primary tumor, local invasion (in the case of breast cancer, usually to the axillary lymph nodes or skin overlying the breast), and evidence for metastatic disease (Fig. 27.22). Classically, axillary adenopathy suggests local advancement, although lymph nodes may be clinically normal. A more conclusive diagnosis is made by conducting a biopsy of lymph nodes that serve that particular part of the breast. The most common sites for metastatic breast

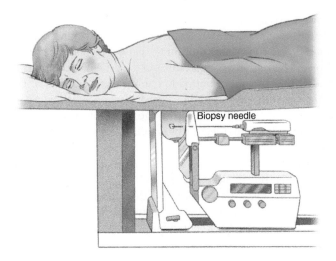

Figure 27.21. Stereotactic breast biopsy. For this procedure, the patient is placed in the prone position on a special table and the breast to be biopsied is compressed firmly between two plates. Sampling is by a needle guided by mammography. (Reprinted with permission from *Lippincott Nursing Advisor February 2014 release*. Philadelphia, PA: Lippincott Williams & Wilkins.)

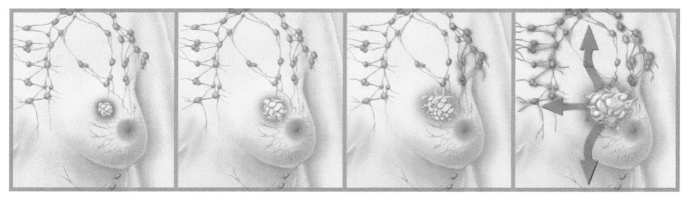

Stage I
T (<2 cm)
N (no axillary metastasis)
M (no metastasis)

Stage II
T (>2 cm)
N (axillary metastasis
nonfixed)
M (no metastasis)

Stage III
T (>5 cm)
N (axillary metastasis fixed)
M (no metastasis)

Stage IV
T (any size)
N (supra- or infraclavicular
nodes)
M (distant metastasis)

Figure 27.22. Stages of breast cancer. Clinical staging is a part of the pretreatment evaluation and is performed by histologic examination of the biopsied tissue and axillary specimen to assess the extent of the disease, lymph node involvement, the status of the other breast, and the possibility of systemic metastasis (passing from one site to another). The most commonly used system is the **Tumor-Nodes-Metastasis system (TNM)**. **T** represents the primary tumor, **N** describes lymph node involvement, and **M** describes metastasis, if any. (Reprinted with permission from *Lippincott Nursing Advisor February 2016 release*. Philadelphia, PA: Lippincott Williams & Wilkins.)

cancer are the lungs (symptoms may include shortness of breath or a cough), the liver (nausea, jaundice, or abdominal pain), and bone (pain at the site of metastases).

Prognosis

Regarding an individual patient's expected clinical outcome related to breast cancer, the healthcare team must consider two different sets of factors: prognostic factors and predictive factors. A prognostic factor is a characteristic of the patient or the patient's disease that provides information at the time of diagnosis about the expected clinical outcome for the patient without treatment. A predictive factor is a characteristic of the patient or the patient's disease that provides information about the likelihood of the patient to clinically respond to a particular treatment.

Prognostic factors include the age and race of the patient, smoking status, tumor stage, tissue markers (the presence of estrogen and/or progesterone receptors, HER2 expression level), gene expression, proliferation markers, tumor assays, and circulating tumor cells (Box 27.8).

Of these prognostic factors, one of the most significant is stage, both in terms of guiding the choice of treatment and in predicting the likelihood of survival. For example, metastatic breast cancer (stage IV) is rarely cured by any means. Treatment for this group is palliative and focused on minimizing complications while maximizing quality of life. Systemic therapy with chemotherapy is the primary treatment for this population, although localized treatments such as mastectomy and radiotherapy may also be part of this process.

Overall, the 5-year survival rate for patients with early-stage disease is 95% to 100%, and for women with locally advanced disease is 72% to 93%. In contrast, women with stage IV metastatic disease have a 22% survival rate over 5 years (American Cancer Society,

2016a). However, staging is only one factor used to prognosticate, and other factors also help guide treatment and inform the prognosis.

Predictive factors inform treatment so that patients can be treated by the modality or modalities most likely to be successful. The most reliable predictive factors to guide treatment are the presence or absence of estrogen receptors and HER2 expression (Box 27.9). Other predictive genomic assays are currently being investigated to guide treatment.

Surgery

Patients with early-stage breast cancer are usually offered **breast-conserving surgery (BCS)** in conjunction with radiation therapy (BCS and radiation therapy combined are referred to as breast-conserving therapy [BCT]). The alternative for women who decline or are not good candidates for BCT is **mastectomy**. A prophylactic mastectomy may be a preferred solution for women with a known high risk of developing breast cancer, most often because of a *BRCA1* or *BRCA2* mutation. Removal of the breasts reduces the chances of developing breast cancer by 90% to 95% (National Cancer Institute, 2013). The types of mastectomy include radical, modified radical, simple, skin-sparing, and nipple- and areola-sparing.

Breast-Conserving Surgery
BCS involves the removal of only the tumor and a border of healthy tissue to insure clear margins. To be successful, the surgical excision of the tumor must be complete. Margins that are not clear suggest that some malignant tissue may have been left behind. This surgery is also referred to as a lumpectomy, segmental mastectomy, or partial mastectomy. Survival with BCT with adequate BCS is now believed to be at least as effective if not more effective for disease treatment than mastectomy (van Maaren et al., 2016).

Box 27.8 Prognostic Factors for Breast Cancer

- *Age:* Women under 35 y old have the worst 5-y survival rate, with a mortality rate of 70%.
- *Ethnicity:* African American women have a lower risk for cancer but a higher mortality rate.
- *Smoking status:* Patients who smoke just prior to and/or after diagnosis have a worse prognosis.
- *Cancer stage:* Cancer is staged according to tumor size, node involvement, and metastasis. Earlier staging is generally correlated with a better prognosis.
- *Tumor grade:* Tumors are graded on the degree of their differentiation from surrounding tissues. The less a

tumor is differentiated from surrounding tissues, the worse the prognosis.
- *Hormone receptors:* Greater estrogen and/or progesterone receptor expression is associated with improved short-term outcomes.
- *Human epidermal growth factor receptor 2 (HER2) expression level:* Overexpression (expression greater than normal) of the protein HER2 indicates a more aggressive tumor, resistance to some forms of chemotherapy, and a poorer prognosis.
- *Circulating tumor cells:* Tumor cells identified in the blood is associated with a poor prognosis.

Adapted from Rack, B., Schindlbeck, C., Juckstock, J., Andergassen, U., Hepp, P., Zwingers, T., . . . Janni, W.; SUCCESS Study Group. (2014). Circulating tumor cells predict survival in early average-to-high risk breast cancer patients. *Journal of the National Cancer Institute, 106*(5). doi:10.1093/jnci/dju066; Passarelli, M. N., Newcomb, P. A., Hampton, J. M., Trentham-Dietz, A., Titus, L. J., Egan, K. M., . . . Willett, W. C. (2016). Cigarette smoking before and after breast cancer diagnosis: Mortality from breast cancer and smoking-related diseases. *Journal of Clinical Oncology, 34*(12), 1315–1322. doi:10.1200/JCO.2015.63.9328; Siegel, R. L., Miller, K. D., & Jemal, A. (2017). Cancer statistics, 2017. *CA: A Cancer Journal for Clinicians, 67*(1), 7–30. doi:10.3322/caac.21387.

Patients are not considered good candidates for BCT if they have any of the following:

- Multiple primary tumors
- An identified tumor that is large in relation to the breast
- Diffuse microcalcifications in the breast (suggesting possible diffuse disease)
- A history of chest radiation
- Current pregnancy
- Margins of the surgically excised lesion remaining positive for malignancy after repeated attempts of BCS

Some patients who do not meet the criteria for BCT, however, may be offered neoadjuvant systemic therapy to elicit a tumor response prior to surgery. Such treatment is most often chemotherapy, although endocrine therapy may be appropriate for some patients, and a HER2-directed agent in addition to chemotherapy may be appropriate for patients with a HER2-positive breast cancer. After neoadjuvant therapy, the patient is reevaluated and a determination made about the eligibility for

BCT. Neoadjuvant therapy is recommended for most women with locally advanced cancer.

Radical Mastectomy

The radical mastectomy is performed only very rarely today. It includes removal of the breast tissue, including skin, the pectoralis major and minor muscles, and all axillary lymph nodes.

Modified Radical Mastectomy

A modified radical mastectomy is preferred for patients who would rather have a mastectomy than a lumpectomy and who have metastases to the axillary lymph nodes as confirmed by biopsy. The surgery includes removal of the entire breast as well as the pectoralis major and most axillary lymph nodes.

Simple Mastectomy

A simple mastectomy preserves the pectoral muscles and axillary lymph nodes while removing the entire breast.

Box 27.9 Predictive Factors for Breast Cancer

- *Estrogen receptor status:* Women who are estrogen receptor–positive respond particularly well to certain medications, such as tamoxifen, which reduces recurrence by 39% and mortality by 30% for these patients but not others.
- *Human epidermal growth factor receptor 2 (HER2) expression level:* Women with cancer cells that overexpress the protein HER2 benefit from medications that target this population, including trastuzumab.

- *21-Gene recurrence score profile:* This measure applies specifically to patients with estrogen receptor–positive, node-negative cancers. Women with a high 21-gene recurrence score are more likely to derive a substantial benefit from chemotherapy. Patients with a low score are less likely.
- *Breast cancer index:* This measure predicts the responsiveness of estrogen receptor–positive cancers to endocrine therapy.

Adapted from Early Breast Cancer Trialists' Collaborative Group, Davies, C., Godwin, J., Gray, R., Clarke, M., Cutter, D., . . . Peto, R. (2011). Relevance of breast cancer hormone receptors and other factors to the efficacy of adjuvant tamoxifen: Patient-level meta-analysis of randomised trials. *The Lancet, 378*(9793), 771–784. doi:10.1016/S0140-6736(11)60993-8; Sgroi, D. C., Carney, E., Zarrella, E., Steffel, L., Binns, S. N., Finkelstein, D. M., . . . Goss, P. E. (2013). Prediction of late disease recurrence and extended adjuvant letrozole benefit by the HOXB13/IL17BR biomarker. *Journal of the National Cancer Institute, 105*(14), 1036–1042. doi:10.1093/jnci/djt146

Skin-Sparing Mastectomy

A skin-sparing mastectomy is an increasingly popular option and has a rate of recurrence comparable to that of a mastectomy in which the skin of the breast is also removed. Reconstruction begins immediately. It is contraindicated for women with inflammatory breast cancer, in which the dermal lymphatics have been invaded by malignant cells.

Nipple- and Areola-Sparing Mastectomy

A nipple- and areolar-sparing mastectomy preserves the skin of the nipple and areola but removes the underlying structures, including ducts, as part of the skin-sparing surgery. This approach is most often taken with prophylactic surgery but may be appropriate for women with tumors distant from the nipple. As with other skin-sparing mastectomies, immediate reconstruction is standard. Although most patients recover without complications, a small percentage experience ischemia and subsequent necrosis of the nipple and areola. The survival rate for this type of surgery is equivalent to that of other mastectomy types (De La Cruz, Moody, Tappy, Blankenship, & Hecht, 2015).

Sentinel Node Biopsy

Lymph nodes that are clinically suspicious by ultrasound or exam are biopsied prior to surgery by fine-needle aspiration, as discussed above. In the event of no clinically suspicious nodes, a sentinel node biopsy is performed at the time of lumpectomy or mastectomy. A **sentinel node biopsy** is a procedure that isolates the lymph nodes fed by the region of the tumor for assessment. The advantage of only removing lymph nodes as needed is to limit the complications of surgery, particularly lymphedema of the upper extremity.

To perform a sentinel node biopsy, a radioactive and/or blue dye is injected into the tumor prior to surgery. During surgery, the lymph nodes are examined for uptake of the dye. Nodes that are dye positive are surgically removed and examined by a pathologist immediately for evidence of malignant cells. If the lymph nodes are free of cancer, the risk of metastasis is low and no further nodes are removed. If the lymph nodes are positive, a complete lymph node dissection of the axilla is indicated. This examination of the lymph nodes also helps guide adjuvant systemic treatment.

Breast Reconstruction

Surgery for breast cancer can have a poor cosmetic outcome. Reconstruction can lead to improved self-esteem, body image, and psychological health. This overall improvement in quality of life from breast reconstruction led to changes in the law in the United States that requires health insurance coverage for breast surgery for cosmetic purposes after mastectomy. Approximately 40% of women who have a mastectomy in the United States elect to have additional surgery for breast reconstruction (Albornoz et al., 2013).

Several different procedure types exist for breast reconstruction. A one-step procedure that places a permanent implant at the time of mastectomy may be appropriate, particularly for women who do not need radiation therapy of the breast. A two-step procedure involves placement of a tissue expander following mastectomy that

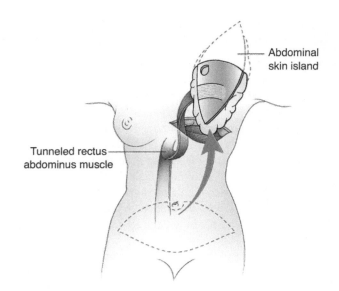

Figure 27.23. Transverse rectus abdominis myocutaneous flap reconstruction of the breast. (Reprinted with permission from Mulholland, M. W., Lillemoe, K. D., Doherty, G. M., Maier, R. V., Simeone, D. M., & Upchurch, G. R. [Eds.]. [2011]. *Greenfield's surgery: Scientific principles and practice* [5th ed., Fig. 45.1]. Philadelphia, PA: Lippincott Williams & Wilkins.)

is gradually filled to the desired volume and then replaced with a permanent implant. Delayed reconstruction occurs at a time distant from the mastectomy. Using tissue from another body site, such as the abdomen or buttocks, may be an option instead of an artificial silicone or saline implant. Artificial implants are placed under the chest muscle rather than on top of it. When the tissue from other body sites is used, it consists of muscle, skin, and fat, which is transplanted to the chest in a "flap" procedure (Fig. 27.23).

If nipple and areola preservation was not possible or advisable at the time of surgery, a new nipple and areola may be constructed from autologous tissue from another donor site. Women may alternatively have a cosmetic tattoo that resembles a nipple and areola (Fig. 27.24).

After a lumpectomy, a woman may opt for oncoplastic reconstruction to minimize asymmetry and contour abnormalities. Oncoplastic surgery, like reconstruction after a mastectomy, may be immediate or delayed and is completed prior to starting radiation therapy. Other procedures that are performed after radiation, including autologous fat transfers and breast reduction, may also minimize contour abnormalities (Losken, Pinell-White, Hodges, & Egro, 2015).

Radiation Therapy

Radiation therapy is done after BCS or mastectomy to eliminate any malignancy that may remain in the breast after surgery to reduce the risk of recurrence and improve survival. Most women who receive BCS receive whole-breast radiation therapy. As discussed previously, radiation may be give prior to BCS (neoadjuvant radiation) if the woman is not initially eligible for BCS in the hope that radiation can adequately shrink a tumor to allow for BCS. Women with lymph node involvement and tumor types with a

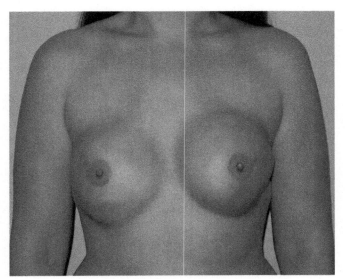

Figure 27.24. Nipple and areola reconstruction. Options include tattoo only, nipple reconstruction with areola tattoo, and nipple reconstruction with areola graft. This patient opted for a "3-D" tattoo created by a professional tattoo artist who specializes in nipple and areola reconstruction tattoos (Vinnie Myers in Finksburg, MD—http://www.vinniemyers.com).

high risk of tumor recurrence (e.g., a triple-negative tumor, which is negative for estrogen and progesterone receptors and HER2 overexpression) may also receive radiation to the regional lymph nodes. Additional "boost" radiation may be administered to the tumor bed after completion of whole-breast radiation. Treatment is delivered by external beam radiation 5 days a week over 5 to 5 ½ weeks or at an alternative dosing that allows completion of therapy over 3 weeks.

An alternative to whole-breast radiation is accelerated partial-breast radiation, which exposes only a portion of the breast to radiation. This type of radiation may, like whole-breast radiation, be delivered by external beam. Alternatively, it may be delivered by brachytherapy, which is the temporary introduction of a radioactive substance into tissue for localized radiation.

Intraoperative radiation is a form of accelerated partial-breast radiation that introduces the entire therapeutic dose to the tumor bed during surgery prior to wound closure. It too may be delivered by brachytherapy or external beam.

Radiation after a mastectomy is given for the same reasons as after a lumpectomy. The decision to perform radiation therapy after a mastectomy is based on the risk of recurrence. Radiation after a mastectomy would be administered to the chest wall and the regional lymph nodes. Radiation after an axillary lymph node dissection would be administered only to the supraclavicular and infraclavicular nodes and chest wall, to limit the risk of edema of the upper extremity.

Radiation therapy is associated with acute toxicity to the skin, muscles, and underlying organs. Many women complain of acute fatigue during radiation therapy. Such complications are sometimes acute and often chronic and long term. Short-term toxicities include edema of the arm, decreased range of motion,

rib fracture, sunburn-like erythema of the skin, burns, and fibrosis of the breast skin. Long-term complications include injury to the lungs and heart, as well as secondary malignancies that result directly from the radiation itself. Such complications can occur many years after the initial treatment (Taylor et al., 2017).

For patients who are also receiving chemotherapy after surgery, radiation therapy is usually administered after the completion of chemotherapy. Patients with estrogen receptor–positive breast cancer who are receiving endocrine therapy may receive radiation therapy at the same time. Alternatively, endocrine therapy may be administered after the completion of radiation therapy if the side effects of endocrine therapy (such as joint pain) make positioning for radiation uncomfortable. Patients with cancers with HER2 overexpression may receive trastuzumab (Herceptin) concurrent with radiation therapy.

Chemotherapy

The decision to implement chemotherapy is guided by the same considerations that inform other treatment decisions. Chemotherapy administered prior to surgery is referred to as neoadjuvant chemotherapy, whereas chemotherapy administered after surgery is referred to as adjuvant chemotherapy.

Neoadjuvant Chemotherapy

The goal of **neoadjuvant** therapy is to minimize the extent of required surgery and complications and to improve cosmetic outcomes. For women with tumors that overexpress HER2, chemotherapy is usually given with an additional biologic therapy (trastuzumab) that targets this tumor type. Patients with tumors that are hormone receptor positive may be treated with endocrine therapy instead of or in conjunction with chemotherapy.

Chemotherapy is usually dosed during six to eight sessions either weekly or every 2 weeks. Surgery is usually scheduled 3 to 6 weeks after completion of chemotherapy to allow time for the patient to recover from the toxicity of the medications. After surgery, the decision to implement adjuvant chemotherapy is based on the HER2 and hormone receptor status of the disease as well as the existence of residual disease after surgery.

Regular assessment of the patient is ongoing during neoadjuvant chemotherapy to determine the tumor response to chemotherapy. A physical examination is performed every 2 to 4 weeks that includes an examination of the breast and axilla. Imaging studies, usually ultrasound or MRI, are performed if disease progression is suspected.

Adjuvant Chemotherapy

Adjuvant chemotherapy is indicated for patients with metastatic disease, early-stage disease, or locally invasive disease with residual disease remaining after surgery, and for patients with certain tumor types, regardless of staging. Women with triple-negative tumors (negative for estrogen and progesterone receptors and HER2 overexpression), for example, have a particularly aggressive tumor type with a high risk of recurrence.

Adjuvant chemotherapy has traditionally been administered every 3 weeks, but newer regimens, referred to as "dose dense," involve dosing every 1 to 2 weeks and are associated with superior outcomes, with fewer adverse events and a shorter duration of therapy. Chemotherapy is usually started 4 to 6 weeks after surgery. Radiation therapy, if indicated, usually occurs after chemotherapy.

Women should be aware that the benefits of adjuvant chemotherapy are real but by no means a guarantee of cure. A 2012 study found the overall risk of recurrence was 39% with chemotherapy and 47% without; the breast cancer–related mortality risk was 29% with chemotherapy and 36% without chemotherapy (Early Breast Cancer Trialists' Collaborative et al., 2012). Chemotherapy risks include significant acute toxicities, including hair loss, nausea, vomiting, bone marrow suppression, and immunosuppression, which can lead to infection. Neuropathy associated with some chemotherapeutic agents may be temporary or irreversible. Cardiotoxicity and leukemia are rare long-term complications associated with chemotherapy.

The monitoring of chemotherapy for patients with metastatic disease may have several components, depending on the area of metastasis and treatment goals. If the goal of therapy is palliative, a careful history may be sufficient to gauge response to therapy. If the area of metastasis is accessible, such as palpable nodules or lymph nodes, a physical examination can be helpful in assessing response. Some tumor markers, such as CA15-3, CEA, and CA27.29, may be helpful for tracking the course of treatment. Imaging using X-ray, CT, MRI, or positron emission tomography can be helpful. The presence of circulating tumor cells in blood samples may be predictive of overall survival. Treatment failure is an indication to switch treatment. Recurrence after treatment has ceased is a reason to start chemotherapy again (Aebi et al., 2014).

Endocrine/Biologic Therapy

Patients with hormone receptor–positive cancer may receive endocrine therapy rather than chemotherapy prior to surgery and, if so, will likely also receive endocrine therapy after surgery for a number of years as well. Endocrine therapy is given over a longer span of time than radiation or chemotherapy. For example, tamoxifen and aromatase inhibitors, such as anastrozole, letrozole, and exemestane, are taken for a total of 5 years, typically.

Tamoxifen is perhaps the best known of the endocrine treatments for breast cancer. It is a selective estrogen receptor modulator that creates an antiestrogenic effect and significantly reduces cancer recurrence and breast cancer–related mortality. The adverse effects of tamoxifen include an increased rate of thromboemboli and endometrial cancer as well as hot flashes, sexual dysfunction, vaginal discharge, and, for women who are not postmenopausal, menstrual irregularities.

Aromatase inhibitors suppress plasma estrogen levels and provide an improved outcome compared with tamoxifen for postmenopausal women with a hormone receptor–positive breast cancer. They reduce recurrence or mortality for women with nonmetastatic hormone receptor–positive cancer (Early Breast Cancer Trialists' Collaborative, 2015). Aromatase inhibitors cause joint pain for 20% to 70% of patients (Beckwee, Leysen, Meuwis, & Adriaenssens, 2017). They are also associated with a higher incidence of carpal tunnel syndrome (Spagnolo, Sestak,

Howell, Forbes, & Cuzick, 2016). Because of the antiestrogenic effect, women are also at an increased risk for sexual dysfunction, vaginal dryness, and dyspareunia. Women using aromatase inhibitors are also more likely to complain of impaired cognition, fatigue, and poor sleep than women who do not use endocrine therapy (Ganz, Petersen, Bower, & Crespi, 2016). They are at a lower risk for thrombosis and endometrial cancer than patients using tamoxifen but at a higher risk for osteoporosis, heart disease, high cholesterol, and fractures (Early Breast Cancer Trialists' Collaborative, 2015).

Tamoxifen and aromatase inhibitors may both be used as a course of tamoxifen followed by a course of an aromatase inhibitor, or vice versa. For women receiving tamoxifen who are not postmenopausal, the use of a nonhormonal form of contraception is important as the medication is a known teratogen.

HER2-Directed Therapy

Women with tumors that overexpress HER2 are usually treated with trastuzumab in addition to chemotherapy. After chemotherapy is completed, trastuzumab is usually continued until a total treatment duration of 52 weeks is reached. Toxicities associated with the use of trastuzumab include congestive heart failure and a decline in left ventricular ejection fraction. Trastuzumab is given intravenously and dosed either weekly or every 3 weeks. The other agents in this class are pertuzumab and neratinib.

Follow-Up

In the United States, three million women have a personal history of breast cancer, accounting for 41% of female cancer survivors (DeSantis et al., 2014). These survivors may experience long-term effects of therapy and are at risk for recurrence. Although most recurrence occurs within 5 years of treatment, it may also occur decades later. Survivors may have long-term psychological, social, and employment issues related to cancer and treatment. Women diagnosed prior to the completion of childbearing may have reproductive issues. Women with a known heritable trait, usually *BRCA1* or *BRCA2* mutation, are living not only with a heightened risk of a new breast cancer, but also with an elevated risk of ovarian, fallopian tube, and peritoneal cancer, as well as the risk of passing the genetic mutation on to offspring.

It is generally recommended that patients be seen every 3 to 6 months during the first 3 years after therapy, then every 6 to 12 months until year 5, and then annually for a history and physical examination (Runowicz et al., 2016). Both are used to assess for recurrence and for long-term consequences of therapy (Box 27.10).

Self-care through a healthy lifestyle that includes regular physical activity, a balanced diet, and avoidance of obesity and alcohol is associated with a decreased rate of cancer recurrence. Moderation in consumption of soy products, which contain plant-based estrogens, is encouraged, as high intake could theoretically increase the risk of recurrence. Complementary therapies such as acupressure reduce fatigue and improve quality of life and sleep (Zick et al., 2016).

Box 27.10 Elements of Follow-Up for Breast Cancer

History

- *Constitutional:* Unintended weight loss, anorexia, fatigue, or malaise
- *Bones:* Presence of pain
- *Pulmonary:* Dyspnea or persistent cough
- *Neurologic:* Confusion, weakness, headache, numbness, or tingling
- *Gastrointestinal:* Nausea, vomiting, tarry or bloody stool, new onset constipation or diarrhea, or right upper quadrant pain
- *Genitourinary:* Pelvic pain, vaginal bleeding, pelvic fullness, or difficulty with urination
- *Psychological:* Insomnia, depression, or anxiety
- *Reproductive/endocrine:* Hot flashes, night sweats, sexual dysfunction, or fertility problems

Physical Examination

- Examination of the breast and/or chest wall
- Examination for lymphedema of the upper extremities
- Palpation of the pelvis, ribs, sternum, and spine for tenderness
- Auscultation of breath sounds and percussion
- Palpation of the right upper quadrant for liver tenderness and/or hepatomegaly
- Evaluation for heart failure
- Neurologic examination, including sensory and motor function as well as balance and gait

Imaging

- Annual mammogram
- Magnetic resonance imaging if at high risk for recurrence
- Dual-energy X-ray absorptiometry scan for osteoporosis

Genetic Counseling

- *Appropriate candidates:* Men with breast cancer, women who were under 40 y old when diagnosed, people of Ashkenazi background, and people with a family history of breast and/or ovarian cancer

Reproductive Considerations

Women with a personal history of breast cancer who become pregnant do not have a worse breast cancer–related prognosis (Iqbal et al., 2017). Women are often advised to wait at least 2 years after completion of treatment to attempt pregnancy, as most cancers that recur do so within the first 2 years. Chemotherapy can cause amenorrhea, which generally reverses within the first few years of treatment but is not necessarily a good predictor of fertility. Women may also ovulate in the absence of menses, and women who do not wish to be pregnant should use a nonhormonal method of birth control.

Women with a new diagnosis of breast cancer who desire a pregnancy in the future should be referred to a reproductive endocrinologist so that fertility-sparing measures may be taken prior to the administration of chemotherapy. Ovarian stimulation is done, usually with an aromatase inhibitor or tamoxifen, and the eggs retrieved, frozen, and stored for future use. For women who require neoadjuvant chemotherapy and thus cannot undergo ovarian stimulation prior to chemotherapy, harvesting immature oocytes is a possibility, although thus far the viable pregnancy yield has been low for these individuals (Practice Committees of the American Society for Reproductive Medicine and the Society for Assisted Reproductive Technology, 2013).

Breast cancer is considered gestational if it is diagnosed during pregnancy, the first year postpartum, or the period of lactation. Approximately 20% of breast cancers diagnosed in women under 30 years old are gestational, as are 5% of the breast cancers diagnosed in women under 50 years old. Approximately 1 in 3,000 women are diagnosed with breast cancer in pregnancy (Hammarberg et al., 2017). Breast cancer detection can be complicated in pregnancy because of the physiologic changes of this period, including breast hypertrophy. Postpartum, the cancer is often found by the identification of a mass. Occasionally, an infant rejects the breast with a cancerous tumor, a rare phenomenon called the milk rejection sign. Mammography, ultrasound, and MRI are not contraindicated in pregnancy. Gestational breast cancer is often diagnosed at an advanced stage and requires additional imaging to locate distant disease.

The treatment of gestational breast cancer is similar to that of nongestational breast cancer, although modifications may be necessary to protect the fetus. Radiation is not advisable in pregnancy, for example, making mastectomy the surgery of choice rather than BCS. Alternatively, BCS may be performed in pregnancy with radiation therapy performed after the birth. An axillary lymph node dissection may be preferred to a sentinel node biopsy because of concerns about exposing the fetus to the dye used for the procedure. Chemotherapy given after the first trimester appears to be relatively safe (Amant et al., 2015). Breastfeeding is contraindicated for women receiving chemotherapy, endocrine therapy, and/or trastuzumab. The use of endocrine therapy and trastuzumab is contraindicated in pregnancy. Termination of the pregnancy does not appear to improve outcomes.

Ductal Carcinoma In Situ

Ductal carcinoma in situ (DCIS) is a form of neoplasm that is limited to the ducts of the breast. It is primarily identified by mammogram and accounts for 25% of the breast cancers identified in the United States (Siegel et al., 2015). The treatment goal for DCIS is to prevent progression from DCIS to invasive cancer. It is considered a stage 0 cancer. Diagnosis is by biopsy. It is treated by mastectomy or BCT. Approximately 50% to 75% of women with DCIS have tumors that are endocrine receptor–positive and are candidates for tamoxifen and/or an aromatase inhibitor. The 20-year mortality risk from breast cancer for women treated with DCIS is 3.3% (Narod, Iqbal, Giannakeas, Sopik, & Sun, 2015).

Atypical Hyperplasia

Atypical hyperplasia is typically found as an incidental biopsy finding. The three types are atypical ductal hyperplasia, atypical lobular hyperplasia, and lobular carcinoma in situ. They are associated with a higher risk for breast cancer, although over 40% of subsequent cancers occur in breasts in which atypical hyperplasia was not found. The risk of developing breast cancer in patients with atypical hyperplasia is 35% over 30 years (Collins et al., 2007).

Because of the higher risk for cancer, women with atypical hyperplasia are often encouraged to get yearly mammograms and twice yearly clinical breast examinations. Hormonal contraception and perimenopausal hormonal therapy are contraindicated. For some women, prophylactic surgery, tamoxifen or an aromatase inhibitor may be considered.

Breast Cysts

Breast cysts are common, particularly in women 35 to 50 years old. On examination they are usually firm and round or ovoid and have clear edges. They may present as clinically palpable breast masses or be localized by mammogram. Simple breast cysts are benign but can cause acute localized pain of sudden onset. They may appear alone or in clusters. Symptoms from breast cysts, including pain and size, usually fluctuate. Although a clinical breast examination may confirm the existence of a presumed cyst, imaging by mammogram, ultrasound, or MRI is necessary to confirm the diagnosis of a mass as cystic. A simple cyst presents no increased cancer risk. A complex cyst, however, may present a cancer risk and should be biopsied. Aspiration of a simple cyst can be performed to relieve breast pain.

Many women of reproductive age have **fibrocystic breasts**, which have a ropey, lumpy texture. The lumps typical of fibrocystic breasts are smooth and mobile and found throughout the breast, although they may be more clustered in the upper, outer quadrant (Fig. 27.25). Premenstrually, fibrocystic breasts are more likely to feel tender, heavy, swollen, and full. The condition typically subsides with menopause. Women with fibrocystic breasts are not at an increased risk for breast cancer.

Mammary Duct Ectasia

Mammary duct **ectasia** is the widening of a breast duct directly beneath the nipple. The wall of the widened duct then thickens and the duct fills with fluid. Women may experience breast tenderness, inflammation, mastitis, or nipple discharge. The discharge from ductal ectasia can be thick and dark, appearing blue under the skin. A lump just under the nipple may be palpable. Surgical intervention may be necessary to remove the duct.

Intraductal Papilloma

Intraductal **papilloma** is a benign breast tumor of the milk duct. It most commonly occurs in women aged 35 to 55 years. There are two types of intraductal papilloma. The most common is a solitary intraductal papilloma that presents frequently as a small

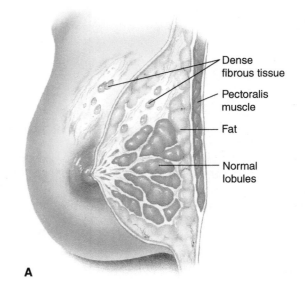

A

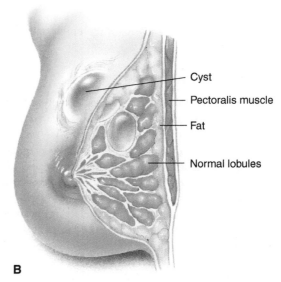

B

Figure 27.25. Fibrocystic breasts. (A) Fibrocystic breast changes. **(B)** Breast cysts. (Reprinted with permission from Anatomical Chart Company. [2002]. *Atlas of pathophysiology.* Philadelphia, PA: Springhouse.)

lump near the nipple. This type of intraductal papilloma may cause nipple discharge or bleeding but is not associated with breast cancer.

A second form of intraductal papilloma occurs in a more peripheral area of the breast, away from the nipple. Rather than a solitary phenomenon, these intraductal papilloma are smaller and grow in clusters. This type of intraductal papilloma is associated with atypical hyperplasia, a potentially precancerous condition.

Intraductal papilloma may manifest as a lump that is 1 to 2 cm wide or may be identified by mammogram, although they are best localized by ultrasound. On occasion, intraductal papilloma may cause discomfort. Papilloma close to the nipple may cause bleeding or nipple discharge. The diagnosis is confirmed after a fine-needle biopsy. If atypical cells are identified, excision is indicated and endocrine therapy may be started to prevent breast cancer.

Breast Pain

Breasts are responsive to cyclic menstrual changes. In the days immediately preceding ovulation, elevated levels of both estrogen and progesterone cause temporary breast growth, water retention, tenderness, and swelling, which can result in breast pain (mastalgia). Regression of these changes occurs after menstruation, and with it the regression of mastalgia. A minority of women report cyclic breast pain significant enough to interfere with social, sexual, physical, or educational activities.

Breast pain may also be noncyclic. This type of breast pain is more likely to be caused by a lesion, such as a breast cyst. Rarely, breast cancer may present as pain. Noncyclic pain is more likely to be unilateral. Large breasts can cause pain from the stretching of ligaments. Nicotine and caffeine may increase breast pain. Some women using hormone therapy after menopause report noncyclic breast pain that resolves spontaneously. Ductal ectasia, which causes painful dilation of the ducts of the breasts, can cause noncyclic breast pain. Mastitis, which is typically associated with lactation but may happen in its absence, is an acute condition and can be quite painful. Inflammatory breast cancer presents as a tender, painful, firm, enlarged breast with overlying erythematous skin. Pregnancy, trauma, some medications, and other conditions can also contribute to breast pain.

What is perceived by the patient as breast pain may instead originate in the chest wall, spine, lungs, gallbladder, or heart.

A careful history is important when assessing breast pain to determine the pain's timing, location, quality, severity, regularity (cyclic or noncyclic), impact on daily activities, and potential causes and associated factors, including the following:

- Use of hormones and other medications
- Recent pregnancies
- Recent activity using the muscles of the upper body
- Injuries to the upper body or spine
- Fever
- Chest trauma

Imaging is typically not indicated for cyclic breast pain. For focal pain, an ultrasound and/or mammogram should be performed.

The treatment of breast pain is in accordance with its cause. Although interventions such as cutting back on caffeine, a low-fat diet, and supplementation with vitamin E and evening primrose are often recommended, little evidence supports their use for reducing mastalgia. A supportive well-fitting bra, warm compresses, ice packs, gentle massage, acetaminophen, and oral or topical NSAIDs may be helpful in reducing breast pain. Rarely, medications such as danazol and tamoxifen are given for breast tenderness, but both have significant side effects. For many women, both cyclic and noncyclic breast pain resolve spontaneously.

Breast pain is associated with breast cancer in only 0.5% to 3.3% of patients, although it is typically an incidental finding, with the actual origin of the pain being a cyst adjacent to the cancerous tumor (Leddy et al., 2013). It should be noted that when breast pain is assessed by mammogram and cancer is discovered, the cancer is just as likely to be in the painful breast as it is to be in the nonpainful breast (Duijm, Guit, Hendriks, Zaat, & Mali, 1998).

Fibroadenomas

A fibroadenoma is a benign tumor that comprises both glandular and stromal tissue. Fibroadenomas may present as solitary or multiple lesions and typically occur in women of reproductive age, regressing after menopause. For most women, fibroadenomas do not indicate a higher risk for breast cancer (Nassar et al., 2015).

Fibroadenomas on examination feel like marbles under the skin. They are mobile and well defined. Masses are generally assessed by ultrasound. A repeat ultrasound is done for a benign-appearing mass after 6 to 12 months to assess for change. A definitive diagnosis is made by biopsy.

Lesions that are asymptomatic are usually left in place to avoid the scarring, changes in breast contour, and changes that may confuse imaging in the future that may result from excision. Patients who are particularly anxious about the fibroadenoma, however, may prefer to have it excised. A symptomatic or enlarging fibroadenoma should be excised. Alternatively, an in-office cryoablation procedure under ultrasound may be used to remove the fibroadenoma.

Nipple Discharge

Most nipple discharge is benign. Discharge is more likely to be physiologic if it is bilateral, involves multiple ducts, and occurs with manipulation of the breasts. Discharge is more likely to be pathologic if it is unilateral; involves a solitary duct; is bloody, spontaneous, or associated with a breast mass; or occurs in women over the age of 40. Note, however, that bloody nipple discharge is common during pregnancy and breastfeeding and is considered a normal finding.

Nipple discharge not associated with lactation is referred to as galactorrhea. Galactorrhea may be caused by medications (particularly serotonin reuptake inhibitors, metoclopramide, and phenothiazines), a pituitary adenoma, endocrine abnormalities, or certain other medical conditions. Galactorrhea is bilateral and involves multiple ducts. Nipple discharge may be white, clear, green, brown, yellow, or gray. Initial laboratory tests for the assessment of physiologic nipple discharge include a pregnancy test, prolactin level testing, thyroid testing, and evaluation of renal function. Ultrasound and mammography with biopsy may be indicated.

The most common source of pathologic nipple discharge is an intraductal papilloma. Malignancy, however, may be the cause a small percentage of pathologic nipple discharge. Pathologic nipple discharge is evaluated by ultrasound and/or mammogram with a surgical evaluation as indicated.

Think Critically

1. What does PALM-COEIN stand for?
2. Identify the different types of pelvic prolapse and treatments.
3. What are the differences between stress, urge, and overflow incontinence?
4. You are caring for a woman in perimenopause who is experiencing hot flashes. She asks you how she will know that she is menopausal. What do you tell her?
5. Explain how functional cysts can become symptomatic and what the natural history is of such cysts.
6. You have a patient who is newly diagnosed with polycystic ovarian syndrome. What are the metabolic concerns for this patient? Are there other health concerns?
7. Why is unopposed endogenous or exogenous estrogen dangerous for people with intact uteri?

8. Your patient is diagnosed with adenocarcinoma in situ. Her physician is recommending a hysterectomy. The patient's sister has a history of abnormal Pap tests that are managed conservatively. How do you explain to your patient how her situation differs from her sister's?
9. What is the difference between a prognostic factor and a predictive factor?
10. Your patient has gestational breast cancer. She is confused about her treatment options. How do you help explain them to her?
11. Your patient is complaining of nipple discharge. What are the important aspects of her history and of the physical examination?

References

Aebi, S., Gelber, S., Anderson, S. J., Lang, I., Robidoux, A., Martin, M., . . . Wapnir, I. L.; CALOR Investigators. (2014). Chemotherapy for isolated locoregional recurrence of breast cancer (CALOR): A randomised trial. *The Lancet. Oncology, 15*(2), 156–163. doi:10.1016/S1470-2045(13)70589-8

Albornoz, C. R., Bach, P. B., Mehrara, B. J., Disa, J. J., Pusic, A. L., McCarthy, C. M., . . . Matros, E. (2013). A paradigm shift in U.S. Breast reconstruction: Increasing implant rates. *Plastic and Reconstructive Surgery, 131*(1), 15–23. doi:10.1097/PRS.0b013e3182729cde

Al-Mukhtar Othman, J., Akervall, S., Milsom, I., & Gyhagen, M. (2017). Urinary incontinence in nulliparous women aged 25-64 years: A national survey. *American Journal of Obstetrics and Gynecology, 216*(2), 149.e1–149.e11. doi:10.1016/j.ajog.2016.09.104

Amant, F., Vandenbroucke, T., Verheecke, M., Fumagalli, M., Halaska, M. J., Boere, I., . . . Van Calsteren, K.; International Network on Cancer, Infertility, and Pregnancy. (2015). Pediatric outcome after maternal cancer diagnosed during pregnancy. *New England Journal of Medicine, 373*(19), 1824–1834. doi:10.1056/NEJMoa1508913

American Cancer Society. (2016a). *Breast cancer survival rates.* Retrieved from https://www.cancer.org/cancer/breast-cancer/understanding-a-breast-cancer-diagnosis/breast-cancer-survival-rates.html

American Cancer Society. (2016b). *Survival rates for ovarian cancer, by stage.* Retrieved from https://www.cancer.org/cancer/ovarian-cancer/detection-diagnosis-staging/survival-rates.html

American College of Obstetricians and Gynecologists. (2013a). ACOG committee opinion no. 557: Management of acute abnormal uterine bleeding in nonpregnant reproductive-aged women. *Obstetrics and Gynecology, 121*(4), 891–896. doi:10.1097/01.AOG.0000428646.67925.9a

American College of Obstetricians and Gynecologists. (2013b). Committee opinion no. 580: von Willebrand disease in women. *Obstetrics and Gynecology, 122*(6), 1368–1373. doi:10.1097/01.AOG.0000438961.38979.19

Barcellos, M. B., Lasmar, B., & Lasmar, R. (2016). Agreement between the preoperative findings and the operative diagnosis in patients with deep endometriosis. *Archives of Gynecology and Obstetrics, 293*(4), 845–850. doi:10.1007/s00404-015-3892-x

Barone, M. A., Widmer, M., Arrowsmith, S., Ruminjo, J., Seuc, A., Landry, E., . . . Gulmezoglu, A. M. (2015). Breakdown of simple female genital fistula repair after 7 day versus 14 day postoperative bladder catheterisation: A randomised, controlled, open-label, non-inferiority trial. *The Lancet, 386*(9988), 56–62. doi:10.1016/S0140-6736(14)62337-0

Beckwee, D., Leysen, L., Meuwis, K., & Adriaenssens, N. (2017). Prevalence of aromatase inhibitor-induced arthralgia in breast cancer: A systematic review and meta-analysis. *Supportive Care in Cancer, 25*(5), 1673–1686. doi:10.1007/s00520-017-3613-z

Blumel, J. E., Chedraui, P., Baron, G., Belzares, E., Bencosme, A., Calle, A., . . . Vallejo, M. S. (2013). Menopause could be involved in the pathogenesis

of muscle and joint aches in mid-aged women. *Maturitas, 75*(1), 94–100. doi:10.1016/j.maturitas.2013.02.012

Breastcancer.org. (2017). *U.S. breast cancer statistics.* Retrieved from http://www.breastcancer.org/symptoms/understand_bc/statistics

Brinton, L. A., Thistle, J. E., Liao, L. M., & Trabert, B. (2017). Epidemiology of vulvar neoplasia in the NIH-AARP Study. *Gynecologic Oncology, 145*(2), 298–304. doi:10.1016/j.ygyno.2017.02.030

Butt, J. L., Jeffery, S. T., & Van der Spuy, Z. M. (2012). An audit of indications and complications associated with elective hysterectomy at a public service hospital in South Africa. *International Journal of Gynaecology and Obstetrics, 116*(2), 112–116. doi:10.1016/j.ijgo.2011.09.026

Chlebowski, R. T., Cirillo, D. J., Eaton, C. B., Stefanick, M. L., Pettinger, M., Carbone, L. D., . . . Wactawski-Wende, J. (2013). Estrogen alone and joint symptoms in the Women's Health Initiative randomized trial. *Menopause, 20*(6), 600–608. doi:10.1097/GME.0b013e31828392c4

Ciavattini, A., Delli Carpini, G., Clemente, N., Moriconi, L., Gentili, C., & Di Giuseppe, J. (2016). Growth trend of small uterine fibroids and human chorionic gonadotropin serum levels in early pregnancy: An observational study. *Fertility and Sterility, 105*(5), 1255–1260. doi:10.1016/j.fertnstert.2016.01.032

Collins, L. C., Baer, H. J., Tamimi, R. M., Connolly, J. L., Colditz, G. A., & Schnitt, S. J. (2007). Magnitude and laterality of breast cancer risk according to histologic type of atypical hyperplasia: Results from the Nurses' Health Study. *Cancer, 109*(2), 180–187. doi:10.1002/cncr.22408

Cote, M. L., Ruterbusch, J. J., Ahmed, Q., Bandyopadhyay, S., Alosh, B., Abdulfatah, E., . . . Ali-Fehmi, R. (2014). Endometrial cancer in morbidly obese women: Do racial disparities affect surgical or survival outcomes? *Gynecologic Oncology, 133*(1), 38–42. doi:10.1016/j.ygyno.2014.01.013

De La Cruz, L., Moody, A. M., Tappy, E. E., Blankenship, S. A., & Hecht, E. M. (2015). Overall survival, disease-free survival, local recurrence, and nipple-areolar recurrence in the setting of nipple-sparing mastectomy: A meta-analysis and systematic review. *Annals of Surgical Oncology, 22*(10), 3241–3249. doi:10.1245/s10434-015-4739-1

de Sanjose, S., Alemany, L., Ordi, J., Tous, S., Alejo, M., Bigby, S. M., . . . Bosch, F. X.; HPV VVAP Study Group. (2013). Worldwide human papillomavirus genotype attribution in over 2000 cases of intraepithelial and invasive lesions of the vulva. *European Journal of Cancer, 49*(16), 3450–461. doi:10.1016/j.ejca.2013.06.033

DeSantis, C. E., Lin, C. C., Mariotto, A. B., Siegel, R. L., Stein, K. D., Kramer, J. L., . . . Jemal, A. (2014). Cancer treatment and survivorship statistics, 2014. *CA: A Cancer Journal of Clinicians, 64*(4), 252–271. doi:10.3322/caac.21235

Duijm, L. E., Guit, G. L., Hendriks, J. H., Zaat, J. O., & Mali, W. P. (1998). Value of breast imaging in women with painful breasts: Observational follow up study. *BMJ, 317*(7171), 1492–1495.

Dumoulin, C., Hay-Smith, E. J., & Mac Habee-Seguin, G. (2014). Pelvic floor muscle training versus no treatment, or inactive control treatments, for urinary incontinence in women. *Cochrane Database of Systematic Reviews, (5)*, CD005654. doi:10.1002/14651858.CD005654.pub3

Early Breast Cancer Trialists' Collaborative Group. (2015). Aromatase inhibitors versus tamoxifen in early breast cancer: Patient-level meta-analysis of the randomised trials. *The Lancet, 386*(10001), 1341–1352. doi:10.1016/S0140-6736(15)61074-1

Early Breast Cancer Trialists' Collaborative Group, Peto, R., Davies, C., Godwin, J., Gray, R., Pan, H. C., . . . Pritchard, K. (2012). Comparisons between different polychemotherapy regimens for early breast cancer: Meta-analyses of long-term outcome among 100,000 women in 123 randomised trials. *The Lancet, 379*(9814), 432–444. doi:10.1016/S0140-6736(11)61625-5

Emons, G., Beckmann, M. W., Schmidt, D., Mallmann, P., & Uterus Commission of the Gynecological Oncology Working Group. (2015). New WHO classification of endometrial hyperplasias. *Geburtshilfe und Frauenheilkd, 75*(2), 135–136. doi:10.1055/s-0034-1396256

Ezendam, N. P., Pijlman, B., Bhugwandass, C., Pruijt, J. F., Mols, F., Vos, M. C., . . . van de Poll-Franse, L. V. (2014). Chemotherapy-induced peripheral neuropathy and its impact on health-related quality of life among ovarian cancer survivors: Results from the population-based PROFILES registry. *Gynecologic Oncology, 135*(3), 510–517. doi:10.1016/j.ygyno.2014.09.016

Figo Committee on Gynecologic Oncology. (2014). FIGO staging for carcinoma of the vulva, cervix, and corpus uteri. *International Journal of Gynaecology and Obstetrics, 125*(2), 97–98. doi:10.1016/j.ijgo.2014.02.003

Ganz, P. A., Petersen, L., Bower, J. E., & Crespi, C. M. (2016). Impact of adjuvant endocrine therapy on quality of life and symptoms: Observational data over 12 months from the mind-body study. *Journal of Clinical Oncology, 34*(8), 816–824. doi:10.1200/JCO.2015.64.3866

Giri, A., Hartmann, K. E., Hellwege, J. N., Velez Edwards, D. R., & Edwards, T. L. (2017). Obesity and pelvic organ prolapse: A systematic review and meta-analysis of observational studies. *American Journal of Obstetrics and Gynecology, 217*(1), 11.e3–26.e3. doi:10.1016/j.ajog.2017.01.039

Glazener, C., Elders, A., Macarthur, C., Lancashire, R. J., Herbison, P., Hagen, S., . . . Wilson, D.; ProLong Study Group. (2013). Childbirth and prolapse: Long-term associations with the symptoms and objective measurement of pelvic organ prolapse. *British Journal of Obstetrics and Gynaecology, 120*(2), 161–168. doi:10.1111/1471-0528.12075

Gleason, C. E., Dowling, N. M., Wharton, W., Manson, J. E., Miller, V. M., Atwood, C. S., . . . Asthana, S. (2015). Effects of hormone therapy on cognition and mood in recently postmenopausal women: Findings from the randomized, controlled KEEPS-cognitive and affective study. *PLoS Medicine, 12*(6), e1001833; discussion e1001833. doi:10.1371/journal.pmed.1001833

Grigoriadis, T., Valla, A., Zacharakis, D., Protopapas, A., & Athanasiou, S. (2015). Vaginal hysterectomy for uterovaginal prolapse: What is the incidence of concurrent gynecological malignancy? *International Urogynecology Journal, 26*(3), 421–425. doi:10.1007/s00192-014-2516-5

Hammarberg, K., Sullivan, E., Javid, N., Duncombe, G., Halliday, L., Boyle, F., . . . Fisher, J. (2017). Health care experiences among women diagnosed with gestational breast cancer. *European Journal of Cancer Care.* doi:10.1111/ecc.12682

Heo, J., Chun, M., Oh, Y. T., Noh, O. K., & Kim, L. (2017). Psychiatric comorbidities among ovarian cancer survivors in South Korea: A nationwide population-based, longitudinal study. *Psychooncology.* doi:10.1002/pon.4628

Hickey, M., Ballard, K., & Farquhar, C. (2014). Endometriosis. *BMJ, 348,* g1752. doi:10.1136/bmj.g1752

Iqbal, J., Amir, E., Rochon, P. A., Giannakeas, V., Sun, P., & Narod, S. A. (2017). Association of the timing of pregnancy with survival in women with breast cancer. *JAMA Oncology, 3*(5), 659–665. doi:10.1001/jamaoncol.2017.0248

Iversen, L., Sivasubramaniam, S., Lee, A. J., Fielding, S., & Hannaford, P. C. (2017). Lifetime cancer risk and combined oral contraceptives: The Royal College of General Practitioners' Oral Contraception Study. *American Journal of Obstetrics and Gynecology, 216*(6), 580.e1–580.e9. doi:10.1016/j.ajog.2017.02.002

Jafri, M. S. (2014). Mechanisms of myofascial pain. *International Scholarly Research Notices, 2014:*523924. doi:10.1155/2014/523924

Joham, A. E., Ranasinha, S., Zoungas, S., Moran, L., & Teede, H. J. (2014). Gestational diabetes and type 2 diabetes in reproductive-aged women with polycystic ovary syndrome. *Journal of Clinical Endocrinology and Metabolism, 99*(3), E447–E452. doi:10.1210/jc.2013-2007

Jordan, S. J., Na, R., Johnatty, S. E., Wise, L. A., Adami, H. O., Brinton, L. A., . . . Webb, P. M. (2017). Breastfeeding and endometrial cancer risk: An analysis from the epidemiology of Endometrial Cancer Consortium. *Obstetrics and Gynecology, 129*(6), 1059–1067. doi:10.1097/AOG.0000000000002057

Jung, M. S., Zhang, M., Askren, M. K., Berman, M. G., Peltier, S., Hayes, D. F., . . . Cimprich, B. (2017). Cognitive dysfunction and symptom burden in women treated for breast cancer: A prospective behavioral and fMRI analysis. *Brain Imaging and Behavior, 11*(1), 86–97. doi:10.1007/s11682-016-9507-8

Khandker, M., Brady, S. S., Stewart, E. G., & Harlow, B. L. (2014). Is chronic stress during childhood associated with adult-onset vulvodynia? *Journal of Women's Health, 23*(8), 649–656. doi:10.1089/jwh.2013.4484

Kurkijarvi, K., Aaltonen, R., Gissler, M., & Makinen, J. (2017). Pelvic organ prolapse surgery in Finland from 1987 to 2009: A national register based study. *European Journal of Obstetrics, Gynecology, and Reproductive Biology, 214,* 71–77. doi:10.1016/j.ejogrb.2017.04.004

Labrie, J., Berghmans, B. L., Fischer, K., Milani, A. L., van der Wijk, I., Smalbraak, D. J., . . . van der Vaart, C. H. (2013). Surgery versus physiotherapy for stress urinary incontinence. *New England Journal of Medicine, 369*(12), 1124–1133. doi:10.1056/NEJMoa1210627

Lavelle, R. S., Christie, A. L., Alhalabi, F., & Zimmern, P. E. (2016). Risk of prolapse recurrence after native tissue anterior vaginal suspension procedure with intermediate to long-term followup. *Journal of Urology, 195*(4 Pt 1), 1014–1020. doi:10.1016/j.juro.2015.10.138

Leddy, R., Irshad, A., Zerwas, E., Mayes, N., Armeson, K., Abid, M., . . . Lewis, M. (2013). Role of breast ultrasound and mammography in evaluating patients presenting with focal breast pain in the absence of a palpable lump. *Breast Journal, 19*(6), 582–589. doi:10.1111/tbj.12178

Lee, B., Hong, S. H., Kim, K., Kang, W. C., No, J. H., Lee, J. R., . . . Kim, Y. B. (2015). Efficacy of the device combining high-frequency transcutaneous electrical nerve stimulation and thermotherapy for relieving primary dysmenorrhea: A randomized, single-blind, placebo-controlled trial. *European Journal of Obstetrics, Gynecology, and Reproductive Biology, 194,* 58–63. doi:10.1016/j.ejogrb.2015.08.020

Legro, R. S., Arslanian, S. A., Ehrmann, D. A., Hoeger, K. M., Murad, M. H., Pasquali, R., & Welt, C. K.; Endocrine Society. (2013). Diagnosis and treatment of polycystic ovary syndrome: An Endocrine Society clinical practice guideline. *Journal of Clinical Endocrinology and Metabolism, 98*(12), 4565–4592. doi:10.1210/jc.2013-2350

Losken, A., Pinell-White, X., Hodges, M., & Egro, F. M. (2015). Evaluating outcomes after correction of the breast conservation therapy deformity. *Annals of Plastic Surgery, 74* Suppl 4, S209–S213. doi:10.1097/SAP.0000000000000443

Mantegna, G., Petrillo, M., Fuoco, G., Venditti, L., Terzano, S., Anchora, L. P., . . . Ferrandina, G. (2013). Long-term prospective longitudinal evaluation of emotional distress and quality of life in cervical cancer patients who remained disease-free 2-years from diagnosis. *BMC Cancer, 13,* 127. doi:10.1186/1471-2407-13-127

Martin-Hirsch, P. P., Paraskevaidis, E., Bryant, A., & Dickinson, H. O. (2013). Surgery for cervical intraepithelial neoplasia. *Cochrane Database of Systematic Reviews,* (12), CD001318. doi:10.1002/14651858.CD001318.pub3

Massad, L. S., Einstein, M. H., Huh, W. K., Katki, H. A., Kinney, W. K., Schiffman, M., . . . Lawson, H. W.; 2012 ASCCP Consensus Guidelines Conference. (2013). 2012 updated consensus guidelines for the management of abnormal cervical cancer screening tests and cancer precursors. *Journal of Lower Genital Tract Disease, 17*(5 Suppl 1), S1–S27. doi:10.1097/LGT.0b013e318287d329

Matthews, C. A., Whitehead, W. E., Townsend, M. K., & Grodstein, F. (2013). Risk factors for urinary, fecal, or dual incontinence in the Nurses' Health Study. *Obstetrics and Gynecology, 122*(3), 539–545. doi:10.1097/AOG.0b013e31829efb8f

Mavaddat, N., Peock, S., Frost, D., Ellis, S., Platte, R., Fineberg, E., . . . Easton, D. F.; EMBRACE. (2013). Cancer risks for BRCA1 and BRCA2 mutation carriers: Results from prospective analysis of EMBRACE. *Journal of the National Cancer Institute, 105*(11), 812–822. doi:10.1093/jnci/djt095

Maybin, J. A., & Critchley, H. O. (2015). Menstrual physiology: Implications for endometrial pathology and beyond. *Human Reproduction Update, 21*(6), 748–761. doi:10.1093/humupd/dmv038

McCabe, M. P., Sharlip, I. D., Atalla, E., Balon, R., Fisher, A. D., Laumann, E., . . . Segraves, R. T. (2016). Definitions of sexual dysfunctions in women and men: A consensus statement from the Fourth International Consultation on Sexual Medicine 2015. *Journal of Sexual Medicine, 13*(2), 135–143. doi:10.1016/j.jsxm.2015.12.019

Michels, K. A., Velez Edwards, D. R., Baird, D. D., Savitz, D. A., & Hartmann, K. E. (2014). Uterine leiomyomata and cesarean birth risk: A prospective cohort with standardized imaging. *Annals of Epidemiology, 24*(2), 122–126. doi:10.1016/j.annepidem.2013.10.017

Morley, L. C., Tang, T. M. H., & Balen, A. H. (2017). Metformin therapy for the management of infertility in women with polycystic ovary syndrome: Scientific impact paper no. 13. *British Journal of Obstetrics and Gynaecology, 124*(12), e306–e313. doi:10.1111/1471-0528.14764

Mowers, E. L., Lim, C. S., Skinner, B., Mahnert, N., Kamdar, N., Morgan, D. M., & As-Sanie, S. (2016). Prevalence of endometriosis during abdominal or laparoscopic hysterectomy for chronic pelvic pain. *Obstetrics and Gynecology, 127*(6), 1045–1053. doi:10.1097/AOG.0000000000001422

Mutch, D. G., & Prat, J. (2014). 2014 FIGO staging for ovarian, fallopian tube and peritoneal cancer. *Gynecologic Oncology, 133*(3), 401–404. doi:10.1016/j.ygyno.2014.04.013

Narod, S. A., Iqbal, J., Giannakeas, V., Sopik, V., & Sun, P. (2015). Breast cancer mortality after a diagnosis of ductal carcinoma in situ. *JAMA Oncology, 1*(7), 888–896. doi:10.1001/jamaoncol.2015.2510

Nassar, A., Visscher, D. W., Degnim, A. C., Frank, R. D., Vierkant, R. A., Frost, M., . . . Ghosh, K. (2015). Complex fibroadenoma and breast cancer risk: A Mayo Clinic Benign Breast Disease Cohort Study. *Breast Cancer Research and Treatment, 153*(2), 397–405. doi:10.1007/s10549-015-3535-8

National Cancer Institute. (2013). *Surgery to reduce the risk of breast cancer.* Retrieved from https://www.cancer.gov/types/breast/risk-reducing-surgery-fact-sheet

National Cancer Institute. Retrieved from https://seer-cancer-gov.ezproxy.uvm.edu/statfacts/html/corp.html

National Cancer Institute. Retrieved from https://seer-cancer-gov.ezproxy.uvm.edu/statfacts/html/vulva.html

National Institutes of Health. (2012). *Evidence-based methodology workshop on polycystic ovary syndrome.* Retrieved from https://www.nichd.nih.gov/news/resources/spotlight/112112-pcos

NCCN Clinical Practice Guidelines in Oncology. (2016). *Cervical cancer.* https://www.nccn.org/professionals/physician_gls/pdf/cervical.pdf.

NCCN Clinical Practice Guidelines in Oncology. (2017). *Uterine neoplasms.* Retrieved from http://www.nccn.org/professionals/physician_gls/pdf/uterine.pdf

Nguyen, J. T., Palladino, H., Sonnema, A. J., & Petty, P. M. (2013). Long-term satisfaction of reduction mammaplasty for bilateral symptomatic macromastia in younger patients. *Journal of Adolescent Health, 53*(1), 112–117. doi:10.1016/j.jadohealth.2013.01.025

Practice Committees of the American Society for Reproductive Medicine and the Society for Assisted Reproductive Technology. (2013). In vitro maturation: A committee opinion. *Fertility and Sterility, 99*(3), 663–666. doi:10.1016/j.fertnstert.2012.12.031

Prat, J., & Mbatani. (2015). Uterine sarcomas. *International Journal of Gynaecology and Obstetrics, 131* Suppl 2, S105–S110. doi:10.1016/j.ijgo.2015.06.006

Rosenfeld, H., & Byard, R. W. (2012). Lower extremity deep venous thrombosis with fatal pulmonary thromboembolism caused by benign pelvic space-occupying lesions—An overview. *Journal of Forensic Sciences, 57*(3), 665–668. doi:10.1111/j.1556-4029.2011.02047.x

Rosenfield, R. L. (2015). The diagnosis of polycystic ovary syndrome in adolescents. *Pediatrics, 136*(6), 1154–1165. doi:10.1542/peds.2015-1430

Rosenfield, R. L., & Ehrmann, D. A. (2016). The pathogenesis of polycystic ovary syndrome (PCOS): The hypothesis of PCOS as functional ovarian hyperandrogenism revisited. *Endocrine Reviews, 37*(5), 467–520. doi:10.1210/er.2015-1104

Runowicz, C. D., Leach, C. R., Henry, N. L., Henry, K. S., Mackey, H. T., Cowens-Alvarado, R. L., . . . Ganz, P. A. (2016). American Cancer Society/American Society of Clinical Oncology breast cancer survivorship care guideline. *Journal of Clinical Oncology, 34*(6), 611–635. doi:10.1200/JCO.2015.64.3809

Salani, R., Puri, I., & Bristow, R. E. (2009). Adenocarcinoma in situ of the uterine cervix: A metaanalysis of 1278 patients evaluating the predictive value of conization margin status. *American Journal of Obstetrics and Gynecology, 200*(2), 182.e1–182.e5. doi:10.1016/j.ajog.2008.09.012

Schmid, D., Behrens, G., Keimling, M., Jochem, C., Ricci, C., & Leitzmann, M. (2015). A systematic review and meta-analysis of physical activity and endometrial cancer risk. *European Journal of Epidemiology, 30*(5), 397–412. doi:10.1007/s10654-015-0017-6

Siegel, R. L., Miller, K. D., & Jemal, A. (2015). Cancer statistics, 2015. *CA: A Cancer Journal for Clinicians, 65*(1), 5–29. doi:10.3322/caac.21254

Siegel, R. L., Miller, K. D., & Jemal, A. (2017). Cancer statistics, 2017. *CA: A Cancer Journal for Clinicians, 67*(1), 7–30. doi:10.3322/caac.21387

Soini, T., Hurskainen, R., Grenman, S., Maenpaa, J., Paavonen, J., & Pukkala, E. (2014). Cancer risk in women using the levonorgestrel-releasing intrauterine system in Finland. *Obstetrics and Gynecology, 124*(2 Pt 1), 292–299. doi:10.1097/AOG.0000000000000356

Spagnolo, F., Sestak, I., Howell, A., Forbes, J. F., & Cuzick, J. (2016). Anastrozole-induced carpal tunnel syndrome: Results from the International Breast Cancer intervention study II prevention trial. *Journal of Clinical Oncology, 34*(2), 139–143. doi:10.1200/JCO.2015.63.4972

Tanner, E. J., Garg, K., Leitao, M. M., Jr., Soslow, R. A., & Hensley, M. L. (2012). High grade undifferentiated uterine sarcoma: Surgery, treatment, and survival outcomes. *Gynecologic Oncology, 127*(1), 27–31. doi:10.1016/j.ygyno.2012.06.030

Taylor, C., Correa, C., Duane, F. K., Aznar, M. C., Anderson, S. J., Bergh, J., . . . McGale, P.; Early Breast Cancer Trialists' Collaborative Group. (2017). Estimating the risks of breast cancer radiotherapy: Evidence from modern radiation doses to the lungs and heart and from previous randomized trials. *Journal of Clinical Oncology, 35*(15), 1641–1649. doi:10.1200/JCO.2016.72.0722

Torre, L. A., Bray, F., Siegel, R. L., Ferlay, J., Lortet-Tieulent, J., & Jemal, A. (2015). Global cancer statistics, 2012. *CA: A Cancer Journal for Clinicians, 65*(2), 87–108. doi:10.3322/caac.21262

Trope, C. G., Abeler, V. M., & Kristensen, G. B. (2012). Diagnosis and treatment of sarcoma of the uterus. A review. *Acta Oncologica, 51*(6), 694–705. doi:10.3109/0284186X.2012.689111

van Maaren, M. C., de Munck, L., de Bock, G. H., Jobsen, J. J., van Dalen, T., Linn, S. C., . . . Siesling, S. (2016). 10 year survival after breast-conserving surgery plus radiotherapy compared with mastectomy in early breast cancer in the Netherlands: A population-based study. *The Lancet. Oncology, 17*(8), 1158–1170. doi:10.1016/S1470-2045(16)30067-5

Vercellini, P., Bracco, B., Mosconi, P., Roberto, A., Alberico, D., Dhouha, D., & Somigliana, E. (2016). Norethindrone acetate or dienogest for the treatment of symptomatic endometriosis: A before and after study. *Fertility and Sterility, 105*(3), 734.e3–743.e3. doi:10.1016/j.fertnstert.2015.11.016

Wu, J. M., Vaughan, C. P., Goode, P. S., Redden, D. T., Burgio, K. L., Richter, H. E., & Markland, A. D. (2014). Prevalence and trends of symptomatic pelvic floor disorders in U.S. women. *Obstetrics and Gynecology, 123*(1), 141–148. doi:10.1097/AOG.0000000000000057

Zick, S. M., Sen, A., Wyatt, G. K., Murphy, S. L., Arnedt, J. T., & Harris, R. E. (2016). Investigation of 2 types of self-administered acupressure for persistent cancer-related fatigue in breast cancer survivors: A randomized clinical trial. *JAMA Oncology, 2*(11), 1470–1476. doi:10.1001/jamaoncol.2016.1867

Suggested Readings

American Congress of Obstetricians and Gynecologists. (2017). *When sex is painful.* Retrieved from https://www.acog.org/Patients/FAQs/When-Sex-Is-Painful

Rosser, M., & Marshall, K. (2015). *A clinical update on endometriosis.* Retrieved from http://www.nursinginpractice.com/article/clinical-update-endometriosis

Stilos, K., Doyle, C., & Daines, P. (2008). Addressing the sexual health needs of patients with gynecologic cancers. *Clinical Journal of Oncology Nursing, 12*(3), 457-463. doi:10.1188/08.CJON.457-463

28 Infections

Infections are a common complaint in women's health. Infections may be fairly benign but annoying, such as vaginal yeast infections, or potentially dangerous, such as certain sexually transmitted infections (STIs) or a urinary tract infection that ascends into or even beyond the kidneys. Many women feel socially conditioned to think of their bodies as unclean and to perceive examinations and interviews about genital health invasive and embarrassing. Such feelings can delay critical assessments and care. It is a role of the nurse to normalize such assessments to encourage greater comfort and access for patients.

Urinary Tract Infections

A **urinary tract infection (UTI)** is an infection that occurs anywhere between the kidneys and the egress of the urethra. Although either men or women can have UTIs, they are more common in women, largely because of anatomic reasons. The male urethra is approximately 7 in long, whereas the female urethra is approximately 2 ½ in long. This shorter urethra allows for quicker transit of bacteria to the bladder, where it can become an infection. Incomplete emptying of the bladder, as can happen with a cystocele, which kinks the bladder (see Chapter 27), is a common cause of recurrent UTIs for older women. Women are often instructed to wipe from front to back and to urinate before and after sex to avoid UTIs. This common-sense advice, however, is not well researched.

In women, UTI typically occurs because of the ascension of fecal flora into the urethra and bladder. In the case of pyelonephritis, these bacteria then ascend to the kidneys by way of the ureters. Because of this, a majority of UTIs are caused by *Escherichia coli*.

Simple Cystitis

Simple cystitis is the most common form of UTI. It is a UTI limited to the bladder itself. Cystitis is considered complex instead of simple if there is a condition that increases the risk for a progressing infection or failure of therapy, such as a drug-resistant pathogen, obstruction, pregnancy, poorly controlled diabetes, a compromised immune system, urinary catheterization, kidney disease, renal transplant, or other urologic dysfunction.

Signs and Symptoms

The common symptoms of cystitis include urinary frequency, urinary urgency, a sensation of incomplete emptying, and pain with urination (dysuria). Women may sometimes also complain of frank hematuria (blood in the urine) or a sensation of pelvic pain or fullness. Approximately half of women reporting one of these symptoms are diagnosed with a UTI, as are a majority of women with dysuria alone. Nurses should be aware that the very young and very old may present differently. In the very old, UTI may present as a change in mental status.

Prognosis

UTIs, although uncomfortable, are rarely life-threatening and often resolve within 3 days of symptom onset without treatment. Progression of simple cystitis to pyelonephritis is rare (Foxman & Buxton, 2013).

Assessment

The initial assessment of a UTI includes a point-of-care urinalysis (Fig. 28.1). Patients must be instructed to collect urine midstream after thoroughly cleansing the genitals per institution protocol. A urinalysis strip may assess for several different values. The values specific to a UTI are leukocytes, nitrites, and blood. The nurse should be aware, however, that a urinalysis is not particularly specific or sensitive. As many as 20% of women with UTIs may have a negative urinalysis (Middelkoop, van Pelt, Kampinga, Ter Maaten, & Stegeman, 2016). Other conditions, such as vaginal atrophy and vaginitis, can cause leukocytes to appear. A more definitive test is a urine culture, which must be done in a laboratory setting, takes several days to return, and is considerably more expensive than simple point-of-care testing. Urine cytology is thus often reserved for cystitis that recurs within a short period of time, is inadequately treated with a first-line antibiotic, has progressed to an ascending infection, or is considered complex for a different reason. Because of these factors, suspected simple cystitis is often treated in the absence of confirmatory laboratory results.

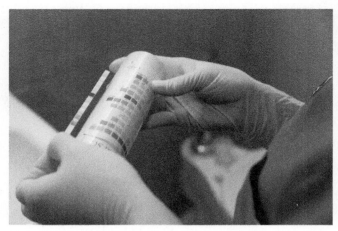

Figure 28.1. Urinalysis. Chemically treated reagent strips are used to test urine for some substances. (Reprinted with permission from Carter, P. J. [2016]. *Lippincott textbook for nursing assistants: A humanistic approach to caregiving* [4th ed., Fig. 24-4]. Philadelphia, PA: Lippincott Williams & Wilkins.)

Treatment

Phenazopyridine is a urinary analgesic that can at least partially manage the symptoms of simple cystitis for a few days. Phenazopyridine is available over the counter, but this medication cannot actually cure the UTI.

Simple cystitis is routinely treated with antibiotics. First-line antibiotics include sulfamethoxazole/trimethoprim twice daily for 3 days and nitrofurantoin twice daily for 7 days. Nurses should be aware that many patients have sulfa allergies, which would make sulfamethoxazole/trimethoprim a poor medication choice. However, sulfamethoxazole/trimethoprim is a much less expensive medication with a shorter course, which may make it a better choice for a patient who does not have a sulfa allergy. Other medications, such as ciprofloxacin, are effective against UTI but are not considered first-line medications because of concerns about bacteria building antibiotic resistance against these medications.

Patients should feel considerably better within 24 to 48 hours of starting antibiotics. As with any course of antibiotics, the nurse should advise patients to complete their medication even if they feel better before the course of medication has been completed. For patients taking phenazopyridine, the nurse should instruct them to take the medication for no more than 2 days, as it masks UTI symptoms. Phenazopyridine changes urine to a bright orange color, which can be alarming to a patient if unexpected. The orange color can also obscure a urinalysis.

Pyelonephritis

Pyelonephritis is a UTI that has ascended to the kidneys. It is often referred to simply as a kidney infection. In addition to cystitis symptoms, people with pyelonephritis will complain of fever and back pain. They often report chills and flu-like symptoms. On exam, costovertebral tenderness is present (Fig. 28.2). Pyelonephritis is much rarer than simple cystitis and also potentially much

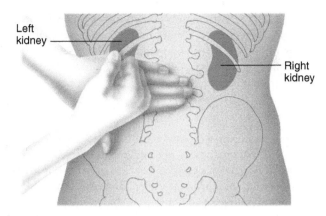

Left kidney

Right kidney

Figure 28.2. Eliciting CVA tenderness. To elicit CVA tenderness, have the patient sit upright facing away from you or have her lie in a prone position. Place the palm of your left hand over the left CVA and then strike the back of your left hand with the ulnar surface of your right fist (as shown). Repeat this percussion technique over the right CVA. A patient with CVA tenderness should experience acute pain as a result of this test. CVA, costovertebral angle. (Reprinted with permission from Lippincott's Nursing Advisor, 2009.)

more dangerous. A diagnosis of pyelonephritis is an indication for a urine culture, as it is important that the right antibiotic is prescribed to avoid long-term consequences of infection, including kidney failure, shock, multiple organ dysfunction, sepsis, and death. Ciprofloxacin and levofloxacin are two common first-line medications that are both prescribed for a week. Patients

should be instructed to check in within 2 or 3 days of starting treatment to verify an improvement of symptoms. If symptoms are not regressing, it is probable that a different antibiotic needs to be prescribed.

Vaginosis and Vaginitis

The term vaginosis refers to any abnormality of the discharge of the vagina. The term vaginitis means inflammation of the mucosa of the vagina. Often, conditions that affect the vaginal discharge, odor, or sensation (particularly pruritus) have less to do with a true infection and more to do with an overgrowth of normally occurring vaginal microbes.

Bacterial vaginosis (BV), candida, and trichomoniasis, account for most cases of vaginitis (Table 28.1). Note that infections may include some, all, or none of the common symptoms or examination findings.

Bacterial Vaginosis

BV is a common complaint and accounts for approximately half of the complaints of abnormal vaginal discharge. It is described as a vaginosis rather than vaginitis because inflammation is not part of the clinical picture.

Etiology

BV is associated with a higher pH environment, in which certain bacteria that occur normally in the vagina can become dominant.

Table 28.1 Evaluation Findings Associated With Vaginitis and Vaginosis

	Normal	Candida	Bacterial Vaginosis	Trichomoniasis
Symptoms	N/A	Acute pruritus, vulvar swelling, dyspareunia, and "soreness"	Mild irritation and "fishy" smelling discharge	Dyspareunia, dysuria, copious "fishy" discharge, and burning
Examination findings	Discharge thin, thick, slippery, sticky, white, or clear	Discharge sparse or white, clumpy, and adherent	Thin white or gray discharge	Vulvovaginal erythema, yellow or green frothy discharge, and strawberry cervix
Vaginal pH	4.0–4.5	4.0–4.5	>4.5	>5.0
Whiff test result (add potassium hydroxide)	Negative	Negative	Positive	Positive
Saline microscopy findings	Squamous epithelial cells, rarely white blood cells, and lactobacilli	Pseudohyphae, spores, lactobacilli, squamous epithelial cells, and rarely white blood cells	Clue cells, few lactobacilli or white blood cells, and some normal squamous cells	White blood cells too numerous to count and motile trichomonads
Potassium hydroxide microscopy findings	Negative	Pseudohyphae and spores	Negative	Negative

N/A, not applicable.

The normal pH of the vagina is approximately 4 to 4.5. This pH level is maintained by lactobacilli in the vagina, which create hydrogen peroxide, leading to the slightly acidic pH. The normal acidity of the vagina can be disrupted by numerous factors, including antibiotics, contraception, bleeding, intercourse, pregnancy, menopause, feminine hygiene products, and foreign objects such as retained tampons.

An overgrowth of lactobacilli is relatively rare and is referred to as cytolytic vaginosis. An undergrowth of lactobacilli is quite common, however. Fewer lactobacilli result in a higher, more alkaline pH, in which other bacteria, particularly those responsible for BV, can thrive. Thus, BV is an overgrowth of diverse normal bacteria in the vagina and an undergrowth of lactobacilli.

Although BV is not sexually transmitted, it is sexually associated. It is rare for women who are not sexually active to be diagnosed with BV, but treating partners is not beneficial for preventing recurrence (Bradshaw & Sobel, 2016). Women in same-sex relationships are particularly prone to BV (Vodstrcil et al., 2015).

Factors that predispose women to BV include douching, removing pubic hair by shaving or waxing, smoking, and having multiple sexual partners (Bradshaw et al., 2014). Women with darker skin are more likely to complain of BV than women with lighter skin, leading to the theory that low levels of vitamin D may also contribute. One sampling of 3,700 women found that 29% of all women and 50% of African American women 14 to 49 years old were positive for BV. Most women who have BV are asymptomatic. Some researchers and clinicians also hypothesize that BV is not pathologic but instead a normal variation (Kenyon, Colebunders, & Crucitti, 2013).

Signs and Symptoms

BV results in a higher pH, a fishy vaginal odor, and thin white/gray vaginal discharge. The extra moisture from the discharge often causes vulvar irritation, but not the acute pruritus often caused by a candidiasis infection.

Prognosis

BV tends to be recurrent, with up to 60% of women who experience it developing the condition again within a year (Marshall, 2015). Although BV is typically a relatively benign condition, women with BV are more likely to contract STIs (Balkus et al., 2014). In pregnancy, BV is associated with preterm labor and infection after invasive procedures such as dilation and curettage.

Assessment

The common means of assessing BV include a combination of history, physical examination, pH, and microscopy. Many women present with vaginal discharge as a sole complaint. It is important for the nurse to know that vaginal discharge is normal, and most women produce 1 to 4 mL of discharge within a 24-hour time period. Normal discharge is white or clear, thin, mucosal, slippery, thick, and/or sticky. It is typically odorless. Normal discharge changes in response to hormones and thus changes throughout the month and throughout the life span. Generally, vaginal discharge is considered normal in the absence of pain, pruritus, abnormal bleeding, irritation, erosions, erythema, or a foul or fishy odor.

The examination of a patient with BV is often unremarkable, although copious, thin discharge may be visualized. The pH of BV is high, above 5.5. A drop of potassium hydroxide added to the vaginal discharge collected at the time of examination elicits an "amine" or fishy odor typical of the condition. Microscopically, no or few lactobacilli are seen. Squamous epithelial cells collected have a "salt and pepper" appearance because of the adherence of bacteria to the cell walls. The edges of the cell have a ragged appearance. These cells are called "clue cells" (Fig. 28.3).

Treatment

Although it often regresses spontaneously, BV may also be treated with oral metronidazole twice weekly for 7 days or with a vaginal cream, either metronidazole or clindamycin. The treatment of asymptomatic BV is not generally indicated unless a procedure is planned. Routine screening and treatment of BV in pregnancy are controversial because of inconsistent evidence about risks and benefits (Thinkhamrop, Hofmeyr, Adetoro, Lumbiganon, & Ota, 2015).

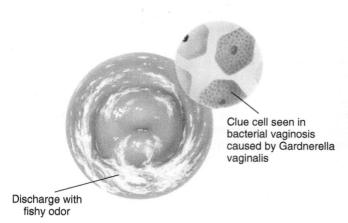

Clue cell seen in bacterial vaginosis caused by Gardnerella vaginalis

Discharge with fishy odor

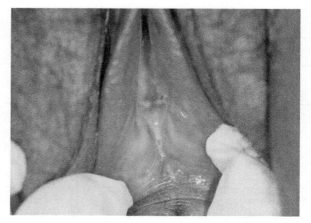

Figure 28.3. Bacterial vaginosis. (Reprinted with permission from Ricci, S. S. [2013]. *Essentials of maternity, newborn, & women's health nursing* [3rd ed., Fig. 5.3]. Philadelphia, PA: Lippincott Williams & Wilkins.)

Candidiasis Vulvovaginitis

Candida vulvovaginitis, commonly known as a yeast infection, is a frequent cause of vaginitis, particularly among women of reproductive age. Candidiasis is the growth of yeast within the vagina and accounts for about a third of cases of vaginosis (Workowski, Bolan, & Centers for Disease Control and Prevention [CDC], 2015).

Etiology

Yeast is a normally occurring vaginal microbe that is typically dormant. Unusual warmth and high levels of glucose, as with diabetes, are factors known to contribute to yeast activation.

Candida albicans is the most common yeast isolated in the vagina, but others, most often *Candida glabrata*, are also identified. All have a different microscopic appearance. Only *C. albicans* has the classic "spaghetti and meatballs" appearance created by the presence of both spores and pseudohyphae (Fig. 28.4). *C. glabrata* and *Candida tropicalis* do not form pseudohyphae.

Like BV, candidiasis is not sexually transmitted. Associated risk factors include the use of some antibiotics that disrupt the balance of vaginal flora; restrictive clothing such as bathing suits, leotards, and underwear made with artificial fibers; and glucose intolerance. Similar to a UTI, candida organisms likely originate in the rectum and migrate to the vagina. It may occasionally be shared sexually.

Signs and Symptoms

Many women are asymptomatically colonized. Symptoms when they occur include acute vaginal and vulvar, and sometimes perineal, pruritus, and erythema and edema of the mucosa. Classically, women also report a thick, cottage cheese–like vaginal discharge. In fact, this discharge is highly adherent to the vaginal walls, and many women report no discharge. Vaginal candidiasis may also manifest as acute vaginal dryness. Upon examination, the vulva may appear excoriated because of scratching of inflamed tissue.

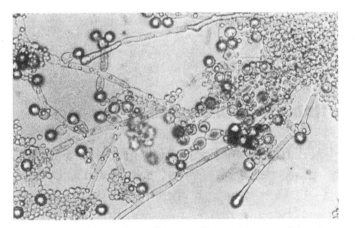

Figure 28.4. *Candida albicans*. Note the pseudohyphae ("spaghetti") and the spores ("meatballs"). (Reprinted with permission from Molle, E. A., Kronenberger, J., & Durham, L. S. [2005]. *Lippincott comprehensive medical assisting* [2nd ed.]. Philadelphia, PA: Lippincott Williams & Wilkins.)

Prognosis

An infection is considered complicated if symptoms are severe; the cause is a non-albicans strain; the patient is pregnant, diabetic, or immunosuppressed; or the infection is recurrent. Candida is considered recurrent when a woman has four or more confirmed symptomatic episodes in a single year. Women with recurrent yeast infections should be assessed for diabetes, although this accounts for only a minority of recurrent infections. Complicated infections may require a longer course of medication or treatment with intravaginal boric acid.

Assessment

Approximately 10% to 20% of asymptomatic women of reproductive age have candida that can be identified, although the disease is diagnosed only in the case of symptoms (Tibaldi et al., 2009).

Treatment

Over-the-counter treatments are effective for most patients with a *C. albicans* infection with mild-to-moderate symptoms. Such treatments are 1-, 3-, 5-, or 7-day over-the-counter vaginal preparations. Most of these preparations, with the exception of tioconazole, are best suited to treating *C. albicans* and may not be as useful for treating *C. tropicalis* or *C. glabrata*. The shorter, 1- and 3-day treatments tend to be more concentrated and may be irritating to already inflamed tissue. They may also not be as effective as the 5- or 7-day treatments. Prescription treatments include fluconazole and other vaginal preparations. Fluconazole is an oral preparation and is often requested by patients because of ease of use. It generally takes a day or two longer to be effective than vaginal treatments.

Trichomoniasis

Trichomoniasis is a sexually transmitted form of vaginitis caused by a microscopic flagellated protozoan, *Trichomonas vaginalis*.

Prevalence

In some parts of the country, trichomoniasis, often called "trich" for short, is the most common nonviral STI. The prevalence of *T. vaginalis* in women aged 14 to 49 years is 8.7% in the general population and 16% in those who are incarcerated or who present at a clinic specializing in STIs (Ginocchio et al., 2012).

Signs and Symptoms

Women with trichomoniasis often complain of symptoms similar to those of BV: thin vaginal discharge, fishy odor, and vulvar irritation. Additional common complaints are pelvic pain, dysuria, urinary frequency, and off-schedule vaginal bleeding. Up to half of women with trichomoniasis are asymptomatic (Van Der Pol, Kraft, & Williams, 2006).

Prognosis

An untreated *T. vaginalis* infection can lead to cystitis, pelvic inflammatory disease (PID), cellulitis, infertility, preterm birth, premature rupture of membranes, and infection of an infant at birth.

Assessment

On examination, inflammation of the vaginal mucosa and cervix is often observed. Classically, the cervix takes on a spotted appearance and is referred to as a "strawberry cervix," although this is rarely observed clinically (Fig. 28.5). The discharge associated with trichomoniasis is typically frothy, yellow, and copious.

Microscopically, copious white blood cells are visualized in the vaginal fluid. The trichomonads themselves can be visualized moving through the fluid, aided by their flagella. Trichomoniasis can be diagnosed only if this movement has been visualized, as a still trichomonad bears close resemblance to a white blood cell and a desquamated nucleus of a squamous epithelial cell. The pH of the vaginal discharge is typically higher for trichomoniasis than for BV. Alternatively, a sample of the vaginal discharge may be sent to a laboratory for analysis. In cases of a high suspicion of disease and negative microscopy, nucleic acid amplification testing may be performed.

Treatment

Trichomoniasis can be treated with a single dose of 2 mg of metronidazole. Topical vaginal metronidazole is not considered curative, as trichomonads may colonize the Bartholin and Skene glands of the vulva, which are not accessed by a localized treatment. Sexual partners must be treated as well or the patient may be reinfected. The reinfection rate is 17% (Workowski et al., 2015).

Sexually Transmitted Infections

STIs are an important public health problem. They impact fertility and quality of life and in some cases are potentially deadly. Routine

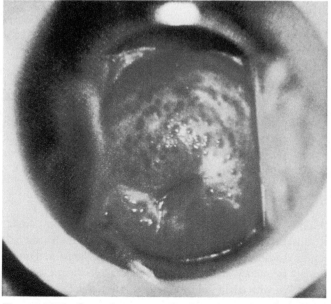

Figure 28.5. Strawberry cervix due to a trichomoniasis infection. With trichomoniasis, the cervical mucosa may reveal punctate hemorrhages with accompanying vesicles or papules, also known as strawberry cervix. (Image courtesy of Centers for Disease Control and Prevention Public Health Image Library ID 5240. Retrieved from http://phil.cdc.gov)

screening is advised for some infections (see Chapter 26). Treatment is well defined for most, although the treatment for HIV is evolving and the treatment for gonorrhea is tenuous.

In Chapter 7, Hannah visited her healthcare provider for STI screening prior to starting a sexual relationship with John. Although John said that STI screening wasn't romantic, Hannah pointed out that neither were STIs.

Many sexually transmitted diseases are reportable to the state health department. Which diseases are reportable varies by state. It is the responsibility of the nurse to be familiar with the reporting laws in the state in which she or he is employed.

The only definitive means of preventing the spread of STIs is complete abstinence. This, however, is not a reasonable or acceptable universal expectation. Condom use can lessen the risk from some infections, such as **chlamydia**, **gonorrhea**, and HIV, but provides imperfect protection. It is important that patients feel safe seeking screening and care for STIs so they may be quickly diagnosed and treated, thus reducing the rate of transmission and individual negative sequelae. The partners of infected individuals should also be offered treatment. In some states, the treatment of select STIs, including chlamydia and trichomoniasis, is available to the partners of individuals with a confirmed STI diagnosis without a visit to a healthcare provider.

Chlamydia

Prevalence

Chlamydia is the most commonly diagnosed bacterial STI in the United States. In 2015, 1,526,548 cases were identified (CDC, 2016c).

Etiology

The causative pathogen of chlamydia is the gram-negative bacterium *Chlamydia trachomatis*. The transmission of chlamydia is almost always sexual. It is not clear how likely transmission is from an infected to uninfected partner after a single or multiple contacts. The prevalence of infection is highest among young women aged 15 to 24 years and young men aged 20 to 24 years (CDC, 2016c). Besides age, risk factors include new and multiple sexual partners, inconsistent condom use, and a previous history of chlamydia or a different STI.

Signs and Symptoms

In men, chlamydia is a common cause of **urethritis** (inflammation of the urethra) and in women it is a common cause of **cervicitis** (inflammation of the cervix), although it is typically asymptomatic. It may also present as dysuria, PID, perihepatitis (inflammation of the liver), proctitis, epididymitis, prostatitis, or reactive arthritis. Reactive arthritis, or Reiter syndrome, is a rare complication that presents as arthritis, urethritis, and uveitis (inflammation of the middle layer of the eye).

Prognosis

Despite a frequent lack of symptoms, chlamydia can devastate a woman's ability to reproduce by causing inflammation of the fallopian tubes, ovaries, and endometrium that results in scarring that, in turn, increases the risk for both infertility and ectopic pregnancy (Davies et al., 2016).

Assessment

Because it is usually asymptomatic, chlamydia is most often detected during screening (see Chapter 26). Screening is typically done by a laboratory analysis of urine for men and women. Vaginal, cervical, or urethral swabs are another option. If a patient is engaging in receptive anal or oral sex, rectal and pharyngeal sampling may be warranted. Urine tests should be gathered without precleansing. It is preferable that the patient not have voided within 2 hours of specimen collection.

Treatment

The treatment of chlamydia is either 1 g of azithromycin in a single dose or doxycycline 100 mg twice daily for a week. Sexual partners must also be treated. It takes approximately a week for the antibiotics to eliminate the disease, and patients should refrain from sexual activity during this time. Reinfection is common, occurring in up to 15% of patients within 3 months after treatment (Hoover, Tao, Nye, & Body, 2013). It is recommended that patients return for retesting approximately 3 months after treatment.

Gonorrhea

Prevalence

Gonorrhea is the second-most prevalent bacterial STI in the United States. In 2015, 395,216 cases were diagnosed (CDC, 2016c).

Etiology

Gonorrhea is caused by the bacterium *Neisseria gonorrhoeae*. Like chlamydia, gonorrhea can be passed by oral and rectal sex, in addition to vaginal intercourse.

Signs and Symptoms

Symptoms, when they occur, are similar to those of chlamydia: urethritis in men and cervicitis in women.

Prognosis

Untreated gonorrhea can lead to PID, which can cause infertility, ectopic pregnancy, and chronic pelvic pain (CDC, 2016c). Other manifestations of the infection may include perihepatitis, bartholinitis (inflammation of the Bartholin glands), pregnancy complications, epididymitis, proctitis, and pharyngitis.

A disseminated form of gonorrhea will be identified in up to 3% of people with the infection (Belkacem et al., 2013). As with chlamydia, disseminated infection most often manifests as reactive arthritis as evidenced by purulent arthritis, joint pain, nonpurulent arthritis, and/or tenosynovitis (inflammation of the sheath that covers tendons). Associated symptoms may include fever, chills, malaise, and a dermatitis that is typically vesiculopustular or pustular but may take other forms (Fig. 28.6). Mucosal symptoms seen with the nondisseminated form of infection typically do not occur with these symptoms. Rare complications include meningitis, osteomyelitis, myopericarditis, and endocarditis (Bunker & Kerr, 2015).

Assessment

Because most people are asymptomatic, routine screening for gonorrhea is recommended for women under the age of 25; men who have sex with men; people with a past history of sexually transmitted disease, current HIV, or new or multiple sexual partners; and women under 35 years and men under 30 years who are entering correctional facilities. Co-testing for chlamydia is standard (Aberg et al., 2014; Workowski et al., 2015). Testing protocols and considerations are similar to those for chlamydia.

Treatment

Once curable with penicillin, gonorrhea has proved to be adaptable, and strains now exist in many different countries that are resistant to all antibiotics. First-line treatment for gonorrhea is 250 mg of ceftriaxone intramuscularly plus 1 g of azithromycin. In cases of azithromycin allergy, doxycycline 100 mg twice daily for a week may be used, instead. Alternative regimens are available but are recommended only in the case of severe allergies or if the preferred treatment is not available. People who receive an alternative regimen should return for a test of cure by culture after 7 days or by nucleic acid amplification testing after at least 14 days (Wind et al., 2016).

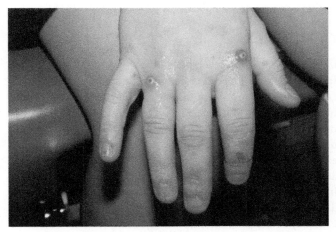

Figure 28.6. Disseminated gonorrhea with hemorrhagic vesiculopustules. (Reprinted with permission from Hall, B. J., & Hall, J. C. [Eds.]. [2017]. *Sauer's manual of skin diseases* [11th ed., Fig. 29.10]. Philadelphia, PA: Lippincott Williams & Wilkins.)

Pelvic Inflammatory Disease

PID is an ascending vaginal infection that targets the uterus, fallopian tubes, and ovaries. It may present as pelvic pain or purulent cervical discharge.

Etiology

PID may be caused by various pathogens, including normal vaginal bacteria, although it is classically caused by chlamydia or gonorrhea. Chlamydia accounts for about a third of cases of PID, and approximately 10% to 15% of cases of chlamydia and gonorrhea progress to PID (CDC, 2016c). However, PID is considered a mixed infection, and in most cases the microbial cause is unknown. Risk factors include past infection with chlamydia, BV, a history of PID, a partner with an STI, multiple partners, and failure to use condoms. Women who are not sexually active are not at risk for PID, and women in long-term monogamous relationships rarely develop the disease. Women aged 15 to 25 years are at highest risk (Kreisel, Torrone, Bernstein, Hong, & Gorwitz, 2017; Sonnenberg et al., 2013).

Signs and Symptoms

PID may be symptomatic or asymptomatic. Patients who are symptomatic may present with just endometritis (inflammation of the endometrium) or endometritis in addition to inflammation of the fallopian tubes, ovaries, and other structures of the pelvis. Acute PID presents as lower abdominal pain and tenderness of the organs on examination. The pain is typically bilateral and of short duration prior to presentation. Pain may be subtle or intense and is most acute with jarring motions, as with intercourse (Workowski et al., 2015). Rarely, women develop an abscess in the pelvis or peritonitis (inflammation of the peritoneum). When this occurs, systemic symptoms such as fever and chills are more common.

Prognosis

Failure to adequately treat can result in permanently compromised fertility, sepsis, and even death (Workowski et al., 2015).

Assessment

On examination, thick yellow discharge can often be observed from the cervix. Under the microscope, numerous white blood cells can be observed when the discharge is examined. Cervical motion tenderness is the term used to describe pain elicited by manipulation of the cervix, although any uterine or adnexal tenderness is suspicious for PID. Pain or tenderness with bimanual examination is considered diagnostic of PID in the absence of another diagnosis. The white blood cells seen microscopically in the presence of the pain or tenderness confirm the diagnosis. The absence of white blood cells suggests an alternative diagnosis. PID may be diagnosed retrospectively. Many women with tubal scarring contributing to infertility have no known past history of PID and are strongly suspected to have had subclinical disease. Laboratory examinations indicated for a woman presenting with suspected PID include gonorrhea, chlamydia, a microscopy of vaginal discharge, a pregnancy test, and HIV and syphilis testing.

Treatment

Early diagnosis and treatment of PID is important for preventing long-term damage from the infection. Treatment of PID is with two or three antibiotics. Outpatient, first-line treatment includes 250 mg intramuscular (IM) ceftriaxone as a single dose and doxycycline twice daily for 14 days. Depending on the clinical picture, metronidazole twice daily for 14 days may also be prescribed. Patients should return within 2 or 3 days after starting medication and again after completing medication to assess for progress and cure.

Indications for hospitalization include failure to respond to or tolerate oral medications, severe illness, pelvic abscess, pregnancy, and the possibility of an alternative diagnosis requiring surgical intervention, such as appendicitis. These patients receive intravenous (IV) antibiotics, often cefoxitin and clindamycin.

Syphilis

Prevalence

The rate of syphilis infection has been rising since 2000. From 2000 to 2015, the number of new infections annually increased from 8,724 to 23,892 nationwide. Of these cases, 90% were in men, and 81% were in men who have sex with men (CDC, 2016c).

Etiology

Syphilis is caused by the bacterium *Treponema pallidum*. It occurs in four stages: primary, secondary, latent, and tertiary. The disease is transmitted as *T. pallidum* invades through microscopic abrasions of the skin from individuals with primary, secondary, or early latent syphilis. The risk of transmission through intact skin is low. The pathogen passes via direct contact with an active or recently active lesion. A chancre of syphilis is established at the site of exposure.

Signs and Symptoms

Syphilis has no single presentation and is sometimes referred to as "the great pretender" because of its varying manifestations and similarities to other diseases. Although, classically, primary syphilis manifests as a single, painless chancre, it may also manifest as multiple or uncomfortable lesions (Fig. 28.7). These lesions resolve within 6 weeks. Primary syphilis may have its onset at any time from 3 to 90 days after infection.

Prognosis

If left untreated, within weeks or months of the development of the chancre, many of those infected develop secondary syphilis. Generalized symptoms are flu-like, including fever, headache, malaise, muscle aches, sore throat, and weight loss. Most patients have palpable lymphadenopathy. Other clinical manifestations can include a "moth-eaten" alopecia and gastrointestinal, musculoskeletal, renal, neurologic, and ocular abnormalities. The rash of secondary syphilis classically is a macular or papular eruption of the trunks and extremities, including the palms of the hands and the soles of the feet (Fig. 28.8). A mucosal rash, referred

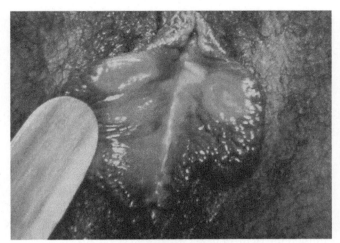

Figure 28.7. A chancre typical of primary syphilis. (Reprinted with permission from Ricci, S. S. [2017]. *Essentials of maternity, newborn, & women's health nursing* [4th ed., Fig. 5.6]. Philadelphia, PA: Lippincott Williams & Wilkins.)

to as condyloma lata, appears most often in areas close to the chancre of primary syphilis, but can form on any mucosal tissue (Fig. 28.9). These manifestations resolve spontaneously.

In a minority of untreated patients, clinical manifestations of late syphilis will present 1 to 30 years after exposure, even in individuals who did not exhibit primary or secondary syphilis. The most common manifestations are cardiovascular, neurologic, and gummatous syphilis. Gummatous syphilis is nodular lesions that can occur anywhere on the body, but most commonly on the skin and bones. When cardiovascular or gummatous manifestations occur, the disease state is referred to as tertiary

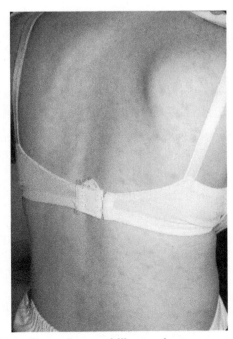

Figure 28.8. Secondary syphilis papulosquamous eruption. (Reprinted with permission from Hall, B. J., & Hall, J. C. [Eds.]. [2017]. *Sauer's manual of skin diseases* [11th ed., Fig. 29.11]. Philadelphia, PA: Lippincott Williams & Wilkins.)

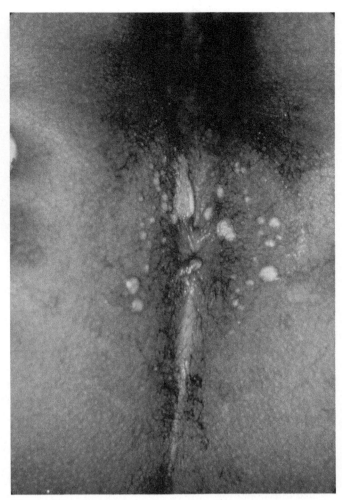

Figure 28.9. Condyloma lata. (Reprinted with permission from Goodheart, H. P. [2011]. *Goodheart's same-site differential diagnosis: A rapid method of diagnosing and treating common skin disorders* [1st ed., Fig. 19.13]. Philadelphia, PA: Lippincott Williams & Wilkins.)

syphilis. When central nervous system manifestations occur, the disease state is referred to as neurosyphilis. Neurosyphilis is not, however, specific to tertiary syphilis, as it may also appear earlier in the disease process.

Latent syphilis is a symptom-free disease state. Early latent syphilis occurs within the first 12 months of clinical manifestations, and late latent syphilis is the symptom-free period after 12 months. Patients with late latent syphilis are not considered infectious, whereas patients with early latent syphilis are. Pregnant women in latent syphilis can transmit syphilis to their fetus for the first 4 years of the latency period.

Although potentially devastating (particularly in neonates, see Chapter 25), syphilis is generally curable with a course of IM penicillin.

Assessment

All individuals with symptoms consistent with syphilis should be tested. All pregnant women, people with partners diagnosed with syphilis, men who have sex with men, people with a diagnosis of

HIV, people engaging in high-risk sexual activities, and people with a history of commercial sex work or incarceration should be screened.

The diagnosis of syphilis can be confusing as multiple tests must be ordered to confirm the diagnosis. The two types of blood test for syphilis are treponemal-specific and nontreponemal. Both tests must be done for a diagnosis to be made. The use of only one test can result in a false positive. If neurosyphilis is suspected, cerebrospinal fluid is also tested.

Nontreponemal tests are nonspecific and thus not definitive but are often used for screening purposes. These tests include rapid plasma test, venereal disease research laboratory test, and toluidine red unheated serum test. These tests are reported as a titer (such as 1:16 or 1:32). After treatment, this titer is used to assess therapeutic response. Over time, responses to a nontreponemal test revert to nonreactive after treatment. In people with early disease, as evidenced by a chancre, early nontreponemal tests may give a false negative. These patients should again be tested after 2 to 4 weeks. A nontreponemal test is obtained just prior to treatment to establish the titer that will help clinicians monitor treatment.

The more complex and expensive treponemal tests are used to confirm reactive nontreponemal testing. These tests include fluorescent treponemal antibody absorption, microhemagglutination test for antibodies to *T. pallidum*, *T. pallidum* particle agglutination assay, *T. pallidum* enzyme immunoassay, and chemiluminescence immunoassay. Although nontreponemal tests are reported as a titer, treponemal tests are reported as reactive or nonreactive. Nurses should be aware that this test generally remains positive for life, so is not useful for detecting a new infection after a prior treated infection.

Treatment

IM penicillin G is the treatment of choice for syphilis. The dosing and duration of treatment are decided on the basis of the stage and, in some cases, the site of the disease (neurosyphilis, for example, has a different treatment). Patients with a reported penicillin allergy may have testing to confirm that it is actually an allergy as opposed to a side effect, desensitization therapy if allergy testing is positive, and/or an alternative therapy with close follow-up for cure. Alternative agents include cephalosporins and tetracyclines. For an account of the controversial Tuskegee syphilis study and the ethics of informed consent, see Box 28.1.

For patients with primary, secondary, or early latent syphilis, a single dose of penicillin G 2.4 million U IM is typically sufficient therapy. Patients with late syphilis are treated weekly for 3 weeks with 2.4 million U of IM penicillin G. Neurosyphilis is generally treated with IV penicillin G, either in multiple 3 to 4 million U doses every 4 hours or 18 to 24 million U daily by continuous infusion for 10 to 14 days (Workowski et al., 2015).

Follow-up is by nontreponemal testing. A change in titer by two dilutions (such as 1:32 to 1:8) is considered adequate response to therapy. Most patients have nonreactive nontreponemal testing within 2 years. Those who do not are considered serofast. Treatment is considered a failure if nontreponemal titers do not decline 4-fold or more. All patients should have a nontreponemal titer drawn just prior to treatment. Patients diagnosed with primary, secondary, or early latent syphilis should have the titer repeated at 6 and 12 months after treatment, or if symptoms recur. Patients with late disease should have additional testing at 24 months (Workowski et al., 2015).

Herpes Simplex Virus

Herpes simplex virus (HSV) is actually two different viruses, type 1 and type 2 (HSV1 and HSV2). Both can cause a periodic localized vesicular rash and nonscarring skin erosions (Fig. 28.10). Most people are carriers of one or both of the viruses, and most people who carry the virus will never have a symptom of the infection (Bernstein et al., 2013; Bradley, Markowitz,

---

Box 28.1   The Tuskegee Syphilis Study

In 1932, the organization that would become the U.S. Department of Health and Human Services began research to study the natural history of syphilis. Recruited were 600 African American men in Tuskegee, Alabama, 399 of whom had syphilis and 201 of whom did not. With no known cure available for the disease, researchers hoped to learn more about the natural course of syphilis. However, the study occurred without the informed consent of the subjects. The recruits were told they were being treated for "bad blood" and, in return for their participation, received free medical examinations, meals, and burial insurance.

The men were never treated for syphilis, even after penicillin became the medication of choice for this disease in 1947. Many died from their disease and many sexual partners also contracted the disease. Female partners passed it on to their offspring in the form of congenital syphilis. And yet, the study was ongoing until 1972, when the Associated Press brought it to light. Only an ad hoc advisory panel formed in response to public outrage stopped the Tuskegee study, which has become a pivotal case in medical ethics.

In 1974, a $10 million dollar settlement was reached on behalf of the study subjects, including medical and burial benefits. Offspring, wives, and widows were included in the settlement in 1975. The last study participant died in 2004. The last widow died in 2009. Twelve surviving offspring still receive settlement benefits (Centers for Disease Control and Prevention, 2016d).

Although the Tuskegee study may have been true to its research goals, it was unquestionably a public health, ethical, moral, and human failure.

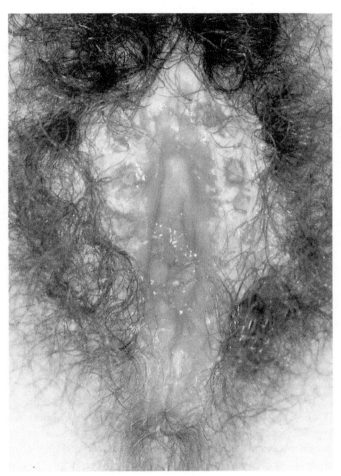

Figure 28.10. Herpes simplex virus vesicles. Multiple tender erosions of approximately 3 days' duration associated with fever and dysuria. (Reprinted with permission from Wilkinson, E. J., & Stone, I. K. [2012]. *Wilkinson and Stone atlas of vulvar disease* [3rd ed., Fig. 8.14]. Philadelphia, PA: Lippincott Williams & Wilkins.)

Gibson, & McQuillan, 2014). It is perhaps the most stigmatized of all STIs despite the limited physical health impact (the exception is the neonate; see Chapter 25).

Etiology

HSV is transmitted by skin-to-skin contact, usually of the mucosa, although it may occasionally infect via broken nonmucosal epithelia. The virus is usually dormant, residing in the basal ganglia. During these times the patient does not have outbreaks and is not contagious. During periods of silent viral shedding, the virus may be present on the mucosa, but no lesion appears. The individual is also contagious just prior to, during, and after an outbreak (Johnston & Corey, 2016).

HSV can only be symptomatic at and contagious from the site of initial contact. After HSV antibodies are present in the blood, the virus cannot be spread to or manifest from any other part of the body. Thus, a person with the HSV virus cannot contract the virus multiple times or on multiple body parts after circulating antibodies are present.

HSV infections are referred to as primary, nonprimary, and recurrent and may be symptomatic or asymptomatic. A primary infection occurs in a person with no preexisting antibodies to either HSV1 or HSV2. Nonprimary infection refers to the acquisition of HSV1 in someone who already has antibodies to HSV2, or acquisition of HSV2 in someone who already has antibodies to HSV1. A recurrent infection is not a new exposure but rather an activation of a previously existing infection.

Signs and Symptoms

The primary infection of genital herpes classically includes a painful vesicular rash and skin erosions, tender inguinal lymphadenopathy, fever, headache, and dysuria. The primary infection, however, is often asymptomatic, subclinical, or so mild as to go unrecognized. Average incubation of the primary infection is 4 days.

Subsequent nonprimary infections (infection with HSV1 with preexisting HSV2 or vice versa) are typically less acute and have a higher likelihood of being asymptomatic. Both primary and nonprimary infections, the average duration of lesions, if they occur, is under 3 weeks.

Recurrent infections (periodic manifestations of a preexisting infection) are the least severe. Lesions, when they occur, persist for an average of 10 days, and viral shedding persists for 2 to 5 days. Although the lesions typically appear as vesicles or erosions, fissures and areas of irritation of intact skin are also possible manifestations. Approximately one quarter of people have recurrent infections that are consistently asymptomatic, and half of those who manifest lesions experience a prodrome prior to the appearance of lesions. The prodromal discomfort is neuropathic and presents as tingling, burning, or shooting pain. HSV1 infections tend to recur less frequently on the genitals. A particularly acute primary infection increases the risk for more frequent recurrence.

HSV1 is most commonly associated with cold sores of the mouth, and HSV2 is most commonly associated with genital lesions. However, either virus can be present on any mucosa, depending on the nature of exposure. In recent decades, as awareness of herpes has increased, the incidence of HSV1 and oral herpes has gone down. Although this may sound like good news, oral HSV1 prevents genital infection with HSV1. As oral sex has become more common in recent decades and as fewer people have been contracting HSV1 orally as children, HSV1 infection of the genitals has become more common. People already infected with HSV1 are more likely to be asymptomatic if they later contract HSV2.

HSV2 is more likely to cause frequent outbreaks and viral shedding; thus, HSV1 is often thought of as the "good" herpes. Either kind of herpes, however, can be unpredictably contagious and cause lesions at the site of exposure.

The further out a person is from his or her initial exposure to HSV, the less likely the person is to have outbreaks or shed virus and thus be contagious. The chance of an infected person passing the virus on to a regular sexual partner in the course of a year is approximately 10% (Mertz, Benedetti, Ashley, Selke, & Corey, 1992). HSV2 is associated with more frequent outbreaks, with an average of four annually and 20% of people infected experiencing more than 10 in the first year after the primary infection. HSV1 recurs approximately once a year. Over time, the frequency of recurrence decreases for both HSV1 and HSV2.

Prognosis

A severe primary infection can very occasionally result in urinary retention requiring catheterization. This is different from urinary hesitancy from dysuria, which can be managed by encouraging the patient to void into water, or to cover the lesions with petroleum jelly prior to voiding to avoid splash burn. The other unusual complications of a primary infection include meningitis and proctitis. Infection with HSV increases the risk for HIV transmission (Johnston & Corey, 2016). See Chapters 20 and 25 for information about HSV in pregnancy and its effect on the neonate.

Assessment

HSV can be diagnosed by direct culture or by assessment by direct fluorescent antibody or polymerase chain reaction of a lesion. Serology testing is available and is accurate within several weeks of the primary infection. Serology testing is not recommended for people who have never had symptoms (U. S. Preventive Services Task Force et al., 2016).

HSV2 serology tests have a high false-positive rate, with a positive predictive value of 50% (Feltner et al., 2016). Patients should be aware that, apart from the risk for a false-positive result, the test does not specify the location of the infection and cannot predict if and when a patient will have lesions or shed virus. Screening for HSV has not been shown to change sexual behavior or limit the spread of the infection. In addition, because there is no cure for herpes, screening does not change the course of the disease. The shame and stigma associated with the diagnosis, the lack of a cure, and the lack of evidence that screening impacts sexual behavior or the spread of the virus all limit the utility of screening in asymptomatic individuals while creating a risk for actual harm (CDC, 2017).

Treatment

Herpes cannot be cured in that the virus cannot be eliminated, but treatment has been available for nearly 40 years that can suppress the virus, prevent outbreaks, reduce viral shedding, and shorten outbreaks. The three medications used, valacyclovir, acyclovir, and famciclovir, are very similar and equally effective. Acyclovir was the first of the medications used to suppress HSV and requires the most frequent dosing. It is also the least expensive. Valacyclovir dosing is less frequent but the medication is considerably more expensive. Famciclovir, the least-used medication in its class, falls between the two.

The medications for HSV suppression may be used episodically or continuously. Continuous, daily use of the medication completely prevents outbreaks in half of patients and reduces the frequency of recurrence for those not completely suppressed. Continuous use of suppressive therapy can significantly decrease the number of days in which the virus is shed, thus reducing the chance of transmitting the virus to a partner. Episodic medication is taken only for a few days with prodromal symptoms or within 72 hours of the appearance of a lesion. Episodic dosing can prevent and shorten outbreaks (Table 28.2).

Care Considerations

A new diagnosis of HSV is often associated with significant psychological distress. Assuring the patient that HSV is by no means uncommon and that the infection does not make her dirty, a pariah, or even unusual may be comforting. It is helpful to give the patient room to discuss her concerns. Many may worry that a new infection is evidence that her partner is cheating. However, the unpredictable and often asymptomatic nature of viral shedding and recurrent infections makes it difficult or impossible to predict when primary infection occurred, and many people with HSV do not get symptoms and do not know they are infected (Bernstein et al., 2013).

Table 28.2 Herpes Therapy

| Agent | Dosage | | |
	Primary Infection	Recurrent Infection, Episodic	Suppressive Therapy
Acyclovir	400 mg three times daily or 200 mg five times daily for 7–10 d	800 mg three times daily for 2 d; "or" 800 mg twice daily for 5 d; "or" 400 mg three times daily for 5 d	400 mg twice daily
Famciclovir	250 mg three times daily for 7–10 d	1,000 mg twice daily for 1 d; "or" 125 mg twice daily for 5 d; "or" 500 mg once plus 250 mg daily for 2 d	250 mg twice daily
Valacyclovir	1,000 mg twice daily for 7–10 d	500 mg twice daily for 3 d; or 1,000 mg daily for 5 d	500 mg or 1,000 mg daily

Adapted from Workowski, K. A., Bolan, G. A., & Centers for Disease Control and Prevention. (2015). Sexually transmitted diseases treatment guidelines, 2015. *MMWR Recommendations and Reports, 64*(RR-03), 1–137.

Viral Hepatitis

The most common types of viral hepatitis are hepatitis types A, B, and C. Although in theory any of the three may be transmitted sexually, hepatitis B is the only form that transmits readily during intercourse.

Hepatitis A

Prevalence

In the United States, 2,500 cases of **hepatitis A** infection were reported in 2014 (CDC, 2016a).

Etiology

Hepatitis A transmits primarily via the fecal/oral route and has an average incubation period of 28 days. Hepatitis A risk factors include illicit drug use, living in a residential facility, exposure to day care centers, and homosexual activity between men (CDC, 2016a).

Signs and Symptoms

Approximately 30% of individuals with hepatitis A have asymptomatic infections. The remainder report acute-onset abdominal pain, flu-like symptoms, nausea, vomiting, and anorexia. Within a week, urine darkens and stool becomes pale. Up to 80% of individuals become jaundiced and report overall pruritus. Individuals are infectious during the incubation until a week after the appearance of jaundice (CDC, 2016a).

Prognosis

The infection is usually self-limiting, with liver failure occurring in very few individuals, typically those with underlying liver disease. Full clinical recovery occurs for most patients within 2 to 3 months. Hepatitis A does not become a chronic condition, and individuals cannot contract the infection more than once (CDC, 2016a).

Assessment

The diagnosis is confirmed by laboratory testing.

Treatment

No specific treatment is required beyond supportive care. Vaccination has been routine for all infants since 2006, for individuals considered at high risk for infection since 1996, and for children in states with the highest incidence since 1999 (CDC, 2016a).

Hepatitis B

Prevalence

Worldwide, approximately two billion people are estimated to have evidence of **hepatitis B** exposure, 248 million are chronic carriers of the disease, and 600,000 die annually from liver disease related to hepatitis B. The incidence in the United States, however, is less than 2% (Schweitzer, Horn, Mikolajczyk, Krause, & Ott, 2015). Chronic disease is much more common with early exposure, with 90% of those infected perinatally and fewer than 5% of those infected as adults developing chronic hepatitis B (Wasley, Grytdal, Gallagher, & CDC, 2008).

Etiology

Although the primary mode of transmission of hepatitis B is perinatal transmission in high-prevalence areas and childhood transmission in intermediate-prevalence areas, in low-prevalence areas such as the United States, the primary modes of transmission are unprotected sexual intercourse and the use of illicit injection drugs. Hepatitis B infection may be acute or chronic. Incubation of the virus is 1 to 4 months. When the virus is transmitted sexually, the risk is highest for individuals with multiple sexual partners and men who have sex with men. In the United States, approximately 35% of new cases of hepatitis B are attributed to sexual transmission (Iqbal et al., 2015).

Signs and Symptoms

The presentation of hepatitis B ranges from asymptomatic to liver failure. A typical course includes a prodromal period that resembles serum sickness followed by right upper quadrant discomfort, nausea and vomiting, anorexia, jaundice, and fatigue. Although the jaundice typically resolves within 3 months, fatigue may be prolonged.

A small minority of adults progress from an acute to chronic infection. Many patients with a chronic infection are asymptomatic, whereas others complain of fatigue or manifest recurrent symptoms of hepatitis or liver failure. Chronic liver disease may present as peripheral edema, ascites, splenomegaly, and encephalopathy. Liver enzymes are generally elevated, even in those who are asymptomatic.

Prognosis

People with chronic hepatitis B are at risk for cirrhosis, liver failure, liver cancer, and death.

Assessment

If an individual is exposed to hepatitis B and her immunization status is unknown, laboratory testing for immunity should be part of the initial visit (Table 28.3). The first dose of the hepatitis B vaccine should be administered prior to the return of results. In addition, hepatitis B immune globulin should be administered within 14 days after sexual exposure. If, following immunity testing, hepatitis B surface antibody (anti-HBs) level positive, no further intervention is necessary. If the anti-HBs level is negative, the vaccination series should be completed.

Treatment

Treatment is primarily supportive and symptomatic. Vaccination is by far the most effective means of avoiding hepatitis B infection. Universal vaccination is recommended for neonates as well as all children and adolescents younger than 19 years who were not previously vaccinated. Adults who were not vaccinated in childhood or adolescence but are considered high risk should also be offered vaccination (CDC, 2016b; Box 28.2). Vaccination is provided in three doses, with the second dose 1 month after the first and the third dose 6 months after the first. The response

Table 28.3 Interpreting Hepatitis B Testing

Test Results No.	Tests Conducted	Test Results	Explanation of Findings
1	HBsAg	Negative	Susceptible to infection
	Anti-HBc	Negative	
	Anti-HBs	Negative	
2	HBsAg	Negative	• Immune due to natural infection or hepatitis B vaccination
	Anti-HBc	Negative	• Not susceptible to infection
	Anti-HBs	Positive	• Not contagious
3	HBsAg	Positive	• Acutely infected
	Anti-HBc	Positive	• Contagious
	IgM anti-HBc	Positive	
	Anti-HBs	Negative	
4	HBsAg	Positive	• Chronically infected
	Anti-HBc	Positive	• Contagious
	IgM anti-HBc	Negative	
	Anti-HBs	Negative	
5	HBsAg	Negative	• Resolved infection
	Anti-HBc	Positive	"or"
	Anti-HBs	Negative	• False-positive anti-HBc finding (susceptible)
			"or"
			• Low-level chronic infection
			"or"
			• Resolving acute infection

HBsAG, hepatitis B surface antigen; Anti-HBc, total hepatitis B core antibody; Anti-HBs, hepatitis B surface antibody; IgM anti-HBc, Immunoglobulin M antibody to hepatitis B core antigen.
Adapted from Centers for Disease Control and Prevention. *Interpretation of hepatitis B serologic test results*. Retrieved from https://www.cdc .gov/hepatitis/hbv/pdfs/serologicchartv8.pdf

Box 28.2 Candidates for Hepatitis B Vaccination

- People whose sex partners have hepatitis B
- Sexually active persons who are not in long-term monogamous relationships
- Persons seeking evaluation or treatment for a sexually transmitted disease
- Men who have sexual contact with other men
- People who share needles, syringes, or other drug-injection equipment
- People who have household contact with someone infected with the hepatitis B virus
- Healthcare and public safety workers at risk for exposure to blood or body fluids
- Residents and staff of facilities for developmentally disabled persons
- Persons in correctional facilities
- Victims of sexual assault or abuse
- Travelers to regions with increased rates of hepatitis B
- People with chronic liver disease, kidney disease, HIV infection, or diabetes
- Anyone who wants to be protected from hepatitis B

HIV; human immunodeficiency virus.
Adapted from Centers for Disease Control and Prevention. (2016b). *Hepatitis B VIS*. Retrieved from https://www.cdc.gov/vaccines/hcp/vis/vis-statements/hep-b.html

rate to the vaccination is approximately 95%, with protection persisting for up to 30 years. Patients who do not respond to the initial vaccination series should have the series repeated (Bruce et al., 2016).

Patients with chronic hepatitis B should use condoms to prevent transmission if their sexual partner is not immune or their immune status is unknown.

Hepatitis C

Etiology
Hepatitis C is almost always a bloodborne disease. The risk of the sexual transmission of hepatitis C is low, although the prevalence is higher among heterosexuals with multiple partners and men who have sex with men. The incidence of transmission by sex for monogamous, heterosexual couples is approximately 0.07% annually. The risk for household transmission in the absence of sexual activity is even lower (Terrault et al., 2013).

Signs and Symptoms
Most patients with hepatitis C are asymptomatic or complain only of fatigue or other nonspecific symptoms.

Prognosis
Up to 85% of people who contract the virus develop a chronic infection (Grebely et al., 2014). Up to 30% of people infected with hepatitis C develop cirrhosis of the liver if left untreated. In addition to cirrhosis, the other risks of chronic infection include liver failure and liver cancer. In the United States, annually 8,000 to 13,000 people die as a result of the hepatitis C virus, most aged 45 to 65 (Ly et al., 2012).

Assessment
Assessment for hepatitis C is by the hepatitis C antibody test.

Treatment
Treatment with new antiviral therapy is curative for over 99% of patients (Simmons, Saleem, Hill, Riley, & Cooke, 2016). The high cost of these medications has made their use controversial, although they are believed to be cost-effective in many populations (Chhatwal, Kanwal, Roberts, & Dunn, 2015).

Human Immunodeficiency Virus

The human immunodeficiency virus (HIV) was first recognized in 1981 as a disease that quickly decimated the immune systems of homosexual men, ultimately killing them. Today we know the virus does not discriminate. Although in the United States a majority of those infected are still men who have sex with men, persons with opposite sex partners living with HIV is a growing population.

Prevalence
Internationally, 70% of the two million people infected with HIV live in sub-Saharan Africa, with women as well represented as men (Maartens, Celum, & Lewin, 2014). With more than

35 million fatalities thus far, the HIV epidemic now ranks with the bubonic plague of the 14th century in terms of the number of fatalities (CDC, 2006). Internationally, 36.7 million people are living with HIV, 2.1 million are newly infected annually, and 1.1 million die as a result of the infection (Joint United Nations Programme on HIV/AIDS [UNAIDS], 2016). In 2014 in the United States, 1.2 million were living with HIV and 44,073 were diagnosed with the virus. By 2013, 673,538 people had died from the disease in the United States alone (CDC, 2015).

Etiology

Worldwide, most cases of transmission of HIV are sexual. The risks for sexual transmission include STIs that cause skin breakdown, such as HSV and syphilis, the presence of other STIs, the lack of penile circumcision, receptive vaginal or anal sex, multiple sexual partners, and the lack of condom use.

In general, those at the highest risk for transmission are people who receive contaminated blood, those with needle sticks from contaminated blood who are not treated prophylactically, IV drug users, and, most commonly, those who have either vaginal or anal receptive sex with an infected individual without a condom. There is no known transmission via kissing or any other contact. In the United States, 80% of those diagnosed are men, primarily men who have sex with men. African Americans and Latinos are more likely to be diagnosed than the people of European descent, and African American men who have sex with men are three times as likely to be infected than European American men who have sex with men (Millett et al., 2012). Heterosexual contact accounts for fewer than a quarter of infections in the United States (CDC, 2012).

Stages

HIV can be effectively tested for from 15 to 60 days after exposure, depending on the type of test done.

Acute Infection
Acute infection is also referred to as recent, primary, or early HIV and encompasses the first 6 months after acquisition of the disease. Clinically, the signs and symptoms of acute infection are flu-like, with fever, headache, lymphadenopathy, sore throat, rash, myalgia, and arthralgia being common. Approximately 50% to 90% of those who contract HIV are symptomatic (Workowskiet al., 2015).

Chronic HIV Without Acquired Immunodeficiency Syndrome
The stage that starts 6 months after acquisition of the HIV virus and lasts until the cluster of differentiation 4 (CD4) count is below 200 is considered HIV without acquired immunodeficiency syndrome (AIDS). A CD4 count below 200 is considered severe immunosuppression and is diagnostic of AIDS. In the absence of therapy, this is a period of time typically lasting a decade or less. Most people in this stage are asymptomatic, although some have persistent generalized lymphadenopathy. During chronic HIV without AIDS, CD4 counts typically decline progressively.

People with a CD4 count that is low, although not low enough to be diagnostic of AIDS, may be susceptible to various conditions, including oral and vaginal thrush, oral hairy leukoplakia, herpes zoster, peripheral neuropathy, idiopathic thrombocytopenia purpura, bacterial folliculitis, and seborrheic dermatitis. Nonspecific constitutional complaints are also common.

AIDS

HIV becomes AIDS when the HIV virus, acting on the immune system, causes the CD4 count to drop below 200 cells/μL, or when the patient with HIV is diagnosed with an AIDS-defining condition. Prior to the advent of antiretroviral therapy (ART), AIDS-defining conditions were the primary cause of death for people infected with HIV (Box. 28.3; Fig. 28.11).

Box 28.3   Acquired Immunodeficiency Syndrome–Defining Illnesses

- Candidiasis of the esophagus, bronchi, trachea, or lungs (but "not" the mouth, which is a condition known as thrush)
- Cervical cancer, invasive
- Coccidioidomycosis, disseminated or extrapulmonary
- Cryptococcosis, extrapulmonary
- Cryptosporidiosis, chronic intestinal (greater than 1 month's duration)
- Cytomegalovirus disease (other than liver, spleen, or nodes)
- Cytomegalovirus retinitis (with loss of vision)
- Encephalopathy, related to HIV
- Herpes simplex: chronic ulcer(s) (more than 1 mo in duration); or bronchitis, pneumonitis, or esophagitis
- Histoplasmosis, disseminated or extrapulmonary
- Isosporiasis, chronic intestinal (more than 1 mo in duration)
- Kaposi sarcoma
- Lymphoma, Burkitt (or equivalent term)
- Lymphoma, immunoblastic (or equivalent term)
- Lymphoma, primary, of the brain
- Mycobacterium avium complex or M kansasii, disseminated or extrapulmonary
- Mycobacterium tuberculosis, any site (pulmonary or extrapulmonary)
- Mycobacterium, other species or unidentified species, disseminated or extrapulmonary
- Pneumocystis jiroveci pneumonia
- Pneumonia, recurrent
- Progressive multifocal leukoencephalopathy
- Salmonella septicemia, recurrent
- Toxoplasmosis of the brain
- Wasting syndrome due to HIV

HIV, human immunodeficiency virus.
Adapted from Centers for Disease Control and Prevention. (1992). 1993 revised classification system for HIV infection and expanded surveillance case definition for AIDS among adolescents and adults. *MMWR Recommendations and Reports, 41*(RR-17), 1–19.

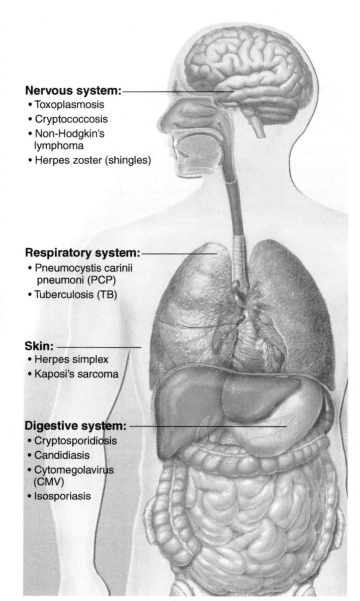

Nervous system:
- Toxoplasmosis
- Cryptococcosis
- Non-Hodgkin's lymphoma
- Herpes zoster (shingles)

Respiratory system:
- Pneumocystis carinii pneumoni (PCP)
- Tuberculosis (TB)

Skin:
- Herpes simplex
- Kaposi's sarcoma

Digestive system:
- Cryptosporidiosis
- Candidiasis
- Cytomegolavirus (CMV)
- Isosporiasis

Figure 28.11. Sites of AIDS-defining illnesses. (Reprinted with permission from Anatomical Chart Company.)

Treatment

Although there is no known cure or vaccine, the treatment for HIV has progressed over the years. For most with access to the disease-modifying medications, HIV is a chronic condition rather than a terminal one. In 1987, ART was introduced, and combination ART became the standard of care, reducing mortality, progression to AIDS, AIDS-defining diagnoses, and hospitalizations by 60% to 80% (Mocroft et al., 2003). As of 2015, of the 36.7 million people living with HIV worldwide, 17 million are treated with ART (UNAIDS, 2016). ART is often started for individuals with a CD4 count below 350, as therapy started at this time has been shown to improve survival and delay the progression of the disease. Other experts advocate for ART therapy whenever the virus is detectable, regardless of CD4 count (Gunthard et al., 2016).

Preexposure Prophylaxis

Although the search continues for a vaccination for the virus and a cure, preexposure prophylaxis (PrEP) has become available in the United States. PrEP is a daily medication that is a combination of tenofovir-disoproxil-fumarate and emtricitabine. This medication, when taken daily, appears to almost eliminate transmission of the HIV virus among people engaging in high-risk sexual behaviors (Box 28.4). To be eligible for PrEP, patients must test negative for HIV prior to the start of therapy and then every 3 months. Tests are also performed to assess for hepatitis B status and renal function prior to PrEP start. The cost of PrEP, however, may be prohibitive for many. In 2013, the monthly cost without insurance was $1,425 per month (Horberg & Raymond, 2013). By 2017, the cost had ranged from $1,600 to $2,100, depending on the retailer (GoodRX). See Chapter 30 for a summary of post exposure prophylaxis (PEP).

Low-Risk Human Papillomavirus

Prevalence

The prevalence of **human papillomavirus (HPV)** infection with subtypes that cause genital warts is 10% to 20% in the unvaccinated population in the United States, with a 0.2% to 5.1% prevalence of warts (Patel, Wagner, Singhal, & Kothari, 2013). See Chapters 26 and 27 for a discussion of high-risk HPV as it relates to cervical cancer prevention, screening, diagnosis, and treatment.

Etiology

Two low-risk forms of HPV, 8 and 11, which are included in the Gardasil vaccine, cause 90% of condylomata acuminata, also referred to as anogenital warts. Transmission is sexual, from direct contact with infected skin or mucosa. The typical incubation period is anywhere from 3 weeks to 8 months. For women, the chance of developing anogenital warts after contact with a low-risk form of HPV is approximately 50% (Arima et al., 2010).

> ### Box 28.4 High-Risk Behaviors for Preexposure Prophylaxis Eligibility
>
> - Condomless penile-anal or penile-vaginal sex with partners other than one's main partner
> - A monogamous relationship with someone who is human immunodeficiency virus–positive
> - Sex while using drugs
> - High number of sexual partners
> - Injection of heroin or cocaine
> - Sharing needles or other drug equipment
> - Injecting in a shooting gallery
> - Use of drugs during sex, reducing the likelihood of using condoms

---

Signs and Symptoms

Genital warts are soft papules or plaques that often have a cauliflower-like appearance, with a single stalk ending in multiple projections (Fig. 28.12). They may occur as single or multiple lesions. They may be seen on the external genitalia, perineum, groin, or perianal mucosa.

Prognosis

Genital warts may resolve spontaneously, advance, or remain unchanged for a period of time. Approximately one third regress spontaneously without treatment within 4 months (Yanofsky, Patel, & Goldenberg, 2012). Genital warts are considered primarily a cosmetic issue with little malignant potential.

Assessment

Warts are almost always diagnosed by clinical examination. Atypical warts or warts that fail to respond to therapy, however, may be removed and sent for assessment by a pathologist.

Treatment

There are two primary strategies for wart removal: the self-administered cream imiquimod, which targets the HPV virus itself, and caustic treatments that destroy the lesions. Caustic treatments such as cryotherapy and topical treatment with trichloroacetic acid are administered in office by a clinician. Multiple treatments may be necessary. An alternative is the cream podophyllotoxin, which is self-administered by the patient over a number of days.

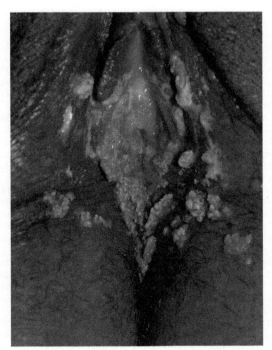

Figure 28.12. Perianal condyloma. (Reprinted with permission from Edwards, L. & Lynch, P. J. [2018]. *Genital dermatology atlas and manual* [3rd ed., Fig. 8.42]. Philadelphia, PA: Lippincott Williams & Wilkins.)

Patients should be aware that the virus may still be present even after the warts have been successfully removed. It takes approximately 6 to 12 months for a healthy immune system to eliminate a low-risk HPV type (de Sanjose, Brotons, & Pavon, 2017). However, there is no clinically routine way to assess for the virus. Although the patient does not currently manifest HPV lesions, she may still be able to pass the virus on to a partner.

Think Critically

1. You are caring for a patient with a urinary tract infection who is wondering what she can do at home to avoid future infections. What do you tell her?
2. A patient with bacterial vaginosis wants to know if her infection is sexually transmitted. What do you tell her?
3. You have a patient who is diagnosed with syphilis. She complains of flu-like symptoms, alopecia, and a rash that appeared about 6 months ago and then resolved. What stage of syphilis do you suspect she is in?
4. Your patient and her partner both have a history of oral cold sores since childhood. Because of this, your patient is concerned about transmitting the herpes simplex virus to her partner's genitals during oral sex. Is this possible? Why or why not?
5. You are caring for a patient whose partner has hepatitis C. What kind of counseling can you offer about her risk of contracting the virus?
6. How is HIV different from AIDS? At what point is a patient determined to have AIDS?
7. How would you describe the difference between low- and high-risk forms of human papillomavirus to a patient?

References

Aberg, J. A., Gallant, J. E., Ghanem, K. G., Emmanuel, P., Zingman, B. S., Horberg, M. A., & Infectious Diseases Society of America. (2014). Primary care guidelines for the management of persons infected with HIV: 2013 update by the HIV medicine association of the Infectious Diseases Society of America. *Clinical Infectious Diseases, 58*(1), e1–e34. doi:10.1093/cid/cit665

Arima, Y., Winer, R. L., Feng, Q., Hughes, J. P., Lee, S. K., Stern, M. E., . . . Koutsky, L. A. (2010). Development of genital warts after incident detection of human papillomavirus infection in young men. *Journal of Infectious Diseases, 202*(8), 1181–1184. doi:10.1086/656368

Balkus, J. E., Richardson, B. A., Rabe, L. K., Taha, T. E., Mgodi, N., Kasaro, M. P., . . . Abdool Karim, S. S. (2014). Bacterial vaginosis and the risk of trichomonas vaginalis acquisition among HIV-1-negative women. *Sexually Transmitted Diseases, 41*(2), 123–128. doi:10.1097/OLQ.0000000000000075

Belkacem, A., Caumes, E., Ouanich, J., Jarlier, V., Dellion, S., Cazenave, B., . . . Patey, O.; Working Group FRA-DGI. (2013). Changing patterns of disseminated gonococcal infection in France: Cross-sectional data 2009–2011. *Sexually Transmitted Infections, 89*(8), 613–615. doi:10.1136/sextrans-2013-051119

Bernstein, D. I., Bellamy, A. R., Hook, E. W., III, Levin, M. J., Wald, A., Ewell, M. G., . . . Belshe, R. B. (2013). Epidemiology, clinical presentation, and antibody response to primary infection with herpes simplex virus type 1 and type 2 in young women. *Clinical Infectious Diseases, 56*(3), 344–351. doi:10.1093/cid/cis891

Bradley, H., Markowitz, L. E., Gibson, T., & McQuillan, G. M. (2014). Seroprevalence of herpes simplex virus types 1 and 2--United States, 1999–2010. *Journal of Infectious Diseases, 209*(3), 325–333. doi:10.1093/infdis/jit458

Bradshaw, C. S., & Sobel, J. D. (2016). Current treatment of bacterial vaginosis-limitations and need for innovation. *Journal of Infectious Diseases, 214* Suppl 1, S14–S20. doi:10.1093/infdis/jiw159

Bradshaw, C. S., Walker, S. M., Vodstrcil, L. A., Bilardi, J. E., Law, M., Hocking, J. S., . . . Fairley, C. K. (2014). The influence of behaviors and relationships on the vaginal microbiota of women and their female partners: The WOW Health Study. *Journal of Infectious Diseases, 209*(10), 1562–1572. doi:10.1093/infdis/jit664

Bruce, M. G., Bruden, D., Hurlburt, D., Zanis, C., Thompson, G., Rea, L., . . . McMahon, B. J. (2016). Antibody levels and protection after hepatitis B vaccine: Results of a 30-year follow-up study and response to a booster dose. *Journal of Infectious Diseases, 214*(1), 16–22. doi:10.1093/infdis/jiv748

Bunker, D., & Kerr, L. D. (2015). Acute myopericarditis likely secondary to disseminated gonococcal infection. *Case Reports in Infectious Diseases, 2015*, 385126. doi:10.1155/2015/385126

Centers for Disease Control and Prevention. (2006). The global HIV/AIDS pandemic, 2006. *MMWR Morbidity and Mortality Weekly Report, 55*(31), 841–844.

Centers for Disease Control and Prevention. (2012). HIV infections attributed to male-to-male sexual contact—Metropolitan statistical areas, United States and Puerto Rico, 2010. *MMWR Morbidity and Mortality Weekly Report, 61*(47), 962–966.

Centers for Disease Control and Prevention. (2015). *Diagnoses of HIV infection in the United States and dependent areas, 2014.* Retrieved from https://www.cdc.gov/hiv/pdf/library/reports/surveillance/cdc-hiv-surveillance-report-us.pdf

Centers for Disease Control and Prevention. (2016a). *Hepatitis A questions and answers for health professionals.* Retrieved from https://www.cdc.gov/hepatitis/hav/havfaq.htm

Centers for Disease Control and Prevention. (2016b). *Hepatitis B VIS.* Retrieved from https://www.cdc.gov/vaccines/hcp/vis/vis-statements/hep-b.html

Centers for Disease Control and Prevention. (2016c). *Sexually transmitted disease surveillance 2015.* Retrieved from https://www.cdc.gov/std/stats15/default.htm

Centers for Disease Control and Prevention. (2016d). *U.S. public health service syphilis study at Tuskegee.* Retrieved from https://www.cdc.gov/tuskegee/timeline.htm

Centers for Disease Control and Prevention. (2017). *Genital herpes screening FAQ.* Retrieved from https://www.cdc.gov/std/herpes/screening.htm

Chhatwal, J., Kanwal, F., Roberts, M. S., & Dunn, M. A. (2015). Cost-effectiveness and budget impact of hepatitis C virus treatment with sofosbuvir and ledipasvir in the United States. *Annals of Internal Medicine, 162*(6), 397–406. doi:10.7326/M14-1336

Davies, B., Turner, K. M., Frolund, M., Ward, H., May, M. T., Rasmussen, S., . . . Westh, H.; Danish Chlamydia Study Group. (2016). Risk of reproductive complications following chlamydia testing: A population-based retrospective cohort study in Denmark. *The Lancet. Infectious Diseases, 16*(9), 1057–1064. doi:10.1016/S1473-3099(16)30092-5

de Sanjose, S., Brotons, M., & Pavon, M. A. (2017). The natural history of human papillomavirus infection. *Best Practice and Research. Clinical Obstetrics and Gynaecology.* doi:10.1016/j.bpobgyn.2017.08.015

Feltner, C., Grodensky, C., Ebel, C., Middleton, J. C., Harris, R. P., Ashok, M., & Jonas, D. E. (2016). Serologic screening for genital herpes: An updated evidence report and systematic review for the US Preventive Services Task Force. *JAMA, 316*(23), 2531–2543. doi:10.1001/jama.2016.17138

Foxman, B., & Buxton, M. (2013). Alternative approaches to conventional treatment of acute uncomplicated urinary tract infection in women. *Current Infectious Disease Reports, 15*(2), 124–129. doi:10.1007/s11908-013-0317-5

Ginocchio, C. C., Chapin, K., Smith, J. S., Aslanzadeh, J., Snook, J., Hill, C. S., & Gaydos, C. A. (2012). Prevalence of Trichomonas vaginalis and coinfection with Chlamydia trachomatis and Neisseria gonorrhoeae in the United States as determined by the Aptima Trichomonas vaginalis nucleic acid amplification assay. *Journal of Clinical Microbiology, 50*(8), 2601–2608. doi:10.1128/JCM.00748-12

GoodRX. *Prices and coupons for 30 tablets of Truvada 200mg/300mg.* Retrieved from https://www.goodrx.com/truvada?drug-name=truvada

Grebely, J., Page, K., Sacks-Davis, R., van der Loeff, M. S., Rice, T. M., Bruneau, J., . . . Prins, M.; InC3 Study Group. (2014). The effects of female sex, viral genotype, and IL28B genotype on spontaneous clearance of acute hepatitis C virus infection. *Hepatology, 59*(1), 109–120. doi:10.1002/hep.26639

Gunthard, H. F., Saag, M. S., Benson, C. A., del Rio, C., Eron, J. J., Gallant, J. E., . . . Volberding, P. A. (2016). Antiretroviral drugs for treatment and prevention of HIV infection in adults: 2016 Recommendations of the International Antiviral Society-USA Panel. *JAMA, 316*(2), 191–210. doi:10.1001/jama.2016.8900

Hoover, K. W., Tao, G., Nye, M. B., & Body, B. A. (2013). Suboptimal adherence to repeat testing recommendations for men and women with positive Chlamydia tests in the United States, 2008–2010. *Clinical Infectious Diseases, 56*(1), 51–57. doi:10.1093/cid/cis771

Horberg, M., & Raymond, B. (2013). Financial policy issues for HIV pre-exposure prophylaxis: Cost and access to insurance. *American Journal of Preventive Medicine, 44*(1 Suppl. 2), S125–S128. doi:10.1016/j.amepre.2012.09.039

Iqbal, K., Klevens, R. M., Kainer, M. A., Baumgartner, J., Gerard, K., Poissant, T., . . . Teshale, E. (2015). Epidemiology of acute hepatitis B in the United States from population-based surveillance, 2006–2011. *Clinical Infectious Diseases, 61*(4), 584–592. doi:10.1093/cid/civ332

Johnston, C., & Corey, L. (2016). Current concepts for genital herpes simplex virus infection: Diagnostics and pathogenesis of genital tract shedding. *Clinical Microbiology Reviews, 29*(1), 149–161. doi:10.1128/CMR.00043-15

Joint United Nations Programme on HIV/AIDS. (2016). *Global AIDS update.* Retrieved from http://www.unaids.org /sites/default/files/media_asset/global-AIDS-update-2016_en.pdf

Kenyon, C., Colebunders, R., & Crucitti, T. (2013). The global epidemiology of bacterial vaginosis: A systematic review. *American Journal of Obstetrics and Gynecology, 209*(6), 505–523. doi:10.1016/j.ajog.2013.05.006

Kreisel, K., Torrone, E., Bernstein, K., Hong, J., & Gorwitz, R. (2017). Prevalence of pelvic inflammatory disease in sexually experienced women of reproductive age—United States, 2013–2014. *MMWR Morbidity and Mortal Weekly Report, 66*(3), 80–83. doi:10.15585/mmwr.mm6603a3

Ly, K. N., Xing, J., Klevens, R. M., Jiles, R. B., Ward, J. W., & Holmberg, S. D. (2012). The increasing burden of mortality from viral hepatitis in the United States between 1999 and 2007. *Annals of Internal Medicine, 156*(4), 271–278. doi:10.7326/0003-4819-156-4-201202210-00004

Maartens, G., Celum, C., & Lewin, S. R. (2014). HIV infection: Epidemiology, pathogenesis, treatment, and prevention. *The Lancet, 384*(9939), 258–271. doi:10.1016/S0140-6736(14)60164-1

Marshall, A. O. (2015). Managing recurrent bacterial vaginosis: Insights for busy providers. *Sexual Medicine Reviews, 3*(2), 88–92. doi:10.1002/smrj.45

Mertz, G. J., Benedetti, J., Ashley, R., Selke, S. A., & Corey, L. (1992). Risk factors for the sexual transmission of genital herpes. *Annals of Internal Medicine, 116*(3), 197–202.

Middelkoop, S. J., van Pelt, L. J., Kampinga, G. A., Ter Maaten, J. C., & Stegeman, C. A. (2016). Routine tests and automated urinalysis in patients with suspected urinary tract infection at the ED. *American Journal of Emergency Medicine, 34*(8), 1528–1534. doi:10.1016/j.ajem.2016.05.005

Millett, G. A., Peterson, J. L., Flores, S. A., Hart, T. A., Jeffries, W. L., Wilson, P. A., . . . Remis, R. S. (2012). Comparisons of disparities and risks of HIV infection in black and other men who have sex with men in Canada, UK, and USA: A meta-analysis. *The Lancet, 380*(9839), 341–348. doi:10.1016/S0140-6736(12)60899-X

Mocroft, A., Ledergerber, B., Katlama, C., Kirk, O., Reiss, P., d'Arminio Monforte, A., . . . Lundgren, J. D.; EuroSIDA Study Group. (2003). Decline in the AIDS and death rates in the EuroSIDA study: An observational study. *The Lancet, 362*(9377), 22–29.

Patel, H., Wagner, M., Singhal, P., & Kothari, S. (2013). Systematic review of the incidence and prevalence of genital warts. *BMC Infectious Diseases, 13*, 39. doi:10.1186/1471-2334-13-39

Schweitzer, A., Horn, J., Mikolajczyk, R. T., Krause, G., & Ott, J. J. (2015). Estimations of worldwide prevalence of chronic hepatitis B virus infection: A systematic review of data published between 1965 and 2013. *The Lancet, 386*(10003), 1546–1555. doi:10.1016/S0140-6736(15)61412-X

Simmons, B., Saleem, J., Hill, A., Riley, R. D., & Cooke, G. S. (2016). Risk of late relapse or reinfection with hepatitis C virus after achieving a sustained virological response: A systematic review and meta-analysis. *Clinical Infectious Diseases, 62*(6), 683–694. doi:10.1093/cid/civ948

Sonnenberg, P., Clifton, S., Beddows, S., Field, N., Soldan, K., Tanton, C., . . . Johnson, A. M. (2013). Prevalence, risk factors, and uptake of interventions for sexually transmitted infections in Britain: Findings from the National Surveys of Sexual Attitudes and Lifestyles (Natsal). *The Lancet, 382*(9907), 1795–1806. doi:10.1016/S0140-6736(13)61947-9

Terrault, N. A., Dodge, J. L., Murphy, E. L., Tavis, J. E., Kiss, A., Levin, T. R., . . . Alter, M. J. (2013). Sexual transmission of hepatitis C virus among monogamous heterosexual couples: The HCV partners study. *Hepatology, 57*(3), 881–889. doi:10.1002/hep.26164

Thinkhamrop, J., Hofmeyr, G. J., Adetoro, O., Lumbiganon, P., & Ota, E. (2015). Antibiotic prophylaxis during the second and third trimester to reduce adverse pregnancy outcomes and morbidity. *Cochrane Database of Systematic Reviews,* (6), CD002250. doi:10.1002/14651858.CD002250.pub3

Tibaldi, C., Cappello, N., Latino, M. A., Masuelli, G., Marini, S., & Benedetto, C. (2009). Vaginal and endocervical microorganisms in symptomatic and asymptomatic non-pregnant females: Risk factors and rates of occurrence. *Clinical Microbiology and Infection, 15*(7), 670–679. doi:10.1111/j.1469-0691.2009.02842.x

U. S. Preventive Services Task Force, Bibbins-Domingo, K., Grossman, D. C., Curry, S. J., Davidson, K. W., Epling, J. W., Jr., . . . Tseng, C. W. (2016). Serologic screening for genital herpes infection: US Preventive Services Task Force Recommendation Statement. *JAMA, 316*(23), 2525–2530. doi:10.1001/jama.2016.16776

Van Der Pol, B., Kraft, C. S., & Williams, J. A. (2006). Use of an adaptation of a commercially available PCR assay aimed at diagnosis of chlamydia and gonorrhea to detect Trichomonas vaginalis in urogenital specimens. *Journal of Clinical Microbiology, 44*(2), 366–373. doi:10.1128/JCM.44.2.366-373.2006

Vodstrcil, L. A., Walker, S. M., Hocking, J. S., Law, M., Forcey, D. S., Fehler, G., . . . Bradshaw, C. S. (2015). Incident bacterial vaginosis (BV) in women who have sex with women is associated with behaviors that suggest sexual transmission of BV. *Clinical Infectious Diseases, 60*(7), 1042–1053. doi:10.1093/cid/ciu1130

Wasley, A., Grytdal, S., Gallagher, K., & Centers for Disease Control and Prevention. (2008). Surveillance for acute viral hepatitis—United States, 2006. *MMWR Surveillance Summaries, 57*(2), 1–24.

Wind, C. M., Schim van der Loeff, M. F., Unemo, M., Schuurman, R., van Dam, A. P., & de Vries, H. J. C. (2016). Test of cure for anogenital gonorrhoea using modern RNA-based and DNA-based nucleic acid amplification tests: A prospective cohort study. *Clinical Infectious Diseases, 62*(11), 1348–1355. doi:10.1093/cid/ciw141

Workowski, K. A., Bolan, G. A., & Centers for Disease Control and Prevention. (2015). Sexually transmitted diseases treatment guidelines, 2015. *MMWR Recommendations and Reports, 64*(RR-03), 1–137.

Yanofsky, V. R., Patel, R. V., & Goldenberg, G. (2012). Genital warts: A comprehensive review. *Journal of Clinical and Aesthetic Dermatology, 5*(6), 25–36.

Suggested Readings

Centers for Disease Control and Prevention. (2018). *Viral hepatitis.* Retrieved from https://www.cdc.gov/hepatitis/index.htm

Centers for Disease Control and Prevention. *2015 Sexually transmitted disease treatment guidelines.* Retrieved from https://www.cdc.gov/std/tg2015/default.htm

East, L., Jackson, D., O'Brien, L., & Peters, K. (2015). Being diagnosed with a sexually transmitted infection (STI): Sources of support for young women. *Contemporary Nurse, 50*(1), 50–57. doi:10.1080/10376178.2015.1013427

Gnann, J. W., Jr., & Whitley, R. J. (2016). CLINICAL PRACTICE. Genital Herpes. *New England Journal of Medicine, 375*(7), 666–674. doi:10.1056/NEJMcp1603178

29 Family Planning

Objectives

1. Compare the different forms of contraception available.
2. Identify important family planning considerations.
3. Describe the different aspects of abortion care.
4. Distinguish how care might differ for a woman who is planning to give a neonate up for adoption.
5. Discuss the different kinds of infertility care available.
6. Explain how contraception, infertility care, and abortion are all important aspects of women's healthcare.

Key Terms

Anovulation
Artificial reproductive technology (ART)
Bilateral tubal ligation (BTL)
Combined oral contraceptive (COC)
Depot medroxyprogesterone acetate (DMPA)
Emergency contraception (EC)
Gamete intrafallopian transfer (GIFT)
Hysterosalpingogram
In vitro fertilization (IVF)

Infertility
Intrauterine contraceptive (IUC)
Long-acting reversible contraception (LARC)
Natural family planning (NFP)
Oligoovulation
Progestin-only pill (POP)
Vasectomy
Zygote intrafallopian transfer (ZIFT)

The term *family planning* includes any educational, social, or healthcare interventions that allow people to plan reproduction. Family planning includes contraception, abortion, and interventions and education when subfertility or infertility occurs. Optimal family planning always involves shared decision making between patients and their healthcare providers. Nurses participating in family planning must be respectful of patients' choices and priorities and be careful not to interject their own biases. Family planning decisions are deeply personal and must be made by the people whose lives are most affected and who understand their lives and situations best: the patients themselves.

Contraception

The goal of contraception is to prevent unwanted or mistimed pregnancies. The goal of contraceptive counseling is to educate a woman about the methods of contraception to facilitate decision making. When counseling a woman regarding contraception, the nurse should consider some key criteria for selecting a method, assess the woman for current pregnancy and future pregnancy plans, and emphasize the correct use of the form of contraception selected, if relevant. The major types of contraception that the nurse should be familiar with include long-acting reversible contraception (LARC); combined oral contraceptives (COCs), progestin only pills (POPs) hormonal patches, and hormonal vaginal rings; barrier methods; spermicide; **natural family planning (NFP)**; withdrawal; and contraceptive injections sterilization.

Selecting a Method of Contraception

The elements of education regarding contraception should include current reproductive needs and plans for the future, patient preference reliability of the method, cost, convenience, safety, side effects, contraindications, patient lifestyle, and any noncontraceptive benefits. Although many nurses and other healthcare providers may have contraceptive methods they personally prefer, it is important not to pressure a patient to choose a particular method but rather to provide her with the best, most accurate information so that she may make the choice that's right for her. The best birth control method is the one that works for the patient.

Current and Future Reproductive Needs

A major factor that should guide a woman's choice of contraception is her current and future plans for reproduction. An important question to guide the discussion is, "Do you plan to become pregnant in the next year?" For women who do, a short-acting method of contraception such as a contraceptive pill may be more appropriate, and preconception counseling is indicated. For women who do not want to be pregnant for some time or ever, a LARC method or sterilization may be more appealing.

Reliability

In terms of reliability or effectiveness, contraceptive methods are often conceptualized in three categories: most effective, effective, and less effective (see Fig. 11.1). The most effective methods include sterilization—**bilateral tubal ligation (BTL)** and **vasectomy**—and methods of LARC (contraceptive implants and intrauterine contraception). The most effective methods do not depend on patient adherence for efficacy and have a less than 1% rate of failure.

Effective methods have a very low associated pregnancy rate but are subject to user error. Although contraceptive pills, rings, patches, and injections all have a less than 1% failure rate when used perfectly, with typical use, the failure rate is from 6% to 9%. The diaphragm, the least reliable of the effective methods, has a 6% failure rate with perfect use and a 12% failure rate with typical use (Curtis, Tepper, et al., 2016).

The least effective methods have a higher rate of failure than those in either the most effective or effective tiers with both perfect and typical use. These methods include cervical caps, sponges, male condoms, female condoms, withdrawal, spermicides, and NFP. With perfect use, these methods have a failure rate from 0.4% to 20%. With typical use, the failure rate is from 14% to 28%. For context, a sexually active woman using no method over the course of a year has on average an 85% chance of pregnancy (Curtis, Tepper, et al., 2016).

Cost, Convenience, and Other Considerations

At the time of this writing, health insurers participating in the Patient Protection and Affordable Care Act exchange are required to pay for contraception without a co-pay. Exceptions are made for employers who cite a religious objection to their employees' use of contraception. A patient who does not have contraception coverage, however, may find the cost of some methods, particularly LARC methods, prohibitive. Convenience may also be a consideration; for example, a patient with poor transportation or an erratic schedule may be concerned about methods that require refills. A patient who is planning to become pregnant in a year may prefer a method other than **depot medroxyprogesterone acetate (DMPA)** or a hormonal **intrauterine contraceptive (IUC)**, which can have a longer return to fertility. A woman who prefers to have her period monthly may not do well with methods that often cause amenorrhea or off-cycle bleeding, such as a DMPA injection, a hormonal implant, or a hormonal IUC. A woman with a heavy menses, however, may find the heavier period typical of the copper IUC intolerable. Women who do not wish for a partner or family member to know she is using contraception may prefer a more private, hidden method, such as DMPA, an IUC, or a hormonal implant.

Safety, Side Effects, and Contraindications

Although most women list effectiveness, affordability, maintenance, and the duration of a contraceptive method as the most important considerations, the nurse should not assume that these are the particular concerns of a particular patient (Madden, Secura, Nease, Politi, & Peipert, 2015). A patient may be concerned with the safety of the hormones in the contraceptive pill or the procedure for the insertion of an IUC. Another patient may be concerned about side effects, such as weight gain from DMPA or breast tenderness from the contraceptive patch.

Lastly, healthcare providers must be aware of contraindications of particular methods. The most commonly contraindicated aspect of contraception is the estrogen in the COC, the ring, and the patch. The supplemental estrogen is contraindicated with migraine with aura, a history of blood clots, hypertension, and other conditions.

Pregnancy Assessment

Traditionally, healthcare providers encouraged women to start birth control at the time of menses or on the Sunday after the first day of menses to rule out the possibility of pregnancy and maintain the woman's existing menstruation schedule. They did this, in part, because of concerns over oral hormone-containing contraceptives causing birth defects or other birth complications, as well as concerns over side effects of the contraceptive masking signs of pregnancy and leading to a delay in diagnosis of the pregnancy. Research has shown, however, that hormonal contraceptives are not teratogens. And although such contraceptives may mask the signs of pregnancy, women who start them without ruling out pregnancy can be asked to return for pregnancy testing after 2 to 4 weeks (Curtis, Jatlaoui, et al., 2016). Pregnancy tests are typically reliable when used at least 2 to 3 weeks after the last episode of unprotected intercourse. Therefore, any type of hormonal or barrier contraceptive that is not inserted into the uterus will not harm the woman or embryo if she is indeed pregnant while using such contraception and can be safely started at any point in the woman's menstrual cycle.

Ruling out pregnancy is important, however, prior to the insertion of an IUC, as insertion of the method in early pregnancy can cause pregnancy complications, including delayed diagnosis of pregnancy. Still, the possibility of pregnancy can be reasonably excluded if women answer yes to any of the following questions (Curtis, Jatlaoui, et al., 2016):

- Have you not had sexual intercourse since your last menstrual period?
- Have you started a normal period within the past week?
- Have you been using a reliable form of birth control correctly every time you've had sex since your last period?
- Have you had a miscarriage or abortion within the past 7 days?
- Have you given birth within the past 4 weeks?
- Have you given birth within the past 6 months *and* are you breastfeeding on demand *and* have you not had your period since the delivery?

Method Continuation

A contraception method is only as good as the patient's adherence to and continued, consistent use of the method once adopted. Careful counseling by the nurse to help the patient find the method she feels is the best fit for her is critical to this process, as is creating a welcoming environment that encourages the patient to return to discuss any concerns and switch methods as necessary.

Generally speaking, IUCs have the best continuation rates at 1 year, including up to 93% of women with a hormonal IUC and 85% of those with a copper IUC. The continuation rate at 1 year for hormonal implants is also high, at up to 84%. In contrast, 33% to 50% of women using estrogen-containing methods—such as the ring, patch, or pill—discontinue the method within a year. Up to 44% of women stop receiving their DMPA injections stop within in a year, and a similar number stop using the diaphragm. More than 50% of women using NFP and almost 60% using male or female condoms for contraception stop using these methods within a year (Birgisson, Zhao, Secura, Madden, & Peipert, 2015b). Women who choose contraception methods with low continuation rates should be particularly carefully counseled about the availability of other methods that they may consider should they rethink their initial choice.

Hormone-Containing Methods

Contraceptives containing hormones may contain just progestin (the artificial form of progesterone) or estrogen and progestin. Progestin-only methods include the **progestin-only pill (POP)**; the hormonal implant, DMPA; and the hormonal IUCs. Estrogen-progestin methods include the COC, the patch, and the ring.

The estrogen component works by suppressing the mid-cycle secretion of the luteinizing hormone (LH), which provokes ovulation, and by suppressing secretion of the follicle-stimulating hormone (FSH) and, in turn, folliculogenesis. The suppression

of FSH, however, is most pronounced with older, higher doses of estrogen and less with modern, lower doses (20- and 35-μg doses are most common today; Golobof & Kiley, 2016).

Progestin works to prevent pregnancy in three ways. The most important mechanism of action is a decrease in the volume and increase in the viscosity of the cervical mucus, which effectively blocks sperm from traveling into the uterus and fallopian tubes. The second mechanism is a suppression of ovulation (although less so than for estrogen). The third mechanism is a thinning of the uterine lining so that, in the event of failure of other mechanisms of action, the implantation of a fertilized ovum is less likely.

Indications, Contraindications, and Risks

Indications

Besides providing contraception, estrogen-progestin methods are used to treat hyperandrogenism (most often polycystic ovary syndrome [PCOS]), acne, dysmenorrhea, amenorrhea, heavy menstrual bleeding, premenstrual dysphoric disorder, and endometriosis. Estrogen-progestin methods can also reduce menstrual migraines, bleeding caused by fibroids, and the formation of functional cysts (although they cannot help cysts resolve faster). The use of these methods is also associated with a reduced risk for endometrial and ovarian cancers (Iversen, Sivasubramaniam, Lee, Fielding, & Hannaford, 2017). The POP is often used to treat dysmenorrhea or heavy periods.

Women using IUCs of either kind are at a considerably reduced risk for cervical cancer and endometrial cancer. A hormonal IUC may also be recommended to treat heavy or dysmenorrhea, anemia related to heavy menses, endometrial hyperplasia, and pain from endometriosis. The hormonal IUC is also protective against pelvic inflammatory disease (PID; Cortessis et al., 2017). Likewise, DMPA may be used to treat anemia related to menses, dysmenorrhea associated with endometriosis, and heavy menses.

Contraindications

There are many contraindications to the use of hormonal contraception (https://www.cdc.gov/reproductivehealth/unintended-pregnancy/pdf/legal_summary-chart_english_final_tag508.pdf). Most are related to the estrogen component of the combined contraceptive, although some are related to progestin-only methods. Common contraindications to estrogen-progestin methods include migraine with aura, hypertension, and smoking after the age of 34. The only absolute contraindications to progestin are a current diagnosis of breast cancer and acute viral hepatitis (Curtis, Jatlaoui, et al., 2016).

Risks

The use of estrogen-progestin contraceptives is associated with many more increased risks than is the use of progestin-only or barrier methods methods but also with some reduced risks for other conditions. For example, the use of estrogen-progestin contraceptives is associated with a small but significant increase in the absolute risk of arterial and venous thrombosis. This risk, however, is much higher for women 35 years and older who smoke 15 or more cigarettes a day, and so, such women should not use an estrogen-progestin method of contraception. Although there is no ongoing increased risk for cardiovascular disease after discontinuation of the method, even low-dose estrogen-progestin methods may induce hypertension in a small minority of patients (Curtis, Jatlaoui, et al., 2016).

An increased risk for stroke is also associated with the use of estrogen-progestin contraceptives. The risk of stroke among women who take a low-dose progestin-estrogen pill is approximately 8.5 out of 100,000, when compared with 4.4 out of 100,000 for those not using a form of hormonal contraception. The risk of stroke among women using a contraceptive patch is approximately 14 out of 100,000 and among those using a contraceptive ring is 11 out of 100,000. For context, the risk of a pregnancy-associated stroke is 18 out of 100,000 (Lidegaard, Lokkegaard, Jensen, Skovlund, & Keiding, 2012; Tate & Bushnell, 2011). Factors that increase the risk for stroke among women using estrogen-progestin methods include smoking, hypertension, migraine with aura, older age, obesity, dyslipidemia, and prothrombotic genetic mutations such as factor V Leiden (Bushnell et al., 2014).

The use of estrogen-progestin methods is also associated with an increased risk of venous thromboembolism (VTE). Although the risk among women not using an estrogen-progestin method is approximately 0.19 to 0.37 per 1,000 woman years, the risk is approximately 0.67 to 1.3 per 1,000 woman years for the users of estrogen-progestin methods of contraception. The highest risk is for formulas containing the progestin drospirenone (de Bastos et al., 2014; Vinogradova, Coupland, & Hippisley-Cox, 2015). The risk for VTE is considerably higher in estrogen-progestin contraceptive users who are obese and/or smokers.

In terms of cancer risk, the results are mixed. As previously mentioned, women using estrogen-progestin methods have a lower risk for endometrial and ovarian cancers. Neither long- nor short-term use of estrogen-progestin methods has demonstrated an increased breast cancer risk in some studies (Vessey & Yeates, 2013), although an increased rate of breast cancer was found in others (Cortessis et al., 2017). However, the risk of cervical cancer appears to be increased among women who are positive for high-risk forms of the human papillomavirus who use estrogen-progestin contraceptives (Iversen et al., 2017).

Although hormonal contraception does not impact future fertility, contraceptives containing estrogen may have a detrimental effect on the milk supply of lactating women, particularly when taken in the first 6 weeks after birth. Although estrogen-progestin methods are known to suppress testosterone levels, the effect on the libido is not clear. Low-dose estrogen-progestin methods do not stimulate fibroid growth, and studies have not found a correlation between the use of estrogen-progestin methods and weight gain (Gallo et al., 2014).

Drug Interactions
Many anticonvulsants, including phenytoin, topiramate, oxcarbazepine, carbamazepine, barbiturates, and primidone, reduce the efficacy of all hormonal methods of birth control except DMPA and the hormonal IUC. The efficacy hormonal implant is only slightly impacted, but estrogen-progestin methods and the POP have a high risk of failure. In addition, estrogen-progestin methods have a high risk of failure when taken with the anticonvulsant

lamotrigine, although it does not impact the efficacy of other hormonal methods, including the POP (Curtis, Jatlaoui, et al., 2016).

Antibiotic use is often thought to interfere with the efficacy of contraception; in fact, the only antibiotic proven to do so is rifampin, a medication used to treat tuberculosis. Women taking rifampin should be encouraged to use a method other than the pill, patch, or ring. The effectiveness of the progestin IUC and DMPA is not affected by concurrent use with rifampin, and the effectiveness of the contraceptive implant is only mildly compromised (Curtis, Jatlaoui, et al., 2016). All antiretroviral therapies have a mild effect on the efficacy of hormonal methods, but the medication fosamprenavir reduces the efficacy of estrogen-progestin methods to such a degree as to outweigh any benefits of their use (Curtis, Jatlaoui, et al., 2016).

Side Effects
The side effects of modern COCs tend to be mild and resolve within a few months after starting the COC. They include breast tenderness, nausea, and bloating. Women who initially experience nausea with a COC may find it helpful to take it at night and with food. Breakthrough bleeding is a common side effect of low-dose estrogen-progestin contraceptives (20, 30, or 35 µg of estrogen) and the POP. Breakthrough bleeding is not a sign that the method of contraception is less effective but is often a side effect of missing pills, which does affect efficacy. Although amenorrhea is the goal of extended-cycle contraceptives (see below), many women taking traditional-cycle, low-dose contraceptives, particularly a 20-µg dose, skip menses. Although this side effect is acceptable to some women, others prefer the reassurance of a monthly menses.

A recent large study found a higher start rate for antidepressants among women who use progestin methods, but a causal relationship has not been established (Skovlund, Morch, Kessing, & Lidegaard, 2016).

Oral Contraceptives

In Chapter 2, Tatiana Bennett was put on a COC to help control her PCOS by regulating her menses and counteracting the androgenic effects of the condition.

Combined Oral Contraceptives
COCs are an extremely effective method of birth control and are often the method that comes to mind first (Fig. 29.1). When taken correctly, their failure rate is 0.1%. However, with typical use, which means missing pills or taking them off schedule, the efficacy of a COC for preventing pregnancy is only about 92% (Curtis, Jatlaoui, et al., 2016).

A thorough physical examination, including a pelvic examination, was once a standard requirement prior to prescribing COCs, but this is no longer the case. A healthcare provider may safely prescribe COCs after taking a careful history and an accurate blood pressure measurement (Curtis, Jatlaoui, et al., 2016).

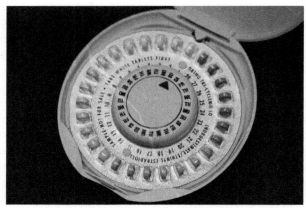

Figure 29.1. A sample pack of combined oral contraceptives. (Reprinted with permission from Evans, R. J., Brown, Y. M., & Evans, M. K. [2014]. *Canadian maternity, newborn, and women's health nursing* [2nd ed., Fig. 8.8]. Philadelphia, PA: Lippincott Williams & Wilkins.)

Most COCs are packages with 21 hormone-containing pills followed by seven placebo pills. These placebo pills serve as place markers to help keep women in the habit of taking a daily pill even during the week of the withdrawal bleed, when they are not taking a hormone. Missing a placebo pill does not affect the efficacy of the method for preventing pregnancy. Missing more than one hormone-containing pill, however, does reduce the efficacy of the method. Women should take missed or late hormone-containing pills as soon as possible. If a woman misses a

dose by 48 hours or more, she should also consider using a backup method of contraception (Patient Teaching 29.1).

When starting the pill, many patients and providers prefer the "quick start" method, which allows the patient to start taking the pill at any point during the menstrual cycle. If the woman starts the COC within 5 days after the first day of her menses, the pill is considered effective immediately. If it has been more than 5 days since her menses started, she should use a backup method (such as condoms or abstinence) for 7 days before relying on the COC to prevent pregnancy (Curtis, Jatlaoui, et al., 2016). Alternate methods have the woman starting the pill the first day of her next period or the Sunday after the start of her next period. The advantage of quick start, however, is that she is protected from an unplanned pregnancy earlier than she would be if she waited to start her COC.

Annual follow-up is indicated for prescription renewal. Optimally, an entire year's worth of COCs is dispensed annually to enhance method adherence. Healthy women who are nonsmokers may continue taking the pill until the age of probable menopause in the absence of other contraindications, which may help control uncomfortable manifestations of perimenopause, such as hot flashes and irregular bleeding.

Extended Cycling. Although most women using COCs elect to take them as traditionally packaged (21 estrogen-progestin pills followed by 7 days of placebo pills), an alternate method is known as extended cycling. Extended cycling increases the number of days of taking estrogen-progestin pills to limit the number of days of withdrawal bleeds during placebo days. Women may choose

---

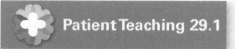 **Patient Teaching 29.1**   **Recommended Actions After Late or Missed Doses of Combined Oral Contraceptives**

If one pill is late (fewer than 24 h since the pill should have been taken) or missed (24–48 h since the pill should have been taken), the patient should do the following:

- Take the late or missed pill as soon as possible.
- Continue taking the remaining pills at the usual time (even if it means taking two pills on the same day).
- No additional contraceptive protection is needed.
- Emergency contraception is not usually needed but can be considered if hormonal pills were missed earlier in the cycle.

If two or more pills are missed consecutively (48 or more hours since pills should have been taken), the patient should do the following:

- Take the most recent missed pill as soon as possible (any other missed pills should be discarded).
- Continue taking the remaining pills at the usual time (even if it means taking two pills on the same day).
- Use backup contraception (e.g., condoms) or avoid sexual intercourse until hormonal pills have been taken for 7 consecutive days.
- If pills were missed in the last week of hormonal pills (e.g., days 15–21 for 28-d pill packs):
  - Omit the hormone-free interval by finishing the hormonal pills in the current pack and starting a new pack the next day.
  - If unable to start a new pack immediately, use backup contraception (e.g., condoms) or avoid sexual intercourse until hormonal pills from a new pack have been taken for 7 consecutive days.
- Emergency contraception should be considered if hormonal pills were missed during the first week and unprotected sexual intercourse occurred in the previous 5 d.
- Emergency contraception may also be considered at other times as appropriate.

Adapted from Curtis, K. M., Jatlaoui, T. C., Tepper, N. K., Zapata, L. B., Horton, L. G., Jamieson, D. J., & Whiteman, M. K. (2016). U.S. selected practice recommendations for contraceptive use, 2016. *MMWR Recommendations and Reports, 65*(4), 1–66. doi:10.15585/mmwr.rr6504a1.

this method of cycling because they wish to have fewer periods or as a strategy to minimize the symptoms of endometriosis, menstrual migraines, hyperandrogenism, or premenstrual dysphoric disorder. The efficacy and safety associated with extended cycling with COCs are identical with those associated with traditional cycling with COCs. There are no known negative health effects of extended cycling.

COCs specifically packaged for extended cycling may include any one of the following combinations of pills: 84 estrogen-progestin pills followed by 7 placebo pills; 84 estrogen-progestin pills followed by 7 low-dose estrogen pills; or only estrogen-progestin pills. Alternatively, traditionally packaged pills may be used for extended cycling by discarding placebo pills and immediately starting a new pill pack after completing the estrogen-progestin pills in the previous pack.

Mono- and Multiphasic Contraceptives. Another choice to consider in COCs is monophasic versus multiphasic pills. Monophasic pills have the same hormone level in each of the 21 estrogen-progestin pills. Current monophasic pills typically contain 20, 30, or 35 μg of estrogen. Occasionally, a pill with 50 μg of estrogen is prescribed. Previous generations of pills contained 80 to 100 μg of estrogen. The lowest-dose formulation currently available contains 10 μg of estrogen. Several different forms of progestin may be coupled with the estrogen, including norgestimate, desogestrel, levonorgestrel, drospirenone, and others. Multiphasic pills vary the estrogen and/or progestin dosing over the course of the month. Although the bleeding profile may be slightly better for multiphasic formulations, any clinical difference is small.

Progestin-Only Pills

In the United States, the only POP formulation currently available is 0.35 mg of the progestin norethindrone daily. This dose is significantly lower than the daily progestin dose in a COC. Patients should be aware that each of the 28 pills in a POP pack contains progestin. There are no placebo pills and there is no scheduled withdrawal bleed as there is with a COC. POPs are commonly prescribed for women for whom estrogen is contraindicated, such as those who are lactating, women with migraine with aura, and women with high blood pressure.

The POP is shorter-acting than a COC. Although there is some flexibility about when in a day a woman takes a COC, the POP must be taken within a 3-hour window every day for it to be effective. If a woman misses a pill at any point in the cycle, she must use a backup method of contraception for the next 7 days.

The primary side effect with the POP is a change in menstrual bleeding. Because there is no placebo week or scheduled withdrawal week, the users of the POP tend to have a less regular period and more breakthrough bleeding. They may also report amenorrhea and prolonged periods of spotting. Although pregnancy is rare in women taking the POP, if a pregnancy does occur, it is more likely to be ectopic because of slowed motility of the cilia of the fallopian tube in response to progestin (Curtis, Jatlaoui, et al., 2016).

In Chapter 6, Rebecca Sweet chose the POP for her contraception because her nurse practitioner informed her that it did not contain any estrogen and only a third of the dose of progestin, and she hoped it would make her less moody than the COC had. She didn't mind having to take it within the same 3-hour window every day because she liked the discipline it required.

Contraceptive Ring

The contraceptive ring available in the United States is marketed under the name Nuva Ring (Fig. 29.2). It is a flexible silicone ring impregnated with estrogen and the progestin etonogestrel that releases a small amount of the hormones into the vaginal mucosa daily. The woman places the ring inside the vagina for 3 weeks, then removes it for a week to create a withdrawal bleed, and then replaces it with a new ring. Alternatively, the woman may leave the ring in place for a full 4 weeks and then immediately replace it with a new ring, thus typically experiencing spotting rather than the period-like withdrawal bleed.

Although most couples do not find the ring uncomfortable during intercourse, the woman may remove it before having intercourse and leave it out for up to 3 hours a day with it still being effective. The location of the ring within the vagina is not important. As long as the ring is in contact with the vaginal mucosa, it is effective (Curtis, Jatlaoui, et al., 2016).

Occasionally, the vaginal ring may be dislodged by bearing-down movements. Therefore, the nurse should encourage patients to check the placement of the ring after a bowel movement.

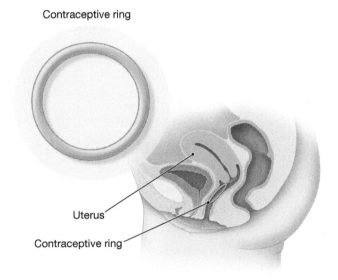

Contraceptive ring

Uterus

Contraceptive ring

Figure 29.2. A contraceptive ring. (Reprinted with permission from Beckmann, C. R., Herbert, W., Laube, D., Ling, F., & Smith, R. [2013]. *Obstetrics and gynecology* [7th ed., Fig. 26.3]. Philadelphia, PA: Lippincott Williams & Wilkins.)

Most women place the ring by simply compressing it and sliding it into the vagina with their fingers. Other women may be more comfortable, however, inserting the ring with the aid of a tampon applicator. To do this, the woman removes the tampon from the applicator and replaces with the ring. The insertion is then similar to a tampon insertion. The woman may remove the ring by reaching into the vagina, hooking a finger around the ring, and pulling.

Contraceptive Patch

The contraceptive patch available in the United States is marketed under the name Xulane (Fig. 29.3). It releases 20 μg of estrogen and 150 μg of the progestin daily. The woman changes the patch weekly for 3 weeks. There is a planned patch-free week during which the user has a withdrawal bleed. Alternatively, the woman may use a fourth patch during the fourth week for extended cycling (Curtis, Jatlaoui, et al., 2016).

The woman should place the patch on the upper back, upper arm, upper buttock, or lower abdomen, but not on the breast. To avoid skin irritation, the woman should rotate the site weekly and always place the patch on clean, dry skin that has not been treated recently with lotions, creams, or oils at least a half hour after bathing. To avoid lint accumulation in the adhesive of the patch, the woman may sprinkle a white powder over the patch immediately after application.

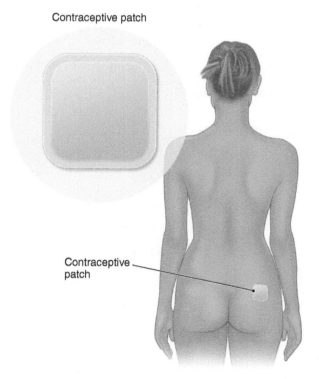

Contraceptive patch

Contraceptive patch

Figure 29.3. A contraceptive patch. (Reprinted with permission from Beckmann, C. R., Herbert, W., Laube, D., Ling, F., & Smith, R. [2013]. *Obstetrics and gynecology* [7th ed., Fig. 26.2]. Philadelphia, PA: Lippincott Williams & Wilkins.)

Emergency Contraception

Emergency contraception (EC) is contraception that a woman implements after coitus to prevent pregnancy. EC, also referred to as the morning-after pill or postcoital contraception, is indicated for women who suspect a failure of their regular contraceptive or had unprotected intercourse. It is not intended as a primary method but rather as an occasional intervention.

EC is available in two forms: medication and copper IUC. EC medications work by delaying ovulation, whereas copper IUCs inhibit sperm viability. Regardless of the mechanism of action, both work primarily by preventing fertilization and perhaps secondarily by preventing implantation. No method of EC causes abortion (American College of Obstetricians and Gynecologists [ACOG], 2015b; Gemzell-Danielsson, Berger, & Lalitkumar, 2013).

Although conception is possible only in the few days near ovulation, EC is generally offered within 5 days of unprotected intercourse for women who were not using contraception. Providing the medication forms of EC to women prior to when it is required has shown an increased use of the method but not increase in unprotected intercourse (ACOG, 2015b).

The copper IUC is the most effective method of EC, preventing 95% of pregnancies when inserted within 72 hours after intercourse. It has the additional benefit of providing a reliable means of long-term, reversible contraception. For more information on copper IUCs, see the section "Intrauterine Contraceptives." Ulipristal, marketed under the brand name Ella, prevents approximately two thirds of pregnancies, and levonorgestrel, marketed as PlanB or NextChoice, prevents approximately 50% of pregnancies when administered within 72 hours after intercourse (Glasier, 2013). Regardless of the method of EC selected, the woman should take a pregnancy test 3 weeks after using the EC if no menses or withdrawal bleeding has occurred.

No deaths have been associated with the use of EC, and the most common side effects with medication EC are nausea, vomiting, headache, and irregular bleeding (ACOG, 2015b). If a woman who has taken levonorgestrel or ulipristal vomits within 3 hours after taking the medication, she may be given an antiemetic and a second dose. Vomiting after 3 hours should not affect the efficacy of the medication.

Levonorgestrel Emergency Contraception

Levonorgestrel EC, which is available over the counter or by prescription, is most effective when taken within 72 hours after unprotected intercourse but does have some reduced effect when taken 72 to 120 hours after intercourse. After taking levonorgestrel as EC, women, on average, experience their next menses a day early, but a delay is not uncommon. The administration of levonorgestrel does not affect an established pregnancy, and no testing for pregnancy is necessary prior to administration. The efficacy of this method may be limited in patients with a body weight above 75 kg (165 lb; Kapp et al., 2015). It is typically packaged as a 1.5-mg single tablet but may be offered as two 0.75-mg tablets that may be taken together or 12 hours apart. Women may start a new method of contraception immediately after taking levonorgestrel. They should use the new method for 7 days before relying on it to prevent pregnancy.

Ulipristal

Ulipristal is an antiprogesterone and can delay ovulation by as much as 5 days. It is more effective than levonorgestrel as EC and may be used within 120 hours of unprotected intercourse. Ulipristal is also more likely to be effective for women with a body weight of greater than 75 kg than levonorgestrel. However, in the United States, it is available by prescription only, administered as a single 30-mg tablet. Patients should be aware that menses after the use of ulipristal usually comes a few days later than expected.

No physical examination is required prior to a woman starting ulipristal. However, because ulipristal—unlike levonorgestrel—may impact an existing pregnancy, a nurse should exclude the possibility of pregnancy on the basis of the woman's history before the woman starts this medication. If pregnancy cannot be excluded, the nurse should administer a pregnancy test prior to the administration of ulipristal to ensure the patient was not already pregnant prior to the unprotected intercourse in question.

Because ulipristal is a progestin blocker, the woman should take care when starting a new method of hormonal contraception or restarting a previous method of hormonal contraception. The woman should use a nonhormonal method of contraception for the first 5 days after administration. If she chooses to start or restart a hormonal method, the woman should begin taking it 5 days after taking ulipristal and use it for 7 days before relying on it for birth control. This means the patient should plan to use abstinence or a barrier method of contraception for 12 days after taking ulipristal.

Contraceptive Injection: DMPA

The DMPA (Depo-Provera) as a method of contraception is a progestin-only injection administered every 3 months until and unless pregnancy is desired. It can be a good choice for women who do not wish to manage their contraception daily, weekly, or monthly or for women who wish to avoid estrogen or for whom estrogen is contraindicated. Women using DMPA often experience less frequent or scant menses or even no menses at all. However, this change typically occurs only after a few injections and is not an immediate benefit.

The benefits of DMPA include the following:

- A reduction of heavy bleeding, dysmenorrhea, and iron deficiency anemia
- Protection of the endometrium, a reduction in the incidence of PID, and a reduction in the incidence of ectopic pregnancy
- Superior hygiene for individuals with special needs, careers, or activities that would make menses particularly challenging
- A reduction in sickle cell crisis for women with the disease
- A reduction in the frequency of seizures in women with epilepsy
- A reduction in the incidence of the vasomotor symptoms of perimenopause (Curtis, Tepper, et al., 2016).

DMPA works by suppressing both FSH and LH, thus inhibiting follicle maturation and ovulation. It also causes atrophy of the endometrium and changes to the cervical mucus that render it inhospitable to sperm, although this is unlikely to be a primary mechanism of action. With perfect use, the failure rate of DMPA is 0.2%. With more typical use, the failure rate is closer to 6%, primarily because of women returning late for their injection (Curtis, Jatlaoui, et al., 2016).

The contraindications to DMPA are few. Women using aminoglutethimide or long-term corticosteroid therapy should avoid DMPA for contraception. Because of an anticipated delay in the return of fertility, DMPA may not be the optimal method for women planning pregnancy in the next year. Women with breast cancer should not be offered DMPA (Curtis, Tepper, et al., 2016).

Optimally, a woman should start DMPA within 7 days after the start of her last menses, although she may start it at any time if the possibility of pregnancy can be reasonably ruled out. However, there is no evidence that DMPA harms a pregnancy (Brent, 2005). DMPA is available in intramuscular and subcutaneous formulations, both of which are administered approximately every 13 weeks. Most clinics allow a 2-week grace period, however, as ovulation does not occur for at least 14 weeks after administration. If a woman presents for injection more than 15 weeks after her last injection, she should take a pregnancy test prior to administration and use a backup method of contraception for 7 days following administration (Curtis, Jatlaoui, et al., 2016). A woman may receive an injection earlier than 13 weeks after her last one to accommodate her schedule or to stop the breakthrough bleeding that is common toward the end of a 3-month DMPA cycle.

Approximately half of women who try to conceive after using DMPA become pregnant within a year after discontinuing it. In a small subset of women, however, ovulation suppression continues until 18 months after the last injection. Women with lower body weights may return to fertility faster than larger women (Schwallie & Assenzo, 1974).

Changes in bleeding are the most common reason for women to switch from DMPA to another method of contraception. Over the course of the first one, two, or more injections, irregular bleeding and spotting are not unusual and become more common in the weeks preceding the next injection. Approximately half of women still using DMPA after a year achieve amenorrhea, and this is usually viewed as one of the benefits of the method (Hubacher, Lopez, Steiner, & Dorflinger, 2009).

Women are often concerned about weight gain related to DMPA. This concern may cause them to not select the method or to switch methods. Multiple studies of DMPA have shown an average weight gain over a year of less than 5 lb, which is similar to that associated with other methods (Lopez et al., 2013).

In Chapter 3, Susan's preferred method of contraception was DMPA. She stopped getting her shot because she was concerned that it was the source of her weight problem and because she thought she might like to be pregnant again.

In a subset of women, DMPA may provoke or worsen head-aches. It may also cause or worsen depression in some women, particularly those with a preexisting history of mood disorders or premenstrual dysphoric disorder.

DMPA is associated with a decrease in bone mass density (BMD). The loss of BMD plateaus after 2 years of using DMPA, however, and is reversed after discontinuation of the method. The fracture risk is equivalent for DMPA users and nonusers (Lanza et al., 2013). The BMD reduction is equivalent to that seen during pregnancy and lactation. Despite a black box warning against using DMPA long term due to BMD concerns, several professional organizations have advocated for an unrestricted use of DMPA by women aged 18 to 45 years. Additionally, DMPA use is not an indication for BMD testing (ACOG, 2014).

Contraceptive Implant

The only hormonal contraceptive implant available in the United States at this time is a 4-cm (1.5-in) long rod of nonestrogen etonogestrel (sold under the brand names Implanon and Nex-planon) that is inserted under the skin of the inner upper arm in a short, office-based procedure. Although approved for use for 3 years, this implant consistently time-releases etonogestrel for at least 4 years at a level adequate for contraception (Ali et al., 2016). As with other progestin-only methods of contraception, the primary mechanisms of action are inhospitable changes to cervical mucus and changes in fallopian tube motility that impede fertilization. Follicle maturation and ovulation are also suppressed. The only absolute contraindication to the etonoges-trel implant is current breast cancer (Curtis, Jatlaoui, et al., 2016). There is no increased risk for myocardial infarction, stroke, or VTE as a result of etonogestrel implant use (Curtis, Jatlaoui, et al., 2016).

Along with sterilization and IUCs, the etonogestrel implant is one of the most effective methods of contraception available today. A BMI greater than 30 does not appear to make this method less effective (Morrell, Cremers, Westhoff, & Davis, 2016). Efficacy may be diminished, however, for women using antiretroviral medications (Curtis, Jatlaoui, et al., 2016).

Unscheduled bleeding is by far the most common side effect of the etonogestrel implant, as well as the most common reason for discontinuation of the method. Although the bleeding profile often improves over time, a favorable change in bleeding is not guaranteed with continued use. Bleeding may be treated with a short course of nonsteroidal anti-inflammatory drugs, COCs, or supplemental estrogen with varying degrees of success. Despite these interventions, nuisance bleeding often persists or resumes after the treatment is complete (Guiahi, McBride, Sheeder, & Teal, 2015).

No physical examination or laboratory testing is indicated prior to etonogestrel implant insertion. The clinician should be reasonably sure that the patient is not pregnant according to the criteria reviewed previously. The woman should use a backup method of contraception if it has been 5 or more days since the start of her last menstrual period.

The etonogestrel implant can be removed at any time during a brief in-office procedure. A vast majority of women ovulate within a month after implant removal, and the nurse should counsel women to consider themselves fertile at the time of the implant removal unless they select a different method of contraception. If the woman selects a different hormonal method, she should use a backup method for 7 days after the start of the new method before relying on it for birth control. If the implant is expired and the patient desires a new one, the new implant may be inserted in the same track as the old. The new implant should be considered immediately effective.

Intrauterine Contraceptives

In Chapter 1, Bess had her IUC removed early in order to conceive.

IUCs—also known as intrauterine devices, or IUDs—are T-shaped plastic devices wrapped in copper or containing progestin that are inserted into the uterus to prevent conception. They are one of the most effective methods of contraception, with the prob-ability of getting pregnancy after 1 year of use being just 0.1% (Heinemann, Reed, Moehner, & Minh, 2015a).

Worldwide, nearly a quarter of women who use contraception use an IUC (Buhling, Zite, Lotke, & Black, 2014). As of 2012, 12% of women in the United States using contraception chose an IUC, up from just 2% in 2002 (Kavanaugh, Jerman, & Finer, 2015).

A number of misconceptions about IUCs are a barrier to uptake of the method in the United States. Misperceptions include the idea that IUCs increase the risk for PID, sexually transmitted infections (STIs), ectopic pregnancy, and future infertility after method discontinuation. Additionally, although it has been well demonstrated that IUCs prevent fertilization and do not cause abortions, this misperception persists and was the cornerstone of a United States Supreme Court ruling that has denied this very effective method of contraception to employees of individuals who do not understand the mechanism of action of this partic-ular form of contraception (Birgisson, Zhao, Secura, Madden, & Peipert, 2015a; Charo, 2017; Frega et al., 2016).

Patient satisfaction and continuation rates for IUCs are the highest of all reversible forms of contraception. In a study of women with a 5-year progestin IUC, at 1 year, 88% still had their IUC and at 5 years, 54% had continued with the method through expiration. In comparison, shorter-acting methods such as the COC, patch, ring, and DMPA have a 30% adherence rate at 3 years (Birgisson et al., 2015b; Diedrich, Zhao, Madden, Secura, & Peipert, 2015).

IUCs fall into two categories: copper IUCs and progestin IUCs.

Copper IUC

The only copper IUC available in the United States, sold under the name brand ParaGard, is approved for use for 10 years, al-though it has been successfully tested to prevent pregnancy for 12 years (Wu & Pickle, 2014).

As noted above, the copper IUC is the most effective form of EC (Fig. 29.4). To be effective as EC, the copper IUC must be

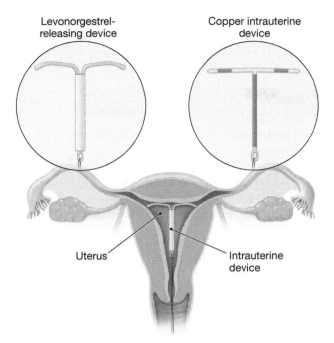

Levonorgestrel-
releasing device

Copper intrauterine
device

Uterus

Intrauterine
device

Figure 29.4. Copper (ParaGard) intrauterine contraceptive device. (Reprinted with permission from Beckmann, C. R., Herbert, W., Laube, D., Ling, F., & Smith, R. [2013]. *Obstetrics and gynecology* [7th ed., Fig. 26.8]. Philadelphia, PA: Lippincott Williams & Wilkins.)

inserted within 5 to 7 days after unprotected intercourse. Access to the method may be challenging, however, as a trained provider must place the IUC within the required window of time. A pregnancy test is required prior to insertion to assess for a pregnancy that predates the unprotected intercourse in question. Many offices do not stock the device for reasons of cost. When offered the option, approximately 11% of women choose the copper IUC as emergency and ongoing contraception (Schwarz et al., 2014). Of the women who choose to use the copper IUC as EC, 60% continue to use the method for ongoing contraception at a year (Sanders et al., 2017).

The copper IUC works primarily by the production of cytotoxic peptides and enzymes that inhibit sperm motility, capacitation, survival, and phagocytosis, thus inhibiting fertilization. This understanding is supported by tubal flushing studies that failed to find evidence of fertilized ovum when fallopian tubes were flushed. In addition, no chemical evidence has been found of fertilized ovum that fail to implant because of the presence of the copper IUC (Curtis & Peipert, 2017).

Progestin IUCs

There are several hormonal IUCs, all of which contain the progestin levonorgestrel. They are sold under the brand names Mirena, Liletta, Kyleena, and Skyla, each of which has a slightly different total amount and/or or release rate of hormone. The Mirena IUC contains 52 mg of levonorgestrel that releases 20 µg a day and is approved for 5 years. The Liletta IUC also contains 52 mg of levonorgestrel but releases 18.6 µg per day over 3 years (although its manufacturer is attempting to extend the approval of the device to 7 years). The Kyleena IUC contains

19.5 mg of levonorgestrel and releases 17.5 µg/d for 5 years. The Skyla IUC contains 13.5 mg of levonorgestrel and releases 14 µg/d over 3 years.

Progestin IUCs have the additional mechanism of causing inhospitable changes to the cervical mucus, endometrial atrophy, and variable effects on ovulation. There is no evidence, however, of any IUC, regardless of the specific mechanism of action, acting as an abortifacient or disrupting an existing pregnancy.

Contraindications

There are relatively few contraindications to the IUC. Neither the copper nor hormonal method should be used routinely in women with abnormalities of the uterine cavity, endometrial cancer, untreated ovarian cancer, persistent gestational trophoblastic disease, current PID or pelvic tuberculosis, current postabortion sepsis, abnormal vaginal bleeding suspicious for malignancy, or pregnancy. Copper IUCs are contraindicated for women with the rare Wilson disease or copper allergy. Although IUCs once were not recommended for use in teenagers or women who had not given birth previously, strong guidelines now recommend the IUC for anyone who desires the method and who has no contraindications (ACOG, 2015a; Curtis, Tepper, et al., 2016).

Side Effects

The most common side effect for both categories of IUC is a change in bleeding pattern. The copper IUC can often result in a longer, heavier, crampier menses, particularly with initial use. The progesterone IUCs can cause spotting, unscheduled bleeding, and amenorrhea, although overall they significantly reduce bleeding and few women discontinue use of the hormonal device because of bleeding concerns.

Partners may occasionally complain of discomfort from the strings of the IUC poking the head of the penis. Strings are generally cut long enough that women can tuck them into the vaginal fornix. The nurse can encourage patients to perform this tucking maneuver with their fingers prior to intercourse. Although the strings can be cut shorter, flush with the external cervical os, doing so can make later removal of the IUC far more challenging for the clinician and uncomfortable for the patient.

There are no systemic side effects of a copper IUC. The progestin IUC works primarily locally at the level of the pelvic organs, and the amount of circulating hormone is one fifth that of women using a COC for contraception. Although some women may be particularly sensitive to even low levels of progesterone, large studies have not found an association between the progestin IUC and weight gain or diminished libido (Boozalis, Tutlam, Chrisman Robbins, & Peipert, 2016; Vickery et al., 2013).

Risks

Perforation of the uterus at the time of IUC insertion is a risk, although rare, occurring with approximately 1 in 1,000 insertions (Heinemann, Reed, Moehner, & Minh, 2015b). When the perforation is recognized at the time of insertion, the insertion tools and device (if placed) are removed, and the uterine wall typically heals spontaneously in less than a month. Women with a suspected intraperitoneal bleed, worsening pain, and unstable vital signs should be transferred to the hospital. Mild-to-moderate cramping or pain is typical in the first week after insertion, however, and can usually be successfully managed with nonsteroidal anti-inflammatory medications.

Women are routinely screened for gonorrhea and chlamydia at the time of insertion or previous to insertion to avoid an ascending infection and PID. With this practice, PID risk for women with IUCs is the same as that for women without IUCs (Birgisson et al., 2015a). The presence of PID after insertion is not an indication for IUC removal (Curtis, Jatlaoui, et al., 2016).

Spontaneous expulsion of the IUC from the uterus through the cervix is another risk. Spontaneous expulsion, if it occurs, typically occurs in the first year of use. The nurse should advise women to report new acute cramping, which may indicate that the IUC has slipped into the cervix. Women were once advised to periodically check their strings to confirm the presence of the IUC. This is no longer recommended, although some women still do so. If women complain that they cannot find their strings or the clinician cannot observe strings during a pelvic exam performed for another reason, the clinician will assess further for the presence of the string. Strings can often be teased out of the cervical os. If the clinician cannot find the strings, an ultrasound may be performed to confirm the presence of the IUC.

Insertion and Removal

The IUC is usually inserted in the office by a nurse practitioner, physician, or physician assistant in a procedure that typically takes less than 10 minutes (Fig. 29.5). A thorough cleansing of the cervix and vagina and the use of sterile tools are important for safe placement. The steps of IUC placement are detailed in Step-by-Step Skills 29.1.

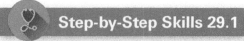

Step-by-Step Skills 29.1

Intrauterine Contraceptive Placement Procedure

1. Perform a bimanual examination to determine the orientation of the uterus.
2. Place and use a speculum in the vagina to visualize the cervix.
3. Swab the cervix and vagina with a cleanser.
4. Administer lidocaine to the cervix or in multiple spots of the vaginal fornix.
5. Place a tenaculum on the cervix, usually on the anterior lip.
6. Apply traction with the tenaculum to straighten the uterine cavity and stabilize the cervix.
7. Measure (sound) the uterus using a metal or plastic uterine sound.
8. Place the intrauterine contraceptive per the manufacturer's instructions.
9. Trim the strings of the intrauterine contraceptive.
10. Remove all tools from the vagina.

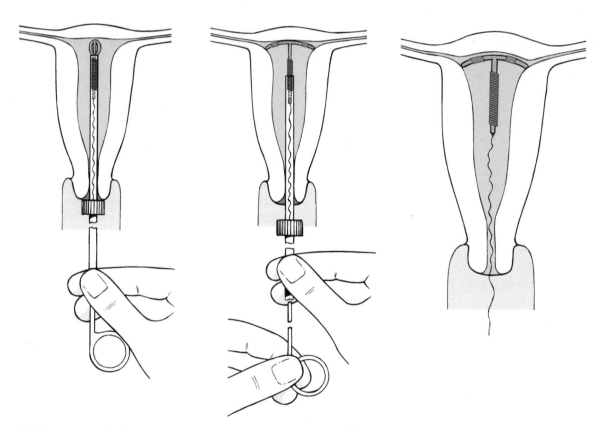

Figure 29.5. Placement of a ParaGard intrauterine contraceptive device. (Reprinted with permission from Callahan, T. L., & Caughey, A. B. [2013]. *Blueprints obstetrics & gynecology* [6th ed., Fig. 24.8]. Philadelphia, PA: Lippincott Williams & Wilkins.)

Removal is usually straightforward. After placing the speculum and visualizing the cervix, the clinician grasps the strings of the IUC with long-handled forceps and pulls the IUC out through the cervix.

Barrier Methods

The barrier methods of contraception are generally less effective as contraceptives but condoms provide the best protection against STIs of any birth control method other than abstinence. The nurse should strongly encourage any patient who is not monogamous, whose partner is not monogamous, or who does not know her own STI status or the STI status of her partner or partners to use either male or female condoms, regardless of what other contraception she may be using.

Barrier methods, particularly condoms and sponges, expire. Prior to use, women should check the expiration dates on packaging and discard expired products. Women should also open packages carefully to avoid compromising the contents.

Male Condom

With typical use and if used as the sole form of contraception, the male condom has a failure rate over the course of a year of 18% (Curtis, Tepper, et al., 2016).

Most male condoms are made of latex. For many women, the first sign of a latex sensitivity or allergy is discomfort after having sex involving a latex condom. Condoms are also often used with the spermicide nanoxynol-9, which is also irritating to the vaginal mucosa. Nonlatex condoms are made from animal intestines or polyisoprene. Patients should be aware that animal-based condoms do not provide protection against STIs. Nonlatex condoms are also generally more expensive than latex condoms.

A woman should use a new condom for each episode of oral, rectal, or vaginal sex with a partner whose STI status is unknown.

The partner should always put on the condom prior to genital contact (Fig. 29.6). The partner should take care with the initial placement of the condom. A common mistake is to place the condom on the head of the penis upside down, which becomes evident when the partner cannot unroll the condom down the shaft of the penis. If this occurs, the partner should then discard the condom. Turning the condom over and restarting the process with the same condom puts the woman at risk for STI exposure.

The partner should remove and safely discard the condom immediately after ejaculation. After ejaculation, the partner should hold the condom at its base while removing the penis from the vagina, rectum, or mouth to avoid spilling semen from the condom.

Condoms are extremely flexible and rarely break with appropriate use. Large condoms are available and may be preferred by men who feel constricted by condom use. Smaller condoms are available for those preferring a snug fit, and variations on ribbed and cobbled are marketed for those seeking a different kind of stimulation.

Female Condom

The female condom is the female-controlled counterpart of the male condom. Although male condoms provide some protection against STIs, particularly gonorrhea and chlamydia, female condoms provide better protection against diseases that are transmitted skin to skin, such as herpes simplex virus, syphilis, and human papillomavirus. Female condoms are approved for use with vaginal sex but may also be used during anal sex. With typical use, the failure rate of the female condom is 21% within a year (Curtis, Tepper, et al., 2016).

The female condom, however, is more expensive and cumbersome to use than the male condom. Although the male condom is a simple flexible sheath, the female condom contains two semirigid

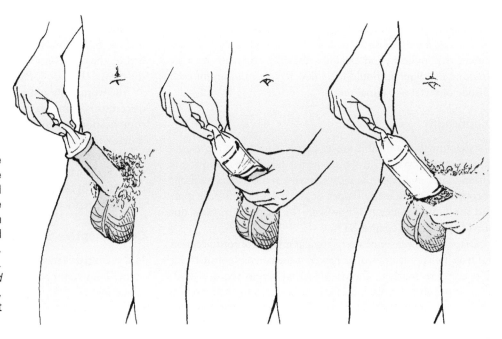

Figure 29.6. Male condom. The male places the condom over the erect penis before making any genital contact with his partner. Some space should be left at the tip of the condom to contain the ejaculate. (Reprinted with permission from Evans, R. J., Brown, Y. M., & Evans, M. K. [2014]. *Canadian maternity, newborn, and women's health nursing* [2nd ed., Fig. 8.2]. Philadelphia, PA: Lippincott Williams & Wilkins.)

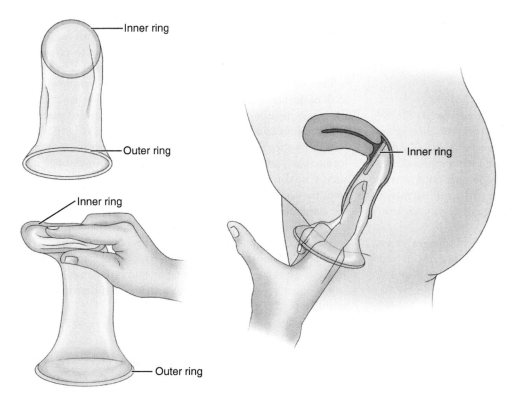

Figure 29.7. **Female condom.** To insert the female condom, hold the inner ring between the thumb and the middle finger. Put the index finger on the pouch between the thumb and other fingers and squeeze the ring. Slide the condom into the vagina as far as it will go. The inner ring keeps the condom in place. (Reprinted with permission from Pellico, L. H. [2013]. *Focus on adult health: Medical-surgical nursing* [1st ed., Fig. 35.1]. Philadelphia, PA: Lippincott Williams & Wilkins.)

rings, one attached to the opening of a nitrile tube and the other inside and at the end of this tube, for facilitating placement and use of the condom (Fig. 29.7).

The placement of the female condom is similar to the placement of a tampon or contraceptive ring. The woman pinches the inner ring (still inside the nitrile tube) between her fingers and slides it into the vagina. She should insert it as high into the vagina as it will go, being careful not to twist the tube. The outer ring remains outside the vagina and covers much of the vulva. The penis goes inside the outer ring and into the nitrile tube. After sex, the woman should twist the outer tube to avoid spilling semen, remove the condom, and carefully discard it. As with the male condom, the woman should use a new female condom for each episode of rectal or vaginal sex.

Diaphragm

The diaphragm is a flexible saucer that is placed into the vagina to cover the cervix. With typical use, it has a 12% failure rate within a year, making it the most effective of the barrier methods of contraception (Curtis, Tepper, et al., 2016). Unlike the male and the female condoms, however, the diaphragm does not provide protection against STIs.

Diaphragms were once a very popular method of contraception but have fallen out of favor as newer, more convenient methods have come to market. The use of a diaphragm requires skill, motivation, and planning. It may be best suited to older women who are subfertile, motivated, and do not require concealment of their method of birth control.

Although originally latex, all diaphragms in the United States are now made of silicone. As the popularity of the method has waned, it has become more difficult to source and is not reliably stocked in pharmacies. Unlike male and female condoms, diaphragms are available by prescription only. They must be used in conjunction with spermicide.

Two different types are currently available, a single-sized diaphragm, marketed under the name Caya, and a sized diaphragm. Sizing of the sized diaphragm is according to the length between the pubic symphysis and the posterior vaginal fornix. This sizing is done by a clinician during an office visit. At the time of a fitting, the clinician must counsel the woman on optimal use of the device (Fig. 29.8; Patient Teaching 29.2).

The woman should replace the diaphragm if she experiences discomfort during sex or frequent urinary tract infections. Other complications can include vaginal irritation and, very rarely, toxic shock syndrome.

The fit of the sized diaphragm should be checked if the woman gives birth, has a miscarriage or abortion, gains or loses more than 10 lb, or has pelvic surgery. Regardless, silicone diaphragms should be replaced every 2 years.

Contraceptive Sponge

In the United States, the contraceptive sponge is sold under the name Today's Sponge and is available over the counter. It is a 2-in round foam disk with a depression in the center on one side for the cervix and a nylon ribbon on the other for easy removal. It is infused with spermicide and comes in only one size. Like the

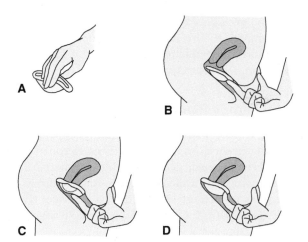

Figure 29.8. Proper insertion of a diaphragm. (A) After spermicidal jelly or cream is applied to the rim, the woman pinches the diaphragm between the fingers and the thumb. **(B)** She then inserts the folded diaphragm into the vagina and pushes it backward as far as it will go. **(C)** To check for proper positioning, the woman should feel the cervix to be certain it is completely covered by the soft rubber dome of the diaphragm. **(D)** To remove the diaphragm, the woman hooks a finger under the forward rim and pulls the diaphragm down and out. (Reprinted with permission from Pillitteri, A. [2014]. *Maternal and child health nursing: Care of the childbearing and childrearing family* [7th ed., Fig. 6-6]. Philadelphia, PA: Lippincott Williams & Wilkins.)

cervical cap, it is more effective in women who have never given birth, having a 12% failure rate over 1 year in this population. In contrast, it has a failure rate over 1 year of 24% in women who have previously given birth (Curtis, Tepper, et al., 2016).

Prior to insertion, the woman wets the sponge with water and squeezes it to distribute the water throughout the sponge. She then folds and inserts the sponge with her fingers to the top of the vagina, fitting the dimple over the cervix. She should take care when inserting it to maintain finger contact with the ribbon side for correct placement and later ease of removal. The sponge may be placed up to 24 hours before sexual intercourse is anticipated to occur but should stay in place no more than 30 hours.

Cervical Cap

The cervical cap, similar to the diaphragm, holds spermicide against the cervix to prevent the passage of sperm. Unlike the diaphragm, it is shaped more like a small cup than a saucer. This method is most effective for women who have not given birth, having a 16% failure rate over the course of a year in this population. For women who have given birth, the failure rate with typical use over a year is 32% (Curtis, Tepper, et al., 2016). In the United States, the cervical cap is marketed under the name FemCap. It comes in three sizes: small, medium, and large. The small size is indicated for women who have never been pregnant, medium for women who have had an abortion or cesarean birth, and large for women who have delivered a pregnancy vaginally.

 Patient Teaching 29.2 **Correct Use and Care of a Diaphragm**

Diaphragm Use
- Before each use, hold the diaphragm up to a light and examine the dome for any puncture marks or cracks. Alternatively, fill the dome with water and check it for leaks.
- Apply 1 tablespoon of spermicide to the hollow of the dome and along the rim. Only use spermicides approved for use with a diaphragm.
- Insert the diaphragm into the vagina and check its position to ensure that the cervix is completely covered within the spermicide-containing dome. The anterior rim should be securely positioned behind the pubic bone.
- After the diaphragm is in place, place an additional applicator of spermicide in the vagina.
- Make sure the diaphragm is inserted into the vagina less than 2 h prior to sexual intercourse.
- If placed 3–6 h before intercourse, insert another applicator full of fresh spermicide into the vagina just before intercourse.
- Check the position of the diaphragm after intercourse. If it has moved out of position, push it back into position and reapply spermicide.
- Before each new episode of intercourse, insert fresh spermicide while the diaphragm is in place.
- Leave the diaphragm in place for at least 6 h after the last episode of intercourse. Remove it by 24 h after the initial placement.
- Do not share diaphragms.
- Do not use a diaphragm during menses because blood will accumulate behind the diaphragm and could increase the risk for infection. The risk of pregnancy is extremely low during the first 5 d after the onset of menses.

Diaphragm Care
- Wash the diaphragm with mild soap and warm water after use.
- Air-dry the diaphragm.
- Do not use silicone-based lubricants or other products with silicone diaphragms, as they may damage the diaphragm.
- Replace the diaphragm after 2 y.

To use this device, the woman places spermicide in the dome and around the edges on one side and in the folds of the device on the other side. She then inserts it so that it covers the cervix (Fig. 29.9). She may insert it up to 6 hours prior to sex and should remove it 6 to 48 hours after intercourse. She should insert additional spermicide into the cap without removing it for each additional episode of intercourse. Care of the cervical cap is similar to that for the diaphragm. Vaginal irritation is possible with use of the cervical cap as with the diaphragm.

Spermicide

Spermicide is a jelly, cream, suppository, or film that contains a chemical that kills sperm and that is inserted into the vagina prior to intercourse to prevent pregnancy. The woman should insert spermicide into the vagina at least 10 minutes prior to intercourse and apply more spermicide prior to every new episode of intercourse. The only spermicide approved by the Food and Drug Administration for use in the United States is nanoxynol-9. Used alone, it has a 20% failure rate over the course of a year (Curtis, Tepper, et al., 2016). It is often used in conjunction with barrier methods, however, such as condoms, diaphragms, cervical caps, and sponges. Nonoxynol-9 can be quite irritating to the mucosa. Women using spermicide are more prone to urinary tract infections and vaginal irritation and inflammation. This inflammation and irritation makes women more vulnerable to infection with STIs, including human immunodeficiency virus.

Natural Family Planning

NFP—also referred to as fertility awareness, the rhythm method, and timed intercourse—is an approach to contraception in which women rely on the predictability of fertile and infertile times of the menstrual cycle to avoid conception. Approximately 1% of contracepting women use NFP in the United States (Freundl, Sivin, & Batar, 2010). The annual efficacy rate is 76% with typical use (Curtis, Tepper, et al., 2016).

Using this approach, a woman avoids having intercourse on and immediately prior to identified fertile days, with the understanding that an ovum can be fertilized only for a maximum of 24 hours after ovulation and that sperm can live for up to 5 days in the upper genital tract. Thus, a woman is fertile from about 5 days prior to ovulation through 24 hours after ovulation. The chance of pregnancy is 4% 3 to 5 days prior to ovulation, 25% to 28% 2 days prior to ovulation, 8% to 10% in the 24 hours after ovulation, and nonexistent during the remaining days of the cycle (Wilcox, Weinberg, & Baird, 1998).

The methods of determining the timing of ovulation include the Standard Days Method, various methods based on the evaluation of cervical secretions, the symptothermal method, and symptohormonal methods. Some of these methods are used in conjunction with computer and smart phone applications that help interpret data provided by the woman. Many women use a combination of methods for greater efficacy.

Standard Days Method

The Standard Days Method requires avoiding intercourse on days 8 through 19 of the menstrual cycle. Unprotected intercourse may occur on the remaining days. This method is most appropriate for the 78% of women with cycles that consistently range from 26 to 32 days. It is not an appropriate method for women with irregular menses, such as women who are perimenopausal or adolescent, recently gave birth, or have PCOS. When used perfectly, fewer than 5 out of 100 women become pregnant within 13 months of beginning this method. With typical use, 12 women out of 100 become pregnant in the same period of time (Curtis, Jatlaoui, et al., 2016). Cycle beads are a convenient tool to help women with this method of NFP (Fig. 29.10).

Cervical Secretion Methods

The Billings and Creighton methods require a woman to evaluate her cervical secretions several times daily and avoid having unprotected intercourse on days when her cervical mucus is of a consistency that indicates fertility. With perfect use, the efficacy of these methods is 97%. With typical use, the efficacy drops to 77% (Bhargava, Bhatia, Ramachandran, Rohatgi, & Sinha, 1996).

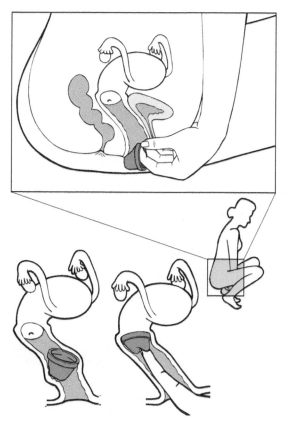

Figure 29.9. Insertion of a cervical cap. (Reprinted with permission from Callahan, T. L., & Caughey, A. B. [2013]. *Blueprints obstetrics & gynecology* [6th ed., Fig. 24.5]. Philadelphia, PA: Lippincott Williams & Wilkins.)

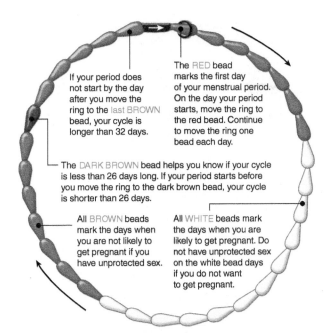

If your period does not start by the day after you move the ring to the last BROWN bead, your cycle is longer than 32 days.

The RED bead marks the first day of your menstrual period. On the day your period starts, move the ring to the red bead. Continue to move the ring one bead each day.

The DARK BROWN bead helps you know if your cycle is less than 26 days long. If your period starts before you move the ring to the dark brown bead, your cycle is shorter than 26 days.

All BROWN beads mark the days when you are not likely to get pregnant if you have unprotected sex.

All WHITE beads mark the days when you are likely to get pregnant. Do not have unprotected sex on the white bead days if you do not want to get pregnant.

Figure 29.10. Cycle beads. With this contraceptive aid, a woman moves one bead every day to predict her fertile days if her menstrual cycles range from 26 to 32 days. (Reprinted with permission from Evans, R. J., Brown, Y. M., & Evans, M. K. [2014]. *Canadian maternity, newborn, and women's health nursing* [2nd ed., Fig. 8.13]. Philadelphia, PA: Lippincott Williams & Wilkins.)

Specifically, these methods require women to avoid having intercourse during the following times:

- On days when menses might obscure secretions
- On days between menses and ovulation following intercourse, to avoid the obscuring of secretions by semen
- On days when secretions are stretchy, transparent, wet, or slippery, and therefore suggestive of ovulation
- For 4 days after the last day of secretions suggestive of ovulation
  Following these rules, unprotected sex is avoided for 14 to 17 days of each cycle.

The TwoDay Method also bases unprotected intercourse decision making on cervical secretions. The users of this method avoid having unprotected intercourse on each day on which they note having cervical secretions and the day following. With this method, 13 days of each cycle require the avoidance of unprotected intercourse. With perfect use, 3 to 4 out of 100 women using this approach become pregnant within a year. With typical use, about 14 out of 100 women become pregnant within a year (Arevalo, Jennings, Nikula, & Sinai, 2004).

Symptothermal Method

The symptothermal method requires a combination of evaluating cervical secretions several times a day and taking a daily temperature prior to rising with a basal body thermometer. A woman's temperature dips slightly on the day of ovulation and then rises sharply after ovulation has occurred. Some users of this method also evaluate the position and consistency of their cervix. The cervical secretions help identify the beginning of the fertile period,

whereas the temperature allows the woman to identify the end of the fertile period. The cervix around the time of ovulation is soft, open, and higher in the vagina than it does at other times in the menstrual cycle. Following this approach, the woman avoids having unprotected intercourse for 12 to 17 days of each month. With perfect use, 2 out of 100 women become pregnant annually. With more typical use, 13 to 20 out of 100 women become pregnant every year (Frank-Herrmann et al., 2007).

Symptohormonal Methods

Other methods of NFP involve measuring hormone levels, alone or in conjunction with assessing other symptoms, to determine fertile days, on which the woman should avoid having unprotected intercourse. One such method, the Marquette Model, includes the use of a device that measures hormones in the urine, which may be combined with an assessment of cervical secretions (Fehring, Schneider, Raviele, Rodriguez, & Pruszynski, 2013).

Withdrawal

Withdrawal is the avoidance of ejaculation into the vagina during intercourse. It is also referred to as the pull-out method or coitus interruptus. It is not an uncommon choice of contraception for established monogamous couples in a trusting relationship who do not want the trouble, side effects, or risks of other forms of contraception. Although many couples have great long-term success with the method, it is not considered a particularly effective method, with a 22% chance of method failure every year (Curtis, Tepper, et al., 2016). Failure occurs if sperm is in the pre-ejaculation fluid that is emitted from the penis during intercourse or if withdrawal is poorly timed. Cleaning the tip of the penis and urinating between ejaculations help remove sperm remaining from a prior ejaculation and may improve efficacy.

Sterilization

Both men and women may be sterilized. The sterilization of a woman is called BTL. The sterilization of a man is referred to as a vasectomy. Contraception failure is rare with sterilization.

Bilateral Tubal Ligation

BTL is the most common form of contraception globally and the second most common form of contraception in the United States (Jones, Mosher, & Daniels, 2012). A BTL may involve the cauterization, suturing, clamping, or removal of a portion the fallopian tubes. A BTL may be performed immediately after a cesarean section or within 24 to 48 hours after a vaginal birth. After the immediate postpartum period, a BTL is usually performed by outpatient laparoscopic surgery or by in-office hysteroscopy. Approximately 6% of hysteroscopic sterilizations are unsuccessful as opposed to 1% of laparoscopic sterilizations (Gariepy, Creinin, Smith, & Xu, 2014).

Hysteroscopic sterilization is performed by the placement of sterile plugs into the fallopian tubes via the cervix (Fig. 29.11). Over the course of 3 months, scar tissue forms around the plugs, occluding them. After 3 months, tubal occlusion is complete and the woman is considered sterile.

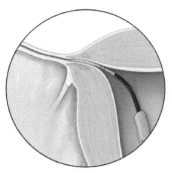

1. The Adiana system involves priming the tube with low-frequency radiowaves.

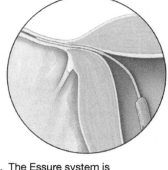

1. The Essure system is introduced hysteroscopically.

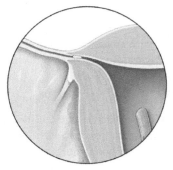

2. The 0.4 cm flexible silicon Adiana system is placed in the tube.

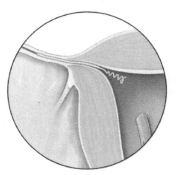

2. The 3.6 cm Essure coil is released in the tube.

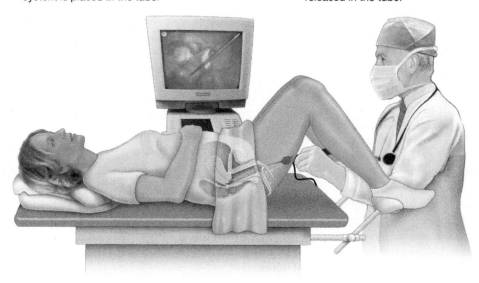

Figure 29.11. Bilateral tubal ligation via hysteroscopic sterilization. (Reprinted with permission from Beckmann, C. R., Herbert, W., Laube, D., Ling, F., & Smith, R. [2013]. *Obstetrics and gynecology* [7th ed., Fig. 27.5]. Philadelphia, PA: Lippincott Williams & Wilkins.)

Regret is a risk of sterilization, although the number of women who request reversal of sterilization or in vitro fertilization (IVF) to achieve pregnancy after sterilization is low. The reported rate of regret is between 1% and 26%, with a higher occurrence among younger women (Curtis, Jatlaoui, et al., 2016).

Vasectomy

Vasectomy is the safest means of permanent sterilization and the most cost-effective. However, although 25% of women in the United States using contraception choose BTL, only 8% of sexually active men have been sterilized (Daniels, Daugherty, Jones, & Mosher, 2015). Approximately 5% regret their choice of vasectomy (Curtis, Jatlaoui, et al., 2016).

A vasectomy is performed by making two openings into the scrotum, removing a portion of the vas deferens on either side, and occluding the resulting ends (Fig. 29.12). It is generally performed in office with only local anesthetic. Testing performed after 3 months confirms sterility. Potential complications include bleeding, infection, and postvasectomy pain.

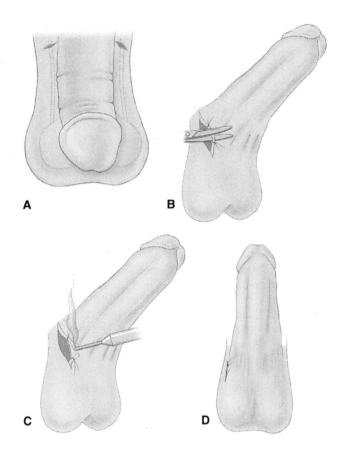

Figure 29.12. Vasectomy. (A) Site of vasectomy incisions. **(B)** The vas deferens is cut with surgical scissors. **(C)** Cut ends of the vas deferens are cauterized to ensure blockage of the passage of sperm. **(D)** Final skin suture. (Reprinted with permission from Chow, J., Ateah, C. A., Scott, S. D., Ricci, S. S., & Kyle, T. [2013]. *Canadian maternity and pediatric nursing* [Fig. 4.19]. Philadelphia, PA: Lippincott Williams & Wilkins.)

Unwanted or Mistimed Pregnancy

Approximately half of pregnancies in this country are unplanned (Finer & Zolna, 2016). Unintended pregnancies are associated with poor outcomes, including late prenatal care, intimate partner violence against the pregnant woman, maternal depression, less breastfeeding, and financial instability (Healthy People 2020).

Reasons women cite for unintended pregnancy are that they did not believe they could get pregnant when conception occurred (33%), they did not mind getting pregnant (30%), their partners did not wish to use contraception (22%), they do not like the side effects of contraception (16%), they believed that they or their partners were sterile (10%), or they have difficulty accessing contraception (18%; Nettleman, Chung, Brewer, Ayoola, & Reed, 2007).

The decisions made regarding an unwanted or mistimed pregnancy are deeply personal. The options include abortion or offspring the pregnancy with the expectation of either raising the continuing or surrendering him or her for adoption. Factors included in the decision-making process may include the woman's current financial, family, work, school, or relationship status, as well as plans and hopes for the future. Pregnancy and childbirth

are by no means risk free or without the potential for long-term effects or consequences.

Abortion

A majority of the 926,200 abortions performed in the United States in 2014 were of unintended pregnancies. Approximately 19% of pregnancies ended in abortion (Finer & Zolna, 2016). Despite the myth that a majority of abortions occur in adolescence, a majority of abortions are performed for women in their 20s (Jerman, Jones, & Onda, 2016). Of the women who seek abortions, 59% have at least one child (Jerman et al., 2016).

Most women cite as reasons for abortion the inability to afford to care for a child, not wanting to be a single parent, problems with the partner of the pregnancy, and the challenge of caring for a child in addition to existing children, school, work, and other responsibilities (Jones, Zolna, Henshaw, & Finer, 2008).

Of women who elected to terminate pregnancies in 2014, 46% reported that they were neither married nor cohabitating (Jerman et al., 2016). Of the women who terminated pregnancies, 75% had incomes of less than 199% of the federal poverty level (Jerman et al., 2016).

A vast majority of abortions are performed in early pregnancy: two thirds occur at or prior to 8 weeks of gestation, and 89% are completed prior to 12 weeks of gestation (Finer & Zolna, 2016). Later abortions are due to difficulty with the expense of the procedure, parental involvement laws, poor access to abortion providers, and a delay in identification of the pregnancy (Jones et al., 2008). A small number of later abortions are indicated because of fetal anomalies or concerns for maternal health.

In addition to obtaining a thorough history in advance of an abortion, it is important to determine if coercion is a factor in the woman's decision to terminate the pregnancy. It is critical that the decision be her own. Any discussion of other options, including parenting and adoption, must be nondirective.

Nurses who participate in abortion care must be aware of state law. Some states require a mandated waiting period between counseling and the procedure, and others require parental notification and consent. Some states mandate what information must be part of patient counseling.

The determination of gestational age is important for planning the procedure. Patients who are up to 70 days of gestation may be offered a medication abortion. Cervical ripening prior to a surgical procedure may be indicated for later gestations. Although most providers use ultrasound to confirm pregnancy dating, particularly when determining eligibility for a medication abortion, menstrual dating with a confirmatory physical examination may be adequate in some situations.

Prior to termination, the woman's hemoglobin level and Rh status must be checked. Women who are very anemic may be ineligible for some procedures or may require more intensive care. Women who are Rh negative require the administration of Rh_o (D) immune globulin at the time of termination. Routine screening of all patients for gonorrhea and chlamydia is standard.

The administration of antibiotics is standard prior to a surgical abortion and common prior to a medication abortion.

Surgical Abortion

Surgical abortion is typically done by uterine aspiration and is also called dilation and curettage, dilation and evacuation, aspiration curettage, and suction curettage. Later abortion is generally by dilation and evacuation. Although uterine aspiration uses suction to empty the uterine contents, evacuation uses surgical tools in addition to the suction.

Cervical Dilation

Dilation of the cervix is necessary prior to abortion and may be facilitated by rigid dilators, osmotic dilators, misoprostol, or, mifepristone, depending on gestation. Mechanical dilation with rigid dilators at the time of procedure is typically sufficient for first trimester abortions, whereas cervical preparation with osmotic dilators, in addition to misoprostol and/or mifepristone, prior to the procedure is required for later procedures.

Rigid dilators are stainless steel or plastic and come in graduated sizes. They are introduced sequentially from smaller sizes to larger sizes to quickly mechanically dilate the cervix. Osmotic dilators, usually made of sterile seaweed or a synthetic material, are placed in the cervix, where they absorb moisture and swell, causing the cervix to dilate more slowly. Osmotic dilators are typically placed 12 to 18 hours prior to the procedure, whereas mechanical dilators are used at the time of the procedure. Misoprostol may be placed in the vagina 2 to 3 hours prior to the procedure to ripen the cervix and aid dilation. The use of mifepristone for this purpose is investigational but promising.

Anesthesia and Analgesia

Local anesthesia is used for most first trimester procedures. Lidocaine is usually injected into the anterior lip of the cervix as well as into multiple areas of the vaginal fornix. Patients who desire conscious sedation or for whom conscious sedation is indicated may receive midazolam or fentanyl intravenously. The administration of ibuprofen 1 hour prior to the procedure may help diminish pain both during and after the abortion. The use of neuraxial or general anesthesia is rare for abortion but may be indicated for certain patients and clinical situations.

Procedure

A majority of abortion procedures are done by either manual or electric vacuum aspiration (Fig. 29.13) after dilation has been achieved. A small minority, particularly later abortions, include curettage (scraping of the walls of the uterus) or extraction of the uterine contents with the aid of forceps. The procedure once started takes only a few minutes and is considered very safe. After the procedure, the clinician examines the uterine contents to make sure the abortion is complete.

Postprocedure Care

The nurse should observe patients for at least 30 minutes after the procedure, with regular monitoring for hemorrhage and intraabdominal bleeding by vital sign, pain assessments, and evaluation of bleeding. Women who are Rh negative in the first trimester generally require only 50 μg of Rh$_o$ (D) immune globulin, although women with later procedures require a 300-μg

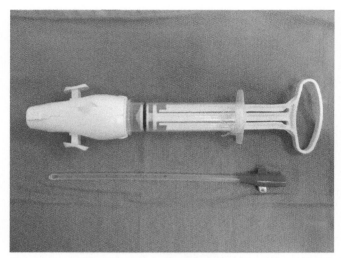

Figure 29.13. Manual vacuum aspiration syringe (above) with flexible suction cannula (below). (Reprinted with permission from Nakajima, S. T., McCoy, T. W., Krause, M. S., & Berek, J. S. [Eds.]. [2017]. *Operative techniques in gynecologic surgery: Reproductive endocrinology and infertility* [1st ed., Fig. 10.1]. Philadelphia, PA: Lippincott Williams & Wilkins.)

dose. Mild lower abdominal cramping is common for a few days after the procedure, as are some bleeding and passage of tissue comparable to that of menses.

The nurse should instruct the patient to call the office where the procedure was performed or other care provider if she experiences fever, heavy bleeding, or worsening of abdominal pain within a week of the procedure. The patient should also be reassessed if pregnancy symptoms such as nausea and breast tenderness do not resolve or if menses has not returned within 6 weeks. The rate of major complications (blood transfusion, surgery, hospital admission) after a first trimester aspiration abortion is 0.16%, and the rate of minor complications is 1.1% (Upadhyay et al., 2015). The mortality rate from legal surgical abortion is 0.8 out of every 100,000 procedures, when compared with 12 maternal deaths out of every 100,000 live births in the United States (Jatlaoui et al., 2016).

The nurse should review contraception options with the patient prior to termination and encourage the patient, if possible, to implement contraception immediately after termination. IUCs may be placed at the time of a surgical procedure.

Medication Abortion

The medication abortion is an option for women who are up to 70 days pregnant. Over 22% of abortions performed at or before 8 weeks are medication abortions (Jatlaoui et al., 2016). The most common regimen includes a 200-mg dose of mifepristone in the office at the time of the visit followed by 800 μg of misoprostol administered vaginally, buccally, or sublingually at home. If taken vaginally, misoprostol may be taken as soon as 6 hours after the mifepristone. If taken buccally or sublingually, misoprostol should be taken 24 to 48 hours after the mifepristone.

The rate of complications associated with medication abortion is similar to that for surgical abortion (Cleland, Creinin,

Nucatola, Nshom, & Trussell, 2013). Women who are Rh negative require Rh$_0$ (D) immune globulin at the time of the first visit. Although the cramping that accompanies a medication abortion is typically well managed with ibuprofen, it is usually appropriate to offer a short course of opioids to the patient. In-office follow-up with ultrasound is required 1 to 2 weeks after the initial visit to ensure the pregnancy has been expelled. Alternatively, the beta-human chorionic gonadotropin (β-hCG) level may be assessed at the time of the first visit and then at follow-up to ensure that levels are dropping appropriately. The medications used for a medication abortion are teratogens. In the case of a failed medication abortion, a surgical procedure is indicated. It is highly recommended that women electing to have a medication abortion identify a friend or family member who can stay with them throughout the experience in the event that aid or support is required.

The experience of a medication abortion is different from that of a surgical abortion. A surgical abortion is an invasive procedure that is finished in the course of a visit. A medication abortion avoids an invasive procedure but typically takes 2 days to complete, most of this time away from healthcare personnel. The uncomfortable effects of cramping and bleeding that occur with a medication abortion are prolonged when compared with those of a surgical abortion. Depending on the gestational age, the products of conception may be recognizable when they pass, and it may be more difficult for the woman emotionally to manage this part of the process. Some women prefer the level of control of a medication abortion, however, and the framing of the procedure as an induced miscarriage.

After an abortion, most women describe some mix of relief, sadness, loss, and transient guilt. There is no evidence that abortion predisposes a woman to depression or other psychiatric illness (Cohen, 2013). Although evidence is mixed, women who have terminated a pregnancy may have a small increased risk of preterm labor and low birth weight infants with future pregnancies, particularly when abortions are provided later in pregnancy. Early term abortions carry no risk to future pregnancies. Abortion does not cause breast cancer (Guttmacher Institute, 2018).

Adoption

A mother who chooses to release a child for adoption is a birth mother. As with the choice to abort, the choice to surrender for adoption is a deeply personal one. A birth mother may struggle with the decision or it may be immediately clear to her. She may change her mind several times before and after giving birth.

The pregnancy goals of a birth mother are likely the same as those of a woman intending to raise the infant: delivery of a healthy baby. Birth mothers should be given every opportunity to access services, such as quality prenatal care, just as with any pregnant woman. Discussion of the adoption should be led by the birth mother. When possible, counseling should be made available during and after the pregnancy to help manage her psychological health. Many women mourn the loss of the mothering role. The birth mother may suffer anticipatory grief as well as grief during the adoption process and after its completion.

A nurse attending the birth of a woman intending to put the infant up for adoption should seek clear instructions from the birth mother, obtaining answers to the following questions: Does she want to hold the baby after the birth? Should the baby be handed to the adoptive parents? Does she wish to see the infant at all? Does she wish to nurse the infant? If she will be spending time with the infant after the birth, does she wish to be alone? Does she wish to have the adoptive parents present during the delivery? During the postpartum period, when possible, the birth mother should be roomed away from mothers with infants unless otherwise requested.

An open adoption includes an agreement of communication between the birth parents and adoptive parents, as consented to by all parties. Today in the United States, most adoptions are open adoptions. Open adoption may create identity issues for the birth mother who now has a part in the child's life but not a parenting role. Adoptions that are closed may still have open records depending on the state in which the adoption occurred. With open records, an adult adoptee may receive his or her adoption records and birth certificate by request.

Adoption facilitation services are usually provided by a public or private agency. Agency services include an evaluation of the potential adoptive family to determine their suitability as adoptive parents. Alternatively, an independent adoption excludes the aid of a specialized agency but may include support by attorneys, healthcare clinicians, and others.

In the United States, 120,000 children are adopted annually, 38% through a private domestic adoption, 37% through the foster care system, 25% through international adoption, and the remainder through the adoption of the child by relatives (Jones & Schulte, 2012).

Infertility

Infertility is not a women's health problem. It is a couple's problem. Of 6% of couples with fertility issues in the United States, 8% have male-factor infertility as the sole cause, whereas 35% experience infertility because of various causes, including male factor (Centers for Disease Control and Prevention [CDC], 2017).

Infertility is the term used to describe a lack of pregnancy after 12 months of well-timed intercourse when the woman is under 35 years old and after 6 months for women 35 years and over. In general, 80% to 90% of apparently normal couples conceive within the first year, and an additional 5% to 15% conceive in the second year, meaning that approximately 95% of couples achieve pregnancy within 24 months (Slama et al., 2012).

Optimizing Fertility

For some couples who are struggling to conceive or are planning conception, education about optimizing pregnancy naturally can be helpful. Many people are unaware of the fertile window of a woman's menstrual cycle. The nurse can instruct women on how to predict ovulation to achieve pregnancy using the same methods they would use to prevent pregnancy: evaluating cervical secretions, estimating standard days, measuring body temperature, and using home ovulation kits. Although couples are most likely to attain pregnancy by having intercourse every day or every other day, intercourse two or three times weekly starting after the cessation of menses is usually sufficient. Nurses should be aware, however, that although these methods give couples some sense of control over conception planning, there is little evidence to suggest that fertility awareness increases their chances of achieving pregnancy (Manders et al., 2015).

Factors often thought to impact the chance of conception, such as lubricant, female orgasm, and position during sex and after ejaculation do not impact a couple's chance of pregnancy (Practice Committee of American Society for Reproductive Medicine in Collaboration With Society for Reproductive Endocrinology and Infertility, 2013). Cigarette smoking, excessive exercise, BMI (high or low), alcohol use, stress, early age at first intercourse and/or many sexual partners for women, and caffeine consumption may have an effect on fertility, although few well-designed studies exist to tease out what may be a true risk factor and what is merely a correlation.

Evaluation for Infertility

Infertility is a source of personal and relationship stress for most couples struggling to achieve pregnancy. For most committed couples, sex is an expression of love and bonding. Infertility can make sex a chore and a source of a sense of failure. Failure to achieve pregnancy, an evaluation for the source of infertility, and treatment can be time-consuming, financially expensive, physically challenging, and psychologically trying. Nurses working with patients coping with infertility should anticipate anxiety, stress, depression, anger, and even lashing out that has little to do with the nurse or the partner. Compassion for the couple is critical at this time.

The timing of the initial evaluation for infertility is based on the age of the woman attempting pregnancy. Timing may be adjusted, however, according to the clinical picture. Some risk factors for infertility, such as endometriosis, chemotherapy, radiation, a history of PID, and infrequent menses, may cue earlier evaluation.

Because of the occurrence of infertility in both men and women, evaluation of the couple should be done simultaneously. The aspects of standard initial testing for infertility are included in Box 29.1.

Female Infertility

The most common female factors contributing to infertility are ovulatory disorders, endometriosis, pelvic adhesions, uterine abnormalities (including fibroids), tubal blockage, tubal abnormalities other than blockage, and hyperprolactinemia. Age also plays a part, as fertility declines with age as a result of a decrease in the quantity and quality of oocytes. Although this process of diminishing fertility naturally accelerates when a woman reaches her mid-thirties, smoking, radiation, and chemotherapy can accelerate this process. The treatment of infertility depends on the root cause, if it can be determined.

Box 29.1   Common Aspects of Initial Evaluation for Infertility

Female
- Menstrual history
- Urine testing for luteinizing hormone (following the anticipated surge) and/or progesterone level (during the luteal phase)
- Hysterosalpingogram to assess the uterine cavity and patency of the fallopian tubes
- Serum follicle-stimulating hormone and estradiol levels on the third day of menses
- Thyroid-stimulating hormone levels

Male
- Semen analysis (of a specimen collected by masturbation 2–7 d after the last ejaculation; at least two samples should be collected at least a week apart)
  - Measurement of semen volume and pH
  - Microscopy of semen for debris and agglutination
  - Assessment of sperm concentration, motility, and morphology
  - Sperm leukocyte count
  - Search for immature germ cells

Oligoovulation and Anovulation

Oligoovulation (infrequent or irregular ovulation) and anovulation (no ovulation) not caused by ovarian failure, which is irreversible, can typically be treated successfully with ovulation induction.

Ovulation Induction

There are several methods of inducing ovulation. Some are low-cost or even free. Some are invasive or expensive. Some provide an excellent chance for conception but an increased risk for a multiple pregnancy.

Ovulation may be induced simply by losing or gaining weight, for women who are overweight or underweight. For others, medications such as clomiphene citrate, aromatase inhibitors, or gonadotropin may be required. A potential risk of medication-induced ovulation, however, is ovarian hyperstimulation syndrome (OHSS).

Weight Loss or Gain

Having too high or too low a BMI can contribute to oligoovulation or anovulation. Women with a BMI of 27 or above who are anovulatory are advised to lose weight. Women with PCOS who lose 5% to 10% of their body weight have at least a 55% chance of inducing ovulation through weight loss alone (Pasquali et al., 2011). Women who are obese and lose weight prior to undergoing fertility treatments are more likely to conceive spontaneously and after fewer fertility treatments. They do not, however, have an overall higher chance of achieving pregnancy (Mutsaerts et al., 2016). Women with a higher BMI are more likely to be insulin resistant. For these women, metformin can enhance the rate of spontaneous ovulation (Legro et al., 2013).

Conversely, women with a BMI below 17 or who have an unusually strenuous exercise regimen or an eating disorder may also be anovulatory. These women are advised to gain weight and exercise less. Such women may be reluctant to gain weight and may benefit from therapy to encourage weight gain and optimize nutritional intake.

Clomiphene Citrate

Clomiphene citrate (Clomid) is a selective estrogen receptor modulator and a common first-line medication used to induce ovulation. Clomiphene citrate is usually started 5 days after the start of a menses. If the patient is not menstruating spontaneously, she may be given a course of progestin for 10 days, with a withdrawal bleed anticipated in the days following completion of the medication.

The usual starting dose for clomiphene citrate is 50 mg a day for 5 days. If ovulation does not occur after one cycle at 50 mg, the dose is increased to 100 mg a day for the next cycle. If 100 mg is insufficient to induce ovulation, the dose may be increased to 150 mg a day. Clomiphene citrate may be administered for 4 to 6 cycles before the strategy is abandoned.

A surge of LH that induces ovulation is expected 5 to 12 days after the completion of the 5-day cycle of clomiphene citrate. Ovulation usually occurs 14 to 26 hours after the LH surge, although it may take up to 48 hours. The LH surge is typically monitored for by testing of the urine. If indicated, a serum progesterone level may be taken a week after the LH surge. A concentration greater than 3 ng/mL indicates that ovulation occurred.

Approximately 80% of women with PCOS ovulate after taking clomiphene citrate, and half of women ovulate at the lowest dose of 50 mg. The rates of miscarriage and ectopic pregnancy with the use of clomiphene citrate are similar to those with spontaneous pregnancies. The risk for multiple gestation is increased by 7% with clomiphene citrate when compared with spontaneous pregnancy (Legro et al., 2014).

Aromatase Inhibitors

Aromatase inhibitors, particularly letrozole, are a common second-line choice after clomiphene citrate failure. This is an off-label use for the medication. A typical starting dose for letrozole is 2.5 mg daily for 4 days starting on day 3 after a spontaneous menses or progestin-induced bleed. If ovulation does not occur, the dose may be doubled for the next cycle. The maximum dose for letrozole is 7.5 mg a day for days 3 through 7 of the menstrual cycle. Letrozole may have a higher rate of ovulation and pregnancy for women with PCOS than does clomiphene citrate. The rate of multiple pregnancy is likely lower (Legro et al., 2014).

Gonadotropin

Gonadotropin therapy is far more intensive than treatment with clomiphene citrate or letrozole. It is more expensive, carries a higher risk of multiple gestation, and has more side effects. Gonadotropin therapy is often used in conjunction with gonadotropin-releasing hormone agonists to optimize cycle control and prevent an LH surge prior to complete maturation of the developing follicles.

Gonadotropin therapy requires the patient to self-inject a FSH or human menopausal gonadotropin preparation either subcutaneously or intramuscularly over a number of days. Every few days a transvaginal ultrasound is done to assess the growth of follicles. The presence of three or more follicles of 15 mm or more is an indication to stop the cycle because of the high risk for a multiple pregnancy. If one or two follicles reach 10 mm, the dose of FSH is usually gradually titrated down as the patient continues to be monitored. When the follicle or follicles reach 18 mm, ovulation is triggered with a preparation of β-hCG. Concurrent serum estrogen monitoring is necessary to monitor for side effects.

The use of gonadotropin therapy to achieve pregnancy in the case of unexplained infertility is successful for about a third of women (Curtis & Peipert, 2017).

Ovarian Hyperstimulation Syndrome

A relatively common side effect of ovarian stimulation is OHSS, which includes the enlargement of the ovaries with multiple cysts and the accumulation of abdominal fluid associated with hypovolemic shock, acute respiratory distress, renal failure, thromboemboli, and death. The development of several follicles and high levels of serum estrogen identify women at a high risk for OHSS. The condition is much more common with the use of injectable fertility medications than with letrozole or clomiphene citrate. The condition is usually successfully treated medically.

Tubal Infertility

Infertility may also be caused by abnormalities of the fallopian tubes, often resulting from an ascending infection, either symptomatic or asymptomatic, that causes inflammation and eventual scarring, adhesions, and occlusion of the tubes. For many women, IVF (see below) may be the option that offers the greatest chance of success. Some women, however, may be successfully treated surgically.

A **hysterosalpingogram** is an imaging test used to assess the fallopian tubes and uterus. During the test, a water- or oil-based contrast medium is introduced into the uterus. Imaging is used to track the path of the contrast medium and determine if there is a structural abnormality of the uterus or fallopian tubes or a blockage of one or both tubes. Almost 40% of women who have a hysterosalpingogram with oil contrast, however, achieve spontaneous pregnancy (Dreyer et al., 2017). For this subset of women, a hysterosalpingogram appears to be both diagnostic and therapeutic.

Luteal Phase Defect

Insufficiencies of the luteal phase were long thought to contribute to infertility and were often treated with progesterone supplementation. There is not enough evidence at this time, however, to identify a luteal phase defect as an independent diagnosis that requires a particular treatment (Practice Committee of the American Society for Reproductive Medicine, 2015).

Cervical Factor Infertility

Cervical factor infertility is the presence of cervical secretions that are thin or scanty or that may otherwise impede the passage of sperm. The cause is often unknown, as is the significance of variations of cervical secretions. Although intrauterine insemination (IUI, see below) is often used to bypass the cervix and thus cervical factor infertility, there is little evidence to support the efficacy of IUI over well-timed intercourse. Postcoital testing was once a common means of evaluating for cervical factor infertility. It has poor diagnostic and predictive value, however, and incorporating its use has not been shown to improve outcomes (Practice Committee of American Society for Reproductive Medicine, 2012).

Male Infertility

Male infertility may be caused by hypothalamic pituitary disease, primary hypogonadism, the disorders of sperm transport, or dysfunction of the seminiferous tubule. Past and current infections may impact fertility, as may drugs and environmental exposures, such as chemotherapy, toxic chemicals, radiation therapy, anabolic steroids, and alcohol. For some men, genetic testing may be helpful, as well as measurement of serum levels of testosterone, LH, and FSH.

Age plays a minor role for men, as well, with fertility diminishing after the age of 50. From 1973 to 2011, the average sperm count of men has declined worldwide by more than half in developed countries for reasons that are not yet clear (Levine et al., 2017).

Fewer treatments are available for male-factor infertility than female factor infertility. Traditional wisdom has suggested that keeping the scrotum cooler by a change in underwear or the avoidance of warm baths or showers improves fertility. Studies have not supported this assumption, however. Transport issues, such as the absence of a vas deferens in men with cystic fibrosis, may be addressed by **artificial reproductive technology** (ART, see below).

Artificial Reproductive Technology

ART is used to treat infertility due to male, female, or mixed factors as well as infertility due to unknown causes. ART accounts for approximately 1.5% of all births and 20% of all multiple births (Ory, 2013).

Intrauterine Insemination

In Chapter 9, Nancy used IUI to get pregnant not because she has any known fertility issues but rather because she was using donated sperm rather than attempting pregnancy through intercourse.

IUI is a procedure in which ejaculated sperm is washed to remove prostaglandins and semen proteins and then concentrated in culture media. This washed sperm is then drawn into a narrow catheter and introduced into the upper uterine cavity by way of the cervix (Fig. 29.14). IUI is optimally done just prior to either natural or induced ovulation. IUI alone without other

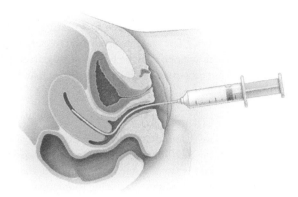

Figure 29.14. Intrauterine insemination technique. (Reprinted with permission from Beckmann, C. R., Herbert, W., Laube, D., Ling, F., & Smith, R. [2013]. *Obstetrics and gynecology* [7th ed., Fig. 42.7]. Philadelphia, PA: Lippincott Williams & Wilkins.)

interventions is marginally more effective than well-timed intercourse or the introduction of washed sperm at the level of the cervix (intracervical insemination) in the case of unexplained fertility (Guzick et al., 1999).

IUI may also be used for couples with severe sexual dysfunction such as vaginismus, which makes sex impossible. IUI is often used to achieve pregnancy using donated sperm.

In Vitro Fertilization

IVF is a cornerstone of ART. It is used to treat infertility due to tubal factors, severe male factors (see the section "Intracytoplasmic Sperm Injection"), low ovarian reserve, unexplained infertility, ovarian failure (using donor eggs), uterine factors, and other causes of infertility. It may be used to achieve pregnancy in a gestational carrier for women who produce oocytes but for whom pregnancy is contraindicated, unwanted, or not possible. It may also be used for sex selection of the embryo and preimplantation genetic diagnosis.

IVF is expensive and often not covered by health insurance. For this reason, less invasive, less expensive strategies are typically tried prior to IVF.

In IVF, the ovaries are stimulated as described previously but with a goal of safely maximizing oocyte recruitment. Ovulation is triggered with β-hCG. Oocytes are retrieved by transvaginal ultrasound-guided follicle aspiration 34 to 36 hours after the administration of β-hCG (Fig. 29.15).

The recovered oocytes are then mixed with cleaned spermatozoa in a culture medium. The spermatozoa may be recently obtained or from a frozen sample. Similarly, eggs may be harvested and frozen before or after fertilization. This process is referred to as fertilization in vitro. Successful fertilization can generally be identified approximately 17 hours later.

If preimplantation genetics are being assessed, a single cell is removed during the blastocyst stage, usually at day 5. Embryo transfer must take place by day 6. This means that if genetic assessment is indicated prior to implantation, the blastocysts will

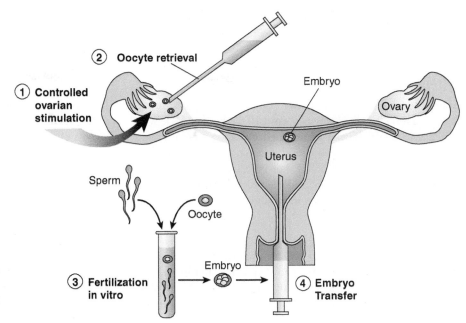

Figure 29.15. In vitro fertilization process. (Reprinted with permission from Alldredge, B. K., Corelli, R. L., Ernst, M. E., Guglielmo, B. J., Jacobson, P. A., Kradjan, W. A., & Williams, B. R. [2013]. *Koda-Kimble & Young's applied therapeutics: The clinical use of drugs* [10th ed., Fig. 48.2]. Philadelphia, PA: Lippincott Williams & Wilkins.)

likely need to be frozen after the removal of the cell for evaluation and prior to transfer to the uterus.

Although in the past approximately 80% of frozen embryos survived the freezing/thawing process, approximately 90% now survive. Children born of frozen embryos have a comparable rate of malformation (Levi Dunietz et al., 2017).

The selection of the embryos to be transferred is based on morphology or genetic testing, if it was done. If genetic testing was not done, most embryos are transferred approximately 72 hours after the eggs are retrieved. If genetic testing was done, a day 5 transfer of a thawed embryo is more common. Later transfer also has the advantage of achieving a similar pregnancy rate as earlier transfers but with fewer embryos, reducing the rate of a multiple pregnancy (Glujovsky, Farquhar, Quinteiro Retamar, Alvarez Sedo, & Blake, 2016).

The embryos to be transferred are loaded into a catheter and deposited near the top of the uterine cavity through the cervix via ultrasound guidance. The catheter is checked immediately after the transfer to ensure it is empty and no embryos remain. It is standard practice for patients to be administered a progesterone supplement intramuscularly or vaginally after embryo transfer until an accurate positive or negative pregnancy test is obtained or through the first trimester.

The number of embryos transferred depends on the maternal age, the number of oocytes retrieved, and the number of embryos that may be frozen for future procedures. The transfer of multiple embryos improves the chances of success but also increases the rate of a multiple pregnancy. In general, the American Society for Reproductive Medicine recommends the transfer of no more than two embryos in young women, no more than three or four in women aged 38 to 40 years, and no more than five in women older than 40 years (Practice Committee of the American Society for Reproductive Medicine, 2017).

Intracytoplasmic Sperm Injection

IVF traditionally introduces semen into the same environment as harvested oocytes to promote fertilization. Intracytoplasmic sperm injection (ICSI), however, is the direct injection of a single spermatozoon into an oocyte (Fig. 29.16). It is used to achieve pregnancy in the case of poor sperm motility, high levels of abnormal sperm morphology, oligospermia, and for men who produce but do not ejaculate sperm. In the case of men who do not ejaculate sperm, sperm is obtained by testicular biopsy or fine-needle aspiration.

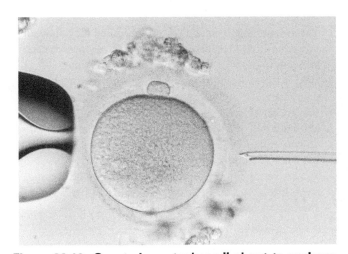

Figure 29.16. Oocyte in metaphase II about to undergo ICSI. The ooplasm is clear, with the first polar body located at 12 o'clock. During ICSI, the introducing pipette (right) places a single sperm (at the tip of the pipette) into the cytoplasm of the egg. The holding pipette (left) holds the egg in place with gentle suction. ICSI, intracytoplasmic sperm injection. (Reprinted with permission from Scott, J. R., Gibbs, R. S., Karlan, B. Y., & Haney, A. F. [2003]. *Danforth's obstetrics and gynecology* [9th ed., Fig. 39-3]. Philadelphia, PA: Lippincott Williams & Wilkins.)

The pregnancy yield of and the rate of multiple pregnancy is approximately equivalent to that of IVF without ICSI (CDC, 2016).

Gamete Intrafallopian Transfer and Zygote Intrafallopian Transfer

Gamete intrafallopian transfer (GIFT) and zygote intrafallopian transfer (ZIFT) are two less-used methods of ART. With GIFT, as with IVF, follicles are recruited, ovulation is induced, and oocytes are retrieved. The oocyte and semen are then transferred to a fallopian tube. With ZIFT, however, fertilization happens in vitro, outside of the body, and the zygote is then transferred to a fallopian tube rather than the uterus.

Oocyte Donation

Donated oocytes are used to achieve pregnancy in the case of ovarian failure, genetic disease, and pregnancy later in life. It is increasingly used by same-sex male partners to create families with the aid of gestational carriers. In the United States, donors are usually recruited from within the community and paid between $2,500 and $10,000 per retrieval cycle. Most donors are from 21 to 34 years old. Donors may also be family members or friends. Potential donors are usually screened for communicable disease, Rh status, and genetic illness. The procedure for follicle recruitment and oocyte harvesting is the same as for IVF.

Sperm Donation

Sperm donation is a viable route to parenthood for single mothers, same-sex female couples, and men with male-factor infertility. Several clinics exist that screen donors. Donor sperm is then cleaned, added to a culture medium, and frozen. In most cases, it can be shipped for insemination according to the specifications of the buyer. Transfer of the sperm may be in a clinic, often by IUI, or at home at the time of ovulation. Sperm donation is also referred to as therapeutic donor insemination. Alternatively, sperm may be donated directly, bypassing clinics.

Gestational Carriers

Gestational carriers are also called "surrogate mothers." Traditionally, the gestational carrier was inseminated with the sperm of the father, making the gestational carrier also the biologic mother. Today, more often a donor egg is used, sometimes the egg of a woman seeking a child. Alternatively, a previously fertilized embryo may be transferred to the gestational carrier. Gestational carriers may be friends or family members. They may also be hired for the purpose. Laws pertaining to gestational carriers vary across states, and the practice raises ethical questions about exploitation, particularly when the gestational carrier lives in a developing country.

Think Critically

1. You are caring for a patient seeking contraception. What questions are important to ask her when determining what contraindications she may have to particular methods, if any?
2. You are rooming a patient who is scheduled for to have an intrauterine contraceptive placed. She is very nervous and asks you to describe the procedure. What do you tell her?
3. Why is it important to ask a woman what her pregnancy plans are when providing contraception counseling?
4. You are caring for a patient who is considering using natural family planning (NFP) to prevent pregnancy. How do you explain NFP to her in a way that helps maximize her chances for success?
5. You are caring for a woman who is pregnant and seeking an abortion. You are opposed to abortion. What is your appropriate course of care at this point?
6. Your patient presents for a medication abortion and tells you she's unwilling to have a surgical procedure. What might you be concerned about in this situation?
7. You are caring for a patient in labor and delivery who is planning to give the infant up for adoption. How do the care considerations differ for this patient?
8. Your patient has a diagnosis of polycystic ovarian syndrome and a body mass index of 30. She is seeking pregnancy. What do you anticipate will be the first-line recommendation for her to achieve pregnancy?
9. A patient has been identified as a good candidate for clomiphene citrate. She's confused by the protocol. How do you explain to her how she should take her medication, when she will most likely ovulate, and when she should have sex to optimize her chances of achieving pregnancy?

References

Ali, M., Akin, A., Bahamondes, L., Brache, V., Habib, N., Landoulsi, S., & Hubacher, D; WHO Study Group on Subdermal Contraceptive Implants for Women. (2016). Extended use up to 5 years of the etonogestrel-releasing subdermal contraceptive implant: Comparison to levonorgestrel-releasing subdermal implant. *Human Reproduction, 31*(11), 2491–2498. doi:10.1093/humrep/dew222

American College of Obstetricians and Gynecologists. (2014). Committee opinion no. 602: Depot medroxyprogesterone acetate and bone effects. *Obstetrics and Gynecology, 123*(6), 1398–1402. doi:10.1097/01.AOG.0000450758.95422.c8

American College of Obstetricians and Gynecologists. (2015a). Committee opinion no. 642: Increasing access to contraceptive implants and intrauterine devices to reduce unintended pregnancy. *Obstetrics and Gynecology, 126*(4), e44–e48. doi:10.1097/AOG.0000000000001106

American College of Obstetricians and Gynecologists. (2015b). Practice bulletin no. 152: Emergency contraception. *Obstetrics and Gynecology, 126*(3), e1–e11. doi:10.1097/AOG.0000000000001047

Arevalo, M., Jennings, V., Nikula, M., & Sinai, I. (2004). Efficacy of the new TwoDay method of family planning. *Fertility and Sterility, 82*(4), 885–892. doi:10.1016/j.fertnstert.2004.03.040

Bhargava, H., Bhatia, J. C., Ramachandran, L., Rohatgi, P., & Sinha, A. (1996). Field trial of billings ovulation method of natural family planning. *Contraception, 53*(2), 69–74.

Birgisson, N. E., Zhao, Q., Secura, G. M., Madden, T., & Peipert, J. F. (2015a). Positive testing for Neisseria gonorrhoeae and Chlamydia trachomatis and the risk of pelvic inflammatory disease in IUD users. *Journal of Women's Health, 24*(5), 354–359. doi:10.1089/jwh.2015.5190

Birgisson, N. E., Zhao, Q., Secura, G. M., Madden, T., & Peipert, J. F. (2015b). Preventing unintended pregnancy: The contraceptive CHOICE project in review. *Journal of Women's Health, 24*(5), 349–353. doi:10.1089/jwh.2015.5191

Boozalis, A., Tutlam, N. T., Chrisman Robbins, C., & Peipert, J. F. (2016). Sexual desire and hormonal contraception. *Obstetrics and Gynecology, 127*(3), 563–572. doi:10.1097/AOG.0000000000001286

Brent, R. L. (2005). Nongenital malformations following exposure to progestational drugs: The last chapter of an erroneous allegation. *Birth Defects Research. Part A, Clinical and Molecular Teratology, 73*(11), 906–918. doi:10.1002/bdra.20184

Buhling, K. J., Zite, N. B., Lotke, P., Black, K., & INTRA Writing Group. (2014). Worldwide use of intrauterine contraception: A review. *Contraception, 89*(3), 162–173. doi:10.1016/j.contraception.2013.11.011

Bushnell, C., McCullough, L. D., Awad, I. A., Chireau, M. V., Fedder, W. N., Furie, K. L., . . . Walters, M. R.; Council for High Blood Pressure Research. (2014). Guidelines for the prevention of stroke in women: A statement for healthcare professionals from the American Heart Association/American Stroke Association. *Stroke, 45*(5), 1545–1588. doi:10.1161/01.str.0000442009.06663.48

Centers for Disease Control and Prevention. (2016). *ART and intracytoplasmic sperm injection (ICSI) in the United States.* Retrieved from https://www.cdc.gov/art/key-findings/icsi.html

Centers for Disease Control and Prevention. (2017, March 30). *Infertility FAQs.* Retrieved from https://www.cdc.gov/reproductivehealth/infertility/index.htm

Charo, R. A. (2017). Alternative science and human reproduction. *New England Journal of Medicine, 377*(4), 309–311. doi:10.1056/NEJMp1707107

Cleland, K., Creinin, M. D., Nucatola, D., Nshom, M., & Trussell, J. (2013). Significant adverse events and outcomes after medical abortion. *Obstetrics and Gynecology, 121*(1), 166–171. doi:10.1097/AOG.0b013e3182755763

Cohen, S. A. (2013). *Still true: Abortion does not increase women's risk of mental health problems.* Retrieved from https://www.guttmacher.org/gpr/2013/06/still-true-abortion-does-not-increase-womens-risk-mental-health-problems

Cortessis, V. K., Barrett, M., Brown Wade, N., Enebish, T., Perrigo, J. L., Tobin, J., . . . McKean-Cowdin, R. (2017). Intrauterine device use and cervical cancer risk: A systematic review and meta-analysis. *Obstetrics and Gynecology, 130*(6), 1226–1236. doi:10.1097/AOG.0000000000002307

Curtis, K. M., Jatlaoui, T. C., Tepper, N. K., Zapata, L. B., Horton, L. G., Jamieson, D. J., & Whiteman, M. K. (2016). U.S. selected practice recommendations for contraceptive use, 2016. *MMWR Recommendations and Reports, 65*(4), 1–66. doi:10.15585/mmwr.rr6504a1

Curtis, K. M., & Peipert, J. F. (2017). Long-acting reversible contraception. *New England Journal of Medicine, 376*(5), 461–468. doi:10.1056/NEJMcp1608736

Curtis, K. M., Tepper, N. K., Jatlaoui, T. C., Berry-Bibee, E., Horton, L. G., Zapata, L. B., . . . Whiteman, M. K. (2016). U.S. Medical eligibility criteria for contraceptive use, 2016. *MMWR Recommendations and Reports, 65*(3), 1–103. doi:10.15585/mmwr.rr6503a1

Daniels, K., Daugherty, J., Jones, J., & Mosher, W. (2015). Current contraceptive use and variation by selected characteristics among women aged 15–44: United States, 2011–2013. *National Health Statistics Reports,* (86), 1–14.

de Bastos, M., Stegeman, B. H., Rosendaal, F. R., Van Hylckama Vlieg, A., Helmerhorst, F. M., Stijnen, T., & Dekkers, O. M. (2014). Combined oral contraceptives: Venous thrombosis. *Cochrane Database of Systematic Reviews,* (3), CD010813. doi:10.1002/14651858.CD010813.pub2

Diedrich, J. T., Zhao, Q., Madden, T., Secura, G. M., & Peipert, J. F. (2015). Three-year continuation of reversible contraception. *American Journal of Obstetrics and Gynecology, 213*(5), 662.e1–662.e8. doi:10.1016/j.ajog.2015.08.001

Dreyer, K., van Rijswijk, J., Mijatovic, V., Goddijn, M., Verhoeve, H. R., van Rooij, I. A. J., . . . Mol, B. W. J. (2017). Oil-based or water-based contrast for hysterosalpingography in infertile women. *New England Journal of Medicine, 376*(21), 2043–2052. doi:10.1056/NEJMoa1612337

Fehring, R. J., Schneider, M., Raviele, K., Rodriguez, D., & Pruszynski, J. (2013). Randomized comparison of two Internet-supported fertility-awareness-based methods of family planning. *Contraception, 88*(1), 24–30. doi:10.1016/j.contraception.2012.10.010

Finer, L. B., & Zolna, M. R. (2016). Declines in unintended pregnancy in the United States, 2008–2011. *New England Journal of Medicine, 374*(9), 843–852. doi:10.1056/NEJMsa1506575

Frank-Herrmann, P., Heil, J., Gnoth, C., Toledo, E., Baur, S., Pyper, C., . . . Freundl, G. (2007). The effectiveness of a fertility awareness based method to avoid pregnancy in relation to a couple's sexual behaviour during the fertile time: A prospective longitudinal study. *Human Reproduction, 22*(5), 1310–1319. doi:10.1093/humrep/dem003

Frega, A., Manzara, F., Schimberni, M., Guarino, A., Catalano, A., Bianchi, P., . . . Caserta, D. (2016). Human papilloma virus infection and cervical cytomorphological changing among intrauterine contraception users. *European Review for Medical and Pharmacological Sciences, 20*(17), 3528–3534.

Freundl, G., Sivin, I., & Batar, I. (2010). State-of-the-art of non-hormonal methods of contraception: IV. Natural family planning. *European Journal of Contraception and Reproductive Health Care, 15*(2), 113–123. doi:10.3109/13625180903545302

Gallo, M. F., Lopez, L. M., Grimes, D. A., Carayon, F., Schulz, K. F., & Helmerhorst, F. M. (2014). Combination contraceptives: Effects on weight. *Cochrane Database of Systematic Reviews,* (1), CD003987. doi:10.1002/14651858.CD003987.pub5

Gariepy, A. M., Creinin, M. D., Smith, K. J., & Xu, X. (2014). Probability of pregnancy after sterilization: A comparison of hysteroscopic versus laparoscopic sterilization. *Contraception, 90*(2), 174–181. doi:10.1016/j.contraception.2014.03.010

Gemzell-Danielsson, K., Berger, C., & Lalitkumar, P. G. L. (2013). Emergency contraception—Mechanisms of action. *Contraception, 87*(3), 300–308. doi:10.1016/j.contraception.2012.08.021

Glasier, A. (2013). Emergency contraception: Clinical outcomes. *Contraception, 87*(3), 309–313. doi:10.1016/j.contraception.2012.08.027

Glujovsky, D., Farquhar, C., Quinteiro Retamar, A. M., Alvarez Sedo, C. R., & Blake, D. (2016). Cleavage stage versus blastocyst stage embryo transfer in assisted reproductive technology. *Cochrane Database of Systematic Reviews,* (6), CD002118. doi:10.1002/14651858.CD002118.pub5

Golobof, A., & Kiley, J. (2016). The current status of oral contraceptives: Progress and recent innovations. *Seminars in Reproductive Medicine, 34*(3), 145–151. doi:10.1055/s-0036-1572546

Guiahi, M., McBride, M., Sheeder, J., & Teal, S. (2015). Short-term treatment of bothersome bleeding for etonogestrel implant users using a 14-day oral contraceptive pill regimen: A randomized controlled trial. *Obstetrics and Gynecology, 126*(3), 508–513. doi:10.1097/AOG.0000000000000974

Guttmacher Institute. (2018). *Induced abortion in the United States.* Retrieved from https://www.guttmacher.org/fact-sheet/induced-abortion-united-states

Guzick, D. S., Carson, S. A., Coutifaris, C., Overstreet, J. W., Factor-Litvak, P., Steinkampf, M. P., . . . Canfield, R. E. (1999). Efficacy of superovulation and intrauterine insemination in the treatment of infertility. National Cooperative Reproductive Medicine Network. *New England Journal of Medicine, 340*(3), 177–183. doi:10.1056/NEJM199901213400302

Healthy People 2020. Retrieved from https://www.healthypeople.gov/2020/topics-objectives/topic/family-planning/objectives

Heinemann, K., Reed, S., Moehner, S., & Minh, T. D. (2015a). Comparative contraceptive effectiveness of levonorgestrel-releasing and copper intrauterine devices: The European Active Surveillance Study for Intrauterine Devices. *Contraception, 91*(4), 280–283. doi:10.1016/j.contraception.2015.01.011

Heinemann, K., Reed, S., Moehner, S., & Minh, T. D. (2015b). Risk of uterine perforation with levonorgestrel-releasing and copper intrauterine devices in the European Active Surveillance Study on Intrauterine Devices. *Contraception, 91*(4), 274–279. doi:10.1016/j.contraception.2015.01.007

Hubacher, D., Lopez, L., Steiner, M. J., & Dorflinger, L. (2009). Menstrual pattern changes from levonorgestrel subdermal implants and DMPA: Systematic review and evidence-based comparisons. *Contraception, 80*(2), 113–118. doi:10.1016/j.contraception.2009.02.008

Iversen, L., Sivasubramaniam, S., Lee, A. J., Fielding, S., & Hannaford, P. C. (2017). Lifetime cancer risk and combined oral contraceptives: The Royal College of General Practitioners' Oral Contraception Study. *American Journal of Obstetrics and Gynecology, 216*(6), 580.e1–580.e9. doi:10.1016/j.ajog.2017.02.002

Jatlaoui, T. C., Ewing, A., Mandel, M. G., Simmons, K. B., Suchdev, D. B., Jamieson, D. J., & Pazol, K. (2016). Abortion surveillance—United States, 2013. *MMWR Surveillance Summaries, 65*(12), 1–44. doi:10.15585/mmwr.ss6512a1

Jerman, J., Jones, R. K., & Onda, T. (2016). *Characteristics of U.S. abortion patients in 2014 and changes since 2008.* Retrieved from https://www.guttmacher.org/report/characteristics-us-abortion-patients-2014

Jones, J., Mosher, W., & Daniels, K. (2012). Current contraceptive use in the United States, 2006–2010, and changes in patterns of use since 1995. *National Health Statistics Reports,* (60), 1–25.

Jones, R. K., Zolna, M. R., Henshaw, S. K., & Finer, L. B. (2008). Abortion in the United States: Incidence and access to services, 2005. *Perspectives on Sexual and Reproductive Health, 40*(1), 6–16. doi:10.1363/4000608

Jones, V. F., Schulte, E. E., & Committee on Early Childhood; Council on Foster Care, Adoption, and Kinship Care. (2012). The pediatrician's role in supporting adoptive families. *Pediatrics, 130*(4), e1040–e1049. doi:10.1542/peds.2012-2261

Kapp, N., Abitbol, J. L., Mathe, H., Scherrer, B., Guillard, H., Gainer, E., & Ulmann, A. (2015). Effect of body weight and BMI on the efficacy of levonorgestrel emergency contraception. *Contraception, 91*(2), 97–104. doi:10.1016/j.contraception.2014.11.001

Kavanaugh, M. L., Jerman, J., & Finer, L. B. (2015). Changes in use of long-acting reversible contraceptive methods among U.S. Women, 2009–2012. *Obstetrics and Gynecology, 126*(5), 917–927. doi:10.1097/AOG.0000000000001094

Lanza, L. L., McQuay, L. J., Rothman, K. J., Bone, H. G., Kaunitz, A. M., Harel, Z., . . . Wolter, K. D. (2013). Use of depot medroxyprogesterone acetate contraception and incidence of bone fracture. *Obstetrics and Gynecology, 121*(3), 593–600. doi:10.1097/AOG.0b013e318283d1a1

Legro, R. S., Arslanian, S. A., Ehrmann, D. A., Hoeger, K. M., Murad, M. H., Pasquali, R., . . . Endocrine Society. (2013). Diagnosis and treatment of polycystic ovary syndrome: An Endocrine Society clinical practice guideline. *Journal of Clinical Endocrinology and Metabolism, 98*(12), 4565–4592. doi:10.1210/jc.2013-2350

Legro, R. S., Brzyski, R. G., Diamond, M. P., Coutifaris, C., Schlaff, W. D., Casson, P., . . . Zhang, H.; NICHD Reproductive Medicine Network. (2014). Letrozole versus clomiphene for infertility in the polycystic ovary syndrome. *New England Journal of Medicine, 371*(2), 119–129. doi:10.1056/NEJMoa1313517

Levi Dunietz, G., Holzman, C., Zhang, Y., Talge, N. M., Li, C., Todem, D., . . . Diamond, M. P. (2017). Assisted reproductive technology and newborn size in singletons resulting from fresh and cryopreserved embryos transfer. *PLoS One, 12*(1), e0169869. doi:10.1371/journal.pone.0169869

Levine, H., Jørgensen, N., Martino-Andrade, A., Mendiola, J., Weksler-Derri, D., Mindlis, I., . . . Swan, S. H. (2017). Temporal trends in sperm count: A systematic review and meta-regression analysis. *Human Reproduction Update, 23*(6):646–659. doi:10.1093/humupd/dmx022

Lidegaard, O., Lokkegaard, E., Jensen, A., Skovlund, C. W., & Keiding, N. (2012). Thrombotic stroke and myocardial infarction with hormonal contraception. *New England Journal of Medicine, 366*(24), 2257–2266. doi:10.1056/NEJMoa1111840

Lopez, L. M., Edelman, A., Chen, M., Otterness, C., Trussell, J., & Helmerhorst, F. M. (2013). Progestin-only contraceptives: Effects on weight. *Cochrane Database of Systematic Reviews,* (7), CD008815. doi:10.1002/14651858.CD008815.pub3

Madden, T., Secura, G. M., Nease, R. F., Politi, M. C., & Peipert, J. F. (2015). The role of contraceptive attributes in women's contraceptive decision making. *American Journal of Obstetrics and Gynecology, 213*(1), 46.e1–46.e6. doi:10.1016/j.ajog.2015.01.051

Manders, M., McLindon, L., Schulze, B., Beckmann, M. M., Kremer, J. A., & Farquhar, C. (2015). Timed intercourse for couples trying to conceive. *Cochrane Database of Systematic Reviews,* (3), CD011345. doi:10.1002/14651858.CD011345.pub2

Morrell, K. M., Cremers, S., Westhoff, C. L., & Davis, A. R. (2016). Relationship between etonogestrel level and BMI in women using the contraceptive implant for more than 1 year. *Contraception, 93*(3), 263–265. doi:10.1016/j.contraception.2015.11.005

Mutsaerts, M. A., van Oers, A. M., Groen, H., Burggraaff, J. M., Kuchenbecker, W. K., Perquin, D. A., . . . Hoek, A. (2016). Randomized trial of a lifestyle program in obese infertile women. *New England Journal of Medicine, 374*(20), 1942–1953. doi:10.1056/NEJMoa1505297

Nettleman, M. D., Chung, H., Brewer, J., Ayoola, A., & Reed, P. L. (2007). Reasons for unprotected intercourse: Analysis of the PRAMS survey. *Contraception, 75*(5), 361–366. doi:10.1016/j.contraception.2007.01.011

Ory, S. J. (2013). The national epidemic of multiple pregnancy and the contribution of assisted reproductive technology. *Fertility and Sterility, 100*(4), 929–930. doi:10.1016/j.fertnstert.2013.06.004

Pasquali, R., Gambineri, A., Cavazza, C., Ibarra Gasparini, D., Ciampaglia, W., Cognigni, G. E., & Pagotto, U. (2011). Heterogeneity in the responsiveness to long-term lifestyle intervention and predictability in obese women with polycystic ovary syndrome. *European Journal of Endocrinology, 164*(1), 53–60. doi:10.1530/EJE-10-0692

Practice Committee of American Society for Reproductive Medicine. (2012). Diagnostic evaluation of the infertile female: A committee opinion. *Fertility and Sterility, 98*(2), 302–307. doi:10.1016/j.fertnstert.2012.05.032

Practice Committee of the American Society for Reproductive Medicine. (2015). Current clinical irrelevance of luteal phase deficiency: A committee opinion. *Fertility and Sterility, 103*(4), e27–e32. doi:10.1016/j.fertnstert.2014.12.128

Practice Committee of the American Society for Reproductive Medicine. (2017). Guidance on the limits to the number of embryos to transfer: A committee opinion. *Fertility and Sterility, 107*(4), 901–903. doi:10.1016/j.fertnstert.2017.02.107

Practice Committee of American Society for Reproductive Medicine in Collaboration With Society for Reproductive Endocrinology and Infertility. (2013). Optimizing natural fertility: A committee opinion. *Fertility and Sterility, 100*(3), 631–637. doi:10.1016/j.fertnstert.2013.07.011

Sanders, J. N., Turok, D. K., Royer, P. A., Thompson, I. S., Gawron, L. M., & Storck, K. E. (2017). One-year continuation of copper or levonorgestrel intrauterine devices initiated at the time of emergency contraception. *Contraception, 96*(2), 99–105. doi:10.1016/j.contraception.2017.05.012

Schwallie, P. C., & Assenzo, J. R. (1974). The effect of depo-medroxyprogesterone acetate on pituitary and ovarian function, and the return of fertility following its discontinuation: A review. *Contraception, 10*(2), 181–202.

Schwarz, E. B., Papic, M., Parisi, S. M., Baldauf, E., Rapkin, R., & Updike, G. (2014). Routine counseling about intrauterine contraception for women seeking emergency contraception. *Contraception, 90*(1), 66–71. doi:10.1016/j.contraception.2014.02.007

Skovlund, C. W., Morch, L. S., Kessing, L. V., & Lidegaard, O. (2016). Association of hormonal contraception with depression. *JAMA Psychiatry, 73*(11), 1154–1162. doi:10.1001/jamapsychiatry.2016.2387

Slama, R., Hansen, O. K., Ducot, B., Bohet, A., Sorensen, D., Giorgis Allemand, L., . . . Bouyer, J. (2012). Estimation of the frequency of involuntary infertility on a nation-wide basis. *Human Reproduction, 27*(5), 1489–1498. doi:10.1093/humrep/des070

Tate, J., & Bushnell, C. (2011). Pregnancy and stroke risk in women. *Women's Health (London, England), 7*(3), 363–374. doi:10.2217/whe.11.19

Upadhyay, U. D., Desai, S., Zlidar, V., Weitz, T. A., Grossman, D., Anderson, P., & Taylor, D. (2015). Incidence of emergency department visits and complications after abortion. *Obstetrics and Gynecology, 125*(1), 175–183. doi:10.1097/AOG.0000000000000603

Vessey, M., & Yeates, D. (2013). Oral contraceptive use and cancer: Final report from the Oxford-Family Planning Association contraceptive study. *Contraception, 88*(6), 678–683. doi:10.1016/j.contraception.2013.08.008

Vickery, Z., Madden, T., Zhao, Q., Secura, G. M., Allsworth, J. E., & Peipert, J. F. (2013). Weight change at 12 months in users of three progestin-only contraceptive methods. *Contraception, 88*(4), 503–508. doi:10.1016/j.contraception.2013.03.004

Vinogradova, Y., Coupland, C., & Hippisley-Cox, J. (2015). Use of combined oral contraceptives and risk of venous thromboembolism: Nested case-control studies using the QResearch and CPRD databases. *BMJ, 350*, h2135. doi:10.1136/bmj.h2135

Wilcox, A. J., Weinberg, C. R., & Baird, D. D. (1998). Post-ovulatory ageing of the human oocyte and embryo failure. *Human Reproduction, 13*(2), 394–397.

Wu, J. P., & Pickle, S. (2014). Extended use of the intrauterine device: A literature review and recommendations for clinical practice. *Contraception, 89*(6), 495–503. doi:10.1016/j.contraception.2014.02.011

Suggested Readings

Hershberger, P. E., & Stevenson, E. L. (2016). Advancing the care of individuals and couples at risk for and diagnosed with infertility. *Journal of Obstetric, Gynecologic, and Neonatal Nursing, 45*(1), 98–99. doi:10.1016/j.jogn.2015.10.002

National Abortion Federation. (2005). *The abortion option: A values clarification guide for health professionals.* Retrieved from https://prochoice.org/resources/the-abortion-option-a-values-clarification-guide-for-health-professionals

Planned Parenthood. Retrieved from https://www.plannedparenthood.org

30 Vulnerable Populations

Objectives

1. Describe priority nursing actions when caring for victims of sexual assault.
2. Identify key safety considerations and resources when caring for the victims of intimate partner violence and human trafficking.
3. Identify issues specific to caring for incarcerated women during pregnancy.
4. Differentiate between the three most common eating disorders in adults.
5. Discuss key nursing behaviors when caring for sexual minority women.

Key Terms

Anorexia nervosa
Binge eating disorder
Bulimia nervosa
Human trafficking
Intimate partner violence

Sexual assault
Sexual assault nurse evaluation
Sexual minority women
Transman
Transwoman

People may be identified as vulnerable for various reasons. They may be victims of intimate partner violence or sexual assault. They may suffer from an eating disorder. They may be victims of human trafficking or identified as members of a sexual minority, such as lesbian, bisexual, or transgender. They may be incarcerated. The members of vulnerable populations often receive poor or infrequent care. They may hesitate to disclose their circumstances and provide healthcare providers with incomplete information that compromises their care. They may not have the resources to complete recommended care and may be lost to follow-up. Vulnerable patients, like all patients, require respectful care and should be treated with dignity and compassion.

Sexual Assault

Over the course of their lifetimes, 43.9% of women and 23.4% of men experience sexual violence, which is defined as unwanted sexual experiences, unwanted sexual contact, and sexual coercion. A further 19.3% of women and 1.7% of men are raped (Breiding et al., 2014). The blanket term sexual assault is used to describe any sexual act performed on another person without that person's consent. The use of force is not necessary to the definition. Instead, a threat of force or the victim's inability to consent is sufficient. Sexual assault is a weapon of control and conquest. There is no place for blaming the victim for "enticing" or "leading on" the attacker.

Only a small number of sexual assaults are reported to authorities. The most common reasons victims cite for not reporting are a prior relationship with the attacker, reluctance to see the attacker incarcerated, and fear that the authorities would blame the victim for the attack (Patterson & Tringali, 2015). Note that mandated reporting varies by state and applies to children, the elderly, and other vulnerable adults. Nurses are mandated reporters, and it is the responsibility of the nurse to be familiar with the reporting requirements in his or her practice state.

Evaluation

Ideally, a trained provider should evaluate a victim of a sexual assault within 72 hours after the crime. In the United States, specially trained nurses often carry out these evaluations. This model is referred to as **sexual assault nurse evaluation** (SANE), and the nurses are often called SANE nurses. These nurses are trained and certified by the International Association of Forensic Nurses to perform thorough, consistent, expedited, high-quality examinations and specimen collection with sensitivity and compassion. Different states have different documentation requirements for the examination, with some requiring a specific form to be used.

History

History taking is critical to the evaluation of a survivor of sexual assault. It is often helpful to have a sexual assault advocate from a rape crisis organization present during history taking. The advocate does not answer for the victim but helps guide the victim through the process. Advocates, as well as any friends or family members present, may be called as witnesses should the victim press charges. Questions pertinent to the evaluation are listed in Table 30.1. Whenever possible, the nurse should conduct the history taking with the victim fully dressed. It is critical that the interviewing nurse use neutral language and take pains to avoid implying blame of the victim.

Examination

Items frequently used during the course of an examination after a sexual assault include a camera to document injuries, a colposcope to identify microinjuries, an ultraviolet light source to identify semen and other foreign objects, and specimen collection tools such as swabs and evidence bags, a ruler or other easily sized item for photographs, and a speculum. The nurse or other healthcare provider should not take any samples or pictures or conduct any physical examination without the explicit consent of the victim.

The victim should undress while on a sheet to collect any evidence that may fall off of her clothing or body during this process. Nurses should be aware that the examination itself can be traumatizing. The patient may feel shame and a loss of control. Nurses should not force any evaluation, treatment, or other course of action. Control should remain with the victim whenever possible.

The nurse should closely examine any body parts the victim identifies as having been subjected to trauma. The TEARS categorization (tears, ecchymoses, abrasions, redness, and swelling) is often used to help organize and describe examination findings (White, 2013).

Table 30.1 Patient History Topics to Address Following Sexual Assault

Topic	Rationale
Personal hygiene activities since the assault (bathing, showering, wiping, changing clothes, eating, brushing teeth, use of tampon or sanitary pad, use of barrier contraception)	Any of these activities can reduce the chances of adequate forensic specimen collection.
Circumstances of the assault	Information about the date, time, and location of the assault, as well as the use of weapons, force, or restraints, can guide the physical examination, investigation, and future care.
Loss of consciousness or memory	Loss of consciousness or memory may indicate the use of flunitrazepam (also called Rohypnol or "the date rape drug"), gamma-hydroxybutyrate, benzodiazepines, or other sedatives in the assault.
Physical description of the assailant	A physical description of the assailant helps guide the investigation and may inform the physical examination.
Specifics of the assault (oral, anal, or vaginal contact; ejaculation; and condom use)	Details about the assault help guide the examination and specimen collection.
Other areas of trauma	Knowledge of injury to other body parts, such as the breasts or neck, helps guide the examination.
Bleeding by the victim or assailant	Bleeding by the victim, the assailant, or both heightens concerns about disease transmission, particularly human immunodeficiency virus and hepatitis. Continuous bleeding of the victim raises concern for an acute, progressive physical injury.
Recent consensual sex	A report of any recent episodes of consensual sex the victim has engaged in helps inform the examination and interpretation of specimens.

Forensic Evaluation

As with all aspects of a sexual assault evaluation, the nurse or other healthcare provider must obtain patient consent before conducting a forensic examination. A forensic evaluation requires the collection of numerous samples for evaluation by a laboratory if indicated (Box 30.1). Special kits are used for this purpose. A victim is under no obligation to pursue police reporting even after specimen collection. At times the nurse may have to conduct a forensic examination of the perpetrator, as well, using a similar methodology.

Documentation is a critical part of forensic nursing. The forensic report is a separate form from the regular medical record. The nurse must securely store evidence gathered even if the victim chooses not to report the sexual assault. Rape kits are often destroyed after a period of time set by the local jurisdiction. The patient must be informed prior to destruction of the evidence should they choose not to report.

Laboratory Testing and Prophylactic Medications

Sexually transmitted infections (STIs) and pregnancy are both concerns for many victims of sexual assault. A pregnancy or STI test taken at the time of the initial evaluation is unlikely to detect a pregnancy or STI resulting from the assault because of incubation periods. On account of this, women are often treated at the time of initial presentation prior to receiving a positive result.

Pregnancy

The risk of pregnancy after a single act of unprotected intercourse varies according to a woman's cycle. The overall risk for pregnancy after rape is approximately 5% (Crawford-Jakubiak, Alderman, & Leventhal, 2017). A woman who is using contraception is clearly not at any greater risk for pregnancy from nonconsensual sex than she would be from consensual sex, although her anxiety about pregnancy may be heightened. Emergency contraception as detailed in Chapter 29 is indicated as soon as possible after the assault for women who are not using reliable contraception. The woman should take a follow-up pregnancy test if she misses her period or 2 to 3 weeks after the assault.

Box 30.1   Forensic Examination Samples

- Clothing
- Swabs of tissue from the buccal mucosa, vagina, rectum, and other areas highlighted by ultraviolet light
- Combed specimens from the scalp and pubic hair
- Fingernail scrapings and clippings
- Control samples of the victim's scalp and pubic hair to compare against other hair collected
- Whole blood sample
- Saliva sample

Sexually Transmitted Infections

The risk of contracting chlamydia or gonorrhea after a sexual assault is as high as 15% and 5%, respectively (Jaureguy, Chariot, Vessieres, & Picard, 2016). Patients who initially present for evaluation and treatment after a sexual assault are often lost to follow-up. Because of these two factors, the high risk for exposure and infrequent follow-up, patients are often treated prophylactically for chlamydia and gonorrhea as well as trichomoniasis (see Chapter 28 for STI treatments).

Hepatitis B Virus

Although many women who are sexually assaulted have been vaccinated for the hepatitis B virus, most have not been tested for immunity against this virus. Like all vaccinations, the vaccination for hepatitis B does not guarantee immunity after the completion of a vaccine series. Because of this, the first of the hepatitis B vaccine series is indicated at the time of initial evaluation. If the patient has tested immune prior to the assault or immediately after the assault, the remaining two vaccinations in the series are not necessary. If the perpetrator of the assault is known to be infected with hepatitis B, the nurse should administer the hepatitis B immune globulin to the woman in addition to the first of the vaccination series (Workowski & Bolan, 2015).

Human Immunodeficiency Virus

The risk of contracting human immunodeficiency virus (HIV) after a single episode of consensual sex with someone who is HIV positive is approximately 0.1% for vaginal sex and 2% for receptive anal sex (Patel et al., 2014). These figures may be higher after a sexual assault if trauma and bleeding have created enhanced entry for the virus.

Patients thought to be at a high risk for HIV transmission may elect to take postexposure prophylaxis (PEP). PEP is most effective if started within 4 hours after exposure and is not effective if started 72 or more hours after exposure. Treatment with PEP lasts for 28 days, although fewer than 40% of patients complete the full course (Ford et al., 2014). PEP consists of medications used to treat HIV. The choice of medications used is usually made in consultation with disease specialists.

Women who have been sexually assaulted should be tested for HIV at 4 to 6 weeks and at 3 months. Syphilis testing is also indicated at these times (Workowski & Bolan, 2015).

Human Papillomavirus

Female victims of sexual assault who meet the age eligibility requirements should receive the vaccine against human papillomavirus. Patients who have already been vaccinated do not need to be revaccinated. For patients who have not been vaccinated, the series should be completed as per the recommendations for the general population (Workowski & Bolan, 2015).

Follow-Up

The nurse should offer all victims of sexual assault access to mental health services. Potential health sequelae of a sexual assault include posttraumatic stress disorder (PTSD), anorexia, insomnia, anxiety, depression, shame, guilt, fear, anger, intrusive thoughts, and pain of the pelvis, abdomen, genitals, and musculoskeletal system. Misuse of prescription medications, suicidality, reduced sexual satisfaction, and irregular menses are all more common in women with a history of sexual assault (Tiihonen Moller, Backstrom, Sondergaard, & Helstrom, 2014). People who have been sexually assaulted often find the provision of sexual healthcare, including pelvic exams, traumatic, and should be encouraged to tell clinicians of their history with assault. The nurse can help people find counselors who specialize in sexual trauma by referring them to sexual crisis organizations. More sexual assault resources for patients can be accessed at RAINN: www.rainn .org, (802) 656-HOPE.

Intimate Partner Violence

Although many people conceptualize it as only physical abuse, **intimate partner violence (IPV)** is any actual or threatened psychological, sexual, or physical harm of one current or past intimate partner by the other. Although both women and men can be victims of IPV, four out of every five victims are women (Catalano, 2015). Up to 36% of women in the United States experience IPV in their lifetimes (Smith et al., 2017). The overall rate of IPV declined 64% from 1994 to 2001. From 2001 to 2010, the rate stabilized (Catalano, 2015).

In Chapter 12, Loretta Hale's partner was abusive. As is common with IPV, the abuse did not start out as physical but rather as psychological. Loretta had a family history of abuse and thought of it as a normal part of being in a relationship.

Factors Contributing to the Perpetuation of IPV

Victims stay in IPV relationships and return to the relationships after leaving for a number of reasons. Perpetrators are controlling and often ensure they have economic control, making the victim dependent. Economic dependence is particularly acute if the victim has children. The abuser often isolates the victim from friends and family members, limiting her ability to seek help and shelter elsewhere. The abuser promises to change and expresses remorse, and the victim, who often still loves the abuser, wants to believe him. The victim and the perpetrator are bonded by the trauma, which manifests itself as a feeling of love. The victim often feels shame and guilt about the abuse, and, prompted by the abuser, believes she deserves it. The victim may be in greater danger from her abuser if she leaves (World Health Organization, 2012).

Role of the Nurse

The dominant feature of IPV is the power one partner has over another (see Chapter 26 for information on IPV screening). Therefore, a critical consideration when caring for victims of IPV is patient empowerment (Box 30.2). The nurse should allow the patient to direct her own care as much as possible. It is not

---

Box 30.2 Principles of Clinician Intervention

- *Safety:* Maximize safety and reduce the risk of harm to victims and their children
- *Empowerment:* Facilitate patient self-determination
- *Abuser accountability:* Hold the perpetrator responsible for the violence and its resolution, not the victim
- *Advocacy:* Advocate within and beyond the healthcare setting for political, legal, and social change
- *Change:* Continuously seek ways to improve the delivery of care to victims

Adapted from Ganley, A. (1998). *The health care response to domestic violence: A trainer's manual for health care providers.* San Francisco, CA: Family Violence Prevention Fund.

the role of the healthcare provider to tell the patient to leave her abuser. The role of the nurse is to build a trusting relationship with the patient and to facilitate patient decisions. The nurse can provide ongoing support, educate women about available resources and services, and, critically, assess patient safety. Care should be nonjudgmental and confidential. Whenever possible, the nurse should discuss IPV privately with the patient, without the presence of friends or family members.

Compassionate support and planning are critical to the care of IPV patients. However, little evidence supports the efficacy of interventions to prevent IPV or stop ongoing IPV. Interventions may be more effective during pregnancy or if a woman has already spent at least one night in a shelter, which indicates a readiness to leave (Ellsberg et al., 2015; Feder, Wathen, & MacMillan, 2013; Jahanfar, Howard, & Medley, 2014; Rivas et al., 2015). That interventions may not prevent or stop violence, however, should not discourage nurses from providing care and support to IPV victims. The offer of help and the knowledge of available support may be therapeutic in and of themselves.

Offering Support

It often takes several encounters before a woman discloses IPV. It may take several more before a woman chooses to act. It is very common for a woman to return to an abusive relationship multiple times, and it is important that the nurse withhold judgment. Expressing empathy, validating the woman's feelings, and offering assistance as appropriate show support. The nurse may pursue avenues for change when the patient expresses readiness. Examples of helpful and unhelpful statements are included in Box 30.3.

The victims of IPV often have a low sense of self-worth. Depression, anxiety, and substance abuse are more common in this population. The nurse should screen the victims of IPV for psychological issues and include counseling in care, which may improve the patient's uptake of safe behavior (Rivas et al., 2015).

Evaluating for Safety

Although most victims of IPV are not in immediate danger, in 2010 at least 39% of homicides of women were by intimate

Box 30.3 Support of the Victim of Intimate Partner Violence

Helpful Statements

- "I'm so sorry this is happening."
- "This must be really hard."
- "How can I be most helpful?"
- "I can help connect you with people and resources that can help you when and if you're ready."
- "This is not your fault."
- "You are a strong woman. It takes courage to tell me what you've told me."
- "I'm so glad you told me."
- "This is not an uncommon problem. You are not alone."

Unhelpful Statements

- "You should leave him."
- "Just kick him out."
- "I'd never let anyone hurt me like that."
- "Why do you let him do that?"
- "I don't understand how women get themselves into these situations."
- "What did you do that made him hurt you?"
- "What do you think is wrong with you that you get into these situations?"
- "If it's so bad, why do you stay?"

Box 30.4 Risk Factors for the Escalation of Intimate Partner Violence

Victim

- Seeks to leave the relationship
- Seeks help
- Is afraid for her life
- Is suicidal
- Is homicidal

Perpetrator

- Is violent outside the home
- Threatens violence outside the home
- Threatens to kill self, victim, or children
- Escalates threats
- Is violent with children
- Uses drugs
- Is abusive in pregnancy
- Is obsessive
- Is controlling
- Has inflicted prior serious injury
- Owns weapons

Adapted from Campbell, J. C., Webster, D. W., & Glass, N. (2009). The danger assessment: Validation of a lethality risk assessment instrument for intimate partner femicide. *Journal of Interpersonal Violence, 24*(4), 653–674. doi:10.1177/0886260508317180.

partners, when compared with 2.8% of homicides of men (Catalano, 2015). With this in mind, the nurse should assess the patient's perception of her safety and a plan for safety with every encounter. Nurses should be aware, however, that, despite the abuse, victims often downplay the danger of their situation because of denial, embarrassment, the difficulties of leaving their abuser, and fear of their abuser, as well as to protect the abuser, whom they often still love.

The nurse should always offer patients resources that may optimize their safety, particularly information on IPV advocacy organizations and shelters. It is important that the patient herself make the decision to seek help. Victims are at an increased risk for escalating violence when they seek outside help or attempt to leave the relationship, so the nurse must respect their judgment about when and whether to leave (Sheehan, Murphy, Moynihan, Dudley-Fennessey, & Stapleton, 2015). Nurses should be alert, however, for signs of escalating violence (Box 30.4).

Safety Planning

Safety planning is an attempt to reduce the risk of escalating violence. A woman may make a safety plan with the help of a nurse and facilitation by a community domestic violence advocate or social worker. The aspects of a safety plan include arrangements for a place to escape to, a signal to alert others to contact emergency services, the avoidance of rooms such as kitchens and bathrooms that contain potential weapons, and the preparation of an emergency kit. The emergency kit includes

essential documents, money, keys, identification, medications, and other items that can be stored outside of the home in the event of an urgent escape.

Although written materials that guide and educate patients about IPV and safety can be helpful, they may endanger the victim if discovered by the abuser. The nurse can coach victims to memorize the phone numbers of local advocacy agencies or to store information where it will not be discovered. Some agencies provide coin-like tokens with their contact information that are more easily hidden or information cards that obfuscate their purpose. The nurse should never confront the perpetrator directly or indirectly as this may endanger the victim, the nurse, or others.

Victims may seek a domestic violence protection order from the courts, often with the help of a community advocate. Evidence as to the efficacy of such orders is mixed. Temporary orders are associated with an uptick of psychological abuse, whereas permanent orders are associated with a reduction in physical violence. Victims, however, may find the use of protection orders empowering, so although the protection order itself may be counterproductive at times, it may also be an important step for some women in the ultimate quest for improved safety (Cattaneo, Grossmann, & Chapman, 2016).

Perpetrator Treatment

Court-mandated treatment of perpetrators is a common legal intervention that decreases the rate of reoffense by approximately 5% to 7%. The dropout rate from such programs is high, and those who fail to complete the programs are most likely to reoffend (Alexander, Morris, Tracy, & Frye, 2010). Other studies suggest that such programs have no impact on the likelihood of a perpetrator of IPV to reoffend (Haggard, Freij, Danielsson, Wenander, & Langstrom, 2015).

Mandated Reporting and Documentation

Nurses are mandated reporters. Which activities must be reported to law enforcement or a state agency varies by state, and it is the responsibility of the nurse to be familiar with state law. Only a few states mandate the reporting of IPV in all cases. More states mandate the reporting of IPV under certain conditions, such as if the abuse is of a disabled person, if a weapon is used in an assault, if the abuse is of an elder, or if a child is either the target of the abuse or a witness to the abuse.

Documentation of abuse is important as the patient may seek legal help in the future through divorce, child custody, or criminal prosecution. The nurse should document any physical examination findings and the patient's report of the nature and timing of abuse and the perpetrator. In the case of sexual assault in the context of IPV, documentation and evidence collection are identical.

Long-Term Consequences

As with victims of sexual assault, IPV victims are subject to long-term health consequences even after the victimization has stopped. Victims are more likely to have chronic and acute physical health complaints, such as pain, gynecologic issues, and infections. The experience of IPV within a year before pregnancy is associated with a higher rate of pregnancy-related complications. Psychological issues include anxiety, depression, insomnia, PTSD, eating disorders, low self-esteem, suicidality, and others (Beydoun, Williams, Beydoun, Eid, & Zonderman, 2017; Bosch, Weaver, Arnold, & Clark, 2015).

Human Trafficking

Human trafficking is often conceptualized as the import of humans from one part of the world to another for unpaid labor. In fact, individuals exploited by human trafficking may not be imported and are often enslaved in their own communities (CdeBaca & Sigmon, 2014). Of the estimated 21 million victims of human trafficking today, 4.5 million are estimated to be commercial sex workers, primarily women and girls (International Labor Organization, 2017). Human trafficking is defined by the United Nations as ". . . the recruitment, transportation, transfer, harboring or receipt of persons, by means of the threat or use of force or other forms of coercion, of abduction, of fraud, of deception, of the abuse of power or of a position of vulnerability or of the giving or receiving of payments or benefits to achieve the consent of a person having control over another person, for the purpose of exploitation. Exploitation shall include, at a minimum, the exploitation of the prostitution of others or other forms of sexual exploitation, forced labor or services, slavery or

practices similar to slavery, servitude, or the removal of organs (United Nations, 2001)."

Among the survivors of sex trafficking, mental and physical health problems are very common. A majority report physical and sexual abuse, and approximately half attempt suicide. The rate of HIV among the victims of sex trafficking is as high as 60%. Problems associated with unprotected sex and sex with multiple partners, including STIs and unwanted pregnancies, are also common (Grace, Ahn, & Macias Konstantopoulos, 2014).

Identification of Victims

Because of their frequent health problems, the victims of trafficking often have contact with healthcare providers, with a majority reporting the use of healthcare services (Chisolm-Straker et al., 2016; Lederer & Wetzel, 2014). Victims rarely self-report trafficking for various reasons. Some may fail to recognize their situation, perceiving themselves to be in a romantic relationship with their trafficker. Others may fear retribution against themselves, their children, or their families. People without paperwork to prove legal residency may fear deportation or criminal prosecution or abuse by law enforcement. Feelings of shame and worthlessness and trauma bonding similar to those experienced with IPV may also prevent reporting (Macias-Konstantopoulos, 2016).

As with all patients, the nurse should interview patients suspected of being victims of human trafficking alone to facilitate disclosure. Questions should be open-ended and not accusatory. The nurse should limit the number of questions asked with the intent to reveal trafficking to avoid the patient feeling badgered or frightened. Confidentiality is paramount. The nurse must use professional interpreters, if an interpreter is necessary, to protect confidentiality and prevent disclosure to the trafficker. Nurses must recognize that the disclosure of human trafficking can be extremely risky for the victim and potentially for family members and is an act of courage.

Generally, victims are more likely to report trafficking after multiple visits during which trust is built. They often delay care and may present late in the course of a disease. The nurse should look for signs of controlling behavior by a person who presents with the patient. The clinical findings are often not consistent with the patient history. A list of red flags associated with human trafficking is included in Box 30.5. Note that this list is not comprehensive or diagnostic.

Care of Victims

The victims of human trafficking and those who care for them are at risk for harm from traffickers. Therefore, the nurse should take care to protect patient confidentiality and clinic security. The nurse should not encourage victims to leave their situation if they are unwilling or feel unsafe doing so.

During a physical examination, the clinician must avoid retraumatizing the patient whenever possible. Patients should guide the examination and be kept covered as much as is feasible.

Box 30.5 Human Trafficking Red Flags in Patients

General Indicators of Human Trafficking

- Shares a scripted or inconsistent history
- Is unwilling or hesitant to answer questions about the injury or illness
- Is accompanied by an individual who does not let the patient speak for himself or herself, refuses to let the patient have privacy, or interprets for the patient
- Exhibits signs of being in controlling or dominating relationships (excessive concerns about pleasing a family member, romantic partner, or employer)
- Demonstrates fearful or nervous behavior or avoids eye contact
- Is resistant to assistance or demonstrates hostile behavior
- Is unable to provide his or her address
- Is not aware of his or her location, the current date, or time
- Is not in possession of his or her identification documents
- Is not in control of his or her own money
- Is not being paid or has wages withheld

Sex Trafficking Indicators

- Is under the age of 18 y and is involved in the commercial sex industry
- Has tattoos or other forms of branding, such as tattoos that say, "Daddy," "Property of . . .," "For sale," etc.
- Reports an unusually high number of sexual partners
- Does not have appropriate clothing for the weather or venue
- Uses language common in the commercial sex industry

Labor Trafficking Indicators

- Has been abused at work or threatened with harm by an employer or supervisor
- Is not allowed to take adequate breaks, food, or water while at work
- Is not provided with adequate personal protective equipment for hazardous work
- Was recruited for different work than he or she is currently doing
- Is required to live in housing provided by the employer
- Has a debt to the employer or recruiter that he or she cannot pay off

Adapted from National Human Trafficking Resource Center. (2016). *Identifying victims of human trafficking: What to look for in a healthcare setting.* Retrieved from https://humantraffickinghotline.org/sites/default/files/What to Look for during a Medical Exam - FINAL - 2-16-16.pdf.

The nurse should query the patient as to what other accommodations can be made to help them feel safer. Examination findings consistent with physical abuse include genital trauma, branding, strangulation injuries, burns, scarring, and others.

Altered mental status may be evidence that drugs were used to facilitate sexual assault as discussed previously. A forensic examination may be indicated and should be executed as detailed earlier in the chapter. The clinician should also offer laboratory testing and STI and pregnancy prophylaxis for the victims of sex trafficking as for other victims of sexual assault. Careful documentation is necessary.

Patients are often not able to leave the trafficking situation even after being identified as victims and being provided them with initial care. As with the victims of IPV, written materials may be inappropriate because of the risk for discovery. The nurse can coach the patient to memorize the phone number for the National Human Trafficking Hotline, which may be best memorized if unconventionally organized: 888-3737-888. When possible, the nurse should schedule the victims of human trafficking for follow-up visits to monitor the situation and facilitate care.

Reporting

The reporting of suspected trafficking of minors is mandated. The reporting of trafficking of mentally and physically abled adults is not mandated. However, if a nurse suspects or has knowledge of trafficking, the nurse can report it and seek guidance from the National Human Trafficking Resource Center by calling the hotline number provided in the last paragraph. Nurses should be aware that patients are protected by the Health Insurance Portability and Accountability Act and that their protected health information should not be disclosed. Internal reporting should be per institution protocol. Whenever possible, the nurse should inform patients of outside reporting to law enforcement or, in the case of minors, protective services.

Eating Disorders

The most commonly identified eating disorders in adults are anorexia nervosa, binge eating disorder, and bulimia nervosa. They are collectively defined as a disturbance in eating with a negative impact on physical or mental health. Screening for eating disorders is reviewed in Chapter 26.

Anorexia Nervosa

A diagnosis of **anorexia nervosa** is made when the patient exhibits each of the three following criteria (Forman, 2018):

- Calorie restriction below that required for weight maintenance.
- A fear and profound anxiety about being overweight despite being underweight.
- A perception of body weight that is distorted and disproportionately important to the patient. Sufferer may deny medical significance of perception and behavior.

The severity of the disease is classified in accordance with the patient's body mass index (BMI). The condition is considered mild if the patient's BMI is 17 to 18.49 kg/m^2, moderate with a BMI from 16 to 15.99 kg/m^2, severe with a BMI from 15 to 15.99 kg/m^2, and extreme with a BMI less than 15 kg/m^2 (Klein & Attia, 2018). Patients may lose or maintain weight by restricting the categories of food, calories, fasting, excessive exercise, vomiting, and the use of laxatives, enemas, or diuretics.

Although the term "anorexia" means loss of appetite, individuals with anorexia nervosa retain their appetite. There are numerous symptoms associated with the condition that are not included in the diagnostic criteria, including perfectionism, preoccupation with food, resistance to treatment, limited insight, food restriction, social withdrawal, and others (Klein & Attia, 2018; Lavender et al., 2015). Comorbid mental and personality disorders are common, including anxiety, depression, obsessive-compulsive disorder, narcissism, substance use disorder, PTSD, borderline personality disorder, and others (Kollei, Schieber, de Zwaan, Svitak, & Martin, 2013).

The mortality rate for people diagnosed with anorexia nervosa is 4% to 14% higher than for the general population, with approximately 60% of deaths resulting from medical complications stemming directly from the anorexia (Fichter & Quadflieg, 2016). To compound this, the lifetime risk of suicidality is 10% to 25% for patients with anorexia, and suicide accounts for approximately a quarter of the deaths, making the risk for suicide in those with anorexia nervosa approximately five times that of the general population (Hoang, Goldacre, & James, 2014; Yao et al., 2016).

People with anorexia often hide their illness, making the prevalence of the illness challenging to assess. Estimates range from 0.6% to 4.2% of the population, with women diagnosed and treated more frequently than men by a ratio as high as 20 to 1 (Brown, Holland, & Keel, 2014; Pedersen et al., 2014).

The treatment of anorexia usually consists of a combination of psychotherapy and nutritional rehabilitation, either inpatient or in the community. In some situations, medication may also be used to promote weight gain, but rarely as a first-line intervention. Antipsychotic medications are used most frequently for this purpose (Kishi, Kafantaris, Sunday, Sheridan, & Correll, 2012).

The medical complications of anorexia may be constitutional, cardiovascular, gynecologic, endocrine, gastrointestinal, renal, electrolyte, pulmonary, hematologic, neurologic, dermatologic, or muscular (Fig. 30.1). The clinician must regularly assess for and treat complications as indicated.

Although normalizing weight is the goal of treatment of anorexia, nutritional therapy can lead to refeeding syndrome, which is potentially fatal. It is the result of a shift in fluids and electrolytes during nutritional rehabilitation. The characteristics of the condition include congestive heart failure, peripheral edema, seizures, hemolysis, rhabdomyolysis, hypophosphatemia, and hypokalemia. Hypophosphatemia, in particular, is a hallmark of the condition. Patients with a BMI under 16 kg/m^2 are at particular risk for refeeding syndrome.

Patients are at the highest risk for refeeding syndrome within the first 2 weeks after starting nutritional therapy. Refeeding syndrome is avoided by a slow restoration of nutrition, a close monitoring for the condition, and a proactive correction of electrolyte imbalances. The treatment for refeeding syndrome is the reduction of nutrition restoration and electrolyte correction.

Binge Eating Disorder

Binge eating disorder is frequent binging—or bouts of overeating—without inappropriate compensatory behaviors, such as purging or excessive exercise. Binging is generally considered to be consuming the equivalent of two or more meals or 2,000 calories or more within a given period of time (such as 2 hours). Binging generally continues until the patient feels physical discomfort or pain (Forman, 2018).

In the United States, the lifetime prevalence of binge eating disorder in women is 3.5% and the median age of onset is 23 years old (Hudson, Hiripi, Pope, & Kessler, 2007; Kessler et al., 2013). Of those diagnosed, nearly 80% have a comorbid mental health diagnosis, most commonly a specific phobia, social phobia, depression, PTSD, or alcoholism (Hudson et al., 2007). Commonly associated physical comorbidities include hypertension, diabetes, and chronic pain. People with binge eating disorder have a higher BMI on average than the general population and are more likely to be obese (Kessler et al., 2013). However, the relationship between binge eating and obesity is unclear.

Treatment goals for patients with binge eating disorder include reducing the number of binge eating episodes and weight loss if indicated. Patients with poor body image may have an additional treatment goal of self-acceptance. Treatment strategies include psychotherapy and pharmacotherapy. The pharmaceuticals most commonly used to treat binge eating disorder are selective serotonin reuptake inhibitors (SSRIs), topiramate (an antiepileptic), and lisdexamfetamine, a medication most often used to treat attention deficit hyperactivity disorder (Brownley et al., 2016). Bariatric surgery may be useful for controlling weight and binge eating in select patients with comorbid obesity.

Bulimia Nervosa

Bulimia nervosa is defined as recurrent binge eating with inappropriate compensatory behaviors (purging, excessive exercise, and the use of medications such as laxatives and diuretics) in an attempt to control weight gain at least once weekly for a minimum of 3 months (Engel, Steffen, & Mitchell, 2018). As with patients with other eating disorders, patients with bulimia nervosa often try to hide their illness. It is estimated that the lifetime prevalence of the condition in the United States is approximately 1%, and the condition is three times as common in women as it is in men. The median age for developing bulimia nervosa is 18 years (Kessler et al., 2013).

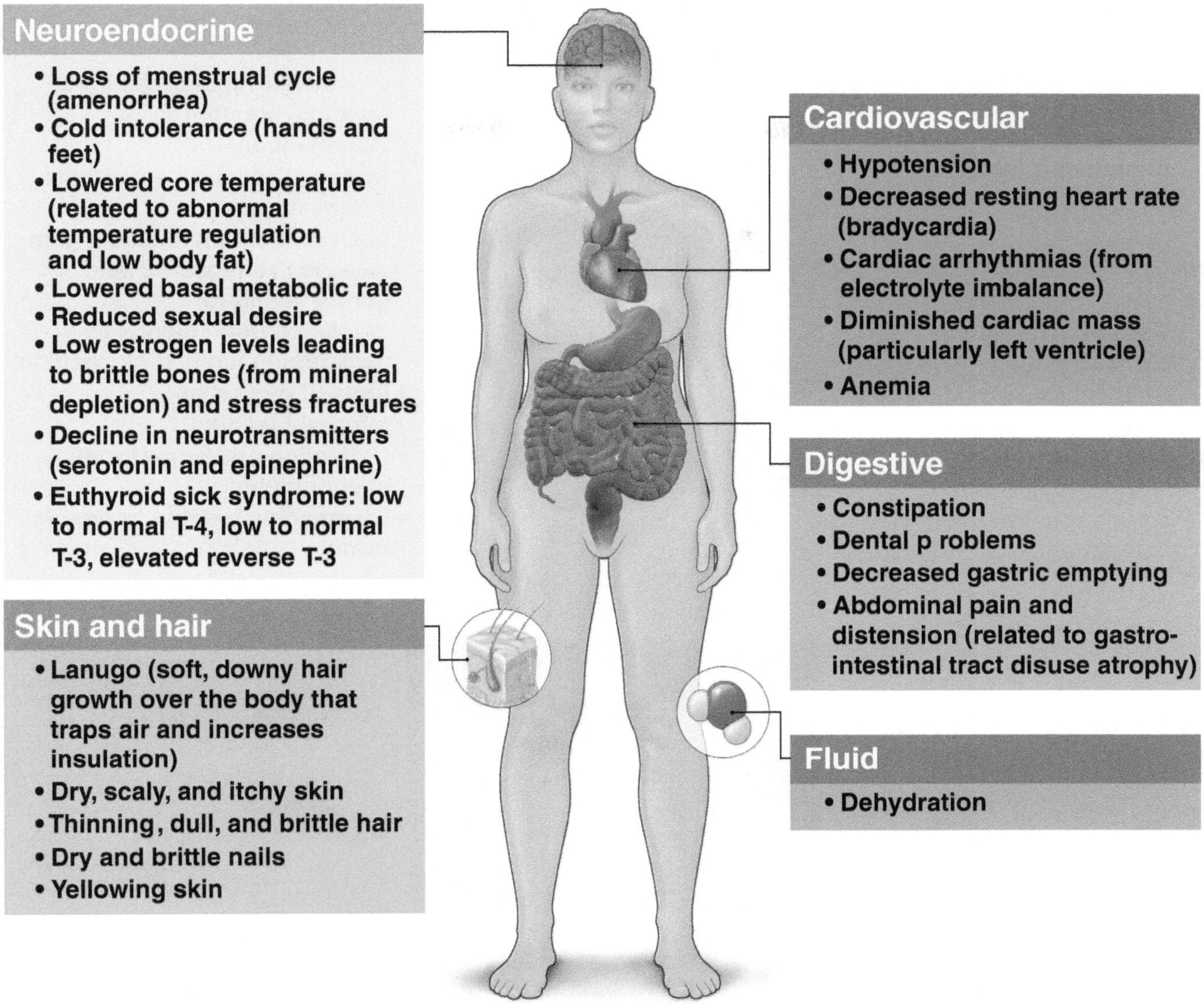

Neuroendocrine

- **Loss of menstrual cycle (amenorrhea)**
- **Cold intolerance (hands and feet)**
- **Lowered core temperature (related to abnormal temperature regulation and low body fat)**
- **Lowered basal metabolic rate**
- **Reduced sexual desire**
- **Low estrogen levels leading to brittle bones (from mineral depletion) and stress fractures**
- **Decline in neurotransmitters (serotonin and epinephrine)**
- **Euthyroid sick syndrome: low to normal T-4, low to normal T-3, elevated reverse T-3**

Skin and hair

- **Lanugo (soft, downy hair growth over the body that traps air and increases insulation)**
- **Dry, scaly, and itchy skin**
- **Thinning, dull, and brittle hair**
- **Dry and brittle nails**
- **Yellowing skin**

Cardiovascular

- **Hypotension**
- **Decreased resting heart rate (bradycardia)**
- **Cardiac arrhythmias (from electrolyte imbalance)**
- **Diminished cardiac mass (particularly left ventricle)**
- **Anemia**

Digestive

- **Constipation**
- **Dental p roblems**
- **Decreased gastric emptying**
- **Abdominal pain and distension (related to gastro-intestinal tract disuse atrophy)**

Fluid

- **Dehydration**

Figure 30.1. Physical and medical consequences of anorexia nervosa. (Reprinted with permission from McArdle, W. D., Katch, F. I., & Katch, V. L. [2013]. *Sports and exercise nutrition* [4th ed., Fig. 15.6]. Philadelphia, PA: Lippincott Williams & Wilkins.)

Bulimia nervosa frequently co-occurs with depression, anxiety, body dysmorphic disorder, PTSD, substance use disorder, specific phobias, social anxiety disorder, and other mental disorders. Personality disorders, including borderline personality disorder, are also more common in this population (Kollei et al., 2013; Nobles et al., 2016).

The physical examination findings of bulimia nervosa can include the erosion of dental enamel, tachycardia, hypotension, xerosis (dry skin), and swelling of the parotid glands (Brown & Mehler, 2013). The complications of the condition may be gastrointestinal, renal, electrolyte, cardiac, endocrine, dental, or related to dehydration (Fig. 30.2).

Bulimia nervosa is associated with an increase in the all-cause mortality of up to eight times that is observed in people without the condition (Hoang et al., 2014). Approximately 17% attempt suicide, twice the rate of the general population (Yao et al., 2016).

The goal of treatment is to stop or significantly reduce the episodes of binge eating and the associated inappropriate compensatory behaviors. Treatment includes psychotherapy, nutritional rehabilitation, and the use of medications. Most are treated on an outpatient basis. SSRIs are the first-line pharmaceutical for this population.

Pregnancy Care for Incarcerated Patients

Although the expectation for care in pregnancy of patients who are incarcerated is the same as that for patients who are not imprisoned, logistics and nursing concerns often differ. Nurses should be aware that the logistics of incarceration can present a barrier to care. Common challenges are related to transportation, communication, timely follow-up, and care of the neonate if the

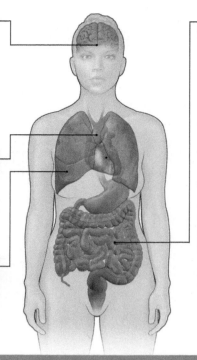

Neuroendocrine
- **Irregular menstrual cycle (erratic estrogen production)**
- **Decreased serotonin and norepinephrine**

Cardiovascular
- **Cardiac arrhythmias (from electrolyte imbalances)**

Pulmonary
- **Aspiration pneumonia (related to regurgitation)**

Digestive
- **Digestive irregularities (gas, bloating, cramps)**
- **Constipation**
- **Reflux of stomach's contents and heartburn**
- **Loss of tooth enamel and gum disease (from gastric acid during vomiting)**
- **Swollen parotid glands in neck region (chipmunk cheeks)**
- **Loss of gag reflex**
- **Internal bleeding**
- **Ulceration and/or perforation of esophagus**
- **Esophagitis (related to gastric acidity)**

Other
- **Bags under eyes**
- **Broken facial blood vessels**
- **Muscle weakness**
- **Fainting**
- **Vision problems**
- **Elevated plasma pH and HCO_3^- (from acid loss with purging)**
- **Electrolyte imbalances (from mineral loss with purging)**

Figure 30.2. Physical and medical consequences of bulimia nervosa. (Reprinted with permission from McArdle, W. D., Katch, F. I., & Katch, V. L. [2013]. *Sports and exercise nutrition* [4th ed., Fig. 15.7]. Philadelphia, PA: Lippincott Williams & Wilkins.)

patient gives birth while incarcerated. All incarcerated individuals are legally entitled to care per the Eighth Amendment of the United States Constitution, although specific policies regarding the care of inmates in pregnancy vary according to state.

From 1980 to 2014, the number of women incarcerated in the United States increased by more than 700% (Carson, 2015). Approximately 1.2 million women are incarcerated at any given time, of whom 6% to 10%, approximately 12,000, are pregnant (American College of Obstetricians and Gynecologists [ACOG], 2012). The American College of Obstetricians and Gynecologists advises all women under the age of 55 to be tested for pregnancy when initially entering the correctional facility, with repeat testing done after 2 weeks (ACOG, 2012).

On-site medical staff, including nurses and other healthcare providers, often do not provide any prenatal care or provide only limited prenatal care, with ultrasounds and the management of high-risk pregnancies occurring off-site. Care provided outside

of the correctional facility is arranged in coordination with prison officers and on-site staff. Time for transport and security precautions must be factored into the plans of care. For reasons of security, inmates are often not told of their schedule of care.

In coordination with outside care providers, on-site care providers may need to intervene to accommodate pregnancy safely, including providing prenatal vitamins, frequent hydration, and small meals. Institutions may have set pregnancy accommodations that include activity restrictions.

When an off-site provider sees a patient, to ensure patient confidentiality, visit records are transported back to the on-site staff by the corrections officer in a sealed folder. Also for reasons of confidentiality, it is important that corrections officers are not used to pass verbal messages that include protected patient information between on-site and off-site staff. After receiving the written records, on-site staff then consult the visit notes to coordinate future visits and any pertinent on-site care. Specific requests made by off-site providers, such as for the provision of extra food, may be considered a special privilege that the on-site team must vet and approve. Just as with a patient who is not incarnated, female inmates retain the right to consent to and refuse treatment, including pregnancy termination.

During a visit with an off-site provider, the corrections officer may be asked to leave the room during the course of the visit to maintain patient privacy. The presence of the officer may be required, however, in situations in which the lack of presence may pose a danger to the healthcare staff or the examination space available offers a flight risk. In some cases the officer may be required to maintain direct visual contact of the inmate at all times (ACOG, 2012).

Care considerations and provision of care are the same as for the nonincarcerated population. Women who are incarcerated are more likely to have a high-risk pregnancy because of a higher incidence of current and past trauma, drug abuse, chronic illness, infections, alcohol abuse, smoking, and poor prenatal care and a lower socioeconomic status. As when caring for other pregnant women, the nurse regularly screens incarcerated pregnant women for STIs, including HIV, and the use of tobacco, drugs, and alcohol. The food made available by the corrections facility may need to be adjusted to exclude food that is unpasteurized as well as cold cuts or undercooked meat, which may contain pathogens dangerous in pregnancy.

Although women who are incarcerated are at a higher risk for pregnancy complications, long incarceration is associated with better outcomes, likely because of consistent access to prenatal care (Shaw, Downe, & Kingdon, 2015).

Intrapartum Care

The recommendations of many organizations, including medical, governmental, and legal bodies, the United Nations, and Amnesty International, call for restraints such as handcuffs only being used during labor and delivery in extreme circumstances. Actual patient experience may differ, particularly when away from the correctional facility, in transit, or at an outside healthcare facility. Nurses should be aware that shackles increase the risk of fall and injury from fall. They limit mobility and can be a dehumanizing and stigmatizing distraction. As with prenatal care, the presence of a corrections officer in the room may be required in some circumstances during labor and delivery.

Postpartum Care

Few correctional facilities have the capability to make accommodations for infants on site. Most infants are separated from their mothers at the time of hospital discharge and placed with family, friends, or a foster family or placed for adoption. These arrangements are typically made prior to the birth but may be delayed until the time of hospitalization.

Because of the separation from the infant, prolonged breast-feeding beyond hospitalization is rarely possible. In the case of an expected imminent release of the mother, however, some facilities may accommodate pumping of breast milk in the short term.

Some facilities may also have programs that allow for milk to be pumped and picked up by the infant's guardian.

As with all pregnant women, the nurse should discuss contraception as part of prenatal care. Women are up to 15 times more likely to start contraception if it is offered during incarceration rather than delaying until after release. Approximately half of incarcerated women become pregnant within 3 months of release from prison, making the provision of contraception prior to release particularly important. Despite this, contraception is often considered nonessential care during incarceration, thus limiting inmate access (Grubb, Beyda, Eissa, & Benjamins, 2018).

Care After Incarceration

Most sentences for women are brief, and release from incarceration is scheduled prior to delivery. Often, they are released without stable finances or housing and limited options for transportation. This immediate chaos of release can compromise access to care. When possible, nurses should facilitate activation or reactivation of outside health insurance. Appointment dates are withheld during incarceration but should be released to the pregnant woman just prior to exiting the facility. If the transfer of outside care providers is required or requested, patient records should be transferred prior to release. Patients should be released with a supply of medications, including prenatal vitamins, sufficient to keep them supplied until their next appointment. For patients receiving opioid-replacement therapy with methadone or buprenorphine, it is particularly essential that there be no lapse in care. Coordination with an outside treatment clinic to avoid a gap in treatment is essential.

Sexual Minority Women

Sexual history taking and screening related to **sexual minority women (SMW)** is reviewed in Chapter 26. The term SMW may be used to describe a woman who identifies as lesbian, bisexual, pansexual, transgender, gay, or polyamorous.

Approximately 3.5% of people in the United States identify as lesbian, gay, or bisexual, and 0.3% identify as transgender (National LGBT Health Education Center, 2017). The nurse should not make assumptions about an individual's gender identity, sexual orientation, or sexual behaviors on the basis of appearance, past history, or a single known factor, such as gender identity or sexual orientation. Although these issues may seem intensely private and the nurse may be hesitant to discuss them, SMW are at an increased risk for STIs, substance abuse, and mental health problems and disclosure can help guide care. Common terms used to discuss sexual minority are defined in Box 30.6.

In Chapter 9, Nancy is married to Missy and by the end of the chapter they have two sons together. Nancy is lucky during the course of the chapter to find acceptance among her friends, family, and healthcare providers.

Box 30.6 Sexual Minority Terminology

- *Gender:* A social construct that attributes a designation of male or female to patterns of behavior, dress, personality, experience, etc.
- *Gender expression:* How masculine or feminine characteristics is manifested in an individual.
- *Gender identity:* A person's self-concept of the person's gender as male, female, or other. Gender identity may or may not align with the person's natal sex.
- *Gender role conformity:* A statement of the degree to which a person conforms to the person's gender identity.
- *Natal sex:* The sex assigned to a person at the time of birth.
- *Sex:* A biologic term relating to the physiologic, hormonal, and anatomic characteristics of a person.
- *Sexual attraction:* Experiencing erotic and/or romantic attraction to one or more genders; commonly categorized as heterosexual, homosexual, bisexual, and pansexual.
- *Sexual behavior:* Actual romantic and/or sexual activities that a person engages in, which may be congruent with the person's stated attraction or may differ. A woman who has sex with other women, for example, may not identify as homosexual. In one study, only 1.3% of women identified as lesbian, but 17.4% reported sexual activity with other women (Copen, Chandra, & Febo-Vazquez, 2016).
- *Transgender:* Having a gender identity that is not concordant with one's natal sex.

Impact on Health

Significant barriers to care for SMW include the lack of insurance, the low income of women relative to men, and a history of poor experiences with healthcare providers related to sexuality or gender (Arbeit, Fisher, Macapagal, & Mustanski, 2016; Austin, 2013).

Health disparities in SMW are due to discrimination, stigma, and civil and human rights violations. Discrimination is a source of considerable stress and limits access to employment, housing, and insurance. SMW are more likely to attempt suicide and become homeless. They are less likely to obtain screening for cervical and breast cancer. SMW are more prone to obesity. Sexual minority individuals have a higher rate of tobacco, alcohol, and drug use than the general population. Transgender individuals are at the highest risk for negative health consequences (Healthy People 2020, 2017).

Stigmatization and rejection by friends, family members, and peers create an enormous source of stress for SMW. Of individuals who identify as lesbian, gay, bisexual, or transgender, 39% report being rejected by a friend or family member because of their sexual minority status, 30% report being physically attacked, and 21% report unfair treatment in the workplace (Pew Research Center, 2013). Eleven percent report healthcare workers refusing to touch them or using excessive precautions, 12% report being blamed by healthcare workers for their health status, and 11% report the use of harsh or abusive language by healthcare providers (Lambda Legal, 2010).

Conversely, the lack of disclosure of gender or sexual orientation is associated with a higher risk for depression and suicidality. SMW who do disclose report overall less stress and depression. Nurses should be aware of the higher rates of anxiety, stress, depression, and suicidality in SMW patients (Makadon, Mayer, Potter, & Goldhammer, 2015).

Creating Safe Spaces

Effective communication is important to all care. A part of communicating effectively is avoiding assumptions and judgment.

The nurse should avoid gendered terms or phrases that pertain to sexual orientation when possible. Rather than referring to a husband, wife, girlfriend, or boyfriend, the nurse should ask about a partner. When reporting to another provider, rather than referring to "he" or "she," the nurse should refer to "the patient" until or unless the patient's gender identity and preferred pronoun use are clear.

Transgender individuals often have a name or gender identity different from that on legal documents such as insurance cards. It is important to refer to the patient by the preferred name and pronouns. The preferred name and pronouns should be prominently visible in the health record and used consistently by all staff. Some people prefer gendered pronouns such as she/her/hers or he/him/his. Others prefer gender-neutral pronouns such as they/them/their, ze/zim/zirs, or sie/hir/hirs. It is not uncommon to accidentally use the wrong pronoun. The best course of action when this happens is a respectful apology.

As with any person, it is important to avoid gossiping about patients or resorting to stereotypes when communicating to or about patients. It is not appropriate to tell people who identify as bisexual that they just haven't made up their minds yet. A person who identifies as a lesbian should not be told that she's too pretty to be a lesbian. A transwoman should not be told she "looks like a real woman" and a transman should not be told, "I never would have guessed you're really a woman." Although these phrases may be intended as complimentary, they can be deeply hurtful and are neither kind nor appropriate.

Care of Transgender Individuals

The terms **transwoman** and male-to-female are often used to describe a person assigned male at birth who identifies as female. The terms **transman** and female-to-male are used to describe a person assigned female at birth who identifies as male. People may also identify as gender fluid or gender queer. People who are not transgender are sometimes referred to as cisgender or cis. As discussed in Chapter 26, being transgender is not a mental health condition, although dysphoria caused by an inability to present as the gender with which the person identifies is (American Psychiatric Association, 2013).

There is no one way to be a transgender person. For some people, a simple change in legal name may be sufficient gender expression. For others, a change in wardrobe or hair may be adequate. Some elect for hormone therapy, and still others may elect for gender-confirming surgery. There is no one choice of medication or surgery. Both are individualized according to the needs of the patient.

Nurses should be aware that of transgender individuals, 61% report being physically attacked because of their gender identity and 55% report losing a job because of employer bias against transgender individuals. Twenty-five percent report harassment in the healthcare setting and 19% report being denied healthcare because they are transgender (Grant et al., 2011). A part of the responsible care of individuals who identify as transgender, as with any patient, is unbiased compassion.

Hormone Therapy

The goal of hormone therapy in transgender individuals is to induce physical change in keeping with gender identity. The priorities for transwomen often include minimization of facial hair and feminization of fat distribution for a slimmer waist, broader hips, and larger breasts. The goals for virilization for transmen include changes in fat distribution, muscle mass, and deepening of the voice. To start hormone therapy, patients must communicate persistent gender dysphoria and a capacity for informed decision-making. Any other physical or mental health conditions should be well managed prior to starting care (World Professional Association for Transgender Health [WPATH], 2015).

All patients contemplating hormone therapy should be aware that in the short term, hormone therapy can diminish but not eliminate fertility. An individual taking virilizing testosterone may still get pregnant. An individual taking feminizing estrogen may still ejaculate viable sperm sufficient for pregnancy. Greater fertility returns with the cessation of hormone therapy. Transmen may become pregnant if the reproductive organs remain intact, and transwomen with intact genitalia may provide the sperm to create pregnancy. Some individuals may elect to harvest and freeze ova or sperm prior to gender-confirming hormone therapy or surgery.

Transwomen

Estrogen is the cornerstone of treatment for most transwomen seeking hormone therapy, typically in the form of transdermal or oral 17-beta estradiol (the ethinyl estradiol used in birth control pills is generally not recommended, as the dosage required is associated with an excess risk of venous thrombosis; Asscheman et al., 2014). Additional antiandrogen treatment is frequently added with the use of spironolactone or, less commonly, gonadotropin-releasing hormone agonist therapy. Should the patient elect for an orchidectomy (removal of testicles), antiandrogen therapy is no longer indicated. Changes are gradual and happen over the course of months to years (Table 30.2). It should be noted that hormone therapy does not change the voice. If the patient was balding prior to starting hormone therapy, scalp hair does not regenerate.

Table 30.2 Onset and Maximum Effect of Hormone Therapy for Transwomen

	Time Since Initiation of Therapy									
	Months						Years			
Change in Body	1	2	3	4	5	6	1	2	3	>3
Decrease in libido	Onset 1–3 mo			ME 2–6 mo						
Decrease in spontaneous erections	Onset 1–3 mo			ME 2–6 mo						
Redistribution of body fat			Onset 3–6 mo					ME 2–3 y		
Decrease in muscle mass and strength			Onset 3–6 mo				ME 1–2 y			
Softening of skin and decrease in oiliness			Onset 3–6 mo				Time of ME unclear			
Breast growth			Onset 3–6 mo					ME 2–3 y		
Decrease in testicular volume			Onset 3–6 mo					ME 2–3 y		
Decrease in the growth of body hair							Onset 6–12 mo			ME>3 y
Sexual dysfunction	Variable									
Decrease in sperm production	Onset unknown									ME>3 y

Abbreviations: ME, maximum effect.
Adapted from Hembree, W. C., Cohen-Kettenis, P., Delemarre-van de Waal, H. A., Gooren, L. J., Meyer, W. J., III, Spack, N. P., . . . Montori, V. M.; Endocrine Society. (2009). Endocrine treatment of transsexual persons: An Endocrine Society clinical practice guideline. *Journal of Clinical Endocrinology and Metabolism, 94*(9), 3132–3154. doi:10.1210/jc.2009-0345.

Table 30.3 Onset and Maximum Effect of Hormone Therapy for Transmen

Change in Body	Time Since Initiation of Therapy										
	Months						Years				
	1	2	3	4	5	6	1	2	3	4	5
Acne and oily skin	Onset 1–6 mo						ME 1–2 y				
Redistribution of body fat	Onset 1–6 mo							ME 2–5 y			
Menses cessation	Onset 2–6 mo and for the duration of therapy. Bleeding may persist in some patients.										
Enlargement of clitoris			Onset 3–6 mo				ME 1–2 y				
Vaginal atrophy			Onset 3–6 mo				ME 1–2 y				
Voice deepening						Onset 6–12 mo	ME 1–2 y				
Facial and body hair growth						Onset 6–12 mo				ME 4–5 y	
Loss of scalp hair						Onset 6–12 mo	Duration and extent in keeping with genetic predisposition				
Increase in strength and muscle mass						Onset 6–12 mo	ME 2–5 y				

ME, maximum effect.
Adapted from Hembree, W. C., Cohen-Kettenis, P., Delemarre-van de Waal, H. A., Gooren, L. J., Meyer, W. J., III, Spack, N. P., . . . Montori, V. M.; Endocrine Society. (2009). Endocrine treatment of transsexual persons: An Endocrine Society clinical practice guideline. *Journal of Clinical Endocrinology and Metabolism, 94*(9), 3132–3154. doi:10.1210/jc.2009-0345

Individuals receiving estrogen for gender confirmation generally follow up every 3 months during the first year and then once or twice yearly. Because spironolactone is a potassium-sparing diuretic, patients using this therapy have their potassium level monitored regularly. Although hormone therapy dosing is generally guided by patient report, some clinicians choose to monitor estrogen with a goal of keeping the estrogen dose sufficient to maintain levels equivalent to physiologic levels of the hormone as seen in natal females.

Because of the risk for venous thromboembolism with estrogen, therapy should be stopped 2 to 4 weeks prior to major surgery and restarted in the month following. Estrogen can cause an elevation in triglyceride levels, particularly in patients with a strong family history of hypertriglyceridemia.

Transmen

Testosterone therapy is the mainstay of treatment for transmen. Testosterone may be delivered as a transdermal gel, buccal tablet, or by intramuscular or subcutaneous injection. As with hormonal therapy for transwomen, the onset and maximum effect for particular changes is variable (Table 30.3).

Follow-up for patients using testosterone is generally every 3 months for the first year and then once or twice a year afterward.

Earlier follow-up is required with dose adjustments. During these visits, the nurse measures the patient's weight and blood pressure, as well as hematocrit level. The most common adverse effect of testosterone therapy for gender confirmation therapy is erythrocytosis. The goal hematocrit level for patients is under 55% (Weinand & Safer, 2015). Although testosterone dosing is most often led by patient report, some clinicians may choose to routinely monitor testosterone with a goal of maintaining levels in the physiologic range for natal men.

Surgery

In addition to meeting the criteria for starting hormone therapy, patients desiring to undergo gender confirmation surgery are generally required to live as their identified gender for at least 1 continuous year prior to surgery (WPATH, 2015). There is no one type of surgery for gender confirmation. "Top" surgery refers to the removal of breast tissue for transmen and the augmentation of breast tissue for transwomen. Genital surgery varies according to the goals and preferences of the patient. Other surgeries may include the alterations of facial features or, in the case of transwomen, feminization of the neck by minimization of the laryngeal prominence.

Think Critically

1. You are caring for a patient who is reporting a sexual assault. Write a short dialogue of the questions you think are important to ask at this time. Consider the best way of posing each question.
2. You are performing the intake for a new patient. The patient's partner is present. You need to ask the patient questions about intimate partner violence. What is your best approach?
3. You are caring for a patient whom you suspect is a victim of human trafficking. List five different red flags that make you suspicious. How would you bring this up with the patient?
4. Find and review the mandated reporting laws for your state: https://www.childwelfare.gov/pubPDFs/manda .pdf#page=5&view=Summaries of State laws

5. You are caring for a woman with a body mass index of 16. What are your concerns? What questions should you ask her to assess her health and safety?
6. You are caring for a woman in labor and delivery. She is in transition and is shackled to the bed. Consider how you might address the situation with the corrections officer.
7. Review the standards for pregnancy care for incarcerated women for your state: https://www.aclu.org/state-standards-pregnancy-related-health-care-and-abortion-women-prison-0
8. You are caring for a patient who is male but was identified as female at birth. You need to ask the patient what reproductive organs are present. How do you ask the question? What if the patient challenges you? How do you explain why the question and answer are important to the provision of care?

References

Alexander, P. C., Morris, E., Tracy, A., & Frye, A. (2010). Stages of change and the group treatment of batterers: A randomized clinical trial. *Violence and Victims, 25*(5), 571–587.

American College of Obstetricians and Gynecologists. (2012). ACOG committee opinion no. 535: Reproductive health care for incarcerated women and adolescent females. *Obstetrics and Gynecology, 120,* 425–429.

American Psychiatric Association. (2013). *Diagnostic and statistical manual of mental disorders* (5th ed.). Arlington, VA: Author.

Arbeit, M. R., Fisher, C. B., Macapagal, K., & Mustanski, B. (2016). Bisexual invisibility and the sexual health needs of adolescent girls. *LGBT Health, 3*(5), 342–349. doi:10.1089/lgbt.2016.0035

Asscheman, H., T'Sjoen, G., Lemaire, A., Mas, M., Meriggiola, M. C., Mueller, A., . . . Gooren, L. J. (2014). Venous thrombo-embolism as a complication of cross-sex hormone treatment of male-to-female transsexual subjects: A review. *Andrologia, 46*(7), 791–795. doi:10.1111/and.12150

Austin, E. L. (2013). Sexual orientation disclosure to health care providers among urban and non-urban southern lesbians. *Women and Health, 53*(1), 41–55. doi:10.1080/03630242.2012.743497

Beydoun, H. A., Williams, M., Beydoun, M. A., Eid, S. M., & Zonderman, A. B. (2017). Relationship of physical intimate partner violence with mental health diagnoses in the nationwide emergency department sample. *Journal of Women's Health, 26*(2), 141–151. doi:10.1089/jwh.2016.5840

Bosch, J., Weaver, T. L., Arnold, L. D., & Clark, E. M. (2015). The impact of intimate partner violence on women's physical health: Findings from the Missouri behavioral risk factor surveillance system. *Journal of Interpersonal Violence.* doi:10.1177/0886260515599162

Breiding, M. J., Smith, S. G., Basile, K. C., Walters, M. L., Chen, J., & Merrick, M. T. (2014). Prevalence and characteristics of sexual violence, stalking, and intimate partner violence victimization—National intimate partner and sexual violence survey, United States, 2011. *MMWR Surveillance Summaries, 63*(8), 1–18.

Brown, C. A., & Mehler, P. S. (2013). Medical complications of self-induced vomiting. *Eating Disorders, 21*(4), 287–294. doi:10.1080/10640266.2013.797317

Brown, T. A., Holland, L. A., & Keel, P. K. (2014). Comparing operational definitions of DSM-5 anorexia nervosa for research contexts. *International Journal of Eating Disorders, 47*(1), 76–84. doi:10.1002/eat.22184

Brownley, K. A., Berkman, N. D., Peat, C. M., Lohr, K. N., Cullen, K. E., Bann, C. M., & Bulik, C. M. (2016). Binge-eating disorder in adults: A systematic review and meta-analysis. *Annals of Internal Medicine, 165*(6), 409–420. doi:10.7326/M15-2455

Carson, E. A. (2015). *Prisoners in 2014.* Retrieved from https://www.bjs.gov/content/pub/pdf/p14.pdf

Catalano, S. (2015). *Intimate partner violence, 1993–2010.* Retrieved from https://www.bjs.gov/content/pub/pdf/ipv9310.pdf

Cattaneo, L. B., Grossmann, J., & Chapman, A. R. (2016). The goals of IPV survivors receiving orders of protection: An application of the empowerment process model. *Journal of Interpersonal Violence, 31*(17), 2889–2911. doi:10.1177/0886260515581905

CdeBaca, L., & Sigmon, J. N. (2014). Combating trafficking in persons: A call to action for global health professionals. *Global Health, Science and Practice, 2*(3), 261–267. doi:10.9745/GHSP-D-13-00142

Chisolm-Straker, M., Baldwin, S., Gaigbe-Togbe, B., Ndukwe, N., Johnson, P. N., & Richardson, L. D. (2016). Health care and human trafficking: We are seeing the unseen. *Journal of Health Care for the Poor and Underserved, 27*(3), 1220–1233. doi:10.1353/hpu.2016.0131

Copen, C. E., Chandra, A., & Febo-Vazquez, I. (2016). Sexual behavior, sexual attraction, and sexual orientation among adults aged 18-44 in the United States: Data from the 2011–2013 National Survey of Family Growth. *National Health Statistics Reports,* (88), 1–14.

Crawford-Jakubiak, J. E., Alderman, E. M., Leventhal, J. M., & Committee on Child Abuse and Neglect; Committee on Adolescence. (2017). Care of the adolescent after an acute sexual assault. *Pediatrics, 139*(3). doi:10.1542/peds.2016-4243

Ellsberg, M., Arango, D. J., Morton, M., Gennari, F., Kiplesund, S., Contreras, M., & Watts, C. (2015). Prevention of violence against women and girls: What does the evidence say? *The Lancet, 385*(9977), 1555–1566. doi:10.1016/S0140-6736(14)61703-7

Engel, S. S., Steffen, K., & Mitchell, J. E. (2018). Bulimia nervosa in adults: Clinical features, course of illness, assessment, and diagnosis. *UpToDate.*

Feder, G., Wathen, C. N., & MacMillan, H. L. (2013). An evidence-based response to intimate partner violence: WHO guidelines. *JAMA, 310*(5), 479–480. doi:10.1001/jama.2013.167453

Fichter, M. M., & Quadflieg, N. (2016). Mortality in eating disorders—Results of a large prospective clinical longitudinal study. *International Journal of Eating Disorders, 49*(4), 391–401. doi:10.1002/eat.22501

Ford, N., Irvine, C., Shubber, Z., Baggaley, R., Beanland, R., Vitoria, M., . . . Calmy, A. (2014). Adherence to HIV postexposure prophylaxis:

A systematic review and meta-analysis. *AIDS, 28*(18), 2721–2727. doi:10.1097/QAD.0000000000000505

Forman, S. F. (2018). Eating disorders: Overview of epidemiology, clinical features, and diagnosis. *UpToDate.*

Grace, A. M., Ahn, R., & Macias Konstantopoulos, W. (2014). Integrating curricula on human trafficking into medical education and residency training. *JAMA Pediatrics, 168*(9), 793–794. doi:10.1001/jamapediatrics.2014.999

Grant, J. M., Mottet, L. A., Tanis, J., Harrison, J., Herman, J. L., & Keisling., M. (2011). *Injustice at every turn: A report of the national transgender discrimination survey.* Washington, DC: National Center for Transgender Equality and National Gay and Lesbian Task Force.

Grubb, L. K., Beyda, R. M., Eissa, M. A., & Benjamins, L. J. (2018). A contraception quality improvement initiative with detained young women: Counseling, initiation, and utilization. *Journal of Pediatric and Adolescent Gynecology.* doi:10.1016/j.jpag.2018.01.002

Haggard, U., Freij, I., Danielsson, M., Wenander, D., & Langstrom, N. (2015). Effectiveness of the IDAP treatment program for male perpetrators of intimate partner violence: A controlled study of criminal recidivism. *Journal of Interpersonal Violence.* doi:10.1177/0886260515586377

Healthy People 2020. (2017). *Lesbian, gay, bisexual, and transgender health.* Retrieved from https://www.healthypeople.gov/2020/topics-objectives/topic/lesbian-gay-bisexual-and-transgender-health

Hoang, U., Goldacre, M., & James, A. (2014). Mortality following hospital discharge with a diagnosis of eating disorder: National record linkage study, England, 2001–2009. *International Journal of Eating Disorders, 47*(5), 507–515. doi:10.1002/eat.22249

Hudson, J. I., Hiripi, E., Pope, H. G., Jr., & Kessler, R. C. (2007). The prevalence and correlates of eating disorders in the National Comorbidity Survey Replication. *Biological Psychiatry, 61*(3), 348–358. doi:10.1016/j.biopsych.2006.03.040

International Labor Organization. (2017). *Forced labor, modern slavery, and human trafficking.* Retrieved from http://www.ilo.org/global/topics/forced-labour/lang--en/index.htm

Jahanfar, S., Howard, L. M., & Medley, N. (2014). Interventions for preventing or reducing domestic violence against pregnant women. *Cochrane Database of Systematic Reviews,* (11), CD009414. doi:10.1002/14651858.CD009414.pub3

Jaureguy, F., Chariot, P., Vessieres, A., & Picard, B. (2016). Prevalence of Chlamydia trachomatis and Neisseria gonorrhoeae infections detected by real-time PCR among individuals reporting sexual assaults in the Paris, France area. *Forensic Science International, 266*, 130–133. doi:10.1016/j.forsciint.2016.04.031

Kessler, R. C., Berglund, P. A., Chiu, W. T., Deitz, A. C., Hudson, J. I., Shahly, V., . . . Xavier, M. (2013). The prevalence and correlates of binge eating disorder in the World Health Organization World Mental Health Surveys. *Biological Psychiatry, 73*(9), 904–914. doi:10.1016/j.biopsych.2012.11.020

Kishi, T., Kafantaris, V., Sunday, S., Sheridan, E. M., & Correll, C. U. (2012). Are antipsychotics effective for the treatment of anorexia nervosa? Results from a systematic review and meta-analysis. *Journal of Clinical Psychiatry, 73*(6), e757–e766. doi:10.4088/JCP.12r07691

Klein, D. A., & Attia, E. (2018). Anorexia nervosa in adults: Clinical features, course of illness, assessment, and diagnosis. *UpToDate.*

Kollei, I., Schieber, K., de Zwaan, M., Svitak, M., & Martin, A. (2013). Body dysmorphic disorder and nonweight-related body image concerns in individuals with eating disorders. *International Journal of Eating Disorders, 46*(1), 52–59. doi:10.1002/eat.22067

Lambda Legal. (2010). *When health care isn't caring: Lambda legal's survey of discrimination against LGBT people and people with HIV.* Retrieved from https://www.lambdalegal.org/publications/when-health-care-isnt-caring

Lavender, J. M., Wonderlich, S. A., Engel, S. G., Gordon, K. H., Kaye, W. H., & Mitchell, J. E. (2015). Dimensions of emotion dysregulation in anorexia nervosa and bulimia nervosa: A conceptual review of the empirical literature. *Clinical Psychology Review, 40*, 111–122. doi:10.1016/j.cpr.2015.05.010

Lederer, L. J., Wetzel, C. A. (2014). The health consequences of sex trafficking and their implications for identifying victims in healthcare facilities. *Annals of Health Law, 23*(1).

Macias-Konstantopoulos, W. (2016). Human trafficking: The role of medicine in interrupting the cycle of abuse and violence. *Annals of Internal Medicine, 165*(8), 582–588. doi:10.7326/M16-0094

Makadon, H. J., Mayer, K. H., Potter, J., & Goldhammer, H. (2015). *The fenway guide to lesbian, gay, bisexual, and transgender health.* Philadelphia, PA: American College of Physicians.

National LGBT Health Education Center (Producer). (2017, August 17). *Providing quality care to lesbian, gay, bisexual, and transgender patients: An introduction*

for staff training. Retrieved from https://www.lgbthealtheducation.org/lgbt-education/learning-modules/

Nobles, C. J., Thomas, J. J., Valentine, S. E., Gerber, M. W., Vaewsorn, A. S., & Marques, L. (2016). Association of premenstrual syndrome and premenstrual dysphoric disorder with bulimia nervosa and binge-eating disorder in a nationally representative epidemiological sample. *International Journal of Eating Disorders, 49*(7), 641–650. doi:10.1002/eat.22539

Patel, P., Borkowf, C. B., Brooks, J. T., Lasry, A., Lansky, A., & Mermin, J. (2014). Estimating per-act HIV transmission risk: A systematic review. *AIDS, 28*(10), 1509–1519. doi:10.1097/QAD.0000000000000298

Patterson, D., & Tringali, B. (2015). Understanding how advocates can affect sexual assault victim engagement in the criminal justice process. *Journal of Interpersonal Violence, 30*(12), 1987–1997. doi:10.1177/0886260514552273

Pedersen, C. B., Mors, O., Bertelsen, A., Waltoft, B. L., Agerbo, E., McGrath, J. J., . . . Eaton, W. W. (2014). A comprehensive nationwide study of the incidence rate and lifetime risk for treated mental disorders. *JAMA Psychiatry, 71*(5), 573–581. doi:10.1001/jamapsychiatry.2014.16

Pew Research Center. (2013). *A survey of LGBT Americans: Attitudes, experiences and values in changing times.* Retrieved from file: http://www.pewsocialtrends.org/files/2013/06/SDT_LGBT-Americans_06-2013.pdf

Rivas, C., Ramsay, J., Sadowski, L., Davidson, L. L., Dunne, D., Eldridge, S., . . . Feder, G. (2015). Advocacy interventions to reduce or eliminate violence and promote the physical and psychosocial well-being of women who experience intimate partner abuse. *Cochrane Database of Systematic Reviews,* (12), CD005043. doi:10.1002/14651858.CD005043.pub3

Shaw, J., Downe, S., & Kingdon, C. (2015). Systematic mixed-methods review of interventions, outcomes and experiences for imprisoned pregnant women. *Journal of Advanced Nursing, 71*(7), 1451–1463. doi:10.1111/jan.12605

Sheehan, B. E., Murphy, S. B., Moynihan, M. M., Dudley-Fennessey, E., & Stapleton, J. G. (2015). Intimate partner homicide: New insights for understanding lethality and risks. *Violence Against Women, 21*(2), 269–288. doi:10.1177/1077801214564687

Smith, S. G., Chen, J., Basile, K. C., Gilbert, L. K., Merrick, M. T., Patel, N., . . . Jain, A. (2017). *The national intimate partner and sexual violence survey (NISVS): 2010–2012 state report.* Retrieved from Atlanta, GA: National Center for Injury Prevention and Control, Centers for Disease Control and Prevention.

Tiihonen Moller, A., Backstrom, T., Sondergaard, H. P., & Helstrom, L. (2014). Identifying risk factors for PTSD in women seeking medical help after rape. *PLoS One, 9*(10), e111136. doi:10.1371/journal.pone.0111136

United Nations. (2001). *Resolution adopted by the general assembly, 55th session, agenda item 105.* Retrieved from https://www-unodc-org.ezproxy.uvm.edu/pdf/crime/a_res_55/res5525e.pdf

Weinand, J. D., & Safer, J. D. (2015). Hormone therapy in transgender adults is safe with provider supervision; A review of hormone therapy sequelae for transgender individuals. *Journal of Clinical and Translation Endocrinology, 2*(2), 55–60. doi:10.1016/j.jcte.2015.02.003

White, C. (2013). Genital injuries in adults. *Best Practice and Research. Clinical Obstetrics and Gynaecology, 27*(1), 113–130. doi:10.1016/j.bpobgyn.2012.08.011

Workowski, K. A., Bolan, G. A., & Centers for Disease Control and Prevention. (2015). Sexually transmitted diseases treatment guidelines, 2015. *MMWR Recommendations and Reports, 64*(RR-03), 1–137.

World Health Organization. (2012). *Understanding and addressing violence against women.* Retrieved from http://apps.who.int/iris/bitstream/10665/77432/1/WHO_RHR_12.36_eng.pdf

World Professional Association for Transgender Health. (2015). *Standards of care for the health of transsexual, transgender, and gender nonconforming people.* Retrieved from https://www.wpath.org/media/cms/Documents/SOC%20v7/SOC%20V7_English.pdf

Yao, S., Kuja-Halkola, R., Thornton, L. M., Runfola, C. D., D'Onofrio, B. M., Almqvist, C., . . . Bulik, C. M. (2016). Familial liability for eating disorders and suicide attempts: Evidence from a population registry in Sweden. *JAMA Psychiatry, 73*(3), 284–291. doi:10.1001/jamapsychiatry.2015.2737

Suggested Readings

Futures Without Violence. Retrieved from www.futureswithoutviolence.org

International Association of Forensic Nurses. Retrieved from http://www.forensicnurses.org

National Human Trafficking Hotline. Retrieved from http://polarisproject.org/national-human-trafficking-hotline

National LGBT Health Education Center. Retrieved from www.lgbthealtheducation.org

Glossary

A

Acceleration: In fetal monitoring after about 32 weeks of gestation, an increase in fetal heart rate of at least 15 beats per minute for at least 15 seconds; prior to 32 weeks of gestation, an increase in fetal heart rate of at least 10 beats per minute for at least 15 seconds

Accessory breast tissue: Breast tissue present in a location on the body other than the breasts

Acme: The peak of intensity of a uterine contraction

Acquired immunodeficiency syndrome (AIDS): An immune system disorder caused by infection with the human immunodeficiency virus and clinically diagnosed on the basis of certain signs and symptoms

Acrosome: A cap on the head of the sperm that aids with the penetration of the ovum

Acute bilirubin encephalopathy (ABE): The acute clinical manifestations of bilirubin-induced neurologic dysfunction

Adenomyosis: The occurrence of endometrial-type tissue within the myometrium (the muscle of the uterus)

Adjuvant therapy: Treatment given in addition to the primary therapy that is designed to help eliminate a disease and prevent its recurrence

Advanced maternal age: The age at or after which the ability to conceive begins to decline and the risk of pregnancy-related complications increases significantly, usually defined as age 35 or greater; may alternately be defined as age 40 or older

Afterpains: Uncomfortable cramping of the uterus postpartum

Aliquots: Samples or portions of blood, as are removed during an exchange transfusion in the treatment of hyperbilirubinemia

Amastia: The absence of breast tissue

Amenorrhea: The lack of menses

Amniocentesis: A diagnostic procedure to remove amniotic fluid during a pregnancy to assess for chromosomal abnormalities, neural tube defects, blood type, infection, fetal sex, and, in late pregnancy, fetal lung development

Amnioreduction: a therapeutic reducing of amniotic fluid to normalize levels

Amnioinfusion: A process of reintroducing amniotic fluid into the amniotic sac

Amnion: The innermost of the fetal membranes, which surrounds the embryo and later the fetus and is filled with amniotic fluid

Amniotic sac: also referred to as fetal membranes or "bag of fluids," it is filled with amniotic fluid and surrounds and protects the developing fetus

Amniotic fluid embolism: A life-threatening complication of pregnancy in which amniotic fluid enters the maternal circulation

Ampulla: The distal third of the fallopian tube, furthest from the uterus

Anencephaly: A neural tube defect resulting in the absence of the major portions of the brain, scalp, and skull

Anorectal atresia: A condition in which the rectum and anus are absent or abnormally placed

Anorexia nervosa: An eating disorder characterized by low body weight due to a pathologic restriction of nutrition

Anovulation: A lack of ovulation

Antiemetics: A class of medications that relieve nausea and vomiting

Apnea: A cessation of breathing for 15 to 20 seconds or more

Approximation: The proximity of wound edges to each other

Arthralgia: Joint pain

Artificial reproductive technology (ART): Fertility treatments, including ovarian stimulation and in vitro fertilization, among other strategies

Athelia: The absence of a nipple

Atony: A condition involving a failure to contract, as may occur in the uterus postpartum

Atopic eruption of pregnancy (AEP): A papular or eczematous dermatitis of pregnancy that usually starts prior to the third trimester

Aura: A temporary sensory alteration, such as visual or tactile, that precedes or accompanies a migraine headache

Autosomal dominant: A type of genetic disorder in which an individual needs to receive only the mutated gene from one parent to have the disorder

Autosomal recessive: A type of genetic disorder in which an individual must receive the mutated gene from both parents to have the disorder

Autosome: a chromosome that is not a sex chromosome

B

Bacterial vaginosis (BV): An imbalance of normally occurring vaginal flora that can cause changes in vaginal odor and discharge

Bandl's ring: A constriction between the upper and lower uterine segments

Basal body thermometer: A thermometer with a finer scale that can sense minor fluctuations in body temperature and is often used to monitor for ovulation

Beta-human chorionic gonadotropin (β-hCG): A hormone produced by the placenta during early pregnancy that helps sustain the growth and development of the fetus; measured as an indicator of pregnancy; in rare cases, may be produced by a cancerous tumor

Bilateral tubal ligation (BTL): A surgical procedure to sterilize females that involves bilateral occlusion of the fallopian tubes (via cauterization, suturing, clamping, or removal of a portion), which prevents ova from traveling from the ovaries to the uterus and sperm from traveling up the fallopian tubes to the ova

Bilirubin: A yellow bile pigment produced by the breakdown of red blood cells

Bilirubin-induced neurological dysfunction (BIND): A complication of severe hyperbilirubinemia that occurs when serum bilirubin crosses the blood–brain barrier and binds to the brain tissue

Binge eating disorder: An eating disorder characterized by frequent overeating without inappropriate compensatory measures

Biochemical pregnancy: A pregnancy that ends shortly after implantation

Biophysical profile: An ultrasound evaluation of fetal well-being in later pregnancy

Blastocoel: The fluid-filled cavity of the blastocyst

Blastocyst: A partially differentiated preembryonic structure

Blastomere: A cell formed during the early cleavage of the fertilized ovum

Bloody show: A small amount of bloody mucus that may be passed from the vagina prior to or during labor

725

Body mass index (BMI): An estimate of body mass calculated on the basis of a person's height and weight that is used to assess for underweight, normal weight, overweight, and obesity

Boggy uterus: A condition in which the uterus is soft to palpation postpartum, which is diagnostic of atony and indicates an increased risk for postpartum hemorrhage

Brachial plexus: A network of nerves in the neck and shoulder

Braxton Hicks contractions: Weak, irregular, nonprogressing uterine contractions that do not cause cervical effacement and dilation

Breast awareness: An approach to breast cancer screening in which the patient becomes familiar with her breasts rather than examining them according to a schedule to detect any changes that might indicate cancer

Breast milk jaundice: A form of typically physiologic jaundice that usually occurs from 4 to 7 days postpartum, may last as long as 4 months, and is associated with breastfeeding

Breast-conserving surgery (BCS): The removal of only the tumor and a border of healthy tissue rather than the breast

Breastfeeding-associated jaundice: A form of jaundice that occurs in the first week postpartum and is caused by ineffective breastfeeding

Bronchopulmonary dysplasia: A chronic lung disorder most common in premature infants treated with mechanical ventilation

Bulimia nervosa: An eating disorder characterized by frequent overeating with inappropriate compensatory measures

C

Calorie: A unit used to measure the amount of energy contained in food and defined as the energy required to raise 1 kg of water 1°C; also known as a kilocalorie

Candida vulvovaginitis: An inflammation of the female genitals caused by an overgrowth of yeast

Capacitation: a biochemical change in the sperm that allows penetration into the egg and increased sperm mobility

Caput succedaneum: Edema of the fetal scalp

Cell-free DNA (cfDNA) screening: A test that assesses fetal DNA fragments extracted from the maternal circulation to determine the risk for chromosomal defects

Cephalhematoma: A hemorrhage between the skull and the periosteum of a newborn resulting from trauma during birth

Cephalopelvic disproportion (CPD): A mismatch between the size of the fetal head and the size of the maternal pelvis, typically resulting in dystocia

Cerebral palsy: A permanent disorder of movement and balance caused by damage to the brain in utero, intrapartum, and/or after birth

Cervical intraepithelial neoplasia (CIN): A condition of abnormal growth in the squamous cells of the cervix

Cervicitis: Inflammation of the cervix

Cesarean section: A method of delivering an infant by making a surgical incision in the mother's abdomen

Chadwick's sign: A bluish discoloration of the female genitalia that is an early sign of pregnancy

Chancre: A painless ulcer that is an early and transient manifestation of syphilis

Chlamydia: The most prevalent bacterial sexually transmitted infection

Chloasma: A condition of hyperpigmentation of the face that commonly occurs in pregnancy as a result of changes in estrogen level

Choanal atresia: A complete blockage of the nose by cartilage or other tissue

Cholestasis: A condition in which the flow of bile from the liver is impaired, one of the causes of which is hormonal changes in pregnancy; symptoms include intense itching, particularly in the palms of the hands and the soles of the feet

Chorioamnionitis: Inflammation of the fetal membranes caused by infection; also known as intraamniotic infection

Choriocarcinoma: A malignancy originating from abnormal placental cells

Chorion: The outermost of the fetal membranes, from which develop the chorionic villi and the placenta

Chorionic villi: Vascular structures of the placenta that attach to the decidua of the uterus and form the exchange border between the maternal and fetal circulations

Chorioretinitis: An inflammation of the eye that can lead to vision loss

Circumoral: Around the mouth

Cisgender: Having a gender identity that aligns with one's anatomic sex at birth

Coagulopathy: A disorder in which the blood's ability to clot is impaired

Cohabitating-parent family: A family in which the parents are partners who live together but are not married

Colostrum: An early type of breast milk that is yellowish and high in protein and that sustains the newborn until the mature breast milk comes in

Colposcopy: An examination of the cervix with a microscope specially designed for this purpose, known as a colposcope

Combined oral contraceptive (COC): A type of oral contraceptive that contains a combination of estrogen and progestin, which can prevent pregnancy and provide other health benefits; also known as "the pill"

Complete molar pregnancy: A pregnancy resulting from the fertilization of an egg that does not contain genetic material

Compression ultrasound (CUS): A method of ultrasound imaging done to assess for deep vein thrombosis in which the probe is used to compress the veins being imaged

Conception: The process of becoming pregnant

Congenital: A condition that exists at or prior to birth

Congenital diaphragmatic hernia: A condition in which the abdominal contents herniate through the diaphragm and into the chest

Continuous positive airway pressure (CPAP): A treatment for infant respiratory distress syndrome that uses a constant stream of air to keep the airways and air sacs open for improved breathing and to deliver supplemental oxygen

Contraction stress test: An assessment for fetal well-being that evaluates fetal response to induced contractions

Cord prolapse: A condition in which the umbilical cord precedes the fetal head in the birth canal, increasing the risk of cord compression and hypoxia to the fetus

Corona radiata: The outermost portion of the ovum

Corpus luteum: A hormone-secreting structure that forms from the follicle from which an egg has been released from the ovary

Cortical reaction: A process by which the ovum prevents penetration from more than one sperm

Couvelaire uterus: A condition of retroplacental bleeding that invades the uterine wall

Crackles: An abnormal lung sound associated with fluid in the lungs, collapsed alveoli, and other disease processes

Cycle of abuse/cycle of violence: A repeating cycle of tension building, acute violence, reconciliation, and calm common to abusive relationships

Cystic fibrosis: A genetic disorder in which excessively thick mucus is secreted by the body, blocking passageways in the lungs and other organs

Cystitis: Inflammation of the urinary bladder

D

Deceleration: In fetal monitoring, a decrease in fetal heart rate below baseline, the significance of which depends on frequency and relation to uterine contractions

Decidua: The endometrium, or innermost layer of the uterus, in pregnancy

Decidua basalis: The portion of the decidua (endometrium) underlying the placenta

Decrement: The relaxation phase of a uterine contraction

Deep vein thrombosis: A condition in which a blood clot forms in a deep vein of the body, typically in the legs, often as a result of inactivity, and causes pain or swelling in the area

Depot medroxyprogesterone acetate (DMPA): A progestin-only hormonal contraceptive given by intramuscular or subcutaneous injection every 3 months; also known by the brand name Depo-Provera

Detrusor muscle: A smooth muscle of the bladder wall

Diabetic ketoacidosis: A life-threatening complication of diabetes mellitus in which ketones accumulate in the blood as a result of the metabolizing of stored fats, causing a state of acidosis

Diabetogenic: Causing diabetes

Diaphragm: A form of barrier contraception consisting of a cup-like silicone device that is inserted into the vagina prior to sex

Diastasis recti: A condition in which the abdominal muscles separate at the midline of the body, commonly occurring during pregnancy

Dilation: The gradual opening of the cervix, which occurs during the first stage of labor

Dilation and curettage (D&C): A procedure to remove remaining fetal tissue from the uterus, typically following a miscarriage or incomplete abortion, in which the cervix is dilated and the contents of the uterus are scraped or suctioned out

Diploid: Having two sets of chromosomes, one from each parent

Dirty Duncan: The side of the placenta that faces and attaches to the uterus, so called because of its rough texture and tendency to bleed on delivery

Disseminated intravascular coagulation (DIC): A condition of clotting and pathologic bleeding that occurs throughout the body because of an underlying pathology, in this case placental abruption

Dizygotic: A type of multiple pregnancy that arises from two fertilized ova, each of which develops into an embryo

Ductus arteriosus: A fetal blood vessel that connects the pulmonary artery and descending aorta

Ductus venosus: A fetal blood vessel that connects the umbilical vein and inferior vena cava

Duration: The time from the beginning of a contraction to the end of that same contraction

Dysmaturity: A disorder of postmature newborns associated with placental insufficiency

Dysmenorrhea: Pain with menses

Dyspareunia: Pain with sexual intercourse

Dyspnea: A feeling of impaired breathing, sometimes called "air hunger"

Dystocia: An abnormally slow intrapartum progression

Dysuria: Pain with urination

E

Eating disorder: A pattern of eating that impairs psychological or physical functioning

Ecchymosis: Bruising

Ectasia: A widening of a breast duct directly beneath the nipple

Ectoderm: The outermost germ layer of an embryo in early development

Ectopic pregnancy: A pregnancy in which the fertilized egg has implanted somewhere other than in the uterus

Effacement: The gradual thinning of the cervix, which occurs late in pregnancy and during labor

Embryo: The human organism in the stage of development from 3 to 12 weeks after conception

Embryoblast: The inner cell mass of a blastocyst, which forms the embryo

Emergency contraception (EC): A medication or intrauterine device used after sexual intercourse to prevent the fertilization of an oocyte

Endoderm: The innermost germ layer of an embryo in early development

Endometrial: Pertaining to the innermost layer or lining of the uterus, which is shed in part during menstruation

Endometrial hyperplasia: A condition involving overgrowth and accumulation of the lining of the uterus, which can occur when menstrual periods are too infrequent

Endometriosis: The occurrence of the endometrial tissue outside of the uterus

Endometritis: A condition of inflammation of the endometrium, usually from infection

Endometrium: The innermost layer or lining of the uterus, which is shed in part during menstruation and is termed decidua in pregnancy

Engage: Referring to the fetal head, to descend into the pelvic cavity

Engagement: The entering of the presenting part of the fetus into the maternal pelvis

Engorgement: The swelling of a woman's breasts with breast milk that occurs initially several days after childbirth and later on occasion if not enough milk is expressed

Enteral tube feeding: A method of feeding that involves the delivery of nutrients to the stomach via a tube that passes through a nostril or the mouth and into the stomach or through a gastrostomy (a surgical opening in the stomach)

Episiotomy: A surgical incision of the posterior aspect of the vulva made during the second stage of labor to prevent third- or fourth-degree perineal tears and to expedite delivery to prevent fetal compromise

Epispadias: A rare birth defect in which the opening of the urethra is on the dorsum of the penis, rather than on the tip

Epstein's pearls: Benign white or yellow epithelial cysts that commonly appear on the gums and roof of the mouth in newborns

Epulis: A benign tumor of the gums

Erb's palsy: An injury of the brachial plexus at the level of vertebrae C5 and C6 that results in weakness or loss of movement in an arm

Exercise: Any activity designed to increase or maintain physical fitness

Extended family: Family beyond the nuclear family

External cephalic version (ECV): A procedure in which an obstetric provider manually rotates the fetus from a breech to a cephalic presentation prior to labor by externally manipulating fetal parts through the mother's abdomen

Extracorporeal membrane oxygenation (ECMO): A process for removing blood from the heart, filtering out carbon dioxide from it, and oxygenating it, thus serving as an artificial heart and lung machine; used in the treatment of severe respiratory failure in neonates

F

Fallopian tubes: Tubes that attach to the uterus and lead to, but do not attach to, the ovaries

False labor: The experience of having weak, irregular, nonprogressing uterine contractions that do not cause cervical effacement and dilation (Braxton Hicks contractions)

Ferguson reflex: An urge to push during labor that is generated by the stretching of the uterus and cervix caused by the low position of the fetus in the pelvis

Fertility awareness–based contraception: A method of birth control that relies on accurately predicting the fertile part of a woman's cycle and abstaining from unprotected sexual intercourse during that time; also known as natural family planning

Fertilization: The fusion of egg and sperm

Fetal attitude: The position of the fetal body parts in relationship to each other

Fetal growth restriction (FGR): A condition in which fetal growth is smaller than expected; also known as intrauterine growth restriction

Fetal lie: The relationship of the fetal spine to the maternal spine

Fetal malposition: Any position of the fetus relative to the maternal pelvis that is not optimal for delivery; that is, any position other than an occiput anterior position

Fetal movement count: The counting of fetal movements by the pregnant woman in the third trimester; also known as a kick count

Fetal pole: The earliest detectable form of the embryo, typically appearing as a thickening on the edge of the yolk sac in early pregnancy ultrasound

Fetal position: The relationship of the presenting part of the fetus to the maternal pelvis

Fetal presentation: The part of the fetus that enters the pelvis first; the presenting part

Fetus: A human in the stage of development from 9 weeks after conception until birth

Fibroadenoma: A benign tumor that comprises both glandular and stromal tissue

Fibrocystic breasts: A condition in which benign, cyclic lumps and thickening occur in the breasts, often causing them to be tender or painful

Fistula: An abnormal passage between adjacent body structures

Folic acid: A B vitamin important in pregnancy, particularly in the earliest part of the first trimester, for the prevention of neural tube defects

Follicle-stimulating hormone (FSH): A hormone produced by the pituitary gland that, in women, regulates the menstrual cycle and recruitment of follicles by the ovaries

Follicular phase: The first half of the ovarian cycle, during which a follicle containing an egg matures on the ovary and which ends with ovulation

Foramen ovale: A hole or shunt that normally occurs in the wall of the fetal heart and that allows blood to flow directly from the right atrium into the left

Fourth stage of labor: The final stage of labor, which begins with the birth of the placenta and ends after 4 hours or with the clinical stabilization of the mother

Fraternal twins: Twins born of two fertilized ova

Frequency: The time from the beginning of one contraction to the beginning of the next contraction

Fundus: The muscular top of the uterus opposite the cervix

G

Galactorrhea: A condition of nipple discharge not associated with lactation

Gamete intrafallopian transfer (GIFT): A method of ART that involves the transfer of oocytes and sperm into the fallopian tube

Gametogenesis: The biologic process whereby cells undergo division to create gametes

Gender: A set of traits determined by culture and one's own personal perception of one's identity that is associated with femaleness or maleness

Gender dysphoria: A condition of distress or discomfort resulting from one's gender identity not aligning with one's anatomic sex; also known as gender incongruence

Gender expression: The manner in which a person presents to the world as male, female, neither, both, or a combination thereof, which may or may not correlate with the person's gender identity

Gender identity: A person's innate sense of being male, female, neither, both, or a combination thereof

Gender role: The set of societal expectations placed on a person on the basis of the person's identified gender, typically either male or female

Genderqueer: Identifying as neither male nor female but as a fluid combination of the two

Germinal matrix: A highly vascular area of the brain of the fetus and preterm neonate adjacent to the lateral ventricles that is susceptible to fluctuations in the cerebral blood flow and subject to bleeding because of the thin walls of the vasculature

Gestational choriocarcinoma: A form of cancer resulting from a molar pregnancy

Gestational diabetes: A type of diabetes that occurs only during pregnancy and that is characterized by insulin resistance and increased blood glucose levels; similar to type 2 diabetes

Gestational sac: The earliest identified structure of pregnancy, which contains the embryo, the amniotic sac and fluid, and the placenta

Gestational trophoblastic disease (GTD): A condition characterized by tumors originating from the trophoblasts of the pregnancy

Gestational trophoblastic invasive mole: A form of choriocarcinoma limited to the muscular wall of the uterus

Gestational trophoblastic neoplasm: A new, malignant tumor originating from the trophoblasts of the pregnancy that may follow a molar pregnancy or a normal pregnancy

Gluconeogenesis: The production of new glucose from noncarbohydrate sources such as protein or fat

Glycemic index: A measure of the effect of a food on blood glucose level, with the value of 100 equaling that of pure glucose

Gonadotropin-releasing hormone (GnRH): A hormone produced by the hypothalamus that, when secreted, triggers the pituitary gland to secrete the gonadotropin hormones, luteinizing hormone and follicle-stimulating hormone, which are involved in regulating the ovarian cycle

Gonorrhea: A common bacterial sexually transmitted infection

Goodell's sign: A softening of the cervix that occurs in pregnancy

Graafian follicle: A mature ovarian follicle from which the secondary oocyte will issue

Graves' disease: An autoimmune disease and the most common cause of hyperthyroidism

Group B streptococcus (GBS): A type of bacteria from the genus *Streptococcus* that can cause sepsis in newborns, which can lead to brain damage and death

H

Haploid: Having one set of chromosomes

Hashimoto thyroiditis: An autoimmune disease that results in the destruction of the thyroid

Hegar's sign: A softening of the isthmus of the uterus that occurs during pregnancy

HELLP syndrome: A syndrome specific to pregnancy involving Hemolysis (destruction of red blood cells), Elevated Liver enzyme levels, and Low Platelets

Hematoma: An accumulation of blood in the tissue

Hematuria: Blood in the urine

Hemoconcentration: A decrease in plasma volume resulting in an increased concentration of red blood cells

Hemodynamic stability: A condition in which a stable blood flow is available to all body parts

Hemoglobin A_{1c}: A laboratory test that indicates the average glucose level in the blood over the past 2 to 3 months to evaluate for the onset and progression of diabetes mellitus and to help manage this condition

Hepatitis A: A form of viral hepatitis that is transmitted primarily by contact with food or water contaminated with fecal matter but that may be transmitted sexually

Hepatitis B: A form of viral hepatitis that is transmitted by contact with infected bodily fluids, including blood, semen, and vaginal secretions

Hepatitis C: A form of viral hepatitis transmitted primarily by contact with infected blood

Heteropaternal superfecundation: A multiple pregnancy involving multiple ova as well as more than one father

Hook effect: A phenomenon by which the human chorionic gonadotropin level is so high that it causes a false negative pregnancy test result

Human chorionic somatomammotropin: A hormone secreted by the placenta during pregnancy that alters maternal metabolism to ensure adequate supply of energy to the fetus

Human immunodeficiency virus (HIV): A chronic but treatable viral infection transmitted by infected blood or genital secretions or vertically from mother to fetus

Human papillomavirus: A family of over 150 related sexually transmitted viruses, key strains of which can cause genital warts or cellular changes that may lead to cervical and other types of cancer

Human trafficking: Illegal exploitation of individuals for sex work and other labor

Hydramnios: A condition of excess amniotic fluid; also known as polyhydramnios

Hydrops: Abnormal fluid accumulation in the body

Hydrops fetalis: Abnormal accumulation of fluid in two or more parts of the fetus

Hygroscopic dilators: Hydrophilic substances used to expand the cervical os in preparation for the induction of labor

Hyperbilirubinemia: A condition of high levels of bilirubin in the blood

Hyperemesis gravidarum: A form of extreme nausea and vomiting in pregnancy that results in weight loss and electrolyte imbalance in the mother

Hyperplasia: A type of tissue growth that results from an increase in the number of new cells being produced

Hypertonic uterine dysfunction: Strong, disorganized uterine contractions in the latent phase of labor

Hypertrophy: A type of tissue growth that results from an increase in the size of existing cells

Hypoglycemia: A condition of low blood glucose

Hypospadias: A rare birth defect in which the opening of the urethra is on the ventral aspect of the penis or in the scrotum, rather than on the tip of the penis

Hypotension: Abnormally low blood pressure, which can be a sign of hemodynamic instability related to blood loss

Hypothalamic–pituitary–ovarian (HPO) axis: An endocrine feedback loop between the hypothalamus, anterior pituitary gland, and ovaries that regulates the ovarian cycle

Hypotonic uterine dysfunction: Infrequent or ineffective uterine contractions in the active phase of the first stage of labor

Hypovolemic shock: A state of shock caused by decreased blood volume

Hypoxia: A condition of oxygen deficiency in the tissues of the body

Hysterectomy: Surgical removal of the uterus

Hysterosalpingogram: An imaging technique to assess the patency of the fallopian tubes

I

Iatrogenic: Caused by a medical examination or treatment

Idiopathic: Of unknown cause

Ileostomy: An opening in the abdomen made during surgery through which an end or loop of the bowel is diverted

Ileus: Cessation of peristalsis of the bowel

Immune thrombocytopenic purpura (ITP): A condition of isolated low platelet count that results in a purple rash

Impedance pneumography: A method of monitoring the activity of breathing via electrical leads placed on the chest

In vitro fertilization (IVF): A procedure in which an oocyte and sperm are harvested and fertilization occurs outside of the body

Increment: The buildup phase of a uterine contraction

Infant mortality rate: The number of infants per 1,000 born alive who die within the first year of life

Infertility: The inability to achieve or induce pregnancy within 6 months or 1 year

Infundibulum: The distal end of the fallopian tube, near the fibria

Infiltrate: The leakage of intravenous fluid into the surrounding tissue

Intensity: The strength of a uterine contraction

Intimate partner violence (IPV): Physical, sexual, economic, verbal, and/or emotional abuse inflicted on someone by a current or former intimate partner

Intracervical insemination: A procedure in which sperm are placed near but not into the cervix to facilitate conception

Intrahepatic cholestasis: A condition in which the flow of bile from the liver is impaired, causing a pruritic dermatitis

Intrapartum: Occurring during labor and delivery

Intrauterine contraceptive (IUC): A reversible form of long-acting contraception in which a device placed in the uterus slowly releases a hormone to prevent pregnancy; also known as an intrauterine device (IUD)

Intrauterine device (IUD): A reversible form of long-acting contraception in which a device placed in the uterus slowly releases a hormone to prevent pregnancy; also known as an intrauterine contraceptive (IUC)

Intrauterine growth restriction (IUGR): A condition in which fetal growth is smaller than expected

Intrauterine insemination: A procedure in which sperm are placed into the uterus via the cervix to facilitate conception

Intrauterine resuscitation: Any intervention that is used to improve fetal oxygenation during labor

Intrauterine system (IUS): A device placed in the uterus that slowly releases progestin to prevent pregnancy; also known as an intrauterine contraceptive (IUC) or intrauterine device (IUD)

Intraventricular hemorrhage: Bleeding into the ventricles of the brain

Intrinsic sphincteric deficiency: A loss of urethral tone

Introitus: The entrance to the vagina

Intubation: The placement of a flexible tube into the trachea to maintain an open airway

Invasive mole: A neoplasia resulting from a molar pregnancy

Involution: The process by which the uterus shrinks postpartum

Ischemia: A condition of restricted blood supply to body tissues

J

Jaundice: A condition of yellowing of the skin and sclera caused by the body's inability to efficiently clear bilirubin

K

Kernicterus: A condition of permanent, irreversible brain damage resulting from extreme hyperbilirubinemia and bilirubin-induced neurologic dysfunction

Ketonuria: A condition of ketones in the urine

L

Laboring down: The use of primary powers in the second stage without pushing for fetal descent

Lamaze: A popular method of childbirth preparation for parents

Lanugo: Soft, fine, and typically unpigmented hair commonly found on the body of the fetus, most abundantly at week 20 of gestation, and often persisting in the newborn

Large for gestational age: A condition in which a newborn weighs more than 90% of all infants (90th percentile) born at the same gestational age

Laryngeal atresia: A complete blockage of the larynx by cartilage or other tissue

Laryngeal webs: A congenital defect in which the two sides of the larynx fail to separate

Laryngomalacia: An overly compliant larynx that collapses with inspiration

Last menstrual period (LMP): The first day of the most recent period; used to calculate the due date in pregnancy and the elements of the menstrual cycle in a nonpregnant woman

Late preterm infant: An infant born between 34 weeks 0 days and 36 weeks 6 days

Leiomyoma: A benign tumor of the uterus

Leopold's maneuvers: The palpation of the abdomen of a pregnant woman by an examiner in four different positions to ascertain fetal position

Leukorrhea: A milky vaginal discharge that is normal during pregnancy

Linea nigra: A temporary dark line that appears on the pregnant abdomen running vertically from the pubis to the umbilicus or all the way up the abdomen and that occurs in most pregnancies

Lochia: A vaginal discharge of mucus, blood, and tissue that occurs for 4 to 6 weeks following birth

Lochia alba: The third stage of vaginal discharge postpartum, which is characterized by white or yellowish-white discharge and may last until the sixth week after birth

Lochia rubra: The first stage of vaginal discharge postpartum, which is characterized by red discharge and typically lasts 3 to 5 days after birth

Lochia serosa: The second stage of vaginal discharge postpartum, which is characterized by brown or pink discharge and lasts for about a week

Long-acting reversible contraception (LARC): An easily reversible, long-term, highly effective method of contraception

Luteinizing hormone (LH): A hormone originating in the anterior pituitary gland that triggers ovulation

M

Macronutrients: Nutrients that the body needs in large quantities to function properly, typically referring to fats, carbohydrates, and protein

Macrosomia: A birth weight greater than 4,000 g (8 lb, 13 oz) regardless of gestational age

Macrosomic: Having a birth weight that is larger than normal, or greater than 4,000 g (8 lb, 13 oz)

Malpresentation: Any presentation of the fetus that is not optimal for delivery; that is, any presentation other than vertex cephalic, such as breech, nonvertex cephalic, and shoulder

Mastalgia: Breast pain

Mastectomy: Removal of the breast

Mastitis: A condition of inflammation of the breast tissue, often due to infection

McRoberts' maneuver: An obstetrical procedure used to facilitate childbirth, particularly in cases of shoulder dystocia, that involves hyperflexing the mother's hips to bring the legs back toward the chest, thus allowing passage of the anterior fetal shoulder from under the pubic symphysis

Membrane sweeping: A manual separation of the fetal membranes from the uterus intended to stimulate labor

Menopause: The cessation of menstrual cycles

Menstrual cycle: Changes to the endometrium during the course of a woman's hormonal cycle

Mesoderm: Middle germ layer

Metaplasia: The transformation of a group of cells from one type to another, as occurs at the transformation zone of the cervix, where columnar cells transition to squamous cells

Microcephaly: A congenital defect resulting from abnormal brain development in which the neonate's head is smaller than normal

Micromastia: A condition of underdevelopment of the breast tissue

Micronutrients: Nutrients that the body needs in only very small quantities to function properly, such as vitamins and minerals

Migraine headache: A type of recurrent headache characterized by throbbing rather than "vice-like" pain and often accompanied by photophobia (light sensitivity) and nausea

Milia: A common benign condition in the newborn characterized by small cysts on the face, appearing as white raised spots

Molar pregnancy: A pregnancy resulting from abnormal fertilization that results in the pathologic development of the placental cells

Monoamniotic-monochorionic (MoMo) twins: Twins that share an amniotic sac and a placenta

Monozygotic: A type of multiple pregnancy that arises from a single fertilized ovum that splits and forms two embryos

Morbidly adherent placenta: Any condition in which the villi of the placenta extend beyond the decidua of the uterus, resulting in a failure of the placenta to detach from the uterus and be delivered; conditions include placenta accreta, placenta increta, and placenta percreta

Morula: An early pre-embryotic structure composed of blastocoels

Mucus plug: A protective plug of mucus that forms in the uterine cervix during pregnancy and that is discharged shortly before labor

Multigenerational household: A household containing three or more generations of a family

Multiple sclerosis (MS): A demyelinating disease that disrupts nerve communication

Multizygotic: A type of multiple pregnancy that arises from multiple fertilized ova, each of which develops into an embryo

N

Naegele's rule: A method of estimating a pregnancy due date that involves adding 7 days to the first day of the last normal menstrual period, going back 3 months from that date, and then going forward 1 year

Nasal flaring: A widening of the nostrils with breathing indicating respiratory distress

Natal sex: The identity of male or female assigned to a person at birth on the basis of that person's genetics, hormone expression, and anatomic characteristics; also known as biologic or anatomic sex

Natural family planning (NFP): A method of birth control that relies on accurately predicting the fertile part of a woman's cycle and abstaining from unprotected sexual intercourse during that time; also known as fertility awareness–based contraception

Necrotizing enterocolitis: A condition, most often occurring in premature neonates, in which the tissues of the intestine become infected and inflamed and die

Neoadjuvant: A type of treatment such as radiation or chemotherapy done prior to a primary therapy, such as surgery

Neonatal apnea: Cessation of breathing in the newborn for more than 15 to 20 seconds

Neonatal death: The death of an infant within the first 28 days after birth

Neonatal period: The stage of infant development from birth to 28 days postpartum

Neonatal respiratory distress syndrome: A breathing disorder that occurs in premature neonates because of a lack of the substance surfactant, which facilitates breathing by lubricating air sacs and allowing them to remain open during respiration

Neural tube defect: A defect of the spine, spinal cord, or brain that develops in the first month of pregnancy

Newborn screening: A panel of tests routinely performed on newborns from 24 hours to 1 week after birth that helps identify congenital disorders

Nikolsky's sign: A test for staphylococcal scalded skin syndrome; a positive finding is indicated when gentle pressure applied to the skin causes separation and sloughing of the epidermis

Nitrazine dye: A dye that indicates a pH level between 4.5 and 7.5 and is thus used in tests to determine whether the fluid present in the vagina is amniotic

Nocturia: Excessive nocturnal urination

Nonnutritive sucking (NNS): Sucking for nonnutritive purposes, such as with a pacifier and to help develop feeding skills

Nonreassuring fetal status: An abnormality of the fetal heart rate or rhythm typically caused by fetal ischemia, such as occurs in cord prolapse

Nonstress test: The monitoring of the fetal heart rate late in pregnancy to assess well-being

Normoglycemic: Having a normal glucose concentration in the blood

Nuchal cord: A common complication of labor and delivery in which the umbilical cord becomes wrapped around the fetal neck

Nuchal translucency ultrasound: An ultrasound screening of the nape of the fetal neck done between weeks 11 and 13 of pregnancy to evaluate the amount of fluid collected there; an increased amount of fluid indicates a greater risk of fetal chromosomal abnormality

Nuclear family: A family consisting of a married heterosexual couple and their children

O

Oligohydramnios: A condition of decreased volume of amniotic fluid

Oligomenorrhea: Infrequent menses, defined as more than 35 days occurring between periods

Oligoovulation: Infrequent or irregular ovulation

Oliguria: A condition of underproduction of urine

Oocyte: An immature ovum cell

Oogenesis: The biologic process whereby cells undergo division to create ova

Open glottis pushing: Maternal pushing during labor in which the breath is not held

Operculum: A mucus plug in the cervix during pregnancy

Ophthalmopathy: An inflammatory condition of the eye that can cause retraction of the eyelid, conjunctivitis, swelling, and bulging eyes associated with Graves' disease

Oral glucose tolerance test: A blood test done in combination with the ingestion of a high-glucose solution to assess for diabetes by evaluating the body's ability to compensate for the glucose

Organogenesis: The biologic process whereby organs are created

Orthostatic hypotension: A decrease in blood pressure (by at least 20 mm Hg systolic or 10 mm Hg diastolic) caused by sitting up or standing that often results in dizziness, lightheadedness, and other symptoms

Ovarian cycle: The phases of a woman's hormonal cycle specific to the ovaries, including the follicular phase, ovulation, and the luteal phase

Oxytocin: A hormone that causes the uterus to contract during labor and milk to release during lactation

P

Palmar erythema: A reddening of the palms of the hands and soles of the feet in pregnancy due to physiologic changes

Pap test: A screening procedure for cervical cancer and cellular changes that can lead to cervical cancer done during a pelvic examination that involves scraping cells from the cervix for laboratory analysis to detect abnormal changes

Papilloma: A benign epithelial tumor

Parenteral feeding: A method of feeding that involves infusing nutrients directly into the bloodstream intravenously, bypassing the gastrointestinal tract; also known as parenteral nutrition and total parenteral nutrition

Partial molar pregnancy: A form of molar pregnancy involving the fertilization of one egg by two sperm

Patent ductus arteriosus (PDA): A condition common in preterm infants in which the blood vessel known as the ductus arteriosus, which connects the pulmonary artery to the proximal descending aorta in the fetus, allowing blood to bypass the fetal lungs, fails to narrow and close soon after birth, as it normally does

Pelvimetry: Assessment and measurement of the bony pelvis of the mother in preparation for childbirth

Pemphigoid gestationis: An autoimmune dermatitis of pregnancy

Perinatal: Occurring around the time of birth—before, during, or after

Perinatal loss: The delivery of a fetus that has no signs of life

Perineal: Referring to the region of the body between the legs, from the pubic symphysis to the coccyx

Periodontal disease: A condition caused by bacterial infection of the structures around the teeth, including the gums, periodontal ligament, and alveolar bone

Periosteum: Connective tissue that lines bones

Periventricular leukomalacia: Injury to the white matter of the brain and the most common cause of cerebral palsy

Pessary: A space-occupying device that may be put into the vagina to optimize the position of pelvic organs

Phenylketonuria (PKU): A genetic amino acid disorder

Physical activity: Any instance in which contraction of the skeletal muscles increases one's energy expended above the level of the basal metabolism

Physiologic jaundice: jaundice due to normal processes typically occurring in the second or third day of life and resolving spontaneously

Pica: An eating disorder characterized by a craving for nonnutritive substances, often occurring during pregnancy

Placenta: An organ of pregnancy that attaches to the uterine wall, connecting the fetus to the mother's blood supply and thereby providing it with nutrition support, gas exchange, protection from infection, and waste elimination, and that produces hormones essential to the maintenance of a pregnancy

Placenta previa: A condition in which the placenta partially or totally overlies the maternal cervix

Placental abruption: The premature detaching of the placenta from the uterine wall prior to the birth of the fetus

Placentation: The formation and arrangement of the placenta

Pneumatosis intestinalis: A condition characterized by the occurrence of cysts of gas in the wall of the bowel; a hallmark of necrotizing enterocolitis

Pneumoperitoneum: The collection of air in the abdominal cavity, as seen with bowel perforation

Polycystic ovarian syndrome (PCOS): An endocrine disorder marked by an imbalance of hormones in women that can produce menstrual irregularities, growth of facial hair, ovarian cysts, and acne

Polycythemia: A condition of increased red blood cells

Polyhydramnios: A condition of excess amniotic fluid

Polymastia: The presence of any accessory breast tissue

Polyp: A fleshy growth projecting from the mucous membrane

Polythelia: The presence of additional nipples

Polyzygotic: A type of pregnancy involving more than one ovum, at least one of which has split into monozygotic twins

Postnatally: Occurring after birth

Postneonatal death: The death of an infant that occurs from 29 days to 1 year after birth

Postpartum angiopathy: A rare vasoconstrictive condition with a presentation similar to that of stroke

Postpartum blues: A transitory self-limiting condition that produces depression-like symptoms in the early postpartum period

Postpartum depression: A form of clinical depression associated with childbearing

Postpartum hemorrhage (PPH): A condition of severe bleeding that occurs following birth

Postpartum psychosis: A condition of pregnancy-associated psychosis

Postterm infant: An infant born at 42 weeks of gestation or later

Precipitous birth: A birth that lasts 3 or fewer hours, from the onset of regular contractions to the delivery of the baby; also known as precipitous labor

Preeclampsia: A disorder specific to pregnancy characterized by high blood pressure and protein in the urine; severe forms can be dangerous to the mother and the fetus

Premature rupture of membranes (PROM): A rupture of the amniotic membranes more than 1 hour before the onset of contractions

Preterm infant: An infant born prior to 37 weeks of gestation

Preterm premature rupture of membranes (PPROM): A rupture of membranes occurring before the start of contractions and before 37 weeks' gestation

Prodrome: An early symptom of disease onset

Progestin: A synthetic form of the naturally occurring hormone progesterone, which plays a role in the menstrual cycle and pregnancy

Progestin-only pill: A form of oral contraceptive that contains only progestin and no estrogen

Prolactin: A hormone that stimulates lactation and suppresses ovulation

Proliferative phase: The first half of the endometrial cycle, during which the endometrial lining thickens prior to ovulation

Pruritic urticarial papules and plaques of pregnancy (PUPPP): A benign dermatitis typically appearing in the last weeks of pregnancy or the first weeks of the postpartum period

Ptyalism: Excessive production of saliva

Pulmonary embolism: A life-threatening condition in which a blood clot forms in a pulmonary artery and occludes blood flow to the lungs

Pustular psoriasis of pregnancy (PPP): A form of dermatitis that typically appears in late pregnancy and presents with systemic symptoms and a risk to the fetus

Pyelonephritis: Inflammation of the kidneys, usually from infection

R

Reactive: In the context of a nonstress test, a condition in which the fetal heart rate accelerates at least twice in 20 minutes without decelerations

Reanastomosis: A surgical reversal of an ileostomy procedure

Relaxin: A hormone secreted by the placenta during pregnancy that relaxes ligaments of the pelvic girdle in preparation for birth

Respiratory distress syndrome (RDS): A breathing disorder that occurs in neonates because of lung immaturity and a lack of the substance surfactant, which facilitates breathing by lowering the surface tension of the walls of the air sacs of the lungs and allowing them to remain open during respiration; also known as neonatal respiratory distress syndrome

Retained placenta: A complication of birth in which the placenta does not detach from the uterine wall within 30 minutes after delivery of the infant

Retinopathy of prematurity: Temporary or permanent damage to the retina of an infant associated with oxygen therapy

Retractions: A pulling in of the intercostal and substernal regions of the chest that causes the bony structures of the chest to become temporarily better defined, which can indicate respiratory distress

Rh₀ (D) immune globulin: A medication containing antibodies to the Rh factor that is injected in Rh-negative women to prevent Rh sensitization; also known by the brand name RhoGAM

Rugae: Folds within the vagina that allow it to stretch during childbirth and that re-form postpartum

S

Salpingoophorectomy: Surgical removal of the ovaries and fallopian tubes

Scotomata: Blind spots within the field of vision

Screening: A type of early, routine evaluation designed to identify the presence of a condition in individuals in the general population or a subgroup

Secretory phase: The phase of the endometrial cycle immediately after ovulation and before menses

Seesaw breathing: An abnormal breathing pattern in which the abdomen rises as the chest falls, typically associated with airway obstruction

Sentinel node biopsy: A procedure in which the lymph nodes fed by the region of a tumor are isolated and excised for assessment

Sepsis: An inflammatory reaction to an infection that can be life-threatening

Sexual assault: An unwelcome sexual act performed on one person by another

Sexual assault nurse evaluation: A nurse-led model of evaluation of victims of sexual assault

Sexual minority women (SMW): Women who identify as lesbian, bisexual, gender queer, or transgender

Sexual orientation: A natural inclination to be sexually attracted to people of a given gender

Shiny Schultze: The side of the placenta that faces the fetus, so called because of its shiny appearance and smooth texture

Shoulder dystocia: A condition of obstructed labor in which the head is delivered but a shoulder, typically anterior, is trapped behind the mother's pubic bone so the fetus cannot pass

Small for gestational age (SGA): A condition in which a newborn weighs less than 90% of all infants (10th percentile) born at the same gestational age

Spermatogenesis: The biologic process whereby cells undergo division to create sperm

Spina bifida: A neural tube defect in which the spine and membranes around the spinal cord do not close completely, resulting in minor or major neurologic and physical problems

Spinnbarkeit: The stringy, elastic, egg-white–like quality of cervical mucus that occurs around the time of ovulation

Spiral arteries: The arteries of the uterus that are converted to supply uteroplacental blood flow in pregnancy

Spontaneous abortion: The spontaneous end of a pregnancy prior to 20 weeks

Squamocolumnar junction (SCJ): An area of the uterine cervix where the squamous cells of the ectocervix meet the columnar epithelium of the endocervix

Station: A measure of the degree of descent of the presenting part of the fetus in the uterine canal

Striae gravidarum: A type of scarring of the skin of the abdomen that commonly occurs in pregnancy as a result of rapid weight gain and stretching of the skin; also known as stretch marks

Stripping of the membranes: A procedure in which a care provider inserts a finger into the cervix of a pregnant woman during a pelvic examination and manually detaches the fetal membranes from the uterine lining to help initiate labor; also known as sweeping of the membranes

Subgaleal hemorrhage: Bleeding between the periosteum and the scalp

Subinvolution: A condition involving the failure of the uterus to shrink postpartum

Surfactant: A pulmonary secretion that lines the alveoli and prevents them from collapsing

Syncytiotrophoblast: A placental membrane through which nutrient, waste, and gas exchange occurs

Systemic lupus erythematosus (SLE): A chronic inflammatory autoimmune disease

T

Tachycardic: Having a rapid pulse of 100 or more beats per minute

Tachypneic: Having a rapid rate of breathing, greater than 20 breaths per minute in adults

Tamponade: A method of stopping bleeding by creating a blockage that applies direct pressure within a canal or cavity; also may refer to a pathologic blockage

Tay-Sachs disease: A genetic neurodegenerative disorder

Teratogen: A substance with the potential to harm a pregnancy

Teratogenic: Having a toxic effect on a pregnancy, typically in reference to an agent or drug

Theca lutein cyst: A type of ovarian cyst that is filled with clear fluid, usually resulting from hyperstimulation with human chorionic gonadotropin

Thrombus: A blood clot

Tidal volume: The volume of air that enters the lungs during normal inhalation

Tocodynamometer (toco): A pressure transducer used to monitor uterine contractions

Tocolytic: An agent that reduces or stops uterine contractions

Tonic-clonic seizure: A seizure involving violent muscle contractions and loss of consciousness

Total parenteral nutrition (TPN): A method of feeding that involves infusing nutrients directly into the bloodstream intravenously, bypassing the gastrointestinal tract

Tracheal atresia: A complete or partial absence of the trachea below the larynx; usually a fatal condition

Tracheomalacia: An overly compliant trachea that collapses with breathing

Transcutaneous bilirubin monitoring: A method of measuring the amount of bilirubin in the blood

Transformation zone: An area of the uterine cervix distal to and surrounding the squamocolumnar junction in which abnormal cells are most likely to develop

Transgender: Having a gender identity that does not align with one's anatomic sex at birth

Transman: A person with a male gender identity who was assigned female sex at birth; also known as a transgender man

Transvaginal transducer: An ultrasound wand device that is inserted into the vagina during an examination in early pregnancy or to examine pelvic structures

Transwoman: A person with a female gender identity who was assigned male sex at birth; also known as a transgender woman

Traumatic bonding: A powerful emotional bond that forms between an abuser and a victim resulting from the cycle of abuse

Trichomoniasis: A common genital infection caused by a protozoan parasite

Trophoblasts: Cells that play an important role in embryonic nutrition, the formation of chorionic villi, the attachment of the placenta to the uterus, and the functioning of the placenta

Tuberous breast: A condition of underdevelopment of the breast and the comparative overdevelopment of the nipple and areola

Twin-to-twin transfusion syndrome (TTTS): A condition that occurs in monochorionic twins sharing a placenta in which one twin receives more of the placental blood supply than the other

Type 1 diabetes: A disease state in which the pancreas produces no insulin, resulting in an increased blood glucose level unless treated with exogenous insulin

Type 2 diabetes: A disease state in which cells are resistant to insulin, resulting in high levels of blood glucose

U

Umbilical cord: The cord attaching the embryonic or fetal umbilicus to the placenta

Urethral hypermobility: A condition of imperfect constriction of the urethra due to pelvic floor weakness

Urethritis: Inflammation of the urethra

Urinary incontinence: Involuntary loss of urine

Urinary tract infection (UTI): An infection that occurs anywhere from the kidneys to the egress of the urethra

Uterine atony: A lack of muscle tone in the uterus following birth, which can result in a failure of the uterus to contract and of the blood vessels to close, leading to postpartum hemorrhage

Uterine inversion: A condition in which the uterus prolapses into the uterine cavity

Uterine rupture: A tear in the wall of the uterus

Uterine tachysystole: Excessive uterine contractions

Uterus: The hollow female reproductive organ in which embryonic and fetal development occur and the site of menstruation, which results from the shedding of its inner layer, the endometrium

V

Vaginitis: Inflammation of the vagina

Vaginosis: Any disease or infection of the vagina

Variability: In fetal heart monitoring, a measure of the change in fetal heart rate from beat to beat

Vasculopathy: A disease affecting the blood vessels

Vasectomy: A surgical procedure to sterilize males that involves occlusion of the vas deferens tube, through which sperm travel to join with seminal fluid to form semen during ejaculation

Vena cava: A large vein that brings deoxygenated blood back to the heart and that, if compressed, can cause maternal hypotension and poor uterine profusion

Vernix: A cheesy, white substance found on the skin of neonates seen primarily on term and premature infants; also known as vernix caseosa

Vertical transmission: The passage of a pathogen from the mother to the fetus or infant via the placenta or during birth or breastfeeding

Very advanced maternal age: Age 45 or older; may alternately be defined as age 50 or older

von Willebrand disease (VWD): A genetic or acquired clotting disorder

Vulvar hematoma: A collection of blood in the vulva

W

Wernicke's encephalopathy: A serious neurologic disorder caused by a thiamine deficiency

Wharton's jelly: A gelatinous substance surrounding the umbilical vessels

Y

Yolk sac: A structure of early pregnancy that is crucial to embryonic blood production

Z

Zona pellucida: The layer of the ovum immediately below the corona radiata

Zygote: A fertilized ovum

Zygote intrafallopian transfer (ZIFT): A method of ART that involves in vitro fertilization followed by transfer of the zygote into the fallopian tube

Index